# HANDBOOK OF APPLIED BEHAVIOR ANALYSIS

# HANDBOOK OF APPLIED BEHAVIOR ANALYSIS

## SECOND EDITION

Edited by
Wayne W. Fisher
Cathleen C. Piazza
Henry S. Roane

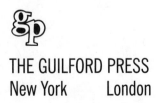

THE GUILFORD PRESS
New York     London

The authors have checked with sources believed to be reliable in their efforts to provide
information that is complete and generally in accord with the standards of practice that are
accepted at the time of publication. However, in view of the possibility of human error or
changes in behavioral, mental health, or medical sciences, neither the authors, nor the editors
and publisher, nor any other party who has been involved in the preparation or publication
of this work warrants that the information contained herein is in every respect accurate or
complete, and they are not responsible for any errors or omissions or the results obtained from
the use of such information. Readers are encouraged to confirm the information contained in
this book with other sources.

**Library of Congress Cataloging-in-Publication Data**

Names: Fisher, Wayne W., editor. | Piazza, Cathleen C., editor. | Roane, Henry S., editor.
Title: Handbook of applied behavior analysis / edited by Wayne W. Fisher, Cathleen C. Piazza,
    Henry S. Roane.
Other titles: Handbook of applied behavior analysis (Guilford Press)
Description:Second edition. | New York, NY : The Guilford Press, [2021] |
    Includes bibliographical references and index.
Identifiers: LCCN 2020057977 | ISBN 9781462543755 (paperback) |
    ISBN 9781462543762 (hardcover)
Subjects: LCSH: Classroom management. | Classroom management—Case studies. |
    Organizational behavior.
Classification: LCC LB3013 .H335 2021 | DDC 371.102/4—dc23
LC record available at https://lccn.loc.gov/2020057977

# About the Editors

**Wayne W. Fisher, PhD, BCBA-D,** is the Henry Rutgers Endowed Professor of Pediatrics at Robert Wood Johnson Medical School and a core faculty member of the Brain Health Institute. He is also inaugural director of the Rutgers Center for Autism Research, Education, and Services (RUCARES) at Rutgers, The State University of New Jersey. His influential research has focused on preference assessment, choice responding, and the assessment and treatment of autism and severe behavior disorders. Dr. Fisher has published over 200 peer-reviewed journal articles. He is a past editor of the *Journal of Applied Behavior Analysis*, past president of the Society for the Experimental Analysis of Behavior (SEAB), and a Fellow of the Association for Behavior Analysis International (ABAI). Dr. Fisher is a recipient of the Bush Leadership Award; the Nathan H. Azrin Distinguished Contribution to Applied Behavior Analysis Award and the SEAB Don Hake Translational Research Award from Division 25 (Behavior Analysis) of the American Psychological Association; and research and mentorship awards from the University of Nebraska.

**Cathleen C. Piazza, PhD, BCBA-D,** is Professor in the Graduate School of Applied and Professional Psychology at Rutgers, The State University of New Jersey, and founding director of the Pediatric Feeding Disorders Program at Children's Specialized Hospital in New Jersey. Dr. Piazza and her colleagues have examined various aspects of feeding disorders—among the most common health problems in children—and have developed a series of interventions to address them. Her research has established strong empirical support for applied-behavior-analytic interventions for feeding disorders. Dr. Piazza is a former editor of the *Journal of Applied Behavior Analysis*, past president of the SEAB, and a Fellow of the ABAI. She is a recipient of the Nathan H. Azrin Distinguished Contribution to Applied Behavior Analysis Award from Division 25 (Behavior Analysis) of the American Psychological Association and the Outstanding Mentor Award from the ABAI.

**Henry S. Roane, PhD, BCBA-D,** is Vice President of Clinical Quality at Sprout Therapy and holds the Gregory S. Liptak, MD, Professorship of Child Development in the Department of Pediatrics at the State University of New York (SUNY) Upstate Medical University. Dr. Roane serves as Chief of the Division of Development, Behavior and Genetics; Director of the Golisano Center for Special Needs; and Chair of the Behavior Analysis Studies Program at Upstate. He is Editor-in-Chief of *Behavioral Development* and has served as an associate editor and editorial board member for journals in the fields of pediatrics, behavior analysis, and school psychology. Dr. Roane has coauthored over 100 research articles and chapters as well as several academic texts on the assessment and treatment of behavior disorders in children with autism and related disorders. He is a Fellow of the ABAI, a member of the Society for Pediatric Research, and a previous recipient of the SUNY Chancellor's Award for Excellence in Faculty Service.

# Contributors

**Scott P. Ardoin, PhD,** Department of Educational Psychology, University of Georgia, Atlanta, Georgia

**Elizabeth Athens, PhD,** ABA Learning Center, and Department of Disability and Community Studies, Douglas College, Vancouver, British Columbia, Canada

**Jonathan C. Baker, PhD,** Department of Psychology, Western Michigan University, Kalamazoo, Michigan

**John C. Begeny, PhD,** Department of Psychology, North Carolina State University, Raleigh, North Carolina

**Samantha C. J. Bergmann, PhD,** Department of Behavior Analysis, University of North Texas, Denton, Texas

**Alison M. Betz, PhD,** Betz Behavioral Consulting, LLC, Highlands Ranch, Colorado

**Kyle Boerke, PhD,** Center for Psychological Studies, Nova Southeastern University, Fort Lauderdale, Florida

**Andy Bondy, PhD,** Pyramid Educational Consultants, New Castle, Delaware

**John C. Borrero, PhD,** Department of Psychology, University of Maryland, Baltimore County, Baltimore, Maryland

**Kelly J. Bouxsein, MS,** CHI Health, Omaha, Nebraska

**Nathan A. Call, PhD,** Marcus Autism Center, Emory University School of Medicine, Atlanta, Georgia

**James E. Carr, PhD,** Behavior Analyst Certification Board, Littleton, Colorado

**A. Charles Catania, PhD,** Department of Psychology, University of Maryland, Baltimore County, Baltimore, Maryland

**Casey J. Clay, PhD,** Thompson Autism Center, Children's Hospital of Orange County and Chapman University, Orange, California

**Robin S. Codding, PhD,** Department of Applied Psychology, Northeastern University, Boston, Massachusetts

**Andrew R. Craig, PhD,** Departments of Pediatrics, Behavior Analysis Studies, and Neuroscience and Physiology, State University of New York Upstate Medical University, Syracuse, New York

**Shannon Crozier, PhD,** Behavior University, Las Vegas, Nevada

**Edward J. Daly III, PhD,** Department of Educational Psychology, University of Nebraska–Lincoln, Lincoln, Nebraska

**Iser G. DeLeon, PhD,** Department of Psychology, University of Florida, Gainesville, Florida

**Nicole M. DeRosa, PsyD,** Departments of Pediatrics and Behavior Analysis Studies, State University of New York Upstate Medical University, Syracuse, New York

**Florence D. DiGennaro Reed, PhD,** Department of Applied Behavioral Science, University of Kansas, Lawrence, Kansas

**John W. Donahoe, PhD,** Department of Psychological and Brain Sciences, University of Massachusetts–Amherst, Amherst, Massachusetts

**Kyle E. Ferguson, PhD,** Department of Family Medicine, University of Washington, Seattle, Washington; Squaxin Island Health Clinic, Shelton, Washington

**Jonathan K. Fernand, PhD,** Department of Applied Behavior Analysis, Aurora University, Aurora, Illinois

**Nathalie Fernandez, MS,** Department of Psychology, University of Florida, Gainesville, Florida

**Wayne W. Fisher, PhD,** Department of Pediatrics and Brain Health Institute, Robert Wood Johnson Medical School, and Rutgers Center for Autism Research, Education, and Services, Rutgers, The State University of New Jersey, New Brunswick, New Jersey

**Patrick C. Friman, PhD,** Clinical Services and Research, Boys Town, Boys Town, Nebraska

**Dana M. Gadaire, PsyD,** Department of Counseling and Human Services, The University of Scranton, Scranton, Pennsylvania

**Kissel J. Goldman, PhD,** Florida Children's Institute, Jacksonville, Florida

**Nicole E. Gravina, PhD,** Department of Psychology, University of Florida, Gainesville, Florida

**Brian D. Greer, PhD,** Department of Pediatrics and Brain Health Institute, Robert Wood Johnson Medical School, and Rutgers Center for Autism Research, Education, and Services, Rutgers, The State University of New Jersey, New Brunswick, New Jersey

**Rebecca A. Groff, MA,** BTEC Behavioral Therapy, Inc., Pensacola, Florida

**Amy C. Gross, PhD,** Department of Pediatrics, University of Minnesota Medical School, Minneapolis, Minnesota

**Laura L. Grow, PhD,** Executive Director, Garden Academy, West Orange, New Jersey

**Lisa M. Hagermoser Sanetti, PhD,** Department of Educational Psychology, University of Connecticut, Storrs, Connecticut

**Gregory P. Hanley, PhD,** FTF Behavioral Consulting, Worcester, Massachusetts

**August F. Holtyn, PhD,** Department of Psychiatry and Behavioral Sciences, Center for Learning and Health, Johns Hopkins University School of Medicine, Baltimore, Maryland

**Einar T. Ingvarsson, PhD,** Virginia Institute of Autism, Charlottesville, Virginia

**Brantley P. Jarvis, PhD,** Knoweiss, LLC, Fairfax, Virginia

**Corina Jimenez-Gomez, PhD,** Center for Autism Research, Treatment, and Training, Department of Psychological Sciences, Auburn University, Auburn, Alabama

**James M. Johnston, PhD,** Department of Psychology, Auburn University, Auburn, Alabama

**Heather J. Kadey, MS,** Department of Pediatrics, Upstate Golisano Children's Hospital, Syracuse, New York

**SungWoo Kahng, PhD,** Department of Applied Psychology, Rutgers, The State University of New Jersey, New Brunswick, New Jersey

**Michael E. Kelley, PhD,** Department of Counseling and Human Services, The University of Scranton, Scranton, Pennsylvania

**Caitlin A. Kirkwood, PhD,** Center for Pediatric Behavioral Health, Wilmington, North Carolina

**Tiffany Kodak, PhD,** Department of Psychology, Behavior Analysis Program, Marquette University, Milwaukee, Wisconsin

**Robert H. LaRue, PhD,** Department of Applied Psychology, Rutgers, The State University of New Jersey, New Brunswick, New Jersey

**Linda A. LeBlanc, PhD,** LeBlanc Behavioral Consulting, Denver, Colorado

**Dorothea C. Lerman, PhD,** Department of Clinical, Health, and Applied Sciences, University of Houston–Clear Lake, Houston, Texas

**Scott D. Lindgren, PhD,** Stead Family Department of Pediatrics, The University of Iowa Carver College of Medicine, Iowa City, Iowa

**F. Charles Mace, PhD,** retired, Sioux Falls, South Dakota

**Brian MacNeill, MA,** Department of Psychology, Western Michigan University, Kalamazoo, Michigan

**Kenneth M. Macurik, PhD,** Spectrum Transformation, Richmond, Virginia

**Brian K. Martens, PhD,** Department of Psychology, Syracuse University, Syracuse, New York

**Caio Miguel, PhD,** Department of Psychology, California State University, Sacramento, California

**Sarah J. Miller, PhD,** Department of Psychology, Children's Hospital of New Orleans, New Orleans, Louisiana

**Raymond G. Miltenberger, PhD,** Department of Child and Family Studies, University of South Florida, Tampa, Florida

**George H. Noell, PhD,** Department of Psychology, Old Dominion University, Norfolk, Virginia

**Melissa R. Nosik, PhD,** Behavior Analyst Certification Board, Littleton, Colorado

**William O'Donohue, PhD,** Department of Psychology, University of Las Vegas–Reno, Reno, Nevada

**Niamh P. O'Kane, MA,** private practice, Arlington, Tennessee

**Heather Penney, MSc,** Aran Hall School, Rhydymain, Dolgellau, Gwynedd, Wales, United Kingdom

**Cathleen C. Piazza, PhD,** Department of Applied Psychology, Rutgers, The State University of New Jersey, New Brunswick, New Jersey

**Christopher A. Podlesnik, PhD,** Department of Psychological Sciences, Auburn University, Auburn, Alabama

**Duncan Pritchard, PhD,** Aran Hall School, Rhydymain, Dolgellau, Gwynedd, Wales, United Kingdom

**Anna M. Quigg, PhD,** Occupational Therapy Program, Cox College, Springfield, Missouri

**Christine L. Ratcliff, MS,** Behavioral Health Center of Excellence and School of Behavior Analysis, Florida Institute of Technology, Melbourne, Florida

**Paige B. Raetz, PhD,** Southwest Autism Research and Resource Center, Phoenix, Arizona

**Derek D. Reed, PhD,** Department of Applied Behavioral Science, University of Kansas, Lawrence, Kansas

**Dennis H. Reid, PhD,** Carolina Behavior Analysis and Support Center, Morganton, North Carolina

**David Reitman, PhD,** College of Psychology, Nova Southeastern University, Fort Lauderdale, Florida

**Billie Retzlaff, PhD,** Intermediate School District 917, Rosemount, Minnesota

**Henry S. Roane, PhD,** Departments of Pediatrics and Psychiatry, State University of New York Upstate Medical University, Syracuse, New York

**Valdeep Saini, PhD,** Department of Applied Disability Studies, Brock University, St. Catherines, Ontario, Canada

**Sindy Sanchez, PhD,** Comprehensive Behavioral Consulting, Tampa, Florida

**Elizabeth Schieber, MS,** Department of Psychology, University of Florida, Gainesville, Florida

**Kelly M. Schieltz, PhD,** Stead Family Department of Pediatrics, University of Iowa Stead Family Children's Hospital, Iowa City, Iowa

**Kimberly E. Seckinger, PhD,** Mary Free Bed Rehabilitation Hospital, Grand Rapids, Michigan

**Kenneth Silverman, PhD,** Department of Psychiatry and Behavioral Sciences, Center for Learning and Health, Johns Hopkins University School of Medicine, Baltimore, Maryland

**Jennifer L. Simon, PhD,** private practice, Lawrence, Kansas

**Richard G. Smith, PhD, LBA-TX,** Department of Behavior Analysis, University of North Texas, Denton, Texas

**Joseph E. Spradlin, PhD,** Department of Applied Behavioral Science (Emeritus), University of Kansas, Lawrence, Kansas

**Shrinidhi Subramaniam, PhD,** Department of Psychology and Child Development, California State University–Stanislaus, Turlock, California

**Alyssa N. Suess, PhD,** Child Psychology, Chatter Pediatric Therapy, Williston, North Dakota

**William E. Sullivan, PhD,** Departments of Pediatrics and Behavior Analysis Studies, SUNY Upstate Medical University, Syracuse, New York

**Heather M. Teichman, MEd,** Beacon Services of Connecticut, Cromwell, Connecticut

**Rachel H. Thompson, PhD,** Department of Psychology, Western New England University, Springfield, Massachusetts

**Jeffrey H. Tiger, PhD,** Department of Psychology, Marquette University, Marquette, Wisconsin

**Matt Tincani, PhD,** Department of Teaching and Learning, Temple University, Philadelphia, Pennsylvania

**Lisa M. Toole, MA,** Douglass Developmental Disabilities Center, Rutgers, The State University of New Jersey, New Brunswick, New Jersey

**Diego Valbuena, PhD,** Comprehensive Behavioral Consulting, Tampa, Florida

**Areti Vassilopoulos, PhD,** Department of Psychiatry, Harvard Medical School and Boston Children's Hospital, Boston, Massachusetts

**Rocío Vegas, PhD,** Institute of Psychology, Universidad Central de Venezuela, Caracas, Venezuela

**Timothy R. Vollmer, PhD,** Department of Psychology, University of Florida, Gainesville, Florida

**David P. Wacker, PhD,** Stead Family Department of Pediatrics, The University of Iowa Carver College of Medicine, Iowa City, Iowa

**David A. Wilder, PhD,** School of Behavior Analysis, Florida Institute of Technology, Melbourne, Florida

# Preface

For the things we have to learn before we can do them,
we learn by doing them.
—ARISTOTLE

Addressing the social and behavior problems that humans display is a daunting task; the first and most important step is the realization that changing behavior inevitably involves *learning by doing* in an environmental context in which the contingencies of reinforcement promote desirable behavior over undesirable behavior. As behavior analysts, we may identify and understand the prevailing contingencies of reinforcement better than most laypersons, but that knowledge does not inoculate us from the potent effects those contingencies have on our own behavior. As applied behavior analysts, in particular, we often find ourselves in contexts involving strong social contingencies in which we are expected to solve complex and socially important behavior problems. Such powerful contingencies are likely to shape and hone our behavior-analytic skills—much more so than reading this or any other book. Nevertheless, an informative text can provide a roadmap that helps us respond to those social contingencies more effectively and rapidly. We have developed and revised this book specifically for that purpose.

As we conceived of and developed the first edition of this book, it occurred to us that there was no single source we would consistently go to when faced with a particularly challenging clinical or applied research problem. Rather, we might start by going to any one of a number of different sources, including (1) consulting with in-house colleagues or those at other institutions, (2) conducting searches of the *Journal of Applied Behavior Analysis* or the *Journal of the Experimental Analysis of Behavior*, or (3) reading sections of the many books covering behavior-analytic topics relevant to the specific clinical or research challenge before us. Thus our central goal for the first edition of this book was to develop a resource for those behavior analysts working in service and applied research settings—one that, we hoped, would be the first source they would turn to when presented with a unique or difficult clinical or applied research problem. In fact, in selecting the authors for each of the chapters, we spent a considerable amount of time asking ourselves whom we would call upon as a first choice for a consultant on the specific topic, and then we invited that person to be the senior author for the chapter. It was exceedingly reinforcing when our first choices accepted our invitation to author the chapters on their specific areas of expertise in almost every case.

In planning the second edition of this book, we relied heavily on the feedback we received from applied behavior analysts who used the first edition, particularly the feedback we received from professors who employed the first edition to aid in the teaching of applied behavior analysis. Based on that feedback, we have worked diligently to update and improve the integration, readability, and relevance of the book's contents. Importantly, we have expanded the number of chapters from 30 to 34, in order to cover topics important to our readers that we did not cover sufficiently in the first edition. We have added two chapters on the quantitative analysis of behavior: one on the matching law and behavioral persistence by Podlesnik et al. (Chapter 6), and another on behavioral economics by DeLeon et al. (Chapter 7). These chapters cover highly relevant topics in applied work, since they address the basic processes that govern how individuals allocate their time to various response options, such as why individuals chose to emit problem behavior over adaptive behavior in certain environmental conditions. We have also added a chapter on the assessment and treatment of pediatric feeding disorders by Piazza and Kirkwood (Chapter 25), one on teacher training by DiGennaro Reed and colleagues (Chapter 27), one on providing in-home behavioral services via telehealth by Wacker et al. (Chapter 31), and one on organizational behavior management by Wilder and Gravina (Chapter 32). These chapters provide important and timely information on topics highly relevant to applied behavior analysts providing services in these areas.

The overall organization of this second edition of the book is similar to that of the first, in that it provides the reader with the foundations of behavior analysis in the early chapters and then ties these basic concepts to applications in subsequent chapters. As such, it strikes a balance between emphasis on research and clinical applications. The book provides a detailed level of analysis for both general and specialized areas of behavior analysis. Its content reflects the breadth of behavior analysis and the expansion of applied behavior analysis into mainstream domains such as pediatric care, psychology, organization management, psychiatry, and drug addiction.

After the book's Introduction (Part I/Chapter 1), Part II of the book devotes six chapters to a concise yet detailed review of the history, philosophy, and basic principles that provide the foundational basis for applied behavior analysis. Part III is devoted to two chapters on measurement, experimental design, and related methodological issues. Part IV consists of four chapters that discuss stimulus preference assessments and both functional and structural approaches to assessing problem behavior, as well as specific chapters on indirect, direct, and controlled functional assessments. Part V of the book describes a variety of concepts and procedures relevant to interventions for increasing desirable behavior. The four chapters in this section cover topics such as differential-reinforcement procedures, building complex repertoires and establishing stimulus control, teaching verbal behavior, and staff training and management. Part VI of the book includes five chapters covering issues related to developing interventions for decreasing problem behavior. Topics in this section include developing antecedent interventions; designing function-based extinction, reinforcement, and punishment interventions; and developing token economies. Part VII describes a variety of important subspecialties within the field of applied behavior analysis, including treatment of autism spectrum disorder, behavioral pediatrics, treatment of pediatric feeding disorders, behavioral approaches to education, teacher training, establishing safety skills in children, behavioral treatment of drug addiction, behavioral gerontology, telehealth delivery of behavioral services, and organizational behavior management. Part VIII, the final section of the book, focuses on professional issues in applied behavior analysis; it includes a chapter on ethics and training, and another on professional certification. Of interest to the reader is that although the topics of each chapter are specific to that content area, there are several overlapping themes across chapters. The discussion of specific principles across different content domains is representative of the breadth of the basic tenets of behavior analysis.

This book can be used as a core or primary textbook for courses in psychology, education, or behavior analysis. The target audiences for the book are practicing behavior analysts and students in graduate classes in psychology, education, or other related fields, and it could serve as a primary source for preparing for professional certification. The quality and comprehensiveness of the book make it a must-have for any behavior analysis library. We hope that our readers will find this text as informative as it was enjoyable for us to edit.

WAYNE W. FISHER
CATHLEEN C. PIAZZA
HENRY S. ROANE

# Contents

# PART I

# INTRODUCTION

In Chapter 1, Fisher, Groff, and Roane introduce the reader to the field of behavior analysis and its three subfields: behaviorism; the experimental analysis of behavior; and applied behavior analysis, the principal topic of this book. The chapter introduces many concepts (e.g., stimulus equivalence) that are discussed in greater depth in subsequent sections of the handbook. Because the history of applied behavior analysis has not changed appreciably since the first edition of this handbook appeared, this introductory chapter has undergone only minor changes for the second edition.

# CHAPTER 1

# Applied Behavior Analysis
## History, Philosophy, Principles, and Basic Methods

Wayne W. Fisher, Rebecca A. Groff, and Henry S. Roane

*Behavior analysis* is a discipline with three primary branches (Morris, Todd, Midgley, Schneider, & Johnson, 1990): (1) behaviorism, which focuses on the worldview or philosophy of behavior analysis; (2) the experimental analysis of behavior, which focuses on identifying and analyzing the basic principles and processes that explain behavior; and (3) applied behavior analysis (ABA), which focuses on solving problems of social importance using the principles and procedures of behavior analysis. Although this third branch is the primary topic of our text, a basic knowledge of the other branches is necessary to appreciate the development and dimensions of ABA fully.

Behavior analysis began as a school or subfield within the discipline of psychology. Some still view behavior analysis as a subspecialty in psychology, whereas others believe that the basic tenets of behavior analysis and traditional psychology are so fundamentally at odds that the two cannot coexist within a single discipline (e.g., Fraley & Vargus, 1986). The basic tenets that distinguish behavior analysis from other areas of psychology include its emphasis on (1) behavior as the basic datum for the field, rather than the *psyche*, the *self*, or other internal mental or metaphysical structures or phenomena; (2) continuity between publicly observable behavior and private events, such as thinking and feeling; (3) prediction and control of the be-

havior of individuals rather than groups; (4) environmental explanations of behavior; and (5) the study of behavior as a natural science. We discuss each of these tenets before turning our attention to the dimensions that specifically define ABA.

## BEHAVIOR AS SUBJECT MATTER

As behavior analysts, we believe that the appropriate subject matter for our field is behavior. We define *behavior* quite broadly to include anything an individual does when interacting with the physical environment (Catania, 2013; Skinner, 1938), including crying, speaking, listening, running, jumping, shifting attention, and even thinking. This behavioral philosophy contrasts with that of mentalists or cognitive psychologists: They view thinking, feeling, and other internal events as activity that occurs within metaphysical entities such as the *self*, the *psyche*, or the *mind*, and they believe that these entities influence or control outward behavior. Mentalists observe behavior to draw inferences about these hypothetical structures, which they view as the appropriate subject matter for the field of psychology. They believe that understanding these inner constructs helps to explain observable behavior. Behaviorists believe that behavior itself is their appropriate subject matter, and that they should study it directly, without references to internal causes. Behaviorists view the brain as real but the mind as an invention, something thought up rather than something that thinks and controls behavior.

Although people in all walks of life talk about the mind as if it were a real entity, when questioned about its location and its characteristics, they find that the mind is difficult if not impossible to locate or describe in precise terms. Another problem that arises when one attempts to explain outward, observable behavior by appealing to causation via internal events is that one then must explain what causes the internal events. Two philosophical arguments illustrate this problem: Ryle's regress and the homunculus fallacy.

Ryle (1949) identified a logical flaw in the traditional (dualist) view of intelligent behavior (see Tanney, 2018). The dualist position, viewing the mind and body as two distinct entities, is that when an individual displays an intelligent act (i.e., an observable response), internal, mental reflection on how to act intelligently must have preceded and directed it. Ryle pointed out that if the logic of the dualist view were accurate, then the internal operation of *reflection* also would be an intelligent act (albeit an internal one) that would need to be preceded and guided by reflection about various alternative ways of reflecting, thus creating a potentially never-ending succession of reflecting about reflecting about reflecting. The endless need for a predecessor and director of every intelligent act is called *Ryle's regress*.

The *homunculus fallacy* is analogous to Ryle's regress, except that it focuses on how we interpret visual stimulation. A mentalist viewpoint is that light projects onto the back of the retina, and that the mind views these images like the way an individual views a motion picture. The mind is thus akin to a little man or homunculus who is metaphorically sitting inside the brain viewing the movie. The question, then, is how the mind or the homunculus sees and interprets the motion picture playing inside the human brain. In keeping with the mentalist hypothesis, another, smaller homunculus inside the first would have to see and interpret its movie, which would need to have an even smaller homunculus inside it to interpret its movie. We call the endless need for another homunculus to explain the visual interpretations of the prior one the *homunculus fallacy* (Uttal, 2000).

These arguments illustrate that proving or disproving the existence of the mind is impossible, much like the impossibility of proving or disproving the existence of ghosts. Modern-day mentalists (e.g., cognitive psychologists) do not often talk about the mind per se, but they are much more likely than behaviorists to look to internal variables (e.g., thoughts and feelings) to explain how behavior and similar logical problems arise. That is, they use observable behavior (e.g., preparing a sandwich) to formulate hypotheses about internal constructs (e.g., the individual is hungry), which they then use to explain the observed behavior (e.g., the person has prepared a sandwich because of the hunger). Skinner (1953, p. 31) pointed out that the two statements "He eats" and "He is hungry" describe a single set of facts. Thus the observer cannot use one statement, "He is hungry," to explain the other, "He eats." Skinner also argued that appeals to such inner causes impede scientific inquiry, because once we identify a supposed cause of behavior (i.e., "He eats because he is hungry"), there is no reason to continue searching for an explanation of the behavior.

By contrast, B. F. Skinner's approach to explaining behavior represents a constantly evolving one in which experimental findings guide theory much more than theory guides experimentation. In fact, revisions and updates of behavior-analytic explanations of behavior are often based on new experimental findings—an approach that some have referred to as "a work in progress" (e.g., Catania, 1988, 2013). One notable example of the way we have updated our conceptualizations of behavior based on new experimental findings is the way we define our subject matter, *behavior*.

Early definitions of *behavior* focused on its physical or topographical characteristics; for example, "thought processes are really motor habits in the larynx, improvements, short cuts, changes, etc." (Watson, 1913, p. 177). Skinner (1938) provided a broader definition of *behavior* and introduced the concept of the three-term contingency (*antecedent–behavior–consequence*) that defines operant behavior. That is, we define *operant behavior* by its topographical features and by its functional properties—namely, the environmental antecedents and consequences functionally related to the specific response topography. The topographical features of a person running to catch a bus may be like those of someone running out of a burning building. The two forms of running, however, are distinctly separate operant responses because they are under the control of different environmental antecedents and consequences, and these environment–behavior relations define operant behavior (Donahoe, 2004).

More recent empirical findings have led to additional refinements regarding what constitutes behavior. For example, research has shown that operant behavior is sensitive to both molecular and molar patterns of reinforcement (e.g., Herrnstein, 1969). Based in part on this empirical finding, teleological behaviorism attempts to explain complex behavior (e.g., building a house, falling in love) by identifying organized patterns of environment–behavior relations that involve both proximal and ultimate causes or consequences. Rachlin (2012, 2018) explains that hammering a nail is a function of not only the immediate consequence of fastening two boards together, but also the larger task of constructing a floor, which in turn is a function of the task of building a house; these nested responses are functions of the ultimate consequence of sheltering and protecting one's family.

Our conception of what constitutes behavior also has expanded because of research on stimulus equivalence and relational-frame theory (Hayes, Barnes-Holmes, & Roche, 2001; Sidman, 2000). Research in this area has shown consistently that when we train certain stimulus relations (e.g., "Mike is heavier than Bill; Bill is heavier than Sam") with verbally competent human participants, other stimulus relations emerge without specific training (e.g., "Sam is lighter than Mike"). These emergent or derived relations are important because they may be prerequisites to and form the basis of generative-language acquisition. They also are potentially important because they require a broader definition of what constitutes operant behavior; that is, equivalence classes or relational frames represent broader units of operant behavior that include both trained (i.e., reinforced) and untrained stimulus relations.

## PRIVATE EVENTS

A common misconception of behavior analysis is that it does not acknowledge or attempt to explain internal, private events such as thoughts and dreams. Many behavior analysts believe that the same laws that govern overt behavior govern private events, and they do not explain these private events by using mentalistic processes (Moore, 2003). The major difference between public and private behavior is that others can observe and verify public behavior, but only the individual performing the behavior can observe private behavior.

Consider the scenario of a married man driving home with his spouse in one car, and a single man driving home alone in another car. The married man looks at his spouse while stopped at a traffic light and says, "Remind me to take the garbage out when we get home." At the same stoplight, the single man thinks silently to himself, "I've got to remember to take the garbage out when I get home."

Behaviorists would view the talking done by the married man and the thinking done by the single man as distinct forms of behavior governed by the same laws, in which talking is a public behavior that others can observe, and thinking is a private behavior that only the single man can observe. Behavior analysts almost exclusively study public behavior because they can observe, quantify, and subject it objectively to the scientific method. However, behaviorists believe that the general principles of behavior derived from the study of public responses (e.g., talking aloud) also apply to and explain private responses (e.g., thinking or talking silently to oneself). They also believe that private events (e.g., pain) often correlate with observable events, thus allowing an individual to *tact* or describe common private events (e.g., skinning a knee; cf. Welsh, Najdowski, Strauss, Gallegos, & Fullen, 2019).

Behaviorists focus on general principles that relate to the function of behavior—that is, its purpose or why it occurs. Behaviorists believe that environmental events that occur in close physical and temporal proximity to the behavior determine the function of a response. Important environmental events that influence behavior include (1) the context in which the response occurs (e.g., teenagers behave differently at home with parents than at a party with peers); (2) motivational factors (e.g., searching for a restaurant is more likely if one has not eaten in a while); (3) antecedents that signal which responses will be successful (e.g., proceeding if a traffic light is green because it signals safety, and stopping if it is red because it signals danger), and (4) the consequences or outcomes of responses that influence whether they will recur (e.g., an individual is more likely to study for a test in the future if he or she gets a better grade as a result).

Applying these general principles to the previous scenario, a behavior analyst might hypothesize that the married man asks his spouse to remind him to take out the trash because (1) stopping at a traffic light provides a signal or cue indicating that it is momentarily safe to shift his attention to matters other than driving the car; (2) the man has experienced a negative outcome associated with forgetting to take out the trash previously, such as trash piling up because the cans would not hold it all; and (3) asking his spouse to remind him to take out the garbage increases the likelihood that he will take out the trash and avoid the negative consequence of the trash piling up. The same three reasons would apply to the single man, except that he has no companion in the car to help him remember to take out the trash, so he says the words silently rather than aloud. Thus, although the two responses in this example (talking aloud and thinking about the trash) are different topographically because others can observe talking but not thinking, they are similar functionally because both are occasioned by the same antecedent (sitting at the stoplight) and reinforced by the same consequence (avoiding the trash piling up).

The only way to identify whether a private event has occurred is through self-report, because others cannot observe an individual's covert behaviors. Self-observation, however, is often unreliable (Skinner, 1953). In fact, Skinner points out the irony in the fact that the verbal community teaches an individual to "know oneself." That is, the two primary ways in which an individual learns to identify and label his or her private events is (1) to "find commonalities between private and public events," or (2) for others to "identify things that usually occasion it [the private event] or behavior that usually co-occurs" (p. 259). For example, if a mother and child both cover their ears as a low-flying jet passes them, and then the parent says, "That hurt my ears," the child may subsequently learn to use the label *hurt* to describe or tact a similar sensation in the ear caused by an ear infection.

Similarly, if a child vomits, refuses to eat food, and has a temperature, a parent might tell the child, "Your stomach hurts." Skinner (1953) explains that if a culture cannot teach an individual to discriminate private events, the individual may never develop the skill of identifying private events, and the individual may not have an extensive knowledge of *self*.

## Studying the Behavior of Individuals

Modern psychology often studies groups to identify patterns of individual differences. Psychological research focused on topics such as personality, intelligence, self-concept, and self-efficacy generally follows this approach. By contrast, behavior analysis generally focuses on the behavior of individuals to identify general principles describing behavior relations that show consistency within and across species such as pigeons, dogs, and humans, and environmental contexts such as laboratory, home, and school (Keller & Schoenfeld,

1950; Mace, 1996). The experimental methods of mainstream psychology, which studies groups, and behavior analysis, which studies individuals, reflect this fundamental difference between the two fields. Most psychological researchers employ group comparison designs and use inferential statistics to identify significant differences between various groups, whereas behavior analysts use single-case designs to study the generality of principles of behavior (e.g., behavioral momentum, delay discounting). Behavior analysts find the prediction and control of the behavior of individuals rather than groups advantageous, because individuals engage in behavior but groups do not (Johnston & Pennypacker, 1993, p. 23).

Researchers using group comparison methods often present their results in terms of statistical means to describe how the average individual in the group behaved, and they use standard deviations to describe how much behavioral variability was present in the group. From a behavioral perspective, these statistics do not describe the behavior of any individual in the group accurately, which is a limitation (Johnston & Pennypacker, 1993, p. 324). Each individual in the group has a unique genetic makeup and an extensive learning history. Consequently, environmental manipulations may evoke different behavior in one individual than in another. To illustrate, one intervention that may be effective for one individual in a group may not be as effective for another.

Conversely, in a single-case design experiment, an individual serves as his or her own experimental control. Thus the experiment accounts for the individual's unique genetic makeup and operant-learning history. Because the individual serves as his or her own control (i.e., the researcher compares his or her behavior in baseline or control conditions to that in intervention conditions), this type of research can determine whether an intervention is effective for an individual.

## Environmental Explanations of Behavior

Behavior analysts identify causes of behavior in the environment. Skinner (1969) proposed that variables influencing behavior fall into two categories: phylogenetic and ontogenetic.

*Phylogenetic variables* are genetic traits passed from parent to offspring through reproduction. *Natural selection*, which Charles Darwin originally described, is the process by which parents pass on the traits most likely to aid their offspring's survival. Individuals with traits that are well adapted to their environment are more likely to survive and procreate; consequently, those adaptive traits are more likely to appear in the next generation than traits that do not facilitate survival and procreation. Natural selection is typically a gradual process. The genetic makeup of an individual evolves gradually over many generations to a point where it is drastically different from the genetic makeup of its ancestors (Skinner, 1969). These genetic variables in conjunction with an individual's environment contribute to both respondent and operant behavior. In fact, Skinner (1981) postulated that "operant behavior is an evolved process" (p. 502); that is, operant behavior evolved and persisted through the phylogenetic process of natural selection because it provided a means by which individuals could acquire behavior that was adaptive to novel and changing environments.

*Ontogenetic variables* are like phylogenetic variables and natural selection, except that the changes occur in an individual's lifetime and often from moment to moment, rather than across multiple generations (Skinner, 1969). *Ontogeny* refers to the natural selection of behaviors resulting from their environmental consequences. If an individual emits a response (such as betting on the most muscular-looking horse in a race) that produces a favorable or reinforcing consequence (such as winning the bet), the probability that he or she will repeat that response in similar environmental contexts increases. That is, the environment selects and shapes the behavior because individuals repeat responses that produce favorable outcomes or consequences in that environment. Similarly, if an individual emits a behavior (such as reaching into a hole in the ground) that produces an unfavorable or punishing consequence (such as being bitten by an unseen animal), the probability that he or she will emit a similar response in the future decreases. Thus both natural selection and operant selection involve selection by consequences. The environment selects traits correlated with survival of the species with natural selection, and changes in such traits evolve slowly over many generations. The environment selects responses correlated with favorable consequences (e.g., satiation of hunger, quenching of thirst, numbing of pain) with operant selection, and changes in response patterns can occur from one moment to the next or over a person's lifetime.

In both phylogeny and ontogeny, some genetic traits and behaviors are not selected directly; rather, they are *spandrels*—by-products or "free riders" of selection of other traits or behaviors (Skinner, 1969). For example, suppose a genetic trait for fast-twitch muscles aids in survival, allowing organisms to outrun predators. These organisms are more likely to survive than are organisms that run more slowly and get eaten by predators. Consequently, the organisms with fast-twitch muscles are more likely to reproduce and pass their fast-twitch-muscle genes to the next generation. By contrast, suppose the organism with fast-twitch muscles also has blue eyes. Blue eyes may not aid in the survival of the organism. The organism's opportunity to reproduce, however, is increased because of its fast-twitch muscles; thus the organism is likely to pass the trait of blue eyes to the next generation. Therefore, blue eyes are a spandrel or by-product of natural selection. Similarly, reading a textbook before taking a test may increase the probability that an individual achieves a good grade on a test; consequently, textbook-reading behavior may increase in the future. The environment directly strengthens this behavior through its consequences. If the individual drinks green tea while reading a textbook, then the behavior of drinking green tea may increase as a by-product of its correlation with the reinforcing consequences associated with reading. The increase in green tea does not cause the individual to do well on his or her test, but the behavior increases as a by-product of the reinforcement associated with reading.

Knowledge of spandrels plays a role in the application of behavior analysis. To illustrate, when a behavior analyst implements an intervention to either decrease or increase a specific target behavior, he or she must consider what other behaviors the intervention will affect as a by-product of the intervention for target behavior and must plan accordingly. For example, *extinction* (i.e., no longer providing reinforcement for a behavior that is maintained by that reinforcer) of disruptive behavior may result in an increase in aggression, even if this latter response did not produce reinforcement in the past. Thus the behavior analyst should add an intervention component to account for this (e.g., providing access to the reinforcer, contingent on an alternative behavior).

## STRUCTURAL VERSUS FUNCTIONAL CLASSIFICATION OF BEHAVIOR

Most approaches for classifying and understanding aberrant behavior emphasize (1) the behavior's topographical features and (2) how certain responses tend to co-occur. For example, a boy who avoids physical contact and eye contact with others and who displays peculiar vocal and motor responses (e.g., referring to himself as "you" and others as "I" and repetitively spinning objects) may receive a diagnosis of autism spectrum disorder (ASD). Clinicians then may use this diagnosis as an explanation of the aberrant behavior that led to the diagnosis (e.g., "He repetitively spins objects because he has ASD"). As discussed earlier in the example provided by Skinner (1953; i.e., "He eats," "He is hungry"), the statements "He has ASD" and "He repetitively spins objects" are two ways of describing the same set of facts; thus one statement does not explain the other.

Behavior analysts frequently work with children with ASD (see, e.g., Kodak, Grow, & Bergmann, Chapter 23, this volume), but they view the diagnosis as descriptive rather than explanative. Because behavior analysts work to identify operant contingencies that are maintaining a behavior, they assess and categorize aberrant behavior according to its function. Other fields of science, such as microbiology, have long understood the importance of analyzing both the structure and function of dynamic entities. Behavior analysts employ a similar practice by categorizing behavior by its structural characteristics and its function. For example, one child with ASD might slap other people because when he does, others are less likely to approach him with schoolwork to complete. In this case, the function of aggression would be to avoid schoolwork. By contrast, another child with ASD might slap other people because when she does, her caregivers are more likely to give her physical attention in the form of tactile stimulation (e.g., sensory integration). In this case, the function of aggression would be to gain a specific form of caregiver attention. Thus, although both cases involve the aggressive act of slapping others, the function of the behavior differs. Analyzing the function of an individual's aberrant behavior allows us to predict the differential effectiveness of interventions more accurately. For example, a time out from attention would be an effective intervention for self-injurious behavior maintained by attention, but it would likely worsen self-injurious behavior maintained by avoidance or escape from social interaction.

## THE STUDY OF BEHAVIOR AS A NATURAL SCIENCE

The final tenet that distinguishes behavior analysis from traditional psychology is that it examines behavior as a natural science (Baum, 2018); thus professionals in the field of behavior analysis conduct research and develop theories in ways similar to those in the natural sciences of chemistry and physics. The behavior of scientists, like that of any other organism, is a consequence of their interaction with the environment. Consequently, behavior analysts must apply the same behavior-analytic principles to themselves as they do to the individuals with whom they conduct research to improve their own behavior (Johnston & Pennypacker, 1993). Skinner (1953) stated that "science is first of all a set of attitudes," and "science [should] reject even its own authorities when they interfere with the observation of nature" (p. 12). Skinner emphasized that "science is a willingness to accept facts even when they are opposed to wishes," and that scientists should "remain without an answer until a satisfactory one can be found" (pp. 12–13). This approach to science and to scientists' attitudes is equally relevant to clinicians who apply the natural science of behavior analysis to problems of social importance.

## DIMENSIONS OF THE EXPERIMENTAL ANALYSIS OF BEHAVIOR

In addition to Skinner's (1969) general views on scientific attitudes, several specific attitudes form the basis of the experimental analysis of behavior as a natural science. These include (1) determinism, (2) experimentation, (3) empiricism, (4) reliability, (5) philosophical doubt, and (6) parsimony. Behavior analysts are more likely to conduct objective research that aids in furthering the theories and principles of behavior analysis if they maintain these attitudes.

### Determinism

*Determinism* is the belief or attitude that all events in the universe including behavioral events are orderly, lawful, predictable, and determined by physical causes (Cooper, Heron, & Heward, 2007; Mazur, 2006; Neuringer, & Englert, 2017). In general, this means that behavior does not spontaneously occur (e.g., a child does not hit a sibling out of the blue); there is always a reason why an individual or organism emits a behavior (e.g., hitting in the past resulted in the sibling's leaving the play area and the child's gaining access to the video game). As behavior analysts, we believe that the phylogenetic and ontogenetic variables described previously determine current behavior, and we focus on current operant contingencies because we can alter them in ways that promote socially important changes (e.g., reducing sibling aggression).

An individual does not have to accept the premise that all behavior is determined to be a behavior analyst and to approach the study of behavior as a natural science. To do so would conflict with *philosophical doubt*, which maintains that we should continually question our assumptions, findings, and conclusions, and with *empiricism*, which requires that we empirically demonstrate determinism before we accept it fully (see discussions below).

Scientists in the field of physics, which is clearly a natural science, have adopted stochastic models and quantum mechanics (which are not deterministic) to explain certain phenomena that classical Newtonian mechanics (which is deterministic) does not explain well. Nevertheless, a general belief in determinism at this juncture in the development of behavior analysis is at least useful, because it focuses our attention on the functional characteristics of behavior. After we identify the functional variables maintaining behavior, we then can manipulate these variables to either increase desirable behavior or decrease aberrant behavior. Scientists would be unable to identify why an individual emits a behavior and would be unable to modify the behavior if the behavior of organisms was not lawful.

### Experimentation

Adopting *experimentation* as the principal method of studying behavior is the only reasonable option if we accept that natural physical events determine behavior, and that the primary goals of a natural science of behavior are the prediction and control of its subject matter. Skinner (1953) speculated that "perhaps the greatest contribution which a science of behavior may make to the evaluation of cultural practices is an insistence upon experimentation" (p. 436).

Behavior analysts are interested in experimentation involving the manipulation of environmental antecedents, consequences, or both as the independent variables, and behavior as the dependent variable. The purpose of this type of experimentation is to identify the specific environmental variables of which a behavior is a function. A *functional relation* exists when a change in an independent behavior reliably produces a defined change in the dependent variable. Describing a functional relation between a response and its reinforcer under a specified environmental context is more precise than saying that the environmental events caused the behavior.

Skinner (1953) acknowledged that other non-experimental methods play a role in the scientific analysis of behavior, including casual, clinical, and controlled observations. He also acknowledged that scientists achieve the rigor and control in the laboratory with nonhuman species at the price of ecological validity or "unreality in conditions" (p. 37). However, the experimental analysis of behavior counters this limitation by focusing on the identification of the basic behavioral processes that underlie both simple animal behavior and complex human behavior.

Skinner (1953) argued that "the commonest objection to a thoroughgoing functional analysis [of complex human behavior] is simply that it cannot be carried out, but the only evidence for this is that it has not yet been carried out" (p. 41). As several chapters in this book show, we have made considerable progress in conducting functional analyses of complex human behavior since Skinner's time, such as self-injurious behavior (Iwata, Dorsey, Slifer, Bauman, & Richman, 1982/1994).

### Empiricism

*Empiricism* is the attitude or viewpoint that the information available to science comes from the senses, and that scientists should base their conclusions primarily on sensory evidence. This means that scientists should be careful observers and believe what they observe the world to be, rather than what others have taught them it should be.

When conducting an experiment, behavior analysts must maintain the attitude of empiricism, which is the practice of making objective scientific decisions based on factual data regarding interventions, research, and theory development. A scientist's behavior is a function of environmental variables (Johnston & Pennypacker, 1993); thus numerous variables are controlling his or her behavior at any given time. These variables may include personal experiences, personal advancement, opinions, or beliefs. As much as possible, a behavior analyst's decisions should be a function of the available empirical data and not of these other variables. Conversely, if variables other than objective data are controlling a scientist's behavior, then the results of the experiment will not be empirical or valid.

### Reliability

Conducting a single experiment does not provide sufficient evidence to determine how an independent variable affects a dependent variable. Behavior analysts hold the attitude that experimental control must be *reliable*. Behavior analysts evaluate reliability at multiple levels. One experiment with only one participant can demonstrate a functional relation between an independent variable, such as contingent praise, and a dependent variable, such as compliance with instructional requests. A behavior analyst can accomplish this by measuring the participant's level of compliance in the absence of praise across multiple sessions until the participant's responding is stable. Next, the behavior analyst introduces the independent variable (e.g., compliance consistently results in praise on a specified schedule) and measures levels of compliance across multiple sessions until the participant's responding is stable. Finally, the behavior analyst repeats these two steps, measuring levels of compliance with and without praise across multiple sessions. Results demonstrate a functional relation between contingent praise and compliance for this individual if levels of compliance are higher in phases in which compliance produced praise than in phases in which compliance did not produce praise. However, demonstrating that contingent praise increased compliance with just one individual does not allow us to draw conclusions about the relation between praise and compliance for other individuals, which requires additional replication. That is, the behavior analyst would enhance the generality of the finding greatly by replicating this same functional relation with multiple participants in one experiment and replicating it across experiments with different types of participants, such as children, adolescents, and adults, in different contexts and over time.

### Philosophical Doubt

The behavior analyst should maintain a reasonable degree of skepticism or *philosophical doubt*, meaning that he or she should "continually question the truthfulness of what is regarded as fact" (Cooper et al., 2007, p. 6), even after reliably demonstrating a relation between an independent and dependent variable numerous times. The behavior analyst should acknowledge the limitations of the obtained data and view them as exploratory, because collection of all data and facts is almost impossible. Philosophical doubt ensures that the field of applied behavior analysis continues to (1) expand its theoretical and behavioral principle base and (2) implement the most efficient and effective behavioral interventions for those it serves.

### Parsimony

Scientists should favor the simpler explanation when two alternative explanations account for the available observations and facts equally well. The medieval philosopher William of Ockham (or Occam) introduced this attitude of *parsimony*, and others have referred to the concept as *Occam's razor* (Smith, 2017). Similarly, one of Einstein's famous sayings, "Make things as simple as possible but no simpler," reflects the principle of parsimony. Parsimony for a behavior analyst involves a preference for explanations that are simple and based on previously established basic principles of behavior analysis before resorting to explanations that require more assumptions and variables to explain the behavior (Johnston & Pennypacker, 1993). The principle of parsimony is also important for applied behavior analysts because caregivers are more likely to implement simple interventions with integrity if they are effective.

## APPLIED BEHAVIOR ANALYSIS

The general principles on which ABA was founded were developed and continue to be refined from the results of laboratory experiments in the experimental analysis of behavior. Thus behavior analysts should also espouse the attitudes emphasized in the experimental analysis of behavior in applied settings. This section briefly describes the basic tenets of the field of ABA.

Applied behavior analysis differs from the experimental analysis of behavior in that it uses the general principles of learning and behavior to solve problems of social relevance. Early in ABA's development, applied behavior analysts worked primarily in the fields of psychology and education. Baer, Wolf, and Risley (1968) described seven dimensions of ABA, to focus our discipline on the central goal of solving problems of social importance: It is (1) applied, (2) behavioral, (3) analytic, (4) technological, (5) conceptually systematic, (6) effective, and (7) generalizable.

Applied behavior analysts select behaviors that are *applied*, meaning that they are important to society, to the individual whose behavior the behavior analyst is modifying, and to his or her family (Baer et al., 1968). For example, teaching a child with a diagnosis of ASD who does not speak or communicate to imitate speech sounds or to request preferred items would represent a socially relevant target of intervention, whereas teaching the child to glue pieces of construction paper together would not. At any point, a behavior analyst might target several response classes, and he or she must prioritize which behaviors are most important to modify.

Consistent with the other two branches of behavior analysis, a principal dimension of ABA is its focus on *behavior*, exemplified through the direct observation, objective measurement, quantification, prediction, and control of behavior (Baer et al., 1968). Behavior analysts typically do not rely on indirect measures of behavior, such as self-reports, interviews, or checklists (Baer, Wolf, & Risley, 1987). In addition, they do not attribute behavior to characteristics of inner qualities, such as personality traits. Instead, they attempt to identify a function of the behavior by manipulating environmental events as independent variables and observing changes in behavior as the dependent variable.

The third dimension of ABA is that it is *analytic*, which means that when we treat behavior, we use objective and controlled single-case designs that permit a believable demonstration of the effectiveness of our intervention. We strive to demonstrate a functional relation between our intervention and any observed changes in the target behavior (Baer et al., 1968), using single-case experimental designs, including reversal, multielement, and multiple-baseline designs (see DeRosa, Sullivan, Roane, Craig, & Kadey, Chapter 9, this volume). Baer et al. (1987) emphasized that behavior analysts should select the design that is best suited for the experimental question, rather than adjust the experimental question to fit a specific experimental design.

Behavior analysts should also be *technological*, which means that they should thoroughly and accurately describe their procedures while conducting research and in clinical practice. They should document this information, which includes a written procedure, operational definitions of target behaviors, and procedural-integrity data, in a way that allows another reasonably competent behavior analyst to replicate the procedure after reading these documents (Baer et al., 1968, 1987).

The assessments and interventions applied behavior analysts implement are applied in nature. However, these interventions and the approaches used to develop the interventions should be *conceptually systematic* (Baer et al., 1968), which means that they should be based on the basic behavior principles validated through empirical research conducted over many years by scientists

involved in the experimental analysis of behavior. Examples of conceptually systematic intervention components are extinction and schedules of reinforcement.

Many experiments that use group designs incorporate inferential statistics to determine whether statistically significant differences between groups exist. Applied behavior analysts rarely use statistics to determine whether a behavior change is significant. Instead, behavior analysts determine the *effectiveness* of their procedures by evaluating their data, often through visual inspection (Fisher, Kelley, & Lomas, 2003)—that is, whether the individual whose behavior was changed and the family, caregivers, and friends of that individual find the behavior change significant. The fact that a behavior change is statistically significant does not mean that the change is socially important. For example, a reduction in a boy's head banging from a rate of 12 per minute to 6 per minute may be statistically significant. However, the boy is still hitting his head over 300 times an hour. Consequently, this is not a socially acceptable reduction in head banging. A more significant reduction needs to occur before the intervention can be classified as effective.

The last principle of ABA is that the findings must be *generalizable* to other settings, caregivers, or behaviors (Baer et al., 1968). If we decrease a child's aggressive behavior to near-zero levels in our clinic, but the child still engages in aggression at school and at home, then the behavior reduction has not generalized. Generalization is important because a decrease in aberrant behavior is not beneficial if the child only spends a few hours a week in the clinic. The behavioral intervention is only beneficial if it decreases the child's behavior across different settings when different caregivers implement it. The most effective way to ensure that generalization occurs is to program it into the intervention (Stokes & Baer, 1977).

## SUMMARY

To summarize, there are three branches of behavior analysis: behaviorism, experimental behavior analysis, and ABA. Each branch is interested in directly studying, predicting, and controlling behavior, rather than observing behavior as a means of making inferences about the *mind*, the *psyche*, the *self*, or other internal mental or metaphysical structures or phenomena. Behaviorists believe that there is continuity between the behavior of human and nonhuman species and between public and private behavior (e.g., thinking, feeling). Behaviorists believe that behavior is lawful, that it occurs for a reason, and that they can study it by using the rigorous scientific methods applied in other natural or "hard" sciences. Finally, behaviorists focus on the function(s) of behavior and believe that they can explain and control behavior by observing and manipulating environmental events that occur in relation to the behavior.

## REFERENCES

Baer, D. M., Wolf, M. M., & Risley, T. R. (1968). Some current dimensions of applied behavior analysis. *Journal of Applied Behavior Analysis, 1,* 91–97.

Baer, D. M., Wolf, M. M., & Risley, T. R. (1987). Some still-current dimensions of applied behavior analysis. *Journal of Applied Behavior Analysis, 20,* 313–327.

Baum, W. M. (2018). Multiscale behavior analysis and molar behaviorism: An overview. *Journal of the Experimental Analysis of Behavior, 110,* 302–322.

Catania, A. C. (1988). The behavior of organisms as a work in progress. *Journal of the Experimental Analysis of Behavior, 50,* 277–281.

Catania, A. C. (2013). *Learning* (5th ed.). Cornwall-on-Hudson, NY: Sloan.

Cooper, J. O., Heron, T. E., & Heward, W. L. (2007). *Applied behavior analysis* (2nd ed.). Upper Saddle River, NJ: Pearson/Merrill–Prentice Hall.

Donahoe, J. W. (2004). Ships that pass in the night. *Journal of the Experimental Analysis of Behavior, 82,* 85–93.

Fisher, W. W., Kelley, M. E., & Lomas, J. E. (2003). Visual aids and structured criteria for improving visual inspection and interpretation of single-case designs. *Journal of Applied Behavior Analysis, 36,* 387–406.

Fraley, L. E., & Vargas, E. A. (1986). Separate disciplines: The study of behavior and the study of the psyche. *Behavior Analyst, 9,* 47–59.

Hayes, S. C., Barnes-Holmes, D., & Roche, B. (2001). Relational frame theory: A precis. In S. C. Hayes, D. Barnes-Holmes, & B. Roche (Eds.), *Relational frame theory: A post-Skinnerian account of human language and cognition* (pp. 141–154). New York: Kluwer Academic/Plenum Press.

Herrnstein, R. J. (1969). Method and theory in the study of avoidance. *Psychological Review, 76,* 49–70.

Iwata, B. A., Dorsey, M. F., Slifer, K. J., Bauman, K. E., & Richman, G. S. (1994). Toward a functional analysis of self-injury. *Journal of Applied Behavior Analysis, 27,* 197–209. (Reprinted from *Analysis and Intervention in Developmental Disabilities, 2,* 3–20, 1982)

Johnston, J. M., & Pennypacker, H. S. (1993). *Strategies and tactics of behavioral research* (2nd ed.). Hillsdale, NJ: Erlbaum.

Keller, F. S., & Schoenfeld, W. N. (1950). *Principles of psychology.* New York: Appleton-Century-Crofts.

Mace, F. C. (1996). In pursuit of general behavioral relations. *Journal of Applied Behavior Analysis, 29,* 557–563.

Mazur, J. E. (2006). *Learning and behavior* (6th ed.). Upper Saddle River, NJ: Pearson/Prentice Hall.

Moore, J. (2003). Explanation and description in traditional neobehaviorism, cognitive psychology, and behavior analysis. In K. A. Lattal & P. N. Chase (Eds.), *Behavior theory and philosophy* (pp. 13–39). New York: Kluwer Academic/Plenum Press.

Morris, E. K., Todd, J. T., Midgley, B. D., Schneider, S. M., & Johnson, L. M. (1990). The history of behavior analysis: Some historiography and a bibliography. *Behavior Analyst, 13,* 131–158.

Neuringer, A., & Englert, W. (2017). Epicurus and B. F. Skinner: In search of the good life. *Journal of the Experimental Analysis of Behavior, 107,* 21–33.

Rachlin, H. (2012). Our overt behavior makes us human. *Behavior Analyst, 35,* 49–57.

Rachlin, H. (2018). Is talking to yourself thinking? *Journal of the Experimental Analysis of Behavior, 109,* 48–55.

Ryle, G. (1949). *The concept of mind.* Chicago: University of Chicago Press.

Sidman, M. (2000). Equivalence relations and the reinforcement contingency. *Journal of the Experimental Analysis of Behavior, 74,* 127–146.

Skinner, B. F. (1938). *The behavior of organisms.* Acton, MA: Copley.

Skinner, B. F. (1953). *Science and human behavior.* New York: Free Press.

Skinner, B. F. (1969). *Contingencies of reinforcement: A theoretical analysis.* Englewood Cliffs, NJ: Prentice-Hall.

Skinner, B. F. (1981). Selection by consequences. *Science, 213,* 501–504.

Smith, T. L. (2017). The epistemologies of parsimony: A review of *Ockham's razors: A user's manual* by Elliott Sober. *Journal of the Experimental Analysis of Behavior, 108,* 485–498.

Stokes, T. F., & Baer, D. M. (1977). An implicit technology of generalization. *Journal of Applied Behavior Analysis, 10,* 349–367.

Tanney, J. (2018). Remarks on the "thickness" of action description: With Wittgenstein, Ryle, and Anscombe. *Philosophical Explorations, 21,* 170–177.

Uttal, W. R. (2000). *The war between mentalism and behaviorism: On the accessibility of mental processes.* Mahwah, NJ: Erlbaum.

Watson, J. B. (1913). Psychology as the behaviorist views it. *Psychological Review, 20,* 158–177.

Welsh, F., Najdowski, A. C., Strauss, D., Gallegos, L., & Fullen, J. A. (2019). Teaching a perspective-taking component skill to children with autism in the natural environment. *Journal of Applied Behavior Analysis, 52,* 439–450.

# PART II

# BASIC PRINCIPLES AND CONCEPTS

A proverb attributed to the Chinese philosopher Lao Tzu is this: "Give a man a fish and you will feed him for a day; teach him to fish and you will feed him for a lifetime." The same can be said for the importance of teaching behavior analysts the basic principles and concepts of our field, rather than only giving them specific procedures for specific problems. Learning the basic principles and concepts of behavior analysis will not only allow applied behavior analysts to address the specific socially significant problems they are likely to face upon graduation (e.g., teaching verbal behavior skills to a child with autism spectrum disorder), but will also provide them with the tools they will need to address novel problems for which no protocols exist (e.g., teaching handwashing skills and social distancing to schoolchildren during a coronavirus pandemic).

In the first chapter of Part II (Chapter 2), Donahoe and Vegas introduce the basic principles of respondent (or classical) conditioning, in which a neutral stimulus that previously had no effect on the target response comes to reliably evoke the target response after the behavior analyst has consistently paired that previously neutral stimulus with a stimulus that consistently and unconditionally evokes the target response. These authors discuss how respondent conditioning is important to the development and amelioration of various clinical disorders, such as drug addiction and panic disorder. Next, Catania introduces the reader in Chapter 3 to basic operant contingencies of reinforcement and punishment, as well as the antecedent stimuli that occasion and establish the effectiveness of those contingencies. Understanding and analyzing operant contingencies in relation to the stimuli that evoke and motivate responding are critical to the development of effective behavioral assessments (e.g., analyzing idiosyncratic functions of problem behavior) and behavioral interventions (e.g., developing novel function-based treatments). In Chapter 4, Mace, Pritchard, and Penney provide a detailed discussion of basic and complex schedules of reinforcement, including differential, compound, and concurrent schedules. They provide a variety of examples illustrating how such reinforcement schedules are pertinent to applied work. Spradlin, Simon, and Fisher introduce the basic processes and principles of stimulus control in Chapter 5, which describes how and why the behavior of individuals changes and adapts to the stimulus conditions present in different situations and at different times (e.g., why spectators at a baseball game sing during the seventh-inning stretch but not during other parts of the game). These authors describe how stimulus control is relevant to a wide variety of clinical applications, ranging from teaching simple discriminations (e.g., only crossing a street when the traffic light is green) to teaching in ways that promote the emergence of generative verbal behavior.

In a new contribution to this edition of the handbook, Chapter 6, Podlesnik, Jimenez-Gomez, and Kelley discuss two quantitative theories of behavior that have considerable relevance to applied work—namely, the generalized matching law and behavioral-momentum theory. The matching law is particularly relevant to how and why individuals allocate their time and responding to adaptive and maladaptive responses, and behavioral-momentum theory is pertinent to understanding and mitigating treatment relapse. In another new addition, Chapter 7, DeLeon and colleagues describe the subarea of behavioral economics, which integrates principles from microeconomics and behavior analysis to demonstrate and analyze how the demand for commodities (i.e., reinforcers) relates to the work or effort an individual puts forth to obtain those reinforcers. They illustrate how these concepts are directly applicable to disorders of impulse control, such as attention-deficit/hyperactivity disorder, and to various health-related behaviors.

# CHAPTER 2

# Respondent (Pavlovian) Conditioning

John W. Donahoe and Rocío Vegas

At the dawn of the 20th century, two scientists—one in St. Petersburg, Russia, and the other in Cambridge, Massachusetts—independently began the search to discover how individual experience produced long-lasting changes in behavior. The first scientist was Ivan Pavlov (1927/1960), a physiologist whose earlier research on digestion would earn a Nobel Prize. The second was Edward Thorndike (1903), a psychologist whose published work would eventually exceed in volume that of any other psychologist—past or present (Jonçich, 1968). The methods these pioneers used differed, but both described themselves as following in Darwin's footsteps: That is, they were trying to explain complex phenomena as the cumulative product of more basic processes. For Darwin, the basic process was evolution through natural selection. For Pavlov and Thorndike, the basic process has come to be known as *selection by reinforcement* or simply *reinforcement*. Darwin primarily studied how changes in *structure* could arise from natural selection. Pavlov and Thorndike studied how changes in *function* could arise from selection by reinforcement. Both shared the belief that even the most complex phenomena could be understood as the cumulative result of selection processes acting over time. The selection process discovered by Darwin usually acted over extremely long periods and could be known largely through naturalistic observation. By contrast, selection by reinforcement could occur rapidly and be studied within the laboratory.

Pavlov's and Thorndike's procedures differed in a critically important respect, but they began from the same starting point—by presenting the learner with a stimulus to which the learner would already reliably respond. Stated more technically, both Pavlov and Thorndike presented an *eliciting stimulus* (say, food) that reliably evoked a behavior (say, eating). Because of natural selection, the taste and smell of food elicit a variety of responses—including salivation, approach, and eating. The experimenter could manipulate an eliciting stimulus easily and readily measure the elicited response. Pavlov and Thorndike differed about the type of event that reliably preceded the eliciting stimulus and its elicited response. In Pavlov's laboratory, a specified *stimulus* (such as the ticking sound of a metronome) preceded the presentation of food to a dog. In Thorndike's procedure, a specified *behavior* (such as moving a rod) allowed a cat to escape from a cage and gain access to food. Figure 2.1 shows the relation between Pavlov's and Thorndike's procedures. As indicated in this figure, the critical difference between the two procedures is that a specific stimulus ($S_i$) reliably preceded the eliciting stimulus in Pavlov's procedure, whereas a specific response ($R_j$) reliably preceded the eliciting stimulus in Thorndike's procedure. B. F. Skinner was the first to appreciate fully that this

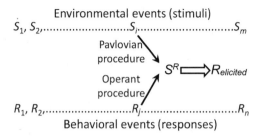

Environmental events (stimuli)

Behavioral events (responses)

**FIGURE 2.1.** The critical events in the Pavlovian (respondent) and operant procedures. In both procedures, the learner is immersed in a stream of environmental (S) events and is responding (R) in their presence. The experimenter introduces a reinforcing stimulus ($S^R$) into the environment in both procedures. The critical difference between the two procedures is that in Pavlov's procedure an environmental stimulus (here, $S_i$) reliably precedes the reinforcing stimulus, whereas in the operant procedure a specific behavior (here, $R_j$) reliably precedes the reinforcing stimulus. The Pavlovian technical terms for the environmental event that precedes the reinforcing stimulus is the conditioned stimulus (CS), for the reinforcing stimulus is the unconditioned stimulus (US), and for the elicited response ($R_{elicited}$) is the unconditioned response (UR).

procedural difference would have a profound effect on the outcome of selection by reinforcement (Skinner, 1935, 1937).

Skinner (1938) extended the analysis of Pavlovian and operant conditioning in his seminal book *The Behavior of Organisms*. He labeled the two procedures, respectively, *Type S* or *respondent* conditioning and *Type R* or *operant* conditioning. Skinner named Pavlov's procedure respondent conditioning to emphasize that the behavior of interest was an elicited response (i.e., a *respondent*) evoked by a specific *stimulus* (the eliciting stimulus). He called Pavlov's procedure Type S conditioning because a specific stimulus evoked the behavior. Type R conditioning was the operant procedure. Skinner introduced the term *operant* to emphasize that the response ($R_j$) operated on the environment to produce the eliciting stimulus. Skinner called the procedure Type R conditioning to emphasize that the relation of the learner's *response* to the reinforcer was paramount, and that this response was not occasioned by a specifiable stimulus. In Skinner's words, "there are two types of conditioned reflex, defined according to whether the reinforcing stimulus is correlated with a stimulus or with a response" (1938, p. 62). "The fundamental difference rests upon the term with

which the reinforcing stimulus . . . is correlated. In Type S it is the stimulus . . . , in Type R the response" (1938, p. 109). Note especially that a procedural distinction defines (his word) the two types of conditioning and does not necessarily imply a fundamentally different conditioning process.

Skinner cited, without dissent, the views of contemporaries who proposed that a common conditioning process was involved in the Pavlovian and operant procedures. "An analysis of differences between the two types has been made by Hilgard (1937), who points out that both types usually occur together and that 'reinforcement' is essentially the same process in both. The present distinctions [Skinner's procedural distinctions] are, however, not questioned" (Skinner, 1938, p. 111). Skinner next cited the following, also without dissent: "Mowrer (1937) holds out the possibility that the two processes may eventually be reduced to a single formula" (p. 111). Skinner noted further that "in Type R . . . the process is very probably that referred to in Thorndike's Law of Effect" (p. 111). (For a presentation of Thorndike's views as they relate to current work on reinforcement, see Donahoe, 1999.)

In summary, Skinner based his prescient distinction between Pavlovian (respondent or Type S) and operant (instrumental or Type R) conditioning on procedural grounds. A unified theoretical treatment of the conditioning process involved in the two procedures was a possibility that Skinner both anticipated and welcomed. The view that one fundamental conditioning process occurs in both procedures may seem inconsistent with Skinner's treatment of conditioning; it is not (Donahoe, Burgos, & Palmer, 1993). We describe the current best understanding of the conditioning process shortly, but we first introduce technical terms associated with the Pavlovian procedure. These terms are necessary to understand the experimental literature on Pavlovian conditioning.

Pavlov devised a technical vocabulary for the stimulus and response events in his procedure. The *conditioned stimulus* (CS) was the environmental event that preceded the eliciting stimulus. The eliciting stimulus was the *unconditioned stimulus* (US), and the elicited response was the *unconditioned response* (UR). In Pavlov's laboratory, the CS might be presentation of the ticking sound of a metronome, the US the presentation of food, and the UR the elicitation of salivation. After several pairings of the CS with the US/UR, the CS evoked a response that resembled the UR in the typical case. In the present example, after the experimenter paired the ticking sound with food, the ticking sound evoked salivation when presented alone. The *conditioned response* (CR) was the response that the CS evoked *after* the experimenter repeatedly paired the CS with the US/UR, and is the behavioral effect scientists usually measure in the Pavlovian procedure. The process whereby the environment acquired its ability to control behavior was called *conditioning* because the ability of the CS to evoke the CR was *conditional* upon (i.e., dependent upon) pairing the CS with the US/UR.

Scientists generally call Pavlov's procedure *classical conditioning* in recognition of his historical priority. Scientists ultimately used the term *conditioning* for Thorndike's procedure—but called it *operant conditioning* to distinguish it from Pavlov's procedure. As already noted, the Thorndike–Skinner procedure differed from Pavlov's in a critical respect: The event that reliably preceded the eliciting stimulus was a response, not a stimulus. Because an increase in the strength of the response was dependent on presentation of an eliciting stimulus in both procedures, we call the eliciting stimulus a *reinforcing stimulus* or simply a *reinforcer*. An eliciting stimulus functions as a reinforcer in either conditioning procedure.

## TOWARD A UNIFIED CONCEPTION OF THE CONDITIONING PROCESS

Skinner realized that Pavlov's procedure permitted an experimental analysis of only the relation between the environment and the reinforcer. Thus the classical procedure was limited to changing the stimulus that could control a response that was already elicited by another stimulus. The operant procedure, in which a reinforcer could follow *any* response without regard to the particular stimulus present at that moment, opened up the possibility of changing the full behavioral repertoire of the learner, not just the elicited response.

### Temporal Relation between the CS and the US/UR

Given an appropriate choice of CS and US, what must take place for conditioning to occur? Research has identified two critical variables: (1) the temporal relation between the CS and US/UR, and (2) a change in the ongoing behavior evoked by the US. Pavlov demonstrated the first variable, the temporal relation between the CS and the US/UR, known as *temporal contiguity*. The

second variable was not identified until the late 1960s, beginning with the work of Leon Kamin (1968, 1969). Kamin used a method developed by Skinner's student William Estes (Estes & Skinner, 1941). Kamin found that temporal contiguity between the CS and US/UR was sometimes not enough to produce conditioning. The US also had to evoke a *change* in ongoing behavior in addition to contiguity with the CS. That is, the US had to evoke behavior that was not already occurring before the experimenter presented the US. A contiguous CS–US/UR relation would produce conditioning only if such a change occurred. We call this second factor a *behavioral discrepancy*.

### Temporal Contiguity

The classical procedure permits an analysis of the effects of the temporal relation between the CS and the US/UR on conditioning (Gormezano & Kehoe, 1981; Kirkpatrick & Balsam, 2016). Experimental analysis is facilitated because the experimenter can control the presentation of both stimuli and can measure the relevant behavior. Figure 2.2 shows a representative effect of varying the temporal relation between the onset of the CS and US (Smith, Coleman, & Gormezano, 1969). Here the CS was a tone, the US was a mild shock given

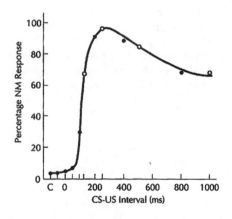

**FIGURE 2.2.** Effect of the CS–US interval on the percentage of CRs with the Pavlovian procedure. Different groups of rabbits were trained at each of the CS–US intervals. The CS was a tone, and the US was a mild shock in the region of the eye. The shock elicited a "blink" of the nictitating membrane (NM). ms, milliseconds. From Donahoe and Palmer (1994/2005), based on findings from Smith, Coleman, and Gormezano (1969). Copyright © 2005 John W. Donahoe. Reprinted by permission.

near a rabbit's eye, and the CR was movement of the nictitating membrane that the shock elicited. (The nictitating membrane is a semitransparent membrane that extends over the eye to protect it. This membrane is present in many animals, such as dogs and cats, but is vestigial in humans, where only the pink tissue in the nasal corner of each eye remains.) The nictitating membrane's response is particularly well suited for experimental analysis, because membrane movement is rare except when the eye is "threatened." Thus any movement of the nictitating membrane following the CS is very likely to be a CR and not the result of other factors.

After CS–US/UR pairings in which the experimenters trained different animals with different intervals between the CS and the US/UR, the major findings shown in Figure 2.2 were these:

1. When the CS came *after* the US/UR, a *backward-conditioning* procedure, conditioning did not occur.
2. As the interval between the CS and the US/UR increased, CR responding became more probable at first and then reached a maximum at a relatively short value (here, less than a half-second, or 500 milliseconds).
3. CR responding declined when the CS–US/UR interval further increased.

To summarize, selection by reinforcement occurs over only a relatively brief interval in a well-controlled Pavlovian procedure. Stimuli (CSs) that reliably precede the US/UR acquire control over the CR due to reinforcement. Conditioning may occur after only one or a few CS–US/UR pairings, depending on the specific training regi-

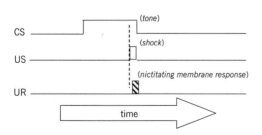

**FIGURE 2.3.** Schematic diagram of the events in a typical Pavlovian (respondent) procedure. A specified environmental stimulus (here, the CS of a tone) precedes an eliciting stimulus (here, the US of a mild shock in the region of the eye of a rabbit) that evokes a response (here, the UR of a brief nictitating membrane response).

men (e.g., Kehoe & Macrae, 1994; Van Willigen, Emmett, Cote, & Ayres, 1987). Longer-term relations between the environment and behavior may occur only by filling the gap between the CS and remote US/URs with more immediate events that sustain conditioning because the conditioning process operates over very short time intervals. We describe how this occurs in a subsequent section on higher-order conditioning and conditioned reinforcement.

### Critical Temporal Relation: CS–US or CS–UR?

The experimenter in the Pavlovian procedure manipulates the relation between stimuli—the CS and the reinforcing US. By contrast, we have seen that the experimenter in the operant procedure manipulates the relation between a response (the operant) and the reinforcing stimulus. Note that although the experimenter directly controls the temporal relation between the CS and US, the relation between the CS and UR necessarily varies as well (see Figure 2.3). Thus whether the CS–US relation or the CS–UR relation is critical for conditioning is unclear. Teasing apart these relations might appear unimportant, except that the difference between the events that the experimenter manipulates in the Pavlovian and operant procedures has led many to interpret the difference as more than a procedural distinction (e.g., Rescorla, 1991). Specifically, the subject in a classical procedure is sometimes said to learn a stimulus–stimulus relation, whereas the subject in an operant procedure learns a stimulus–response relation. Figure 2.1 illustrates the stimulus–response relation of the operant procedure. Note that the reinforced operant necessarily occurs in the presence of *some* environmental stimulus. Scientists call the stimulus that guides behavior in the operant procedure a *discriminative stimulus*. As Skinner (1937) noted, "It is the nature of [operant] behavior that . . . discriminative stimuli are practically inevitable" (p. 273; see also Catania & Keller, 1981; Dinsmoor, 1995; Donahoe, Palmer, & Burgos, 1997). Thus some environmental stimulus is likely to acquire control over behavior in the operant procedure, even though the experimenter may not manipulate this relation directly. The idea that the participant acquires different *kinds* of relations in the two procedures rests upon the fact that the experimenter manipulates different kinds of events in the two procedures. Whether the CS–US relation, a relation between two stimuli, or the CS–UR relation, a relation between a stimulus and a response, is fundamental in the Pavlovian procedure becomes important to determine.

Donahoe and Vegas (2004) developed an experimental procedure in which the UR occurred with enough delay after the US that they could separate the effects of the CS–UR relation from the CS–US relation. The experimenters injected water into a pigeon's mouth as a US and identified the throat movements that accompanied swallowing as a UR. The advantage of this procedure is that throat movements, the UR, begin about 500 milliseconds after the injection of water, the US, and these movements continued for several seconds. Thus the CS could be introduced *after* the onset of the US, but *before* or *during* the UR. This produced a backward CS–US relation—a relation that does not promote conditioning with brief-duration URs, such as the nictitating membrane response. Also, experimenters could introduce the CS *after* the onsets of both the US and UR but still overlap the UR, because the swallowing UR continued for some seconds. The central finding was that the CS, a light, came to evoke the CR, swallowing, independently of the relation of the CS to the US as long as the CS preceded or overlapped the UR. Thus conditioning in the Pavlovian procedure varied more systematically with the temporal relation between the CS and UR than between the CS and US. The inference that the learner acquired a different *kind* of relation with the Pavlovian procedure—a relation between two environmental events (CS–US) instead of an environment–behavior relation (CS–UR)—arose from a misinterpretation of the finding that variations in the CS–US relation affected conditioning. Varying the temporal relation between the CS and US also varied the CS-UR relation, and this is the relation that appears critical.

The finding that the relation of the CS to the *behavior* evoked by the US allowed us to understand certain previously puzzling findings. For example, conditioning of the nictitating membrane does not occur if a CS occurs *after* a shock US presented near the rabbit's eye, which is a backward-conditioning procedure. However, conditioning of a change in heart rate does occur with this same preparation (Schneiderman, 1972). If conditioning is dependent on the CS-UR relation, these different results may be explained as follows: The nictitating membrane UR is very rapid and of very brief duration, whereas the heart rate UR is more delayed and longer lasting. Thus the backward-conditioning procedure allowed the CS to precede and overlap the heart rate UR but not the nicti-

tating membrane UR. The autonomic nervous system governs heart rate, which is important in emotional responding. We may anticipate that the more delayed and longer-lasting emotional responses mediated by the autonomic nervous system may be acquired and maintained under circumstances in which more rapidly occurring and shorter-duration responses are not.

## Behavioral Discrepancy Produced by the Reinforcing Stimulus

As noted earlier, experiments conducted by Leon Kamin in the late 1960s showed that something in addition to contiguity between the CS and US/ UR was needed for conditioning. Many subsequent experiments confirmed and extended these findings by using both Pavlovian and operant procedures (e.g., Fam, Westbrook, & Holmes, 2017; Rescorla & Wagner, 1972; Vom Saal & Jenkins, 1970). Some previous studies had pointed in a similar direction, but their significance was not fully appreciated (e.g., Johnson & Cumming, 1968; Rescorla, 1967).

Kamin devised a multiphase Pavlovian procedure known as the *blocking design*, which is summarized in Table 2.1. Kamin conditioned the CRs to CS1 in the experimental group of animals during Phase 1. He continued to pair CS1 with the US in Phase 2, but CS1 was now accompanied by CS2, a stimulus that came on and went off at the same time as CS1. Note that the temporal relation of CS2 to the US/UR should also support conditioning if CS–US/UR contiguity were the only requirement: The temporal relation of CS2 to the US was the same as for CS1. To determine whether each stimulus had acquired the CR, Kamin presented CS1 and CS2 separately in a test phase. As shown in Table 2.1, the CR occurred to CS1 but was attenuated or eliminated to CS2. An otherwise effective temporal relation of CS2 to the US/ UR did not condition a CR. Prior conditioning to CS1 had *blocked* conditioning to CS2.

One possible interpretation of the blocking of conditioning to CS2 is that two CSs cannot be conditioned simultaneously to the same US. Various control experiments eliminated this possibility. For example, experimenters first conditioned animals to an unrelated stimulus CS3 during Phase 1 (see Table 2.1). These animals then received the same training as the experimental group. The experimenters simultaneously presented CS1 and CS2 followed by the US/UR during Phase 2. Then, when the experimenters presented

**TABLE 2.1. The Experimental Design Used to Demonstrate Blocking of Conditioning**

|  | Experimental group | Control group |
|---|---|---|
| Conditioning phase 1 | CS1 (tone) ⟶ US (food) | CS3 (click) ⟶ US (food) |
| Conditioning phase 2 | CS1 (tone) plus<br>CS2 (light) } ⟶ US (food) | CS1 (tone) plus<br>CS2 (light) } ⟶ US (food) |
| Test phase | CS1 (tone) presented alone—CR<br>CS2 (light) presented alone—no CR | CS1 (tone) presented alone—CR<br>CS2 (light) presented alone—CR |

CS1 and CS2 separately to the control animals during the test phase, each stimulus evoked a CR. Thus two stimuli could be conditioned to the same US simultaneously, and the explanation of blocking had to be sought elsewhere.

Robert Rescorla and Allan Wagner (1972) first offered a compelling explanation of blocking. Stated in behavioral terms instead of in the associationist language of the original formulation, a stimulus becomes a CS when the UR that is evoked by the US differs from the behavior occurring just before the US was presented, given an appropriate temporal relation to the UR (Donahoe, Crowley, Millard, & Stickney, 1982; Mizunami, Terao, & Alvarez, 2018; Stickney & Donahoe, 1983). Technically speaking, the US must evoke a *behavioral change* or *discrepancy* for it to function as a reinforcer. In the experimental group, the experimenter blocked conditioning to CS2 during Phase 2, because CS1 was already evoking the CR (e.g., salivation) *before* the US evoked the UR (also salivation). The UR did not constitute a sufficient change in ongoing behavior to produce new conditioning. In the control group, however, when CS2 occurred during Phase 2, it accompanied a stimulus (CS1) that did *not* already evoke a CR, and both CS1 and CS2 became effective conditioned stimuli.

The significance of the behavioral-discrepancy requirement is that a stimulus must evoke a *change* in behavior for it to function as a reinforcer. In everyday language, the learner must be *surprised* to make the elicited response. Natural selection has chosen neural mechanisms of conditioning that function only when the would-be reinforcer evokes a behavioral change. As a possible everyday example, parents who lavish praise on a child independently of the child's behavior may find that their praise becomes ineffective as a reinforcer. Frequent and indiscriminate praise is not surprising. Conversely, sparingly delivered parental praise may

continue to be an effective reinforcer. The more deprived the learner is of contact with a stimulus, the more vigorous is the behavior evoked by that stimulus, and the more effectively it can function as a reinforcer (cf. Donahoe, 1997a; Premack, 1959; Seaver & Bourret, 2020; Timberlake & Allison, 1974). Food for a food-deprived animal evokes vigorous eating; food for a satiated animal does not.

## A Unified Principle of Reinforcement

Our present understanding of the conditions required for selection by reinforcement may be summarized as follows: If a stimulus evokes a change in ongoing behavior (behavioral discrepancy), then that stimulus functions as a reinforcer for the environment–behavior events that accompany the discrepancy (temporal contiguity; Donahoe et al., 1982, 1993).

Figure 2.1 shows that in the Pavlovian procedure, the stimulus that reliably precedes the discrepancy is the CS, and the behavior that reliably instantiates the discrepancy is the UR. Figure 2.1 also shows that in the simplest operant procedure, no particular stimulus reliably precedes the discrepancy, and the events that accompany the discrepancy are the operant and the UR. Thus both the operant and the CR are acquired in the operant procedure. The basic conditioning process, selection by reinforcement, appears to be the same in both the classical and operant procedures. However, the events that reliably accompany the discrepancy in the two procedures are different, and the outcomes of the two procedures are therefore different. In the Pavlovian procedure, a specific stimulus, the CS, gains control over a specific response, the CR, but whatever other responses occur at the time of the discrepancy are uncontrolled. In the operant procedure, two specific responses, the operant and the CR, are acquired, but the antecedent stimuli that accompany the operant are uncontrolled. (Note that a discriminated operant procedure does specify the antecedent stimuli.) Because the reinforcement process appears to be fundamentally the same in the Pavlovian and operant procedures, we call it the *unified reinforcement principle* (Donahoe et al., 1982).

In the Pavlovian procedure, no specified response necessarily precedes the UR-instigated discrepancy, and in the simple operant procedure, no specified environmental stimulus necessarily precedes the discrepancy. However, this does not mean that a response other than the CR cannot be acquired in the classical procedure, or that no stimulus acquires control of behavior in the operant procedure (Donahoe et al., 1997). To the extent that conditioning is promoted by only a single occurrence of a discrepancy, other responses may become conditioned in the Pavlovian procedure, and some stimuli may acquire control of the operant in the operant procedure. Indeed, Skinner (1948) demonstrated that an operant response may be conditioned when reinforcers occur independently of behavior. The responses the participant acquired are those that happen by chance to precede the reinforcer. Thus a pigeon that is given occasional presentations of food independently of its behavior may nevertheless acquire behavior such as pecking screw heads on the wall of the test chamber or pacing in front of the feeder (Staddon & Simmelhag, 1970; Timberlake & Lucas, 1985). Once such a response happens to precede food, it can be further strengthened by later presentations of food that also follow that response. Skinner referred to this phenomenon as *superstitious conditioning.* Experimenters discovered an analogous phenomenon in the Pavlovian procedure (Benedict & Ayres, 1972). When an experimenter presents a CS and a US independently, chance conjunctions of the CS with the US may allow the CS to acquire control of the CR, especially when the chance pairings occur early in training.

The conditioning process cannot distinguish between a chance and a nonchance contiguity of an event with a reinforcer on a single occasion. Perhaps Pavlov's dog perked up its ears after hearing the metronome when the experimenter presented food. The procedure might then strengthen the behavior of raising the ears in the presence of the sound of the metronome and not merely the CR of salivating. Similarly, Skinner's rat likely looked at the bar when about to press it, or his pigeon looked at the disk when about to peck it before the response produced the food. The conditioning process can discriminate between chance and nonchance relations between events only through repeated experience. A unified reinforcement principle accommodates the different behavioral outcomes produced by the respondent and operant procedures, while also allowing for the occasional emergence of superstitious conditioning in either procedure. Natural selection has produced a conditioning process that is sensitive to *reliable* relations between the environment and behavior, but the process is not infallible.

## CONDITIONED REINFORCEMENT AND COMPLEX BEHAVIOR

In the larger world outside the laboratory, many stimuli that serve as effective reinforcers do not elicit responses that are readily detectable at the behavioral level of observation. Talking with another person continues when the other person engages in that subtle behavior we call *paying attention.* But paying attention is not an elicited behavior and includes barely perceptible and highly variable behavior such as maintaining eye contact. In addition, stimuli that serve as reinforcers in the real world often seem delayed far beyond the time that experimental analysis indicates is effective: The worker who comes to the job on Monday may not receive a paycheck until Friday. How, then, are we to understand the conditioning and maintenance of human behavior when it apparently does not satisfy the requirements for conditioning revealed through experimental analysis? The phenomenon of *conditioned reinforcement* provides a major part of the answer.

### Higher-Order and Conditioned-Reinforcement Procedures

The experimental analysis of conditioning with the Pavlovian and operant procedures uses reinforcers that elicit a readily measured response, such as salivating or eating. The ticking sound of a metronome was followed by food, and salivation came to be evoked by the ticking sound. The experimenter presented food that elicited eating after a rat pressed the lever, which conditioned both bar pressing and salivation (cf. Shapiro, 1962). Stimuli that function as reinforcers when the learner does not have specific prior experience with those stimuli are called *unconditioned reinforcers.* These stimuli evoke behavior that has benefited survival of the species over evolutionary time. Stimuli such as sweet-tasting substances, which are generally rich in calories, and sexual stimuli, which are linked to reproductive behavior, are prime examples.

However, other stimuli acquire the ability to function as reinforcers only after they have been paired with existing reinforcers. These are *conditioned reinforcers*, whose reinforcing function is dependent on individual experience. A stimulus functions as a conditioned reinforcer in the Pavlovian procedure after it has been paired with an unconditioned reinforcer. A CS can then function as a reinforcer for another stimulus if the new stimulus is followed by a CS that already evokes behavior (the CR) due to prior conditioning. We can observe such effects in humans as when the thought of a stimulus that has been paired with food, such as the sight of food, may function as an effective CS. Imagine seeing food that you intend to eat at your next meal, particularly if you are hungry. Can you detect an increase in salivation? Imagining a favored food evokes conditioned salivation through previous experience with that food.

A *higher-order conditioning procedure* is a Pavlovian experimental arrangement in which the experimenter pairs a previously neutral stimulus with an established CS. As a laboratory example, the experimenter first pairs a CS1, such as a tone, with food. After CS1 evokes a salivary CR, the experimenter then introduces a CS2, such as a light, that precedes CS1 alone. As a result, CS2 also acquires the ability to evoke a salivary CR, even though CS2 was never paired with food. CS1 has functioned as a conditioned reinforcer. If the experimenter continues the higher-order procedure, but the CS2–CS1 sequence is never followed by food, then CS1 will cease to function as a conditioned reinforcer. In laboratory experiments on higher-order conditioning, responding to CS2 is usually maintained by occasionally presenting CS1 alone, followed by food (cf. Rescorla, 1980).

We also can study conditioned reinforcers using operant procedures (Williams, 1994a, 1994b). For example, if the experimenter has previously followed the sound of operation of the feeder with access to food, then rats may acquire lever pressing when pressing is followed by that sound (Skinner, 1938). This procedure is called a *conditioned* or *secondary reinforcement procedure*, because the sound of feeder operation, not food, has strengthened the operant. Skinner appreciated that a reinforcer must follow almost immediately after an operant if the operant is to be acquired. Therefore, the clicking sound of the feeder mechanism was paired with food before introducing the response lever into the experimental chamber. The click occurred *immediately* after the rat pressed the lever and served as a conditioned reinforcer for lever pressing.

Temporal contiguity and behavioral discrepancy are required for both conditioned and unconditioned reinforcement. In support of the contiguity requirement for conditioned reinforcement, after a stimulus (CS1) has become a CS by pairing it with an unconditioned reinforcer, another stimulus (CS2) will become a CS only if it precedes CS1 by no more than a few seconds (Kehoe, Gibbs, Garcia, & Gormezano, 1979). Findings obtained with the blocking design show that behavioral discrepancy is also required for conditioned reinforcement: The experimenter first paired a CS1, such as a tone, with food for a pigeon. Then a CS2, such as a light, accompanied the tone, and the experimenter continued to pair the compound light–tone stimulus with food. When the experimenter later presented the pigeon with two disks, pecking the disk that produced the tone increased, but pecking the disk that produced the light did not. The light was blocked from becoming a conditioned reinforcer (Palmer, 1987). To summarize, conditioned and unconditioned reinforcement both require temporal contiguity and behavioral discrepancy.

## Role of Conditioned Reinforcement in Complex Behavior

Human behavior is increasingly acquired and maintained by conditioned reinforcers. Consider the following example: Assume that a child has already learned the alphabet. Stated more technically, the visual stimuli provided by letters have become discriminative stimuli that control saying the names of the letters; B controls /bee/, C controls /see/, D controls /dee/, and so on. Keller and Schoenfeld (1950) proposed that discriminative stimuli can function as conditioned reinforcers when they follow other responses. Dinsmoor (1950) demonstrated experimentally that this conjecture was correct. (For reviews, see Williams, 1994a, 1994b.) Given these findings, suppose that an experimenter asks children who have learned to say letter names when they see a written letter are then asked to write letters when the experimenter says each letter's name. The closer their writing approaches the appearance of the letter the experimenter has instructed them to write, the greater the conditioned reinforcement provided by the visual stimuli produced by their own writing. In short, writing a letter produces immediate conditioned reinforcement, the magnitude of which increases as the writing more closely approximates the correct appearance of the letter. Learning to say letters has allowed the children to write letters with little or no reliance on external reinforcers from others. Conditioned reinforcers that shape behavior in this manner illustrate the process of *automatic conditioned reinforcement* and play an especially important role in the acquisition of verbal behavior (Donahoe & Palmer, 1994/2005; Petursdottir & Lepper, 2015; Sundberg, Michael, Partington, & Sundberg, 1996; Vaughan & Michael, 1982).

Behavior analysts appreciate the central role of reinforcement in understanding behavior, and automatic conditioned reinforcement provides a persuasive account of the acquisition of some aspects of complex behavior. However, for many psychologists, the concept of conditioned reinforcement seems to appeal to something akin to magic. The reluctance to accept conditioned reinforcement arises in part because the conditioned reinforcer often evokes no measurable behavior. We can observe only an increase in the behavior that precedes the conditioned reinforcer. We can document the occurrence of conditioned reinforcement independently, however, by moving from the behavioral to the neural level of observation. The following brief sketch of the neural sys-

tems involved in unconditioned and conditioned reinforcement indicates that both classes of reinforcers engage the same basic neural system.

## Neural Systems of Unconditioned and Conditioned Reinforcement

Figure 2.4 displays a side view of the human cerebral cortex. The shapes outlined by dashed lines indicate the subcortical structures and pathways *beneath* the cortex that are critical for reinforcement. All unconditioned reinforcers, including drugs of abuse, food, and sexual stimuli, activate brain cells (neurons) that are in a subcortical area called the *ventral tegmental area* (see Figure 2.4). Neurons whose cell bodies are in the ventral tegmental area send widely distributed projections (axons) to the prefrontal cortex. The curved arrow between the ventral tegmental area and the prefrontal cortex indicates these pathways in Figure 2.4. The prefrontal cortex receives projections from sensory areas of the brain that converge on neurons that lead ultimately to behavior via their connections to the motor cortex. The prefrontal cortex is thus the area of the brain in which inputs from the environment converge on neurons that lead to behavior. Because of this, connections between these neurons are prime targets for selection by reinforcement.

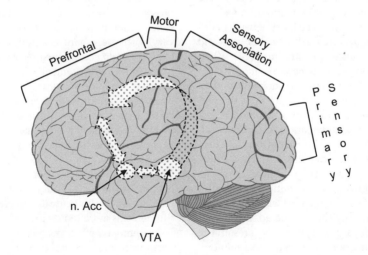

**FIGURE 2.4.** Side view of the left side of the human cerebral cortex. The front of the brain is toward the left portion of the figure. The cortical regions are labeled for purposes of this chapter and are not intended to be complete. For example, the region designated as primary sensory cortex is concerned with vision and does not include other sensory areas such as temporal cortex, which concerns audition. The forms outlined with dashed lines represent subcortical structures and pathways involved in the reinforcement of behavior. VTA, ventral tegmental area; n. Acc, nucleus accumbens. See the text for further information.

How do the projections from the ventral tegmental area to the prefrontal cortex affect the connectivity of prefrontal neurons upon which sensory inputs converge and from which behavioral (motor) outputs arise? Axons from the ventral tegmental area liberate a *neuromodulator* called dopamine. Dopamine is called a neuromodulator because it regulates the effects of other *neurotransmitters*. If dopamine is present when a neuron is activated by neurotransmitters from its input neurons, then the specific connections between the activated input neurons and the activated target neuron are strengthened. In brief, the connections between co-active neurons are strengthened if dopamine is also present. The result is that the next time the environment stimulates the same connections to those prefrontal neurons, the target neurons are more likely to be activated. The effect of this sequence of events is that the behavior that preceded the unconditioned reinforcer becomes more likely to recur in that environment. The neural process that strengthens the connectivity between neurons is called *long-term potentiation* (see Donahoe, 2017, for a review). Research has shown that reinforcement-instigated dopamine is effective for only a few seconds, which is consistent with behavioral research on the importance of temporal contiguity (Yagishita et al., 2014).

The upper panel (A) of Figure 2.5 shows the frequency of activation (firing) of dopamine neurons in the ventral tegmental area (VTA) after orange juice was introduced into the mouth of a monkey (Schultz, 1997). Note that the burst of firing of dopamine neurons occurred a fraction of a second after the orange juice was administered. When dopamine neurons enter a bursting mode, their axons liberate dopamine. The dopamine then briefly diffuses throughout large areas of the prefrontal and motor cortex before being degraded. The brief widespread distribution of dopamine allows dopamine to affect the strengths of connections between co-active neurons throughout these areas. The middle panel (B) of Figure 2.5 shows the frequency of firing of dopamine neurons after many pairings of the CS (a light) with the US (orange juice). Note that the CS caused an increase in the firing of dopamine neurons. As a result, the CS could now function as a conditioned reinforcer. Both conditioned and unconditioned reinforcers activate the *same* dopamine system.

Conditioned and unconditioned reinforcers activate the same dopamine system, but by different routes. Unconditioned reinforcers activate the ventral tegmental area by relatively direct path-

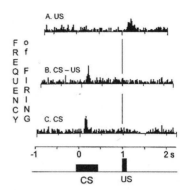

**FIGURE 2.5.** The frequency of firing of dopamine-producing neurons in the ventral tegmental area (VTA). (A) Activation of VTA neurons when a US (orange juice) was introduced into the mouth of a monkey. (B) Activation of VTA neurons during a paired CS–US trial after a number of pairings of the CS (a light) with the US, showing an increase in firing to the CS. (C) Activation of VTA neurons when presented with the CS alone after a number of paired CS–US trials. Note the increase in firing to the CS and the depression of firing during the interval when the US normally occurred. From Donahoe (1997b), based on findings from Schultz (1997).

ways from evolutionarily critical receptors, such as those for taste, smell, and sexual contact. Inputs from these receptors have been important for survival and reproduction, and hence subject to natural selection over evolutionary time. By contrast, stimuli that function as conditioned reinforcers vary with the organism's individual experience. How, then, do conditioned reinforcers gain access to the VTA reinforcement system used by unconditioned reinforcers? As indicated in Figure 2.4, when connections from neurons in the prefrontal cortex to motor neurons are strengthened (thereby making the behavior more likely), connections to neurons in another subcortical structure, called the *nucleus accumbens*, are also strengthened. Neurons in the nucleus accumbens then project to neurons in the VTA. Thus conditioned reinforcers gain access to the ventral tegmental area system through this more indirect route.

In summary, when dopamine strengthens connections from prefrontal neurons to neurons that promote behavior, it also strengthens connections to neurons in the nucleus accumbens and from there to the VTA. The neural mechanisms of reinforcement strengthen both the guidance of behavior by environmental stimuli and the ability of those stimuli to function as conditioned reinforcers. Although stimuli that function as conditioned reinforcers can also serve other functions (Bullock & Hackenberg, 2014; Russell, Ingvarsson, Haggar, & Jessel, 2018; Shahan, 2010), their reinforcing function is clear.

We should mention one additional aspect of the neural mechanisms of reinforcement. The lower panel (C) of Figure 2.5 shows the response of dopamine neurons when the experimenter presented the CS but did not follow it by the US. The CS produced a burst of firing of dopamine neurons, but then a *decrease* in firing at the time when the US would normally occur. At that time, the CS briefly inhibited the dopamine neurons in the VTA. This had the effect of preventing the US from serving as a reinforcer at that moment. The inhibition of dopamine activity by a CS in the Pavlovian procedure, or by a discriminative stimulus in the operant procedure during the time when the US occurs, is the neural basis of blocking (Donahoe et al., 1993; cf. Schultz, 1997, 2001; Waelti, Dickinson, & Schultz, 2001). Thus behavioral and neuroscientific research agree that both temporal contiguity and discrepancy are required for conditioning. Neuroscience complements behavior analysis (Donahoe. 2017). As Skinner (1988) recognized, "The . . . gap between behavior and the variables of which it is a function can be filled only by neuroscience, and the sooner . . . the better" (p. 460).

Finally, consider how the neural mechanisms of conditioned reinforcement help us understand the acquisition of complex behavior by experienced learners. Let us return to the example of children learning to *write* their letters after having learned to *speak* their letters. When the children's writing behavior produces a visual stimulus that approximates the appearance of a well-formed letter, that stimulus then presumably initiates a brief burst of dopamine firing proportional to how closely the visual stimulus corresponds to the letter that controls saying its name. The cumulative effect of this process is that the children produce a progressively well-formed letter. The same process occurs with the behavior of an office worker who receives a paycheck only at the end of the week. Behavior is acquired and maintained not by the delayed paycheck, but by immediate conditioned reinforcers. The sources of these conditioned reinforcers vary and include concurrent social stimuli (such as praise from colleagues) and stimuli produced by the worker's own behavior (such as seeing that he or she has done a job well). A well-done job is one that produces stimuli in whose presence past be-

havior has been reinforced. For a learner with an appropriate history of reinforcement, stimuli that engage the neural mechanisms of conditioned reinforcement continuously and immediately reinforce temporally extended sequences of behavior.

## FACTORS THAT AFFECT BEHAVIORAL CHANGE IN THE CLASSICAL PROCEDURE

The classical procedure is best suited for the experimental analysis of the effects of varying the characteristics of the CS and the reinforcer (the US) and of the temporal relation between them. By contrast, the operant procedure is best suited for the experimental analysis of the effects of varying the characteristics of the response, the reinforcer, and the temporal relation between them. Discriminated operant conditioning, which is considered by Catania in Chapter 3 of this volume, permits the experimental analysis of all three events—the environmental stimulus, the behavior that occurs in the presence of the stimulus, and the reinforcer.

### Characteristics of the CS

Experimenters have used many types of stimuli as CSs in the classical procedure. They include the usual *exteroceptive* stimuli—visual, auditory, and tactile stimuli—but also *interoceptive* stimuli, or those produced by stimulation of internal receptors. Indeed, Pavlovian conditioning influences the regulation of many intraorganismic responses, such as blood pressure, glucose levels, and other behavior mediated by the autonomic nervous system (Dworkin, 1993). Emotional behavior is especially affected by the variables manipulated in the Pavlovian procedure because of their pervasive effects on autonomic responses (Skinner, 1938). As one example of interoceptive conditioning, stimuli from inserting a hypodermic needle into the skin precede the effects of an injected drug, and these stimuli then become CSs for drug-related responses. The effects of such CSs can be complex. When internal receptors on neurons sense the increased concentration of the injected compound, the level of that compound normally produced by neurons decreases. For example, cocaine raises the level of circulating dopamine, and receptors on neurons that release dopamine in the brain detect this increase. These neurons then reduce their production of dopamine. Thus the true UR is not an increase in dopamine from the injection of cocaine, but a decrease in the production of dopamine by neurons whose receptors detect the increased levels of dopamine. As a result, for someone addicted to cocaine, neurons show a conditioned *decrease* in the production of dopamine when the person is given a placebo (i.e., an injection CS that is not followed by cocaine) or presented with stimuli that have previously accompanied drug intake. Decreases in dopamine induce withdrawal symptoms, because the stimulus of the injection produces a conditioned reduction in the internal production of dopamine (Eikelboom & Stewart, 1982; see also Sokolowska, Siegel, & Kim, 2002). Classical conditioning plays an important role in dysfunctional behavior, such as drug addiction.

Classical conditioning can also affect panic disorder (e.g., Bouton, Mineka, & Barlow, 2001). The life histories of those afflicted with panic disorder often include pairings of the feared stimulus with an aversive US (Acierno, Hersen, & Van Hasselt, 1993).

Although many stimuli can function as CSs, all stimuli are not equally effective with all USs. As a laboratory example, if the experimenter presents food to a pigeon following a localized visual stimulus, the pigeon will begin to peck the visual stimulus (Brown & Jenkins, 1968). This procedure, known as *autoshaping*, meets the definition of a classical procedure. Pecking, which was initially elicited by the sight of food, is now directed to a stimulus—the localized light—that reliably precedes the food. However, if the experimenter pairs food with a stimulus that is not spatially localized, such as a sound, pecking is not observed, although other measures indicate that conditioning has occurred (Leyland & Mackintosh, 1978). The expression of the CR depends in part on the CS with which the US is paired. Some instances of this phenomenon—called *differential associability*—arise from the history of the individual. For example, presenting the textual stimulus *DON'T BLINK* to a human as a CS before a puff of air to the eye impairs conditioning of the eye blink relative to a neutral stimulus, such as the presentation of a geometric form. Conversely, conditioning is facilitated if the CS is *BLINK* (Grant, 1972). Research has also shown interactions between the CS and US in the conditioning of phobias. Stimuli that are often the objects of phobias, such as spiders, become CSs more rapidly when they are paired with an aversive US, such as a moderate electric shock (Ohman, Fredrikson, Hugdahl, & Rimmo, 1976; Lindström, Golkar, & Olsson, 2015). When we examine the histories of persons with phobic behavior, they often contain experiences in which the object of the phobia has been paired with an aversive stimulus (Merckelbach & Muris, 1997).

Instances of differential associability also arise from the history of the species of which the individual is a member. Taste (gustatory) or smell (olfactory) stimuli more readily become CSs when paired with food and the consequences of ingestion than do visual or auditory stimuli (Garcia, Erwin, & Koelling, 1966). If nausea is a consequence of ingestion, as occurs with poisons, then an aversion to that food is conditioned. This phenomenon is called *taste aversion* and undoubtedly owes its occurrence to the special status that olfactory and gustatory stimuli have with respect to the ingestion of food. Over evolutionary time, such stimuli have come came immediately before the ingestion of food, thus providing the relative constancy of environmental conditions required for natural selection to operate. Under constant conditions, special neural circuitry is selected between these sensory modalities and the behavior associated with food intake. Taste aversions are generally affected by the same variables as other CRs, although conditioning may take place over longer intervals between the nominal CS and the US, because the UR (e.g., nausea) is delayed (LoLordo & Droungas, 1989). Conditioned aversions to food eaten before chemotherapy often occur because of the nausea-inducing effects of the treatment. Appropriate conditioning regimens, such as pairing the treatment with a nonpreferred food, reduce aversions to other foods. In this way, taste aversions develop toward the nonpreferred food and not the food normally eaten (Bernstein, 1991; Wang, Lee, He, & Huang, 2017).

## Characteristics of the US/UR

The stimuli used as USs vary almost as widely as those used as CSs. Generally, we may divide USs into two classes: those that are *appetitive*, or stimuli that elicit approach behavior; and those that are *aversive*, or stimuli that elicit escape behavior. Appetitive USs, such as food or water, evoke a range of behaviors, including approaching the stimulus and a variety of consummatory responses, when they are presented to an appropriately deprived animal. Similarly, aversive stimuli elicit a range of behavior, including escaping or attacking and freezing when the organism cannot escape the stimulus. The CRs conditioned to environmental stimuli can either facilitate or interfere with operants when the reinforcers occur in an operant procedure. To interpret possible interactions of respondents with operants, we should remember that the total CR is not necessarily restricted to the CRs that we measure. USs generally elicit many URs, some of which are detected less easily at the behavioral level of measurement, such as heart rate changes mediated by the autonomic nervous system.

## SOME PHENOMENA ASSOCIATED WITH THE PAVLOVIAN (RESPONDENT) CONDITIONING PROCEDURE

Thus far, we have been concerned with the *acquisition* of environment–behavior relations via the Pavlovian procedure, and with the process of *reinforcement* that produces acquisition. In this section, we examine several phenomena encountered during the acquisition of CS–CR relations.

### Maintenance of Conditioning

The acquisition of conditioning proceeds most rapidly when every presentation of the CS is followed by a reinforcer—whether an unconditioned or conditioned reinforcer. However, behavior can be maintained at high levels with less frequent reinforcement once it has been acquired. The left panel of Figure 2.6 shows the acquisition of CRs with the nictitating membrane preparation in

rabbits. During acquisition, every presentation of the CS was followed by the US/UR. The three groups of animals then received different percentages of CS–US/UR pairings. One group received reinforcers after 100% of CS presentations, and responding was maintained at the same high level as during acquisition. The remaining two groups received a *gradually* reduced percentage of reinforcement. The US/UR ultimately followed the CS on only 50% of the trials in one group and only 25% of the trials in the other group. As the middle panel of Figure 2.6 shows, performance was relatively unchanged, even though the percentage of reinforced CSs was very substantially reduced. The procedure is called *continuous* reinforcement when the US/UR follows every CS presentation, and *intermittent* (or *partial*) reinforcement when the US/UR follows only some CSs. In these terms, efficient acquisition of CRs requires continuous reinforcement, but the gradual introduction of intermittent reinforcement can maintain responding.

### Stimulus Generalization

The stimulus that reliably precedes the reinforcer during acquisition is the CS. However, the CS is not the only stimulus whose control of the CR is affected by conditioning. Other stimuli that share properties in common with the CS also come to evoke the CR, although with less strength. For

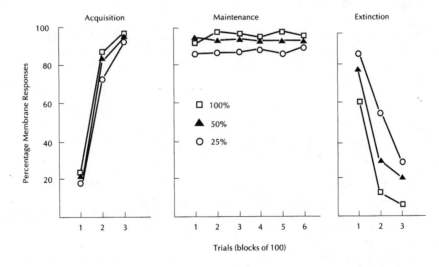

**FIGURE 2.6.** Acquisition, maintenance, and extinction of a Pavlovian nictitating membrane CR in the rabbit. During acquisition, 100% of the CSs were followed by the US. During maintenance, different groups of animals received either 100%, 50%, or 25% CS–US pairings. During extinction, CS presentations were not followed by the US. From Donahoe and Palmer (1994/2005), based on findings from Gibbs, Latham, and Gormezano (1978). Copyright © 2005 John W. Donahoe. Reprinted by permission.

example, if the CS is a tone with a frequency of 1,000 Hertz (Hz), then tones of 800 Hz are likely to evoke CRs, although to a lesser degree. Similarly, tones of 600 Hz may also evoke CRs, but to an even lesser degree. Other stimuli acquire the ability to evoke CRs in proportion to their physical similarity to the training CS. Many classical procedures with human and nonhuman participants have documented this phenomenon, known as *stimulus generalization* (e.g., Gynther, 1957; Hupka, Liu, & Moore, 1969). The experimental analysis of neuroscience is consistent with the behavioral analysis. Responding to a generalization stimulus occurs to the extent that the generalization stimulus activates the same sensory neurons as the training stimulus (Thompson, 1965).

A second source of stimulus generalization arises from the other stimuli that accompany the CS. These stimuli define the stimulus context. The stimulus context seldom evokes the CR by itself, because the more reliably present CS blocks control by contextual stimuli. However, the CS and the contextual stimuli furnish the full stimulus compound with which the US/UR is paired, and the context can also affect responding (Burns, Burgos, & Donahoe, 2011; Donahoe et al., 1997). Contextual stimuli are sometimes said to function as *occasion setters* (Grahame, Hallam, & Geier, 1990).

### Control by CR-Related Interoceptive Stimuli

As conditioning proceeds, the CR begins to occur during the CS before the presentation of the US/UR (Shapiro, 1962). Thus CR-produced stimuli may begin to appear before acquisition is complete. As a result, these interoceptive events bear a temporal relation to the behavioral discrepancy that permits them also to acquire control of the CR. In an illustrative study, the experimenter paired an appetitive US, food, with an aversive stimulus, a moderate electric shock, after the experimenter had previously paired the CS with food alone. (Pairing eliciting stimuli that evoke competing URs is called a *counterconditioning procedure*; cf. Richardson & Donahoe, 1967.) Food-related CRs were weakened when the experimenter presented the CS after the experimenter had paired the food with shock (Colwill & Rescorla, 1985; Donahoe & Burgos, 2000; Holland & Rescorla, 1975). Note that food-related CRs were weakened even though the experimenter had never paired the CS itself with shock. This phenomenon is known as *revaluation*, so called because pairing food with shock

lessened the *value* of the food US. An interpretation of this finding is that pairing food with shock changed the interoceptive stimuli that the CR and the CS jointly controlled during conditioning, and that this change weakened food-related CRs. Clearly, a complex array of stimuli, including the effects of stimulus generalization and control by contextual and interoceptive stimuli, may affect the CR.

### Extinction

After a CS has acquired control of a CR, presenting the CS but omitting the US weakens control, which is an *extinction* procedure. The right panel of Figure 2.6 shows the effect of an extinction procedure on a CR. The percentage of CS presentations that evoked a CR decreased more slowly after intermittent reinforcement than after continuous reinforcement. The responding of animals that received 100% reinforcement declined most rapidly, followed by animals receiving 50% and then 25% reinforcement.

### Punishment

*Punishment* is a term that, strictly speaking, applies only to the operant procedure. In a punishment procedure, the operant response produces a stimulus that decreases the strength of the operant. As a laboratory example, food-reinforced lever pressing can be punished by the occasional presentation of a moderate electric shock. Food-reinforced lever pressing declines under this procedure, and we say that shock functions as a punisher. By contrast, conditioning with the Pavlovian procedure always produces an increase in responding, which is an increase in the behavior that the US elicits. Although punishment occurs only in operant procedures, conditioning in the classical procedure is relevant because CRs contribute to punishment. Specifically, participants acquire CRs and operants together in the operant procedure. These CRs can decrease the operant if the operant and the CR are incompatible (Donahoe & Palmer, 1994/2005). In the preceding example, food conditions lever pressing, whereas shock conditions escape from the lever as well as autonomic responses (Borgealt, Donahoe, & Weinstein, 1972). Because the organism cannot press the lever while simultaneously escaping from the region with the lever, lever pressing declines. The recovery of lever pressing from punishment depends on the extinction of escape responses (Estes & Skinner, 1941).

We can understand certain paradoxical effects of punishment procedures as the product of interactions between operants and respondents. In one line of research, monkeys restrained in a chair were first trained to bite a rubber hose for food. This was an operant task, with biting as the operant and food as the reinforcer. The experimenter then altered the procedure so that biting the hose continued to produce food, but also an occasional electric shock to the tail. Electric shock to the tail of a monkey elicited hose biting. Biting is a component of aggressive behavior that is often elicited by aversive stimuli. Instead of reducing the rate of hose biting, the addition of shock increased it, particularly at the times when shock was most likely. In some cases, the experimenter could eliminate food altogether, and the monkey would continue to bite the hose, the only consequence of which was now the occasional delivery of shock (Branch & Dworkin, 1981; Morse & Kelleher, 1977). This masochistic behavior is understandable, at least in part, as a case in which the operant that produced food and the respondent evoked by shock were similar—biting.

## SOME IMPLICATIONS OF RESPONDENT CONDITIONING FOR APPLIED BEHAVIOR ANALYSIS

Most human behavior involves operant as well as respondent contingencies—that is, contiguity of a response with a reinforcer, and also contiguity of a stimulus with a reinforcer. As a result, techniques that researchers use to modify dysfunctional behavior implement both operant and respondent procedures. An understanding of the conditioning process by the Pavlovian procedure is important for two principal reasons. First, operant contingencies necessarily include stimulus–reinforcer contiguities. Some environmental stimulus always precedes the reinforcing stimulus (or US; see Figure 2.1). Thus reinforcer-evoked responses (CRs) are acquired inevitably in operant procedures. Second, current accounts of operant and Pavlovian procedures indicate that both procedures engage the same fundamental conditioning process. That is, whatever stimuli precede the behavioral discrepancy acquire control over whatever responses accompany the discrepancy. In the Pavlovian procedure, these stimuli are the CS and the context in which the CS occurs, and the behavior is the CR (generally components of the UR). In the operant procedure, the stimuli are those that precede the discrepancy (discriminative stimuli in dis-

criminated operant procedures), and the behavior is the operant plus the CR. The remainder of this chapter describes some implications of the reinforcement process for understanding dysfunctional behaviors that reflect both Pavlovian and operant contingencies.

## What Is the Role of Conditioned Reinforcement in Dysfunctional Behavior?

Conditioned reinforcement plays a critical role in the acquisition and maintenance of temporally extended sequences of behavior. Skinner (1938) illustrated this with rats whose bar presses immediately produced a clicking sound that had been previously paired with food, thereby bridging the time before food was actually ingested. The effect of conditioned reinforcement has also been illustrated with the example of children whose attempts to write their letters produce stimuli that immediately approximate the appearance of letters they have previously learned to speak. The click produced by bar pressing and the visual stimuli produced by writing provide immediate conditioned reinforcers for the behavior. Conditioned reinforcement is mediated by the neural pathways between the prefrontal cortex and the nucleus accumbens and from there to the ventral tegmental area. (See Figure 2.4.) In this section, we consider some of the possible effects on conditioned reinforcement produced by decreases in the functionality of connections from the prefrontal cortex to the nucleus accumbens. A stimulus acquires its ability to function as a conditioned reinforcer through the stimulus–reinforcer relations manipulated in Pavlovian procedures.

### Attention-Deficit/Hyperactivity Disorder

One of the behavioral characteristics of attention-deficit/hyperactivity disorder (ADHD) is difficulty sustaining activity on a task in which the reinforcer is delayed. The conditioned reinforcers that ordinarily maintain temporally extended behavior are relatively ineffective, which allows other concurrently available stimuli to control behavior that competes with the task at hand. In the vernacular, a person with ADHD is easily distracted. Because conditioned reinforcers play an important role in maintaining temporally extended environment–behavior relations, a deficit in conditioned reinforcement is a likely contributor to ADHD. In support of this conjecture, studies have found that the introduction of a conditioned reinforcer, especially if it occurs immediately after the behavior, facilitates choice of a larger but delayed unconditioned reinforcer (Williams, 1994c). Gradually increasing the time between the response and the reinforcer increases the choice of delayed reinforcement by children (Schweitzer & Sulzer-Azaroff, 1988). A gradual introduction of the delay permits stimuli in the delay period to become conditioned reinforcers. Studies of the neural basis of ADHD are consistent with the hypothesis that a deficit in the neural mechanisms of conditioned reinforcement is involved (Donahoe & Burgos, 2005; Johansen et al., 2009).

### Autism Spectrum Disorder

Autism spectrum disorder (ASD; see Kodak, Grow, & Bergmann, Chapter 23, this volume) is a focus of applied behavior analysis because its methods are the only empirically supported procedures that potentially remediate this often debilitating range of behavioral dysfunctions. Experimental evidence suggests that deficits in conditioned reinforcement and its neural mechanisms play an important role in ASD (Donahoe, 2018). The behavioral phenomena seen in ASD may include repetitive behaviors such as hand flapping, verbal deficits such as delayed or absent speech, and social challenges such as lack of eye contact when interacting with others. How might malfunctioning of conditioned reinforcement provide insights into this diverse set of behavioral deficits?

To study the effect of conditioned reinforcers on the behavior of persons with ASD, the experimenter placed participants in an apparatus that monitored the activation levels of various brain regions during a choice task (Dichter et al., 2012; Knutson, Adams, Fong, & Hammer, 2001). When neurons are activated, their demand for oxygen increases, which increases the blood flow in that region. Functional magnetic resonance imaging detects the increase in blood flow. In the experiment, a correct choice was immediately followed by either a dollar sign ($) or a brief view of a picture. The $ indicated that the participant would receive $1.00 at the end of the experimental session, and was intended to serve as a conditioned reinforcer. For participants with ASD, the $ activated neurons in the nucleus accumbens much less than for control participants, where it served as an effective conditioned reinforcer. By contrast, activity in the nucleus accumbens did not differ between participants with ASD and controls when a picture of an object with known attention-demand-

ing properties for persons with ASD immediately followed a correct response. The effective images were mostly of machines, automobiles, computers, and other nonsocial objects that the researchers used because they evoked eye movement fixations from participants with ASD during a pretest. In summary, the $ served as an effective conditioned reinforcer for controls but not for participants with ASD, as measured by choice behavior and by the activation level of neurons in the nucleus accumbens. No deficits were observed in the activation of prefrontal neurons by their multisynaptic inputs from sensory areas. Thus the nucleus accumbens neurons would have been activated if the normal prefrontal connections to the nucleus accumbens had been present. Possible causes of such neurodevelopmental deficits in ASD are under current investigation (e.g., Choi et al., 2016; Donahoe, 2018).

A deficit in the responsiveness of nucleus accumbens neurons to neurons in the prefrontal cortex provides a possible mechanism whereby we may understand the variability of ASD symptoms. If the number and origins of connections from regions in the prefrontal neurons to nucleus accumbens neurons differ for those with ASD, then the potential for the stimuli that activate these neurons to serve as conditioned reinforcers will differ. For example, suppose that during neural development connections are missing from some of the neurons in the premotor cortex to neurons in the nucleus accumbens. Instead, projections form from neurons in adjacent premotor areas that govern arm and hand movements to the nucleus accumbens. Under these circumstances, hand flapping would activate the ventral tegmental area via the nucleus accumbens and would be reinforced. As another example, suppose that projections from the region of the prefrontal cortex activated by speech movements that normally go to the nucleus accumbens are absent or diminished. In this scenario, the articulatory movements that produce speech sounds could not benefit from the automatic conditioned reinforcement that normally aids the acquisition of verbal behavior. Deficits in verbal behavior would result. Finally, suppose that neurons in the region of the prefrontal cortex that receive inputs from the sensory areas involved in face perception do not have connections to the nucleus accumbens. Under these circumstances, seeing a human face could not serve as a source of conditioned reinforcement. Instead, individuals might perceive direct eye contact with another person as a threat gesture, which is the typical reaction in other primates (Emery, Lorincz, Perrett, Oram, & Baker, 1997).

If alterations in the usual connectivity of prefrontal regions to the nucleus accumbens occur with ASD, then the neural mechanisms that mediate conditioned reinforcement would be affected. Experimental analysis suggests some potentially remedial actions if this is the case. For individuals with especially severe deficits, we could use stimuli that function as unconditioned reinforcers because they access the dopaminergic reinforcement system directly through the ventral tegmental area. These stimuli include food and drink (Lovaas, 1987). Other stimuli that are attention-demanding, such as certain visual displays, could also be effective. Baseline preferences for various displays would need to be determined to identify stimuli that could function as conditioned reinforcers (e.g., Mitchell & Stoffelmayr, 1973; Premack, 1959).

The establishment of conditioned reinforcers requires Pavlovian higher-order and compound-conditioning procedures or operant conditioned-reinforcement procedures. Research indicates that if we pair two stimuli with a reinforcer, then some neurons in sensory association areas of the cortex become activated *equally* by either stimulus. These neurons are called *pair-coded neurons* (Sakai & Miyashita, 1991). If one of the stimuli in the pair becomes a conditioned reinforcer, then the other stimulus can also become a conditioned reinforcer, even though it might not become a conditioned reinforcer if it were separately paired with the unconditioned reinforcer. Ideally, the two stimuli become equivalent in their ability to engage the conditioned-reinforcement system.

Matching-to-sample is an operant procedure that promotes the formation of pair-coded neurons. Behavioral evidence demonstrates that matching-to-sample procedures produce stimuli that form equivalence classes for at least some participants with ASD (McLay et al., 2013; cf. Sidman, 2000). In this way, a stimulus that could not function as a conditioned reinforcer when separately paired with a reinforcer may become a conditioned reinforcer through its equivalence with another stimulus that has acquired that function.

## What Stimuli Control Behavior in the Natural Environment?

The stimuli that guide behavior are those that have reliably occurred prior to reinforcers. Although we cannot know all of the stimuli in the natural environment that reliably occurred before reinforcers in the learner's past, we can identify these stimuli by noting the situations in which the behavior now habitually occurs. We must identify these stimuli if the behavioral changes produced by a therapeutic environment are to persist. Three guidelines are useful:

1. To the extent possible, the remedial environment should include some stimuli that control the target behavior in the natural environment. In this way, we maximize stimulus generalization from the remedial to the natural environment (Stokes & Baer, 1977). We must identify the conditions in the natural environment that precede dysfunctional behavior to identify these controlling stimuli.

2. We must introduce stimuli that control behavior in the remedial environment into the natural environment if those stimuli do not occur in the natural environment. This applies whether the intervention seeks to establish appropriate behavior or to establish behavior that competes with the dysfunctional behavior. Reinforcers do not select responses alone; they select environment–behavior relations (Donahoe et al., 1997).

3. We must supplement or remove the reinforcement contingencies that maintain dysfunctional behavior in the natural environment with alternative contingencies that maintain the behavior acquired in the remedial environment. To do this, the conditions in the natural environment that follow dysfunctional behavior and serve as reinforcers must be determined. Such reinforcers must be removed, or competing behavior must be acquired that minimizes contact with them. No behavioral intervention can *inoculate* a person against the effect of reinforcers of dysfunctional behavior encountered in the natural environment.

We can introduce controlling stimuli for alternative behavior from the remedial environment into the natural environment in several ways. These stimuli may be explicitly introduced into the natural environment. For example, we might pair a red card with an aversive stimulus (US) in the remedial environment as a first step to control profligate spending. We then would insert the card into the profligate spender's wallet so that the card is visible before money is accessible. We also can condition verbal responses to stimuli present in the natural environment, and these responses may in turn generate verbal stimuli that control alternative behavior. Continuing with the example of profligate spending, every time the wallet is opened, reinforcers are provided in the remedial environment when the spender verbalizes, "Do I really need to buy this?"

Verbal stimuli are potentially among the most effective stimuli to control behavior in the natural environment, because verbal responses are not dependent on external support in the same way as most nonverbal responses. Verbal responses—and hence the stimuli they produce—are potentially in the behavioral repertoire of a person in any environment. A second advantage of verbal stimuli is that they can be produced by subvocal verbal behavior, and subvocal behavior is not subject to contingencies of reinforcement instituted by others (Palmer, 2012). Others can ask why the red card is in the wallet, because they too can see the red card. But others cannot ask why a *thought* occurred, because a thought is a subvocal verbal response. Subvocal behavior is private behavior—that is, behavior whose stimulus properties are detectable only by the person emitting them (Donahoe & Palmer, 1994/2005; Skinner, 1957). If the goal is to maintain verbal vocal or subvocal responses, they too must be followed by reinforcers. Private behavior, sometimes called *cognitive behavior,* is not immune to the conditioning processes that affect all behavior.

## What Behavior Is Maintained by the Natural Environment?

As we have seen, behavior is maintained in an environment to the extent that the environment contains stimuli in whose presence the behavior has been previously reinforced. In the absence of reinforcement, an extinction procedure is implemented, and responding decreases. Intermittent reinforcement during conditioning increases resistance to the effects of extinction, but responding will not continue indefinitely. Thus the natural environment must contain reinforcers for the behavior established in the remedial environment. If dysfunctional environment–behavior relations continue to be reinforced in the natural environment, then the dysfunctional behavior will recur and persist, and more immediate reinforcers will maintain it even if its *long-term* consequences are maladaptive. Behavior that has undergone extinction in the remedial environment will reappear in the natural environment if the remedial environment does not contain *all* the stimuli that control

dysfunctional behavior in the natural environment.

To be effective, the extinction procedure should be continued substantially beyond the time when the environment first ceases to occasion the behavior. So-called "extinction below zero" increases the likelihood that all of the stimuli controlling the behavior have lost their control (Welker & McAuley, 1978). If effective stimuli remain, they foster resurgence of the maladaptive behavior, and it may be reinforced again (Epstein & Skinner, 1980). The recurrence of behavior after extinction is called *spontaneous recovery* (Estes, 1955; Pavlov, 1927/1960; Skinner, 1938). Again, the remedial environment cannot *inoculate* behavior against the effects of reinforcers for dysfunctional behavior provided by the natural environment.

Addiction provides a particularly striking example of the recurrence of dysfunctional behavior. Research with the classical procedure has shown that CRs evoked early in the conditioning process give rise to stimuli that acquire control over the CR jointly with the CS. The phenomenon of *revaluation* documents the existence of control by CR-related stimuli (Holland & Rescorla, 1975; Wyvell & Berridge, 2000). In the treatment of addiction, we may eliminate *physical dependence* by withholding the substance in the remedial environment. However, drug-related CRs will recur to the extent that the remedial environment differs from the environment in which the person acquired the addiction. Moreover, drug-related operant behavior will recur if it is controlled by interoceptive stimuli from drug-related CRs. To reduce resurgence of drug-related CRs and the untoward effects of the stimuli they produce, the remedial environment must gradually introduce stimuli that are CSs for these CRs, possibly including the sight of drug paraphernalia, and withhold reinforcement in their presence.

Environment–behavior relations that we select in the remedial environment will endure if the reinforcers that previously maintained the dysfunctional behavior are no longer encountered and, in addition, newly established immediate reinforcers are available for alternative behavior. Eliminating previously encountered reinforcers requires changing the natural environment—often a daunting task—or establishing behavior in the remedial environment that reduces contact of the dysfunctional behavior with these reinforcers. For someone with an alcohol addiction, a simplistic example of the latter would be taking a route that does not pass the local pub and being greeted by an adoring partner upon arrival at home. Important sources of immediate reinforcement for behavior that was established in a remedial environment are the stimuli such behavior produces. For example, behavior such as fluently reading or facilely writing a passage produces stimuli that are discriminated as characteristic of *a job well done*. The stimuli produced by such behavior have occurred previously in the remedial environment and have been the occasion for praise (a reinforcer) from others. Because these stimuli have been paired with praise, they become CSs and can function as conditioned reinforcers (Catania, 1975). However, we must continue to pair them with other reinforcers to maintain their status as conditioned reinforcers. Being literate may enhance one's ability to get a job, but the environment must provide jobs if such stimuli are to endure as conditioned reinforcers. Environment–behavior relations track the momentary contingencies of reinforcement, not remote consequences. In the long run, remedial interventions cannot overcome the contingencies repeatedly encountered in the natural environment. To be otherwise would contradict all that we know from the experimental analysis of respondent and operant procedures—efforts begun by Pavlov and Thorndike over 100 years ago.

## REFERENCES

Acierno, R. E., Hersen, M., & Van Hasselt, V. B. (1993). Interventions for panic disorder: A critical review of the literature. *Clinical Psychology Review, 6,* 561–578.

Benedict, J. O., & Ayres, J. J. (1972). Factors affecting conditioning in the truly random control procedure in the rat. *Journal of Comparative and Physiological Psychology, 78,* 323–330.

Bernstein, I. L. (1991). Aversion conditioning in response to cancer and cancer treatment. *Clinical Psychology Review, 2,* 185–191.

Borgealt, A. J., Donahoe, J. W., & Weinstein, A. (1972). Effects of delayed and trace components of a compound CS on conditioned suppression and heart rate. *Psychonomic Science, 26,* 13–15.

Bouton, M. E., Mineka, S., & Barlow, D. H. (2001). A modern learning theory perspective on the etiology of panic disorder. *Psychological Review, 108,* 4–32.

Branch, M. N., & Dworkin, S. I. (1981). Effects of ratio contingencies on responding maintained by schedules of electric-shock presentation (response-produced shock). *Journal of the Experimental Analysis of Behavior, 36,* 191–205.

Brown, P. L., & Jenkins, H. M. (1968). Auto-shaping of the pigeon's key-peck. *Journal of the Experimental Analysis of Behavior, 11,* 1–8.

Bullock, C. E., & Hackenberg, T. D. (2014). The several roles of stimuli in token reinforcement. *Journal of the Experimental Analysis of Behavior, 99,* 1–19.

Burns, R., Burgos, J. E., & Donahoe, J. W. (2011). Pavlovian conditioning: Pigeon nictitating membrane. *Behavioural Processes, 86,* 102–108.

Catania, A. C. (1975). The myth of self-reinforcement. *Behaviorism, 3,* 192–199.

Catania, A. C., & Keller, K. J. (1981). Contingency, contiguity, correlation, and the concept of causality. In P. Harzem & M. D. Zeiler (Eds.), *Predictability, correlation, and contiguity* (pp. 125–167). New York: Wiley.

Choi, G. B., Yim, Y. S., Wong, H., Kim, S., Kim, H., Kim, S. V., et al. (2016). The maternal interleukin-17a pathway in mice promotes autism-like phenotypes in offspring. *Science, 351,* 933–937.

Colwill, R. M., & Rescorla, R. A. (1985). Postconditioning devaluation of a reinforcer affects instrumental responding. *Journal of Experimental Psychology: Animal Behavior Processes, 11,* 120–132.

Dichter, G. S., Felder, J. N., Green, S. R., Ritenberg, A. M., Sasson, N. J., & Bodfish, J. W. (2012). Reward circuitry function in autism spectrum disorders. *Social Cognitive and Affective Neuroscience, 7,* 160–172.

Dinsmoor, J. A. (1950). A quantitative comparison of the discriminative and reinforcing function of a stimulus. *Journal of Experimental Psychology, 40,* 458–472.

Dinsmoor, J. A. (1995). Stimulus control: Part I. *Behavior Analyst, 18,* 51–68.

Donahoe, J. W. (1997a). Positive reinforcement: The selection of behavior. In J. R. O'Donohue (Ed.), *Learning and behavior therapy* (pp. 169–187). Boston: Allyn & Bacon.

Donahoe, J. W. (1997b). Selection networks: Simulation of plasticity through reinforcement learning. In J. W. Donahoe & V. P. Dorsel (Eds.), *Neural-network models of cognition: Biobehavioral foundations* (pp. 336–357). Amsterdam: Elsevier Science.

Donahoe, J. W. (1999). Edward L. Thorndike: The selectionist connectionist. *Journal of the Experimental Analysis of Behavior, 72,* 451–454.

Donahoe, J. W. (2017). Behavior analysis and neuroscience: Complementary disciplines. *Journal of the Experimental Analysis of Behavior, 107,* 301–320.

Donahoe, J. W. (2018). *Autism spectrum disorder: Biobehavioral mechanisms and remediation procedures.* Presentation at the Berkshire Association for Behavior Analysis and Therapy, Amherst, MA. Retrieved from *http://lcb-online.org/Autism-Spectrum_Disorder_Biobehavioral_Mechanisms.wmv.*

Donahoe, J. W., & Burgos, J. E. (2000). Behavior analysis and revaluation. *Journal of the Experimental Analysis of Behavior, 74,* 331–346.

Donahoe, J. W., & Burgos, J. E. (2005). Selectionism: Complex outcomes from simple processes. *Behavioural and Brain Sciences, 28,* 429–430.

Donahoe, J. W., Burgos, J. E., & Palmer, D. C. (1993). Selectionist approach to reinforcement. *Journal of the Experimental Analysis of Behavior, 60,* 17–40.

Donahoe, J. W., Crowley, M. A., Millard, W. J., & Stickney, K. A. (1982). A unified principle of reinforcement. In M. L. Commons, R. J. Herrnstein, & H. Rachlin (Eds.), *Quantitative analyses of behavior: Vol. 2. Matching and maximizing accounts* (pp. 493–521). Cambridge, MA: Ballinger.

Donahoe, J. W., & Palmer, D. C. (2005). *Learning and complex behavior.* Richmond, MA: Ledgetop. (Original work published 1994)

Donahoe, J. W., Palmer, D. C., & Burgos, J. E. (1997). The S-R issue: Its status in behavior analysis and in Donahoe and Palmer's *Learning and complex behavior. Journal of the Experimental Analysis of Behavior, 67,* 193–211.

Donahoe, J. W., & Vegas, R. (2004). Pavlovian conditioning: The CS–UR relation. *Journal of Experimental Psychology: Animal Behavior Processes, 30,* 17–33.

Dworkin, B. R. (1993). *Learning and physiological regulation.* Chicago: University of Chicago Press.

Eikelboom, R., & Stewart, J. (1982). Conditioning of drug-induced physiological responses. *Psychological Review, 89,* 507–528.

Emery, N. J., Lorincz, E. N., Perrett, D. I., Oram, M. W., & Baker, C. I. (1997). Gaze following and joint attention in rhesus monkeys (*Macaca mulatta*). *Journal of Comparative Psychology, 111,* 286–293.

Epstein, R., & Skinner, B. F. (1980). Resurgence of responding after the cessation of response-independent reinforcement. *Proceedings of the National Academy of Sciences of the USA, 77,* 6251–6253.

Estes, W. K. (1955). Statistical theory of spontaneous recovery and regression. *Psychological Review, 62,* 145–154.

Estes, W. K., & Skinner, B. F. (1941). Some quantitative properties of anxiety. *Journal of Experimental Psychology, 29,* 390–400.

Fam, J., Westbrook, R. F., & Holmes, N. M. (2017). An examination of changes in behavioral control when stimuli with different associative histories are conditioned in compound. *Journal of Experimental Psychology: Animal Learning and Cognition, 43*(3), 205–218.

Garcia, J., Erwin, F. R., & Koelling, R. A. (1966). Learning with prolonged delay in reinforcement. *Psychonomic Science, 5,* 121–122.

Gibbs, C. M., Latham, S. B., & Gormezano, I. (1978). Classical conditioning of the rabbit nictitating membrane response: Effects of reinforcement schedule on response maintenance and resistance to extinction. *Animal Learning and Behavior, 6,* 209–215.

Gormezano, I., & Kehoe, E. J. (1981). Classical conditioning and the law of contiguity. In P. Harzem & M. D. Zeiler (Eds.), *Predictability, correlation, and contiguity* (pp. 1–45). New York: Wiley.

Grahame, N. J., Hallam, S. C., & Geier, L. (1990). Context as an occasion setter following either CS acquisition and extinction or CS acquisition alone. *Learning and Motivation, 21,* 237–265.

Grant, D. A. (1972). A preliminary model for processing information conveyed by verbal conditioned stimuli in classical conditioning. In A. H. Black & W. F. Prokasy (Eds.), *Classical conditioning: II. Current research and theory* (pp. 64–99). Englewood Cliffs, NJ: Prentice-Hall.

Gynther, M. D. (1957). Differential eyelid conditioning as a function of stimulus similarity and strength of response to the CS. *Journal of Experimental Psychology, 53,* 408–416.

Hilgard, E. R. (1937). The relationship between the conditioned response and conventional learning experiments. *Psychological Bulletin, 34,* 61–102.

Holland, P. C., & Rescorla, R. A. (1975). The effect of two ways of devaluing the unconditioned stimulus after first- and second-order appetitive conditioning. *Journal of Experimental Psychology: Animal Behavior Processes, 1,* 355–363.

Hupka, R. B., Liu, S. S., & Moore, J. W. (1969). Auditory differential conditioning of the rabbit nictitating membrane response: V. Stimulus generalization as a function of the position of CS+ and CS– on the frequency dimension. *Psychonomic Science, 15,* 129–131.

Johansen, E. B., Killeen, P. R., Russell, V. A., Tripp, G., Wickens, J. R., Tannock, R., et al. (2009). Origins of altered reinforcement effects in ADHD. *Behavioral and Brain Functions, 5,* 1–15.

Johnson, D. F., & Cumming, W. W. (1968). Some determiners of attention. *Journal of the Experimental Analysis of Behavior, 11,* 157–166.

Jonçich, G. (1968). *The sane positivist: A biography of Edward L. Thorndike.* Middleton, CT: Wesleyan University Press.

Kamin, L. J. (1968). Attention-like processes in classical conditioning. In M. R. Jones (Ed.), *Miami symposium on the prediction of behavior* (pp. 9–31). Miami, FL: University of Miami Press.

Kamin, L. J. (1969). Predictability, surprise, attention and conditioning. In B. A. Campbell & R. M. Church (Eds.), *Punishment and aversive behavior* (pp. 279–296). New York: Appleton-Century-Crofts.

Kehoe, E. J., Gibbs, C. M., Garcia, E., & Gormezano, I. (1979). Associative transfer and stimulus selection in classical conditioning of the rabbit's nictitating membrane response to serial compound CSs. *Journal of Experimental Psychology: Animal Behavior Processes, 5,* 1–18.

Kehoe, E. J., & Macrae, M. (1994). Classical conditioning of the rabbit nictitating membrane response can be fast or slow: Implications of Lennartz and Weinberger's (1992) two-factor theory. *Psychobiology, 22,* 1–4.

Keller, F. S., & Schoenfeld, W. N. (1950). *Principles of psychology.* New York: Appleton-Century-Crofts.

Kirkpatrick, K., & Balsam, P. D. (2016). Associative learning and timing. *Current Opinion in Behavioral Sciences, 8,* 181–185.

Knutson, B., Adams, C. M., Fong, G. W., & Hammer, D.

G. (2001). Anticipation of increasing monetary reward selectively recruits nucleus accumbens. *Journal of Neuroscience, 21*(16), RC159.

Leyland, C. M., & Mackintosh, N. J. (1978). Blocking of first- and second-order autoshaping in pigeons. *Animal Learning and Behavior, 6*, 392–394.

Lindström, B., Golkar, A., & Olsson, A. (2015). A clash of values: Fear-relevant stimuli can enhance or corrupt adaptive behavior through competition between Pavlovian and instrumental valuation systems. *Emotion, 15*, 668–676.

LoLordo, V. M., & Droungas, A. (1989). Selective associations and adaptive specializations: Taste aversions and phobias. In S. B. Klein & R. R. Mowrer (Eds.), *Contemporary learning theories: Instrumental conditioning theory and the impact of biological constraints on learning* (pp. 145–179). Hillsdale, NJ: Erlbaum.

Lovaas, I. (1987). Behavioral treatment and normal educational and intellectual functioning in young children with autism. *Journal of Consulting and Clinical Psychology, 55*, 3–9.

McLay, L. K., Sutherland, D., Church, J., & Tyler-Merrick, G. (2013). The formation of equivalence classes in individuals with autism spectrum disorder: A review of the literature. *Research in Autism Spectrum Disorders, 7*, 418–431.

Merckelbach, H., & Muris, P. (1997). The etiology of childhood spider phobia. *Behaviour Research and Therapy, 35*, 1031–1034.

Mitchell, W. S., & Stoffelmayr, B. E. (1973). Application of the Premack principle to the behavioral control of extremely inactive schizrophrenics. *Journal of Applied Behavior Analysis, 6*, 419–423.

Mizunami, M., Terao, K., & Alvarez, B. (2018). Application of a prediction error theory to Pavlovian conditioning in an insect. *Frontiers in Psychology, 9*, 1272.

Morse, W. H., & Kelleher, R. T. (1977). Determinants of reinforcement and punishment. In W. K. Honig & J. E. R. Staddon (Eds.), *Handbook of operant behavior* (pp. 174–200). Englewood Cliffs, NJ: Prentice-Hall.

Ohman, A., Fredrikson, M., Hugdahl, K., & Rimmo, P. A. (1976). The premise of equipotentiality in human classical conditioning: Conditioned electrodermal responses to potentially phobic stimuli. *Journal of Experimental Psychology: General, 105*, 313–337.

Palmer, D. C. (1987). *The blocking of conditioned reinforcement.* Unpublished doctoral dissertation, University of Massachusetts, Amherst, MA.

Palmer, D. C. (2012). The role of atomic repertoires in the interpretation of complex behavior. *Behavior Analyst, 36*, 59–73.

Pavlov, I. P. (1960). *Conditioned reflexes.* New York: Dover. (Original work published 1927)

Petursdottir, A. I., & Lepper, T. L. (2015). Inducing novel vocalizations by conditioning speech sounds as reinforcers. *Behavior Analysis in Practice, 8*, 223–232.

Premack, D. (1959). Toward empirical behavioral laws: I. Positive reinforcement. *Psychological Review, 66*, 219–233.

Rescorla, R. A. (1967). Pavlovian conditioning and its proper control group. *Psychological Review, 74*, 71–80.

Rescorla, R. A. (1980). *Pavlovian second-order conditioning: Studies in associative learning.* Hillsdale, NJ: Erlbaum.

Rescorla, R. A. (1991). Associative relations in instrumental learning: The 18th Bartlett Memorial Lecture. *Quarterly Journal of Experimental Psychology, 43B*, 1–23.

Rescorla, R. A., & Wagner, A. R. (1972). A theory of Pavlovian conditioning: Variations in the effectiveness of reinforcement and nonreinforcement. In A. H. Black & W. F. Prokasy (Eds.), *Classical conditioning: II. Current research and theory* (pp. 64–99). New York: Appleton–Century–Crofts.

Richardson, W. K., & Donahoe, J. W. (1967). A test of the independence of the approach and avoidance gradients. *Psychonomic Science, 9*, 569–570.

Russell, D., Ingvarsson, E. T., Haggar, J. L., & Jessel, J. (2018). Using progressive-ratio schedules to evaluate tokens as generalized conditioned reinforcers. *Journal of Applied Behavior Analysis, 51*, 40–52.

Sakai, K., & Miyashita, Y. (1991). Neural organization for the long-term memory of paired associates. *Nature, 254*, 152–159.

Schneiderman, N. (1972). Response system divergencies in aversive classical conditioning. In A. H. Black & W. F. Prokasy (Eds.), *Classical conditioning: II. Current theory and research* (pp. 313–376). New York: Appleton-Century-Crofts.

Schultz, W. (1997). Adaptive dopaminergic neurons report value of environmental stimuli. In J. W. Donahoe & V. P. Dorsel (Eds.), *Neural-network models of cognition: Biobehavioral foundations* (pp. 317–335). Amsterdam: Elsevier Science.

Schultz, W. (2001). Reward signaling by dopamine neurons. *Neuroscientist, 7*, 293–302.

Schweitzer, J. B., & Sulzer-Azaroff, B. (1988). Self-control: Teaching tolerance for delay in impulsive children. *Journal of the Experimental Analysis of Behavior, 50*, 173–186.

Seaver, J. P., & Bourret, J. C. (2020). Producing mands in concurrent operant environments. *Journal of Applied Behavior Analysis, 53*, 366–384.

Shahan, T. A. (2010). Conditioned reinforcement and response strength. *Journal of the Experimental Analysis of Behavior, 93*, 269–289.

Shapiro, M. M. (1962). Temporal relationship between salivation and lever pressing with differential reinforcement of low rates. *Journal of Comparative and Physiological Psychology, 55*, 567–571.

Sidman, M. (2000). Equivalence relations and the reinforcement contingency. *Journal of the Experimental Analysis of Behavior, 74*, 127–140.

Skinner, B. F. (1935). Two types of conditioned reflex

and a pseudo type. *Journal of General Psychology, 12,* 66–77.

Skinner, B. F. (1937). Two types of conditioned reflex: A reply to Konorski and Miller. *Journal of General Psychology, 16,* 272–279.

Skinner, B. F. (1938). *The behavior of organisms.* New York: Appleton-Century-Crofts.

Skinner, B. F. (1948). "Superstition" in the pigeon. *Journal of Experimental Psychology, 38,* 168–172.

Skinner, B. F. (1957). *Verbal behavior.* New York: Appleton-Century-Crofts.

Skinner, B. F. (1988). Comments and consequences. In A. C. Catania & S. Harnad (Eds.), *The selection of behavior: The operant behaviorism of B. F. Skinner* (pp. 382–461). New York: Cambridge University Press.

Smith, M. C., Coleman, S. R., & Gormezano, I. (1969). Classical conditioning of the rabbit's nictitating membrane response at backward, simultaneous, and forward CS–US intervals. *Journal of Comparative and Physiological Psychology, 69,* 226–231.

Sokolowska, M., Siegel, S., & Kim, J. A. (2002). Intra-administration associations: Conditional hyperalgesia elicited by morphine onset cues. *Journal of Experimental Psychology: Animal Behavior Processes, 28,* 309–320.

Staddon, J. E., & Simmelhag, V. L. (1970). The "superstition" experiment: A reexamination of its implications for the principles of adaptive behavior. *Psychological Review, 78,* 3–43.

Stickney, K., & Donahoe, J. W. (1983). Attenuation of blocking by a change in US locus. *Animal Learning and Behavior, 11,* 60–66.

Stokes, T. F., & Baer, D. M. (1977). An implicit technology of generalization. *Journal of Applied Behavior Analysis, 10,* 349–367.

Sundberg, M. L., Michael, J., Partington, J. W., & Sundberg, C. A. (1996). The role of automatic reinforcement in early language acquisition. *Analysis of Verbal Behavior, 13,* 21–37.

Thompson, R. F. (1965). The neural basis of stimulus generalization. In D. I. Mostofsky (Ed.), *Stimulus generalization* (pp. 154–178). Stanford, CA: Stanford University Press.

Thorndike, E. L. (1903). *Elements of psychology.* New York: Seiler.

Timberlake, W., & Allison, J. (1974). Response deprivation: An empirical approach to instrumental performance. *Psychological Review, 81,* 146–164.

Timberlake, W., & Lucas, G. A. (1985). The basis of superstitious behavior: Chance contingency, stimulus substitution, or appetitive behavior? *Journal of the Experimental Analysis of Behavior, 44,* 279–299.

Van Willigen, F., Emmett, J., Cote, D., & Ayres, J. J. B. (1987). CS modality effects in one-trial backward and forward excitatory conditioning as assessed by conditioned suppression of licking in rats. *Animal Learning and Behavior, 15,* 201–211.

Vaughan, M. E., & Michael, J. (1982). Automatic reinforcement: An important but ignored concept. *Behaviorism, 10,* 217–227.

Vom Saal, W., & Jenkins, H. M. (1970). Blocking the development of stimulus control. *Learning and Motivation, 1,* 52–64.

Waelti, P., Dickinson, A., & Schultz, W. (2001). Dopamine responses comply with basic assumptions of formal learning theory. *Nature, 412,* 43–48.

Wang, Y., Lee, H., He, A. B., & Huang, A. C. W. (2017). Examinations of CS and US preexposure and postexposure in conditioned taste aversion: Applications in behavioral interventions for chemotherapy anticipatory nausea and vomiting. *Learning and Motivation, 59,* 1–10.

Welker, R. L., & McAuley, K. (1978). Reductions in resistance to extinction and spontaneous recovery as a function of changes in transportational and contextual stimuli. *Learning and Behavior, 6,* 451–457.

Williams, B. A. (1994a). Conditioned reinforcement: Neglected or outmoded explanatory construct? *Psychonomic Bulletin and Review, 1,* 457–475.

Williams, B. A. (1994b). Conditioned reinforcement: Experimental and theoretical issues. *Journal of the Experimental Analysis of Behavior, 17,* 261–285.

Williams, B. A. (1994c). Context specificity of conditioned-reinforcement effects on discrimination acquisition. *Journal of the Experimental Analysis of Behavior, 62,* 157–167.

Wyvell, C. L., & Berridge, K. C. (2000). Intra-accumbens amphetamine increases the conditioned incentive salience of sucrose reward: Enhancement of reward "wanting" without enhanced "liking" or response reinforcement. *Journal of Neuroscience, 20,* 8122–8130.

Yagishita, S., Hayashi-Takagi, A., Ellis-Davies, G. C. R., Urakubo, H., Ishii, S., & Kasai, H. (2014). A critical time window for dopamine actions on the structural plasticity of dendritic spines. *Science 345,* 1616–1620.

# CHAPTER 3

# Basic Operant Contingencies
## *Main Effects and Side Effects*

### A. Charles Catania

Handbooks are often consulted as resources for information about specific topics, so this chapter is organized as a set of somewhat independent sections. It opens with a discussion of operant contingencies, then considers some aspects of the basic contingencies known as *reinforcement* and *punishment* and their positive and negative variants, and closes with some implications of these contingencies and brief surveys of a few related issues. For more detailed treatments, see Skinner (1938, 1953, 1999); Iversen and Lattal (1991a, 1991b); Catania (2013); various volumes of the *Journal of the Experimental Analysis of Behavior* and *The Behavior Analyst*; and two special issues of the *European Journal of Behavior Analysis*, one devoted to contingencies (Arntzen, Brekstad, & Holth, 2006) and the other devoted to noncontingent reinforcement (Arntzen, Brekstad, & Holth, 2004).

## RESPONSE–CONSEQUENCE CONTINGENCIES

Contingencies relating responses to their consequences are properties of environments. They are probability relations among events. When a response changes the probability of some event, we say that the change is contingent on the response; when the change is from a relatively low probability to a probability of 1.0, we usually say that the

response has produced the event. An organism is said to *come into contact with a contingency* when its behavior produces some consequences of the contingency. Unless otherwise stated, for convenience the term *contingency* here implies a response–consequence contingency, rather than contingencies more broadly conceived (e.g., stimulus–stimulus contingencies).

When responses produce stimuli, the contingent relation is defined by two conditional probabilities: probability of the stimulus (1) given a response and (2) given no response. Without both probabilities specified, the contingent relations cannot be distinguished from incidental temporal *contiguities* of responses and stimuli that are occurring independently over time.

Response–reinforcer relations involve two terms (the *response* and the *reinforcer*), but when correlated with *discriminative* stimuli (stimuli that set the occasion on which responses have consequences), they produce a *three-term contingency*, which involves antecedents, behavior, and consequences. For example, a child's touch of a card might be reinforced with an edible if the card is green, but not if it is any other color. In this case, green, as the discriminative stimulus, is the first term; the touch, as the response, is the second term; and the edible, as the reinforcer, is the third term. Antecedents typically include establishing

37

conditions as well as discriminative stimuli. For example, the edible might not serve as a reinforcer if the child has eaten very recently.

Conditional discriminations add a fourth term, a fifth, and so on, for other contingency relations of various orders of complexity. For example, if a child is presented with green or red balls or blocks, then the appropriate color name might be reinforced given the question "What color?", whereas the appropriate shape name might be reinforced given the question "What shape?" In this example, the questions are the fourth terms that set the occasion for whether the operative three-term contingency is the one involving color, color name, and reinforcer, or that involving shape, shape name, and reinforcer.

When a response for which a contingency operates produces a stimulus, the stimulus is sometimes called a *contingent* stimulus. The term *consequence* may refer to such a stimulus, but stimuli are not the only kinds of consequences. The term encompasses stimulus presentations or removals, changes in contingencies, or any other environmental alterations that follow a response. For example, food produced by a response is both a stimulus and a consequence, but food presented independently of behavior is a stimulus only; shock prevented by a response is a stimulus, but the consequence of the response is the absence of shock, which is not a stimulus; replacing a defective light switch does not turn on the light, but it changes the consequences of operating the switch. The term *consequence* is particularly useful when the status of a stimulus as a possible reinforcer or punisher is unknown. Contingencies can also be arranged based on context, as when responses are reinforced based on their variability (e.g., Neuringer, 2004), or as when, in learned helplessness, organisms exposed to environments in which their responses lack consequences become insensitive to new contingencies (e.g., Maier, Albin, & Testa, 1973).

## Contingencies, Establishing Events, and Multiple Causation

An establishing or motivational event is any environmental circumstance that changes the effectiveness of a stimulus as a reinforcer or punisher. Here are some examples: deprivation; satiation; procedures that establish formerly neutral stimuli as conditional reinforcers or as conditional aversive stimuli; and stimulus presentations that change the reinforcing or punishing status of other stimuli, as when an already available screwdriver becomes a reinforcer in the presence of a screw that needs tightening (Michael, 1982).

A *conditional* or *conditioned reinforcer* is a stimulus that functions as a reinforcer because of its contingent relation to another reinforcer. If a conditional reinforcer is based on several different primary reinforcers, then it will be more effective than one based on a relation only to a single primary reinforcer. Such a reinforcer is called a *generalized reinforcer*. For example, the sound of a clicker may serve as a generalized reinforcer of a pet's behavior if this sound has been often followed by food, opportunities for play, and other significant consequences.

With regard to establishing events, whether one is in the light or in the dark, a flashlight usually lights when one turns it on, but turning it on usually matters only when it is dark. Thus a change from indoor lighting to the darkness of a power outage is an establishing event with regard to whether one is likely to turn on the flashlight. It is not a discriminative stimulus because one can turn the flashlight on even if there is no power outage.

The consequences change, however, if one's flashlight battery dies. The flashlight no longer works, so now finding a fresh battery is important. Once one finds a battery to replace the dead battery, one's flashlight becomes functional again. In other words, the battery going dead has two effects: It has not only a consequential effect because it changes what happened when one tries to turn on the flashlight, but also an establishing effect because it makes finding a fresh battery important.

Any particular instance of behavior has multiple causes, though some may be more important than others. In behavior analysis, we examine the multiple causes of behavior one at a time and assess their relative contributions. Multiple causation operates in the flashlight example because establishing events ordinarily go together with consequential effects, but it is important to be clear about which behavior is related to each. In these examples, turning on the flashlight is behavior with consequences, but the lighting conditions establish whether it is important to turn the flashlight on; similarly, when the battery goes dead, replacing the battery is behavior with consequences, but the failure of the flashlight to work establishes whether it is important to change the battery (cf. Michael, 1989).

## Distinguishing between Causal Antecedents and Causal Contingencies

Some stimuli have their effects as antecedents of behavior; other stimuli have their effects as its consequences; and sometimes stimuli can serve both roles simultaneously. In chaining, for example, the stimulus produced by a response early in a sequence both reinforces that response and sets the occasion for the next one, as when the opening of a door both reinforces the turn of the doorknob and allows the behavior of stepping through to the next room. Stimuli that reinforce or punish some responses can also elicit or occasion others, so choices among such consequences in reinforcement applications must take into account both the main reinforcing or punishing effects and their eliciting or occasioning side effects.

It may be necessary to determine whether behavior is maintained by its consequences or is produced more directly by stimuli. Imprinting provides a case in point. A newly hatched duckling ordinarily follows the first moving thing it sees; this imprinted stimulus is usually its mother. The duckling's following is sometimes said to be elicited by the imprinted stimulus, but to speak of elicitation is misleading. A natural consequence of walking is changing the duckling's distance from its mother. If closeness is important and requires behavior other than walking, that other behavior should replace the walking.

In one early experiment, when a dark compartment containing a moving imprinted stimulus was on one side of a one-way window and a response was available on the other side that lit up the dark side so the duckling could see it, behavior incompatible with following (such as pecking a stationary disk on the wall or standing still on a platform) was readily shaped (Peterson, 1960). In imprinting, therefore, presentations of the to-be-imprinted stimulus are establishing events, not eliciting stimuli. Imprinted stimuli, which acquire their significance by being presented under appropriate circumstances, begin as stimuli toward which the duckling is relatively indifferent but end as ones that function as reinforcers. Imprinted stimuli do not elicit following; rather, they become important enough that they can reinforce a variety of responses, including following, pecking, and standing still. The point should have been obvious to early researchers on imprinting. In natural environments, swimming replaces walking when the duckling follows its mother into a body of water. If walking were mere elicited behavior, it should not do so.

Analogous relations can have profound implications in clinical settings. For example, interpreting a hospitalized child's problem behavior as elicited behavior when it has its source in reinforcement contingencies might prevent appropriate treatment options from being considered.

But misdiagnosis can go either way. For example, if such behavior has its source in eliciting stimuli, perhaps for neurological reasons, interpreting it as shaped by reinforcement contingencies could similarly lead to ineffective treatment. And it can get even more difficult. In multiple causation, eliciting stimuli and reinforcement contingencies may operate at the same time, so identifying the role of one should not rule out assessments of the other.

## REINFORCEMENT

A reinforcer is a type of stimulus, but reinforcement is neither stimulus nor response. The term *reinforcement* names a relation between behavior and environment. The relation includes at least three components: (1) Responses must have consequences; (2) their probability must increase (i.e., they must become more probable than when they do not have those consequences); and (3) the increase must occur *because* they have those consequences and not for some other reason. For example, if we knew only that responding increased, we could not say that the response must have been reinforced; maybe it was elicited. It would not even be enough to know that the response was now producing some stimulus it had not been producing before. We would still have to know whether responding increased *because* the stimulus was its consequence.

Assume that an abusive parent gets annoyed whenever an infant cries and tries to suppress the crying by hitting the child. The infant cries and then gets hit, which produces even more crying. Here the consequence of crying is getting hit, and getting hit produces more crying, but we cannot argue that the hitting reinforces the crying. Two criteria for reinforcement are satisfied, but not the third. Stimuli may have other effects along with or instead of their effects as consequences of responding. Crying does not increase here because getting hit is a consequence; getting hit brings on crying even if the infant is not crying at the outset. Probably the infant will eventually learn to suppress the crying. At that point, we will know that the crying was punished rather than reinforced.

In earlier days, scientists would have discussed the relation between a response and its reinforcer in terms of associations—a principle with substantial precedent in psychology and philosophy—rather than in terms of contingencies. In this discussion, learning was said to occur through the association of ideas, and the conditional reflexes of Pavlov (1927) seemed to be cases of such associations. In one example of Pavlov's work, the sound of a metronome consistently preceded the delivery of food to a dog, and the dog came to salivate at the sound of the metronome. Scientists assumed that learning occurred through the *temporal contiguity* of events, or their occurrence together in time. However, we cannot interpret this learning as an association or as simply substituting one stimulus for another. Pairings in time or contiguities are not equivalent to contingencies, and pairings alone are not sufficient to produce respondent conditioning. Two stimuli can occur together not only when one never occurs without the other, but also when either can sometimes occur independent of the other. We must specify a contingency, or the probability of one given the other. An account solely in terms of association or contiguity is inadequate (e.g., Catania, 1971; Donahoe & Vegas, 2004).

## Specificity of Reinforcers

By definition, reinforcement always increases responding relative to what it would have been like without reinforcement. Also by definition, that increase must be specific to the response that produces the consequence. For example, if a rat's lever presses produce shock and only the rat's jumping increases, it would be inappropriate to speak of either pressing or jumping as reinforced.

As an operation, reinforcement is presenting a reinforcer when a response occurs; it is carried out on responses, so we speak of reinforcing responses rather than of reinforcing organisms. We may say that a pigeon's key peck was reinforced with food, but not that food reinforced the pigeon or that the pigeon was reinforced for pecking. The main reason for this restriction is that it is too easy to be ambiguous by omitting the response or the reinforcer, or both, when we speak of reinforcing organisms. The restriction forces us to be explicit about what is reinforced by what. For example, if we have been told only that a child has been reinforced, we do not know much about actual contingencies. Although this grammatical restriction forces us to be explicit about which response has been reinforced, it does not prevent us from identifying the organism whose behavior had consequences.

## Function and Topography of Reinforced Responses

Reinforcement creates response classes defined by their functions and not by their forms or topographies. Common contingencies select the members of operant classes, and they do so even if the relations among members are arbitrary. A lever press is a lever press, whether the rat presses with right paw, left paw, chin, or rump.

The distinction between function and topography is particularly crucial when it enters into diagnostic categories. The self-injurious behavior of two children may be similar in topography, but if one child's behavior is reinforced socially by attention and the other's is reinforced by avoidance of compliance with simple requests, effective treatment programs designed for the two children will have to be radically different (Iwata, Pace, Kalsher, Cowdery, & Cataldo, 1990). The first child must be taught more effective ways of engaging the attention of others and must be brought into situations where attention is more readily available. Requests must be selected for the second child that are appropriate to the child's competence, and the child's compliance with those requests must be reinforced (perhaps in the past, such behavior has instead been punished). What behavior does is more important than what it looks like.

## Assessing Reinforcers

Events that are effective as reinforcers are often described in terms of positive feelings or strong preferences. Such descriptions are subject to the inconsistent practices of verbal communities, so we must be wary of using them to predict whether particular events will serve as reinforcers. It is tempting to equate reinforcers with events colloquially called "rewards." But reinforcers do not work because they make the organism "feel good," or because the organism "likes" them. Our everyday language does not capture what is important about reinforcers. For example, staff predictions of the reinforcers that might be effective in managing the behavior of people with profound disabilities were inconsistent with reinforcers identified by systematically assessing each individual's nonverbal preferences among those events (Fisher et al., 1992; Green et al., 1988).

We sometimes make good guesses about what will be effective reinforcers, because reinforcers often involve events of obvious biological significance. But reinforcers are not limited to such events. For example, sensory stimuli, such as flashing lights, can powerfully reinforce the behavior of children along the autism spectrum (Ferrari & Harris, 1981). Restraint also seems an unlikely reinforcer, but in an analysis of self-injurious behavior, restraints that prevented children with severe developmental disabilities from poking or biting themselves were effective in reinforcing arbitrary responses, such as putting marbles in a box (Favell, McGimsey, & Jones, 1978).

In the final analysis, the primary criterion for reinforcement remains whether the consequences of behavior have raised the likelihood of that behavior. Reinforcers may be correlated with other properties, such as reported feelings or preferences, but they are defined solely by their behavioral effects.

## Delay of Reinforcement

The effects of a reinforcer depend on other responses that preceded it besides the one, usually most recent, that produced it. Thus, when one response is followed by a different reinforced response, the reinforcer may strengthen both. Clinicians and teachers need to take this effect into account, because it is important to recognize that reinforcing a single correct response after a long string of errors may strengthen errors along with the correct response.

Assume that a task involves a child's correct responses and errors over trials. Reinforcing every correct response and repeating any trial with an error until the child gets it right guarantees that any sequence of errors will eventually be followed by a reinforced correct response. Correct responses will probably dominate eventually, because the reinforcer most closely follows them. But errors may diminish only slowly and perhaps even continue indefinitely at a modest level, though they never actually produce the reinforcer, because they are reliably followed after a delay by a reinforced correct response. Thus always reinforcing a single correct response after a sequence of errors will probably maintain errors.

Teachers and clinicians must be alert for such situations. A reinforcer that follows a sequence of correct responses will probably do a lot more good than a reinforcer that follows a single correct response after several errors. Thus a teacher must judge whether correct responses are so infrequent that they should be reinforced even though preceded by errors, or so frequent that the reinforcer can wait until the student has made several correct responses in a row. Another way to reduce the strengthening of errors is to extend the time to the next trial after every error.

Many practical applications of reinforcement include other behavior that precedes the behavior we target for reinforcement. When such behavior shares in the effect of the reinforcer, we may mistakenly conclude that the reinforcer is not doing its job very well. But if the reinforced behavior includes response classes that we did not intend to reinforce, it may simply be doing very well a job other than the one we wanted it to do. When one response is followed by a different reinforced response, the reinforcer may strengthen both, so we should keep behavior that we do not want to reinforce from getting consistently close to reinforcers produced by other responses.

An intervention for children with autism spectrum disorder who displayed persistent errors illustrates this principle (Fisher, Pawich, Dickes, Paden, & Toussaint, 2014). The children repeated errors during baseline, even though each correct response produced an edible reinforcer (FR 1). To test whether intermittent errors persisted because the errors frequently preceded a correct response followed immediately by a reinforcer, the investigators implemented a second-order schedule in which they placed an edible reinforcer into one of three small glass containers in front of a child. After three consecutive correct responses, the therapist delivered the three accumulated reinforcers to the child, but after an error, the therapist emptied any accumulated reinforcers from the containers and the child had to start over. This procedure reduced errors by ensuring that reinforcers followed only sequences of three correct responses and thus were not presented soon after errors.

## Relativity of Reinforcement

Reinforcement is relative in the sense that it depends on relations between the reinforced response and the reinforcer. A less probable response may be reinforced by an opportunity to engage in a more probable response. The inverse relation does not hold. For example, food is not always a reinforcer. When a parent allows a child to go out and play with friends only after the child has eaten, the opportunity to play may reinforce the eating.

The reversibility of the reinforcement relation has been amply demonstrated (Premack, 1962). For example, levels of food and water deprivation can be selected so that drinking is reinforced by an opportunity to eat at one time, and eating is reinforced by an opportunity to drink at another. In providing an a priori means for predicting whether an opportunity to engage in one response will reinforce some other response, the relativity of reinforcement also avoids the problems of circular definition inherent in some earlier definitions of reinforcement.

The significance of reinforcers is based on the opportunities for behavior that they allow. For example, when time spent in isolation was used in an attempt to punish the tantrums of a 6-year-old girl with autism spectrum disorder, her tantrums increased substantially instead of decreasing. This child often engaged in self-stimulation, such as waving her fingers over her eyes to create visual flicker, but that behavior was frequently interrupted by the staff. Time in the isolation room reinforced rather than punished her tantrums, because the isolation room allowed her to engage in self-stimulation without interruption (Solnick, Rincover, & Peterson, 1977). Similarly, a number of investigators have shown that contingent access to stereotypic and repetitive behavior can be used to reinforce socially appropriate responses (Charlop, Kurtz, & Casey, 1990; Fisher, Rodriguez, & Owen, 2013).

The relativity of reinforcement reminds us that we should not expect the effectiveness of reinforcers to be constant across different reinforced responses, different individuals, or even different time samples of the behavior of a single individual. When a reinforcer is effective on some behavior in some context, we must not assume that it will be effective on other behavior or even on the same behavior in other contexts.

### Reinforcement and Extinction: Response Rate versus Momentum

The effects of reinforcers are not permanent. Reinforcers have temporary effects; when reinforcement stops, responding returns to its earlier, lower levels. The decrease in responding during extinction does not require a separate treatment; rather, it is simply one property of reinforcement. But reinforcement does not merely maintain rates of responding, which are reduced when it is discontinued. It also produces resistance to change, or momentum (Nevin, 1992). Two different responses with two different histories may be maintained at similar rates, but one may decrease more rapidly in extinction than the other. Responding that is more resistant to change is said to have greater momentum. Extinction is just one type of change, and other sources that may be used to assess momentum include reinforcement of competing responses, establishing conditions, and delay of reinforcement.

If the effects of reinforcement are temporary, then once we have created new behavior with reinforcers, we cannot count on its maintenance after our intervention ends. Consider children learning to read. Only long after they have learned to name letters of the alphabet and to read whole words are they perhaps ready to read stories, so that reading can become "its own reward." Until that happens, teachers have no choice but to arrange artificial contingencies, using extrinsic consequences such as praise to shape the components of reading. Responsible teaching adds extrinsic reinforcers only when there are no effective intrinsic consequences. It is important to build momentum, but if we want to maintain behavior after we terminate artificial consequences, we should do so only if natural consequences are in place that will take over that maintenance.

### Side Effects of Reinforcement and Extinction

Discontinuing reinforcement in extinction has two components: (1) It terminates a contingency between responses and reinforcers, and (2) reinforcers are no longer delivered. Because of the former, the previously reinforced responding decreases. Because of the latter, unwelcome side effects of extinction may appear. For example, aggressive responding is sometimes a major side effect of extinction (e.g., Lerman, Iwata, & Wallace, 1999). If food is suddenly taken away from a food-deprived rat that has been eating, the rat may become more active and perhaps urinate or defecate. If the food was produced by lever presses, the rat may bite the lever. If other organisms are in the chamber, the rat may attack them (Azrin, Hutchinson, & Hake, 1966). These effects and others, though observed in extinction, are not produced by the termination of the reinforcement contingency because they also occur upon the termination of response-independent food deliveries, where there had been no reinforcement contingency. In either case, a rat that had been eating stops getting food. The termination of a reinforcement contingency in extinction necessarily entails the termination of reinforcer deliveries, and the effects of the latter are necessarily superimposed on the decrease in previously reinforced responding.

Even if reinforcers have produced problem behavior, taking them away may still produce undesired side effects. That is why extinction is not the method of choice for getting rid of behavior that has been created by reinforcement. Suppose a developmentally delayed boy engages in severe self-injurious behavior such as head banging or eye poking, and we discover that his behavior is in large part maintained by staff attention as a reinforcer. Because of the harm he might do to himself if the self-injurious behavior is ignored, extinction may be ill advised. Giving him attention independently of the self-injurious behavior is one possibility (*noncontingent* reinforcement, sometimes also called *free* reinforcement) (Catania, 2005; Lattal, 1974; Sizemore & Lattal, 1977); another is to use attention to reinforce alternative responses, and especially ones incompatible with the self-injury. The self-injury will decrease as alternative responses increase.

These side effects are one reason why extinction has fallen out of favor in applied settings, compared to procedures such as noncontingent reinforcement. The *Journal of Applied Behavior Analysis* has published relatively few examples of extinction with humans. In general, the solution is not to take the reinforcers away. The better way to reduce misbehavior is to reinforce good behavior, but sometimes we inadvertently encourage the use of extinction (the less effective alternative)—especially when we present just a few basic facts about behavior, as in an introductory psychology course. Generations of students seem to have taken from cursory accounts of behavioral methods in introductory textbooks the message that if one sees a child doing something one does not approve of, then one should not reinforce that behavior. Instead, one should just ignore it. Left unanswered are the inevitable subsequent questions, such as how parents should handle things when other problematic behavior maintained by the same reinforcer emerges. Rather than teaching parents to ignore the behavior of their children, we should teach them how to use reinforcers more productively, but that alternative is more difficult. Free noncontingent reinforcement coupled with the shaping of other behavior should be recommended to parents or other caregivers, but doing so poses problems of both communication and implementation (Hagopian, Crockett, van Stone, DeLeon, & Bowman, 2000).

Why has extinction for so long remained the primary way to study the effects of terminating contingencies? One concern is that accidental contiguities of responses and noncontingent reinforcers may have effects similar to those of the contiguities that are scheduled when reinforcers are contingent on responding. If noncontingent and contingent reinforcers have similar effects on behavior early in the transition to noncontin-

gent reinforcement, then responding may decrease more slowly than in extinction. But such effects are usually transient, so this is not a big enough concern to rule noncontingent reinforcement out of consideration in either experimental or applied settings. If higher or lower rates of noncontingent reinforcement are available as options, this concern favors the lower rates. If behavior persists for long periods of time under such arrangements, it is more appropriate to look for other sources of the behavior than to attribute it to adventitious correlations of responses and reinforcers.

## Positive Reinforcement and Positive Psychology

Positive reinforcement can be used to change a developmentally delayed child who engages extensively in self-injurious behavior into one who has learned communicative skills and has therefore been empowered to deal in more constructive ways with his or her caregivers. If reinforcers are implicated in the development and maintenance of the self-injurious behavior, then taking them away is not the solution. Reinforcement isn't everything, but extinction isn't anything. If the reinforcers are already there, they should not be wasted; they should instead be used constructively. We all shape each other's behavior, and the more we know about how positive reinforcement works, the more likely we will be to use it productively and avoid pitfalls such as the coercive practices that can occur if the control over reinforcers remains one-sided. For these reasons, it might be thought that positive reinforcement would be especially important to the practitioners of the approach called *positive psychology*. Unfortunately, they eschew it, along with the establishing events that make it effective; their rhetoric implies that contingent acts of kindness should always be replaced by random ones (cf. Catania, 2001; Seligman & Csikszentmihalyi, 2000, 2001).

## Self-Reinforcement as Misnomer

An organism's delivery of a reinforcer to itself based on its own behavior has been called *self-reinforcement*, but any effect such an activity might have cannot be attributed to the action of the specific reinforcers delivered by the organism to itself. In so-called "self-reinforcement," the contingencies and establishing events that modify the behavior purportedly to be reinforced cannot be separated from those that modify the behavior of self-reinforcing. For example, a student who has made a commitment to watch television only after completing a study assignment might think that this arrangement will reinforce studying. But any increase in studying that follows cannot be attributed to the student's contingent watching of television: The student has made the commitment to deal with studying this way because studying has already become important for other reasons. Whatever has brought the student to commit to "self-reinforce" studying in the first place has probably by itself made studying more likely. It is impossible to pull these variables apart.

What was once called *self-reinforcement* is now more properly called *self-regulation* (Bandura, 1976, 1995; Catania, 1975, 1995; Mahoney & Bandura, 1972). To the extent that the activity has effects, it must do so because the individual who appears to "self-reinforce" can discriminate behavior that qualifies for the reinforcer from behavior that does not.

This usage also finesses the problem that the language of self-reinforcement implies reinforcement of the organism rather than reinforcement of behavior. For example, the commitment to reinforce one's own studying involves setting standards for the discrimination between adequate and inadequate studying, so students who try to deal with their study habits in this way are discriminating properties of their own behavior that have become important to them. The contingencies that generate these discriminations are complex and probably involve verbal behavior. The language of self-reinforcement obscures rather than clarifies these phenomena.

## PUNISHMENT

Paralleling the vocabulary of reinforcement, a punisher is a type of stimulus, but punishment is neither stimulus nor response. The term *punishment* names a relation between behavior and environment. The relation includes at least three components. First, responses must have consequences. Second, their probability must decrease (i.e., they must become less probable than when they do not have those consequences). Third, the decrease must occur *because* they have those consequences and not for some other reason. For example, if we knew only that responding decreased, we could not say that it must have been punished; maybe it was previously reinforced responding that had since been extinguished. It would not even be enough to know that the response was now producing some

stimulus it had not produced before. We would still have to know whether responding decreased *because* that stimulus was its consequence.

As defined, punishment is the inverse of reinforcement; it is defined by decreases in consequential responding, whereas reinforcement is defined by increases. The vocabulary of punishment parallels that of reinforcement in its object: Responses, not organisms, are said to be punished. If a rat's lever pressing produces shock and lever pressing decreases, it is appropriate to say that the rat was shocked and that the lever press was punished; it goes against colloquial usage, but it is not appropriate to say that the rat was punished. As with reinforcement, this grammatical distinction discourages ambiguities in the observation and description of behavior.

## Parameters of Punishment

As with reinforcement, the effectiveness of punishment varies with parameters such as magnitude and delay (Azrin & Holz, 1966). For example, the more intense and immediate the punisher, the more effectively it reduces behavior. A punisher introduced at maximum intensity reduces responding more effectively than one introduced at low intensity and gradually increased to maximum intensity. The effectiveness of the punisher may change over time, such as when a punisher of low intensity gradually becomes ineffective after many presentations. As with extinction, it is easier to reduce the likelihood of a response when some other response that produces the same reinforcer is available than when no alternative responses produce that reinforcer. And in a parametric relation especially relevant to human applications, punishers delivered after short delays are more effective than those delivered after long ones; with either pets or children, aversive consequences delivered at some point long after unwanted behavior occurs are not likely to be very effective. If verbal specification of the behavior on which the punisher is contingent matters at all, it can do so only given an extensive and sophisticated verbal history on the part of the individual at the receiving end (Skinner, 1957).

A reduction in responding can be studied only if some responding already exists. A response that is never emitted cannot be punished. Experiments on punishment therefore usually superimpose punishment on reinforced responding. But the effects of punishment then also depend on what maintains responding. For example, punishment by shock probably will reduce food-reinforced lever pressing less if a rat is severely food-deprived than if it is only mildly food-deprived.

## Recovery from Punishment

There are ethical constraints on using punishment to change behavior. The use of punishment as a component of clinical interventions has decreased in recent years (cf. Greer, Fisher, Saini, Owen, & Jones, 2016), but punishment cannot be eliminated from natural environments (Perone, 2003). Without punishment, a child who has been burned upon touching a hot stove or bitten upon approaching an unfamiliar barking dog will remain undeterred from doing so again later on. Artificial punishment contingencies, however, are also constrained by practical considerations. Like reinforcement, the effects of punishment are ordinarily temporary; responding usually recovers to earlier levels after punishment is discontinued. This means that just as behavior analysts must plan for what will maintain the behavior when reinforcement ends, they also must plan for environments in which the relevant contingencies may be absent. It may do little long-term good to eliminate a child's self-injurious behavior with punishment in a hospital setting if the punishment contingency does not exist when the child returns home. The reinforcement of alternative behavior might be easier to maintain.

## Relativity of Punishment

The effectiveness of punishers, like that of reinforcers, is determined by the relative probabilities of the punished response and the responses occasioned by the punisher; punishment occurs when a more probable response forces the organism to engage in a less probable response. Even stimuli that ordinarily serve as reinforcers can become punishers under appropriate conditions. For example, food that is reinforcing at the beginning of a holiday feast may become aversive by the time the meal has ended. On the other hand, events that superficially seem aversive, such as falling from a height, may be reinforcing under some circumstances (consider skydiving). Like reinforcers, punishers cannot be defined in absolute terms or in terms of common physical properties. Rather, they must be assessed in terms of the relation between punished responses and the responses occasioned by the punisher.

Any given state of affairs may be reinforcing or aversive, depending on its context. Suppose a rat receives shocks during a tone, but during a buzzer nothing happens. If chain pulls turn off the tone and turn on the buzzer, the onset of the buzzer will reinforce chain pulls; by pulling the chain, the rat escapes from the tone and its accompanying shock deliveries. Suppose, however, that the rat instead receives food during the tone, but during the buzzer nothing happens. Now if chain pulls turn off the tone and turn on the buzzer, the onset of the buzzer will punish chain pulls; by pulling the chain, the rat produces a time out from the tone and its accompanying food deliveries. In other words, the buzzer serves as reinforcer or as punisher, depending on its context, even though nothing happens during the buzzer in either context. Similarly, as gauged by absenteeism, whether a school environment is punishing or reinforcing may depend on the conditions that prevail at home—as when going to school is punished for one child because it means having to deal with an abusive school bully, but is reinforced for another because it is a convenient way to escape from an even more abusive parent.

## Side Effects of Punishment: Eliciting and Discriminative Effects

Aversive stimuli are likely to have other effects besides those that depend on the punishment contingency (e.g., Azrin, Hutchinson, & McLaughlin, 1965). As with reinforcement, punishment necessarily includes both stimulus presentations and a contingency between responses and stimuli, so the effects of the stimulus presentations must be distinguished from those of the contingency. If an organism is shocked or pinched, some of its responses to those stimuli may have little to do with whether they have been brought on by the organism's own behavior. To qualify as punishment, the reduction in responding must depend on the contingent relation between responses and punishers, and not simply on the delivery of punishers.

A comparison of the effects of response-produced and response-independent shock on food-reinforced lever pressing in rats (Camp, Raymond, & Church, 1967) showed that both procedures reduced lever pressing relative to no-shock conditions, but that response-produced shock had substantially larger effects than response-independent shock. Given that both response-produced and response-independent shocks reduced responding, it would not have been possible to assess the effect of the punishment contingency without the comparison. The difference made it appropriate to call the response-produced shock a punisher. For example, had response-produced shock instead produced only the same reduction as response-independent shock, the appropriate conclusion would have been that the reduction depended wholly on the eliciting effects of shock, and that the punishment contingency was irrelevant. Just as we must distinguish between effects of reinforcer deliveries and effects of the contingent relation between responses and reinforcers, so also we must distinguish between effects of punisher deliveries and effects of the contingent relation between responses and punishers.

Punishers can also acquire discriminative properties, as when a response is reinforced only when it is also punished. For example, one experiment alternated a condition in which a pigeon's key pecks had no consequences with another condition in which every peck produced shock and some produced food reinforcers (Holz & Azrin, 1961). A low rate of pecking was maintained when pecks produced no shock, because then they never produced food either; pecking increased once pecks began to produce shock, however, because only then did they occasionally produce food.

We can ask whether these shocks should really be called punishers. In fact, here we must conclude that the shock had become a conditional reinforcer. The main difference between the shock and other, more familiar reinforcers was that it acquired its power to reinforce through its relation to food; if that relation had been discontinued, it would have lost that power. As an example of a possible source of masochism, these procedures may be relevant to human behavior. For example, a battered child might provoke a parent to the point of a beating because the beatings are often followed by more attention from the then-remorseful parent than ever follows less traumatic parent–child interactions. A parent's attention can be a potent reinforcer and may sometimes override the effects of consequences that would otherwise serve as punishers.

### Passive Avoidance as Misnomer

It has been argued that punishment is reducible to avoidance, in the sense that all behavior other than the punished response avoids the punisher. For example, if a rat is placed on a platform above an electrified grid, then not stepping down onto the grid might be called passive avoidance of shock; by not responding, the rat passively avoids what would otherwise be a punisher. But where-

as punishment is a robust phenomenon that can occur within a short time course (the abrupt introduction of a strong punisher reduces responding quickly), the literature on avoidance shows that though avoidance is robust once in place, it is difficult and time-consuming to get it started. Passive avoidance is therefore best regarded as a misnomer for punishment. It is implausible to say that hypothetical behavior presumed to come from relations that are difficult to establish can explain behavior that is easy to establish. Even if punishment did work this way, so that we learn not to stick our hands into a fire because by so doing we avoid the aversive proprioceptive stimuli occasioned by approaching the fire, it would make little practical difference. For those who have to make decisions about whether or when to use punishers, punishment works pretty much the same way whichever theoretical position one assumes.

### NEGATIVE REINFORCEMENT: ESCAPE AND AVOIDANCE

Organisms not only produce stimuli; they also get rid of them. Without negative reinforcement, a child would not learn to escape from the cold by coming indoors or to avoid others who might cheat at games, bully, or lie. A rat does not ordinarily expose itself to shock, and if shock does occur, the rat escapes from it given the opportunity. If presenting a contingent aversive stimulus punishes a response, removing or preventing that stimulus may reinforce a response. When a response terminates or prevents an aversive stimulus and becomes more probable for that reason, the stimulus is called a *negative reinforcer*, and the operation is called *negative reinforcement*.

In traditional usage, *positive* and *negative*, as modifiers of the term *reinforcement*, refer to whether the consequence produced by responding adds something to the environment or takes something away—but we will see later that there are other, better criteria for the distinction. *Negative reinforcer* refers to the stimulus itself and not to its removal; if removal of shock reinforces a rat's lever press, then shock, not the shock-free period that follows the response, is the negative reinforcer. Negative reinforcement involving the removal of a stimulus that is already present is called *escape*. When it involves the postponement or prevention of a stimulus that has not yet been delivered, it is called *avoidance*. This vocabulary is consistent with everyday usage: We escape from aversive circumstances that already exist, but we avoid potential aversive circumstances that have not yet happened. In clinical situations, escape (e.g., from a medical unit) is often called *elopement*.

Stimuli that can reinforce by their presentation can punish by their removal, and vice versa. If we know that a stimulus is effective as a punisher, then we can reasonably expect it to be effective as a negative reinforcer, and vice versa; this consistency is part of our justification for calling the stimulus aversive. Consistencies are to be expected because these categories have their origins in relations among the probabilities of different response classes. But we must not take too much for granted. The fact that we may easily reinforce jumping with shock removal, whereas we may not so effectively punish it with shock presentation, shows that the symmetry of reinforcement and punishment has limits. Reinforcement is most effective if the reinforced response is compatible with the responding occasioned by the reinforcer. Inversely, punishment is most effective if the punished response is incompatible with, or at least independent of, the responding occasioned by the punisher. Thus it may be easy to reinforce jumping with shock removal (escape), but hard to punish it with shock presentation.

### Escape: Competition between Contingencies and Elicited Behavior

In escape, an organism's response terminates an aversive stimulus. In institutional settings, developmentally delayed children sometimes behave aggressively, in that way escaping from simple demands placed upon them, such as tasks designed to teach them how to fasten and unfasten clothing buttons. For two such children, aggression dropped to near-zero levels when they could escape from demand situations by engaging in other behavior incompatible with aggression (Carr, Newsom, & Binkoff, 1980). But such cases of escape might, of course, imply that typical demand situations in such settings do not provide enough reinforcers.

In positive reinforcement, the reinforcer is absent when the reinforced response is emitted. After the response, the reinforcer is presented and occasions other responses. For example, if a rat's lever press is the reinforced response and food is the reinforcer, food is absent while the rat presses; eating does not occur until food is presented after the press. Thus lever pressing and eating do not directly compete with each other. In escape, however, the negative reinforcer is present before the

reinforced response is emitted; it is removed only after the response. For example, if the negative reinforcer is bright light from which the rat can escape by pressing a lever, the rat may reduce the effects of the light by closing its eyes and hiding its head in a corner. Any movement from that position is punished by greater exposure to the light, so the rat is not likely to come out of the corner and press the lever. Getting a rat to escape from light by lever pressing requires procedures that reduce the likelihood of such competing responses (Keller, 1941).

### Avoidance: Hard to Initiate but Easy to Maintain

Avoidance involves the prevention of an aversive stimulus by a response; the aversive stimulus is not present when the reinforced response occurs. The two major varieties of avoidance procedures are *deletion* and *postponement*. Deletion procedures are analogous to swatting a mosquito before it gets to where it can bite: Once swatted, that mosquito is permanently prevented from biting. Postponement procedures are analogous to putting coins in a parking meter: One postpones the violation flag as long as one puts coins in the meter and resets it, but without additional coins the meter eventually runs out.

In *discriminated* or *signaled avoidance*, a stimulus (sometimes called a *warning stimulus*) precedes the aversive stimulus; a response in the presence of this stimulus prevents the aversive stimulus on that trial. In *continuous* or *Sidman avoidance*, no exteroceptive stimulus is arranged. Each response postpones the aversive stimulus (usually, brief shock) for a fixed time period called the *response–shock (R–S) interval*; in the absence of responses, shocks are delivered regularly according to a *shock–shock (S–S) interval* (Sidman, 1953). Shock can be postponed indefinitely, provided that no R–S interval ends before a response has been emitted.

Success with avoidance procedures sometimes depends on whether the experimenter chooses a response that the organism is likely to emit in aversive situations. With rats, for example, responses such as jumping a hurdle or running from one side of the chamber to the other are likely to be elicited by aversive stimuli even in the absence of a response–shock contingency. Once responding has been produced by shock, it may continue when shock is absent. Thus the rat's first few avoidance responses may occur mainly because of their earlier elicitation by shock.

Avoidance behavior may be persistent after a long history of avoidance; it can be slow to extinguish. But the consequence of effective avoidance is that nothing happens: The aversive event is successfully avoided. Given that an avoidance response is not closely followed by shock, avoidance contingencies implicitly involve delays between responses and their consequences. Thus, despite the persistence of avoidance behavior once it is adequately in place, it is often hard to get it started.

This may explain why safety measures and other preventive procedures are not often shaped by natural contingencies. Someone who has never had a bad experience with fire may be less likely to install a smoke detector than someone who has. One significant problem in medicine is the compliance of patients with regimens such as taking prescribed medications. Many patients stop taking their medications once their symptoms have disappeared, even though further doses may have continued benefits. And with preventive medication, such as vaccination, taking a dose is followed by nothing happening right from the start. This problem exists over a wide range of preventive measures, from immunizations to safe sex, and from using sterile surgical equipment to purifying drinking water. Given what we know about avoidance contingencies, it is no surprise that such measures are sometimes difficult to shape up and maintain.

### Behavioral Criteria for Distinguishing Positive from Negative Reinforcement

Whether stimuli are presented or removed may be a less important criterion for distinguishing positive from negative reinforcement than whether responses generated by the reinforcer occur at times when they can compete with the reinforced response. Consider escape from cold (Weiss & Laties, 1961). In a cold chamber, a rat's lever presses turn on a heat lamp. Because presses add energy in the form of heat, this procedure could be called positive reinforcement. But cold stimulates temperature receptors in the rat's skin, and turning on the heat lamp terminates this effect of cold. Cold is a potent aversive event, so by this interpretation the procedure should be called negative reinforcement.

The justification for choosing the vocabulary of negative reinforcement lies not with questions of physics, such as whether something is presented or removed, but with the behavioral effects of the stimuli presented before and after emission of the reinforced response. Consider the behavior of the rat in the cold. Before the reinforced lever press, it

huddles in a corner and shivers. These responses reduce the likelihood that it will press the lever. Once its lever press turns on the heat lamp, these competing responses become less likely, but a rat that is no longer cold cannot escape from cold. Responses that competed with the reinforced response occurred before rather than after reinforcement, so this example is more like escape from shock or bright light than like production of food or water. In general, the language of negative reinforcement is appropriate when establishing events produce behavior that is likely to compete with the responding to be reinforced.

Another possible criterion is whether one reinforcement situation is preferred over another. In applied areas, such as management, it is useful to distinguish between two management task contingencies: Managers get employees to carry out tasks either by threatening or criticizing until tasks are completed, or, more rarely, by providing praise and recognition after tasks are completed. Given a choice, employees are likely to move from settings in which they receive criticism to those in which they receive praise. Assuming that reductions in threats maintain task completion, we may call that contingency negative reinforcement. Assuming that recognition for completing tasks maintains task completion, we may call that contingency positive reinforcement. The preferences of employees for task contingencies justify this classification.

### The Reinforcer in Negative Reinforcement

When a successful avoidance response occurs, its important consequence is that nothing happens. How can the absence of an event affect behavior? According to one view, avoidance responding is maintained because the organism escapes from some properties of the situation that accompanied past aversive stimuli. This view evolved from earlier procedures in which a warning stimulus preceded shock, and the organism prevented shock by responding in the presence of the warning stimulus. Avoidance was most easily acquired when the avoidance response both terminated the warning stimulus and prevented the shock.

In the context of occasional shocks, a shock-free period can serve as a reinforcer. Avoidance contingencies can be arranged in which the organism can either reduce the total number of shocks in a session or postpone individual shocks, even though the same number of shocks is eventually delivered in both cases. Either condition can maintain avoidance. Situations can be created in which a rat postpones shocks within trials even though it does not reduce the overall shock rate, or in which it reduces the overall shock rate even though responding shortens the time to the next shock (Herrnstein & Hineline, 1966; Hineline, 1970).

## Establishing Events in Negative Reinforcement

An establishing event that makes positive reinforcers more effective is deprivation. Food is less likely to reinforce the behavior of a rat that has recently eaten than of one that has not eaten for some time. The analogous event for negative reinforcers is *presentation* (it would be called *satiation* were the stimulus food instead of shock); the presentation of aversive stimuli makes their removal reinforcing. As with positive reinforcement, these establishing effects must be distinguished from discriminative, eliciting, and other effects of stimuli. Issues of multiple causation may be even more prevalent in cases of aversive control than in cases of positive reinforcement (for examples, see Sidman, 1958).

The aversive stimulus is the establishing event because there is no reason to escape or avoid an aversive stimulus unless it is either actually or potentially present. It is tempting to think of the aversive stimulus as signaling a contingency, but contingencies in which responses turn off shock cannot exist in the absence of shock. When responses produce food in positive reinforcement, that contingency can be signaled whether or not the rat has been food-deprived.

An example may be relevant. Shock is delivered to a rat when a light is either on or off; when the light is on, a lever press removes the shock for a while, but when the light is off, a lever press has no effect (Bersh & Lambert, 1975). Under such circumstances, the rat comes to press the lever when the light is on, but not when it is off. The discriminative stimulus here is the light, because the contingency between lever presses and shock removal is signaled by whether the light is on or off. The shock makes shock-free periods reinforcing, and its presentation is therefore an establishing event; it does not function as a discriminative stimulus because it does not signal the operation of a contingency.

Note that the contingencies that operate in the dark in this example are properly called *extinction* contingencies. Lever presses remove shock when the light is on but not when it is off; but given appropriate contingencies, shock absence would be an effective reinforcer during either. This would

not be so were shock never present when the light was off. In all of these cases, contingencies are about the consequences of responding, whereas establishing or motivating events are about whether those consequences are important enough to serve as reinforcers.

## Extinction after Negative Reinforcement

As with positive reinforcement and punishment, the effects of negative reinforcement are temporary. And as with those other operations, the effects of terminating contingencies between responses and aversive stimuli must be distinguished from those of simply terminating the aversive stimuli. In shock escape, turning off the shock eliminates responding simply because there is no occasion for escape in the absence of the shock. But in avoidance, turning off the shock source has often been considered an extinction operation. If avoidance responding is maintained at such a rate that shocks are rare, the absence of shocks will make little difference, and responding will continue for a long time. In fact, one widely acknowledged property of avoidance responding is its persistence after aversive stimuli are discontinued. For that reason, avoidance has sometimes been regarded as relevant to cases of the persistence of human behavior, as in compulsions.

Consider the alternatives. With food reinforcement, we can arrange extinction by either turning off the feeder or breaking the connection between responses and the feeder. Both have the same effect: Food is no longer delivered. That is not so with negative reinforcement. In escape or avoidance of shock, shock continues if responses can no longer remove or prevent it. This procedure discontinues the response–shock contingency, but it also increases the number of shocks if responding has kept shock rate low. Thus, by itself, this procedure cannot separate the effects of changing the rate of shock from those of changing the contingency.

Discontinuing the aversive stimulus has been the more common extinction procedure in avoidance, but in terms of contingencies, presenting the aversive stimulus while discontinuing the consequences of responding more closely parallels extinction after positive reinforcement. The time course of extinction depends on which operation is used and on how it changes the rate at which aversive stimuli occur (e.g., Hineline, 1981). In any case, extinction after negative reinforcement shows that the effects of negative reinforcement are temporary.

## NEGATIVE PUNISHMENT: TIME OUT

The distinction between positive and negative reinforcement is easily extended to positive and negative punishment (though here too, ambiguous cases are possible). Responses can be punished by some events, such as shock or forced running in a running wheel. Responses also can be punished by the termination of events. For example, removing food contingent on a food-deprived rat's lever presses is likely to reduce the rate of pressing. The problem is that it may be hard to demonstrate negative punishment. If the rat is food-deprived and food is available, it will probably eat rather than press, so we will have few opportunities to punish lever pressing by removing food. For this reason, studies of negative punishment usually have not removed the positive reinforcer itself; paralleling the emphasis on avoidance rather than escape in studies of negative reinforcement, the stimulus in the presence of which responses are reinforced has been removed instead.

For example, suppose that two levers are available to a monkey, and that presses on one lever produce food whenever a light is on. We can expect presses on the other lever, but we can punish them by making each one produce a time period during which the light turns off and presses on the first lever do nothing. Such periods are called *time out*, and the procedure is *punishment by time out from positive reinforcement* (e.g., Ferster, 1958). Time out originated in experiments like these with pigeons, rats, and monkeys, but now is probably best known in its human applications (e.g., Wolf, Risley, & Mees, 1964). For example, time in an isolation room has sometimes been used to punish the problem behavior of institutionalized children. In the casual use of time out as a punisher by parents and teachers, contingencies are often inconsistently applied, and behavior that occurs during the time out is too often neglected. The term is occasionally extended to other cases (e.g., *time out from avoidance*, during which no shocks are delivered).

## REINFORCEMENT AS SELECTION: THE SHAPING OF OPERANT CLASSES

A class of responses created by its consequences is called an *operant*. It is defined by its function and not by its physical or physiological properties (Skinner, 1935). The class depends on *differential reinforcement*, or the reinforcement of only those responses falling within the class. Differential reinforcement makes responding correspond more and more closely to the defining properties of an operant class. It can be based on any dimension of responding, though the dimension cannot always be unambiguously defined. For example, originality and other complex dimensions of behavior may define operant classes, even though we sometimes have difficulty measuring them.

Key pecks by pigeons and lever presses by rats are examples of operant classes, but so are our presses of elevator buttons or our asking someone's name. Sometimes such classes are created naturally by contingencies, but sometimes we create them artificially. If we put a pigeon in an experimental chamber, it may or may not peck a key. Instead of waiting for a peck, we can generate one by *shaping* (i.e., by successively reinforcing other responses that more and more closely approximate it). We start the shaping process by operating a feeder only when the pigeon turns toward the key. After two or three movements toward the key, we then reinforce not just any movement toward the key, but only those including forward motions of the beak. Soon the pigeon's beak movements are full-fledged pecks, and one strikes the key. At this point, our apparatus takes over, and further pecks operate the feeder automatically.

No set of rules for shaping can substitute for what one learns by actually doing it. It is crucial to be sensitive to the moment-to-moment interactions of the organism's behavior and the delivery of reinforcers. Shaping is an art applicable to many skills: gymnastics; playing a musical instrument; seduction; handwriting; and setting someone up as a victim of a con game. In other words, it can be put to either good use or bad, and many use it without even knowing they are doing so. As with reinforcement and punishment, when shaping is put to good use, it might as well be done effectively; when it is put to bad use, the best defense against it is knowing how it works.

An experienced experimenter can shape a pigeon's key peck with just 8–10 reinforcer deliveries. A shaper who works close to the limits of extinction—thereby not reinforcing lots of responses now that will have to be extinguished later, when behavior has moved closer to the target response—will probably finish shaping more quickly than one who is generous with reinforcers but risks satiation before reaching the target.

Shaping works because behavior is variable. In this respect, shaping is analogous to selection in biological systems: Evolution occurs when environments select individual organisms from populations that vary genetically (e.g., Donahoe, Burgos, & Palmer, 1993). Shaping is most obvious when used by a human trainer, as in the teaching of skills to a service dog, but it can also occur as a result of natural contingencies. For example, male cowbirds in different parts of the United States sing different dialects of birdsong (as is usual among songbirds, the female cowbird doesn't sing). A female is most likely to respond with mating-pattern postures to songs that sound most like the ones she heard in her youth, which were in the dialect of local males. When a foreign male is introduced, he begins singing in his own dialect. But he sings with variations, and the more time he spends in her presence, the more his song takes the form of the local dialect. Her differential reactions are reinforcers, and they shape his song (e.g., King & West, 1985).

Shaping can be hard to see if one does not know what to look for; someone who has actually done shaping is more apt to notice it in natural environments than someone who has only read about it. Thus parents who always wait a while before attending to a crying child may not notice that they have gradually shaped louder and more annoying cries. The attention reinforces the crying, and annoying cries are, by definition, the ones most likely to get attention. If one watches what a parent does when a child throws tantrums, it is often easy to guess where the tantrums have come from. The contingencies that produce such problem behavior seldom occur in isolation, so other behavior or other reinforcers may eventually displace the problem behavior, but the spontaneous disappearance of problem behavior must not be taken as evidence that the behavior's source has been independent of shaping.

Shaping can be demonstrated over minutes rather than over days, years, or millennia. If reinforcers can do so much to behavior when contingencies are deliberately arranged over relatively short periods of time, it is reasonable to assume that they also affect behavior when natural contingencies operate over substantial periods throughout an organism's lifetime, as in the acquisition of verbal behavior by children. Many contingencies may take hold of behavior over the course of months or years in the life of a young child. Some may be subtle, especially given the very broad range of events that can serve as reinforcers. Some may produce desirable behavior, and others may do the opposite. The self-injurious behavior of an institutionalized 9-year-old child may seem resistant to

change, but 9 years is a very long time over which contingencies can operate. This does not mean that all such behavior is solely a product of contingencies. In the face of such possibilities, however, it is certainly more appropriate to be alert for the effects of such contingencies than to assume that they do not exist.

## HIGHER-ORDER CLASSES AND OPERANT CONTINGENCIES

Contingencies can operate in combination and present particular challenges when some contingencies are nested in others, in higher-order classes. Sometimes when a response class appears insensitive to its consequences, it is part of a larger class whose other members continue to have the consequences it once shared with them. In such cases, the contingencies operating on the higher-order class may override those arranged for the original class. For example, once generalized imitation has been established, a child may continue to imitate some instance even though that particular imitation is never reinforced. That imitation may seem insensitive to operant contingencies, but it will be maintained by the contingencies that operate on the higher-order class as long as the higher-order class maintains its integrity.

We would ordinarily expect subclasses for which reinforcement has been discontinued to be differentiated from their higher-order classes, but this may not happen if the integrity of the higher-order class depends on its membership in other, interlocking higher-order classes that still include the subclass (e.g., playing the game "Simon Says" on the playground may help to maintain generalized imitation in the classroom, even if imitative responses in the classroom are never reinforced). In some cases this may be a problem, but in others it may instead be advantageous, such as when new behavior emerges as a novel instance of the higher-order class (e.g., the generalized imitation of a movement the child has never seen before).

Now consider a boy whose self-injurious behavior is reinforced by attention. Suppose we try to extinguish his self-injurious behavior by ignoring it. We may have trouble from the start, because we cannot tolerate the damage he may do to himself. We nevertheless persevere and discover that his self-injurious behavior does not decrease. One possibility is that we have not adequately identified the relevant response class. If the function of this behavior is to produce attention, it may be part of a much larger class of behavior that includes shouting obscenities, acting up, hitting or otherwise abusing the caregivers in the treatment center, and any number of other responses that might get attention (Lalli, Mace, Wohn, & Livezey, 1995). This tells us how important attention is to this child. We must consider a treatment program that uses attention to reinforce more effective and appropriate behavior, but the example also reminds us that we cannot define response classes by what they look like.

Related topographies within higher-order classes may also enter into hierarchies in which some subclasses are more likely than others. For example, with severe self-injurious behavior or other dangerous forms of problem behavior, functional analyses may involve risks of injury. But they may also reveal precursors of dangerous behavior within such a hierarchy. Reducing the likelihood of the precursors may also reduce the likelihood of the more dangerous forms of behavior that follow them (Fritz, Iwata, Hammond, & Bloom, 2013). Assessments of hierarchical response classes therefore can lead to function-based interventions that reduce the risks of functional analyses by reducing the likelihood of the most dangerous topographies within the hierarchy.

The criterion for defining response classes is function, and common consequences are the glue that holds classes of behavior together. The larger class is held together by the common consequences of its members, just as the various topographies of a rat's lever presses (left or right paw, both paws, rump) are held together by the common consequence of producing food. But the human case is distinguished by the embedding of one response class within another. The self-injurious behavior in the example above is embedded in the larger class of attention-getting behavior. When a response class seems insensitive to its consequences, such as when the self-injurious behavior seems not to extinguish, we must entertain the possibility that we have improperly specified the class, and that it is part of a larger class whose other members continue to have the consequences it once shared with them. The hierarchical structure of some classes of behavior may sometimes make it appear that reinforcement is not working, but it may be working on a response class larger than the one in which we have been interested. When reinforcement seems not to be working, we should consider whether the response class in which we are interested is part of another larger class (Catania, 1995).

## Verbal Behavior and the Hidden Costs of Reward

Reinforcement may be obscured when human verbal and nonverbal behavior interact. For example, instruction-following behavior is more than the following of particular instructions; it is a higher-order class of behavior held together by common contingencies (e.g., Shimoff & Catania, 1998). Following orders in the military is a product of extensive and powerful social contingencies, often based on aversive consequences, but in actual combat, the long-term contingencies that maintain instruction following in general as a higher-order class may be pitted against the immediate consequences of following a particular order (Skinner, 1969).

Verbal behavior is involved in the distinction between intrinsic and extrinsic reinforcers. An *intrinsic* reward or reinforcer is one that has a natural relation to the responses that produce it, whereas an *extrinsic* one has an arbitrary relation to those responses (e.g., music is an intrinsic consequence of playing an instrument, but the music teacher's praise is an extrinsic one). Events presumed to function as reinforcers because their function has been instructed have been called *extrinsic reinforcers* (e.g., as when a child is told that it is important to earn good grades), but labeling them so does not guarantee their effectiveness. It has been argued that extrinsic consequences undermine the effectiveness of intrinsic ones, and despite much evidence to the contrary, the argument has persisted and continues to influence the use of operant contingencies in schools and other settings (Cameron, Banko, & Pierce, 2001; Cameron & Pierce, 1994; Eisenberger & Cameron, 1996).

In one experiment (Lepper, Greene, & Nisbett, 1973), one group of children received gold stars for artwork such as finger painting; after the gold stars were discontinued, children in this group did less artwork than those in a second group that never received gold stars. The gold stars, extrinsic reinforcers, were said to have undermined the intrinsic reinforcers, the natural consequences of painting. The children had been told to earn the gold stars, however, and the experiment did not test the stars' effectiveness as reinforcers. There were no data to show that children painted more when they got gold stars.

The claimed deleterious effects are only inconsistently demonstrable, and they are small and transient when they do occur (Cameron et al., 2001; Cameron & Pierce, 1994). Problems are more likely to arise with extrinsic reward that is not contingent on performance than with contingent reward (Eisenberger & Cameron, 1996). In any case, if there is an effect, its transience and small size are hardly consistent with the argument that extrinsic reinforcement may ruin the lives of children. Nonverbal effects of reinforcers must be distinguished from the social contingencies that maintain the verbal governance of behavior. When situations involve verbal behavior, there is a good chance that verbal governance will override more direct effects of reinforcement.

## Reinforcers versus Bribes

In the literature of the "hidden costs of reward," reinforcers have sometimes been equated with bribes (Kohn, 1993), but it is unlikely that the arrangements described as bribes by such critics of the practice of reinforcement involve the direct effects of reinforcers. The language of bribery has an extensive history in law and ethics as an offer of goods or favors in exchange for favorable treatment in business, politics, or other human endeavors. Critics of the practice of reinforcement have extended this language to the common parental practice of specifying a consequence when asking a child to do something (e.g., "If you put away your toys, you can watch television"). There are good reasons to advise parents against the practice of bribery in this sense, but the reasons are different from those offered by the critics. They have correctly recognized the potentially different effects of natural and artificial consequences, but they have also seriously conflated cases of verbal stimulus control with those involving other varieties of contingencies.

Parents sometimes complain that their child only cooperates with requests when there is an immediate and explicit payoff. This problem is one of stimulus control. The parent may sometimes say, "It is time to put your toys away," and at other times may say, "If you put away your toys, you can watch television." But unless the child who has complied with the request gets an opportunity to watch television whether or not the contingency has been explicitly stated, the child will learn to comply only when the parent states it.

Given that a bribe specifies behavior and its consequences, offers of bribes instead function as stimuli that set the occasion for particular contingencies. The child who is frequently bribed in this sense will learn to discriminate between conditions in which bribes are in effect and those in which they are not, so the parent who often uses

bribes will no doubt eventually find that the child complies only when a bribe is offered.

The child will not learn to initiate appropriate behavior if the initiation rests with the one who offers the bribe. Over the long run, therefore, compliance with bribes will probably interfere with the effects of more constructive contingencies. If reinforcement works at all in such cases, it is in strengthening compliance with bribes, which is hardly the best way to make use of reinforcers. When such unintended stimulus control develops, it is important to teach the parent to reinforce compliance without explicitly stating the contingency, or at least to reinforce compliance both when the contingency is explicitly stated and when it is not.

As for the parent who has heard the language of bribes applied to the practice of reinforcement and is therefore reluctant to deliver reinforcers, it is crucial to teach that parent not to accompany the arrangement of contingencies for a child's behavior with statements of those contingencies. And that is probably good advice for teachers and clinicians, too.

## REINFORCER CLASSES AND REINFORCER-SPECIFIC EFFECTS

Operant contingencies involve consequences, and like responses, they can profitably be studied in terms of classes (Cuvo, 2000). Successive reinforcers arranged in experimental settings are ordinarily similar but not identical. For example, individual pieces of grain made available when a pigeon's pecks operate its feeder will differ slightly in shape and color; a parent's hugs or smiles or positive comments that reinforce a child's behavior will undoubtedly vary from one instance to the next.

The discussion of higher-order classes has examined the different responses that may produce attention and thereby maintain the self-injurious behavior of children with severe developmental disabilities. Because it shares its consequences with other responses, such as shouting obscenities or throwing things, the self-injurious behavior may be part of a larger class we might call *attention-getting behavior*. Within this class, some types of responses may be more probable than others or may be differently available in different settings (Lalli et al., 1995). For example, a child may be more likely to engage in self-injury if nothing to throw is close at hand, or more likely to shout obscenities given one audience than given another. Nevertheless, their membership in a common class makes it likely that these responses will vary together as a function of establishing events or other variables.

But what if attention from staff members on this child's hospital unit does not function like attention from the child's mother when she visits the unit? If we find that one kind of attention cannot substitute for the other, we might best treat attention from these two different sources as two separate reinforcer classes (cf. Kelly, Roscoe, Hanley, & Schlichenmeyer, 2014). This is important to know, because assessments of problem behavior on the unit may yield different results from those taken at the child's home; therefore, therapeutic interventions shaped by staff attention on the unit may be incompatible with the kinds of behavior shaped by the mother's attention at home. An effective treatment program must deal with the mother's behavior as well as the child's, or the treatment gains realized on the unit will be lost soon after the child's discharge.

The significance of reinforcer classes has been especially demonstrated in research on the acquisition of arbitrary matching by children and by nonhuman organisms (Dube & McIlvane, 1995; Dube, McIlvane, Mackay, & Stoddard, 1987; Kastak, Schusterman, & Kastak, 2001; Urcuioli, 1991, 2005). Experiments on arbitrary matching typically incorporate correction procedures and other features that reduce the proximity of errors to later reinforcers, and that reduce the likelihood that the organism will attend to dimensions of the environment that are irrelevant to the task. Nevertheless, some children, as well as some pigeons, learn slowly.

In a typical matching study, all correct responses, whether to one comparison stimulus or the other, produce the same reinforcer. But if the reinforcers as well as the stimuli and responses of the arbitrary matching tasks enter into functional classes, this may be a mistake. While the contingencies may work to separate the different matching classes, such as green peck given square sample and red peck given circle sample, the common reinforcers may work to keep them together. With the matching task modified for children so that correct responses from the different problem classes each produce a different visual reinforcer (e.g., different cartoon pictures displayed on a video monitor), the acquisition of accurate arbitrary matching usually proceeds far more rapidly than when all responses produce the same reinforcer (e.g., Urcuioli, 2005; Urcuioli & Swisher,

2015). The moral is that whenever possible, we should arrange different reinforcers rather than a single reinforcer for the maintenance or the shaping of different response classes.

## REINFORCEMENT AND CULTURAL SELECTION

The relations among behavior and its consequences in operant contingencies seem simple, but they have subtle properties, some of which become evident only in special contexts. For example, when side effects are not taken into account, contingencies can appear to be ineffective. Side effects of operant contingencies may have affected their acceptance because they allow the effects of contingencies to be masked in various ways. It is therefore prudent to consider the circumstances in which the properties of operant contingencies may mislead us as we deploy them and evaluate their effects. In the interests of preventing misconceptions and misunderstandings, it is probably even more important to remind ourselves of them whenever we present what we know about operant contingencies to those outside behavior analysis. To those who argue that these contingencies should not be studied because they can be misused, the appropriate rejoinder is that detailed familiarity with their properties may be the best defense against their misuse. Alone or in combination, the factors considered here may sometimes give the appearance that operant contingencies do not work. On examination, we might instead conclude that they work more ubiquitously and more profoundly than we had originally imagined.

*Phylogenic* selection is Darwinian selection as it operates in the evolution of species. *Ontogenic* selection is operant selection as it operates in the shaping of behavior within an individual lifetime. A third level of selection is *sociogenic* or *cultural* selection, which involves the selection of behavior as it is passed on from one individual to another (Skinner, 1981). Selection at any one of these levels need not be consistent with selection at the other two. For example, it may not matter how valuable one way of doing things is relative to some other way, if one is easy to pass on from one individual to another, whereas the other can be passed on only with difficulty. The one that is easier to pass on may spread quickly and come to dominate in a culture relative to the other, even if the other would be more beneficial in the long term.

A case in point is the application of techniques of reinforcement relative to those of punishment. Unfortunately, the advantages of reinforcement do not make it more likely than punishment to spread through a culture (Catania, 2000). The problem is that delivering a punisher typically produces more immediate effects on behavior than delivering a reinforcer. Whatever else happens over the long term, a parent who shouts at or strikes a child thought to be misbehaving is likely to see some immediate change in the child's behavior, such as the onset of crying. That change will usually include the termination of the behavior of concern to the parent, even though it may have little to do with whether the behavior will reappear on later occasions, especially in the parent's absence. If stopping the child's behavior is part of what reinforces the parent's application of punishment, the immediacy of that reinforcer will be an important factor in maintenance of the use of punishment by the parent.

With reinforcement, on the other hand, the effects of delivering a reinforcer may not show up until some time has elapsed. In shaping, if a current reinforced response is closer to the target response than any other response seen before by the shaper, the likelihood of similar responses will increase. Even so, many other responses may go by before the shaper sees another one like it. Unlike the punishment case, in which an immediate effect is typically that the target behavior stops, any immediate effect of reinforcement involves behavior unrelated to the target response (e.g., consuming an edible reinforcer). The time periods over which reinforcers change subsequent responding probably play a crucial role in determining how long it takes to teach shaping to students. If this makes it easier to teach aversive techniques than to teach those of reinforcement, perhaps this is also why punitive measures are so commonly used to maintain civil order in so many cultures.

Even as reinforcement begins to be more widely appreciated in our culture, we must not be complacent about teaching what we know about it. Despite the advantages of reinforcement, it is easier to teach the use of punishers than to teach the use of reinforcers, and reinforcement can be misunderstood or be obscured by other processes in various ways. Some people are very good at shaping even without explicit instruction, but for most individuals the effective use of reinforcers has to be carefully taught.

## REFERENCES

Arntzen, E., Brekstad, A., & Holth, P. (Eds.). (2004). Special issue on noncontingent reinforcement. *European Journal of Behavior Analysis, 5*, 1–108.

Arntzen, E., Brekstad, A., & Holth, P. (Eds.). (2006). Special issue on contingent reinforcement. *European Journal of Behavior Analysis, 7*, 99–185.

Azrin, N. H., & Holz, W. C. (1966). Punishment. In W. K. Honig (Ed.), *Operant behavior: Areas of research and application* (pp. 380–447). New York: Appleton-Century-Crofts.

Azrin, N. H., Hutchinson, R. R., & Hake, D. F. (1966). Extinction-induced aggression. *Journal of the Experimental Analysis of Behavior, 9*, 191–204.

Azrin, N. H., Hutchinson, R. R., & McLaughlin, R. (1965). The opportunity for aggression as an operant reinforcer. *Journal of the Experimental Analysis of Behavior, 8*, 171–180.

Bandura, A. (1976). Self-reinforcement: Theoretical and methodological considerations. *Behaviorism, 4*, 135–155.

Bandura, A. (1995). Comments on the crusade against the causal efficacy of human thought. *Journal of Behavior Therapy and Experimental Psychiatry, 26*, 179–190.

Bersh, P. J., & Lambert, J. V. (1975). The discriminative control of free-operant avoidance despite exposure to shock during the stimulus correlated with nonreinforcement. *Journal of the Experimental Analysis of Behavior, 23*, 111–120.

Cameron, J., Banko, K. M., & Pierce, W. D. (2001). Pervasive negative effects of rewards on intrinsic motivation: The myth continues. *Behavior Analyst, 24*, 1–44.

Cameron, J., & Pierce, W. D. (1994). Reinforcement, reward, and intrinsic motivation: A meta-analysis. *Review of Educational Research, 64*, 363–423.

Camp, D. S., Raymond, G. A., & Church, R. M. (1967). Temporal relationship between response and punishment. *Journal of Experimental Psychology, 74*, 114–123.

Carr, E. G., Newsom, C. D., & Binkoff, J. A. (1980). Escape as a factor in the aggressive behavior of two retarded children. *Journal of Applied Behavior Analysis, 13*, 101–117.

Catania, A. C. (1971). Elicitation, reinforcement and stimulus control. In R. Glaser (Ed.), *The nature of reinforcement* (pp. 196–220). New York: Academic Press.

Catania, A. C. (1975). The myth of self-reinforcement. *Behaviorism, 3*, 192–199.

Catania, A. C. (1995). Higher-order behavior classes: Contingencies, beliefs, and verbal behavior. *Journal of Behavior Therapy and Experimental Psychiatry, 26*, 191–200.

Catania, A. C. (2000). Ten points every behavior analyst needs to remember about reinforcement. In J. C. Leslie & D. E. Blackman (Eds.), *Experimental and ap-*

*plied analyses of human behavior* (pp. 23–37). Reno, NV: Context Press.

Catania, A. C. (2001). Positive psychology and positive reinforcement. *American Psychologist, 56,* 86–87.

Catania, A. C. (2005). The nonmaintenance of behavior by noncontingent reinforcement. *European Journal of Behavior Analysis, 6,* 89–94.

Catania, A. C. (2013). *Learning* (5th ed.). Cornwall-on-Hudson, NY: Sloan.

Charlop, M. H., Kurtz, P. F., & Casey, F. G. (1990). Using aberrant behaviors as reinforcers for autistic children. *Journal of Applied Behavior Analysis, 23,* 163–181.

Cuvo, A. J. (2000). Development and function of consequence classes in operant behavior. *Behavior Analyst, 23,* 57–68.

Donahoe, J. W., Burgos, J. E., & Palmer, D. C. (1993). A selectionist approach to reinforcement. *Journal of the Experimental Analysis of Behavior, 60,* 17–40.

Donahoe, J. W., & Vegas, R. (2004). Pavlovian conditioning: The CS–UR relation. *Journal of Experimental Psychology: Animal Behavior Processes, 30,* 17–33.

Dube, W. V., & McIlvane, W. J. (1995). Stimulus–reinforcer relations and emergent matching to sample. *Psychological Record, 45,* 591–612.

Dube, W. V., McIlvane, W. J., Mackay, H. A., & Stoddard, L. T. (1987). Stimulus class membership established via stimulus–reinforcer relations. *Journal of the Experimental Analysis of Behavior, 47,* 159–175.

Eisenberger, R., & Cameron, J. (1996). Detrimental effects of reward: Reality or myth? *American Psychologist, 51,* 1153–1166.

Favell, J. E., McGimsey, J. F., & Jones, M. L. (1978). The use of physical restraint in the treatment of self-injury and as positive reinforcement. *Journal of Applied Behavior Analysis, 11,* 225–241.

Ferrari, M., & Harris, S. L. (1981). The limits and motivating potential of sensory stimuli as reinforcers for autistic children. *Journal of Applied Behavior Analysis, 14,* 339–343.

Ferster, C. B. (1958). Control of behavior in chimpanzees and pigeons by time out from positive reinforcement. *Psychological Monographs, 72*(8, Whole No. 461).

Fisher, W. W., Pawich, T. L., Dickes, N., Paden, A. R., & Toussaint, K. (2014). Increasing the saliency of behavior–consequence relations for children with autism who exhibit persistent errors. *Journal of Applied Behavior Analysis, 47,* 738–748.

Fisher, W. W., Piazza, C. C., Bowman, L. G., Hagopian, L. P., Owens, J. C., & Slevin, I. (1992). A comparison of two approaches for identifying reinforcers for persons with severe and profound disabilities. *Journal of Applied Behavior Analysis, 25,* 491–498.

Fisher, W. W., Rodriguez, N., & Owen, T. (2013). Functional assessment and treatment of perseverative speech about restricted topics in an adolescent with Asperger syndrome. *Journal of Applied Behavior Analysis. 46,* 307–311.

Fritz, J. N., Iwata, B. A., Hammond, J. L., & Bloom, S. E.

(2013). Experimental analysis of precursors to severe problem behavior. *Journal of Applied Behavior Analysis, 46,* 101–129.

Green, C. W., Reid, D. H., White, L. K., Halford, R. C., Brittain, D. P., & Gardner, S. M. (1988). Identifying reinforcers for persons with profound handicaps: Staff opinion versus systematic assessment of preferences. *Journal of Applied Behavior Analysis, 21,* 31–43.

Greer, B. D., Fisher, W. W., Saini, V., Owen, T. M., & Jones, J. K. (2016). Improving functional communication training during reinforcement schedule thinning: An analysis of 25 applications. *Journal of Applied Behavior Analysis, 49,* 105–121.

Hagopian, L. P., Crockett, J. L., van Stone, M., DeLeon, I. G., & Bowman, L. G. (2000). Effects of noncontingent reinforcement on problem behavior and stimulus engagement: The role of satiation, extinction, and alternative reinforcement. *Journal of Applied Behavior Analysis, 33,* 433–449.

Herrnstein, R. J., & Hineline, P. N. (1966). Negative reinforcement as shock-frequency reduction. *Journal of the Experimental Analysis of Behavior, 9,* 421–430.

Hineline, P. N. (1970). Negative reinforcement without shock reduction. *Journal of the Experimental Analysis of Behavior, 14,* 259–268.

Hineline, P. N. (1981). The several roles of stimuli in negative reinforcement. In P. Harzem & M. D. Zeiler (Eds.), *Predictability, correlation, and contiguity* (pp. 203–246). New York: Wiley.

Holz, W. C., & Azrin, N. H. (1961). Discriminative properties of punishment. *Journal of the Experimental Analysis of Behavior, 4,* 225–232.

Iversen, I. H., & Lattal, K. A. (1991a). *Experimental analysis of behavior: Part 1.* Amsterdam: Elsevier.

Iversen, I. H., & Lattal, K. A. (1991b). *Experimental analysis of behavior: Part 2.* Amsterdam: Elsevier.

Iwata, B. A., Pace, G. M., Kalsher, M. J., Cowdery, G. E., & Cataldo, M. F. (1990). Experimental analysis and extinction of self-injurious escape behavior. *Journal of Applied Behavior Analysis, 23,* 11–27.

Kastak, C. R., Schusterman, R. J., & Kastak, D. (2001). Equivalence classification by California sea lions using class-specific reinforcers. *Journal of the Experimental Analysis of Behavior, 76,* 131–158.

Keller, F. S. (1941). Light aversion in the white rat. *Psychological Record, 4,* 235–250.

Kelly, M. A., Roscoe, E. M., Hanley, G. P., & Schlichenmeyer, K. (2014). Evaluation of assessment methods for identifying social reinforcers. *Journal of Applied Behavior Analysis, 47,* 113–135.

King, A. P., & West, M. J. (1985). Social metrics of song learning. *Learning and Motivation, 15,* 441–458.

Kohn, A. (1993). *Punished by rewards.* Boston: Houghton Mifflin.

Lalli, J. S., Mace, F. C., Wohn, T., & Livezey, K. (1995). Identification and modification of a response-class hierarchy. *Journal of Applied Behavior Analysis, 28,* 551–559.

Lattal, K. A. (1974). Combinations of response reinforcer dependence and independence. *Journal of the Experimental Analysis of Behavior, 22,* 357–362.

Lepper, M. R., Greene, D., & Nisbett, R. E. (1973). Undermining children's intrinsic interest with extrinsic reward: A test of the "overjustification" hypothesis. *Journal of Personality and Social Psychology, 28,* 129–137.

Lerman, D. C., Iwata, B. A., & Wallace, M. D. (1999). Side effects of extinction: Prevalence of bursting and aggression during the treatment of self-injurious behavior. *Journal of Applied Behavior Analysis, 32,* 1–8.

Mahoney, M. J., & Bandura, A. (1972). Self-reinforcement in pigeons. *Learning and Motivation, 3,* 293–303.

Maier, S. F., Albin, R. W., & Testa, T. J. (1973). Failure to learn to escape in rats previously exposed to inescapable shock depends on nature of escape response. *Journal of Comparative and Physiological Psychology, 85,* 581–592.

Michael, J. (1982). Distinguishing between discriminative and motivational functions of stimuli. *Journal of the Experimental Analysis of Behavior, 37,* 149–155.

Michael, J. (1989). *Concepts and principles of behavior analysis.* Kalamazoo, MI: Association for Behavior Analysis.

Neuringer, A. (2004). Reinforced variability in animals and people. *American Psychologist, 59,* 891–906.

Nevin, J. A. (1992). An integrative model for the study of behavioral momentum. *Journal of the Experimental Analysis of Behavior, 57,* 301–316.

Pavlov, I. P. (1927). *Conditioned reflexes* (G. V. Anrep, Trans.). London: Oxford University Press.

Perone, M. (2003). Negative effects of positive reinforcement. *Behavior Analyst, 26,* 1–14.

Peterson, N. (1960). Control of behavior by presentation of an imprinted stimulus. *Science, 132,* 1395–1396.

Premack, D. (1962). Reversibility of the reinforcement relation. *Science, 136,* 255–257.

Seligman, M. E. P., & Csikszentmihalyi, M. (2000). Positive psychology: An introduction. *American Psychologist, 55,* 5–14.

Seligman, M. E. P., & Csikszentmihalyi, M. (2001). Reply to comments. *American Psychologist, 56,* 89–90.

Shimoff, E., & Catania, A. C. (1998). The verbal governance of behavior. In K. A. Lattal & M. Perone (Eds.), *Handbook of research methods in human operant behavior* (pp. 371–404). New York: Plenum Press.

Sidman, M. (1953). Two temporal parameters in the maintenance of avoidance behavior by the white rat. *Journal of Comparative and Physiological Psychology, 46,* 253–261.

Sidman, M. (1958). By-products of aversive control. *Journal of the Experimental Analysis of Behavior, 1,* 265–280.

Sizemore, O. J., & Lattal, K. A. (1977). Dependency, temporal contiguity, and response-independent reinforcement. *Journal of the Experimental Analysis of Behavior, 27,* 119–125.

Skinner, B. F. (1935). The generic nature of the concepts of stimulus and response. *Journal of General Psychology, 12,* 40–65.

Skinner, B. F. (1938). *The behavior of organisms: An experimental analysis.* New York: Appleton-Century-Crofts.

Skinner, B. F. (1953). *Science and human behavior.* New York: Macmillan.

Skinner, B. F. (1957). *Verbal behavior.* New York: Appleton-Century-Crofts.

Skinner, B. F. (1969). *Contingencies of reinforcement.* New York: Appleton-Century-Crofts.

Skinner, B. F. (1981). Selection by consequences. *Science, 213,* 501–504.

Skinner, B. F. (1999). *Cumulative record* (V. G. Laties & A. C. Catania, Eds.). Cambridge, MA: B. F. Skinner Foundation.

Solnick, J. V., Rincover, A., & Peterson, C. R. (1977). Some determinants of the reinforcing and punishing effects of timeout. *Journal of Applied Behavior Analysis, 10,* 415–424.

Urcuioli, P. J. (1991). Retardation and facilitation of matching acquisition by differential outcomes. *Animal Learning and Behavior, 19,* 29–36.

Urcuioli, P. J. (2005). Behavioral and associative effects of differential outcomes in discrimination learning. *Learning and Behavior, 33,* 1–21.

Urcuioli, P. J., & Swisher, M. J. (2015). Transitive and anti-transitive emergent relations in pigeons: Support for a theory of stimulus-class formation. *Behavioural Processes, 112,* 49–60.

Weiss, B., & Laties, V. G. (1961). Behavioral thermoregulation. *Science, 133,* 1338–1344.

Wolf, M., Risley, T., & Mees, H. (1986). Application of operant conditioning procedures to the behavior problems of an autistic child. *Behaviour Research and Therapy, 1,* 305–312.

# CHAPTER 4

# Schedules of Reinforcement

F. Charles Mace, Duncan Pritchard, and Heather Penney

Rules that describe the relation between responses and reinforcer deliveries are known as *schedules of reinforcement*. Researchers can arrange these rules deliberately in the context of an experiment or behavioral treatment, or they can surmise them from the pattern of responses to reinforcer deliveries that occur naturally. In either case, schedules of reinforcement are important for applied behavior analysts to consider, because each schedule has predictable effects on one or more dimensions of behavior. With this knowledge, applied behavior analysts can describe the conditions of reinforcement that maintain undesirable behavior, and design interventions that have a higher likelihood of increasing desirable behavior.

This chapter discusses the dimensions of behavior that schedules of reinforcement can affect, and presents descriptions and examples of basic and combined schedules of reinforcement.

## SCHEDULES OF REINFORCEMENT IN CONTEXT

Understanding the effects schedules of reinforcement have on behavior in the broader context in which they operate is important. The basic unit of analysis in applied behavior analysis (ABA) is the *discriminated operant,* which is a class of responses defined by both the effect the responses have on the environment and the stimuli present when responses occur (Catania, 2013). Events that

motivate the occurrence of discriminated operants are known as *motivating operations* (Laraway, Snycerski, Michael, & Poling, 2003). Motivating operations are events preceding occurrences of discriminated operants that can have *evocative* or *abative* effects on behavior; that is, they increase or decrease their occurrence. They alter the effectiveness of consequences of behavior by establishing or abolishing their reinforcing or punishing effects. *Discriminative stimuli* are antecedent occurrences of stimuli or events that correlate with or signal the increased or decreased availability of reinforcement or punishment and affect discriminated operants. Behavior analysts say that discriminative stimuli set the occasion for operants to occur, because they predict the likely consequences of responses. However, the effects of discriminative stimuli on behavior depend on the presence or absence of related motivating operations (Laraway et al., 2003).

In natural human environments, individuals are free to engage in any of several concurrently available discriminated operants. Each one produces one or more consequences, and the individual has a *choice* to engage in any alternative (Fisher & Mazur, 1997; Mace & Roberts, 1993). Investigators have studied the variables that influence choice extensively and have quantified them in the *generalized matching law* (Baum, 1974), which we briefly discuss later. However, one of the variables that affects choice is the relative schedule of reinforcement operating for each concurrently available alternative. We also provide a conceptual framework for understanding how changes in relative motivation and relative history of reinforcement or punishment influence concurrent discriminated operants in a dynamic manner (i.e., behavioral mass; Mace, Gritter, Johnson, Malley, & Steege, 2007; see Figure 4.1). Learning histories affect the relative resistance to change or momentum each discriminated operant has, and can affect the relative value of concurrently available alternatives and the choices individuals make. Nevin and Grace (2000) refer to these histories as *behavioral mass* in the context of their formulation of *behavioral-momentum theory*.

The purpose of this preface to our discussion of schedules of reinforcement is to emphasize that the effects of reinforcement schedules on behavior are *relative*, not absolute (Herrnstein, 1961, 1970). That is, the influence of any given schedule of reinforcement on a discriminated operant will depend on the relative factors that affect choice, including reinforcer rate, quality, and delay, as well as response effort, motivation, and behavioral mass. The practical significance of this conceptual model is that applied behavior analysts may need to consider many factors that influence both desirable and undesirable behavior to maximize the effectiveness of their interventions.

## BEHAVIOR DIMENSIONS AFFECTED BY SCHEDULES OF REINFORCEMENT

In ABA practice, clinicians and researchers deliver reinforcers contingently. There are three general types of contingencies. First, a *ratio contingency* is one between the number of responses that occur and the delivery of a reinforcer. Second, an *interval contingency* is one between the occurrence of responses and the passage of time. Third, a *time contingency* is the passage of time with no relation to the occurrence of responses. The arrangement of ratio, interval, and time contingencies can affect the response's rate, periodicity, and resistance to change.

### Response Rate

*Response rate* is the ratio of the number of responses per time, or response count divided by time. Its synonym is *frequency*. An alternative expression of response rate is the average time between responses, or *interresponse time* (IRT), which is the mean for the elapsed time between the offset of one response and the onset of the next response in the response class. Response rate and IRT have a perfect inverse correlation, such that a unit increase in response rate will have a corresponding unit decrease in interresponse time. In ABA practice, response rate is often an important dimension that the behavior analyst aims to alter—generally by attempting to increase the frequency of desirable behaviors, to decrease the frequency of undesirable ones, or both. Thus knowing the effects of different schedules of reinforcement on response rate is important in the design of interventions.

### Response Periodicity

*Response periodicity* is the pattern of responses in relation to the passage of time. Whereas interre-

## Concurrent Discriminated Operants

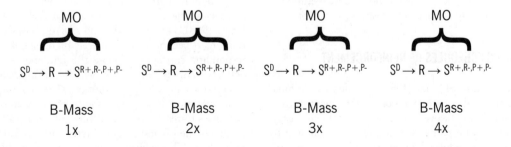

**FIGURE 4.1.** Framework for conceptualizing discriminated operants in context: The dynamic interplay between motivating operations, behavioral mass, and the classic three-term contingency.

sponse time expresses the average time between responses, response periodicity is the pattern of times between individual responses or individual IRTs during a period. In general, schedules of reinforcement promote four patterns of response periodicity. The first pattern is a *constant* time between responses with little variability in individual IRTs, which is characteristic of variable-ratio (VR) and variable-interval (VI) schedules. A second pattern is a *pause* in responding after a comparatively higher response rate. Both fixed-ratio (FR) and fixed-interval (FI) schedules can promote temporary pauses in responding after reinforcement delivery before responding resumes. A third pattern is the *suspension* of responding after a given response pattern. Time, extinction, and differential reinforcement of other behavior (DRO) can produce reductions in response rates to zero or near-zero. Finally, response periodicity can show a pattern of *celeration* (Johnston & Pennypacker, 2009), which refers to a progressive change in individual IRTs. Progressively shorter IRTs reflect *acceleration* in response rate, and progressively longer IRTs reflect *deceleration*. Many schedules of reinforcement can promote these response patterns, as we discuss in the following sections.

### Resistance to Change

An important dimension of behavior that applied behavior analysts increasingly consider is its *resistance to change*, which is the rate of deceleration in responding after the introduction of some *response disruptor* (Nevin, 1974; Nevin, Mandell, & Atak, 1983). Common events that disrupt the response–reinforcer relation include extinction, satiation, alternative reinforcement, punishment, dark-key or between-session reinforcement, and distraction. Each operation can decelerate responding. This dimension of behavior is particularly relevant to ABA work aimed at strengthening the resistance to change of desirable behavior and weakening the resistance to change of undesirable behavior.

## BASIC SCHEDULES OF REINFORCEMENT

Ferster and Skinner (1957) provided the foundational work for schedules of reinforcement in their compilation of over 100 experimental demonstrations of the patterns of responding promoted by various schedules. Numerous applications of various schedules of reinforcement in ABA have demonstrated the relevance of these schedules to the assessment and treatment of human behavior.

Basic schedules are single schedules of reinforcement applied to one class of responses, which form the building blocks for the more complex, combined schedules of reinforcement. Table 4.1 summarizes the basic schedules discussed in this chapter, schedule definitions, the response patterns each schedule promotes, and applications of the schedule in ABA work.

### Ratio Schedules

Ratio schedules of reinforcement specify the number of responses the organism must emit to effect delivery of reinforcement, independent of the time the organism takes to complete the schedule requirement. However, because slow response rates delay the time to reinforcement, ratio schedules generally promote relatively high response rates with relatively constant individual IRTs, with some exceptions noted below. Two schedule features influence the response patterns promoted by ratio schedules: (1) the ratio of responses to reinforcers and (2) the predictability of this ratio.

#### FR Schedules

In an FR schedule, the number of responses required to produce a reinforcer is constant (e.g., inputting a three-digit area code and seven-digit phone number to make a call is an example of an FR 10 schedule). When the ratio of responses to reinforcers is very low, as in the case of the FR 1 schedule or *continuous-reinforcement* (CRF) schedule, responses rates are typically low. However, as reinforcer deliveries become less frequent (e.g., FR 5), the response rates the schedule promotes increase rapidly and eventually support comparatively high rates of responding. As the ratio of responses to reinforcers increases, pauses in responding after the reinforcer delivery, or *postreinforcement pauses*, also increase (Felton & Lyon, 1966). Finally, as the ratio of responses to reinforcers becomes comparatively high, pauses in responding can appear before the reinforcement delivery. This is *ratio strain*, which can produce either the temporary interruption of responding or its cessation. The predictability of the ratio of responses to reinforcers in FR schedules generally promotes the highest response rates with uniform individual IRTs. However, humans may show FR response patterns even when the ratio of responses

**TABLE 4.1.  Basic Schedules of Reinforcement, ABA Example, and the Response Patterns Promoted**

| Schedule | Definition | ABA example | Response pattern promoted |
|---|---|---|---|
| FR—fixed ratio | Reinforcers are contingent on every *i*th response (e.g., FR 4—every fourth response) | Cohen et al. (2001) demonstrated FR patterns by measuring muscle contractions emitted by undergraduate students. | High response rate with comparatively short and uniform IRTs. Pause in responding follows reinforcer deliveries. |
| VR—variable ratio | Reinforcers are contingent on a variable number of responses; the average number of responses defines the schedule. | DeLuca and Holburn (1992) showed VR patterns by measuring obese children's rate of stationary bike revolutions. | High response rate with comparatively short and uniform IRTs. |
| FI—fixed interval | Reinforcers are contingent on the first response following a fixed time interval. | Critchfield et al. (2003) analyzed the bill-passing behavior of the U.S. Congress. | Possible cumulative record scalloping when measurement of the passage of time is unavailable. |
| VI—variable interval | Reinforcers are contingent on the first response following a variable interval of time; the average of these intervals defines the schedule. | Martens, Lockner, and Kelly (1992) demonstrated VI response patterns in the academic engagement of typically developing 8-year-olds. | Moderate response rates with uniform but longer IRTs than ratio schedules. |
| EXT—extinction | Discontinuation of a reinforcement contingency either by withholding contingent reinforcement or delivering reinforcers independently of behavior according to FT or VT schedules. | Magee and Ellis (2001) demonstrated the extinction process for several challenging behaviors (e.g., out-of-seat behavior, hand mouthing, yelling, and property destruction) exhibited by children with developmental disabilities. | When contingent reinforcement is withheld—a sudden increase in response rate (burst) followed by a reduction to zero. When the reinforcement contingency is discontinued but reinforcers are delivered on FT or VT schedules—a sharp drop in response rate to near-zero or zero levels. |
| FT–VT—fixed or variable time schedules | Reinforcers are delivered independently of any behavior at FT or VT intervals. | Vollmer et al. (1998) used FT schedules to reduce problem behaviors (i.e., aggression, self-injurious behavior, disruption, and tantrums) displayed by both children and adults with intellectual disability disorder. Mace and Lalli (1991) used VT schedules to reduce bizarre vocalizations emitted by an adult with moderate intellectual disability disorder. | When combined with EXT, sharp drop in response rate to near-zero or zero levels. When combined with ratio or interval schedules, a reduction in the reinforced class of behaviors. |
| DRA—differential reinforcement of alternative behavior | Reinforcers are contingent on specific topographies of behavior and *not* others. Combines ratio or interval schedules with extinction. | Harding et al. (2004) used DRA schedules to increase adults' correct execution of various martial arts techniques. | Comparatively higher response rates for behaviors that produce reinforcers than for those that do not. |

*(continued)*

**TABLE 4.1.** *(continued)*

| Schedule | Definition | ABA example | Response pattern promoted |
|---|---|---|---|
| DRH–DRL—differential reinforcement of high- or low-rate behavior | Reinforcers are delivered after a specified time interval if response rates are at or above (DRH) or at or below (DRL) a specified rate. | Lane et al. (2007) used DRH schedules to increase a child's class participation (i.e., rates of hand raising and question answering). Wright and Vollmer (2002) used a DRL schedule to reduce rapid eating in an adolescent with intellectual developmental disorder. | DRH schedules promote response rates higher than the specified criterion. DRL schedules promote response rates below the criterion. |
| DRO—differential reinforcement of other behavior | Reinforcers are contingent on the absence of specified behavior(s) during a specified time interval. Also called omission training. | Heard and Watson (1999) used an interval DRO schedule to reduce wandering behavior exhibited by geriatric patients. Kahng, Abt, and Schonbachler (2001) used a momentary DRO schedule to reduce the rate of aggression displayed by a woman with developmental disabilities. | Low or zero rates of the target behavior omitted from reinforcement. Behaviors other than the target behavior increase in rate. |

to reinforcers is not constant. For example, a parent may tell a child that he or she may engage in a leisure activity after the child completes a math homework assignment. Because the child knows how many math problems he or she must complete, the ratio of responses to reinforcers is predictable, and the characteristic FR response pattern may occur.

Cohen, Richardson, Klebez, Febbo, and Tucker (2001) provided undergraduate psychology majors with auditory and visual biofeedback for electromyography readings from their forearms. Investigators instructed participants to alternately tense and relax their forearms. Different groups of students received feedback on whether their electromyography values moved from below a threshold to above the threshold, which were the responses. Investigators provided feedback for these responses according to five different schedules of reinforcement. Two of the schedules were FR schedules: FR 1 and FR 4. The FR 4 schedule generated the highest rates of responding, whereas the FR 1 schedule produced response rates that were approximately half the higher ratio of responses to reinforcers.

### VR Schedules

Like FR schedules, VR schedules or *random-ratio* (RR) schedules deliver reinforcers contingent on the number of responses the organism emits. However, in VR schedules, the interreinforcement response criterion varies for each reinforcer delivery. The *schedule value* is the average ratio of responses to reinforcers over the course of the VR condition. For example, reinforcers delivered after the second response, then after the sixth response, and then after four more responses would be a VR 4 schedule. Examples of human behaviors maintained by VR schedules include sampling restaurants in search of ones that suit one's taste, purchasing lottery tickets, looking for misplaced items, and answering a teacher's questions.

VR schedules generally promote high rates of responding, with short and uniform individual IRTs. However, when the ratio of responses to reinforcers exceeds a threshold, response rates decline as the ratio of responses to reinforcers increases. This value can exceed 200 key pecks per minute in pigeons (Brandauer, 1958). In addition, ratio strain can occur at lower ratios of response to reinforcer values when single interreinforcement intervals become quite large. Finally, the unpredictability of the individual ratio of responses to reinforcers tends to promote short postreinforcement pauses.

DeLuca and Holburn (1992) reinforced revolutions on an exercise bicycle with preferred objects on a VR schedule for three obese children. After calculation of baseline pedal revolutions per minute, the investigators set an initial VR schedule value at 15% above baseline. Investigators implemented two additional increases in VR values after participants demonstrated stability in each VR condition. The progressive arrangement of the VR schedule value, also known as a *progressive VR schedule*, produced an approximate doubling of pedal revolution rates.

## Interval Schedules

Interval schedules of reinforcement define the time that responses become eligible for reinforcement. The *interval value* indicates the minimum time that must elapse before a response produces reinforcement. Unlike ratio schedules, the rate of responding does not affect the rate of reinforcement; response rate and reinforcement rate are independent, in that higher response rates do not produce higher rates of reinforcement in interval schedules. The contingency is between the response periodicity and the delivery of reinforcement. Thus interval schedules generally support lower response rates than ratio schedules (Cohen et al., 2001).

An *adjunctive* procedure, *limited hold*, is needed sometimes for interval schedules to support a consistent response pattern. A limited hold specifies the time that reinforcement is available once the schedule sets it up. Thus a 5-second limited hold means that if a response does not occur within 5 seconds of becoming eligible for reinforcement, the organism forfeits the opportunity for reinforcement. This procedure promotes a consistent pattern of behavior that maximizes obtaining the reinforcement that is available in a period.

### FI Schedules

In an FI schedule of reinforcement, the first response that occurs after the expiration of a constant time produces reinforcement. For example, reinforcement is available every 5 minutes on an FI 5-minute schedule. The predictability of reinforcement availability can promote a pattern of behavior that is sensitive to this periodicity. In the laboratory, especially with nonhuman participants, FI schedules tend to promote an escalation in response rates toward the end of the interval. When expressed in a cumulative record of responses, the pattern has a *scalloped* appearance. A postreinforcement pause that can last more than half the interreinforcement interval occurs after delivery of each reinforcer.

Researchers have speculated whether FI scalloping occurs in humans in natural environments. For example, Critchfield, Haley, Sabo, Colbert, and Macropoulis (2003) analyzed the bill-passing behavior of the U.S. Congress over a 52-year period. Each 2-year Congress comprises two sessions of approximately equal duration. Critchfield et al. graphed bill passing in cumulative records, which showed that bill passing escalated toward the end of each session, in accord with the FI scalloping in laboratory experiments with nonhuman species. However, FI scalloping is a productive response pattern only when there is no external means of discriminating time. When the preparation clearly signals the end of an FI schedule, the most parsimonious response pattern would be to emit a single response at the end of the interval. In the case of Congressional behavior, the contingency would appear to be between the number of bills passed and the production of the reinforcing consequence of reelection or campaign donations, rather than the timing of the completion of any one legislative act. The consensus of other investigators is that FI scalloping in humans is a rare occurrence (Hyten & Madden, 1993; Ninness, Ozenne, & McCuller, 2000).

### VI Schedules

VI schedules or *random-interval* (RI) schedules make responses eligible for reinforcement based on a mean time interval that elapses. For example, a VI 15-second schedule would program reinforcement delivery after the 10th second, then after 20 more seconds, and then after 15 more seconds. Hantula and Crowell (1994) provided a BASIC program for deriving interval values based on the formula by Fleshler and Hoffman (1962), such that the time between reinforcer deliveries is truly random. Because the interreinforcement interval is unpredictable, VI schedules promote consistent response rates with uniform individual IRTs.

Teachers often deliver attention on a VI schedule based on when they can deliver attention, rather than on the number of responses a student makes. Martens, Lochner, and Kelly (1992) provided praise contingent on academic engagement for two 8-year-old students with low baseline rates of academic engagement. The investigator delivered praise alternately on VI 5-minute and VI 2-minute schedules. Both schedules improved academic engagement; however, the VI 2-minute schedule consistently produced higher levels of engagement for both students—a finding consistent with basic research with nonhuman species (Catania & Reynolds, 1968).

## Extinction Schedules

Extinction schedules withhold reinforcement for specified response topographies during certain times. Extinction schedules come in two general forms. First, we can arrange an extinction schedule in which we discontinue reinforcement for responses that we reinforced in the past. Scientists use EXT+ to denote extinction that follows positive reinforcement, and EXT– to denote extinction following negative reinforcement. Second, we can arrange an extinction schedule for responses we have not reinforced explicitly in the past, and we should not reinforce during the process of teaching a new skill. For example, when teaching a child with autism spectrum disorder (ASD) to say the word *apple*, we would not reinforce vocalized sounds unrelated to *a*, *p*, and *l*.

Magee and Ellis (2001) used extinction alone to reduce multiple undesirable behaviors for two children. A functional analysis showed that one child's out-of-seat behavior occurred at high levels when a therapist discontinued instructions contingent on the behavior. Escape extinction (EXT–) consisted of the continuous presentation of instructions every 10 seconds, regardless of occurrences of undesirable behavior. The second child's functional analysis showed that adult attention maintained his object mouthing. Positive reinforcement extinction (EXT+) for this child involved withholding attention following any undesirable responses. Both extinction schedules were effective in reducing out-of-seat behavior and hand mouthing. However, Magee and Ellis found that when they placed these two behaviors on extinction, other topographies of undesirable behaviors emerged—first yelling for one child, and then property destruction for the other. When Magee and Ellis placed these behaviors on extinction, additional topographies of undesirable behaviors began occurring. The sequential emergence of multiple undesirable behaviors demonstrated that the behaviors were members of a response class hierarchy (Lalli, Mace, Wohn, & Livezey, 1995).

Magee and Ellis (2001) illustrated that extinction schedules can have collateral effects, in addition to the reduction of responses subject to extinction. These include the extinction burst (initial increases in responding), extinction-induced aggression (violent acts both related and unrelated to the source of reinforcement), agitated or emotional behavior, resumption of previously reinforced behaviors, behavioral contrast (increased occurrences of undesirable behavior in settings in which individuals do not use extinction), and spontaneous recovery (recurrence of the extinguished target behavior). Lerman, Iwata, and Wallace (1999) examined the prevalence of extinction bursts and extinction-induced aggression for 41 individuals with self-injurious behavior who received treatment using extinction alone or extinction plus additional treatment components. They found that response bursting was evident in 39% of cases, 22% showed increased aggression, and 58% showed neither side effect. However, of the cases treated with extinction alone, 69% showed response bursting and 29% showed increased aggression, compared to only 15% for either side effect when treated with extinction plus another treatment component. These findings suggest the importance of combining extinction with other schedules to avoid unwanted side effects.

## Time Schedules

Time schedules arrange occurrences of reinforcer deliveries contingent on the passage of time and independently of behavior. These reinforcers are *response-independent* and delivered *noncontingently*.[1] In ABA, investigators and clinicians use time schedules (1) to *enrich* an environment and alter the motivation of individuals to engage in undesirable behavior to obtain reinforcement (Horner, 1980); (2) to serve as an experimental control procedure to demonstrate the effects of a contingency between a response and a reinforcer (Thompson & Iwata, 2005); and (3) to reduce undesirable behavior. Our discussion here focuses on this last application of time schedules.

### Fixed- or Variable-Time Schedules

We can deliver reinforcers in time schedules at regular or fixed intervals (FT schedules) or at random or variable intervals (VT schedules). Numer-

---

[1]Researchers introduced the term *noncontingent reinforcement* (NCR) to describe fixed-time (FT) and variable-time (VT) schedules (Vollmer, Iwata, Zarcone, Smith, & Mazaleski, 1993). However, Poling and Normand (1999) questioned the technical accuracy of the term to describe the noncontingent delivery of reinforcement. Because noncontingent delivery of reinforcement does not constitute a reinforcement operation or process (i.e., nothing is reinforced), the term NCR does appear to be a misnomer, and we do not use it in our discussion of the topic.

ous studies have demonstrated that time schedules are effective and efficient for reducing many undesirable behaviors maintained by both positive and negative reinforcement (Vollmer, Marcus, & Ringdahl, 1995; for reviews, see Saini, Miller, & Fisher, 2016; Vollmer & Hackenberg, 2001; Wallace, Iwata, Hanley, Thompson, & Roscoe, 2012). Investigators have used time schedules to reduce the duration and the frequency of exposure to aversive behavioral intervention. For example, Luiselli, Pace, and Dunn (2006) compared behavior-contingent release from therapeutic physical restraint with FT release from restraint to reduce aggressive behavior. The FT release substantially reduced the duration of individual restraints and in some instances the frequency with which the investigators applied restraint.

In an interesting variation of time schedules to reduce undesirable behavior, Marsteller and St. Peter (2014) effectively reduced problem behavior maintained by social contingencies and increased an alternative prosocial behavior, using a differential reinforcement of alternative behavior (DRA) schedule with four children with disabilities. However, after effective DRA treatment, they compared the effects of extinction to FT reinforcement. Extinction after DRA produced a marked resurgence of problem behavior. By contrast, the FT schedule after DRA treatment prevented resurgence despite the discontinuation of the contingency between reinforcement and prosocial alternative behavior.

Time schedules are an attractive treatment alternative for several reasons. First, they often produce rapid suppression of undesirable behavior when the reinforcement maintaining undesirable behavior is time-contingent (Lalli, Casey, & Kates, 1997; Mace & Lalli, 1991). Second, adding time-contingent reinforcement to a context can reduce the motivation to engage in extreme acts, such as undesirable behavior, to obtain reinforcement. This also may increase the probability of prosocial alternative behaviors that require less effort to effect reinforcement (Ecott & Critchfield, 2004). Third, relative to extinction schedules, time schedules often obviate an extinction burst. For example, Vollmer et al. (1998) compared FT deliveries of maintaining reinforcement with withholding that reinforcement (i.e., extinction). A burst was evident during extinction for the three participants in their study. By contrast, the FT schedule produced rapid or immediate suppression of undesirable behavior without response bursting. We note that investigators have reported response bursting when they have faded the rate of reinforcement delivery via time schedules, and it apparently becomes too lean. Vollmer, Ringdahl, Roane, and Marcus (1997) found that undesirable behavior escalated to approximately five times the baseline rate during FT schedule thinning; Mace et al. (2008) reported similar findings.

There are several procedural variations of time schedules to consider in designing interventions. First, the investigator or clinician must select a time-schedule value that is sufficiently dense to suppress undesirable behavior. For example, Ringdahl, Vollmer, Borrero, and Connell (2001) evaluated the effectiveness of initial time-schedule values when they were similar or dissimilar to the rates of baseline reinforcement. They found that FT schedule values that were like baseline rates of reinforcement for undesirable behavior were less effective than those that were dissimilar. This finding held even when the FT schedule values were four to nine times leaner than the baseline reinforcement rates. This counterintuitive finding may be attributed to dissimilar rates being easier to discriminate from baseline. A second procedural question is whether time schedules must be used in conjunction with extinction to be effective. Lalli et al. (1997) compared FT schedules with and without extinction and found that they were comparably effective at reducing undesirable behavior; however, this finding was based on only one participant receiving FT intervention without extinction. Third, most clinical studies using time schedules have evaluated FT rather than VT schedules, but studies comparing the efficacy of FT versus VT schedules have found similar effectiveness (Carr, Kellum, & Chong, 2001; Van Camp, Lerman, Kelley, Contrucci, & Vorndran, 2000). We suggest the initial use of FT schedules and a shift to VT schedules after initial treatment effects are established. The predictability of reinforcement delivery in FI and VI schedules and the characteristic response patterns they promote may logically extend to time schedules.

There is some theoretical interest in which behavioral process or processes are invoked in time schedules to make them effective. The shift from contingent baseline reinforcement to time-contingent reinforcement delivery involves two simultaneous operations. First, the response–reinforcement contingency in baseline is discontinued, constituting a procedural variation of extinction. Second, the motivating operations change by supplying reinforcement on a time schedule. This presumably abolishes the consequence as effective reinforcement for undesirable behavior and abates those same responses. Kahng, Iwata, Thompson, and Hanley (2000) examined response patterns in the time immediately after FT intervention. They reasoned that if FT effects were due to extinction, responding would not resume after FT treatment, because they did not reinstate the response–reinforcement contingency. Alternatively, if FT effects were the result of altered motivating operations, they could expect response rates to resume when reinforcement shifted from being available to unavailable. The findings of Kahng et al. were mixed, with one participant each supporting the extinction and motivating-operations accounts, and a third showed a change in response patterns over time, from supporting the motivating-operations account to the extinction account. Finally, Ecott and Critchfield (2004) suggested that time schedules may be effective because reinforcement delivery may coincide temporally with other behaviors and result in adventitious reinforcement of those responses. In a laboratory demonstration with undergraduate students, the investigators concurrently reinforced two behaviors with points. The investigators reinforced target behavior on a VI 10-second schedule and the alternative behavior on a VI 30-second schedule (see discussion of concurrent schedules of reinforcement below). After responding was stable in this baseline phase, they systematically varied the proportion of reinforcement delivery for the target behavior that was response-contingent from 100 to 66 to 33 to 0%. Results showed that as the proportion of time-contingent reinforcement delivery increased, the response rates for the alternative behavior increased. Ecott and Critchfield suggested that adventitious reinforcement of alternative behavior is one possible account of the behavioral process involved in treatment effects of time schedules.

## Differential-Reinforcement Schedules

Differential schedules of reinforcement specify the dimensions of behavior that are and are not eligible for reinforcement. They also may define the stimuli that must be present when responses produce reinforcement (i.e., an $S^D$), and the stimuli that must be present when responses do not produce reinforcement (i.e., an $S^\Delta$), thus defining the discriminated operant. As such, differential-reinforcement schedules implicitly involve two types of operations: (1) positive or negative reinforcement and (2) extinction. The dimensions of behavior subject to reinforcement and extinction

include specific forms or topographies of responses, response rates and the periodicity of responding, and the time spent engaging in specific behaviors.

In ABA practice, the behavior analyst may change the criteria for reinforcement systematically to promote gradual and progressive changes in responding toward a target criterion. When this involves the discriminative stimuli correlated with reinforcement, the operation is known as *fading*. For example, Flood and Wilder (2004) used differential reinforcement and fading to increase the time an 11-year-old boy with separation anxiety disorder spent away from his mother without distress behavior, such as crying, whining, or other emotional behavior. The investigators provided access to preferred items contingent on the boy's meeting his goals for time spent away from his mother without distress behavior. The investigators faded the time goals from 3 minutes to 90 minutes over 27 treatment sessions. The investigators used a similar fading and differential-reinforcement procedure to increase the distance the boy's mother was from the therapy room.

When changes in specific response topographies or in response rates are subject to changing criteria for reinforcement, the operation is known as *shaping*. Gillis, Hammond Natof, Lockshin, and Romanczyk (2009) used differential reinforcement and gradual exposure with 18 children with ASD who showed extreme fear of medical procedures to increase cooperation with physical examinations. The school nurse used a 17-step procedure to expose the children gradually to the examination room and to the medical instruments, such as a stethoscope, a sphygmomanometer, a thermometer, and an otoscope. The nurse delivered various positive reinforcers for completion of each step in which a child showed minimal or no fear responses. Eighty-three percent of the children completed the 17 steps showing minimal or no fear responses. Tiger and Hanley discuss differential-reinforcement procedures and their application more fully in Chapter 14 of this book.

## COMBINED SCHEDULES OF REINFORCEMENT

Combined schedules of reinforcement comprise two or more basic schedules. Each basic schedule is a *schedule component*. Investigators may arrange these components to alternate, to be available at the same time, to occur in a sequence, or in some combination of these arrangements. Combined schedules are particularly relevant to ABA, because they better represent the circumstances humans encounter in everyday life. Our coverage of combined schedules includes definitions, examples, and a discussion of the relation between certain combined schedules and contemporary developments in ABA, such as behavioral contrast, matching theory, and behavioral momentum. Table 4.2 summarizes the combined schedules discussed here, schedule definitions, response patterns promoted by each schedule, and applications in ABA work.

## Multiple and Mixed Schedules

In multiple and mixed schedules, two or more schedule components alternate in a random, counterbalanced, or natural-temporal sequence. The difference between multiple and mixed schedules is that schedule components are correlated with distinct stimuli in multiple schedules but not in mixed schedules. As an individual experiences the multiple schedules, the correlated stimuli acquire stimulus control over responding and become discriminative stimuli. To the extent that the schedule components differ, differential responding in the schedule components usually occurs more rapidly and is more pronounced in multiple schedules than in mixed schedules.

Humans encounter multiple schedules regularly. Students in school who attend a sequence of classes throughout the day experience a multiple schedule. Each class is a schedule component and is correlated with distinct stimuli, such as different teachers, textbooks, classrooms, and seating arrangements. The teachers in each class undoubtedly reinforce students' participation in classroom activities on different schedules; some use ratio schedules, others use interval schedules, and still others use differential reinforcement of high-rate behavior (DRH) schedules. Humans also encounter mixed schedules frequently. The first time we read a novel, watch a film, or drive through unfamiliar countryside, our points of interest (i.e., the availability of reinforcement) for attention to the activity vary from one time to another. However, there is no indication that the reinforcing properties of the novel, film, or drive are about to shift. Because we usually do not repeat these activities, any stimuli correlated with changes in reinforcement do not develop stimulus control (i.e., the mixed schedule does not become a multiple schedule).

Mace, Pratt, Prager, and Pritchard (2011) used a mixed schedule to evaluate the effectiveness of al-ternative methods of saying no to a child's request for tangible reinforcement. The child approached an adult using a computer and requested to play a computer game. During a functional analysis, denied access to the computer produced high rates of aggressive and disruptive behavior. During treatment, a single therapist in a constant setting denied computer access, but alternately offered another reinforcing activity or delayed access to reinforcement contingent on completing a non-preferred math worksheet. Use of a single therapist in a constant setting did not correlate distinct stimuli with the two alternative methods of denying computer access, making the arrangement a mixed schedule.

We (Pritchard, Hoerger, Mace, Penney, & Harris, 2014) used a multiple schedule to evaluate the effects of different rates of reinforcement on treatment relapse. A functional analysis showed that attention maintained an adolescent's problem behavior. Treatment consisted of withholding attention for problem behavior and providing attention for communication responses or providing attention on a VI VT schedule. One therapist provided VI VT attention at a rate four times greater than that of a second therapist. Both rates of reinforcement reduced problem behavior, but when the two therapists discontinued treatment and provided reinforcement for problem behavior at equal rates, the magnitude of treatment relapse was much higher for the therapist who used the higher rates of VI VT reinforcement during treatment.

Tiger and Hanley (2005) used multiple and mixed schedules to study variables that promoted discriminative control of social-approach responses in preschool children. Two children sat facing the experimenter at tables containing academic materials. The experimenter looked down except when he or she delivered 5 seconds of attention contingent on social-approach responses. The experimenter alternated presentation of three schedule components in a randomized order to each child. In the FR 1 component, the experimenter provided reinforcement in the form of attention for each social-approach response. In the extinction$_1$ component, the experimenter provided reinforcement for one child's social approaches but not for the other child's. In the extinction$_2$ component, the experimenter did not provide reinforcement for either child's social approaches. In the multiple schedule, denoted MULT FR 1 extinction$_1$ extinction$_2$, the experimenter wore a different-colored floral lei during each component. The experimenter did not wear the leis during the mixed

**TABLE 4.2. Combined Schedules of Reinforcement, ABA Example, and the Response Patterns Promoted**

| Schedule | Definition | ABA example | Response pattern promoted |
|---|---|---|---|
| Multiple/mixed schedules | Alternation of two or more schedules of reinforcement. In a multiple schedule, each schedule is correlated with a distinct stimulus (e.g., a VR schedule in context A alternates with a DRL schedule in context B). In a mixed schedule, no distinct stimuli are correlated with each schedule (e.g., a VR schedule and DRL schedule alternate in the same context). | Tiger and Hanley (2005) used MULT and MIX FR 1 $EXT_1$ $EXT_2$ schedules to produce differential rates of social approach responses emitted by preschoolers. | Schedule-specific patterns of behavior are observed in each component. Schedule-specific response patterns are more pronounced in multiple than in mixed schedules. |
| Concurrent/ conjoint schedules | Two or more schedules of reinforcement are available at the same time. In a concurrent schedule, each schedule is correlated with a distinct stimulus (e.g., a choice between VR reinforcement from source A and VI reinforcement from source B in the same context). In a conjoint schedule, no distinct stimuli are correlated with each schedule (e.g., behavior A produces VR reinforcement and behavior B produces DRH reinforcement in the same context). | Conger and Killeen (1974) employed CONC VI VI schedules to demonstrate college students' allocation of attending responses. | Concurrent interval schedules promote allocation of responding to each schedule in proportion to relative rates of reinforcement obtained on each schedule. Concurrent ratio schedules promote exclusive responding on the relatively denser schedule of reinforcement. |
| Chained/tandem schedules | Two or more schedules of reinforcement are available. Completion of schedule A produces schedule B, and completion of schedule B produces reinforcement. In a chained schedule, each schedule component is correlated with a distinct stimulus. In a tandem schedule, no distinct stimuli are correlated with each schedule component. | Hoerger and Mace (2006) used concurrent-chain schedules to measure impulsive versus self-controlled choices made by male children with and without symptoms of ADHD. | Schedule-specific patterns of behavior are observed in each component. Schedule-specific response patterns are more pronounced in chained than in tandem schedules. |
| Conjunctive schedule | Two or more schedules of reinforcement are arranged. All schedule requirements must be completed to receive reinforcement. | Vollmer et al. (1997) used a conjunctive FT DRO schedule to reduce aggression in an adolescent with intellectual developmental disorder. | Schedule-specific patterns of behavior are observed in each component. |
| Alternative schedule | Two or more schedules of reinforcement are available concurrently. The first schedule completed produces reinforcement. | Bowman et al. (1997) utilized an ALT FR 1 FR 1 EXT schedule to evaluate the reinforcer preferences of children with intellectual developmental disorder. | Responding reflects a preference for one schedule component. |

schedule (MIX FR 1 extinction$_1$ extinction$_2$). The students first experienced the mixed schedule, and their social-approach responses were undifferentiated across the three components, indicating that the children were unaware of when the experimenter would and would not provide reinforcement for approach responses. In the subsequent multiple schedule, approach responses became somewhat differentiated for one child, showing more approaches during the FR 1 component than the extinction components. However, approaches remained undifferentiated for the second child. To enhance stimulus control, the experimenter then described the rules of reinforcement and extinction for each schedule component and how each was correlated with a different-colored lei, resulting in a multiple schedule with rules. This condition produced the greatest differential responding, which continued after a return to the mixed schedule.

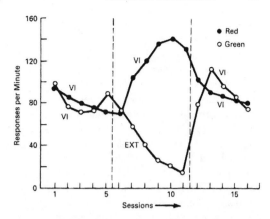

**FIGURE 4.2.** Reynold's (1961) illustration of behavioral contrast in the multiple-schedule arrangement: MULT VI 3-minute VI 3-min schedules followed by MULT VI 3-minute EXT schedules resulted in relative increases in response rates in the unchanged VI 3-minute component.

## Behavioral Contrast

Behavioral contrast is a phenomenon that results from an interaction among schedule components in a multiple schedule; that is, events in one schedule component affect responding in the other components. Reynolds (1961) first described this interaction in an experiment with pigeons exposed to two different multiple schedules. In the first schedule, key pecking was reinforced on a VI 3-minute schedule when the response keys were alternately illuminated red and green, resulting in a multiple VI 3-minute VI 3-minute schedule. After stable responding in this schedule, the experimenter introduced the second multiple schedule. In this schedule, the experimenter changed the green component from VI 3 minutes to extinction, resulting in a multiple VI 3-minute extinction schedule. Figure 4.2 shows the results of Reynolds's experiment. Behavioral contrast is evident in the second multiple schedule. Whereas responding declined as expected during the extinction component, responding in the unchanged VI 3-minute component increased substantially. Note that the increased response rate evident in the unchanged component did not produce an increased rate of reinforcement, because response rate and reinforcement rate are largely independent in interval schedules. Behavioral contrast in interval schedules represents an irrational expenditure of responses and calories. This would not be the case in multiple ratio schedules, in which increased responding in the unchanged component would

compensate for the loss of reinforcement in the extinction component. There are numerous accounts for behavioral contrast (see Catania, 2013, p. 221).

There is growing evidence that humans show behavioral contrast. For example, Hantula and Crowell (1994) presented undergraduate students with a computerized investment task in which they managed money for an investment group with the goal of maximizing financial returns. The experimenters gave the students numerous opportunities to invest between $100 and $10,000 in $100 increments in two different markets. Investments either gained or lost money. Phases 1 and 3 were equal multiple VI VI schedules. Phase 2 was a multiple VI extinction schedule, and Phase 4 was a multiple extinction VI schedule. During the equal VI VI schedules, investments were comparable in the two markets. However, when investments in one market no longer made money (i.e., extinction), behavioral contrast occurred in the market with an unchanged rate of reinforcement.

Tarbox and Parrot Hayes (2005) exposed undergraduate college students to multiple equal VI VI, multiple VI extinction, multiple VI VI, and multiple VI extinction schedules. They observed behavioral contrast consistently only when they provided participants with rules describing the contingencies in the extinction component only. They did not observe contrast when they did not give participants rules or when they gave participants rules for all components. The findings are counterintuitive, but suggest that verbal behavior interacts with direct contingencies in ways that are not well understood yet.

Behavioral contrast can be relevant in clinical ABA work (see Koegel, Egel & Williams, 1980, for an illustration). Interventions typically involve the discontinuation of reinforcement for undesirable behavior. When a caregiver provides reinforcement for the undesirable behavior at a high rate and then places the behavior on extinction in one context (e.g., at school), contrast effects may emerge in other contexts in which the caregiver has not implemented extinction (e.g., home). This may be more likely if the reinforcement of prosocial alternative behavior does not compensate fully for the reduction in reinforcement from the extinction schedule. This possibility should guide the selection of reinforcement schedules for the prosocial behavior and the provision of advice to parents, for example, about the possible side effects of intervention.

## Concurrent and Conjoint Schedules

Concurrent and conjoint schedules arrange for the simultaneous availability of two or more schedule components, such that the individual is free to alternate among the components. This arrangement permits the assessment of the relative preference for the schedule components and the study of choice. As with multiple and mixed schedules, the difference between concurrent and conjoint schedules is that components in concurrent schedules correlate with distinct stimuli, but components in conjoint schedules do not. Concurrent schedules are characteristic of human environments where numerous alternatives are available and generally are correlated with distinct stimuli. For example, a woman commuting to work with a friend on a subway will have many different concurrently available alternatives. She can converse with her friend, read a newspaper, do a crossword puzzle, listen to music, people watch, plan her work day, and so on. Each of these activities is correlated with distinct stimuli, and each provides reinforcement according to some schedule. Because concurrent schedules of reinforcement characterize human environments, this is our emphasis in this chapter.

Experimenters can arrange concurrent schedules for any combination of interval, ratio, or differential schedules of reinforcement (Davison & McCarthy, 1988). However, most studies with concurrent schedules have used concurrent VI VI schedules. This is because concurrent-ratio schedules ordinarily produce exclusive responding on the richer of the two schedules (Herrnstein & Loveland, 1975). The arrangement of asymmetrical schedules, such as concurrent VI FR, can produce a preference for the qualitative features of one schedule that is independent of the amount of reinforcement from the schedule (Baum, 1974). Experiments arranging concurrent VI VI schedules generally include an adjunctive procedure known as a *change-over delay*, which imposes a brief interval during which responses cannot be reinforced immediately after the organism switches from one schedule to another. The change-over delay reduces the likelihood that schedule switching will be reinforced accidentally, relative to the probability of accidental reinforcement when the first response after the schedule switch is eligible for reinforcement.

### Matching Theory

Concurrent schedules promote a pattern of response allocation that is very orderly. Herrnstein (1961, 1970) formulated the *matching law*, which quantitatively describes the functional relation between relative response rates for concurrent alternatives and relative obtained rates of reinforcement. The matching law states that relative response rate will match or be equal to relative reinforcement rate. In its simplest form, the matching law is expressed as $B1/B1 + B2 = r1/r1 + r2$, where $B1$ and $B2$ are response rates for two behaviors, and $r1$ and $r2$ are the obtained reinforcement rates for the two behaviors. We can reduce this equation to $B1/B2 = r1/r2$, and we can fit a line to logarithmic transformations of the obtained data in the form of $\log (B1/B2) = a \log (r1/r2) + \log k$, where $a$ is the slope of the line and $\log k$ is its intercept at the y-axis (see Baum, 1974, and McDowell, 1989, for full descriptions of mathematical transformations of the simplified form of the matching law). When there is perfect matching, $a = 1.0$ and $\log k = 0$. Values of $a > 1.0$ show *overmatching*, and values of $a < 1.0$ show *undermatching*, reflecting the individual's sensitivity to relative reinforcement rate. Values of $\log k > 0$ reflect a bias for $B1$, and values of $\log k < 0$ show a bias for $B2$ due to variables other than relative reinforcement rate (see below).

Conger and Killeen (1974) provided one of the first demonstrations of the matching law involving human social behavior. Participants engaged in conversation with two experimenters, who provided comments of approval contingent on participants' statements. The experimenters provided comments on different sets of concurrent VI VI schedules. The results of the study showed that the relative amount of time participants directed verbal statements to the two experimenters closely matched the relative rates of experimenter attention. Numerous studies have established the generality of the matching law to human behavior in the laboratory (Pierce & Epling, 1984) and to many socially relevant human behaviors, from academic engagement (Martens et al., 1992) to the performance of basketball players (Vollmer & Bourret, 2000). Although these findings are generally robust, results of some studies show human performance departing from matching (Pierce & Epling, 1984). For example, Mace, Neef, Shade, and Mauro (1994) needed to use several adjunctive procedures, a 15-second limited hold, and a change-over delay for adolescents to allocate their time to arithmetic problems in accordance with matching.

Choices are *symmetrical* when they differ only by relative rate of reinforcement. However, human choices in natural environments are most often *asymmetrical*. Response alternatives can differ along several parameters of reinforcement, including reinforcement quality, reinforcement delay, reinforcement amount, reinforcement schedule features, and control of reinforcement. The response requirements or effort to obtain reinforcement can also differ. Baum (1974) proposed a matching equation that accommodated independent variables other than relative reinforcement rate. The *generalized matching law* expresses that $B1/B2 = V1/V2$, where $V$ refers to the *value* of the given alternative as defined by the sum of the relative reinforcement parameters and response effort.

Mace and Roberts (1993) illustrated the applied relevance of the generalized matching law. They provided a conceptual framework to guide the functional assessment of undesirable behaviors and the selection of behavioral treatments. They recommended using a descriptive analysis of undesirable behavior under natural conditions to identify the quality of the reinforcing consequence, the magnitude of delay to reinforcement, the amount of reinforcement provided, and the response requirement to produce reinforcement, and to estimate the operative schedule of reinforcement. The behavior analyst can use information from the descriptive analysis to design an intervention that should effectively compete with the parameters of reinforcement and response effort that maintain undesirable behavior. Mace and Roberts suggested

that this tool affords a more refined approach to develop interventions based on variables that affect choice.

## Chained and Tandem Schedules

Chained and tandem schedules organize sequences of behavior that produce reinforcement. Both schedules comprise two or more components arranged in a sequence. In a two-component example, completion of the schedule requirements for the *initial link* produces the onset of the second component or *terminal link*. Completion of the terminal-link schedule requirements produces delivery of a reinforcer. Schedule components in chained schedules correlate with distinct stimuli, whereas components in tandem schedules do not. Human behavior contacts chained and tandem schedules regularly. For example, numerous sequences of behavior required to experience a vacation constitute a chained schedule, such as planning the vacation (initial link), booking transportation (interim link), and transportation to the desired location (terminal link). Completion of these schedule components produces access to the reinforcing events available during the vacation.

As is true of the basic schedules of reinforcement discussed earlier, chained and tandem schedules rarely operate in isolation. The more common characteristic of natural human environments is for initial links to consist of a concurrent schedule; that is, humans typically have a choice of sequential activities and terminal reinforcers. This arrangement is known as a *concurrent-chain schedule*. In laboratory experiments, the initial-link schedule requirements are usually identical (e.g., concurrent VI 20-seconds VI 20-seconds). However, terminal-link reinforcers and sometimes schedule requirements differ. Completion of the initial-link alternative produces the discriminative stimulus for the terminal link associated with that alternative. For example, completion of initial link A produces presentation of the discriminative stimulus for terminal link A, and completion of this schedule requirement produces reinforcer A. A parallel sequence meets the schedule requirements for initial link B.

### Self-Control

One contemporary development in ABA that uses concurrent-chain schedules is the behavioral model of self-control. Rachlin and Green (1972) formally developed the model in an experiment with pigeons. Figure 4.3 diagrams the concurrent-chain procedure they used. The initial link was a concurrent FR 25 FR 25 schedule with both response keys illuminated white. Completion of the right FR 25 schedule (top sequence) darkened the response keys and house light for *T* seconds. After the blackout, they illuminated the right response key green and the left response key red. The terminal link was a concurrent CRF CRF schedule in which a single key peck on green produced a 4-second blackout followed by 4-second access to food, and a single key peck on red produced immediate access to 2-second access to food followed by a 6-second blackout. Thus completion of the right FR 25 initial link produced later exposure to a choice between small immediate reinforcement and large delayed reinforcement. By contrast, completion of the left initial-link FR 25 schedule produced a similar blackout for *T* seconds, followed by the illumination of the green-key alternative only with the large-delayed-reinforcement contingency. When the time between completion of the initial link and onset of the terminal link was short (e.g., 0.5 second), the pigeons reliably chose the red-key alternative. Rachlin and Green described this choice as *impulsive*, because pigeons forfeited an additional 2-second access to food available for pecking the green key. Thus the delay to reinforcement discounted the value of the large

delayed reinforcement. When the experimenters varied the value of *T*, pigeons showed a shift in their preference on the initial link. In general, as the value of *T* increased, so did the probability of choosing the left initial-link FR 25 schedule that later produced no choice and the large-delayed-reinforcement contingency only. Rachlin and Green called choosing the left initial-link key a *commitment response*—one that avoided the temptation of small immediate reinforcement and exposed the pigeon to the large-delayed-reinforcement contingency only. *Self-control* is said to occur when an individual (1) chooses the large delayed reinforcement over the small immediate reinforcement when exposed to both, or (2) makes the commitment response in the initial link.

Numerous applied studies have used concurrent-chain schedules to study impulsivity and self-control. The behavior of children with attention-deficit/hyperactivity disorder (ADHD) is particularly relevant to this procedure, because a defining characteristic of this disorder is impulsivity, and a primary clinical goal is the development of self-control. For example, numerous studies have found that children with ADHD are more likely than their typically developing peers to choose small immediate reinforcement over large delayed reinforcement (e.g., Hoerger & Mace, 2006; Neef, Marckel, et al., 2005; Schweitzer & Sulzer-Azaroff, 1988). Other studies have shown that impulsive behavior is sensitive to variables other than delayed reinforcement, such as response effort (Hoerger & Mace, 2006). Finally, investigators have used this paradigm to guide the development of interventions to promote self-control, such as delay fading and commitment training (Binder, Dixon, & Ghezzi, 2000; DuPaul & Ervin, 1996), and to evaluate response to stimulant medication (Neef, Bicard, Endo, Coury, & Aman, 2005). Thus the concurrent-chain schedule has provided a conceptual model for understanding impulsivity and self-control; a procedure for objectively assessing an individual's sensitivity to delayed reinforcement and other variables; and a model for identifying specific interventions to promote self-control and evaluating pharmacological interventions.

### Behavioral-Momentum Theory

*Behavioral momentum* is a metaphor used by Nevin et al. (1983) to describe the tendency for baseline response rates to persist after some response disruptor (see the earlier discussion of resistance to change). As in Newton's second law of motion, behavioral momentum is the product of behavior-

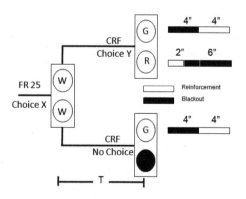

**FIGURE 4.3.** Rachlin and Green's (1972) concurrent-chain schedule illustrates a behavioral model of self-control. The initial link (CONC FR 25 FR 25) presented a choice between access to the terminal link schedules. Completion of the top (right) link produced a *T*-second delay followed by CONC CRF CRF schedules that presented a choice between small immediate reinforcement and large delayed reinforcement. Completion of the bottom (left) link produced a *T*-second delay followed by CONC CRF EXT schedules and the option only for large delayed reinforcement.

al mass and behavioral velocity, where *behavioral velocity* is baseline response rate and *behavioral mass* is the resistance of baseline response rate to change after application of varying amounts of some response disruptor. When we graph response rates across varying amounts of the response disruptor, such as sessions of extinction or amounts of presession food, the height of the curve or function on the *y*-axis is behavioral velocity, and the slope of the function across the *x*-axis is resistance to change; the total area under the curve represents a response's behavioral momentum.

Investigators have used various schedules of reinforcement to study behavioral momentum, including multiple schedules (Nevin et al., 1983), multiple concurrent schedules (Nevin, Tota, Torquato, & Shull, 1990), and concurrent-chain schedules (Grace & Nevin, 1997). Numerous studies have shown that resistance to change is a function of the reinforcement conditions for these schedules. For example, Nevin (1974) and Nevin et al. (1983) used a two-component multiple schedule to demonstrate that resistance to change is a positive function of baseline rate of reinforcement. Different pairs of MULT VI VI schedules arranged a higher rate of reinforcement in one component than in the other. During conditions of extinction, satiation, and dark-key food, key pecking in pigeons was more persistent in the component with the higher baseline reinforcement rate. In a subsequent series of experiments, Nevin et al. (1990) tested the competing hypotheses that resistance to change is a function of baseline response–reinforcer relations versus baseline stimulus–reinforcer relations. In their Experiment 2, baseline consisted of a three-component multiple concurrent schedule (MULT). In each component of the MULT, two concurrent schedules operated, where the left key was the first concurrent schedule and the right key the second: concurrent VI 45/hour VI 15/hour (green), concurrent extinction VI 15/hour (red), and concurrent extinction VI 60/hour (white). In this arrangement, the response–reinforcer contingencies were equal in the green- and red-key components (15/hour each) and less than in the white-key component (60/hour). By contrast, the stimulus–reinforcer contingencies (i.e., the total reinforcers delivered in the presence of each color) were equal in the green- and white-key components (60/hour each) and less than in the red-key component (15/hour). Tests of the resistance of right-key pecking to extinction and satiation showed that resistance to change was a positive function of the total number of reinforcers delivered in each component (color-reinforcer

contingency), rather than the number of reinforcers delivered on the right key (peck-reinforcer contingency). Several researchers have replicated Nevin et al.'s general findings with humans (e.g., Cohen et al., 2001; Dube & McIlvane, 2001; Mace et al., 1990; Pritchard et al., 2014).

Ahearn, Clark, Gardenier, Chung, and Dube (2003) illustrated the relevance of the Nevin et al. (1990) findings to clinically important human behavior. A functional analysis of the stereotypical behavior of three children with ASD suggested that automatic reinforcement maintained stereotypy. Next, investigators identified preferred objects via a preference assessment. They compared levels of stereotypical behavior in a test sequence of conditions and a control sequence. The test sequence consisted of baseline (no play materials available) → VT delivery of a preferred item → test (continuous access to a second preferred item) → baseline. The control sequence consisted of baseline → baseline → test → baseline. Ahern et al. found that although both the VT and test conditions reduced stereotypical behavior relative to baseline, due to the availability of alternative reinforcement, levels of stereotypy were higher in the test condition that followed VT reinforcer deliveries than in the test condition that followed baseline with no toys available. Mace (2000) and Ahern et al. pointed out that although interventions based on DRA and FT or VT schedules reliably reduce occurrences of undesirable behavior, these same interventions can have persistence-strengthening effects on undesirable behavior.

Grace and Nevin (2000) proposed a unifying theory of choice and behavioral momentum in which the variables functionally related to preference or choice were the same as those related to resistance to change. Grace and Nevin (1997) conducted one study forming the basis of this theory. Grace and Nevin (1997) randomly alternated a concurrent-chain procedure and a multiple-schedule procedure in a single experimental session. Three response keys were mounted on a wall above a food magazine. In the concurrent-chain procedure, the side keys illuminated white in the initial link consisting of equal concurrent VI 20-second VI 20-second schedules. Initial-link reinforcement consisted of terminal-link entry and darkening of the side keys, and illumination of the center key (either green or red, depending on whether terminal-link entry was contingent on a left or a right initial-link key peck). The terminal-key colors correlated with a higher- or lower-rate VI schedule. Investigators presented 36 cycles of the concurrent-chain arrangement in each session. Thus the concurrent-chain procedure assessed preference for the terminal link as a function of choice in the initial link. The multiple-schedule procedure in the experimental session involved the usual alternation of green and red keys correlated with the same VI schedules used in the concurrent-chain procedure. After this baseline arrangement, investigators tested resistance to change by dark-key food deliveries between components in the multiple schedule. Grace and Nevin found that relative rate of reinforcement comparably predicted preference in the concurrent-chain schedule and resistance to change in the multiple schedule.

Mace, Mauro, Boyajian, and Eckert (1997) demonstrated the applied significance of Grace and Nevin's work. They modified the high-*p* procedure, a behavioral-momentum-inspired procedure, to increase its effectiveness. Knowing that reinforcer quality affects choice, Mace et al. reasoned that supplying a higher-quality reinforcer (food) contingent on compliance to high-*p* instructions would increase the resistance of compliance to change when they presented a low-*p* instruction. The high-*p* procedure with food increased compliance to low-*p* instructions that were unresponsive to the high-*p* procedure without food.

## Conjunctive and Alternative Schedules

Both conjunctive and alternative schedules comprise two or more schedule components. In conjunctive schedules, the subject must satisfy schedule requirements for *all* components to produce a reinforcer delivery. Unlike chained schedules, the order of schedule completion is irrelevant in conjunctive schedules. By contrast, alternative-schedule components are available concurrently. Reinforcement is contingent on completion of *either* component, whichever occurs first.

Vollmer et al. (1997) evaluated the effectiveness of FT schedules to reduce the severe aggressive behavior of a 13-year-old girl with severe intellectual developmental disorder for whom tangible reinforcement maintained aggression. After a functional-analytic baseline, investigators delivered access to a preferred magazine continuously, resulting in zero occurrences of aggression. Aggression reemerged when the investigators attempted to implement an FT schedule to thin the reinforcement schedule. A within-session analysis of the temporal relation between FT reinforcer deliveries and occurrences of aggression showed that scheduled reinforcer deliveries often coincided (within 10 seconds) with aggressive acts. This suggested

that the FT schedule could have adventitiously reinforced aggressive behavior. To avoid this possibility, Vollmer et al. introduced a conjunctive FT DRO 10-second schedule. The FT schedule set up access to the preferred magazine; however, investigators delivered the magazine only if the participant had not engaged in aggression during the last 10 seconds of the FT interval. That is, the participant had to satisfy both the FT and DRO schedule requirements to gain access to the magazine. After an initial response burst, the conjunctive schedule reduced aggression to low levels, and the investigators then thinned the FT schedule to a conjunctive FT 5-minute DRO 10-second schedule.

Tiger, Hanley, and Hernandez (2006) used an alternative schedule of reinforcement in the context of a concurrent-chain schedule. In a concurrent-chain schedule, two response alternatives (A and B) are available concurrently in the initial link. The participant can choose one alternative. Completion of the schedule requirements for initial link A leads to terminal link A, and completion of the schedule requirements for terminal link A produces a reinforcer. The same is true for initial and terminal link B. In general, the choice to complete initial link A versus B reflects a preference for the reinforcer associated with the respective terminal link. Tiger et al. evaluated preschool children's preference for *choice* as a reinforcer independent of food reinforcers. The initial link presented three different-colored worksheets, each with an identical academic task. Worksheet choice in the initial link was followed by a terminal-link worksheet. Correct responses produced the consequences associated with each colored worksheet: (1) a choice of one of five identical food reinforcers (choice), (2) a single food reinforcer identical to the choice option (no choice), and (3) no material reinforcer. Five of the six children showed a preference for the choice alternative in the initial link, although this preference did not persist for two of the five children. Although the study used a concurrent-chain procedure, it also represented an alternative schedule, because completion of all schedule requirements for each alternative led to the reinforcers associated with each alternative.

## SUMMARY AND CONCLUSION

We have reviewed basic and combined schedules of reinforcement, and have provided definitions for each schedule and illustrations of the applications of the schedules in the ABA research literature. Schedules of reinforcement promote specific patterns of responding, but do so only in a broader context of available concurrent discriminated operants. This broader context includes the temporary motivational conditions for each discriminated operant and its particular history of reinforcement or behavioral mass. We have provided an overview of some contemporary developments in ABA, such as behavioral contrast, matching theory, self-control, and behavioral-momentum theory, and have illustrated that these topics are related directly to specific schedules of reinforcement. Deliberate use of schedules of reinforcement offers applied behavior analysts a powerful tool to understand the conditions that maintain behavior and to design highly effective interventions.

# REFERENCES

Ahearn, W. H., Clark, K. M., Gardenier, N. C., Chung, B. I., & Dube, W. V. (2003). Persistence of stereotypic behavior: Examining the effects of external reinforcers. *Journal of Applied Behavior Analysis, 36,* 439–448.

Baum, W. M. (1974). On two types of deviation from the matching law: Bias and undermatching. *Journal of the Experimental Analysis of Behavior, 22,* 231–242.

Binder, L. M., Dixon, M. R., & Ghezzi, P. M. (2000). A procedure to teach self-control to children with attention deficit hyperactivity disorder. *Journal of Applied Behavior Analysis, 33,* 233–237.

Bowman, L. G., Piazza, C. C., Fisher, W. W., Hagopian, L. P., & Kogan, J. S. (1997). Assessment of preference for varied versus constant reinforcement. *Journal of Applied Behavior Analysis, 30,* 451–458.

Brandauer, C. (1958). *The effects of uniform probabilities of reinforcement on the response rate of the pigeon.* Unpublished doctoral dissertation, Columbia University.

Carr, J. E., Kellum, K. K., & Chong, I. M. (2001). The reductive effects of noncontingent reinforcement: Fixed-time versus variable-time schedules. *Journal of Applied Behavior Analysis, 34,* 505–509.

Catania, A. C. (2013). *Learning* (5th ed.). Cornwall-on-Hudson, NY: Sloan.

Catania, A. C., & Reynolds, G. S. (1968). A quantitative analysis of the responding maintained by interval schedules of reinforcement. *Journal of the Experimental Analysis of Behavior, 11,* 327–383.

Cohen, S. L., Richardson, J., Klebez, J., Febbo, S., & Tucker, D. (2001). EMG biofeedback: The effects of CRF, FR, VR, FI, and VI schedules of reinforcement on the acquisition and extinction of increases in forearm muscle tension. *Applied Psychophysiology and Biofeedback, 26,* 179–194.

Conger, R., & Killeen, P. (1974). Use of concurrent operants in small group research: A demonstration. *Pacific Sociological Review, 17,* 399–416.

Critchfield, T. S., Haley, R., Sabo, B., Colbert, J., & Macropoulis, G. (2003). A half century of scalloping in the work habits of the United States Congress. *Journal of Applied Behavior Analysis, 36,* 465–486.

Davison, M., & McCarthy, D. (1988). *The matching law: A review.* Hillsdale, NJ: Erlbaum.

DeLuca, R. B., & Holburn, S. W. (1992). Effects of a variable-ratio reinforcement schedule with changing criteria on exercise in obese and nonobese boys. *Journal of Applied Behavior Analysis, 25,* 671–679.

Dube, W. V., & McIlvane, W. J. (2001). Behavioral momentum in computer presented discriminations in individuals with severe mental retardation. *Journal of the Experimental Analysis of Behavior, 75,* 15–23.

DuPaul, G. J., & Ervin, R. A. (1996). Functional assessment of behaviors related to attention-deficit/hyperactivity disorder: Linking assessment to intervention design. *Behavior Therapy, 27,* 601–622.

Ecott, C. L., & Critchfield, T. S. (2004). Noncontingent reinforcement, alternative reinforcement, and the matching law: A laboratory demonstration. *Journal of Applied Behavior Analysis, 37,* 249–265.

Felton, M., & Lyon, D. O. (1966). The post-reinforcement pause. *Journal of the Experimental Analysis of Behavior, 9,* 131–134.

Ferster, C. B., & Skinner, B. F. (1957). *Schedules of reinforcement.* New York: Appleton-Century-Crofts.

Fisher, W. W., & Mazur, J. E. (1997). Basic and applied research on choice responding. *Journal of Applied Behavior Analysis, 30,* 387–410.

Fleshler, M., & Hoffman, H. S. (1962). A progression for generating variable-interval schedules. *Journal of the Experimental Analysis of Behavior, 5,* 529–530.

Flood, W. A., & Wilder, D. A. (2004). The use of differential reinforcement and fading to increase time away from a caregiver in a child with separation anxiety disorder. *Education and Treatment of Children, 27,* 1–8.

Gillis, J. M., Hammond Natof, T., Lockshin, S. B., & Romanczyk, R. G. (2009). Fear of routine physical exams in children with autism spectrum disorders. *Focus on Autism and Other Developmental Disabilities, 24,* 156–168.

Grace, R. C., & Nevin, J. A. (1997). On the relation between preference and resistance to change. *Journal of the Experimental Analysis of Behavior, 67,* 43–65.

Grace, R. C., & Nevin, J. A. (2000). Comparing preference and resistance to change in constant- and variable-duration schedule components. *Journal of the Experimental Analysis of Behavior, 74,* 165–188.

Hantula, D. A., & Crowell, C. R. (1994). Matching and behavioral contrast in a two-option repeated investment simulation. *Journal of Applied Behavior Analysis, 27,* 607–617.

Harding, J. W., Wacker, D. P., Berg, W. K., Rick, G., & Lee, J. F. (2004). Promoting response variability and stimulus generalization in martial arts training. *Journal of Applied Behavior Analysis, 37,* 185–196.

Heard, K., & Watson, T. S. (1999). Reducing wandering by persons with dementia using differential reinforcement. *Journal of Applied Behavior Analysis, 32,* 381–384.

Herrnstein, R. J. (1961). Relative and absolute strength of a response as a function of frequency of reinforcement. *Journal of the Experimental Analysis of Behavior, 4,* 267–272.

Herrnstein, R. J. (1970). On the law of effect. *Journal of the Experimental Analysis of Behavior, 13,* 243–266.

Herrnstein, R. J., & Loveland, D. H. (1975). Maximizing and matching on concurrent ratio schedules. *Journal of the Experimental Analysis of Behavior, 24,* 107–116.

Hoerger, M. L., & Mace, F. C. (2006). A computerized test of self-control predicts classroom behavior. *Journal of Applied Behavior Analysis, 39,* 147–159.

Horner, R. D. (1980). The effects of an environmental enrichment program on the behavior of institutionalized profoundly retarded children. *Journal of Applied Behavior Analysis, 13,* 473–491.

Hyten, C., & Madden, G. J. (1993). The scallop in fixed-interval research: A review with data description. *Psychological Record, 43,* 471–500.

Johnston, J. M., & Pennypacker, H. S., Jr. (2009). *Strategies and tactics of behavioral research* (3rd ed.). New York: Routledge.

Kahng, S., Abt, K. A., & Schonbachler, H. E. (2001). Assessment and treatment of low-rate high-intensity problem behavior. *Journal of Applied Behavior Analysis, 34,* 225–228.

Kahng, S., Iwata, B. A., Thompson, R. H., & Hanley, G. P. (2000). A method for identifying satiation versus extinction effects under noncontingent reinforcement schedules. *Journal of Applied Behavior Analysis, 33,* 419–432.

Koegel, R. L., Egel, A. L., & Williams, J. A. (1980). Behavioral contrast and generalization across settings in the treatment of autistic children. *Journal of Experimental Child Psychology, 30,* 422–437.

Lalli, J. S., Casey, S. D., & Kates, K. (1997). Noncontingent reinforcement as treatment for severe problem behavior: Some procedural variations. *Journal of Applied Behavior Analysis, 30,* 127–137.

Lalli, J. S., Mace, F. C., Wohn, T., & Livezey, K. (1995). Identification and modification of a response-class hierarchy. *Journal of Applied Behavior Analysis, 28,* 551–559.

Lane, L. L., Rogers, L. A., Parks, R. J., Weisenbach, J. L., Mau, A. C., Merwin, M. T., et al. (2007). Function-based interventions for students who are nonresponsive to primary and secondary efforts: Illustrations at the elementary and middle school levels. *Journal of Emotional and Behavioral Disorders, 15,* 169–183.

Laraway, S., Snycerski, S., Michael, J., & Poling, A. (2003). Motivating operations and terms to describe them: Some further refinements. *Journal of Applied Behavior Analysis, 36,* 407–414.

Lerman, D. C., Iwata, B. A., & Wallace, M. D. (1999). Side effects of extinction: Prevalence of bursting and aggression during the treatment of self-injurious behavior. *Journal of Applied Behavior Analysis, 32,* 1–8.

Luiselli, J. K., Pace, G. M., & Dunn, E. K. (2006). Effects of behavior-contingent and fixed-time release contingencies on frequency and duration of therapeutic restraint. *Behavior Modification, 30,* 442–455.

Mace, F. C. (2000). The clinical importance of choice and resistance to change. *Behavioral and Brain Sciences, 23,* 105–106.

Mace, F. C., Gritter, A. K., Johnson, P. E., Malley, J. L., & Steege, M. W. (2007). Contingent reinforcement in context. *European Journal of Behavior Analysis, 7,* 115–120.

Mace, F. C., & Lalli, J. S. (1991). Linking descriptive and experimental analyses in the treatment of bizarre speech. *Journal of Applied Behavior Analysis, 24,* 553–562.

Mace, F. C., Lalli, J. S., Shea, M. C., Lalli, E. P., West, B. J., Roberts, M., et al. (1990). The momentum of human behavior in a natural setting. *Journal of the Experimental Analysis of Behavior, 54,* 163–172.

Mace, F. C., Mauro, B. C., Boyajian, A. E., & Eckert, T. L. (1997). Effects of reinforcer quality on behavioral momentum: Coordinated applied and basic research. *Journal of Applied Behavior Analysis, 30,* 1–20.

Mace, F. C., Neef, N. A., Shade, D., & Mauro, B. C. (1994). Limited matching on concurrent schedule reinforcement of academic behavior. *Journal of Applied Behavior Analysis, 27,* 585–596.

Mace, F. C., Pratt, J. L., Prager, K. L., & Pritchard, D. (2011). An evaluation of three methods of saying 'no' to avoid an escalating response class hierarchy. *Journal of Applied Behavior Analysis, 44,* 83–94.

Mace, F. C., & Roberts, M. L. (1993). Factors affecting selection of behavioral interventions. In J. Reichle & D. Wacker (Eds.), *Communicative alternatives to challenging behavior: Integrating functional assessment and intervention strategies* (pp. 113–133). Baltimore: Brookes.

Mace, F. C., Zangrillo, A. N., Prager, K., Carolan, E., Hoerger, M., Thomas, K., et al. (2008). A methodology for maintaining low levels of attention-maintained problem behaviors following variable-time schedule thinning. *European Journal of Behavior Analysis, 9,* 149–156.

Magee, S. K., & Ellis, J. (2001). The detrimental effects of physical restraint as a consequence for inappropriate classroom behavior. *Journal of Applied Behavior Analysis, 34,* 501–504.

Marsteller, T. M., & St. Peter, C. C. (2014). Effects of fixed-time reinforcement schedules on resurgence of problem behavior. *Journal of Applied Behavior Analysis, 47,* 455–469.

Martens, B. K., Lochner, D. G., & Kelly, S. Q. (1992). The effects of variable-interval reinforcement on academic engagement: A demonstration of matching theory. *Journal of Applied Behavior Analysis, 25,* 143–151.

McDowell, J. J. (1989). Two modern developments in matching theory. *Behavior Analyst, 12,* 153–166.

Neef, N. A., Bicard, D. F., Endo, S., Coury, D. L., & Aman, M. G. (2005). Evaluation of pharmacological treatment of impulsivity in children with attention deficit hyperactivity disorder. *Journal of Applied Behavior Analysis, 38,* 135–146.

Neef, N. A., Marckel, J., Ferreri, S. J., Bicard, D. F., Endo, S., Aman, M. G., et al. (2005). Behavioral assessment of impulsivity: A comparison of children with and without attention deficit hyperactivity disorder. *Journal of Applied Behavior Analysis, 38,* 23–37.

Nevin, J. A. (1974). Response strength in multiple schedules. *Journal of the Experimental Analysis of Behavior, 21,* 389–408.

Nevin, J. A., & Grace, R. C. (2000). Preference and resistance to change with constant-duration schedule components. *Journal of the Experimental Analysis of Behavior, 74,* 79–100.

Nevin, J. A., Mandell, C., & Atak, J. R. (1983). The analysis of behavioral momentum. *Journal of the Experimental Analysis of Behavior, 39,* 49–59.

Nevin, J. A., Tota, M. E., Torquato, R. D., & Shull, R. L. (1990). Alternative reinforcement increases resistance to change: Pavlovian or operant contingencies? *Journal of the Experimental Analysis of Behavior, 53,* 359–379.

Ninness, H. A. C., Ozenne, L., & McCuller, G. (2000). Fixed-interval responding during computer interactive problem solving. *Psychological Record, 50,* 387–401.

Pierce, W. D., & Epling, W. F. (1984). On the persistence of cognitive explanation: Implications for behavior analysis. *Behaviorism, 12,* 15–27.

Poling, A., & Normand, M. (1999). Noncontingent reinforcement: An inappropriate description of time-based schedules that reduce behavior. *Journal of Applied Behavior Analysis, 32,* 237–238.

Pritchard, D., Hoerger, M., Mace, F. C., Penney, H., & Harris, B. (2014). Clinical translation of animal models of treatment relapse. *Journal of the Experimental Analysis of Behavior, 101,* 442–449.

Rachlin, H., & Green, L. (1972). Commitment, choice and self-control. *Journal of the Experimental Analysis of Behavior, 17,* 15–22.

Reynolds, G. S. (1961). Behavioral contrast. *Journal of the Experimental Analysis of Behavior, 4,* 57–71.

Ringdahl, J. E., Vollmer, T. R., Borrero, J. C., & Connell, J. E. (2001). Fixed-time schedule effects as a function of baseline reinforcement rate. *Journal of Applied Behavior Analysis, 34,* 1–15.

Saini, V., Miller, S. A., & Fisher, W. W. (2016). Multiple schedules in practical application: Research trends and implications for future investigation. *Journal of Applied Behavior Analysis, 49,* 1–24.

Schweitzer, J. B., & Sulzer-Azaroff, B. (1988). Self-control: Teaching tolerance for delay in impulsive children. *Journal of the Experimental Analysis of Behavior, 50,* 173–186.

Tarbox, J., & Parrot Hayes, L. (2005). Verbal behavior and behavioral contrast in human subjects. *Psychological Record, 55,* 419–437.

Thompson, R. H., & Iwata, B. A. (2005). A review of reinforcement control procedures. *Journal of Applied Behavior Analysis, 38,* 257–278.

Tiger, J. H., & Hanley, G. P. (2005). An example of discovery research involving the transfer of stimulus control. *Journal of Applied Behavior Analysis, 38,* 499–509.

Tiger, J. H., Hanley, G. P., & Hernandez, E. (2006). An evaluation of the value of choice with preschool children. *Journal of Applied Behavior Analysis, 39,* 1–16.

Van Camp, C. M., Lerman, D. C., Kelley, M. E., Contrucci, S. A., & Vorndran, C. M. (2000). Variable-time reinforcement schedules in the treatment of socially maintained problem behavior. *Journal of Applied Behavior Analysis, 33,* 545–557.

Vollmer, T. R., & Bourret, J. (2000). An application of the matching law to evaluate the allocation of two- and three-point shots by college basketball players. *Journal of Applied Behavior Analysis, 33,* 137–150.

Vollmer, T. R., & Hackenberg, T. D. (2001). Reinforcement contingencies and social reinforcement: Some reciprocal relations between basic and applied research. *Journal of Applied Behavior Analysis, 34,* 241–253.

Vollmer, T. R., Iwata, B. A., Zarcone, J. R., Smith, R. G., & Mazaleski, J. L. (1993). The role of attention in the treatment of attention-maintained self-injurious behavior: Noncontingent reinforcement and differential reinforcement of other behavior. *Journal of Applied Behavior Analysis, 26,* 9–21.

Vollmer, T. R., Marcus, B. A., & Ringdahl, J. E. (1995). Noncontingent escape as a treatment for self-injurious behavior maintained by negative reinforcement. *Journal of Applied Behavior Analysis, 28,* 15–26.

Vollmer, T. R., Progar, P. R., Lalli, J. S., Van Camp, C. M., Sierp, B. J., Wright, C. S., et al. (1998). Fixed-time schedules attenuate extinction-induced phenomena in the treatment of severe aberrant behavior. *Journal of Applied Behavior Analysis, 31,* 529–542.

Vollmer, T. R., Ringdahl, J. E., Roane, H. S., & Marcus, B. A. (1997). Negative side effects of noncontingent reinforcement. *Journal of Applied Behavior Analysis, 30,* 161–164.

Wallace, M. D., Iwata, B. A., Hanley, G. P., Thompson, R. H., & Roscoe, E. M. (2012). Noncontingent reinforcement: A further examination of schedule effects during treatment. *Journal of Applied Behavior Analysis, 45,* 709–719.

Wright, C. S., & Vollmer, T. R. (2002). Evaluation of a treatment package to reduce rapid eating. *Journal of Applied Behavior Analysis, 35,* 89–93.

# CHAPTER 5

# Stimulus Control and Generalization

Joseph E. Spradlin, Jennifer L. Simon, and Wayne W. Fisher

A teenage boy may readily acquiesce to his mother's request for a hug and a kiss in the privacy of their home but vehemently refuse the same request in front of his peers. We often yell and cheer at sporting events, sit quietly but periodically sing during a church service, and whisper when we wish to convey information to one individual without being overheard by others. These examples illustrate how the behavior of humans and other species often changes, depending on the circumstances. When our behavior changes in response to such environmental circumstances, we say that it is under *stimulus control*. Stimulus control is highly relevant to applied behavior analysts because most behavior is under some degree of stimulus control. As such, in this chapter we discuss a broad range of phenomena that fall within the topic of stimulus control. These include discriminations that are learned through direct training or experience, such as simple discriminations and conditional discriminations; they also include ones learned through generalization processes, such as stimulus generalization, stimulus equivalence, and recombinative generalization.

Researchers have used the term *stimulus control* in many ways, which have broad connotations. We may define stimulus control in terms of the changes in the probability of a form or rate of a behavior that occur due to the presentation of a stimulus. Defined in this way, stimulus control would include discriminative, eliciting, and rein-

forcing functions of stimuli (Skinner, 1938). We have restricted the discussion for this chapter primarily to discriminative control—the stimulus control that develops when we present positive reinforcement or withdraw negative reinforcement contingent on a response in the presence of a stimulus.

It is difficult to discuss the topic of stimulus discrimination without also discussing its countereffect—generalization. Researchers have used the term *generalization* in many ways. Basic researchers working with nonhumans in the laboratory typically refer to primary stimulus generalization. For example, Jenkins and Harrison (1960) conditioned a response to occur when they presented a 1,000-cycles-per-second (1,000-cps) tone and showed that the response also occurred when they presented a 1,500- or a 670-cps tone. Applied behavior analysts have used the term *generalization* in a much broader sense. Stokes and Baer (1977) defined generalization as "any occurrence of relevant behavior under nontraining conditions (i.e., across subjects, settings, people, behaviors, and/or time) without the scheduling of the same events in those conditions as had been scheduled in the training conditions" (p. 350). We use the term *generalization* in the current chapter in a slightly different way. Generalization for us includes more rapid learning of new discriminations, based on the learning of similar discriminations in the past (i.e., learning to learn; Harlow, 1949).

Individuals continuously contact contextual or background stimuli, such as visual, auditory, tactile, gustatory, and olfactory stimuli. These stimuli can be external or produced by the individual's own body. Whether a specific stimulus gains control over a specific response depends on many factors. First, it depends on the saliency of the stimulus, or how different the stimulus is from background stimuli (Dinsmoor, 1995b). A shout in a quiet library would be salient. By contrast, a whisper at a basketball game would not be salient. Researchers in typical laboratory studies of stimulus control design the environment to control the background stimuli by reducing any extraneous auditory or visual stimuli. For example, a researcher might place a nonhuman subject in a closed chamber, present white noise at a constant level, and eliminate any distracting visual stimuli. The level of experimental control may not be as complete for studies involving human participants, yet researchers should attempt to eliminate changes in the background stimuli that may be distracting to humans.

Second, a stimulus must be associated with differential consequences to gain control over a specific response. A salient stimulus that occurs before any conditioning will evoke responses, such as turning in the direction of a loud noise. The stimulus becomes part of the background if differential contingencies do not occur for specific responses in the repeated presence of the stimulus. For example, a neighbor's barking dog may evoke a startle response, such as turning toward the source of the barking, initially. However, the barking becomes part of the background stimuli and will no longer evoke the initial responses if barking continues without differential consequences following the barking.

Third, the response must be a part of the individual's behavioral repertoire for a stimulus to gain control over a response. For example, we often teach other forms of verbal behavior, such as sign language or picture exchange, to individuals without speech (Landa & Hanley, 2016). We typically select the alternative form of verbal behavior on the basis of responses that the individual already emits, such as pointing or touching; that is, we select a response that is already in the individual's repertoire (e.g., fine motor) instead of a response that the individual has not emitted (e.g., speech).

This chapter begins with establishing simple discriminations and proceeds to more complex stimulus control. The first section on simple stimulus control may initially seem quite removed from the types of complex discriminations required in daily human life. However, the importance of simple discriminations may become more apparent in later sections on more complex discriminations.

## ESTABLISHING CONTROL BY A SINGLE STIMULUS

Establishing stimulus control requires a salient stimulus, a somewhat controlled environment, and a target response that is part of the individual's repertoire. We can bring the target response under the control of a salient stimulus if (1) a reinforcing consequence immediately follows each target response that occurs in the presence of the stimulus, (2) reinforcement of target responding does not occur in the absence of the stimulus, and (3) there are no other conditions correlated with reinforcement and nonreinforcement. We want to ensure that the relevant stimulus is controlling the target response, and that target responding is not based on temporal patterns. For example, target responding could be based on time rather than the presentation of the stimulus if we present a stimulus once every minute for 30 seconds. Therefore, we should present the stimulus on a variable-time schedule.

In some situations, stimulus presentation may function as reinforcement for target responding that occurs before stimulus presentation, particularly when we present the stimulus on a response-independent schedule. The sequence in this case is as follows: target response, stimulus presentation, target response, reinforcement. Stimulus presentation functions as reinforcement for target responding before stimulus presentation when we deliver reinforcement for the target response in the presence of the stimulus. Such reinforcement may impede discriminative responding. Therefore, we should delay the presentation of the stimulus if a target response occurs just before the scheduled presentation of the stimulus, to allow for extinction of the target response during the absence of the stimulus (Ferster & Perrott, 1968). We use the term *change-over delay* or *momentary differential reinforcement of other behavior* to refer to delayed stimulus presentation contingent on responding before stimulus presentation. Applied research on stimulus control of functional communication responses during treatment of problem behavior has included such contingencies to prevent adventitious reinforcement (e.g., Fisher, Greer, Fuhrman, & Querim, 2015).

We should determine whether target responding is under the control of the discriminative properties of the relevant stimulus after target responding occurs primarily when the stimulus is present and not when it is absent. One possibility is that reinforcement may have developed discriminative properties, because reinforcement of target responding is likely to be followed by more reinforcement, and nonreinforcement is likely to be followed by more nonreinforcement. In this case, target responding may occur more after reinforcement delivery than following a response that was not reinforced if the delivery of the reinforcer functions as a discriminative stimulus (Blough, 1966). We can be more confident that the relevant stimulus controls target responding if responding begins immediately after stimulus presentation and stops immediately after stimulus termination.

Even when we use a salient stimulus and have established control over a response, other, similar stimuli also may control the response. Stimulus generalization allows for the reinforcement of responses in the presence of stimuli that initially may have been difficult to condition. For example, Fulton and Spradlin (1971) initially established control over a button-pressing response to a 70-decibel, 500-Hertz tone, which is a salient stimulus for people with normal hearing, to assess the hearing of children with intellectual developmental disorder. Control occurred for a target 70-decibel, 500-Hertz tone for most participants, and less intense tones also controlled responding. Responding to less intense tones than the target 70-decibel tone allowed the researchers to provide reinforcement of responses to lower-intensity tones. Generalization occurred to tones of still lower intensity after researchers provided reinforcement for responses to lower-intensity tones. The tone maintained stimulus control over button pressing due to stimulus generalization and reinforcement of responses to tones with progressively lower intensity until the tone reached a threshold level, which is the magnitude level at which responding is no longer discriminative.

Researchers have conducted most studies of simple stimulus control like those described above with auditory and visual stimuli. We also can use these procedures to establish control with tactile, gustatory, and olfactory stimuli. Although control with a single stimulus has few parallels in individuals' daily lives, single-stimulus control is useful for conducting hearing evaluations for people with intellectual developmental disorder (Fulton & Spradlin, 1971) and for teaching dogs and rats to find people, narcotics, and explosives by smell (e.g., Edwards, La Londe, Cox, Weetjens, & Pol-

ing, 2016). The odors of narcotics and explosives are salient stimuli for dogs and rats, and researchers have trained these animals to respond to the odors by reinforcing a specific response, such as sit and stay, when the odor is present and not when it is absent.

## DIFFERENTIAL STIMULUS CONTROL BY STIMULI PRESENTED SUCCESSIVELY

Although the mere detection of a stimulus is important under some conditions, stimulus control more often involves a discrimination between two stimuli: a positive stimulus correlated with reinforcement, and a negative stimulus correlated with nonreinforcement. The researcher alternates the positive stimulus (such as a red light) with a negative stimulus (such as a green light) of the same intensity and presentation duration, to establish a successive discrimination. We use the term *successive discrimination* because the positive and negative stimuli are present at different times. However, discriminative responding under this condition can be slow and may not occur for all experimental participants.

Fading is likely to establish a more rapid discrimination among the stimuli (Terrace, 1966), because we can maximize the difference between the positive and negative stimuli initially and then decrease the differences between stimuli gradually. Methods for increasing the difference between the stimuli include maximizing the saliency of the positive stimulus (such as a bright red light) and minimizing the saliency of the negative stimulus (such as a faint green light), and presenting the positive stimulus for a long duration and the negative stimulus for a brief duration. Maximizing the differences between the stimuli increases the probability of responding in the presence of the positive stimulus and not responding in the presence of the negative stimulus. Fading initially requires a salient positive stimulus (such as a bright red light) and a nonsalient negative stimulus (such as a faint green light). We establish responding in the presence of the positive stimulus and not in the presence of the negative stimulus. We then increase the intensity of the negative stimulus (such as increasing the brightness of the green light) until the intensity of the positive and negative stimuli is equal, and responding occurs only in the presence of the positive stimulus. We then gradually increase the duration of the negative-stimulus presentation until the durations of positive- and negative-stimulus presentations are equal, and responding occurs only in the presence of the positive stimulus.

Macht (1971) used a similar procedure to teach a discrimination between forward and reversed E's to children with intellectual developmental disorder. He taught each child to press a lever when he presented the letter E (which was the positive stimulus) and not to press the lever when he presented a solid black square (which was the negative stimulus). Initially, presentations of the E's were long in duration, and he presented the black square for a brief period when responding paused. He increased the duration of subsequent black-square presentations and punished responses in its presence. He established discrimination between the forward E and the reversed E by using variations of this procedure after responding between the E and the square was discriminative. He then evaluated each child's vision by moving the child farther and farther from the apparatus that presented the forward and reversed E's.

When we establish the first discrimination (e.g., forward and reversed E's in Macht's experiment) by using a fading technique, the next discrimination we establish (e.g., A vs. F) may not require extensive programming, or we may be able to establish it in fewer stimulus presentations. In addition, we may establish future discriminations (e.g., N vs. M) more quickly even without fading. Dinsmoor (1995a) attributed this type of improvement in discriminative learning to the control of attending responses. We also may consider it as a special case of learning to learn or a learning set (Harlow, 1949).

Even though establishing discrimination between a forward and reversed E may be sufficient for the evaluation of subjective vision, it is insufficient for most educational purposes. For example, teaching the discrimination between a forward and reversed E is unlikely to establish a discrimination between the letters E and F. Therefore, we should use several different negative stimuli, such as F, P, B, and I, and variations of the positive stimulus when teaching such a discrimination, such as E and **E** (see Engelmann & Carnine, 1982, for a more complete discussion).

## DIFFERENTIAL STIMULUS CONTROL BY TWO OR MORE SIMULTANEOUSLY PRESENTED STIMULI

A simple simultaneous discrimination involves the discrimination between two or more stimuli presented at the same time. Sidman and Stoddard (1967) established fine circle–ellipse discriminations by using a fading procedure with an apparatus with eight translucent keys on which they projected light and figures. Initially, there was great disparity between the positive stimulus (a circle on a fully illuminated white key) and the negative stimulus (no figures and nonilluminated keys). Training began with the presentation of one positive and seven negative stimuli. Touching the positive stimulus produced reinforcement, whereas touching any negative stimulus did not. The researchers reinstated the previous fading step when participants made errors. Gradually, the researchers illuminated the seven negative stimuli until they were the same intensity as the positive stimulus. Next, the researchers introduced a horizontal line on the negative-stimulus keys. After participants were responding to the positive stimulus, the researchers gradually changed the negative-stimulus figure (i.e., the horizontal line morphed into a very narrow ellipse). The ellipse morphed into an ellipse-like circle like that on the positive-stimulus key after the researchers illuminated the negative-stimulus keys with an ellipse. Eventually, they established the threshold for the circle–ellipse discrimination.

Sometimes extending stimulus control from stimuli that already control differential responding to stimuli that currently do not is desirable. One method researchers have used to transfer control from existing stimulus dimensions to novel ones is a delayed-prompting procedure (Touchette, 1971). Touchette (1971) demonstrated the delayed-prompting procedure with three adult students with intellectual developmental disorder. He established a discrimination between the positive stimulus (a red key) and the negative stimulus (a white key) by reinforcing responses to the red key and not reinforcing responses to the white key. Next, he established a new discrimination between two stimuli with minimal disparity (a horizontal E with the legs pointing up vs. a horizontal E with the legs pointing down). Initially he superimposed the positive and negative stimuli on the red and white stimuli, which already controlled behavior. He delayed the onset of the red background light behind the positive stimulus for 0.5 second after the first correct response. He delayed the onset of the red background stimulus by an additional 0.5 second and decreased its presentation duration by 0.5 second for each incorrect response on each additional trial. Correct responding occurred before the delivery of the prompt (i.e., the red light) in 10 trials with all three students. However, such rapid acquisition of correct responding does not always occur. Subsequent research suggests that the students may have been atypical (e.g., Oppenheimer, Saunders, & Spradlin, 1993).

Oppenheimer et al. (1993), using a similar procedure with 30 adults with intellectual developmental disorder, obtained three different outcomes. First, some participants were like Touchette's (1971) participants who responded before the onset of the red light and were correct. Second, some participants responded before the onset of the red light, but were correct on only 50% of trials. Third, some participants never responded before the onset of the red light. The researchers conducted further testing with this last group to determine (1) whether responding did not occur because they had not established discrimination between the horizontal E's; or (2) whether they had established the discrimination between the two horizontal E's, but the participants were waiting until the red light came on before responding. Oppenheimer et al. presented the red light simultaneously on the keys behind both the correct and the incorrect E. Some participants did not respond before the red light came on because they did not make the discrimination; that is, their performance was at chance level when the researcher projected the red light on both keys. However, other participants responded correctly when the researcher projected the red light on both E's. Therefore, the red light functioned as a "go" stimulus for discriminative responding between the E's for some participants.

The procedure just described is useful in the laboratory study of discrimination and sensory processes. However, many discrimination situations involve making different responses to different stimuli. Researchers have used variants of the delayed-prompt technique, such as progressive and constant time or prompt delay, to teach a two-choice visual discrimination (e.g., Handen & Zane, 1987). Researchers have used delayed-prompt procedures to teach skills such as selection of letters and numbers (e.g., Bradley-Johnson, Sunderman, & Johnson, 1983; Touchette & Howard, 1984), sight word reading (e.g., Gast, Ault, Wolery, Doyle, & Belanger, 1988; Knight, Ross, Taylor, & Ramasamy, 2003), and naming and requesting (Charlop, Schreibman, & Thibodeau, 1985; Charlop & Walsh, 1986; Halle, Baer, & Spradlin, 1981; Halle, Marshall, & Spradlin, 1979; Knight et al., 2003).

A behavior analyst could present the printed numeral 1 while simultaneously presenting the auditory stimulus "one" to teach a child with imitative speech to name printed numerals. The behavior analyst could present reinforcement for the vocalization when the child imitates the auditory stimulus "one." The behavior analyst should present the auditory stimulus "one" after a few-second delay after presenting the printed numeral 1 on subsequent trials. The behavior analyst should present reinforcement if the child names the numeral before the behavior analyst presents the auditory stimulus; ideally, the probability of reinforcement would be greater for such preemptive responses (Touchette & Howard, 1984). Training on the numeral 2 could begin after the child consistently names the numeral 1. Initially, the behavior analyst should present the auditory stimulus "two" simultaneously with the printed numeral 2. The behavior analyst should provide reinforcement when the child imitates "two." Presentations of the printed numeral 2 should continue with a brief delay before the auditory stimulus. This procedure should continue until the child consistently responds before the auditory stimulus. Then the behavior analyst should present the printed numerals 1 and 2 in a random order. Initially, the behavior analyst should present the auditory stimuli simultaneously with the printed numerals to prevent initial errors. Then the behavior analyst should present the printed numerals (1 or 2) 4–5 seconds before the auditory stimulus. This procedure should produce the discrimination quite rapidly for most children. The behavior analyst can introduce other printed numerals with this same procedure. In many cases, the behavior analyst may begin by intermixing the printed numerals when he or she uses the delayed-prompt technique. In fact, tact training, in which researchers intersperse three targets simultaneously, produced rapid acquisition of multiple target responses and promoted generalization in children with autism spectrum disorder and intellectual developmental disorder (e.g., Leaf et al., 2016; Marchese, Carr, LeBlanc, Rosati, & Conroy, 2012; Wunderlich, Vollmer, Donaldson, & Phillips, 2014).

## CONDITIONAL STIMULUS CONTROL

The discriminations we have discussed previously have been either simple successive or simple simultaneous discriminations, which are essential in daily life. Many discriminations that individuals make during their daily activities, however, are *conditional discriminations*, in which reinforcement of a response in the presence of a stimulus depends on the presence or absence of other stimuli. An example of a conditional discrimination is passing the salt when someone asks you to pass the salt, and passing the bread when someone asks you to pass the bread. That is, the discriminated behavior is conditional because the positive stimulus (e.g., salt, bread) changes, depending on the request (Serna, Dube, & McIlvane, 1997).

Simultaneous identity matching is a very simple conditional-discrimination procedure. Researchers have studied this procedure widely in laboratories with humans and nonhumans. In the laboratory, the typical procedure involves presenting a visual sample stimulus (e.g., the numeral 2) to which the experimental participant must respond. The researcher then presents two or more comparison stimuli (such as 2 and 3, or 2, 3, 4, and 5) after the participant's response to the sample. One of the comparison stimuli (e.g., 2) is identical to the sample stimulus; the remaining stimulus (e.g., 3) or stimuli (e.g., 3, 4, and 5) differ from the sample stimulus. The disparity between the correct comparison stimulus and the other stimuli may be large or small. The researcher presents different stimuli as samples from trial to trial; thus the correct comparison stimulus is conditional on which sample is present. Identity-matching experiments have involved simple trial-and-error procedures (Saunders, Johnson, Tompkins, Dutcher, & Williams, 1997; Saunders & Sherman, 1986) and fading procedures (Dube, Iennaco, & McIlvane, 1993). The researcher may present only the single comparison stimulus that matches the sample stimulus, or the other comparisons may be blank on the first few trials of an identity-matching-to-sample task using a fading procedure. The researcher may begin to fade in the nonmatching stimulus or stimuli after a few trials. The nonmatching stimuli become more visible until the intensity of the nonmatching stimuli matches that of the sample stimulus with each successive trial of correct responding. Participants typically match new stimuli on their first presentation after they have matched a few comparison stimuli to samples; that is, they exhibit generalized identity matching. Nonhuman participants and some participants with intellectual developmental disorder do not exhibit generalized matching readily. Researchers have used video modeling, error correction, and fading from a simple tabletop sorting task to compound identity matching on a computer screen with participants with autism spectrum disorder and intellectual developmental disorder to facilitate generalized identity matching (Alexander, Ayres, Smith, Shepley, & Mataras, 2013; Farber, Dube, & Dixon, 2016).

We consider generalized identity matching as another example of generalization. Preacademic workbooks use identity matching extensively to teach letter and number discrimination to students. Usually, the workbook presents the sample letter or number at the left margin, and the choice letters or numbers in a row to the right of the sample. The student's response is to mark the correct choice. This workbook task is an example of identity matching; however, it is not an ideal teaching technique, because it involves delayed reinforcement for correct responses.

Simultaneous identity matching requires discrimination of the sample stimuli from the remaining comparison stimuli. It neither requires nor ensures successive discrimination among sample stimuli, because the sample stimulus remains available throughout the trial. However, it is a delayed-matching-to-sample procedure if the teacher removes the sample after the onset of the comparisons and probably requires successive discrimination of the sample stimuli (e.g., Constantine & Sidman, 1975).

Closely related to the identity-matching task is the oddity procedure. In this discrimination, the teacher presents the student with an array of three or more stimuli, one of which is different. Sidman and Stoddard (1967) presented such a display to their students; however, they used only one stimulus (a circle) as the correct odd stimulus. Other researchers have presented a series of trials on which the odd stimulus (i.e., the positive stimulus) was different on various trials (e.g., Dickerson & Girardeau, 1971; Ellis & Sloan, 1959; Smeets & Striefel, 1974; Soraci et al., 1987; Stromer & Stromer, 1989). For example, the researcher might present the numeral 1 as the single positive stimulus, with two or more numeral 2's as the negative stimuli on one trial. The researcher might present a single 2 with two or more 1's on other trials. In that case, the oddity task is a conditional-discrimination task, because the stimulus designated as correct depends on the other stimuli. Preacademic workbooks have used the oddity procedure extensively.

A more complex type of conditional discrimination is one in which the comparison stimuli are not similar physically to the sample stimulus. Auditory–visual matching (e.g., receptive labeling) consists of the presentation of an auditory sample, such as dictated object names, with visual comparisons, such as an array of objects. For example, the correct response is conditional on the pre-sented sample if a teacher is training a student to touch specific printed numerals (e.g., *1* and *2*) in response to corresponding auditory samples (e.g., "one" or "two"). That is, the answer is the numeral *1* if the auditory sample is "one," and the correct response is the numeral *2* if the auditory sample is "two." Such a conditional discrimination depends on (1) a successive discrimination of the audi-tory stimuli "one" and "two," (2) a simultaneous discrimination between the printed numerals *1* and *2*, and (3) the correspondence of the auditory stimulus "one" with the numeral *1*. Not all typi-cally developing children learn such conditional discriminations without first learning the compo-nent discriminations. In those cases, the behavior analyst can establish conditional responding by teaching each component discrimination in isola-tion (see Saunders & Spradlin, 1993).

The first component of a component-teaching procedure is to establish successive discrimina-tions among the auditory number samples. A teacher may have the student echo the auditory stimuli if the student emits vocal behavior. The second component is to establish discriminated re-sponding to the comparison stimuli (e.g., printed numerals). The teacher can conduct a matching-to-sample probe with the numerals. The teacher can implement the third component if the student exhibits matching (e.g., *1* to *1*, and *2* to *2*). If not, the teacher should establish the discrimination be-tween the printed numerals. The third component is to establish the relation between the auditory stimulus (e.g., "one") and the corresponding nu-meral comparison (e.g., *1*). The teacher may train this conditional discrimination by using a delayed-prompt procedure (Grow, Carr, Kodak, Jostad, & Kisamore, 2011; Grow, Kodak, & Carr, 2014; Touchette & Howard, 1984) or a blocking proce-dure (Saunders & Spradlin, 1993; Saunders, Wil-liams, & Spradlin, 1995; Smeets & Striefel, 1994).

The teacher typically teaches the second con-ditional discrimination with less careful program-ming and fewer trials after he or she has taught the first conditional discrimination (e.g., between "one" and *1* and "two" and *2*). The teacher can then teach the next discrimination between the printed numeral (e.g., *3*) and the corresponding auditory sample (e.g., "three"), intermixed with trials of the previously discriminated numer-als. The selection of the novel comparison may emerge without direct training when the teacher presents the novel sample and comparison stimuli (e.g., the auditory sample "three" and the numeral

3) with previously trained comparisons (e.g., the numeral *1* or *2*). Researchers have called this type of performance *exclusion* (Dixon, 1977; McIlvane, Kledaras, Lowry, & Stoddard, 1992). Researchers have demonstrated the emergence of exclusion-ary relations between three-dimensional visual and auditory stimuli (e.g., McIlvane & Stoddard, 1981, 1985), between two-dimensional visual and auditory stimuli (e.g., Wilkinson & Green, 1998; Wilkinson & McIlvane, 1994), and between text and auditory stimuli (e.g., de Rose, de Souza, & Hanna, 1996). However, testing for control by the emerged relation under different conditions (e.g., multiple trials with more than two previously unknown comparisons) is necessary to ensure control by the sample (Carr, 2003). The teacher may train new relations by using a variation of the procedure used to teach the initial conditional discrimination if exclusion does not establish the discrimination.

## EQUIVALENCE CLASSES

Configurations of shared physical properties deter-mine many stimulus classes (e.g., balls, cars, cats, humans, men, women, red objects). The actual configurations of shared physical characteristics determining class membership have been the focus of research by psycholinguists, cognitive psy-chologists (Medin & Smith, 1984; Rosch, 1973), and behavior analysts (e.g., Fields et al., 2002; Fields & Reeve, 2001; Galizio, Stewart, & Pilgrim, 2004). However, shared physical properties do not define many important stimulus classes (e.g., lawyers, letters, medical doctors, numbers, tools, toys). Whether each member is substitutable, and whether they evoke new, untrained responses in certain contexts, define the members of these classes (Saunders & Green, 1992; Urcuioli, 2013). For example, we may define toys as a stimulus class because they are items that children manipulate, and we may store them in a toy box. In addition, a child is likely to engage in exploratory and novel play behavior without any direct training when he or she finds a new item in the toy box. Medi-cal doctors are a stimulus class because we call them *doctor,* and any member with the appropri-ate credentials may practice medicine. In addition, people are much more likely to follow the health-related advice of someone called *doctor* than some-one called *waiter.*

Sidman (1971) established an equivalence class using a symbol-matching procedure with a 17-year-old student with microcephaly and intellectual developmental disorder. The student selected 20 pictures when the researcher presented their corresponding dictated words (AB), and could name 20 pictures when the researcher presented the pictures (BD) before the study. However, he did not name the 20 printed words related to the pictures (CD), select printed words in response to their dictated names (AC), select printed words that named the pictures (BC), or select the pictures when presented with the printed words (CB). Sidman trained selection of printed words when he presented corresponding dictated words (AC) to the student. He conducted probes after training to test whether the student would select printed words when given the respective pictures (BC), and whether the student would select the pictures when given the respective printed words (CB). Not only did the student select the printed words when Sidman presented dictated words, but the BC and CB relations between pictures and printed words emerged, regardless of whether Sidman presented the printed words as sample or comparison stimuli. In addition, the student named many of the printed words (CD) after the initial AC training. This training established 20 stimulus classes; each class consisted of the spoken word, the printed word, and the pictures.

Although the results of Sidman's (1971) study were remarkable, the design was less than ideal for demonstrating the development of new stimulus classes, because the stimuli were common (e.g., *car, cat, dog*) and only one student participated. Sidman's experiment led to a flurry of research directed toward the development of stimulus classes comprising stimuli that shared no defining physical properties (Saunders, Saunders, Kirby, & Spradlin, 1988; Saunders, Wachter, & Spradlin, 1988; Sidman, Cresson, & Willson-Morris, 1974; Sidman, Kirk, & Willson-Morris, 1985; Sidman & Tailby, 1982; Spradlin, Cotter, & Baxley, 1973; Spradlin & Saunders, 1986; Wetherby, Karlan, & Spradlin, 1983). These studies and others led to numerous theoretical discussions concerning the necessary and sufficient conditions for the development of such classes (Baer, 1982; Fields & Verhave, 1987; Hayes, Barnes-Holmes, & Roche, 2001; Horne & Lowe, 1996; Saunders & Green, 1992; Sidman, 1994, 2000; Sidman & Tailby, 1982).

Most matching-to-sample studies after Sidman (1971) used procedures with better experimental control (Sidman et al., 1974; Sidman & Tailby, 1982; Spradlin et al., 1973). Experimental stimuli are typically abstract forms (e.g., #, @, ?)

or nonsense stimuli (e.g., *vek, zog*; Fields & Verhave, 1990; Sidman et al., 1974; Sidman & Tailby, 1982; Spradlin et al., 1973). A general procedure consists of teaching an AB conditional discrimination (i.e., present sample stimulus A1, provide reinforcement for selection of comparison stimulus B1; present sample stimulus A2, provide reinforcement for selection of comparison stimulus B2). The researcher teaches a new discrimination (BC) after he or she establishes the AB discrimination. In this case, the researcher presents the stimuli, B1 and B2, as samples and introduces two new comparison stimuli, C1 and C2. The researcher intermixes the AB and BC conditional-discrimination trials after the student demonstrates the BC discrimination. The researcher introduces probe trials when discrimination is nearly perfect on the AB and BC discriminations. The researcher usually introduces probe trials without reinforcement or differential feedback and in a series of AB and BC trials. The first probes are often for *symmetry* (i.e., A1 is the correct comparison when B1 is the sample stimulus, and A2 is the correct comparison when B2 is the sample). In addition, the researcher conducts the CB probe to determine whether the student will select the appropriate comparison, B1 and B2, when presented with the samples C1 and C2. Typically, the student demonstrates symmetry (Fields & Verhave, 1990; Pilgrim & Galizio, 1990).

The researcher conducts another probe to test for *transitivity* (e.g., C1 is the correct comparison when A1 is the sample, and C2 is the correct comparison when A2 is the sample). In addition, the researcher conducts probes to determine whether the student will select A1 as the comparison when C1 is the sample, and whether the student will select A2 as the comparison when C2 is the sample. This final probe is a combined test for symmetry and transitivity, because it cannot be positive unless both symmetry and transitivity are present. The student demonstrates *equivalence* when these tests are positive (Sidman & Tailby, 1982). Most students given this training pass these tests, even though some percentage of students who learn the AB and BC conditional discriminations fail the equivalence tests.

AB and BC training can establish an equivalence class; however, these are not the only combinations that produce an equivalence class. Training AB and AC conditional discriminations or BA and CA conditional discriminations also produces equivalence classes. In fact, some research suggests that teaching students to select a single comparison in response to multiple samples is a more effective procedure for demonstrating stimulus equivalence than the other two procedures (Spradlin & Saunders, 1986). The teacher can use all of the tests for equivalence when the stimuli are visual. However, the teacher typically does not present A1 and A2 as comparisons if they are auditory stimuli, because of problems in presenting and discriminating two auditory stimuli simultaneously.

When we are studying the development of equivalence classes in a laboratory, the procedures and outcomes may appear quite remote from the problems encountered in our daily lives. However, they may not appear quite as remote with an example of equivalence we encounter daily: number equivalence. Although many students learn to select the numerals 1 through 4 in response to dictated number names and to name the numerals 1 through 4, some do not. We can teach these students three conditional discriminations (AB, AC, and AD), and perhaps nine additional conditional discriminations will emerge through symmetry and transitivity (BA, BC, CA, CB, CD, DA, DC, BD, and DB). Additionally, naming numerals, sets (i.e., quantity), and words (BE, CE, DE) may emerge. Naming responses are likely if a student names either the numerals or the sets before training (Gast, VanBiervliet, & Spradlin, 1979). There are many ways that we can establish equivalence classes with numbers. For example, a teacher might teach the student to select (1) the numerals in response to their dictated names (AB), (2) sets in response to their printed numerals (BC), and (3) printed words in response to their respective sets (CD). An effective procedure for establishing the performances if the student is verbal would be to teach the (1) selection of printed numerals in response to presentation of dictated words (AB), (2) names of the printed numerals (BE), (3) selection of sets in response to presentation of printed numerals (BC), (4) selection of the printed words in response to presentation of sets (CD), and (5) appropriate responding to an intermix of trials from the trained discriminations (1, 2, and 3). This procedure may be redundant if students name printed numerals after learning to select printed numerals in response to dictated number names (AB). However, this procedure ensures a student's familiarity with the generalization-testing formats, and the naming response is in the student's repertoire. In addition, intermixing trials maintains prerequisite conditional discriminations (Saunders, Wachter, et al., 1988; Spradlin et al., 1973). There are numerous ways of establishing equivalence classes via conditional discriminations. In addition, four new conditional discriminations (BC, CB, BA, and CA) may emerge when there are three visual stimuli in each class, and we train AB and BC conditional discriminations. Teaching three conditional discriminations (AB, AC, AD) may produce nine new emergent discriminations (BC, CB, BD, DB, CD, DC, BA, CA, DA) when the number of visual stimuli in each class increases to four stimuli; that is, the number of potential untaught discriminations increases dramatically as the number of stimuli in each class increases. Moreover, Saunders, Wachter, et al. (1988) have established equivalence classes with as many as nine members in each class.

Researchers have established equivalence classes with stimuli that have potential social use, including equivalence among printed names, dictated names, and faces of therapists (Cowley, Green, & Braunling-McMorrow, 1992); among dictated words, objects, and manual signs (Van-Biervliet, 1977); among reading-relevant stimuli (de Rose et al., 1996; de Rose, de Souza, Rossito, & de Rose, 1992; Wultz & Hollis, 1980); in prearithmetic skills (Gast et al., 1979); in money relations (Stoddard, Brown, Hurlbert, Manoli, & McIlvane, 1989); and in spelling and reading (Mackay, 1985; Mueller, Olmi, & Saunders, 2000; Stromer & Mackay, 1992).

Research has demonstrated several interesting findings about subsequent performances after the establishment of equivalence classes. First, we can add new members readily to a class (e.g., Gast et al., 1979; Saunders, Wachter, et al., 1988). For example, Saunders, Wachter, et al. (1988) established two eight-member classes of visual stimuli by using procedures analogous to those described earlier. Researchers taught the students to select two visual stimuli, one member from each equivalence class, in response to two different auditory stimuli (i.e., nonsense syllables) after they had established the two classes of eight stimuli each. Three of the four students selected the seven remaining stimuli in each class in response to their respective spoken nonsense syllables when the researchers presented probe trials. They taught the fourth student to select a second stimulus in response to each auditory stimulus. Students selected the remaining six stimuli of each class in response to their respective auditory stimuli after this training.

Second, equivalence classes are durable. After training and probing, Saunders, Wachtel, et al. (1988) dismissed their students for 2–5 months and then retested to see whether the auditory stimuli still controlled the selection of the same comparison stimuli. They provided no differential reinforcement during the pretest for baseline training or for probe trials. Correct selections occurred immediately for three of four students. Responding for the fourth student gradually recovered to prebreak levels, even though the researchers did not deliver differential reinforcement for baseline training or for probe trials.

Third, performances that indicate equivalence are resistant to change as a function of changes in baseline reinforcement conditions (Pilgrim & Galizio, 1990; Saunders, Saunders, et al., 1988). Pilgrim and Galizio (1990) taught five college students AB and AC conditional discriminations, and students demonstrated equivalence after training. The researchers then reversed the contingencies for the AC discrimination (i.e., selecting C2 was reinforced when a student was presented with sample A1, and selecting C1 was reinforced when a student was presented with sample A2). Symmetry responding to CA relations was reversed for some students, but no BC or CB responses were reversed. Saunders, Saunders, et al. (1988) found that equivalence classes were difficult to disrupt once they had established them.

Fourth, conditioning an operant response in the presence of a member of the class produces generalization to other members of the class after the establishment of an equivalence class. Barnes and Keenan (1993) demonstrated the transfer of operant responding from one member of an equivalence class to other members. The researchers established two equivalence classes (A1, B1, and C1; A2, B2, and C2) by training AB and AC relations with college students. The researchers trained the students to respond slowly when they presented one stimulus (B1) and rapidly when they presented the second stimulus (B2) after the students demonstrated equivalence classes. Then the researchers presented the four remaining stimuli (A1, C1, A2, and C2). Students emitted slow responses in the presence of A1 and C1, and rapid responses in the presence of A2 and C2. Gast et al. (1979) demonstrated a similar transfer of control from some members of an equivalence class to a remaining member of that class.

Fifth, if we condition one or more members of an equivalence class to elicit an emotional response, other members of that class will elicit that response (Dougher, Auguston, Markham, Wulfert, & Greenway, 1994). Dougher et al. (1994) established two four-member equivalence classes (A1, B1, C1, and D1; A2, B2, C2, and D2) by training AB, AC, and AD conditional discriminations

with eight students. The researchers used two stimuli (B1 and B2) in a separate classical-conditioning setting after they had established the two four-member equivalence classes. They presented B1 and B2 successively during this phase. Shock always followed B1, but never followed B2. B1 came to elicit a galvanic skin response; B2 did not. Six of the eight students exhibited galvanic skin responses to the stimulus class of which B1 was a member, and did not exhibit galvanic skin responses to the stimulus class including B2, when the researchers presented the six remaining stimuli from the two classes. This study demonstrated that emotional responses can develop without direct conditioning if stimuli that evoke those responses are members of an equivalence class.

The preceding text provides a sample of equivalence studies and some of their implications for understanding the development of stimulus control. Procedures other than conditional discriminations have also resulted in the development of equivalence classes. For example, if we teach a student to say a specific word in response to a set of previously unrelated stimuli, those stimuli are likely to function as a class (Reese, 1972). Researchers have demonstrated that stimuli presented in the same position in a sequence of stimuli function as ordinal-equivalence classes (Mackay, Stoddard, & Spencer, 1989; Sigurdardottir, Green, & Saunders, 1990). For example, if we teach a student to place three stimuli (N, B, and X) in a one–two–three sequence while we teach him or her to place stimuli E, L, and Z in a one–two–three sequence, stimuli N and E are likely to become members of one equivalence class. Stimuli B and L will probably become members of another, and stimuli X and Z will become members of a third class. In addition, stimuli that occur contiguously also may come to function as members of an equivalence class (Stromer & Stromer, 1990a, 1990b).

Finally, researchers have shown that adding stimuli to a previously established equivalence class is possible merely on the basis of shared consequences (Dube & McIlvane, 1995). In summary, there are many ways that we can establish equivalence classes. We would venture that two or more stimuli will become members of the same equivalence class in a context without a change in contingencies if those stimuli are substitutable.

Note that context determines the formation of a stimulus class. For example, if a teacher asks a student to put toys in one box and tools in another, the student will respond differently than if the teacher asks the student to put soft items in one box and hard items in another. Bush, Sidman, and de Rose (1989) demonstrated such contextual control over equivalence class membership with traditional matching-to-sample procedures.

Research on the applied implications of procedures that promote the formation of stimulus classes has proceeded somewhat slowly in comparison to the basic research on this topic (McLay, Sutherland, Church, & Tyler-Merrick, 2013; Rehfeldt, 2011). However, a randomized clinical trial showed that college students learned the generic and brand names of 32 pharmacological agents in both written and spoken forms more quickly when equivalence-based instruction than when a more traditional approach based on flash card instruction was used (Zinn, Newland, & Ritchie, 2015). In addition, research on increasing complex verbal behavior has increasingly examined the extent to which various training procedures affect consistent and rapid improvement in the specifically targeted responses and in the emergence of novel responses (DeSouza, Akers, & Fisher, 2017; Tincani, Miguel, Bondy, & Crozier, Chapter 16, this volume).

As noted earlier, this is far from a complete discussion of stimulus equivalence and related phenomena. We refer the reader to Hayes (1991), Hayes et al. (2001), Horne and Lowe (1996), and Sidman (1994, 2000) for extensive discussions and theoretical interpretations of the necessary and sufficient conditions for the development of such stimulus control.

## STIMULUS CONTROL BASED ON RECOMBINATION OF STIMULUS–RESPONSE COMPONENTS

One of the remarkable characteristics of human behavior is the degree to which responding to complex stimuli occurs without previous direct experience. For example, young children develop generalized imitation so that their behavior can approximate that of a model, even though they have never had direct training on imitating the specific model (e.g., Baer, Peterson, & Sherman, 1967; Peterson, 1968). In addition, individuals may respond appropriately to specific verbal instructions they have never encountered previously (e.g., Stewart, McElwee, & Ming, 2013; Striefel, Wetherby, & Karlan, 1976). *Recombinative generalization* occurs when a student recombines responses targeted during training in novel ways. For example, a student may "push car" and "drop glass" if we teach him or her to "push glass" and "drop car."

Striefel et al. (1976, 1978) extended previous work by demonstrating recombinative generalization of stimulus–response units with nonvocal children with intellectual developmental disorder. They conducted a series of studies to establish instruction following with verb–noun combinations (e.g., "Push glass," "Drop car"). They first taught imitative responding by using instructions, models, reinforcement, and time out. They presented simultaneous vocal instructions (e.g., "Push glass") and modeling after the participants displayed imitation independently. They used a delayed-prompt procedure to train independent responding after consistent performance. They taught new nouns using the same procedure (e.g., "Push glass," then "Push car") after independent responding occurred for the first instruction. They intermixed the two instructions after observing accurate responding with each instruction in isolation. They introduced a new verb instruction with the first trained noun and later intermixed it with the previously taught verb instruction (e.g., "Drop glass" vs. "Push glass"). Training continued with other nouns until responding was accurate with all 12 nouns for both verb instructions. They trained novel verbs by using the same procedure.

Other researchers have extended recombinative generalization to more complex forms of instruction following and accompanying grammatical verbal phrases describing actions (e.g., Frampton, Wymer, Hansen, & Shillingsburg, 2016; Goldstein & Mousetis, 1989) and reading skills and spelling (Mueller et al., 2000; Saunders, O'Donnell, Vaidya, & Williams, 2003). See Goldstein (1984), Saunders (2011), and Wetherby and Striefel (1978) for a more complete discussion of research on recombinative generalization and its potential value in understanding the development of complex behavior and guiding teaching programs.

Studies on the recombination of stimulus–response units (instruction following) with nonvocal children with intellectual developmental disorder may suggest a model for understanding the development of generalized imitation. Baer et al. (1967) taught imitation of several different behaviors to three children with intellectual developmental disorder. The children imitated novel behaviors after training, and they demonstrated generalized imitation. The researchers discussed these phenomena in terms of behavior similarity and response classes. However, the similarity interpretation acknowledges that the similarity only occurs for a third person who observes both the response modeled by the training and the imitative response of the child. From the perspective of the child learning to imitate, little similarity exists between the modeled stimuli and the child's response, because the child only observes the model's behavior. In fact, a more recent study found that allowing the child to observe him- or herself using a mirror during imitation training might facilitate acquisition of imitation skills (Miller, Rodriguez, & Rourke, 2015).

In a sense, imitation training is another instruction-following task. However, the instructional stimuli are visual rather than auditory. Siegel and Spradlin (1978) speculated that generalized imitation might involve a similar process to that demonstrated by Striefel et al. (1976); that is, children learn individual components and then recombine them when they imitate a novel motor response after receiving imitation training with specific motor responses. Siegel and Spradlin noted that 21 of the 131 motor imitations taught to a student, who required the most exemplars before showing generalized imitations, involved the action of tapping. They suggested that the student might tap new objects or body parts without additional training after they taught him to tap a few objects or body parts. In addition, the researchers suggested that generalized imitation occurs only for models in the general training domain (e.g., vocal, motor). Therefore, children may not imitate fine motor movements if training involves following gross motor movements, and children may not imitate vocal models if training involves nonvocal motor movements.

## SOME CONCLUDING REMARKS

Nearly every act throughout the day requires some sort of stimulus discrimination, and teaching each discrimination by direct reinforcement would be an impossible task. Yet we make many discriminations throughout the day, which allow us to respond appropriately in a complex world. The pages of this chapter perhaps provide a less puzzling account of the acquisition of such a vast repertoire of discriminations. In our discussion of simple successive discriminations, we have noted that even though we might condition a single stimulus to control a response, other, physically similar stimuli could also control that response. Fulton and Spradlin's (1971) research on auditory stimulus control demonstrated that if a student learns to press a button in response to a 500-Hertz, 70-decibel tone, pressing the button also may occur in response to

tones with other frequencies and volumes. Hence extending the stimulus control across a total range of frequencies and volumes accessible to human hearing is easy. Therefore, more learning occurs than what we teach directly even in simple successive discriminations. However, the equivalence paradigm provides even more examples of how an extensive repertoire of discriminations can emerge from very little teaching. In the hypothetical number example, researchers only teach three conditional discriminations before the nine additional conditional discriminations, and potentially three stimuli names emerge. Saunders, Wachter, et al. (1988) taught seven conditional discriminations, and a total repertoire of 56 conditional discriminations emerged. In other words, they taught seven conditional discriminations, and 49 emerged.

Recombinative generalization provides an additional example of how a little training produces an extensive repertoire. Striefel et al. (1976) taught 31 noun–verb instructions to a student with intellectual developmental disorder, and 113 emerged without training. The recombination of letter–sound units makes it possible for students to respond appropriately to almost any new printed English word after being taught only a limited number of letter–sound units. Kohler and Malott (2014) recently replicated these finding with children with autism spectrum disorder.

In short, research on primary stimulus generalization, stimulus equivalence, and recombinative generalization provides examples of how behavioral repertoires are acquired rapidly and suggests methods for the effective teaching of such vast repertoires.

## ACKNOWLEDGMENTS

We wish to acknowledge the support of the Schiefelbusch Institute for Life Span Studies and the Department of Applied Behavioral Science of the University of Kansas. We also want to thank Pat White for superb editorial assistance.

## REFERENCES

Alexander, J. L., Ayres, K. M., Smith, K. A., Shepley, S. B., & Mataras, T. K. (2013). Using video modeling on an iPad to teach generalized matching on a sorting mail task to adolescents with autism. *Research in Autism Spectrum Disorders, 7*(11), 1346–1357.

Baer, D. M. (1982). Applied behavioral analysis. In C. T. Wilson & C. M. Franks (Eds.), *Contemporary behavior therapy* (pp. 277–309). New York: Guilford Press.

Baer, D. M., Peterson, R. F., & Sherman, J. A. (1967). The development of imitation by reinforcing behavioral similarity to a model. *Journal of the Experimental Analysis of Behavior, 10,* 405–416.

Barnes, D., & Keenan, M. (1993). A transfer of functions through derived arbitrary and nonarbitrary stimulus relations. *Journal of the Experimental Analysis of Behavior, 59,* 61–81.

Blough, D. S. (1966). The study of animal sensory processes by operant methods. In W. K. Honig (Ed.), *Operant behavior: Areas of research and application* (pp. 345–379). New York: Appleton-Century-Crofts.

Bradley-Johnson, S., Sunderman, P., & Johnson, C. M. (1983). Comparison of delayed prompting and fading for teaching preschoolers easily confused letters and numbers. *Journal of School Psychology, 21,* 327–335.

Bush, K. M., Sidman, M., & de Rose, T. (1989). Contextual control of emergent equivalence relations. *Journal of the Experimental Analysis of Behavior, 51,* 29–45.

Carr, D. (2003). Effects of exemplar training in exclusion responding on auditory–visual discrimination tasks with children with autism. *Journal of Applied Behavior Analysis, 36,* 507–524.

Charlop, M. H., Schreibman, L., & Thibodeau, M. G. (1985). Increasing spontaneous verbal responding in autistic children using a time delay procedure. *Journal of Applied Behavior Analysis, 18,* 155–166.

Charlop, M. H., & Walsh, M. E. (1986). Increasing autistic children's spontaneous verbalizations of affection: An assessment of time delay and peer modeling procedures. *Journal of Applied Behavior Analysis, 19,* 307–314.

Constantine, B., & Sidman, M. (1975). The role of naming in delayed matching to sample. *American Journal of Mental Deficiency, 79,* 680–689.

Cowley, B. J., Green, G., & Braunling-McMorrow, D. (1992). Using stimulus equivalence procedures to teach name–face matching to adults with brain injuries. *Journal of Applied Behavior Analysis, 25,* 461–475.

de Rose, J. C., de Souza, D. G., & Hanna, E. S. (1996). Teaching reading and spelling: Exclusion and stimulus equivalence. *Journal of Applied Behavior Analysis, 29,* 451–469.

de Rose, J. C., de Souza, D. G., Rossito, A. L., & de Rose, T. M. S. (1992). Stimulus equivalence and generalization in reading after matching to sample by exclusion. In S. C. Hayes & L. J. Hayes (Eds.), *Understanding verbal relations* (pp. 69–82). Reno, NV: Context Press.

DeSouza, A. A., Akers, J. S., & Fisher, W. W. (2017). Empirical application of Skinner's verbal behavior to interventions for children with autism: A review. *Analysis of Verbal Behavior, 33,* 229–259.

Dickerson, D. S., & Girardeau, F. L. (1971). Oddity preference by mental retardates. *Journal of Experimental Child Psychology, 10,* 28–32.

Dinsmoor, J. A. (1995a). Stimulus control: Part 1. *Behavior Analyst, 18,* 51–68.

Dinsmoor, J. A. (1995b). Stimulus control: Part 2. *Behavior Analyst, 18,* 253–269.

Dixon, L. S. (1977). The nature of control by spoken words over visual stimulus selection. *Journal of the Experimental Analysis of Behavior, 29,* 433–442.

Dougher, M. J., Auguston, E. M., Markham, M. R., Wulfert, E., & Greenway, D. E. (1994). The transfer of respondent eliciting and extinction functions through stimulus equivalence classes. *Journal of the Experimental Analysis of Behavior, 62,* 331–351.

Dube, W. V., Iennaco, F. M., & McIlvane, W. J. (1993). Generalized identity matching to sample of two-dimensional forms in individuals with intellectual disabilities. *Research in Developmental Disabilities, 14,* 457–477.

Dube, W. V., & McIlvane, W. J. (1995). Stimulus–reinforcer relations and emergent matching to sample. *Psychological Record, 45,* 591–612.

Edwards, T. L., La Londe, K. B., Cox, C., Weetjens, B., & Poling, A. (2016). Effects of schedules of reinforcement on pouched rats' performance in urban search-and-rescue training. *Journal of Applied Behavior Analysis, 49,* 199–204.

Ellis, N. R., & Sloan, W. (1959). Oddity learning as a function of mental age. *Journal of Comparative and Physiological Psychology, 52,* 228–230.

Engelmann, S., & Carnine, D. (1982). *Theory of instruction: Principles and applications.* New York: Irvington.

Farber, R. S., Dube, W. V., & Dickson, C. A. (2016). A sorting-to-matching method to teach compound matching to sample. *Journal of Applied Behavior Analysis, 49,* 294–307.

Ferster, C. B., & Perrott, M. C. (1968). *Behavior principles.* New York: New Century.

Fields, L., Matneja, P., Varelas, A., Belanich, J., Fitzer, A., & Shamoun, K. (2002). The formation of linked perceptual classes. *Journal of the Experimental Analysis of Behavior, 78,* 271–290.

Fields, L., & Reeve, K. F. (2001). A methodological integration of generalized equivalence classes, natural categories, and crossmodal perception. *Psychological Record, 51,* 67–87.

Fields, L., & Verhave, T. (1987). The structure of equivalence classes. *Journal of the Experimental Analysis of Behavior, 48,* 317–332.

Fields, L., & Verhave, T. (1990). The effects of nodality on the formation of equivalence classes. *Journal of the Experimental Analysis of Behavior, 53,* 345–358.

Fisher, W. W., Greer, B. D., Fuhrman, A. M., & Querim, A. C. (2015). Using multiple schedules during functional communication training to promote rapid transfer of treatment effects. *Journal of Applied Behavior Analysis, 48,* 713–733.

Frampton, S. E., Wymer, S. C., Hansen, B., & Shillingsburg, M. A. (2016). The use of matrix training to promote generative language with children with autism. *Journal of Applied Behavior Analysis, 49,* 869–883.

Fulton, R. T., & Spradlin, J. E. (1971). Operant audiometry with severely retarded children. *Audiology, 10,* 203–211.

Galizio, M., Stewart, K. L., & Pilgrim, C. (2004). Typicality effects in contingency-shaped generalization classes. *Journal of the Experimental Analysis of Behavior, 82,* 253–273.

Gast, D. L., Ault, M. J., Wolery, M., Doyle, P. M., & Belanger, S. (1988). Comparison of constant delay and the system of least prompts in teaching sight word reading to students with moderate retardation. *Education and Training in Mental Retardation, 23,* 117–128.

Gast, D. L., VanBiervliet, A., & Spradlin, J. E. (1979). Teaching number–word equivalences: A study of transfer. *American Journal of Mental Deficiency, 83,* 524–527.

Goldstein, H. (1984). Enhancing language generalization using matrix and stimulus equivalence training. In S. F. Warren & A. K. Rogers-Warren (Eds.), *Teaching functional language* (Vol. 9, pp. 225–249). Baltimore: University Park Press.

Goldstein, H., & Mousetis, L. (1989). Generalized language learning by children with severe mental retardation: Effects of peers' expressive modeling. *Journal of Applied Behavior Analysis, 22,* 245–259.

Grow, L. L., Carr, J. E., Kodak, T. M., Jostad, C. M., & Kisamore, A. N. (2011). A comparison of methods for teaching receptive labeling to children with autism spectrum disorders. *Journal of Applied Behavior Analysis, 44,* 475–498.

Grow, L. L., Kodak, T. M., & Carr, J. E. (2014). A comparison of methods for teaching receptive labeling to children with autism spectrum disorders: A systematic replication. *Journal of Applied Behavior Analysis, 47,* 600–605.

Halle, J. W., Baer, D. M., & Spradlin, J. E. (1981). Teachers' generalized use of delay as a stimulus control procedure to increase language use in handicapped children. *Journal of Applied Behavior Analysis, 14,* 398–409.

Halle, J. W., Marshall, A. M., & Spradlin, J. E. (1979). Time delay: A technique to increase language use and facilitate generalization in retarded children. *Journal of Applied Behavior Analysis, 12,* 431–439.

Handen, B. J., & Zane, T. (1987). Delayed prompting: A review of procedural variations and results. *Research in Developmental Disabilities, 8,* 307–330.

Harlow, H. F. (1949). The formation of learning sets. *Psychological Review, 56,* 51–65.

Hayes, S. C. (1991). A relational control theory of stimulus equivalence. In L. J. Hayes & P. N. Chase (Eds.), *Dialogues on verbal behavior* (pp. 19–40). Reno, NV: Context Press.

Hayes, S. C., Barnes-Holmes, D., & Roche, B. (Eds.). (2001). *Relational frame theory: A post-Skinnerian account of language and cognition.* New York: Kluwer Academic/Plenum.

Horne, P. J., & Lowe, C. F. (1996). On the origins of naming and other symbolic behavior. *Journal of the Experimental Analysis of Behavior, 65,* 185–241.

Jenkins, H. M., & Harrison, R. H. (1960). Effects of discrimination training on auditory generalization. *Journal of Experimental Psychology, 59,* 246–253.

Knight, M. G., Ross, D. E., Taylor, R. L., & Ramasamy, R. (2003). Constant time delay and interspersal of known items to teach sight words to students with mental retardation and learning disabilities. *Education and Training in Developmental Disabilities, 38,* 179–191.

Kohler, K. T., & Malott, R. W. (2014). Matrix training and verbal generativity in children with autism. *Analysis of Verbal Behavior, 30*(2), 170–177.

Landa, R., & Hanley, G. P. (2016). An evaluation of multiple-schedule variations to reduce high-rate requests in the picture exchange communication system. *Journal of Applied Behavior Analysis, 49,* 388–393.

Leaf, J. B., Townley-Cochran, D., Mitchell, E., Milne, C., Alcalay, A., Leaf, J., et al. (2016). Evaluation of multiple-alternative prompts during tact training. *Journal of Applied Behavior Analysis, 49,* 399–404.

Macht, J. (1971). Operant measurement of subjective visual acuity in nonverbal children. *Journal of Applied Behavior Analysis, 4,* 23–36.

Mackay, H. A. (1985). Stimulus equivalence in rudimentary reading and spelling. *Analysis and Intervention in Developmental Disabilities, 5,* 373–387.

Mackay, H. A., Stoddard, L. T., & Spencer, T. J. (1989). Symbols and meaning classes: Multiple sequence production and the emergence of ordinal stimulus classes. *Experimental Analysis of Human Behavior Bulletin, 7,* 16–17.

Marchese, N. V., Carr, J. E., LeBlanc, L. A., Rosati, T. C., & Conroy, S. A. (2012). The effects of the question "What is this?" on tact-training outcomes of children with autism. *Journal of Applied Behavior Analysis, 45,* 539–547.

McIlvane, W. J., Kledaras, J. B., Lowry, M. W., & Stoddard, L. T. (1992). Studies of exclusion in individuals with severe mental retardation. *Research in Developmental Disabilities, 13,* 509–532.

McIlvane, W. J., & Stoddard, L. T. (1981). Acquisition of matching-to-sample performances in severe mental retardation: Learning by exclusion. *Journal of Mental Deficiency Research, 25,* 33–48.

McIlvane, W. J., & Stoddard, L. T. (1985). Complex stimulus relations and exclusion in mental retardation. *Analysis and Intervention in Developmental Disabilities, 5,* 307–321.

McLay, L. K., Sutherland, D., Church, J., & Tyler-Merrick, G. (2013). The formation of equivalence classes in individuals with autism spectrum disorder: A review of the literature. *Research in Autism Spectrum Disorders, 7*(2), 418–431.

Medin, D. L., & Smith, E. E. (1984). Concepts and concept formation. *Annual Reviews of Psychology, 35,* 113–138.

Miller, S. A., Rodriguez, N. M., & Rourke, A. J. (2015). Do mirrors facilitate acquisition of motor imitation in children diagnosed with autism? *Journal of Applied Behavior Analysis, 48,* 194–198.

Mueller, M., Olmi, J., & Saunders, K. J. (2000). Recombinative generalization of within-syllable units in prereading children. *Journal of Applied Behavior Analysis, 33,* 515–531.

Oppenheimer, M., Saunders, R. R., & Spradlin, J. E. (1993). Investigating the generality of the delayed-prompt effect. *Research in Developmental Disabilities, 14,* 425–444.

Peterson, R. F. (1968). Some experiments on the organization of a class of imitative behaviors. *Journal of Applied Behavior Analysis, 1,* 225–235.

Pilgrim, C., & Galizio, M. (1990). Relations between baseline contingencies and equivalence probe performances. *Journal of the Experimental Analysis of Behavior, 54,* 213–224.

Reese, H. W. (1972). Acquired distinctiveness and equivalence of cues in young children. *Journal of Experimental Child Psychology, 13,* 171–182.

Rehfeldt, R. A. (2011). Toward a technology of derived stimulus relations: An analysis of articles published in the *Journal of Applied Behavior Analysis,* 1992–2009. *Journal of Applied Behavior Analysis, 44,* 109–119.

Rosch, E. H. (1973). Natural categories. *Cognitive Psychology, 4,* 328–350.

Saunders, K. J. (2011). Designing instructional programming for early reading skills. In W. W. Fisher, C. C. Piazza, & H. S. Roane (Eds.), *Handbook of applied behavior analysis* (pp. 92–109). New York: Guilford Press.

Saunders, K. J., Johnson, M. D., Tompkins, B. F., Dutcher, D. L., & Williams, D. C. (1997). Generalized identity matching of two-dimensional forms by individuals with moderate to profound mental retardation. *American Journal of Mental Retardation, 102,* 285–291.

Saunders, K. J., O'Donnell, J., Vaidya, M., & Williams, D. C. (2003). Recombinative generalization of within-syllable units in non-reading adults with mental retardation. *Journal of Applied Behavior Analysis, 36,* 95–99.

Saunders, K. J., & Spradlin, J. E. (1993). Conditional discrimination in mentally retarded subjects: Programming acquisition and learning set. *Journal of the Experimental Analysis of Behavior, 60,* 571–585.

Saunders, K. J., Williams, D. C., & Spradlin, J. E. (1995). Conditional discrimination by adults with mental retardation: Establishing relations between physically identical stimuli. *American Journal on Mental Retardation, 99,* 558–563.

Saunders, R. R., & Green, G. (1992). The nonequivalence of behavioral and mathematical equivalence. *Journal of the Experimental Analysis of Behavior, 57,* 227–241.

Saunders, R. R., Saunders, K. J., Kirby, K. C., & Spradlin, J. E. (1988). The merger and development of equivalence classes by unreinforced conditional selection of comparison stimuli. *Journal of the Experimental Analysis of Behavior, 50,* 145–162.

Saunders, R. R., & Sherman, J. A. (1986). Analysis of the "discrimination failure hypothesis" in generalized matching and mismatching behavior. *Analysis and Intervention in Developmental Disabilities, 6,* 89–107.

Saunders, R. R., Wachter, J., & Spradlin, J. E. (1988). Establishing auditory stimulus control over an eight-member equivalence class via conditional discrimination procedures. *Journal of the Experimental Analysis of Behavior, 49,* 95–115.

Serna, R. W., Dube, W. V., & McIlvane, W. J. (1997). Assessing same/different judgments in individuals with severe intellectual disabilities: A status report. *Research in Developmental Disabilities, 18,* 342–368.

Sidman, M. (1971). Reading and auditory–visual equivalences. *Journal of Speech and Hearing Research, 14,* 5–13.

Sidman, M. (1994). *Equivalence relations and behavior: A research story.* Boston: Authors Cooperative.

Sidman, M. (2000). Equivalence relations and the reinforcement contingency. *Journal of the Experimental Analysis of Behavior, 74,* 127–146.

Sidman, M., Cresson, O., Jr., & Willson-Morris, M. (1974). Acquisition of matching to sample via mediated transfer. *Journal of the Experimental Analysis of Behavior, 22,* 261–273.

Sidman, M., Kirk, B., & Willson-Morris, M. (1985). Six-member stimulus classes generated by conditional-discrimination procedures. *Journal of the Experimental Analysis of Behavior, 43,* 21–42.

Sidman, M., & Stoddard, L. T. (1967). The effectiveness of fading in programming a simultaneous form discrimination for retarded children. *Journal of the Experimental Analysis of Behavior, 10,* 3–15.

Sidman, M., & Tailby, W. (1982). Conditional discrimination vs. matching-to-sample: An expansion of the testing paradigm. *Journal of the Experimental Analysis of Behavior, 37,* 5–22.

Siegel, G. M., & Spradlin, J. E. (1978). Programming for language and communication therapy. In R. L. Schiefelbusch (Ed.), *Language intervention strategies* (pp. 357–398). Baltimore: University Park Press.

Sigurdardottir, Z. G., Green, G., & Saunders, R. R. (1990). Equivalence classes generated by sequence training. *Journal of the Experimental Analysis of Behavior, 53,* 47–63.

Skinner, B. F. (1938). *The behavior of organisms.* New York: Appleton-Century-Crofts.

Smeets, P. M., & Striefel, S. (1974). Oddity and match-to-sample tasks as the components of a chained schedule with retarded children. *American Journal of Mental Deficiency, 4,* 462–470.

Smeets, P. M., & Striefel, S. (1994). A revised blocked-trial procedure for establishing arbitrary matching in children. *Quarterly Journal of Experimental Psychology, 47B,* 241–261.

Soraci, S. A., Jr., Deckner, C. W., Haenlein, M., Baumeister, A. A., Murata-Soraci, K., & Blanton, R. L. (1987). Oddity performance in preschool children at risk for mental retardation: Transfer and maintenance. *Research in Developmental Disabilities, 8,* 137–151.

Spradlin, J. E., Cotter, V. W., & Baxley, N. (1973). Establishing a conditional discrimination without direct training: A study of transfer with retarded adolescents. *American Journal of Mental Deficiency, 77,* 556–566.

Spradlin, J. E., & Saunders, R. R. (1986). The development of stimulus classes using match-to-sample procedures: Sample classification versus comparison classification. *Analysis and Intervention in Developmental Disabilities, 6,* 41–58.

Stewart, I., McElwee, J., & Ming, S. (2013). Language generativity, response generalization, and derived relational responding. *Analysis of Verbal Behavior, 29,* 137–155.

Stoddard, L. T., Brown, J., Hurlbert, B., Manoli, C., & McIlvane, W. J. (1989). Teaching money skills through stimulus class formation, exclusion, and component matching methods: Three case studies. *Research in Developmental Disabilities, 10,* 413–439.

Stokes, T. F., & Baer, D. M. (1977). An implicit technology of generalization. *Journal of Applied Behavior Analysis, 10,* 349–367.

Striefel, S., Wetherby, B., & Karlan, G. R. (1976). Establishing generative verb–noun instruction-following skills in retarded children. *Journal of Experimental Child Psychology, 22,* 247–260.

Striefel, S., Wetherby, B., & Karlan, G. R. (1978). Developing generalized instruction-following behavior in severely retarded people. In C. E. Meyers (Ed.), *Quality of life in severely and profoundly mentally retarded people: Research foundations for improvement* (Vol. 3, pp. 267–326). Washington, DC: American Association on Mental Deficiency.

Stromer, R., & Mackay, H. A. (1992). Delayed constructed–response identity matching improves the spelling performance of students with mental retardation. *Journal of Behavioral Education, 2,* 139–156.

Stromer, R., & Stromer, J. B. (1989). Children's identity matching and oddity: Assessing control by specific and general sample-comparison relations. *Journal of the Experimental Analysis of Behavior, 51,* 47–64.

Stromer, R., & Stromer, J. B. (1990a). The formation of arbitrary stimulus classes in matching to complex samples. *Psychological Record, 41,* 51–66.

Stromer, R., & Stromer, J. B. (1990b). Matching to complex samples: Further study of arbitrary stimulus classes. *Psychological Record, 40,* 505–516.

Terrace, H. S. (1966). Stimulus control. In W. K. Honig (Ed.), *Operant behavior: Areas of research and application* (pp. 271–344). New York: Appleton–Century–Crofts.

Touchette, P. E. (1971). Transfer of stimulus control: Measuring the moment of transfer. *Journal of the Experimental Analysis of Behavior, 15,* 347–354.

Touchette, P. E., & Howard, J. S. (1984). Errorless learning: Reinforcement contingencies and stimulus control transfer in delayed prompting. *Journal of Applied Behavior Analysis, 17,* 175–188.

Urcuioli, P. J. (2013). Stimulus control and stimulus class formation. In G. J. Madden, W. V. Dube, T. D. Hackenberg, G. P. Hanley, & K. A. Lattal (Eds.), *APA handbook of behavior analysis* (Vol. 1, pp. 361–386). Washington, DC: American Psychological Association.

VanBiervliet, A. (1977). Establishing words and objects as functionally equivalent through manual sign training. *American Journal of Mental Deficiency, 82,* 178–186.

Wetherby, B., Karlan, G. R., & Spradlin, J. E. (1983). The development of derived stimulus relations through training in arbitrary-matching sequences. *Journal of the Experimental Analysis of Behavior, 40,* 69–78.

Wetherby, B., & Striefel, S. (1978). Application of miniature linguistic system or matrix-training procedures. In R. L. Schiefelbusch (Ed.), *Language intervention strategies* (pp. 317–356). Baltimore: University Park Press.

Wilkinson, K. M., & Green, G. (1998). Implications of fast mapping for vocabulary expansion in individuals with mental retardation. *Augmentative and Alternative Communication, 14,* 162–170.

Wilkinson, K. M., & McIlvane, W. J. (1994). Stimulus organization and learning by exclusion: A preliminary experimental analysis. *Experimental Analysis of Human Behavior Bulletin, 12,* 21–25.

Wultz, S. V., & Hollis, J. H. (1980). Word identification and comprehension training for exceptional children. In R. L. Schiefelbusch (Ed.), *Nonspeech language and communication: Analysis and intervention* (pp. 359–387). Baltimore: University Park Press.

Wunderlich, K. L., Vollmer, T. R., Donaldson, J. M., & Phillips, C. L. (2014). Effects of serial and concurrent training on acquisition and generalization. *Journal of Applied Behavior Analysis, 47,* 1–15.

Zinn, T. E., Newland, M. C., & Ritchie, K. E. (2015). The efficiency and efficacy of equivalence-based learning: A randomized controlled trial. *Journal of Applied Behavior Analysis, 48,* 865–882.

# CHAPTER 6

# Matching and Behavioral Momentum
## Quantifying Choice and Persistence

Christopher A. Podlesnik, Corina Jimenez-Gomez,
and Michael E. Kelley

The matching law and behavioral momentum theory are quantitative theoretical frameworks developed to understand how reinforcement affects behavior. The matching law describes how changes in relative reinforcement variables influence the allocation of operant behavior or choice. Behavioral momentum theory asserts that the matching law governs the allocation of operant behavior, but proposes that Pavlovian processes govern the persistence of behavior. This chapter describes matching and behavioral momentum as quantitative frameworks for understanding variables influencing behavior. We also discuss their implications for behavioral treatments.

The primary goal of behavioral science is to identify systematic relations between environmental events and behavior (e.g., Nevin, 1984). Essentially, one asks how changing something in the environment (i.e., the independent variable) affects behavior (i.e., the dependent variable). Reinforcement is one of the primary tools of environmental change that applied behavior analysts use to effect behavior change. Contingencies between behavior and reinforcement can have powerful effects, as demonstrated by the many ways behavior analysts use it in treatments to increase desirable behavior and decrease problem behavior.

With all the ways practitioners might manipulate reinforcement contingencies, those contingencies can influence behavior in complex ways. In some cases, the immediate effects of contingencies differ from long-term effects. To address these different effects of reinforcement, the purpose of the present chapter is to describe research showing how reinforcement contingencies affect (1) the *allocation* of behavior, (2) the *persistence* of behavior, and (3) the allocation and persistence of behavior *in different and perhaps counterintuitive ways*. Thus we will argue that behavior analysts should attend to both the allocation and persistence of behavior, which they can understand through two distinct but related areas of research. Research on choice and the matching law provides insight into the variables influencing the allocation of behavior. Research on persistence and behavioral momentum theory provides insight into variables influencing both the allocation and persistence of behavior. The literature on the matching law and behavioral momentum are extensive, and the present review is quite selective and directed toward introducing these areas.[1]

---

[1] Those interested in a contemporary theoretical integration of choice and persistence should find the framework described by Shahan and Craig (2017) informative.

# RESPONSE ALLOCATION, CHOICE, AND THE MATCHING LAW

The job of applied behavior analysts is to alter the allocation of behavior by increasing desirable behavior and decreasing problematic behavior. The most commonly used behavioral treatment, differential reinforcement of alternative behavior (DRA), reduces or eliminates reinforcement contingent on problem behavior and provides functionally equivalent reinforcement for an alternative behavior (Petscher, Rey, & Bailey, 2009). Because these techniques are so frequently used, precisely understanding how reinforcement variables determine the allocation of behavior is extremely important for applied researchers and practitioners. Research on choice, including theoretical work on the matching law and related frameworks, provides equations for describing, explaining, or describing and explaining how the behavioral processes underlying reinforcement contingencies determine the allocation of behavior. Before introducing these equations, however, we describe findings that provide general support that behavior allocation tracks reinforcement in clinical settings.

Borrero et al. (2010) assessed whether the allocation of functionally equivalent problem and appropriate behavior would follow the allocation of reinforcement in a clinical situation. Three individuals diagnosed with intellectual developmental disorder engaged in severe problem behavior in either hospital or school settings. Functional analyses (Iwata, Dorsey, Slifer, Bauman, & Richman, 1982/1994) identified the reinforcers maintaining the problem behavior (e.g., attention, escape from demands, tangibles). The researchers provided these reinforcers intermittently contingent on problem and appropriate behavior. In doing so, Borrero et al. assessed whether the rates of the two behaviors precisely matched the changes in the allocation of reinforcement between problem and appropriate behavior. That is, as the reinforcement rate for problem behavior increased relative to appropriate behavior, did problem behavior similarly increase relative to appropriate behavior and vice versa?

Borrero et al. (2010) arranged two independent and concurrently available variable-interval (VI) reinforcement schedules for the two behaviors to determine whether problem and appropriate behavior closely tracked changes in relative reinforcement rate. VI schedules present reinforcers for the first response after an average duration elapses (e.g., 60 seconds). However, the availability of those reinforcers varies in time from one reinforcer to the next, with an unpredictable duration between reinforcer availability. Thus some reinforcers become available only moments after the previous reinforcer, and others after a longer time. Importantly, VI schedules allow for the obtained reinforcement rates to approximate the arranged reinforcement rates, which is important when reinforcement rate is the primary independent variable, as is commonly the case in these kinds of choice studies (see Davison & McCarthy, 1988). Reinforcers for problem and alternative behaviors in Borrero et al. consisted of 30 seconds of access to the reinforcer demonstrated to maintain problem behavior during functional analyses.

Borrero et al. (2010) arranged 10-minute sessions with the concurrent VI VI schedules of reinforcement for problem and appropriate behavior. They manipulated the relative reinforcement rates for problem and alternative behavior across successive conditions, with each condition maintaining a constant reinforcement rate for numerous sessions (i.e., between 3 and 20 sessions). When the investigators programmed higher reinforcement rates for problem behavior (e.g., VI 20 seconds) than for alternative behavior (e.g., VI 60 seconds), rates of problem behavior tended to be higher than rates of alternative behavior. Conversely, when Borrero et al. arranged a greater reinforcement rate for alternative behavior than for problem behavior, rates of alternative behavior increased, and rates of problem behavior decreased. These findings showed that changes in the relative reinforcement rates for problem and appropriate behavior determined the participants' allocation to each behavior. Thus the rate of each response depended on the reinforcement rate for that response (e.g., problem behavior) and on the reinforcement rate for the other response (e.g., appropriate behavior). The implication is that behavior in treatment situations is related positively to the reinforcement schedule for that response and negatively related to the reinforcement schedule for other responses. The degree of treatment success depends not only on reinforcement allocated to the target response, but on the allocation of reinforcement to all potential responses in a situation.

At this point, some readers might ask what the use is of providing reinforcement for problem behavior when any treatment will attempt to eliminate problem behavior by eliminating its reinforcement (i.e., extinction). Moreover, readers also might wonder about the relevance of not reinforcing every instance of appropriate behavior. In routine clinical settings (e.g., homes), caregivers might inadvertently reinforce instances of problem behavior and not reinforce instances of appropriate behavior (Athens & Vollmer, 2010). Therefore, these methods of arranging intermittent reinforcement of problem and appropriate behavior simulate situations in which treatment integrity is compromised (St. Peter Pipkin, Vollmer, & Sloman, 2010).

These methods also promote understanding of how reinforcement processes influence the allocation of problem and appropriate behavior. After all, the variables that influence behavioral phenomena do so at the level of fundamental processes. Any treatment or corresponding decrease in treatment integrity affects clients' behavior at the level of behavioral processes, which is the level at which studies of choice and quantitative analyses, beginning with the matching law, become relevant.

## THE STRICT MATCHING LAW

The findings of Borrero et al. (2010) fit not only with the general notion that reinforcement influences clinically relevant behavior, but also with quantitative assessments of choice behavior. Specifically, the proportion of responding allocated between problem behavior ($B_1$) and appropriate behavior ($B_2$) approximately matched the proportion of reinforcement allocated between problem behavior ($R_1$) and appropriate behavior ($R_2$). Figure 6.1 shows an idealized version of such findings, to which we refer as we go along. As $R_1$ increased

relative to $R_2$, $B_1$ increased relative to $B_2$, as described by Equation 1:

$$\frac{B_1}{B_1 + B_2} = \frac{R_1}{R_1 + R_2} \qquad (1)$$

Herrnstein (1961) introduced Equation 1 to describe pigeons' choices in situations resembling those arranged by Borrero et al. (2010). Specifically, pigeons pecked between two lighted keys, with food reinforcement concurrently available on VI VI schedules (i.e., $R_1$ vs. $R_2$) that changed across conditions. Parametric manipulations of relative reinforcement rates (i.e., across a range of different levels of the independent variable) produced proportional rates of behavior that approximately matched the obtained relative reinforcement rates; these findings were generally consistent with Figure 6.1. Thus Borrero et al.'s findings in a clinical setting resembled those with pigeons in a controlled laboratory setting.

Equation 1 suggests that both the rate of reinforcement for the target response and the rate of reinforcement for other responses controls the rate of the target behavior. The effects of a given reinforcement rate ($R_1$) depend on the context of other concurrently available sources of reinforcement. Response rates might be high or low, depending on whether an alternative source of reinforcement is low or high, respectively (e.g., Findley, 1958; Herrnstein, 1961, 1970).

## THE QUANTITATIVE LAW OF EFFECT

$R_2$ is the only alternative source of reinforcement for which Equation 1 accounts. Nevertheless, most environments will include multiple sources of reinforcement; even in experimental situations, there are likely to be sources of reinforcement other than those arranged explicitly. For a pigeon in a largely barren operant chamber, these might include reinforcers for grooming or tending to other bodily functions. Humans might whistle or daydream. Under natural conditions, the possible alternative sources of reinforcement are endless. Herrnstein's important insight was that even simple schedules of reinforcement—situations with only one explicitly arranged reinforcement schedule—necessarily involve choice between the scheduled source of reinforcement and all other sources of reinforcement. That is, organisms choose whether to engage in the target response or in an undefined number of other responses.

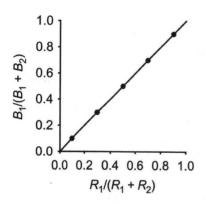

**FIGURE 6.1.** The basic matching relation predicted from Equation 1. The equation predicts that the proportion of responses ($B$) should equal the proportion of reinforcers ($R$).

Herrnstein (1970) built upon Equation 1 to quantify the effect of alternative sources of reinforcement in his quantitative law of effect:

$$B = \frac{kR}{R + R_e} \qquad (2)$$

In this equation, $B$ is the absolute response rate for a target response, $R$ is the contingent reinforcement rate, $k$ is a parameter representing maximal asymptotic response rates, and $R_e$ represents the rate of alternative reinforcement *not* contingent on the target response. Equation 2 states that $B$ is a hyperbolic function of the reinforcement rate, $R$, but that the rate in which $B$ increases with $R$ depends on alternative sources of reinforcement.

Figure 6.2 shows three hyperbolic functions resulting from Equation 2. Equation 2 would be fitted to a range of response rates plotted as a function of a range of reinforcement rates, as shown in Figure 6.2. $R_e$ and $k$ are free parameters determined by using nonlinear regression: The equation determines the form of the line, and regression adjusts the free parameters to best fit the data based on the constraints of the equation. Equation 2, fitted to data points generally following a hyperbolic form, involves nonlinear regression reducing the difference between the data and predictions of Equation 2 by adjusting $R_e$ and $k$. In other words, fitting nonlinear regression functions to data obtained experimentally determine the values of the free parameters. All three hypothetical functions in Figure 6.2 have the same maximum or asymptote of 100, which the parameter $k$ represents. Thus the highest possible rate at which the organism can emit this response is 100 per minute. $k$ depends on how rapidly the organism can emit the response; target responses that take longer for the organism to emit will produce a lower $k$ than those the organism can emit rapidly. Easy and difficult responses might include key pecking and lever pressing, respectively, for a pigeon, or addition and multiplication, respectively, for young students.

In Figure 6.2, the three curves approach $k$ at different rates due to differences in $R_e$. Importantly, $R_e$ is in units of reinforcement for the target response, $R$. In a situation in which a child can engage in a free-operant behavior, such as completing math problems for edibles, the availability of toys would be likely to decrease the rate of completing math problems. $R_e$ provides an index of the effectiveness of toy availability in units of the edible reinforcer for completing math problems. In Figure 6.2, an $R_e$ of 1 means that $B$ will reach 50% of $k$ with 1

alternative reinforcer per minute; an $R_e$ of 20 means that $B$ will reach 50% of $k$ with 20 alternative reinforcers per minute. Thus $R_e$ characterizes how alternative reinforcement rates affect target response rates, with greater alternative reinforcement rates slowing the approach of response rates to maximal asymptotic responding as target reinforcement rate increases. Simply speaking, greater rates of reinforcement for alternative behavior will decrease target response rates, as predicted by Equation 1.

Generality in matching relations across situations and species suggests that the allocation of behavior is in lawful relation with the allocation of reinforcement (Baum, 1979; Davison & McCarthy, 1988; Kollins, Newland, & Critchfield, 1997; Wearden & Burgess, 1982; Williams, 1988). Such consistent regularities in the relation between response and reinforcement rate prompted some to suggest that Equation 2 quantifies the behavioral process underlying reinforcement, which traditionally has been response strength (e.g., Skinner, 1938; Herrnstein, 1970). Moreover, these regularities provide justification for behavior analysts to make principled decisions about treatment. For example, these findings perfectly justify the use of DRA treatments that arrange high reinforcement rates for appropriate behavior ($R_2$) and eliminate reinforcement for problem behavior ($R_1$). Equation 1 predicts that such DRA treatments should produce high rates of appropriate behavior and eliminate problem behavior, which is generally consistent with the literature on DRA (Petscher et al., 2009) and demonstrated in later conditions of Borrero et al. (2010). Furthermore, if $R_2$ from Equation 1 quantifies the effect of reinforcement rate for alternative behavior on rate of problem behavior, then $R_e$ from Equation 2 quantifies the

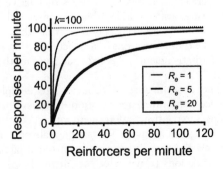

**FIGURE 6.2.** Predictions from Herrnstein's hyperbola (Equation 2), with different free parameters; $k$ is set to 100 with three values of $R_e$.

effect of noncontingent reinforcement (NCR) on the rate of problem behavior in units of target reinforcement rate. In either case, an alternative source of reinforcement decreases problem behavior by providing reinforcement for behavior other than the target response.

Regularities in the relation between independent and dependent variables like those shown in Figures 6.1 and 6.2 allow scientists to evaluate controlling variables to develop a theory. Theories allow scientists to organize findings and develop principled studies testing the adequacy of the theory by examining a range of variables potentially controlling the dependent variable. For these pursuits, we cannot overstate the importance of Herrnstein's (1961, 1970) work; it generated a profound amount of research and theory in the field.

## THE GENERALIZED MATCHING LAW

Researchers call Equation 1 the *strict matching law* because the equation only predicts that the proportion of behavior strictly equals the proportion of reinforcement. Equation 1 makes a very precise prediction, and only one possible data pattern supports the strict matching law. As such, it did not take long after Herrnstein (1961) introduced Equation 1 for studies to prove that it was inadequate in many circumstances (e.g., Baum, 1974, 1979; Davison & McCarthy, 1988; Fantino, Squires, Delbrück, & Peterson, 1972; Staddon, 1968). Inadequacies in the strict matching law set the stage for the development of different approaches for describing and explaining choice. Baum (1974) described two systematic deviations from strict matching relevant to applied-choice situations and to the development of a more adequate description of choice. Specifically, choice behavior often (1) is not perfectly sensitive to changes in relative reinforcement rate and (2) is biased consistently in favor of one reinforced option over another. We describe these deviations from strict matching and a quantitative model proposed to account for them next.

The determinants of behavior are complex. Choice conforming to Equation 1 suggests that changes in relative reinforcement rate accounts for all changes in behavior. This simple state of affairs is rarely the case, even in well-controlled laboratory situations (Davison & McCarthy, 1988). In the previous example, Borrero et al. (2010) observed cases in which changes in relative rates of problem and appropriate behavior changed less than changes in relative reinforcement rates. In addition, they observed cases in which participants' behavior was biased toward either problem or appropriate behavior across all reinforcement ratios. Fortunately, the variables producing deviations from the simple predictions of Equation 1 are becoming understood. To account for deviations from Equation 1, Baum (1974) proposed the *generalized matching law*:

$$\log\left(\frac{B_1}{B_2}\right) = a_r \log\left(\frac{R_1}{R_2}\right) + \log b \qquad (3)$$

Equation 3 is algebraically identical to Equation 1, because the relative rate of behavior ($B_1$ vs. $B_2$) remains a function of changes in the relative rate of reinforcement ($R_1$ vs. $R_2$). The changes from Equation 1 are (1) that Equation 3 is transformed logarithmically to produce a straight line despite deviations from strict matching, and (2) that two free parameters ($a_r$ and log $b$) have been added to characterize deviations from strict matching as changes in the slope and y-intercept of the straight line (Jacobs, Borrero, & Vollmer, 2013; McDowell, 1989; Reed & Kaplan, 2011).

Figure 6.3 shows typical deviations from strict matching and illustrates how Equation 3 characterizes those deviations as changes of the straight line in slope, y-intercept, or both. Specifically, after plotting the log–reinforcement ratios along the x-axis and the log–response ratios along the y-axis, we use linear regression to fit a straight line to the data. This line has a particular slope and y-intercept, given the relation between the ranges of log–response and log–reinforcer ratios. The $a_r$ parameter in Equation 3 is the slope of the line and provides an index of how sensitive the behavior ratio is to changes in the reinforcer ratio. The

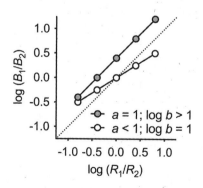

**FIGURE 6.3.** Bias toward $B_1$ (gray points) and undermatching (white points) produced by Equation 3.

log $b$ parameter in Equation 3 is the $y$-intercept of the line and provides an index of bias of the behavior ratio toward one source of reinforcement over another.

If the log–behavior ratios on the $y$-axis approximately equal the log–reinforcement ratios on the $x$-axis, this is strict matching, as the dotted line in Figure 6.3 shows. Log axes represent each 10-fold increase with equal spacing: A ratio of 1:10 equals –1, 1:1 equals 0, 10:1 equals 1, 100:1 equals 2, and so forth. With strict matching, (1) the $a_r$ parameter, indicated by the slope, equals 1; and (2) the log $b$ parameter, indicated by the $y$-intercept, equals 0. The other functions in Figure 6.3 reveal deviations from strict matching. If the range of log–behavior ratios is less than the range of log–reinforcement ratios, the $a$ parameter is less than 1, and log $b$ equals 0 (white data points). We often call this function *undermatching*, because the log–behavior ratios are less extreme than the log–reinforcer ratios. For example, Borrero et al. (2010) arranged 3 times more reinforcement for appropriate behavior than problem behavior in some conditions and vice versa; undermatching would have occurred if the behavior ratio was less than 3 times greater (e.g., only 2:1). A *bias* for $B_1$ occurs if the range of log–behavior ratios spans the same range as log–reinforcement ratios, and the function shifts toward $B_1$ and log $b$ is greater than 0 (gray data points).

Figure 6.3 reveals only two of the most basic deviations from strict matching. Specifically, the slope of the equation can be greater than 1, which is called *overmatching*; the $y$-intercept can be negative (bias for $B_2$); and Equation 3 can describe multiple deviations from strict matching. That is, both slope and $y$-intercept might deviate simultaneously from the dotted line in Figure 6.3 (e.g., $a_r < 1$ and log $b > 1$). When we use Equation 3 to plot deviations from strict matching, changes in slope and $y$-intercept characterize these deviations. Plotting the same data using Equation 1 produces curvilinear functions that are very difficult to characterize intuitively. Thus the added complexity of introducing logarithms with Equation 3 is more than justified by simplifying the data paths and the interpretations and conclusions stemming from them.

Finally, fitting any equation to data requires some assessment of how well the model accounts for the data. This aspect of model fitting can become rather complex because a model fit to data can be less than perfect for multiple reasons. Assessing models involves assessing how much variance in a dataset a model accounts for with measures like $r^2$. An imperfect model fit could be due to random variation in behavior, but a model also could make systematic errors in prediction, thereby indicating that the model makes incorrect assumptions. Another important consideration is whether a model's parameters make sense, and thus whether we can use them to say something meaningful about the variables controlling behavior. That is, do the free parameters reflect a relevant and realistic aspect of behavior, or the environment that guides the endeavors of behavior analysts? These issues are beyond the scope of this chapter, but others have discussed them in detail elsewhere (e.g., Dallery & Soto, 2013; Davison & McCarthy, 1988; Shull, 1991).

Much of our discussion of choice and matching thus far has focused on clarifying how the equation works. Now we discuss which variables can influence choice, how the equation accounts for variables influencing choice, and why an understanding of matching can be useful to behavioral clinicians.

## Variables Affecting Sensitivity

The slope of a function when fitting the generalized matching equation to data expresses sensitivity of choice to reinforcement conditions (Equation 3). In Borrero et al. (2010), one participant, Greg, engaged in problem behavior and appropriate behavior within 1 second of each other when both behaviors produced access to tangibles. The researchers observed that the responses formed a chain, even though they had arranged separate VI schedules for the two responses. That is, the VI schedules did not require the successive emission of both responses to produce reinforcement. In Equation 1, rapid alternation between two responses produces a slope approaching 0, despite parametric changes in relative reinforcement rates. Borrero et al. introduced a 5-second changeover delay to separate the two VI reinforcement schedules for problem and appropriate behavior in time. Introducing the change-over delay successfully increased sensitivity of choice to the different VI schedules (Herrnstein, 1961; Shull & Pliskoff, 1967). In general, researchers believe that changeover delays increase the discriminability between the two concurrently available reinforcement schedules (Davison & Nevin, 1999) and function analogously to increasing the spatial separation between responses (Baum, 1982). Longer duration change-over delays (Shull & Pliskoff, 1967) and more obstructive barriers between responses (e.g., Aparicio & Baum, 1997; Baum, 1982) increase sensitivity to changes in relative reinforcement rates.

Antecedent conditions also can influence sensitivity. An increase in the discriminability between antecedent stimuli that signals the response alternatives also increases sensitivity to changes in relative reinforcement rate (Alsop & Davison, 1991; Miller, Saunders, & Bourland, 1980). When a change-over response controlled pigeons' choices between VI schedules in these studies, greater differences between discriminative stimuli signaling the two VI schedules increased sensitivity to changes in relative reinforcement rate. These findings with change-over requirements and differences in antecedent stimuli suggest that manipulations increasing the discriminability between reinforcement contingencies will increase sensitivity to changes in relative reinforcement rates (Davison & Nevin, 1999; Fisher, Pawich, Dickes, Paden, & Toussaint, 2014).

Lastly, organismic variables influence sensitivity to changes in relative reinforcement rates. For example, Oscar-Berman, Heyman, Bonner, and Ryder (1980) parametrically assessed a range of concurrently available VI schedules of monetary reinforcement between participants with Korsakoff syndrome versus control participants. Relative response rates for participants with Korsakoff syndrome showed less sensitivity to changes in relative reinforcement rates than those of the control participants did. Similarly, Buckley and Rasmussen (2012) assessed matching in two strains of rats: obese and lean Zucker rats. Obese Zucker rats express an obese phenotype and eat more when freely fed than lean Zucker rats. Buckley and Rasmussen found that obese Zucker rats' relative response rates were more sensitive to parametric changes to concurrently available VI schedules of food reinforcement. These findings reveal the usefulness of the sensitivity parameter from Equation 3 for characterizing differences in responsiveness to changes in reinforcement conditions due to organismic variables, such as differences in genes or chronic versus acute drug effects (e.g., Newland, Reile, & Langston, 2004).

## Variables Affecting Bias

The y-intercept of a function when the generalized matching equation is fitted to data expresses bias for one reinforced alternative over others (Equation 3). Thus the log–response ratio remains sensitive to changes in the log–reinforcer ratio, but there is a shift in choice toward one alternative. In Borrero et al. (2010), the relative rate of problem and appropriate behavior with the participant named Greg showed sensitivity to changes in relative reinforcement rates. However, Greg reliably engaged in a higher rate of appropriate behavior than problem behavior than Equation 1 predicted. Thus bias expressed by the y-intercept shifted toward appropriate behavior. Interestingly, escape from demands maintained a different topography of Greg's problem behavior, and relative response rates showed bias toward problem behavior over appropriate behavior. Thus bias can differ between problem and appropriate behaviors, depending on the circumstances—even for the same individual. How does the matching framework inform us about variables producing bias toward one response over another?

The cause of bias for Greg in Borrero et al. (2010) for one response over another might not be clear. It could have been due to differences between problem and appropriate behavior in response variables (e.g., effort) or reinforcer variables, such as magnitude, immediacy, and quality. In these cases, log $b$ in Equation 3 quantifies any inherent bias for one response over another. When we know the differences in response and reinforcement variables, we can expand Equation 3 to account for the effects of variables other than changes in relative reinforcer rate (Baum & Rachlin, 1969; Davison & McCarthy, 1988; Grace & Hucks, 2013; Killeen, 1972):

$$\log\left(\frac{B_1}{B_2}\right) = a_r \log\left(\frac{R_1}{R_2}\right) + \left[a_x \log\left(\frac{X_1}{X_2}\right)\right] + \log b \quad (4)$$

Note that the only difference between Equation 3 and Equation 4 is the addition of the bracketed portion of Equation 4. With $R$ representing reinforcer rate, $X$ is a generic variable that may represent differences in the response and reinforcer variables mentioned above (e.g., response effort, reinforcer magnitude). The $X$ variable may also represent differences in reinforcement history (Davison & McCarthy, 1988) in the sense that problem behavior could have a longer history of reinforcement than appropriate behavior, thereby causing the bias for problem behavior over appropriate behavior. As with relative reinforcer rate, the equation includes a sensitivity parameter, $a_x$, to account for sensitivity to the difference in $X_1$ and $X_2$. Assuming no inherent bias (log $b = 0$), if the relative reinforcer magnitude is 4 times greater for $X_1$ than $X_2$, but the relative response ratio is only 2 times greater for $B_1$ than $B_2$, the estimated sensitivity to reinforcer magnitude (i.e., $a_m$) from log $b$ would be 0.5.

The important point is that Equation 4 can account for how differences in independent variables can bias responding toward or away from one response alternative or another when we manipulate some other independent variable parametrically. We often manipulate $R_1$ and $R_2$ parametrically across conditions, and hold other variables constant and equal. We should hold only one variable constant and different (e.g., relative reinforcer magnitude) while parametrically manipulating another (e.g., relative reinforcer rate) to determine whether variables influence bias Note that we can hold $R_1$ and $R_2$ constant while we vary $X_1$ and $X_2$ parametrically to obtain an estimate of sensitivity to the changes in a variable characterized by $X$ in Equation 4 (e.g., response effort, reinforcer magnitude).

## CHALLENGES TO GENERALIZED MATCHING

Equations 3 and 4 have been useful for describing how changes to response and reinforcement variables influence choice. However, these equations predict only data falling along straight lines because they use linear regression. Several findings produce functions that violate this required relation between response and reinforcer ratios. Researchers have used such findings to evaluate processes potentially underlying choice.

In one example, Davison and Jones (1995) assessed a range of reinforcer ratios beyond what researchers typically examine. A straight line with sensitivity estimates approaching 1.0 characterized the data well when they assessed a typical range of reinforcer–rate ratios from 1:10 to 10:1 (i.e., log values of –1 to +1). However, arranging a very rich versus a very lean reinforcement schedule extended the reinforcer ratios well beyond the normal range—out to 1:100 and 100:1 (i.e., log values of –2 to 2). This produced a flattening of the function between log values of ±1 to ±2. Davison and Jones suggested that discrimination of the response–reinforcer contingencies decreased at these more extreme ratios. Specifically, reinforcers obtained from the currently richer alternative became misallocated to the leaner alternative (see Davison & Jenkins, 1985). This contingency–discriminability interpretation suggests that stimulus control processes play a fundamental role in

choice, but are missing entirely from Equations 1–4. The requirement for nearly perfectly discriminated response–reinforcer contingencies to observe log–response ratios closely matching log–reinforcer ratios is directly relevant to the findings described above from Alsop and Davison (1991). Reducing differences in antecedent stimuli signaling two response alternatives reduced sensitivity to changes in relative reinforcement rates. Thus, despite the fact that Equations 3 and 4 provide adequate descriptions of choice across an impressive range of conditions (Davison & McCarthy, 1988; Grace & Hucks, 2013), these variables affecting bias and sensitivity show that the matching relation between behavior and reinforcement is not the only process governing choice. Researchers continue to debate whether other processes are necessary and, if so, what those processes might be (Baum, 2010; Cording, McLean, & Grace, 2011; Elliffe, Davison, & Landon, 2008; Sutton, Grace, McLean, & Baum, 2008); this debate goes beyond the scope of this chapter.

## CHOICE AND PERSISTENCE

Matching, characterized by Equations 1–4, describes how reinforcement variables influence the allocation of behavior in an environment. Thus matching provides a general framework for understanding how behavior becomes distributed among existing sources of reinforcement. We observe that a given response rate depends on reinforcement contingent on that response (e.g., reinforcement rate or magnitude) and on all other available sources of reinforcement (e.g., Herrnstein, 1961, 1970). Thus a given response, such as problem behavior, will decrease in rate if an alternative response, such as appropriate behavior, produces a greater reinforcement rate (e.g., Borrero et al., 2010). The allocation of behavior relative to available sources of reinforcement is only one consideration, especially when we are planning for the long-term effectiveness of behavioral treatments. What are the factors determining whether problem behavior will persist or relapse, or whether treatments will continue to be effective? The theoretical framework of behavioral momentum primarily concerns the role of learning or training conditions in how likely reinforced behavior is to continue, despite disruptive challenges to treatment.

Mace et al. (2010) arranged reinforcement rates for problem behavior and appropriate behavior like those Borrero et al. (2010) arranged. Rate of appropriate behavior was greater when reinforcement rate for appropriate behavior was greater than for problem behavior. These findings generally are consistent with the predictions of the matching law: Relative response rates track relative reinforcement rates. In addition, these findings are consistent with the goals of DRA treatments to reduce problem behavior. Thus DRA treatments are successful in altering the allocation of appropriate and problem behavior, as the matching law describes.

Mace et al. (2010) assessed another important component of behavior: persistence. Mace et al. arranged baseline conditions in which problem behavior produced reinforcement and appropriate behavior produced no differential consequence. After baseline, Mace et al. then arranged a sequence of phases in which a phase of extinction for problem and appropriate behavior followed either a baseline phase of reinforcement for problem behavior and extinction for appropriate behavior, or a phase of DRA plus reinforcement for problem behavior. The researchers counterbalanced the order of phases so that each participant experienced an extinction phase preceded by a phase of either baseline or DRA plus reinforcement for problem behavior. Problem behavior decreased to near-zero rates in approximately 10 sessions in extinction phases that followed baseline phases. By contrast, problem behavior persisted nearly 3 times longer and occurred at higher rates in extinction phases that followed DRA plus reinforcement for problem behavior phases. Thus rates of problem behavior during DRA plus reinforcement for problem behavior were lower than those in baseline, but the DRA inadvertently increased the persistence of problem behavior during an extinction challenge.

Ahearn, Clark, Gardenier, Chung, and Dube (2003) observed similar response persistence when they used NCR schedules to treat automatically maintained stereotypy in three children with intellectual developmental disorder. They provided participants with intermittent access to a preferred toy independently of behavior during the NCR schedule, which decreased levels of stereotypy relative to the absence of NCR. Equation 2 predicts the reduction in stereotypy with NCR. Specifically, NCR increased $R_e$, which was in competition with reinforcement for engaging in stereotypy, $R$. Ahearn et al. then assessed the persistence of stereotypy in the presence and absence of the NCR schedule. During the assessment of this persistence, they provided participants with intermittent access to a different preferred toy independently of behavior during an NCR schedule. Even though levels of stereotypy decreased during the initial NCR schedule, levels of stereotypy were higher when the persistence assessment followed a phase of NCR versus a phase of baseline. These findings resemble those of Mace et al. (2010) with DRA treatment: Additional reinforcement presented either contingent on a different response (DRA) or noncontingent on response (NCR) decreased the rate or level of problem behavior during treatment implementation, but enhanced the persistence of problem behavior when exposed to a disruptor. Therefore, two very commonly implemented behavioral treatments appeared effective initially, but compromised long-term treatment effectiveness by making problem behavior more resistant to other environmental challenges to treatment.

The findings of Mace et al. (2010) and Ahearn et al. (2003) are similar because they appear to reflect common behavioral processes. Nevertheless, these findings on their own might not convince readers of the reliability or importance of these effects. However, researchers have obtained similar effects repeatedly across many experimental arrangements and species—from fish, rats, and pigeons, to humans with intellectual developmental disorder and to neurotypical humans (e.g., Cohen, 1996; Igaki & Sakagami, 2004; Mace et al., 1990; Mauro & Mace, 1996; Nevin, Tota, Torquato, & Shull, 1990; Nevin & Wacker, 2013; Shahan & Burke, 2004). Moreover, several studies with human and nonhumans also have shown that even when alternative reinforcement decreases behavior, that behavior is likely to relapse later in the absence of the contingencies for the alternative reinforcement (e.g., Kuroda, Cançado, & Podlesnik, 2016; Miranda-Dukoski, Bensemann, & Podlesnik, 2016; Podlesnik & Shahan, 2009, 2010). Therefore, arranging alternative sources of reinforcement that decrease the rate of a target behavior but enhance its persistence is a common and robust finding. Behavioral momentum theory provides a framework within which to understand these effects and potential ways to ameliorate them.

## BEHAVIORAL MOMENTUM THEORY

Behavioral momentum theory assumes that two separate environmental relations govern behavior in the same way that two separate variables govern the movement of physical objects: mass and velocity. Just as objects of high or low mass can move at high or low velocity, behaviors also have properties like mass and velocity. The *rate* of a behavior is analogous to the *velocity* of an object, and the *persistence* of a behavior is analogous to the *mass* of an object. Thus different behaviors can occur at high or low rates that are easy or difficult to disrupt. Research on behavioral momentum evaluates the variables influencing response rates (behavioral velocity) and persistence (behavioral mass).

## Response Rate and Operant Response–Reinforcer Relations

The discriminated operant is the fundamental unit of operant behavior, which includes a discriminative stimulus, a response, and a consequence, according to Skinner (1969). Behavioral momentum theory proposes that the operant relation between responding and consequences govern response rate in a manner consistent with the matching law (Nevin, 2015; Nevin & Grace, 2000). As described in Equations 1–4, the rate of an operant behavior depends on the reinforcement rate for that response and the reinforcement rate for all other responses. Consistent with Equation 1, Mace et al. (2010) observed that decreases in rates of problem behavior ($B_1$) were reinforced at low rates ($R_1$) when appropriate alternative behavior ($B_2$) was reinforced at a higher rate ($R_2$). Consistent with Equation 2, Ahearn et al. (2003) observed decreases in rates of stereotypy ($B$) maintained by automatic reinforcement ($R$) when providing response-independent access to a toy ($R_e$). Therefore, available alternative sources of reinforcement degrade the effectiveness of the operant *response–reinforcer relation*. Specifically, they reduce the proportion of reinforcers delivered contingently on the target response, and thereby decrease the correlation between the response and the reinforcer. The velocity of behavior is an operant process.

Furthermore, response–reinforcer contingencies can shape different patterns of responding (see Morse, 1966). For example, differential reinforcement of low behavior rates (DRL) produces low rates of responding by arranging reinforcement with sufficiently spaced interresponse times. Thus DRL schedules increase the likelihood of pausing between responses. On the other hand, differential reinforcement of high behavior rates (DRH) produces high rates of responding by arranging reinforcement with little or no pausing or

bursts of responses. The patterns with DRL and DRH schedules reflect the effects of the different contingencies in shaping response rates. Essentially, the contingencies alter the functional unit of responding. DRL schedules result in a *pause-then-respond* response unit, and DRH produces bursts of responses as a unit. These units could change in frequency with changes in reinforcement rate, as described by the matching law (Staddon, 1968). Similarly, variable-ratio (VR) and VI schedules produce different response rates even when reinforcement rate is controlled. The important consideration for the present purpose is the idea that response rate itself is a conditionable dimension of behavior (Nevin, 1974). Again, behavioral velocity is an operant process.

As Equation 2 describes, the increases in response rates with increases in reinforcement rates led some to conclude that response rate provides an inappropriate measure of the fundamental processes underlying reinforcement effects, *response strength* (Herrnstein, 1961, 1970; Nevin & Grace, 2000). For these reasons, Nevin (1974) offered a different approach to assessing the processes underlying reinforcement.

## Persistence and Pavlovian Stimulus–Reinforcer Relations

Nevin (1974) suggested that a more appropriate method for evaluating response strength is to assess the way responding changes when some disruptive event challenges it—a measure he called *resistance to change* (see also Nevin & Wacker, 2013). Resistance to change assesses response rates during conditions of disruption compared to previous baseline response rates; it is a measure of behavioral persistence. For example, introducing extinction, distracting stimuli, or providing additional food before or during sessions can disrupt food-maintained responding under steady-state conditions (e.g., Mace et al., 1990, 2010; Nevin et al., 1990). These disruptive events decrease response rates, which we can compare among multiple responses. Persistent responses are ones that decrease less rapidly with more disruptive events (e.g., greater amounts of additional food or successive sessions of extinction), and we call those responses *resistant to change*.

As mass and velocity are separable aspects of physical momentum, response rates and persistence are products of separable processes in behavioral momentum (Bell, 1999; Grace, Schwendiman, & Nevin, 1998; Podlesnik, Jimenez-Gomez,

Ward, & Shahan, 2006; Podlesnik & Shahan, 2008). Behavioral momentum theory asserts that the persistence of behavior results from a Pavlovian process (i.e., respondent or classical conditioning). In Pavlovian conditioning, a conditioned response (CR) occurs to a conditioned stimulus (CS) when the CS forms a predictive relation with an evolutionarily relevant unconditioned stimulus (US; Domjan, 2005, 2016; Lattal, 2013; Rescorla, 1988). A dog salivates (CR) in the presence of a tone (CS) when the tone reliably predicts access to food (US). Similarly, behavioral momentum theory proposes that behavioral persistence is functionally a CR expressed in the presence of the environmental discriminative-stimulus context governing the target behavior. As CSs that more reliably predict USs produce more robust CRs, environmental stimuli more predictive of reinforcement will produce greater persistence. From the discriminated operant, behavioral momentum theory asserts that Pavlovian stimulus–reinforcer relations govern persistence (Nevin & Shahan, 2011):

$$\frac{B_x}{B_0} = 10^{\frac{-x}{r^b}} \qquad (5)$$

$B_x$ is response rate during disruption, and $B_0$ is training response rate; these terms represent the change in behavioral velocity from baseline to disruption. On the right side of the equation, any terms in the numerator of the exponent contribute to the disruption of target responding relative to training response rates; this is disruptive force, represented by the generic term $x$. Terms in the denominator contribute to countering those disruptive effects; this is behavioral mass and is a function of the baseline reinforcement rate, $r$. As described above, $r$ can be contingent on the target response or from other sources. The free parameter $b$ is the sensitivity parameter, which scales the persistence-enhancing effects of $r$ on resistance to change on the left side of the equation. Therefore, greater values of $x$ (e.g., time in extinction or greater satiation) increase the disruptive impact of terms in the numerator, and these effects are countered by all sources of reinforcement in the denominator. Importantly, Equation 5 accounts for data that Equation 2 cannot. Specifically, one could conceptualize the effects of disruptors as increases in $R_e$ in Equation 2, especially common disruptors like free access to the reinforcer maintaining behavior. However, Equation 2 fails to account for the common finding that response rates

that are lower in baseline when alternative reinforcement is available than when it is not available can be greater under conditions of disruption (e.g., Ahearn et al., 2003; Grimes & Shull, 2001; Mace et al., 2010; Nevin et al., 1990).

Mace et al. (2010) compared resistance to extinction following a DRA schedule that arranged low reinforcement rates for problem behavior and greater reinforcement rates for appropriate behavior. Problem behavior persisted more during extinction following the DRA schedule than following the baseline condition when only problem behavior produced reinforcement. Thus adding alternative reinforcement decreased the rate of problem behavior as described by matching in Equation 2, but only by degrading the operant response–reinforcer relation. The additional alternative reinforcement with the DRA schedule increased the total overall reinforcement rate in the current environment, compared with the absence of the DRA schedule. Because the DRA schedule increased the extent to which the current environmental context predicted reinforcement overall, DRA *enhanced* the Pavlovian stimulus–reinforcer relation, compared to the absence of the DRA schedule (see Nevin, 1997; Nevin & Wacker, 2013). According to Equation 5, the DRA increased $r$, thereby countering the disruptive effects of extinction more than when $r$ was lower during the baseline without DRA. Similarly, Ahearn et al. (2003) showed that NCR decreased the ongoing rate of stereotypy but increased its persistence. The addition of a preferred toy as NCR increased the total overall reinforcement rate in the current environment, compared to the environment without NCR (i.e., $r$ in the denominator in Equation 5). As with DRA in Mace et al., Ahearn et al. increased persistence by enhancing the Pavlovian stimulus–reinforcer relation with NCR. Greater reinforcement rates in the presence of discriminative stimuli reliably produce greater persistence when we arrange (1) all reinforcers presented dependently on the target response, (2) a proportion of reinforcers independently of responding, and (3) a proportion of reinforcers dependently on engaging in a different response (Nevin & Wacker, 2013; Podlesnik & DeLeon, 2015). Thus behavioral mass is a Pavlovian process and can be accounted for quantitatively with models like Equation 5. The clinical implications of the findings from Mace et al. and Ahearn et al. are considerable: Common behavioral treatments like DRA and NCR can decrease the rate of problem behavior, but inadvertently increase its persistence. We can understand how behavioral treatments like DRA and NCR can reduce the rate of a problem behavior while simultaneously enhancing its persistence by separating response–reinforcer and stimulus–reinforcer relations.

## Behavioral Momentum and Matching

Despite the response–reinforcer relation governing response rate and stimulus–reinforcer relations governing persistence, response rate and persistence are functions of situational reinforcement parameters. Equation 4 describes how relative response rates match the distribution of reinforcer parameters between two options. For example, parametrically manipulating relative reinforcement rate produces a positive relation between the log–response ratio and log–reinforcer ratio—the slope of the function expressed as $a_r$. Simultaneously arranging a larger reinforcer for Alternative 1 ($x_1$) than Alternative 2 ($x_2$) will produce a shift in the y-intercept through a shift in responding toward $B_1$ (see Cording et al., 2011). We observe similar effects with persistence.

In a study by Grace, Bedell, and Nevin (2002), food reinforcement maintained pigeons' responding. The researchers manipulated relative reinforcement rates parametrically between two alternating discriminative stimuli. Thus sometimes one discriminative stimulus would signal a higher reinforcement rate than the other, and vice versa. At each relative reinforcer rate, Grace et al. disrupted responding by presenting an alternative source of reinforcement response independently during time outs from the procedure. As with sensitivity in choice, persistence between the discriminative stimuli was related positively to reinforcement rate. Moreover, when the different discriminative stimuli arranged constant but different reinforcer magnitudes across relative reinforcement rates, persistence was biased toward the discriminative stimulus presenting the larger-magnitude reinforcer. Moreover, arranging choices between the two discriminative stimuli with concurrent-chain schedules produced changes in the log–response ratio consistent with Equation 4 and correlated with relative persistence, as just described. Therefore, preference for discriminative stimuli and persistence within discriminative stimuli appear to correlate as a function of the current stimulus–reinforcer relations. As such, Grace et al. suggested that preference and persistence provide converging expressions of the same underlying construct of response strength or behavioral mass. Thus we

might use a concurrent-chain schedule to assess client preference among discriminative stimuli (Tiger, Hanley, & Heal, 2006) as a relatively rapid way for determining which environments or treatment approaches might produce more persistent behavior.

## Behavioral Momentum and Relapse

Persistence correlates with another measure of importance concerning outcomes of behavioral treatments for problem behavior: relapse. When behavioral treatments eliminate problem behavior, environmental circumstances can produce a recurrence of problem behavior, or *treatment relapse* (Mace et al., 2010; Pritchard, Hoerger, & Mace, 2014). Many events contribute to treatment relapse under natural conditions, which explains why many preclinical models exist for assessing treatment relapse (Bouton, Winterbauer, & Todd, 2012; Marchant, Li, & Shaham, 2014; Podlesnik & Kelley, 2015; Wathen & Podlesnik, 2018). We discuss a model with direct relevance to behavioral treatments arranging alternative sources of reinforcement—a model called *resurgence*.

Resurgence is the return of a previously reinforced and extinguished target response when we extinguish a more recently reinforced alternative response (Epstein, 1983; Podlesnik & Kelley, 2014). For example, Volkert, Lerman, Call, and Trosclair-Lasserre (2009) reinforced instances of problem behavior according to a fixed-ratio (FR) 1 schedule in children diagnosed with autism spectrum disorder or intellectual developmental disorder. Next, extinction of problem behavior and reinforcement of a functional communication response essentially eliminated problem behavior. Volkert et al. then introduced extinction of the communication response and continued extinction of problem behavior, which produced an increase in problem behavior. That is, problem behavior increased or resurged when the researchers discontinued reinforcement for the appropriate alternative response. Therefore, resurgence models the relapse of problem behavior due to treatment-integrity-produced errors of omission—specifically, failures to reinforce appropriate communication responses or other alternative behavior (St. Peter Pipkin et al., 2010).

Obviously, most omission errors likely will not be as extreme as complete extinction, as in resurgence procedures. However, any decrease in treatment integrity increases the likelihood problem behavior will return and potentially contact reinforcement. Additionally, similar effects occur when response-independent reinforcement is removed, suggesting that removal of NCR will also produce resurgence (Marsteller & St. Peter, 2014; Saini, Fisher, & Pisman, 2017; Winterbauer & Bouton, 2010). Therefore, the findings with resurgence and those described earlier show that behavioral treatments enhance the persistence of problem behavior (Ahearn et al., 2003; Mace et al., 2010). Behavioral momentum theory reconciles these different effects through the same behavioral processes (Nevin & Shahan, 2011; Sweeney & Shahan, 2011).

Behavioral momentum theory asserts that reinforcement obtained in the presence of a discriminative stimulus contributes to the persistence of the responses occasioned by that discriminative stimulus, even when some reinforcement sources might decrease response rates. During DRA and NCR treatments, the participant obtains differential or noncontingent reinforcement in the same context as he or she obtains reinforcement for problem behavior, thereby enhancing the stimulus–reinforcer relation. Additionally, DRA and NCR treatments serve as disruptors of problem behavior, along with the extinction contingency (when we implement one).[2] Thus, greater rates of alternative reinforcement tend to be more effective in decreasing target problem behavior (e.g., Carr & Durand, 1985; Kelley, Lerman, & Van Camp, 2002; Leitenberg, Rawson, & Mulick, 1975; Sweeney & Shahan, 2013), which explains why DRA and NCR decrease problem behavior. During the extinction challenge of resurgence procedures, removing DRA or NCR functionally eliminates a disruptor for problem behavior, according to behavioral momentum theory. Thus problem behavior *resurges* in the absence of the disruptive force of DRA or NCR, which previously suppressed responding.

Shahan and Sweeney (2011) developed a quantitative model of resurgence based on behavioral momentum theory, building on Equation 5. This model asserts the following: (1) Baseline reinforcement rate in Phase 1 of a resurgence procedure enhances the Pavlovian stimulus–reinforcer relation

of the target response; (2) alternative reinforcement (e.g., DRA, NCR) arranged during extinction of target responding in Phase 2 disrupts target responding (i.e., weakens the response–reinforcer relation); (3) alternative reinforcement arranged during Phase 2 (e.g., DRA, NCR) also enhances the Pavlovian stimulus–reinforcer relation of the target response; and (4) removing the alternative reinforcement removes a disruptor of target behavior, thereby producing resurgence of target responding. Thus alternative reinforcement (e.g., DRA, NCR) can both strengthen and disrupt target responding. Shahan and Sweeney's quantitative model of resurgence formalizes these assertions in Equation 6:

$$\frac{B_t}{B_0} = 10^{\frac{-t(kR_a + c + dr)}{(r + R_a)^b}} \tag{6}$$

$B_t$ is response rate at time $t$ in extinction (Phases 2 and 3), and $B_0$ is the training response rate (Phase 1). As in Equation 5, terms in the numerator of the exponent contribute to the disruption of target responding, and terms in the denominator counter those disruptive effects. In effect, Equation 6 expands on the factors contributing to persistence and relapse, compared to Equation 5. During extinction of target responding, $c$ is the effect of removing the contingency between responding and reinforcement; $d$ scales the generalization decrement from eliminating the training reinforcement rate $r$ as stimuli (i.e., the salience of removing reinforcement); and $k$ scales the disruptive effect of alternative reinforcement, $R_a$. In the denominator, $b$ is the sensitivity parameter scaling the persistence-enhancing effects of $r$ and $R_a$ on resistance to extinction and resurgence. Therefore, time in extinction increases the disruptive impact of terms in the numerator, but all sources of reinforcement in the denominator counter those disruptive effects. Equation 6 accounts for resurgence of target responding by (1) setting $R_a$ to the alternative reinforcement rate in the numerator and denominator during Phase 2, and (2) setting $R_a$ only in the numerator to zero when alternative reinforcement is removed in Phase 3. Researchers have used Equation 6 to describe resurgence across a range of experiments involving rats, pigeons, and children (Nevin et al., 2017; Shahan & Sweeney, 2011). By contrast, Shahan and Craig (2017) is a useful resource describing limitations in applying behavioral momentum theory to resurgence.

Overall, Equation 6 provides a set of assumptions based on behavioral momentum theory from

---

[2] Note that conceptualizing DRA and NCR as disruptors of problem behavior differs from the assumptions of the matching law. With the matching law, alternative reinforcement competes with problem behavior by increasing the allocation of behavior toward the alternative response. With behavioral momentum, the alternative reinforcement itself disrupts problem behavior directly.

which to assess the environmental factors contributing to resurgence. Specifically, we can make and test predictions about how common and novel aspects of behavioral treatments influence the persistence and relapse of problem behavior. For example, Equation 6 predicts that higher rates of DRA or NCR will produce greater resurgence because they enhance stimulus–reinforcer relations more than lower rates of DRA or NCR, which is what happens (Leitenberg et al., 1975; Sweeney & Shahan, 2013). For instance, Pritchard, Hoerger, Mace, Penney, and Harris (2014) reinforced aggressive behavior maintained by attention according to a VI 60-second schedule in children with intellectual developmental disorder in the presence of two different therapists. Later, they extinguished reinforcement for problem behavior, and two different therapists reinforced a communication response either every 30 seconds or every 120 seconds on average ($R_a$ in Equation 6) in a multielement design. The researchers discontinued reinforcement for the communication response after problem behavior decreased by setting $R_a = 0$ in the numerator, which produced resurgence in problem behavior with both therapists. Resurgence was greater with the therapist whose reinforcement rate for the communication response was higher in the previous phase, due to greater $R_a$. Thus the common practice of delivering alternative sources of reinforcement with DRA and NCR treatments at higher rates effectively decreases problem behavior (Carr & Durand, 1985), but it may make resurgence more likely. Given these problems with common behavioral treatments, we next discuss some approaches for decreasing the persistence and relapse of problem behavior with DRA and NCR treatments.

## Procedures for Mitigating the Persistence and Relapse of Problem Behavior

Translational researchers have developed several approaches to mitigate the persistence and relapse of problem behavior that DRA and NCR treatments cause. These approaches manipulate reinforcement contingencies and environmental stimuli.

### Methods Focusing on Reinforcement Contingencies

Manipulating reinforcement contingencies is a general method of reducing the likelihood that problem behavior will resurge. One specific approach is to fade the reinforcement schedule for

the alternative response (e.g., Hagopian, Toole, Long, Bowman, & Lieving, 2004). Specifically, researchers have gradually increased the response requirement for reinforcement of the alternative response to produce more manageable reinforcement schedules for alternative behavior. Unfortunately, these methods have not eliminated resurgence in clinical and translational studies (Hagopian et al., 2004; Lieving & Lattal, 2003; Sweeney & Shahan, 2013; Volkert et al., 2009; Winterbauer & Bouton, 2012). Resurgence tends to occur as the reinforcement schedule for the alternative response becomes leaner; this has prompted translational researchers to identify ways to decrease persistence and the likelihood of relapse of problem behavior (DeLeon, Miller, & Podlesnik, 2015; Nevin & Wacker, 2013; Podlesnik & DeLeon, 2015).

Wacker et al. (2011) demonstrated another approach to reduce relapse of problem behavior by manipulating reinforcement contingencies (Leitenberg et al., 1975). They provided differential reinforcement for communication responses and implemented extinction for the problem behavior of eight children with intellectual developmental disorder. They assessed resurgence repeatedly across sessions by arranging extinction for communication responses. Importantly, resurgence generally decreased across successive resurgence sessions (Shahan & Sweeney, 2011). These findings suggest that more extensive exposure to differential reinforcement for alternative or communication behavior reduces the likelihood of resurgence. These findings suggest that maintaining DRA treatments for extended periods may improve the maintenance of treatment gains. Behavioral momentum theory suggests that the disruptive effects of extinction and alternative reinforcement increase with additional exposure to those contingencies. In other words, the disruptive force of DRA treatment increases with additional exposure, thereby increasing the long-term effectiveness of such treatment. We do not know whether the same effects would occur for NCR treatments combined with extinction.

One limitation of this approach is that doing the treatment must involve few or no errors of commission or instances of reinforcing problem behavior. Otherwise, prior stimulus–reinforcer relations might reinstate responding, thereby eliminating progress with DRA treatment. Clearly, treatment-integrity-produced errors are not always predictable in clinical situations, so maintaining high treatment fidelity for long periods could prove difficult or impossible in certain circumstances and with certain caregivers. Nevertheless, these data suggest that extending exposure to DRA treatments could increase their long-term effectiveness, but the conditions under which this is a useful approach remain to be elucidated.

## Methods Focusing on Environmental Stimuli

Mace et al. (2010) introduced an approach that relied primarily on contextual stimulus control to mitigate the persistence-enhancing effects of DRA treatments. Because reinforcing an alternative response in the presence of the same discriminative stimulus as problem behavior enhances the Pavlovian stimulus–reinforcer relation, Mace et al. reasoned that training alternative responding separately from problem behavior could be an effective approach. Specifically, providing reinforcement for the alternative response in a context separate from the context in which problem behavior produces reinforcement allows us to teach the alternative response without enhancing the Pavlovian stimulus–reinforcer relation. After we train the alternative response in the alternative stimulus context, we can combine the alternative stimulus context with a stimulus context associated with problem behavior. Combining stimulus contexts should disrupt problem behavior and provide the individual with the opportunity to engage in appropriate alternative responses and receive reinforcement. Mace et al.'s results provided support for this approach, and researchers have replicated and extended these findings in studies with pigeons (Podlesnik & Bai, 2015; Podlesnik, Bai, & Elliffe, 2012; Podlesnik, Bai, & Skinner, 2016; Podlesnik, Miranda-Dukoski, Chan, Bland, & Bai, 2017) and through telehealth with children diagnosed with ASD (Suess, Schieltz, Wacker, Detrick, & Podlesnik, 2020).

A multiple schedule is another stimulus control approach researchers have used to reduce the persistence of problem behavior. This approach has preliminary support from clinical studies and laboratory models with pigeons (Bland, Bai, Fullerton, & Podlesnik, 2016; Fuhrman, Fisher, & Greer, 2016; Nevin et al., 2016). Fuhrman et al. (2016) found that signaling periods in which functional-communication responses would and would not produce reinforcement could mitigate resurgence of problem behavior, compared to traditional functional-communication training. Therapists reinforced two children's functional-communication responses according to VI 20-second schedules, and extinguished problem behavior during the traditional-training condition. In the modified-training procedure, therapists wore lanyards with different-colored cards to signal a multiple schedule. Signaled components alternated between 60 seconds of reinforcement for functional-communication responses (S+) and 30 seconds of extinction of functional-communication responses (S−). The duration of S− intervals increased across sessions until the extinction component was 240 seconds and the reinforcement component was 60 seconds. During the resurgence test, the therapists extinguished functional-communication responses and presented NCR according to a VT 200-second schedule to decrease discrimination of the extinction contingency. Therapists only presented the S− stimulus during the resurgence test in the modified-training condition. In most cases, the modified procedure reduced resurgence to a greater extent than the traditional procedure did. Therefore, thinning reinforcement schedules for functional-communication responses while incorporating signaled periods of S− could promote generalization and maintenance of behavioral treatments.

In a related laboratory study with pigeons, Bland et al. (2016) reinforced an alternative response in the presence of the same discriminative stimulus as a target response in two different ways. In the first, a distinct stimulus change occurred when alternative reinforcement was available according to a VI schedule. In the other, no stimulus change accompanied the availability of alternative reinforcement. Although target response rates were higher with the signaled alternative reinforcement, target responding was less persistent in the component with the signaled alternative. Thus signaling alternative reinforcement appears to have separated the stimulus–reinforcer relation of the alternative reinforcement from that of the target response. Therefore, these findings and those of Fuhrman et al. (2016) show that discriminable periods of nonreinforcement during functional-communication training may reduce the persistence and relapse of problem behavior during behavioral treatments (Nevin et al., 2016). Nevertheless, future research should assess methods for also reducing the rate of the target response in the presence of the signaled alternative reinforcement, which is a key component of behavioral treatments aimed at reducing problem behavior. The methods of Fuhrman et al. (2016) provide a promising avenue to explore (see also Fisher, Fuhrman, Greer, Mitteer, and Piazza, 2020).

The findings from these studies highlight an important point. Translational and applied studies produce evidence for individual procedures that show promise as effective treatment. Most effective treatments, however, are likely to incorporate multiple approaches developed in parallel, like those described here and elsewhere (e.g., DeLeon et al., 2015). Determining the best methods to incorporate into behavioral treatments with the goal of mitigating the persistence and likelihood of treatment relapse is an important aim for translational researchers.

## Additional Problems to Address in Future Research

The matching law and behavioral momentum theory provide translational researchers and clinicians with powerful tools to understand and assess factors contributing to the effectiveness of behavioral treatments. Nevertheless, the science behind the factors contributing to treatment effectiveness remains incomplete. We discuss two areas in detail in which additional basic and translational research could improve our capacity to understand and effectively implement behavioral treatments.

Typically, researchers assessing persistence and relapse from the framework of behavioral momentum theory use multiple schedules of reinforcement (see Nevin, 1974; Nevin & Grace, 2000). Analogous to multielement designs, multiple schedules rapidly alternate conditions, such as different reinforcement rates in the presence of dramatically different antecedent stimuli. These methods are effective for establishing strong antecedent discriminative stimulus control, but are dissimilar to the delivery of many behavioral treatments. Several researchers arranged different reinforcement rates between multiple-schedule components and assessed the persistence of responding in studies with pigeons (Cohen, 1998; Cohen, Riley, & Weigle, 1993) and in translational research with children with intellectual developmental disorder (Lionello-DeNolf & Dube, 2011). When resistance to disruption between components of a multiple schedule was assessed, persistence was greater in the component arranging greater reinforcement rates. However, arranging the same reinforcement rates between extended conditions did not produce reliable differences in persistence as a function of reinforcement rate (Shull & Grimes, 2006). Nevertheless, researchers assessed the greater persistence in the presence of NCR (Ahearn et al., 2003) and DRA (Mace et al., 2010) across successive conditions arranging reinforcement for problem behavior in the absence of those treatments. Given that most behavior analysts implement behavioral treatments in conditions separate from nontreatment, this issue has implications for the long-term efficacy of behavioral treatments. Therefore, the conditions in which persistence and relapse are reliably functions of reinforcement rate remains an important question for additional research.

Another area of concern is the partial-reinforcement extinction effect (Mackintosh, 1974; Nevin, 1988). This effect occurs when responses reinforced intermittently produce more responding during extinction than responses reinforced continuously on an FR 1 schedule do. These findings appear counter to behavioral momentum theory, because FR 1 schedules should enhance Pavlovian stimulus–reinforcer relations more than any intermittent-reinforcement schedule. Behavioral momentum theory (e.g., Equation 6) accounts for the partial-reinforcement extinction effect as follows. Extinction terminates the contingency between responding and reinforcement with parameter $c$. In addition, the removal of reinforcement is more salient following FR 1 than following intermittent reinforcement, parameter $d$. The *generalization decrement* is the discriminable change in stimulus conditions and is a disruptive force in Equation 6 because it is in the numerator (Nevin, McLean, & Grace, 2001). Despite the many instances of the partial-reinforcement extinction effect in within-participant designs assessing operant behavior (e.g., Nevin & Grace, 2005; Shull & Grimes, 2006), there are many examples in which FR 1 reinforcement produces greater resistance to extinction than intermittent-reinforcement schedules (e.g., Lerman, Iwata, Shore, & Kahng, 1996; Schmid, 1988; Theios, 1962). Exactly which features contribute to changes in resistance to extinction following continuous or intermittent reinforcement is not entirely evident. Given the prevalent use of extinction and continuous-reinforcement schedules in behavioral treatments, understanding the factors contributing to the persistence of behavior during extinction is important. Nevertheless, extinction is only one source of disruption, and behavioral momentum theory predicts that continuously reinforced behavior should be more resistant to all sources of disruption other than extinction (e.g., satiation, distraction).

## CONCLUSIONS

The matching law and behavioral momentum theory provide two quantitative frameworks to describe and explain operant behavior. Readers may want to choose between the two frameworks or conclude whether one is superior. However, theories are like different tools; we use theories for different things. We use a lawn mower to cut a larger section of grass, but a weed whacker to get the edges. Neither one is better in general; they do related things (i.e., shorten grass), but have different purposes. As suggested by Killeen (1999),

> If you think models are about the truth, or that there is a best timing model, then you are in trouble. There is no best model, any more than there is a best car model or a best swimsuit model, even though each of us may have our favorites. It all depends on what you want to do with the model. (p. 275)

Thus matching and behavioral momentum theory both have limitations, but we should not evaluate them for how poorly they account for behavior outside the relevant domain—which is the allocation of behavior for the matching law, and the persistence and relapse of behavior for behavioral momentum theory. Instead, we should evaluate them for how well they account for behavior in the relevant domains (Mazur, 2006). They also serve as frameworks for understanding behavior and posing questions regarding variables that may be relevant to the effectiveness of behavioral treatments (Critchfield & Reed, 2009).

## REFERENCES

Ahearn, W. H., Clark, K. M., Gardenier, N. C., Chung, B. I., & Dube, W. V. (2003). Persistence of stereotypic behavior: Examining the effects of external reinforcers. *Journal of Applied Behavior Analysis, 36*, 439–448.

Alsop, B., & Davison, M. (1991). Effects of varying stimulus disparity and the reinforcer ratio in concurrent-schedule and signal-detection procedures. *Journal of the Experimental Analysis of Behavior, 56*, 67–80.

Aparicio, C. F., & Baum, W. M. (1997). Comparing locomotion with lever-press travel in an operant simulation of foraging. *Journal of the Experimental Analysis of Behavior, 68*, 177–192.

Athens, E. S., & Vollmer, T. R. (2010). An investigation of differential reinforcement of alternative behavior without extinction. *Journal of Applied Behavior Analysis, 43*, 569–589.

Baum, W. M. (1974). On two types of deviation from the matching law: Bias and undermatching. *Journal of the Experimental Analysis of Behavior, 22*, 231–242.

Baum, W. M. (1979). Matching, undermatching, and overmatching in studies of choice. *Journal of the Experimental Analysis of Behavior, 32*, 269–281.

Baum, W. M. (1982). Choice, changeover, and travel. *Journal of the Experimental Analysis of Behavior, 38*, 35–49.

Baum, W. M. (2010). Dynamics of choice: A tutorial. *Journal of the Experimental Analysis of Behavior, 94*, 161–174.

Baum, W. M., & Rachlin, H. C. (1969). Choice as time allocation. *Journal of the Experimental Analysis of Behavior, 12*, 861–874.

Bell, M. C. (1999). Pavlovian contingencies and resistance to change in a multiple schedule. *Journal of the Experimental Analysis of Behavior, 72*, 81–96.

Bland, V. J., Bai, J. Y. H., Fullerton, J. A., & Podlesnik, C. A. (2016). Signaled alternative reinforcement and the persistence of operant behavior. *Journal of the Experimental Analysis of Behavior, 106*, 22–33.

Borrero, C. S., Vollmer, T. R., Borrero, J. C., Bourret, J. C., Sloman, K. N., Samaha, A. L., et al. (2010). Concurrent reinforcement schedules for problem behavior and appropriate behavior: Experimental applications of the matching law. *Journal of the Experimental Analysis of Behavior, 93*, 455–469.

Bouton, M. E., Winterbauer, N. E., & Todd, T. P. (2012). Relapse processes after the extinction of instrumental learning: Renewal, resurgence, and reacquisition. *Behavioural Processes, 90*, 130–141.

Buckley, J. L., & Rasmussen, E. B. (2012). Obese and lean Zucker rats demonstrate differential sensitivity to rates of food reinforcement in a choice procedure. *Physiology and Behavior, 108*, 19–27.

Carr, E. G., & Durand, V. M. (1985). Reducing behavior problems through functional communication training. *Journal of Applied Behavior Analysis, 18*, 111–126.

Cohen, S. L. (1996). Behavioral momentum of typing behavior in college students. *Journal of Behavior Analysis and Therapy, 1*, 36–51.

Cohen, S. L. (1998). Behavioral momentum: The effects of the temporal separation of rates of reinforcement. *Journal of the Experimental Analysis of Behavior, 69*, 29–47.

Cohen, S. L., Riley, D. S., & Weigle, P. A. (1993). Tests of behavioral momentum in simple and multiple schedules with rats and pigeons. *Journal of the Experimental Analysis of Behavior, 60*, 255–291.

Cording, J. R., McLean, A. P., & Grace, R. C. (2011). Testing the linearity and independence assumptions of the generalized matching law for reinforcer magnitude: A residual meta-analysis. *Behavioural Processes, 87*, 64–70.

Critchfield, T. S., & Reed, D. D. (2009). What are we doing when we translate from quantitative models? *Behavior Analyst, 32*(2), 339–362.

Dallery, J., & Soto, P. L. (2013). Quantitative description of environment–behavior relations. In G. J. Madden (Ed.) & W. V. Dube, T. Hackenberg, G. P. Hanley, & K. A. Lattal (Assoc. Eds.), APA handbook of behavior analysis: Vol. 1. Methods and principles (pp. 219–249). Washington, DC: American Psychological Association.

Davison, M., & Jenkins, P. E. (1985). Stimulus discriminability, contingency discriminability, and schedule performance. *Animal Learning and Behavior, 13,* 77–84.

Davison, M., & Jones, B. M. (1995). A quantitative analysis of extreme choice. *Journal of the Experimental Analysis of Behavior, 64,* 147–162.

Davison, M., & McCarthy, D. (1988). *The matching law: A research review.* Hillsdale, NJ: Erlbaum.

Davison, M., & Nevin, J. A. (1999). Stimuli, reinforcers, and behavior: An integration. *Journal of the Experimental Analysis of Behavior, 71,* 439–482.

DeLeon, I. G., Podlesnik, C. A., & Miller, J. R. (2015). Applied research on resistance to change: Implications for treatment in autism spectrum disorders. In F. D. DiGennaro Reed & D. D. Reed (Eds.), *Bridging the gap between science and practice in autism service delivery* (pp. 353–374). New York: Springer.

Domjan, M. (2005). Pavlovian conditioning: A functional perspective. *Annual Review of Psychology, 56,* 179–206.

Domjan, M. (2016). Elicited versus emitted behavior: Time to abandon the distinction. *Journal of the Experimental Analysis of Behavior, 105,* 231–245.

Elliffe, D., Davison, M., & Landon, J. (2008). Relative reinforcer rates and magnitudes do not control concurrent choice independently. *Journal of the Experimental Analysis of Behavior, 90,* 169–185.

Epstein, R. (1983). Resurgence of previously reinforced behavior during extinction. *Behaviour Analysis Letters, 3,* 391–397.

Fantino, E., Squires, N., Delbrück, N., & Peterson, C. (1972). Choice behavior and the accessibility of the reinforcer. *Journal of the Experimental Analysis of Behavior, 18,* 35–43.

Findley, J. D. (1958). Preference and switching under concurrent scheduling. *Journal of the Experimental Analysis of Behavior, 1,* 123–144.

Fisher, W. W., Fuhrman, A. M., Greer, B. D., Mitteer, D. R., & Piazza, C. C. (2020). Mitigating resurgence of destructive behavior using the discriminative stimuli of a multiple schedule. *Journal of the Experimental Analysis of Behavior, 113,* 263–277.

Fisher, W. W., Pawich, T. L., Dickes, N., Paden, A. R., & Toussaint, K. (2014). Increasing the saliency of behavior-consequence relations for children with autism who exhibit persistent errors. *Journal of Applied Behavior Analysis, 47,* 1–11.

Fuhrman, A. M., Fisher, W. W., & Greer, B. D. (2016). A preliminary investigation on improving functional communication training by mitigating resurgence of destructive behavior. *Journal of Applied Behavior Analysis, 49,* 884–899.

Grace, R. C., Bedell, M. A., & Nevin, J. A. (2002). Preference and resistance to change with constant- and variable-duration terminal links: Independence of reinforcement rate and magnitude. *Journal of the Experimental Analysis of Behavior, 77,* 233–255.

Grace, R. C., & Hucks, A. D. (2013). The allocation of operant behavior. In G. J Madden (Ed.) & W. V. Dube, T. Hackenberg, G. P. Hanley, & K. A. Lattal (Assoc. Eds.), *APA handbook of behavior analysis: Vol. 1. Methods and principles* (pp. 219–249). Washington, DC: American Psychological Association.

Grace, R. C., Schwendiman, J. W., & Nevin, J. A. (1998). Effects of unsignaled delay of reinforcement on preference and resistance to change. *Journal of the Experimental Analysis of Behavior, 69,* 247–261.

Grimes, J. A., & Shull, R. L. (2001). Response-independent milk delivery enhances persistence of pellet-reinforced lever pressing by rats. *Journal of the Experimental Analysis of Behavior, 76,* 179–194.

Hagopian, L. P., Toole, L. M., Long, E. S., Bowman, L. G., & Lieving, G. A. (2004). A comparison of dense-to-lean and fixed-lean schedules of alternative reinforcement and extinction. *Journal of Applied Behavior Analysis, 37,* 323–338.

Herrnstein, R. J. (1961). Relative and absolute strength of response as a function of frequency of reinforcement. *Journal of the Experimental Analysis of Behavior, 4,* 267–272.

Herrnstein, R. J. (1970). On the law of effect. *Journal of the Experimental Analysis of Behavior, 13,* 243–266.

Igaki, T., & Sakagami, T. (2004). Resistance to change in goldfish. *Behavioural Processes, 66,* 139–152.

Iwata, B. A., Dorsey, M. F., Slifer, K. J., Bauman, K. E., & Richman, G. S. (1994). Toward a functional analysis of self-injury. *Journal of Applied Behavior Analysis, 27,* 197–209. (Reprinted from *Analysis and Intervention in Developmental Disabilities, 2,* 3–20, 1982)

Jacobs, E. A., Borrero, J. C., & Vollmer, T. R. (2013). Translational applications of quantitative choice models. In G. J. Madden (Ed.) & W. V. Dube, T. D. Hackenberg, G. P. Hanley, & K. A. Lattal (Assoc. Eds.), *APA handbook of behavior analysis: Vol. 2. Translating principles into practice* (pp. 165–190). Washington, DC: American Psychological Association.

Kelley, M. E., Lerman, D. C., & Van Camp, C. M. (2002). The effects of competing reinforcement schedules on the acquisition of functional communication. *Journal of Applied Behavior Analysis, 35,* 59–63.

Killeen, P. (1972). The matching law. *Journal of the Experimental Analysis of Behavior, 17,* 489–495.

Killeen, P. R. (1999). Modeling modeling. *Journal of the Experimental Analysis of Behavior, 71,* 275–280.

Kollins, S. H., Newland, M. C., & Critchfield, T. S. (1997). Human sensitivity to reinforcement in operant choice: How much do consequences matter? *Psychonomic Bulletin and Review, 4,* 208–220.

Kuroda, T., Cançado, C. R. X., & Podlesnik, C. A. (2016). Resistance to change and resurgence in humans engaging in a computer task. *Behavioural Processes, 125,* 1–5.

Lattal, K. M. (2013). Pavlovian conditioning. In G. J. Madden (Ed.) & W. V. Dube, T. D. Hackenberg, G. P. Hanley, & K. A. Lattal (Assoc. Eds.), *APA handbook of behavior analysis: Vol. 1. Methods and principles* (pp. 283–306). Washington, DC: American Psychological Association.

Leitenberg, H., Rawson, R. A., & Mulick, J. A. (1975). Extinction and reinforcement of alternative behavior. *Journal of Comparative and Physiological Psychology, 88,* 640–652.

Lerman, D. C., Iwata, B. A., Shore, B. A., & Kahng, S. W. (1996). Responding maintained by intermittent reinforcement: Implications for the use of extinction with problem behavior. *Journal of Applied Behavior Analysis, 29,* 153–171.

Lieving, G. A., & Lattal, K. A. (2003). Recency, repeatability, and reinforcer retrenchment: An experimental analysis of resurgence. *Journal of the Experimental Analysis of Behavior, 80,* 217–233.

Lionello-DeNolf, K. M., & Dube, W. V. (2011). Contextual influences on resistance to disruption in children with intellectual disabilities. *Journal of the Experimental Analysis of Behavior, 96,* 317–327.

Mace, F. C., Lalli, J. S., Shea, M. C., Lalli, E. P., West, B. J., Roberts, M., et al. (1990). The momentum of human behavior in a natural setting. *Journal of the Experimental Analysis of Behavior, 54,* 163–172.

Mace, F. C., McComas, J. J., Mauro, B. C., Progar, P. R., Taylor, B., Ervin, R., et al. (2010). Differential reinforcement of alternative behavior increases resistance to extinction: Clinical demonstration, animal modeling, and clinical test of one solution. *Journal of the Experimental Analysis of Behavior, 93,* 349–367.

Mackintosh, N. J. (1974). *The psychology of animal learning.* New York: Academic Press.

Marchant, N. J., Li, X., & Shaham, Y. (2013). Recent developments in animal models of drug relapse. *Current Opinion in Neurobiology, 23,* 675–683.

Marsteller, T. M., & St. Peter, C. C. (2014). Effects of fixed-time reinforcement schedules on resurgence of problem behavior. *Journal of Applied Behavior Analysis, 47,* 455–469.

Mauro, B. C., & Mace, F. C. (1996). Differences in the effect of Pavlovian contingencies upon behavioral momentum using auditory versus visual stimuli. *Journal of the Experimental Analysis of Behavior, 65,* 389–399.

Mazur, J. E. (2006). Mathematical models and the experimental analysis of behavior. *Journal of the Experimental Analysis of Behavior, 85,* 275–291.

McDowell, J. J. (1989). Two modern developments in matching theory. *Behavior Analyst, 12,* 153–166.

Miller, J. T., Saunders, S. S., & Bourland, G. (1980). The role of stimulus disparity in concurrently available reinforcement schedules. *Animal Learning and Behavior, 8,* 635–641.

Miranda-Dukoski, L., Bensemann, J., & Podlesnik, C. A. (2016). Training reinforcement rates, resistance to extinction, and the role of context in reinstatement. *Learning and Behavior, 44,* 29–48.

Morse, W. H. (1966). Intermittent reinforcement. In W. K. Honig (Ed.), *Operant behavior: Areas of research and application* (pp. 52–108). New York: Appleton-Century-Crofts.

Nevin, J. A. (1974). Response strength in multiple schedules. *Journal of the Experimental Analysis of Behavior, 21,* 389–408.

Nevin, J. A. (1984). Quantitative analysis. *Journal of the Experimental Analysis of Behavior, 42,* 421–434.

Nevin, J. A. (1988). Behavioral momentum and the partial reinforcement effect. *Psychological Bulletin, 103,* 44–56.

Nevin, J. A. (1997). Choice and momentum. In W. O'Donohue (Ed.), *Learning and behavior therapy* (pp. 230–251). Boston: Allyn & Bacon.

Nevin, J. A. (2015). *Behavioral momentum: A scientific metaphor.* Vineyard Haven, MA: Author.

Nevin, J. A., Craig, A. R., Cunningham, P. J., Podlesnik, C. A., Shahan, T. A., & Sweeney, M. M. (2017). Quantitative models of persistence and relapse from the perspective of behavioral momentum theory: Fits and misfits. *Behavioural Processes, 141,* 92–99.

Nevin, J. A., & Grace, R. C. (2000). Behavioral momentum and the law of effect. *Behavioral and Brain Sciences, 23,* 73–130.

Nevin, J. A., & Grace, R. C. (2005). Resistance to extinction in the steady state and in transition. *Journal of Experimental Psychology: Animal Behavior Processes, 31,* 199–212.

Nevin, J. A., Mace, F. C., DeLeon, I. G., Shahan, T. A., Shamlian, K. D., Lit, K., et al. (2016). Effects of signaled and unsignaled alternative reinforcement on persistence and relapse in children and pigeons. *Journal of the Experimental Analysis of Behavior, 106,* 34–57.

Nevin, J. A., McLean, A. P., & Grace, R. C. (2001). Resistance to extinction: Contingency termination and generalization decrement. *Animal Learning and Behavior, 29,* 176–191.

Nevin, J. A., & Shahan, T. A. (2011). Behavioral momentum theory: Equations and applications. *Journal of Applied Behavior Analysis, 44,* 877–895.

Nevin, J. A., Tota, M. E., Torquato, R. D., & Shull, R. L. (1990). Alternative reinforcement increases resistance to change: Pavlovian or operant contingencies? *Journal of the Experimental Analysis of Behavior, 53,* 359–379.

Nevin, J. A., & Wacker, D. P. (2013). Response strength and persistence. In G. J. Madden (Ed.) & W. V. Dube, T. D. Hackenberg, G. P. Hanley, & K. A. Lattal (Assoc. Eds.), *APA handbook of behavior analysis: Vol. 2. Translating principles into practice* (pp. 109–128). Washington, DC: American Psychological Association.

Newland, M. C., Reile, P. A., & Langston, J. L. (2004). Gestational exposure to methylmercury retards choice in transition in aging rats. *Neurotoxicology and Teratology, 26,* 179–194.

Oscar-Berman, M., Heyman, G. M., Bonner, R. T., & Ryder, J. (1980). Human neuropsychology: Some differences between Korsakoff and normal operant performance. *Psychological Research, 41,* 235–247.

Petscher, E. S., Rey, C., & Bailey, J. A. (2009). A review of empirical support for differential reinforcement of alternative behavior. *Research in Developmental Disabilities, 30,* 409–425.

Podlesnik, C. A., & Bai, J. Y. H. (2015). Method of stimulus combination impacts resistance to extinction. *Journal of the Experimental Analysis of Behavior, 104,* 30–47.

Podlesnik, C. A., Bai, J. Y. H., & Elliffe, D. (2012). Resistance to extinction and relapse in combined stimulus contexts. *Journal of the Experimental Analysis of Behavior, 98,* 169–189.

Podlesnik, C. A., Bai, J. Y. H., & Skinner, K. A. (2016). Greater alternative response and reinforcement rates increase disruption of target responding when combining stimuli. *Journal of the Experimental Analysis of Behavior, 105,* 427–444.

Podlesnik, C. A., & DeLeon, I. G. (2015). Behavioral momentum theory: Understanding persistence and improving treatment. In F. D DiGennaro Reed & D. D. Reed (Eds.), *Bridging the gap between science and practice in autism service delivery* (pp. 327–351). New York: Springer.

Podlesnik, C. A., Jimenez-Gomez, C., Ward, R. D., & Shahan, T. A. (2006). Resistance to change of responding maintained by unsignaled delays to reinforcement: A response-bout analysis. *Journal of the Experimental Analysis of Behavior, 85,* 329–347.

Podlesnik, C. A., & Kelley, M. E. (2014). Resurgence: Response competition, stimulus control, and reinforcer control. *Journal of the Experimental Analysis of Behavior, 102,* 231–240.

Podlesnik, C. A., & Kelley, M. E. (2015). Translational research on the relapse of operant behavior. *Mexican Journal of Behavior Analysis, 41,* 226–251.

Podlesnik, C. A., Miranda-Dukoski, L., Chan, J. C. K., Bland, V. J., & Bai, J. Y. H. (2017). Generalization of the disruptive effects of alternative stimuli when combined with target stimuli in extinction. *Journal of the Experimental Analysis of Behavior, 108,* 255–268.

Podlesnik, C. A., & Shahan, T. A. (2008). Response–reinforcer relations and resistance to change. *Behavioural Processes, 77,* 109–125.

Podlesnik, C. A., & Shahan, T. A. (2009). Behavioral momentum and relapse of extinguished operant responding. *Learning and Behavior, 37,* 357–364.

Podlesnik, C. A., & Shahan, T. A. (2010). Extinction, relapse, and behavioral momentum. *Behavioural Processes, 84,* 400–411.

Pritchard, D., Hoerger, M., & Mace, F. C. (2014). Treatment relapse and behavioral momentum theory. *Journal of Applied Behavior Analysis, 47,* 814–833.

Pritchard, D., Hoerger, M., Mace, F. C., Penney, H., & Harris, B. (2014). Clinical translation of animal models of treatment relapse. *Journal of the Experimental Analysis of Behavior, 101,* 442–449.

Reed, D. D., & Kaplan, B. A. (2011). The matching law: A tutorial for practitioners. *Behavior Analysis in Practice, 4,* 15–24.

Rescorla, R. A. (1988). Pavlovian conditioning: It's not what you think it is. *American Psychologist, 43,* 151–160.

Saini, V., Fisher, W. W., & Pisman, M. D. (2017). Persistence during and resurgence following noncontingent reinforcement implemented with and without extinction. *Journal of Applied Behavior Analysis, 50,* 377–392.

Schmid, T. L. (1988). A comparison of two behavior reduction procedures: Traditional extinction alone and interpolated reinforcement followed by extinction. *Journal of Mental Deficiency Research, 32,* 289–300.

Shahan, T. A., & Burke, K. A. (2004). Ethanol-maintained responding of rats is more resistant to change in a context with added non-drug reinforcement. *Behavioral Pharmacology, 15,* 279–285.

Shahan, T. A., & Craig, A. R. (2017). Resurgence as choice. *Behavioural Processes, 141,* 100–127.

Shahan, T. A., & Sweeney, M. M. (2011). A model of resurgence based on behavioral momentum theory. *Journal of the Experimental Analysis of Behavior, 95,* 91–108.

Shull, R. L. (1991). Mathematical description of operant behavior: An introduction. In I. H. Iversen & K. A. Lattal (Eds.), *Experimental analysis of behavior (Part 2)* (pp. 243–282). Amsterdam: Elsevier.

Shull, R. L., & Grimes, J. A. (2006). Resistance to extinction following variable-interval reinforcement: Reinforcer rate and amount. *Journal of the Experimental Analysis of Behavior, 85,* 23–39.

Shull, R. L., & Pliskoff, S. S. (1967). Changeover delay and concurrent schedules: Some effects on relative performance measures. *Journal of the Experimental Analysis of Behavior, 10,* 517–527.

Skinner, B. F. (1938). *The behavior of organisms: An experimental analysis.* New York: Appleton-Century.

Skinner, B. F. (1969). *Contingencies of reinforcement.* Englewood Cliffs, NJ: Prentice-Hall.

St. Peter Pipkin, C., Vollmer, T. R., & Sloman, K. N. (2010). Effects of treatment integrity failures during differential reinforcement of alternative behavior: A translational model. *Journal of Applied Behavior Analysis, 43,* 47–70.

Staddon, J. E. R. (1968). Spaced responding and choice: A preliminary analysis. *Journal of the Experimental Analysis of Behavior, 11,* 669–682.

Suess, A. N., Schieltz, K. M., Wacker, D. P., Detrick, J., & Podlesnik, C. A. (2020). An evaluation of resurgence following functional communication training conducted in alternative antecedent contexts via telehealth. *Journal of the Experimental Analysis of Behavior, 113,* 278–301.

Sutton, N. P., Grace, R. C., McLean, A. P., & Baum, W. M. (2008). Comparing the generalized matching law and contingency discriminability model as accounts of concurrent schedule performance using residual meta-analysis. *Behavioural Processes, 78,* 224–230.

Sweeney, M. M., & Shahan, T. A. (2013). Behavioral momentum and resurgence: Effects of time in extinction and repeated resurgence tests. *Learning and Behavior, 41*, 414–424.

Theios, J. (1962). The partial reinforcement effect sustained through the blocks of ontinuous reinforcement. *Journal of Experimental Psychology, 64*, 1–6.

Tiger, J. H., Hanley, G. P., & Heal, N. A. (2006). The effectiveness of and preschoolers' preferences for variations of multiple-schedule arrangements. *Journal of Applied Behavior Analysis, 39*, 475–488.

Volkert, V. M., Lerman, D. C., Call, N. A., & Trosclair-Lasserre, N. (2009). An evaluation of resurgence during treatment with functional communication training. *Journal of Applied Behavior Analysis, 42*, 145–160.

Wacker, D. P., Harding, J. W., Berg, W. K., Lee, J. F., Schieltz, K. M., Padilla, Y. C., et al. (2011). An evaluation of persistence of treatment effects during long-term treatment of destructive behavior. *Journal of the Experimental Analysis of Behavior, 96*, 261–282.

Wathen, S. N., & Podlesnik, C. A. (2018). Laboratory models of treatment relapse and mitigation techniques. *Behavior Analysis: Research and Practice, 18*(4), 362–387.

Wearden, J. H., & Burgess, I. S. (1982). Matching since Baum (1979). *Journal of the Experimental Analysis of Behavior, 38*, 339–348.

Williams, B. A. (1988). Reinforcement, choice, and response strength. In R. C. Atkinson, R. J. Herrnstein, G. Lindzey, & R. D. Luce (Eds.), *Stevens' handbook of experimental psychology: Vol. 2. Learning and cognition* (pp. 167–244). New York: Wiley.

Winterbauer, N. E., & Bouton, M. E. (2010). Mechanisms of resurgence of an extinguished instrumental behavior. *Journal of Experimental Psychology: Animal Behavior Processes, 36*, 343–353.

Winterbauer, N. E., & Bouton, M. E. (2012). Effects of thinning the rate at which the alternative behavior is reinforced on resurgence of an extinguished instrumental response. *Journal of Experimental Psychology: Animal Behavior Processes, 3*, 279–291.

# CHAPTER 7

# Behavioral Economics
## Principles and Applications

Iser G. DeLeon, Nathalie Fernandez, Kissel J. Goldman,
Elizabeth Schieber, Brian D. Greer, and Derek D. Reed

It often happens that the development of two different fields of science
goes on side by side for long periods, without either of them exercising
influence on the other. On occasion, again, they may come into closer
contact, when it is noticed that unexpected light is thrown on the
doctrines of one by the doctrines of another.

—ERNST MACH (1914)

*Behavioral economics* is the application of psychological and behavioral principles to understand choice or decision making, but the specific principles differ according to the school of thought and the direction of the flow of influence. The behavioral economics most familiar to behavior analysts draws principally from the integration of microeconomic theory and operant psychology (Kagel & Winkler, 1972). This approach extends both concepts from microeconomic theory to study consumption in various species in the laboratory, and concepts of operant conditioning to understand demand for economic commodities (Hursh, Madden, Spiga, DeLeon, & Francisco, 2013). In this chapter, we concentrate on operant behavioral economics and use the term *behavioral economics* in the operant and not the traditional vein.

One appeal of importing microeconomic theory into behavior analysis is that it gives behavior analysts a framework for understanding choices among concurrently available but *asymmetrical* alternatives (i.e., comparing "apples to oranges"). This may be more relevant in applied contexts, because human decisions about response allocation more often involve responses leading to qualitatively different outcomes (Fuqua, 1984); thus microeconomic and operant theories converge at multiple points. For example, both are concerned with the factors that influence choice under conditions of constraint and the relative value of goods (Hursh et al., 2013; Hursh & Roma, 2016). The parallels between microeconomic theory and behavior analysis suggest a wealth of relations only heretofore considered by economists—new phenomena previously ignored and functional relations previously unnamed by behavior analysts.

In this chapter, we begin by describing those concepts and tools, translating from the language of microeconomics to the language of behavior analysis when necessary. We then review how behavior analysts have applied those concepts and tools to understand and promote beneficial choices. Much of our discussion describes applications to persons with neurodevelopmental disorders because of the predominance of research on this population in applied behavior analysis. We also reference basic or other applied research in which behavioral economics has gained a foothold, such as studies of addictions and health-related behavior.

## EFFORT AS COST: TERMS, CONCEPTS, AND METHODS

Behavioral economists assume that how individuals behave to procure and consume reinforcers follows certain microeconomic principles that govern population dynamics. Behavior analysts have adopted principles largely concerned with *stimulus value*, or whether a reinforcer will maintain responding under varying constraint conditions. In this context, *value* involves the contextual variables that affect the reinforcing efficacy of the stimulus, not an intrinsic stimulus feature. *Constraint* involves contingencies that dictate how, how many, when, and if reinforcers will be delivered. This approach assumes that the effectiveness of a reinforcer is not a static, inherent property of the stimulus; many factors can influence its effectiveness. Below, we define some of the more critical microeconomic terms and principles in this behavioral context.

### Commodities and Unit Price

In behavioral economics, a *commodity* is a reinforcer purchased with behavior. That is, an individual pays the cost of the reinforcer by meeting a behavioral contingency. *Unit price* describes the cost–benefit ratio of a commodity. In behavioral terms, unit price describes the number of responses to the amount of a reinforcer. For example, a person might earn one token (benefit) for five correct responses (cost) on a worksheet; thus the unit price of one token is five responses.

### Consumption

*Consumption* in a behavioral-economic context is a measurement of the quantity of a reinforcer earned during a given time, like an observation session. Consumption often reflects the number of reinforcers earned per day in basic behavioral-economic research. Assessing consumption throughout a day or during long periods in applied settings

with humans may not be feasible. Thus investigators often evaluate consumption during smaller time units or until a participant earns a maximum number of reinforcers available.

### Assessing Stimulus Value with Demand Functions

A *demand function* relates consumption of a reinforcer to its cost. Specifically, demand functions quantify reinforcer consumption amidst increasing costs. We derive this function by varying the reinforcer price (i.e., the schedule requirement) and measuring how much of that reinforcer an individual consumes at each price. Thus a behavior analyst can examine how changes in the amount of work the individual must complete to produce a reinforcer alters how much of that reinforcer the individual earns. For example, if a single response produces the reinforcer on a fixed-ratio (FR) 1 schedule, the demand analysis would quantify how consumption decreases as reinforcer availability decreases (i.e., as the reinforcement schedule shifts from FR 1 to increasingly intermittent schedules). We could vary the response requirement from FR 5, to FR 10, FR 15, FR 20, and so on. The resulting demand function would show the mean number of reinforcers earned at each FR value. Behavioral economists often interpret the resulting demand function as the degree to which an individual will *defend consumption* during increased prices versus when the same reinforcer was inexpensive (i.e., at the FR 1 schedule).

The left panel of Figure 7.1, reproduced from Hursh and Roma (2013), depicts demand functions for food pellets and units of saccharin solution as a function of the number of responses required to earn a unit of each reinforcer, aggregated for two monkeys. Consumption (reinforcers per day) decreased for each reinforcer as price (the FR requirement) increased for both functions. Behavioral economists characterize such a relation as the *law of demand*, which describes the characteristic inverse relation between consumption and unit price. This inverse relation implies that higher unit prices produce less consumption. Stated more simply, consumption of a reinforcer decreases as the number of responses required to earn that reinforcer increases, and vice versa.

Figure 7.1 shows that the slopes of the generated functions are nonlinear, as is typical of demand functions. Initial price increases may have little effect, producing only small decreases in consumption. The effect of additional price in-

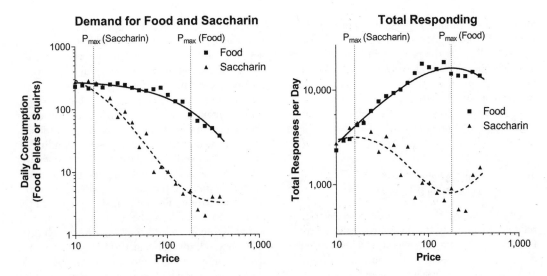

**FIGURE 7.1.** Demand functions (left panel) and work functions (right panel) for food and saccharin across a range of prices for two rhesus monkeys. From Hursh and Roma (2013). Copyright © 2013 Society for the Experimental Analysis of Behavior. Reprinted by permission.

creases is greater as the price increases. In the left panel of Figure 7.1, changes from FR 10 to FR 100 produced small decreases in the number of food pellets earned per day. Consumption began to decrease more steeply as the cost exceeded FR 100. Graphing demand functions on double-logarithmic axes facilitates visual and quantitative analysis of the proportional relation between changes in price and changes in consumption (Hursh et al., 2013).

*Price elasticity of demand* is a measure of the change in consumption that accompanies a price change. When the decrease in consumption is proportionally less than the increase in price, the slope of the double-logarithmic demand function is shallower than –1. Across this range of price increases, we describe demand as *inelastic*. In contrast, the portion of the food function after FR 100 in Figure 7.1 shows *elastic demand*. At higher costs, further increases in price produce supraproportional changes in consumption. We should expect more rapid decreases in consumption with further increases in price after demand elasticity shifts from inelastic to elastic. In Figure 7.1, the lines labeled $P_{max}$ indicate the price at which demand shifted from inelastic to elastic for each reinforcer. This shift in demand corresponded to the price at which consumption became highly sensitive to further price increases. Knowing the price at which such a shift in demand occurs ensures that

we do not set reinforcement schedules that maintain responding too high or too low.[1]

The effect of price changes on consumption can differ across reinforcers. In Figure 7.1, saccharin and food pellets have different demand profiles; consumption of saccharin decreased more rapidly than consumption of food pellets across similar price increases. Thus a subject may consume two reinforcers similarly when both are inexpensive, but consumption of one may decrease more rapidly than consumption of the other as prices increase. The rate at which consumption decreases depends upon the necessity and initial value of the reinforcer and external factors, like the availability of alternative reinforcers and constraints in the economies.

The right panel of Figure 7.1 depicts *work functions*, or total responding for the two reinforcers across unit prices. The work function characteristically shows a positive slope at low prices as the monkeys emitted more responses to defend consumption (i.e., to earn the same number of rein-

---

[1]Readers interested in the important topics of quantifying and extrapolating the shape of demand functions, deriving $P_{max}$, and so on should see Hursh et al. (2013) and Hursh and Silberberg (2008). Those interested in relevant treatments related to neurodevelopmental disorders should see Reed, Kaplan, and Becirevic (2015) and Gilroy, Kaplan, and Leader (2018).

forcers), even though it became increasingly expensive. The demand function turns from inelastic to elastic ($P_{max}$) at the peak of the work function, which begins to slope downward with additional price increases. Thus work functions generally assume an inverted-U shape. Work functions may estimate how high an applied behavior analyst could set a reinforcement schedule requirement before negatively affecting levels of responding.

## Assessing Stimulus Value with Progressive-Ratio Schedules

A related method for assessing stimulus value in relation to price is the *progressive-ratio schedule* (Hodos, 1961). Progressive-ratio schedules, like demand curves, determine reinforcer strength by measuring the amount of work an individual will complete to earn a reinforcer. However, cost increases in progressive-ratio schedules usually occur within an experimental session after each reinforcer delivery (but see Jarmolowicz & Lattal, 2010). The response requirement might begin at FR 1 in each session and then increase after each successive reinforcer delivery, often in arithmetic or geometric progressions. The *step size* is the number of or formula for additionally required responses. The *breakpoint* is the principal dependent measure, which is the last schedule value the individual completes before responding stops for a specified time (e.g., 2 or 5 minutes). We might reasonably conclude that Stimulus A is a more effective reinforcer than Stimulus B if responding stops after completion of an FR 20 schedule for Stimulus A and after an FR 10 schedule for Stimulus B.

Investigators have shown the results of progressive-ratio schedules in applied research by depicting (1) the breakpoint of each progressive-ratio session as a line graph across sessions and conditions (e.g., Francisco, Borrero, & Sy, 2008, Figure 3; Jerome & Sturmey, 2008; Russell, Ingvarsson, Haggar, & Jessel, 2018, Figure 2); (2) the total response output per session (e.g., Fiske et al., 2015; Tiger, Toussaint, & Roath, 2013); (3) the mean breakpoint across repeated progressive-ratio sessions (Call, Trosclair-Lasserre, Findley, Reavis, & Shillingsburg, 2012, Figure 7.3; DeLeon, Frank, Gregory, & Allman, 2009); and (4) the proportion of opportunities that a participant or group of participants earned reinforcement at each schedule value across multiple progressive-ratio sessions (Hoffmann, Samaha, Bloom, & Boyle, 2017; Roane, Lerman, & Vorndran, 2001; Trosclair-Lasserre, Lerman, Call, Addison, & Kodak, 2008). For example, Goldberg et al. (2017) used progressive-ratio schedules to compare the reinforcing efficacy of a solitary or a social activity. Children with autism spectrum disorder earned 30 seconds to do an activity alone on a progressive-ratio schedule that began at one response for the first unit of reinforcement, but increased arithmetically by a step size of 10 responses for each additional unit. The progressive-ratio schedule continued until a child stopped responding for 30 seconds or verbally indicated that he or she was finished responding. Investigators repeated the procedure, but the reinforcer was doing the activity with a parent. The investigators presented the proportion of children who "purchased" each additional 30-second reinforcement unit at each price in each condition. This method of presenting the data is similar to a survival analysis. Figure 7.2 shows the data, which resembles a demand function relating consumption (proportion of children paying each price) to increasing prices. A higher proportion of children paid most prices to do the activity with a parent, perhaps contradicting conventional notions of the value of social interaction in children with autism spectrum disorder.

Progressive-ratio schedules are a quick and effective way to assess stimulus value. Behavior analysts can identify breakpoints across progressive-ratio schedules, directly compare the reinforcing efficacy of two or more stimuli, and use this information to develop more robust reinforcement-based procedures. Behavior analysts can construct progressive-ratio schedules in a variety of ways, and depicting the results graphically can show useful economic relations between behavior and the environment.

## Factors That Influence Demand

When prices increase, demand for some goods is generally more elastic than demand for others. The two curves in Figure 7.1 reflect this relation. In this figure, consumption of food pellets remained relatively unaffected through price increases as high as FR 100. By contrast, saccharin consumption decreased more rapidly across equal price increases. Behavioral economists have evaluated several influences on the shape of these curves, including the nature of the economy (open vs. closed) and the substitutability of reinforcers.

### Open versus Closed Economies

In a *closed* economy, the reinforcer or a close substitute is only available in the earning environment

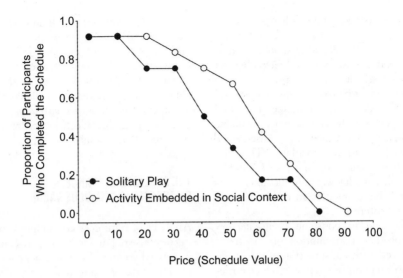

**FIGURE 7.2.** Survivor analysis of solitary play and social play as a proportion of participants who completed each schedule requirement. Data replotted from Goldberg et al. (2017).

(Reed, Niileksela, & Kaplan, 2013). For example, a child can earn access to a highly preferred movie for finishing schoolwork, but that movie is never available otherwise in a closed economy. In an *open* economy, the reinforcer or a close substitute is available in and out of the earning environment. For example, a child in an open economy can earn Skittles candies by touching a communication card in the clinic, but the caregiver allows free access to Skittles at home. Human environments are typically open economies with multiple sources of reinforcement.

Several applied behavioral-economic studies have examined the effects of economy type on responding across price increases. In the open economy in Roane, Call, and Falcomata (2005), correct responding produced reinforcement; however, the investigators gave the participants supplemental reinforcement if they did not earn the maximum number of possible reinforcers during the session. Correct responding was the only way participants accessed reinforcement in the closed economy. Both arrangements increased adaptive responding relative to baseline; however, demand was more elastic in the open economy. Participants were less likely to work for reinforcement at the higher-response requirements when reinforcement was available outside the work environment in the open economy. Kodak, Lerman, and Call (2007) found that mean progressive-ratio breakpoints in a condition without postsession reinforcement

were about twice as high as those in a condition with postsession reinforcement. These results suggest that reinforcers will sustain more responding if they are only available in the earning environment versus when reinforcement is available elsewhere.

## The Continuum of Substitutability

*Substitutability* is a variable that influences demand elasticity on a continuum (Green & Freed, 1993). Stimuli are highly substitutable when decreased consumption of one stimulus results in increased consumption of the other stimulus when income constrains choice or the number of reinforcers an individual can earn. For example, decreased consumption of coffee may be associated with increased consumption of tea. Demand for commodities with many substitutes tends to be more elastic than demand for commodities with few or no substitutes. Thus many people may switch to tea if the price of coffee increases dramatically. By contrast, consumption of heating oil tends to remain relatively stable regardless of price, because it has no close substitute.

We can only determine substitutability by examining changes in consumption experimentally. Specifically, we increase the price of one reinforcer, hold the price of the other constant, and measure relative consumption of each reinforcer at each concurrent-schedule value. Lea and Roper (1977) examined rats' demand for mixed-diet pellets during increases in ratio-schedule requirements (FR 1, FR 6, FR 11, and FR 16), and separate responses produced no food, sucrose, or mixed-diet pellets on a constant FR 8 schedule. As the price of pellets increased, demand for pellets decreased most, and demand for the alternative reinforcer increased most, when pellets were concurrently available and least when the most dissimilar consequence (no food) was concurrently available. Thus the identical edible stimulus was most substitutable, the other edible stimulus was intermediately substitutable, and the absence of an edible stimulus provided no substitute.

Individuals tend to consume *complementary* reinforcers together; consumption of one tends to vary positively with consumption of the other. Increased consumption of tea may produce corresponding increases in consumption of sugar. If the price of one complement decreases its consumption, consumption of the other will also decrease. Increases in the price of tea may produce both decreased tea and sugar consumption. Complementary reinforcers can influence stimuli hypothesized to function as reinforcers in several ways. The removal of one stimulus that was reinforcing behavior may decrease the reinforcing effectiveness of other stimuli also present. For example, a child may play with a basketball when a hoop is available, but not when it is unavailable. The basketball alone may not maintain responding if the basketball and hoop are complementary reinforcers. Similarly, when a reinforcer has many different stimulus properties, removal of one property may alter the stimulus's reinforcing value. For example, attention from one therapist may function as a reinforcer, but attention from another therapist may not. Alternatively, praise with tickles may function as a reinforcer, but praise with a pat on the back may not. In these examples, the combination of stimuli or stimulus features interact in such a way that an increase in effort required to gain access to either stimulus will decrease responding towards both stimuli. Conversely, a decrease in effort required to gain access to either stimulus will increase responding toward both stimuli.

*Independent* commodities are those in which the price of one commodity has no effect on the consumption of another. Increasing the response requirements to earn access to a tablet should not change the effectiveness of food as a reinforcer, so consumption of food will remain constant. Independence is often desired in application. For example, using a doll as a reinforcer would be easier than using a doll and a dollhouse. However, using the doll and dollhouse may be necessary if they are complementary, and the doll is reinforcing only with the dollhouse or another independent stimulus. Similar problems exist when substitutable reinforcers are readily available. For example, acquisition may be slower with popcorn as the programmed reinforcer if other salty snacks (i.e., close substitutes) are available freely.

## THE APPLIED RELEVANCE OF ASSESSING STIMULUS VALUE

Analyses of reinforcer consumption under differing response requirements are particularly relevant in applied settings. Reinforcement schedule thinning from rich contingencies to more stringent response requirements improves treatment practicality and is a common activity for behavior analysts. Essentially, the behavior analyst has created a demand function when the response requirements to produce the same reinforcer increase across sessions.

### Implications for Selecting Reinforcers

Investigators have used demand curves and progressive-ratio schedules to validate predictions of the relative value of stimuli identified with other preference assessment procedures (e.g., Glover, Roane, Kadey, & Grow, 2008; Martin, Franklin, Perlman, & Bloomsmith, 2018; Penrod, Wallace, & Dyer, 2008). For example, DeLeon et al. (2009) showed that stimuli identified as highly preferred in a paired-stimulus preference assessment produced higher mean break points in a progressive-ratio schedule than stimuli identified as less preferred. Fiske et al. (2015) showed that total response output and breakpoints in progressive-ratio schedules matched for token reinforcers and the primary reinforcers with which they had paired the tokens. By contrast, response output and breakpoints for unpaired tokens approximated those of the no-reinforcement control conditions, which were much lower. Researchers have also used demand curves and progressive-ratio schedules to evaluate the accuracy of different preference assessment formats (e.g., Call et al., 2012; Reed et al., 2009).

Choice responses in stimulus-preference assessments typically require minimal effort from subjects, like a reaching response (DeLeon & Iwata, 1996; Fisher et al., 1992; Pace, Ivancic, Edwards, Iwata, & Page, 1985; Roane, Vollmer, Ringdahl, &

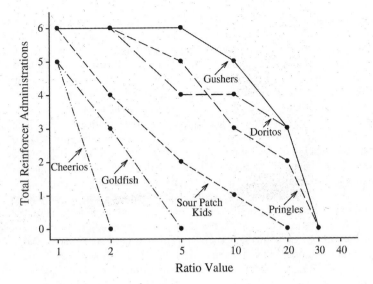

**FIGURE 7.3.** Own-price demand functions showing total number of reinforcer deliveries across various prices (ratio values) of each stimulus. From Reed et al. (2009). Reprinted by permission of the publisher (Taylor & Francis Ltd, *www.tandfonline.com*).

Marcus, 1998). Unfortunately, relative reinforcer effectiveness identified under such low-cost conditions does not always remain constant when response requirements increase. Investigators have used demand curves and progressive-ratio schedules to determine relative value among reinforcers when the effort required to produce them increases. Some studies have shown that distinct reinforcers can maintain equivalent response levels when unit price is low, but increases in unit price reveal important differences across stimuli in maintaining responding, as in Figure 7.1. For example, Reed et al. (2009) evaluated six edible reinforcers independently during progressive-ratio schedules that began with FR 1 and increased after every second reinforcer. The participant had six opportunities to earn each reinforcer.[2] Figure 7.3 shows that the participant earned Cheerios and Goldfish five times, and the other foods six times at FR 1. Notable differences in responding between Cheerios, Goldfish, and Sour Patch Kids and the other edibles began at FR 2, with no responding at FR 2 for Cheerios, at FR 5 for Goldfish, and at FR 20 for Sour Patch Kids. Pringles, Doritos, and Gushers maintained a decreasing number of responses until FR 30, when responding stopped. Results of

Reed et al. (2009) and other studies of participants with neurodevelopmental disabilities (e.g., DeLeon, Iwata, Goh, & Worsdell, 1997; Tustin, 1994, 2000) suggest that behavior analysts should evaluate reinforcer effectiveness under conditions that approximate their use in practice.

Tustin (1994) was the first to explicitly use a behavioral-economic framework with participants with a neurodevelopmental disorder. The demand function for a visual reinforcer had a steeper slope when an auditory reinforcer was concurrently available relative to the demand function for the same visual reinforcer when 5 seconds of social interaction were concurrently available. This finding suggested that the two sensory reinforcers were more substitutable than the sensory reinforcer and attention.

Individuals with neurodevelopmental disorders in DeLeon et al. (1997) could press two different microswitch panels to produce two different reinforcers according to progressively increasing, concurrent-ratio schedules. Participants did not show a clear preference for one reinforcer over the other when the two were functionally dissimilar, like an edible item and a toy. By contrast, participants showed a clear preference for one reinforcer as the schedule requirements increased from FR 1 to FR 5 or FR 10 when the concurrently available reinforcers were functionally similar, like two food items. DeLeon et al. (1997) suggested that the sub-

---

[2]Evaluations of this sort (i.e., assessing demand for each reinforcer independently of other reinforcers) determine *own-price demand.*

stitutability between functionally similar but not functionally dissimilar reinforcers produced this effect. They also proposed that increased schedule requirements may magnify small differences in relative preference for reinforcers that share physical characteristics (like the two food items) because they are also likely to share functional properties, like hunger reduction. Participants could exclusively consume the more preferred or less costly reinforcer without experiencing deprivation when the two concurrently available reinforcers served the same function (e.g., either food reduced hunger). By contrast, when the two stimuli served different functions, exclusive consumption of one reinforcer resulted in deprivation of the other (e.g., sustenance, but no fun or leisure). If each reinforcer is important or valued, individuals may continue to allocate responding to both options as schedule requirements increase.

### Implications for Weakening Undesirable Behavior

Investigators have adopted economic concepts to treat problem behavior through parametric evaluations of differential consequences for problem and appropriate behaviors (DeLeon, Fisher, Herman, & Crosland, 2000; DeLeon, Neidert, Anders, & Rodriguez-Catter, 2001; Delmendo, Borrero, Beauchamp, & Francisco, 2009; Kerwin, Ahearn, Eicher, & Burd, 1995; Perry & Fisher, 2001). Some researchers have manipulated the costs and benefits of responding to treat problem behavior or to maintain treatment effects across unit-price changes when the reinforcers for problem and alternative behaviors are symmetrical. Others have used substitutability concepts. We consider these approaches in separate sections.

#### Unit-Price Manipulations

Investigators have manipulated the cost and benefit components of unit price and assessed its effects on problem behavior. For example, Roane, Falcomata, and Fisher (2007) showed that a schedule for differential reinforcement of other behavior (DRO) in which a 10-second absence of inappropriate vocalizations produced 20 seconds of reinforcement was effective. Next, they increased the DRO interval and held the amount of reinforcement constant. The DRO became ineffective when the interval reached 23 seconds. A behavioral-economic interpretation suggests that the participant was "paying" with a longer delay for the same amount of the reinforcer (i.e., the

unit price had increased). In a second analysis, they again increased the DRO interval, but also proportionally increased the reinforcement component. Problem behavior was maintained at low rates up to a 180-second DRO interval and a corresponding 360-second reinforcement interval. Thus a strategy for increasing the effectiveness of behavioral treatments across price increases involves corresponding changes in the magnitude of the reinforcer to preserve unit price.

Others have similarly manipulated unit price parametrically by varying either the schedule requirements or reinforcer magnitude to produce more favorable response–reinforcer ratios (Borrero, Francisco, Haberlin, Ross, & Sran, 2007; Trosclair-Lasserre et al., 2008). Trosclair-Lasserre et al. (2008) showed less elastic demand for larger-magnitude reinforcers (120 seconds of attention) than smaller-magnitude reinforcers (10 seconds of attention) for two of four children whose problem behavior was maintained by attention. Other investigators have used unit-price manipulations to inform treatment development (DeLeon et al., 2000; Roane et al., 2001; Wilson & Gratz, 2016). DeLeon et al. (2000) used an abbreviated progressive-ratio schedule to accurately predict the difference between reinforcement schedules for aggressive and alternative behaviors needed to maintain more alternative behavior than aggression. Roane et al. (2001) showed that reinforcers with less elastic demand profiles were generally more effective as reinforcers in DRO schedules used to treat problem behavior than were reinforcers with more elastic profiles.

#### Stimulus Substitutability

Numerous human and nonhuman behavioral pharmacology and addiction studies have used economic analyses to examine whether certain compounds can be substituted for drugs of abuse (e.g., Johnson & Bickel, 2003; Petry & Bickel, 1998; Pope et al., 2019; Shahan, Odum, & Bickel, 2000; Smethells, Harris, Burroughs, Hursh, & Lesage, 2018). For example, Pope et al. (2019) recently used demand curves to examine the substitutability of nicotine gum, chewing tobacco, and e-liquid to cigarettes. Only e-liquid, the substance in electronic cigarettes, substituted for actual cigarettes. Substitutability increased as the nicotine concentration in the e-liquid increased, but the overall substitution effects were marginal.

Investigators have also examined whether foods that promote obesity and either healthier foods or activity reinforcers are substitutable. For example, Salvy, Nitecki, and Epstein (2009) examined whether social activities with a friend or with an unfamiliar peer would substitute for food in overweight and nonoverweight children. Social interaction with an unfamiliar but not a familiar peer substituted for food when the cost of food increased for overweight and nonoverweight children. Temple, Legierski, Giacomelli, Salvy, and Epstein (2008) evaluated demand for food on an escalating reinforcement schedule versus nonfood activities on a constant, low schedule. Generally, overweight children completed higher schedule values for food as the price increased than nonoverweight children did. In addition, demand was less elastic for food in overweight children as prices increased when alternative activities were concurrently available.

Shore, Iwata, DeLeon, Kahng, and Smith (1997) were perhaps the first to explicitly examine substitutability in treating problem behavior for individuals with neurodevelopmental disorders. Participants switched from self-injurious behavior (SIB) to engagement with preferred leisure items that were available continuously and noncontingently, suggesting that leisure items were substitutable for the automatic reinforcement from SIB. In a second experiment, participants had leisure-item access on a DRO schedule, and SIB increased. In a third experiment, the investigators tied the leisure item to a string and measured item engagement as a proportion of string length. Thus string length was the measure of effort (i.e., how far a participant had to reach to procure the item). SIB increased and leisure-item engagement decreased when the string was half of its original length.

Similarly, Zhou, Goff, and Iwata (2000) assessed preference for automatically reinforced problem behavior versus preferred leisure-item engagement. Participants engaged in problem behavior when both responses were freely available. Leisure-item engagement substituted for problem behavior when the participants wore a restrictive sleeve that increased response effort for problem behavior. Results of these studies demonstrate that increases in effort for one response will likely increase responding that produces a substitutable reinforcer.

Frank-Crawford, Castillo, and DeLeon (2018) examined whether edible reinforcers would substitute for escape from instructional activities. Participants could choose to complete a task and earn an edible reinforcer, or to take a 30-second break with no edible reinforcer. The response requirements for the edible reinforcer increased after every fifth trial. Some participants chose work regardless of the reinforcement schedule or the specific reinforcer. Others chose to work when the response requirements were low, but switched to escape as the response requirements increased. Furthermore, different edible reinforcers produced different demand profiles, as in Figure 7.1. Results suggested that behavior analysts could use this procedure to predict the relative effectiveness of reinforcers to treat escape-maintained problem behavior during reinforcement schedule thinning.

## DELAY AND PROBABILITY AS COST

Thus far, we have mostly considered cost as the effort required to produce a reinforcer. *Delay* to reinforcement is another "cost" in choice arrangements. In fact, the few studies that have directly compared effort and delay as costs have found parallel effects: Increases in either can result in decreased reinforcer consumption (e.g., Bauman, 1991). Thus, just as increases in response requirements can shift responding away from more expensive items, increases in delay can have the same effect.

### Assessing Delay Discounting

Much of what is known about the impact of delay has been determined in experiments on *delay discounting*. This term usually refers to the decrease in a reinforcer's present subjective value as delay increases (Mazur, 1987; Critchfield & Kollins, 2001). In other words, the efficacy of a reinforcer may decrease as a function of delays to its delivery. A delay-discounting task assesses preferences between a smaller–sooner reward and a larger–later reward at variable delays. Often participants choose the larger–later reward when the delivery of both the smaller–sooner reward and larger–later reward are set in the future. Investigators often observe a change in preference to the smaller–sooner reward as its delivery time draws closer. For example, given a choice between $50 in 9 months or $100 in 1 year, most participants would prefer the larger-magnitude reward. By contrast, *preference reversal* occurs when, given a choice between $50 now or $100 in 3 months, preference for the smaller, more immediate reward emerges (Tversky & Thaler, 1990).

Investigators have replicated the results described above across species (e.g., Kirby & Herrnstein, 1995; Mazur, 1987; Mazur & Biondi, 2009;

Rachlin, Raineri, & Cross, 1991); among individuals with substance abuse (e.g., Bickel, Odum, & Madden, 1999; Coffey, Gudleski, Saladin, & Brady, 2003); and across monetary gains and losses (Odum, Madden, & Bickel, 2002), which are predicted by a hyperbolic discounting function. Mazur (1987) was one of the first investigators to assess delay-discounting rates in pigeons by using an adjusting-delay procedure. Mazur held the amounts of the smaller and larger rewards constant and adjusted the delay to the larger reward delivery across trials. Pigeons selected between 2-second access to grain with a 2-second delay and 6-second access with an adjusted delay. The delay to the larger–later reward in the next trial increased if a pigeon selected the larger–later reward and decreased if the pigeon selected the smaller–sooner reward. This procedure continued until the pigeon reached an *indifference point*, in which it selected either alternative 50% of the time. Thus the subjective value for the smaller–sooner reward and larger–later reward were about equal at the indifference point. Mazur observed that indifference points follow a hyperbolic function, and suggested the following hyperbolic discounting equation:

$$V = \frac{A}{1 + kD}$$

where $V$ is the subjective value of a reward; $A$ is the amount of the reward; $d$ is the delay to the reward; and $k$ is a free parameter that describes how much the delay affects the value of a reward, also called the *discounting rate*. The discounting rate describes how steeply delay decreases the value of a reward, as measured by response rate or choice for one reward over another. In other words, the subjective value of a reward decreases as a function of the delay to the delivery of that reward as $k$ increases. As a fitted parameter, $k$ often serves as the dependent variable in delay-discounting studies and may be considered an individual-differences parameter, sensitive to both state and trait influences (see Odum, 2011).

Alternatively, investigators sometimes hold the delay and amount of the larger–later reward constant and adjust the amount of the smaller–sooner reward until an individual demonstrates indifference in the *adjusting-amount procedure*. For example, Rachlin et al. (1991) assessed choices between large delayed and small immediate hypothetical rewards. Participants could choose between receiving $1,000 delivered at delays from 1 month to 50 years, or an amount that varied from $1 to $1,000 delivered immediately. These investigators additionally examined *probability discounting,* or the extent to which the odds of actually receiving the larger reinforcer would influence choices against certain, but smaller rewards. Participants in the probability-discounting group could choose between receiving $1,000 in probabilities that varied from 5 to 100%, or an amount that varied from $1 to $1,000 delivered for certain. For example, investigators asked participants to choose between having a 50% chance of receiving $1,000 or receiving $1 for certain. Results showed that the hyperbolic discounting function described discounting for both delayed choices and choices with probabilistic outcomes.

## Determinants of Delay Discounting

The *magnitude effect* is the effect of reward magnitude on delay and probability discounting and is a robust finding in the discounting literature. In delay discounting, individuals discount smaller reward magnitudes more steeply than larger ones, with responding for smaller rewards decreasing more rapidly across similar increases in delay (Green, Fry, & Myerson, 1994; Green, Myerson, & McFadden, 1997; Odum, Baumann, & Rimington, 2006). In other words, the decrease in the subjective value of smaller delayed rewards is greater than the decrease in the subjective value of larger delayed rewards. Investigators have observed the opposite effect when rewards are probabilistic: Individuals discount smaller probabilistic rewards less steeply than larger ones (Estle, Green, Myerson, & Holt, 2007). Investigators often use hypothetical rewards in these procedures, to facilitate assessment of large-magnitude rewards that investigators typically cannot pay due to financial constraints (e.g., $1,000). Hypothetical rewards also allow investigators to assess long delays (e.g., 50 years) that may be impractical with real rewards. Importantly, studies have not found differences in discounting between real and hypothetical rewards across preparations (Kirby & Maraković, 1995; Johnson & Bickel, 2002; Lagorio & Madden, 2005).

The *domain effect*, or the type of rewards evaluated, can also influence discounting. The hyperbolic function also describes discounting of nonmonetary rewards like alcohol (Petry, 2001; Estle et al., 2007), cigarettes (Bickel et al., 1999; Odum et al., 2002; Reynolds, Richard, Horn, & Karraker, 2004), food (Charlton & Fantino, 2008; Odum & Rainaud, 2003), and sexual outcomes (Johnson &

Bruner, 2012; Lawyer, Williams, Prihodova, Rollins, & Lester, 2010), but differences in the rate of discounting can be observed across reinforcer classes. For example, Odum and Rainaud (2003) found that participants discounted money less steeply than preferred food and alcohol, which they discounted at similar rates. Charlton and Fantino (2008) theorized that the domain effect observed across consumable commodities was due to metabolic function. They observed that participants discounted money less steeply than entertainment media, and discounted entertainment media less steeply than preferred food. Thus participants tend to discount more steeply those rewards that have a direct metabolic function (e.g., food, water, drugs) relative to those that do not (e.g., money, entertainment media). However, Charlton and Fantino also offered that domain effects may be related to commodity *fungibility*, or the degree to which a commodity is exchangeable for other commodities. Money, for example, is exchangeable for various primary and secondary reinforcers, which may account for the shallower rate of discounting for money versus less fungible commodities, like food and commodity-specific gift cards (Holt, Glodowski, Smits-Seeman, & Tiry, 2016).

## Delay Discounting in Clinical Populations

Studies have shown that populations with substance use disorders discount their preferred drugs more steeply than monetary rewards (Coffey et al., 2003; Madden, Petry, Badger, & Bickel, 1997). Delay-discounting studies with obese adults have found that they discount monetary rewards more steeply than average-weight adults do (Weller, Cook, Avsar, & Cox, 2008; Epstein et al., 2014; Bickel, Wilson, et al., 2014). These results suggest that individuals with substance use disorders and obesity prefer immediate over delayed rewards more than their non-substance-misusing and non-overweight peers.

Characteristics like age (Green et al., 1994; Scheres et al., 2006), IQ (de Wit, Flory, Acheson, McCloskey, & Manuck, 2007), and diagnosis (Demurie, Roeyers, Baeyens, & Sonuga-Barke, 2012) can affect discounting rates. Individuals with impulse-control disorders may be particularly affected by delays to reinforcement; thus studying discounting with this population is important. Research using hypothetical and real monetary rewards delivered in real-time have found that children diagnosed with attention-deficit/hyperactivity disorder, combined type (ADHD-C; combi-

nation hyperactive/impulsive) display steeper discounting rates for monetary rewards than children diagnosed with ADHD, inattentive type (ADHD-I) and their typically developing peers (Scheres, Tontsch, Thoeny, & Kaczkurkin, 2010; Scheres, Tontsch, & Thoeny, 2013; Sonuga-Barke, Taylor, Sembi, & Smith, 1992). Rosch and Mostofsky (2016) assessed discounting for leisure activities in children with ADHD-C and typically developing children. They found that girls with ADHD-C displayed a greater discounting rate for leisure activities than boys with ADHD-C and the typically developing group.

Delays in the delivery of reinforcers are ubiquitous in the natural environment. For example, teachers often use tokens to bridge the delay between the target response and reinforcer delivery (Hackenberg, 2009). Reed and Martens (2011) conducted a discounting assessment for hypothetical monetary rewards with 46 typically developing sixth graders. They then implemented a classwide intervention where students could earn tokens exchangeable for preferred items for on-task behavior. Token exchange occurred immediately after the session or at the beginning of the next day's session. Reed and Martens found that discounting rates correlated with on-task behavior during the intervention. Students who displayed higher scores on the discounting assessment engaged in less on-task behavior when it produced delayed token exchange. Therefore, the delay-discounting assessment for hypothetical rewards was predictive of the effects of delayed rewards on classroom behavior. Investigators have used similar delay-discounting preparations with young children; results suggest that these assessments may be useful for examining developmental progressions, academic disorders, and/or neurodevelopmental disorders in children (see Staubitz, Lloyd, & Reed, 2018)

Leon, Borrero, and DeLeon (2016) assessed the effects of delays for primary and conditioned reinforcers on the responding of individuals with neurodevelopmental disorders. Responding was maintained at high levels when the investigators delivered food or tokens immediately after the response or exchanged tokens for food immediately after a participant earned the token. Responding decreased most as delays to token delivery increased, followed by delays to token exchange. Delays to food reinforcers maintained responding at longer delays than delays to token delivery or token exchange.

Delayed reinforcement may also affect skill acquisition in individuals with neurodevelopmental disorders. Sy and Vollmer (2012) found that al-though some participants learned conditional dis-criminations during delayed-reinforcement condi-tions, others did not. Similarly, Carroll, Kodak, and Adolf (2015) showed that delays to reinforce-ment decreased the efficiency and effectiveness of discrete-trial instruction for a receptive-identifica-tion task.

In summary, delays to reinforcement may have a negative effect on some individuals with neuro-developmental disorders. Investigators have used progressive schedules to teach such individuals to tolerate delay to reinforcement. For example, Dixon et al. (1998) gave three adults with neuro-developmental disorders a concurrent choice be-tween a smaller- and larger-magnitude reward, and asked these adults to engage in a concurrent activ-ity (e.g., exercise) during the delay to the larger reward. Dixon et al. gradually increased the delay to the larger reward, and found that selection of the larger delayed reward and the time engaging in the concurrent activity increased for the three participants. Further research demonstrated that individuals with autism spectrum disorder pre-ferred the activity over waiting without an activity (Dixon & Cummings, 2001; Dixon, Rehfeldt, & Randich, 2003).

## EMERGING THEMES IN BEHAVIORAL ECONOMICS

### Hypothetical Purchase Tasks

Recent research has studied hypothetical choices among commodities with different prices rather than delays (see discussion by Roma, Reed, Di-Gennaro Reed, & Hursh, 2017). Investigators have used a *hypothetical purchase task*, which asks par-ticipants to indicate the quantity of a commodity they would purchase at varying price points. Hy-pothetical purchase tasks demonstrate adequate relations with actual consumption (e.g., Amlung, Acker, Stojek, Murphy, & MacKillop, 2012), pre-dictive validity (e.g., MacKillop & Murphy, 2007), construct validity (e.g., MacKillop et al., 2010), and temporal stability (e.g., Few, Acker, Murphy, & MacKillop, 2012). Behavioral-economic find-ings with hypothetical purchase tasks reproduce those observed in operant laboratories, suggesting that they reflect real-world behavior. For example, these tasks appear sensitive to economy type (e.g., Kaplan et al., 2017) and availability of substitutes (e.g., Grace, Kivell, & Laugesen, 2014); they also demonstrate consistent elasticity across differing price densities (e.g., Reed, Kaplan, Roma, & Hursh, 2014) and sequences (e.g., Amlung & MacKillop, 2012). The sound psychometric properties and correspondence of hypothetical purchase tasks with known behavioral-economic variables is im-portant, because these procedures are helpful in studies that would be unethical or infeasible to do otherwise.

Investigators have used hypothetical purchase tasks to predict how consumption for various com-modities change as a function of price. For ex-ample, Kaplan and Reed (2018) used an alcohol purchase task to examine the effects of happy-hour drink pricing on excessive alcohol consumption. Higgins et al. (2017) demonstrated the utility of cigarette purchase tasks in simulating effects of cigarette nicotine content regulations and pric-ing policies on cigarette smokers. These studies and others show that hypothetical purchase tasks provide a safe simulation of various clinically im-portant consumer behaviors and open the door for large-scale applications of behavioral economics at the policy level.

### Reinforcer Pathology

Investigators have used a *reinforcer pathology* model to characterize some forms of maladaptive behav-ior. This model classifies maladaptive behavior based on responses to reinforcers and manipula-tion of reinforcement parameters, such as exces-sive demand (i.e. willingness to pay much higher prices for a commodity) or excessive sensitivity to delay (i.e., discounting functions for the commod-ity that indicate excessive value of immediacy) relative to the norm (Bickel, Jarmolowicz, Mueller, & Gatchalian, 2011).

Reinforcer pathology has only recently been de-fined as the combined effects of (1) a consistent high valuation of a particular reinforcer or com-modity and (2) excessive preference for immediate reinforcement despite possible negative outcomes (Carr, Daniel, Lin, & Epstein, 2011). For example, cigarette smokers' demand for nicotine is inelastic under conditions of deprivation (Madden & Bick-el, 1999); current cigarette smokers also discount the value of delayed money more steeply than never- and ex-smokers, and more so for delayed cigarettes than for delayed money (Bickel et al., 1999). Therefore, the relation between excessive discounting and demand for the misused com-modity may account for substance use disorders, but research on this relation has been inconclusive

(Bickel, Johnson, Koffarnus, MacKillop, & Murphy, 2014). Rats with steep delay discounting for food demonstrated inelastic demand for nicotine self-administration (Diergaarde, van Mourik, Pattij, Schoffelmeer, & De Vries, 2012). Conversely, Field, Santarcangelo, Sumnall, Goudie, and Cole (2006) found that human participants demonstrated steeper delay discounting for monetary rewards, but that demand for cigarettes was unaffected during nicotine deprivation.

According to the reinforcer pathology model, intervening in substance use should produce change in measures of demand and discounting. Madden and Kalman (2010) monitored smokers' cigarette demand by using a purchase task during a course of either bupropion, a medication that dampens the reinforcing effects of nicotine, or counseling treatment. Shifts in simulated demand after 1 week of either treatment predicted eventual cessation. In a related study, McClure, Vandrey, Johnson, and Stitzer (2013) found that participants receiving varenicline (a medication that reduces nicotine craving and withdrawal) demonstrated greater demand elasticity for simulated cigarette purchases in a programmed relapse period than those receiving a placebo. Additional research on the effects of substance use treatment on simulated demand is needed.

### On Other Variants of Behavioral Economics

We would like to end by emphasizing that behavior analysts should not ignore the very interesting findings of more cognitively oriented behavioral economists. Popular books written from this perspective, such as *Predictably Irrational* (Ariely, 2008), *Thinking, Fast and Slow* (Kahneman, 2011), and *Nudge: Improving Decisions about Health, Wealth, and Happiness* (Thaler & Sunstein, 2008), contain a wealth of information about the factors that influence choice and tactics for changing human behavior in meaningful ways. For example, Thaler and Sunstein introduce the concept of *choice architecture,* which involves how we can arrange environments to promote choices that are beneficial to humans and our cultures. Behavior analysts have begun to deconstruct many of these principles from more behavioral perspectives, like sunk costs (e.g., Navarro & Fantino, 2005), framing effects (e.g., Naudé, Kaplan, Reed, Henley, & DiGennaro Reed, 2018), and prospect theory (e.g., Rachlin et al., 1991). Despite the fact that the interpretation of such phenomena may differ depending upon whether one is a cognitively or behaviorally oriented theorist, behavior analysts should always be interested in procedures that reliably influence human choice.

### CONCLUSION

Behavioral economics represents the intersection of microeconomic concepts and behavioral psychology. Both traditional and operant behavioral economics are gaining notoriety in mainstream media and policy making (Hursh & Roma, 2013), in part due to the face-valid approaches and socially significant outcomes across a range of applications (see the bibliometric analysis by Costa, Carvalho, & Moreira, 2019). The operant approach to behavioral economics is entirely compatible with the dimensions of behavior analysis and offers a unique lens to aid in basic (Hursh & Roma, 2016) and practical (Reed et al., 2013) issues. Although behavior analysis has increasingly used behavioral economics to address applied issues (see Gilroy et al., 2018), the field remains relatively small. Emerging concepts in behavioral economics, like reinforcer pathology theory (e.g., Bickel et al., 2011) and hypothetical purchase tasks (e.g., Roma et al., 2017), provide exciting new frontiers for behavioral-economic approaches to societal concerns. Given the unique insights afforded by behavioral economics, behavior analysts can affect meaningful change that is conceptually systematic with behavior-analytic principles.

### ACKNOWLEDGMENTS

Grant Nos. 5R01HD079113, 5R01HD083214, and 1R01HD093734 from the National Institute of Child Health and Human Development provided partial support to Brian D. Greer for this work.

### REFERENCES

Amlung, M. T., Acker, J., Stojek, M. K., Murphy, J. G., & MacKillop, J. (2012). Is talk "cheap"?: An initial investigation of the equivalence of alcohol purchase task performance for hypothetical and actual rewards. *Alcoholism: Clinical and Experimental Research, 36,* 716–724.

Amlung, M., & MacKillop, J. (2012). Consistency of self-reported alcohol consumption on randomized and sequential alcohol purchase tasks. *Frontiers in Psychiatry, 3,* 65.

Ariely, D. (2008). *Predictably irrational: The hidden forces that shape our decisions.* New York: Harper Perennial.

Bauman, R. (1991). An experimental analysis of the cost of food in a closed economy. *Journal of the Experimental Analysis of Behavior, 56,* 33–50.

Bickel, W. K., Jarmolowicz, D. P., Mueller, E. T., & Gatchalian, K. M. (2011). The behavioral economics and neuroeconomics of reinforcer pathologies: Implications for etiology and treatment of addiction. *Current Psychiatry Reports, 13,* 406–415.

Bickel, W. K., Johnson, M. W., Koffarnus, M. N., MacKillop, J., & Murphy, J. G. (2014). The behavioral economics of substance use disorders: Reinforcement pathologies and their repair. *Annual Review of Clinical Psychology, 10,* 641–677.

Bickel, W. K., Odum, A. L., & Madden, G. J. (1999). Impulsivity and cigarette smoking: Delay discounting in current, never, and ex-smokers. *Psychopharmacology, 146,* 447–454.

Bickel, W. K., Wilson, A. G., Franck, C. T., Mueller, E. T., Jarmolowicz, D. P., Koffarnus, M. N., et al. (2014). Using crowdsourcing to compare temporal, social temporal, and probability discounting among obese and non-obese individuals. *Appetite, 75,* 82–89.

Borrero, J. C., Francisco, M. T., Haberlin, A. T., Ross, N. A., & Sran, S. K. (2007). A unit price evaluation of severe problem behavior. *Journal of Applied Behavior Analysis, 40,* 463–474.

Call, N. A., Trosclair-Lasserre, N. M., Findley, A. J., Reavis, A. R., & Shillingsburg, M. A. (2012). Correspondence between single versus daily preference assessment outcomes and reinforcer efficacy under progressive-ratio schedules. *Journal of Applied Behavior Analysis, 45,* 763–777.

Carr, K. A., Daniel, T. O., Lin, H., & Epstein, L. H. (2011). Reinforcement pathology and obesity. *Current Drug Abuse Reviews, 4,* 190–196.

Carroll, R. A., Kodak, T., & Adolf, K. J. (2016). Effect of delayed reinforcement on skill acquisition during discrete-trial instruction: Implications for treatment-integrity errors in academic settings. *Journal of Applied Behavior Analysis, 49,* 176–181.

Charlton, S. R., & Fantino, E. (2008). Commodity specific rates of temporal discounting: Does metabolic function underlie differences in rates of discounting? *Behavioural Processes, 77,* 334–342.

Coffey, S. F., Gudleski, G. D., Saladin, M. E., & Brady, K. T. (2003). Impulsivity and rapid discounting of delayed hypothetical rewards in cocaine-dependent individuals. *Experimental and Clinical Psychopharmacology, 11,* 18–25.

Costa, D. F., Carvalho, F. D. M., & Moreira, B. C. D. M. (2019). Behavioral economics and behavioral finance: A bibliometric analysis of the scientific fields. *Journal of Economic Surveys, 33,* 3–24.

Critchfield, T. S., & Kollins, S. H. (2001). Temporal discounting: Basic research and the analysis of so-cially important behavior. *Journal of Applied Behavior Analysis, 34,* 101–122.

de Wit, H., Flory, J. D., Acheson, A., McCloskey, M., & Manuck, S. B. (2007). IQ and nonplanning impulsivity are independently associated with delay discounting in middle-aged adults. *Personality and Individual Differences, 42,* 111–121.

DeLeon, I. G., Fisher, W. W., Herman, K. M., & Crosland, K. C. (2000). Assessment of a response bias for aggression over functionally equivalent appropriate behavior. *Journal of Applied Behavior Analysis, 33,* 73–77.

DeLeon, I. G., Frank, M. A., Gregory, M. K., & Allman, M. J. (2009). On the correspondence between preference assessment outcomes and progressive-ratio schedule assessments of stimulus value. *Journal of Applied Behavior Analysis, 42,* 729–733.

DeLeon, I. G., & Iwata, B. A. (1996). Evaluation of a multiple-stimulus presentation format for assessing reinforcer preferences. *Journal of Applied Behavior Analysis, 29,* 519–533.

DeLeon, I. G., Iwata, B. A., Goh, H., & Worsdell, A. S. (1997). Emergence of reinforcer preference as a function of schedule requirements and stimulus similarity. *Journal of Applied Behavior Analysis, 30,* 439–449.

DeLeon, I. G., Neidert, P. L., Anders, B. M., & Rodriguez-Catter, V. (2001). Choices between positive and negative reinforcement during treatment for escape-maintained behavior. *Journal of Applied Behavior Analysis, 34,* 521–525.

Delmendo, X., Borrero, J. C., Beauchamp, K. L., & Francisco, M. T. (2009). Consumption and response output as a function of unit price: Manipulation of cost and benefit components. *Journal of Applied Behavior Analysis, 42,* 609–625.

Demurie, E., Roeyers, H., Baeyens, D., & Sonuga-Barke, E. (2012). Temporal discounting of monetary rewards in children with ADHD and autism spectrum disorders. *Developmental Science, 15,* 791–800.

Diergaarde, L., van Mourik, Y., Pattij, T., Schoffelmeer, A. N., & De Vries, T. J. (2012). Poor impulse control predicts inelastic demand for nicotine but not alcohol in rats. *Addiction Biology, 17,* 576–587.

Dixon, M. R., & Cummings, A. (2001). Self-control in children with autism: Response allocation during delays to reinforcement. *Journal of Applied Behavior Analysis, 34,* 491–495.

Dixon, M. R., Hayes, L. J., Binder, L. M., Manthey, S., Sigman, C., & Zdanowski, D. M. (1998). Using a self-control training procedure to increase appropriate behavior. *Journal of Applied Behavior Analysis, 31,* 203–210.

Dixon, M. R., Rehfeldt, R. A., & Randich, L. (2003). Enhancing tolerance to delayed reinforcers: The role of intervening activities. *Journal of Applied Behavior Analysis, 36,* 263–266.

Epstein, L. H., Jankowiak, N., Fletcher, K. D., Carr, K. A., Nederkoorn, C., Raynor, H. A., et al. (2014).

Women who are motivated to eat and discount the future are more obese. *Obesity, 22*, 1394–1399.

Estle, S. J., Green, L., Myerson, J., & Holt, D. D. (2007). Discounting of monetary and directly consumable rewards. *Psychological Science, 18*, 58–63.

Few, L. R., Acker, J., Murphy, C., & MacKillop, J. (2012). Temporal stability of a cigarette purchase task. *Nicotine Tobacco Research, 14*, 761–765.

Field, M., Santarcangelo, M., Sumnall, H., Goudie, A., & Cole, J. (2006). Delay discounting and the behavioural economics of cigarette purchases in smokers: The effects of nicotine deprivation. *Psychopharmacology, 186*, 255–263.

Fisher, W., Piazza, C. C., Bowman, L. G., Hagopian, L. P., Owens, J. C., & Slevin, I. (1992). A comparison of two approaches for identifying reinforcers for persons with severe and profound disabilities. *Journal of Applied Behavior Analysis, 25*, 491–498.

Fiske, K. E., Isenhower, R. W., Bamond, M. J., Delmolino, L., Sloman, K. N., & LaRue, R. H. (2015). Assessing the value of token reinforcement for individuals with autism. *Journal of Applied Behavior Analysis, 48*, 448–453.

Francisco, M. T., Borrero, J. C., & Sy, J. R. (2008). Evaluation of absolute and relative reinforcer value using progressive-ratio schedules. *Journal of Applied Behavior Analysis, 41*, 189–202.

Frank-Crawford, M. A., Castillo, M. I., & DeLeon, I. G. (2018). Does preference rank predict substitution for the reinforcer for problem behavior?: A behavioral economic analysis. *Journal of Applied Behavior Analysis, 51*, 276–282.

Fuqua, R. W. (1984). Comments on the applied relevance of the matching law. *Journal of Applied Behavior Analysis, 17*, 381–386.

Gilroy, S. P., Kaplan, B. A., & Leader, G. (2018). A systematic review of applied behavioral economics in assessments and treatments for individuals with developmental disabilities. *Review Journal of Autism and Developmental Disorders, 5*, 247–259.

Glover, A. C., Roane, H. S., Kadey, H. J., & Grow, L. L. (2008). Preference for reinforcers under progressive- and fixed-ratio schedules: A comparison of single and concurrent arrangements. *Journal of Applied Behavior Analysis, 41*, 163–176.

Goldberg, M. C., Allman, M. J., Hagopian, L. P., Triggs, M. M., Frank-Crawford, M. A., Mostofsky, S. H., et al. (2017). Examining the reinforcing value of stimuli within social and non-social contexts in children with and without high-functioning autism. *Autism, 21*, 881–895.

Grace, R. C., Kivell, B. M., & Laugesen, M. (2014). Estimating cross-price elasticity of e-cigarettes using a simulated demand procedure. *Nicotine and Tobacco Research, 17*, 592–598.

Green, L., & Freed, D. E. (1993). The substitutability of reinforcers. *Journal of the Experimental Analysis of Behavior, 60*, 141–158.

Green, L., Fry, A. F., & Myerson, J. (1994). Discounting of delayed rewards: A life-span comparison. *Psychological Science, 5*, 33–36.

Green, L., Myerson, J., & McFadden, E. (1997). Rate of temporal discounting decreases with amount of reward. *Memory and Cognition, 25*, 715–723.

Hackenberg, T. D. (2009). Token reinforcement: A review and analysis. *Journal of the Experimental Analysis of Behavior, 91*, 257–286.

Higgins, S. T., Heil, S. H., Sigmon, S. C., Tidey, J. W., Gaalema, D. E., Hughes, J. R., et al. (2017). Addiction potential of cigarettes with reduced nicotine content in populations with psychiatric disorders and other vulnerabilities to tobacco addiction. *JAMA Psychiatry, 74*, 1056–1064.

Hodos, W. (1961). Progressive ratio as a measure of reward strength. *Science, 134*, 943–944.

Hoffmann, A. N., Samaha, A. L., Bloom, S. E., & Boyle, M. A. (2017). Preference and reinforcer efficacy of high- and low-tech items: A comparison of item type and duration of access. *Journal of Applied Behavior Analysis, 50*, 222–237.

Holt, D. D., Glodowski, K., Smits-Seemann, R. R., & Tiry, A. M. (2016). The domain effect in delay discounting: The roles of fungibility and perishability. *Behavioural Processes, 131*, 47–52.

Hursh, S. R., Madden, G. J., Spiga, R., DeLeon, I. G., & Francisco, M. T. (2013). The translational utility of behavioral economics: The experimental analysis of consumption and choice. In G. J. Madden (Ed.) & W. V. Dube, T. D. Hackenberg, G. P. Hanley, & K. A. Lattal (Assoc. Eds.), *APA handbook of behavior analysis: Vol. 2. Translating principles into practice* (pp. 109–128). Washington, DC: American Psychological Association.

Hursh, S. R., & Roma, P. G. (2013). Behavioral economics and empirical public policy. *Journal of the Experimental Analysis of Behavior, 99*, 98–124.

Hursh, S. R., & Roma, P. G. (2016). Behavioral economics and the analysis of consumption and choice. *Managerial and Decision Economics, 37*, 224–238.

Hursh, S. R., & Silberberg, A. (2008). Economic demand and essential value. *Psychological Review, 115*, 186–198.

Jarmolowicz, D. P., & Lattal, K. A. (2010). On distinguishing progressively increasing response requirements for reinforcement. *Behavior Analyst, 33*, 119–125.

Jerome, J., & Sturmey, P. (2008). Reinforcing efficacy of interactions with preferred and nonpreferred staff under progressive-ratio schedules. *Journal of Applied Behavior Analysis, 41*, 221–225.

Johnson, M. W., & Bickel, W. K. (2002). Within-subject comparison of real and hypothetical money rewards in delay discounting. *Journal of the Experimental Analysis of Behavior, 77*, 129–146.

Johnson, M. W., & Bickel, W. K. (2003). The behavioral economics of cigarette smoking: The concurrent presence of a substitute and an independent reinforcer. *Behavioural Pharmacology, 14,* 137–144.

Johnson, M. W., & Bruner, N. R. (2012). The sexual discounting task: HIV risk behavior and the discounting of delayed sexual rewards in cocaine dependence. *Drug and Alcohol Dependence, 123,* 15–21.

Kagel, J. H., & Winkler, R. C. (1972). Behavioral economics: Areas of cooperative research between economics and applied behavioral research. *Journal of Applied Behavior Analysis, 5,* 335–342.

Kahneman, D. (2011). *Thinking, fast and slow.* New York: Farrar, Straus & Giroux.

Kaplan, B. A., & Reed, D. D. (2018). Happy hour drink specials in the alcohol purchase task. *Experimental and Clinical Psychopharmacology, 26,* 156–167.

Kaplan, B. A., Reed, D. D., Murphy, J. G., Henley, A. J., Reed, F. D. D., Roma, P. G., et al. (2017). Time constraints in the alcohol purchase task. *Experimental and Clinical Psychopharmacology, 25*(3), 186–197.

Kerwin, M. E., Ahearn, W. H., Eicher, P. S., & Burd, D. M. (1995). The costs of eating: A behavioral economic analysis of food refusal. *Journal of Applied Behavior Analysis, 28,* 245–260.

Kirby, K. N., & Herrnstein, R. J. (1995). Preference reversals due to myopic discounting of delayed reward. *Psychological Science, 6,* 83–89.

Kirby, K. N., & Maraković, N. N. (1995). Modeling myopic decisions: Evidence for hyperbolic delay-discounting within subjects and amounts. *Organizational Behavior and Human Decision Processes, 64,* 22–30.

Kodak, T., Lerman, D. C., & Call, N. (2007). Evaluating the influence of postsession reinforcement on choice of reinforcers. *Journal of Applied Behavior Analysis, 40,* 515–527.

Lagorio, C. H., & Madden, G. J. (2005). Delay discounting of real and hypothetical rewards: III. Steady-state assessments, forced-choice trials, and all real rewards. *Behavioural Processes, 69,* 173–187.

Lawyer, S. R., Williams, S. A., Prihodova, T., Rollins, J. D., & Lester, A. C. (2010). Probability and delay discounting of hypothetical sexual outcomes. *Behavioural Processes, 84,* 687–692.

Lea, S. E. G., & Roper, T. J. (1977). Demand for food on fixed-ratio schedules as a function of the quality of concurrently available reinforcement. *Journal of the Experimental Analysis of Behavior, 27,* 371–380.

Leon, Y., Borrero, J. C., & DeLeon, I. G. (2016). Parametric analysis of delayed primary and conditioned reinforcers. *Journal of Applied Behavior Analysis, 49,* 639–655.

Mach, E. (1914). *The analysis of sensations and the relation of the physical to the psychical.* Chicago: Open Court.

MacKillop, J., & Murphy, J. G. (2007). A behavioral economic measure of demand for alcohol predicts brief intervention outcomes. *Drug and Alcohol Dependence, 89,* 227–233.

MacKillop, J., O'Hagen, S., Lisman, S. A., Murphy, J. G., Ray, L. A., Tidey, J. W., & Monti, P. M. (2010). Behavioral economic analysis of cue-elicited craving for alcohol. *Addiction, 105,* 1599–1607.

Madden, G. J., & Bickel, W. K. (1999). Abstinence and price effects on demand for cigarettes: A behavioral-economic analysis. *Addiction, 94,* 577–588.

Madden, G. J., & Kalman, D. (2010). Effects of bupropion on simulated demand for cigarettes and the subjective effects of smoking. *Nicotine and Tobacco Research, 12,* 416–422.

Madden, G. J., Petry, N. M., Badger, G. J., & Bickel, W. K. (1997). Impulsive and self-control choices in opioid-dependent patients and non-drug-using control patients: Drug and monetary rewards. *Experimental and Clinical Psychopharmacology, 5,* 256–262.

Martin, A. L., Franklin, A. N., Perlman, J. E., & Bloomsmith, M. A. (2018). Systematic assessment of food item preference and reinforcer effectiveness: Enhancements in training laboratory-housed rhesus macaques. *Behavioural Processes, 157,* 445–452.

Mazur, J. E. (1987). An adjusting procedure for studying delayed reinforcement. In M. L. Commons, J. E. Mazur, J. A. Nevin, & H. Rachlin (Eds.), *Quantitative analysis of behavior: Vol. 5. The effect of delay and of intervening events on reinforcement value* (pp. 55–73). Hillsdale, NJ: Erlbaum.

Mazur, J. E., & Biondi, D. R. (2009). Delay–amount tradeoffs in choices by pigeons and rats: Hyperbolic versus exponential discounting. *Journal of the Experimental Analysis of Behavior, 91,* 197–211.

McClure, E. A., Vandrey, R. G., Johnson, M. W., & Stitzer, M. L. (2012). Effects of varenicline on abstinence and smoking reward following a programmed lapse. *Nicotine and Tobacco Research, 15,* 139–148.

Naudé, G. P., Kaplan, B. A., Reed, D. D., Henley, A. J., & DiGennaro Reed, F. D. (2018). Temporal framing and the hidden-zero effect: Rate-dependent outcomes on delay discounting. *Journal of the Experimental Analysis of Behavior, 109,* 506–519.

Navarro, A. D., & Fantino, E. (2005). The sunk cost effect in pigeons and humans. *Journal of the Experimental Analysis of Behavior, 83,* 1–13.

Odum, A. L. (2011). Delay discounting: I'm a k, you're a k. *Journal of the Experimental Analysis of Behavior, 96,* 427–439.

Odum, A. L., Baumann, A. A., & Rimington, D. D. (2006). Discounting of delayed hypothetical money and food: Effects of amount. *Behavioural Processes, 73,* 278–284.

Odum, A. L., Madden, G. J., & Bickel, W. K. (2002). Discounting of delayed health gains and losses by current, never- and ex-smokers of cigarettes. *Nicotine and Tobacco Research, 4,* 295–303.

Odum, A. L., & Rainaud, C. P. (2003). Discounting of delayed hypothetical money, alcohol, and food. *Behavioural Processes, 64,* 305–313.

Pace, G. M., Ivancic, M. T., Edwards, G. L., Iwata, B. A., & Page, T. J. (1985). Assessment of stimulus preference and reinforcer value with profoundly retarded individuals. *Journal of Applied Behavior Analysis, 18,* 249–255.

Penrod, B., Wallace, M. D., & Dyer, E. J. (2008). Assessing potency of high- and low-preference reinforcers with respect to response rate and response patterns. *Journal of Applied Behavior Analysis, 41,* 177–188.

Perry, A. C., & Fisher, W. W. (2001). Behavioral economic influences on treatments designed to decrease destructive behavior. *Journal of Applied Behavior Analysis, 34,* 211–215.

Petry, N. M. (2001). Delay discounting of money and alcohol in actively using alcoholics, currently abstinent alcoholics, and controls. *Psychopharmacology, 154,* 243–250.

Petry, N. M., & Bickel, W. K. (1998). Polydrug abuse in heroin addicts: A behavioral economic analysis. *Addiction, 93,* 321–335.

Pope, D. A., Poe, L., Stein, J. S., Kaplan, B. A., Heckman, B. W., Epstein, L. H., et al. (2019). Experimental tobacco marketplace: Substitutability of e-cigarette liquid for cigarettes as a function of nicotine strength. *Tobacco Control, 28,* 206–211.

Rachlin, H., Raineri, A., & Cross, D. (1991). Subjective probability and delay. *Journal of the Experimental Analysis of Behavior, 55,* 233–244.

Reed, D. D., Kaplan, B. A., & Becirevic, A. (2015). Basic research on the behavioral economics of reinforcer value. In F. D. DiGennaro Reed & D. D. Reed (Eds.), *Autism service delivery: Bridging the gap between science and practice* (pp. 279–306). New York: Springer.

Reed, D. D., Kaplan, B. A., Roma, P. G., & Hursh, S. R. (2014). Inter-method reliability of progression sizes in a hypothetical purchase task: Implications for empirical public policy. *Psychological Record, 64,* 671–679.

Reed, D. D., Luiselli, J. K., Magnuson, J. D., Fillers, S., Vieira, S., & Rue, H. C. (2009). A comparison between traditional economical and demand curve analyses of relative reinforcer efficacy in the validation of preference assessment predictions. *Developmental Neurorehabilitation, 12,* 164–169.

Reed, D. D., & Martens, B. K. (2011). Temporal discounting predicts student responsiveness to exchange delays in a classroom token system. *Journal of Applied Behavior Analysis, 44,* 1–18.

Reed, D. D., Niileksela, C. R., & Kaplan, B. A. (2013). Behavioral economics. *Behavior Analysis in Practice, 6,* 34–54.

Reynolds, B., Richards, J. B., Horn, K., & Karraker, K. (2004). Delay discounting and probability discounting as related to cigarette smoking status in adults. *Behavioural Processes, 65,* 35–42.

Roane, H. S., Call, N. A., & Falcomata, T. S. (2005). A preliminary analysis of adaptive responding under open and closed economies. *Journal of Applied Behavior Analysis, 38,* 335–348.

Roane, H. S., Falcomata, T. S., & Fisher, W. W. (2007). Applying the behavioral economics principle of unit price to DRO schedule thinning. *Journal of Applied Behavior Analysis, 40,* 529–534.

Roane, H. S., Lerman, D. C., & Vorndran, C. M. (2001). Assessing reinforcers under progressive schedule requirements. *Journal of Applied Behavior Analysis, 34,* 145–167.

Roane, H. S., Vollmer, T. R., Ringdahl, J. E., & Marcus, B. A. (1998). Evaluation of a brief stimulus preference assessment. *Journal of Applied Behavior Analysis, 31,* 605–620.

Roma, P. G., Reed, D. D., DiGennaro Reed, F. D., & Hursh, S. R. (2017). Progress of and prospects for hypothetical purchase task questionnaires in consumer behavior analysis and public policy. *Behavior Analyst, 40,* 329–342.

Rosch, K. S., & Mostofsky, S. H. (2016). Increased delay discounting on a novel real-time task among girls, but not boys, with ADHD. *Journal of the International Neuropsychological Society, 22,* 12–23.

Russell, D., Ingvarsson, E. T., Haggar, J. L., & Jessel, J. (2018). Using progressive ratio schedules to evaluate tokens as generalized conditioned reinforcers. *Journal of Applied Behavior Analysis, 51,* 40–52.

Salvy, S. J., Nitecki, L. A., & Epstein, L. H. (2009). Do social activities substitute for food in youth? *Annals of Behavioral Medicine, 38,* 205–212.

Scheres, A., Dijkstra, M., Ainslie, E., Balkan, J., Reynolds, B., Sonuga-Barke, E., et al. (2006). Temporal and probabilistic discounting of rewards in children and adolescents: Effects of age and ADHD symptoms. *Neuropsychologia, 44,* 2092–2103.

Scheres, A., Tontsch, C., & Thoeny, A. L. (2013). Steep temporal reward discounting in ADHD-combined type: Acting upon feelings. *Psychiatry Research, 209,* 207–213.

Scheres, A., Tontsch, C., Thoeny, A. L., & Kaczkurkin, A. (2010). Temporal reward discounting in attention-deficit/hyperactivity disorder: The contribution of symptom domains, reward magnitude, and session length. *Biological Psychiatry, 67,* 641–648.

Shahan, T. A., Odum, A. L., & Bickel, W. K. (2000). Nicotine gum as a substitute for cigarettes: A behavioral economic analysis. *Behavioural Pharmacology, 11,* 71–79.

Shore, B. A., Iwata, B. A., DeLeon, I. G., Kahng, S., & Smith, R. G. (1997). An analysis of reinforcer substitutability using object manipulation and self-injury as competing responses. *Journal of Applied Behavior Analysis, 30,* 21–40.

Smethells, J. R., Harris, A. C., Burroughs, D., Hursh, S. R., & LeSage, M. G. (2018). Substitutability of nicotine alone and an electronic cigarette liquid using a concurrent choice assay in rats: A behavioral economic analysis. *Drug and Alcohol Dependence, 185,* 58–66.

Sonuga-Barke, E. J. S., Taylor, E., Sembi, S., & Smith, J. (1992). Hyperactivity and delay aversion: 1. The effect of delay on choice. *Journal of Child Psychology and Psychiatry, 33,* 387–398.

Staubitz, J. L., Lloyd, B. P., & Reed, D. D. (2018). A summary of methods for measuring delay discounting in young children. *Psychological Record, 68,* 239–253.

Sy, J. R., & Vollmer, T. R. (2012). Discrimination acquisition in children with developmental disabilities under immediate and delayed reinforcement. *Journal of Applied Behavior Analysis, 45,* 667–684.

Temple, J. L., Legierski, C. M., Giacomelli, A. M., Salvy, S. J., & Epstein, L. H. (2008). Overweight children find food more reinforcing and consume more energy than do nonoverweight children. *American Journal of Clinical Nutrition, 87,* 1121–1127.

Thaler, R. H., & Sunstein, C. R. (2008). *Nudge: Improving decisions about health, wealth, and happiness.* New Haven, CT: Yale University Press.

Tiger, J. H., Toussaint, K. A., & Roath, C. T. (2010). An evaluation of the value of choice-making opportunities in single-operant arrangements: Simple fixed- and progressive-ratio schedules. *Journal of Applied Behavior Analysis, 43,* 519–524.

Trosclair-Lasserre, N. M., Lerman, D. C., Call, N. A., Addison, L. R., & Kodak, T. (2008). Reinforcement magnitude: An evaluation of preference and reinforcer efficacy. *Journal of Applied Behavior Analysis, 41,* 203–220.

Tustin, D. (2000). Revealed preference between reinforcers used to examine hypotheses about behavioral consistencies. *Behavior Modification, 24,* 411–424.

Tustin, R. D. (1994). Preference for reinforcers under varying schedule arrangements: A behavioral economic analysis. *Journal of Applied Behavior Analysis, 27,* 597–606.

Tversky, A., & Thaler, R. H. (1990). Anomalies: Preference reversals. *Journal of Economic Perspectives, 4,* 201–211.

Weller, R. E., Cook, E. W., III, Avsar, K. B., & Cox, J. E. (2008). Obese women show greater delay discounting than healthy-weight women. *Appetite, 51,* 563–569.

Wilson, A. N., & Gratz, O. H. (2016). Using a progressive ratio schedule of reinforcement as an assessment tool to inform treatment. *Behavior Analysis in Practice, 9,* 257–260.

Zhou, L., Goff, G. A., & Iwata, B. A. (2000). Effects of increased response effort on self-injury and object manipulation as competing responses. *Journal of Applied Behavior Analysis, 33,* 29–40.

# PART III

# MEASUREMENT, DESIGN, AND METHODOLOGICAL ISSUES

Adherence to the core analytical foundations of our science is one of the essential underpinnings of applied behavior analysis. Whereas various parts of this text focus on issues related to conceptual principles and application, Part III focuses more narrowly on the core methodological features that define the field of applied behavior analysis. These topics include developing operational definitions, data collection, and experimental design. All of these topics have a well-established literature base associated with their foundational principles and general procedures. In these chapters, the authors have endeavored to present novel developments in these areas, while also offering a summary of the supporting theoretical and historical literature.

Part III begins with Chapter 8 by Kahng et al. on the procedures involved in defining and measuring target behaviors. In this chapter, the authors review the core techniques involved in behavioral measurement (e.g., developing operational definitions, types of bias, measures of interobserver agreement), as well as different observation and data collection procedures. Although these basic procedures have developed little since the first edition of this handbook appeared, Kahng and colleagues have updated their content with new information, particularly in the areas of recent use of direct observation data collection.

Chapter 9 describes the underlying logic and applied use of single-case experimental designs. In this chapter, DeRosa, Sullivan, Roane, Craig, and Kadey deliver content on those designs that are commonly used in applied behavior analysis (e.g., reversals, multiple-baseline), and on related topics such as data collection and visual inspection. The authors offer an extension of their chapter in the first edition by expanding their discussion of visual inspection to include new developments, discussing the effects of observational settings on design, and (most significantly) providing a new discussion related to combined designs and component/parametric analyses.

# CHAPTER 8

# Defining and Measuring Behavior

SungWoo Kahng, Einar T. Ingvarsson, Anna M. Quigg,
Kimberly E. Seckinger, Heather M. Teichman, and Casey J. Clay

A hallmark of applied behavior analysis is the precise measurement of observable behavior (Baer, Wolf, & Risley, 1968). Measurement precision involves the reliable and accurate quantification of some dimension of the target behavior. The response dimensions, which provide the basis for systems of measurement, encompass specific characteristics of behavior such as frequency, duration, and latency. An observation system consists of formalized rules for extracting information from a behavior stream. These rules specify the target behavior; the way the behavior analyst samples the events; the dimensions of the events that the behavior analyst assesses; the way the behavior analyst records the data; and other pragmatic issues, such as observational setting, observers, and cost (Hartmann & Wood, 1982).

Three characteristics of a measurement system—accuracy, validity, and reliability—gauge its predictive value (Poling, Methot, & LeSage, 1995). A measurement system is *accurate* if the yielded values reflect the true values of the target behavioral dimension. Any discrepancy between the obtained values and the true values constitutes *measurement error*. Implications of this relation are considerable, because observational systems that are high in measurement error produce data that fail to reflect true behavioral events and may lead

to ineffective action. *Validity* of a measurement system refers to the extent to which the system measures what it purports to measure. In general, direct observation of the target behavior is likely to yield highly valid measures. However, validity can suffer if (1) the behavior analyst uses indirect measures, (2) the behavior analyst infers the target behavior from other events, or (3) operational definitions specify irrelevant aspects of behavior. For example, measuring headache frequency by counting how often the participant complains of headaches may not be a valid measure, because the participant may not always complain when a headache is present and may sometimes complain when no headache is present. Finally, we define *reliability* as the extent to which a measurement system yields consistent outcomes. A measurement is reliable if it produces the same outcome when we apply it to the same behavior, or when different observers produce the same measurement outcomes while independently scoring the same behavior (Johnston & Pennypacker, 1993; Poling et al., 1995).

Given that multiple factors (e.g., expectation bias, effects of agreement checking, adequacy of behavioral definitions, complexity of coding systems) can affect the measurement of behavior, one of the primary challenges for behavior analysts is to obtain a record of an individual's behavior that is both complete and accurate (Johnston & Pennypacker, 1993). The purpose of this chapter is to provide descriptions of observation and measurement systems and rationales for their use.

## OPERATIONALLY DEFINING BEHAVIOR

### General Characteristics of Behavioral Definitions

Behavioral definitions or observational codes are descriptions of target behaviors that should control observers' scoring behavior. Generally, we should judge the adequacy of behavioral definitions by how consistently and accurately they control observing behavior and whether the resulting data allow the behavior analyst to take effective action (i.e., gain control of socially meaningful behavior). Attention to the following three aspects can help to increase the adequacy of behavioral definitions: (1) *objectiveness,* or whether definitions refer to observable events with which two or more observers can agree (i.e., behavioral definitions should refer to observable behavior such as hitting, rather than abstract concepts such as anger); (2) *clarity,* or the ability of observers to read and paraphrase the definition accurately; and (3) *completeness,* or the inclusion of relevant aspects and exclusion of irrelevant aspects in the definition (Cooper, Heron, & Heward, 2020).

Additionally, definitions might include a description of the conditions under which the target behavior occurs. For example, question answering can occur only when an individual asks a question, and hitting another individual as an instance of aggression can occur only when another individual is in physical proximity. Finally, we can enhance the effectiveness of behavioral definitions by including relevant examples and nonexamples of target behavior, potentially improving the control over observers' scoring behavior (Cooper et al., 2020).

### Topographical versus Functional Definitions

We may define behavior according to either function or topography. *Functional* definitions describe the effects of responding on some aspect of the environment. For example, a behavior analyst might define opening a door solely by the result of door-opening behavior (e.g., the distance between the door and the door frame is at least 2 meters). The movements that bring this result about are not relevant with functional definitions; an individual could open the door with his or her toes, teeth, or hands. *Topographical* definitions describe the form of behavior and specify the physical properties of responding. For instance, we might define door opening as using one's hands to turn the doorknob while standing upright and facing forward (Johnston & Pennypacker, 1993).

Topographical definitions are often important in applied behavior analysis, because socially appropriate and inappropriate behavior may be functionally identical but topographically distinct. To demonstrate, aggressive behavior and appropriate verbal requests may each produce increased control over the social environment, including the behavior of others and access to preferred items and activities (e.g., Bowman, Fisher, Thompson, & Piazza, 1997; Torres-Viso, Strohmeier, & Zarcone, 2018). Topographical definitions that differentiate these two response categories are important, because appropriate requesting is more socially appropriate than aggression. Nevertheless, functional definitions are often useful in applied behavior analysis. For example, researchers might place behavior that produces property destruction, regardless of topography, in a single definitional category (e.g., Fisher, Lindauer, Alterson, & Thompson, 1998). Behaviors that are different topographically, such as crying and throwing toys, may produce the same consequence, such as parent attention (e.g., Fritz, Iwata, Hammond, & Bloom, 2013). We can group these behaviors into the same response class when we define them by function.

## HUMANS AND MACHINES AS OBSERVERS

### Humans as Observers

In applied behavior analysis, we commonly use human observers to collect data. Human observers can collect data in many ways, including marking data sheets with a pencil (e.g., Taravella, Lerman, Contrucci, & Roane, 2000), operating a stopwatch (e.g., Hoch, McComas, Johnson, Faranda, & Guenther, 2002), or pressing keys on a computer keyboard (e.g., Fuhrman, Fisher, & Greer, 2016). Humans as opposed to machines as data collectors have the advantage of greater flexibility, because we can train humans to take data on many responses, and humans can adapt to novel environments relatively easily (Page & Iwata, 1986). However, human observers are prone to the influence of numerous errors and biases that can produce unreliable and inaccurate data collection. We describe the most common potential biases in the following sections.

## Expectancy Bias

Observer expectations about desirable outcomes may bias scoring toward congruence with hypothesized outcomes (Repp, Nieminen, Olinger, & Brusca, 1988). This is particularly likely if supervisor feedback to observers corresponds to changes in behavior rather than reliability and accuracy of measurement (O'Leary, Kent, & Kanowitz, 1975). We can reduce the risk of expectancy bias by ensuring that observers are unaware of the experimental questions and conditions. However, this is often difficult in behavior-analytic research, because the independent variables are frequently apparent through behavior or environmental arrangements. Periodic reliability checks by novel observers who are trained in the behavioral code, but not familiar with the experiment or the field of study, can minimize this bias. Supervisors should also avoid giving feedback that describes how well the obtained data conform to expected outcomes; rather, feedback should focus on the accuracy and reliability of data collection.

## Observer Bias

The presence of a second observer, who is often present to assess the reliability of the data collection procedure, may affect the accuracy and reliability of data (Kent, Kanowitz, O'Leary, & Cheiken, 1977), Specifically, reliability and accuracy may increase when a second observer conducts such checks, but remain lower at other times. One solution to this problem is to have a second observer present during all or most observations; however, this may not be practical. Alternatively, we might conduct covert or unpredictable reliability checks (Kazdin, 1977). One way to accomplish these reliability checks is to video-record sessions and conduct subsequent reliability checks for a randomly selected sample of sessions.

## Reactivity

*Reactivity* is a change in a participant's behavior as a function of being observed (e.g., Hartmann, 1984; Repp et al., 1988). For instance, an employee participating in a project involving organizational behavior management may work harder and generate a higher-quality product as a function of being observed. This is undesirable for two reasons: (1) The behavior analyst cannot be sure that his or her intervention had an effect independent of reactivity, and (2) intervention gains may disappear

when observation stops. One solution is to use unobtrusive measures (i.e., arranging observations in such a way that participants are unaware of being watched) or to reduce the obtrusiveness of observation (e.g., using one-way observation). Another solution is to allow participants time to adapt to the presence of data collectors before beginning the evaluation.

## Observer Drift

The control that behavioral definitions have over observers' behavior may erode over time. We refer to this phenomenon as *observer drift* (Kazdin, 1977), which can result from boredom, fatigue, or illness, and may negatively affect accuracy and reliability of observation. We can reduce observer drift and other scoring errors via additional observer training (calibration), using standard behavior samples (Mudford, Zeleny, Fisher, Klum, & Owen, 2011) and intermittent checks by newly trained observers (Hartmann, 1984). Furthermore, supervisors should limit the number and length of observations, and should ensure that observers feel free to take a break from observational sessions when fatigued.

# Observer Training

Nonmechanical data collection requires human observers to react to behavior as it occurs and convert it to written or computerized form. Ensuring that observers are trained properly will reduce the previously discussed risks. The goals of observer training are to increase the control exerted by the observation code and the participants' behavior over the observers' scoring behavior, and to reduce the likelihood of control by irrelevant sources. A simple training method is to have a novice observer score a representative sample of behavior and make comparisons with an experienced observer's record. The trainer should deliver corrective feedback until the observer achieves sufficient interobserver agreement for a specified number of sessions (Hartmann & Wood, 1982). For purposes of training, observers might benefit from scoring behavior samples from videos, so that they can view instances of behavior repeatedly if necessary. Indeed, researchers have found that using videos to train human observers is as effective as *in vivo* instruction (Dempsey, Iwata, Fritz, & Rolider, 2012). The trainer can obtain behavior samples from pilot studies or preliminary observations, or can generate them from role play. Use of standard behavior samples on videos (e.g., role-played sessions) can be helpful, because the trainer can evaluate observers' accuracy by comparing their scores to predetermined values. The trainer then can calibrate observers' scoring behavior by conducting training to improve accuracy, if needed (Johnston & Pennypacker, 1993; Mudford et al., 2011). Computer technology may also facilitate observer training. For example, Bass (1987) described a computerized system in which observers watched videotapes and received automatic and immediate feedback on their scoring.

## Interobserver Agreement

Applied behavior analysts expect that researchers will report interobserver agreement whenever they use human observers (Page & Iwata, 1986). To obtain interobserver agreement scores, two persons, a primary and a secondary observer, independently but simultaneously score the same behavior episode and calculate agreement between the two records. A common recommendation is to obtain interobserver agreement for a minimum proportion of sessions (e.g., 25–30%) across conditions or phases (Bailey & Burch, 2002; Poling et al., 1995). High interobserver agreement scores (e.g., above 80–90%) do not in and of themselves indicate the accuracy of a measurement system, because both observers could be inaccurate but still agree (Johnston & Pennypacker, 1993). However, low interobserver agreement scores indicate the need for adjustments (e.g., additional observer training, more specific definitions) before observers can produce useful data (Poling et al., 1995). Therefore, applied behavior analysts should assess interobserver agreement scores early in the process. Waiting to calculate interobserver agreement after many sessions or after the study, if observers score sessions from videos, is risky. If researchers discover serious flaws in the measurement system after the conclusion of the manipulation, the only option may be to discard the data and start over. Thus researchers should use interobserver agreement as a proactive way to improve the measurement system and as a retroactive method to evaluate its adequacy. The following are several common methods of calculating interobserver agreement.

### Total Agreement

The simplest index of interobserver agreement is *total agreement*, calculated by dividing the smaller by the larger number of occurrences the two ob-

servers scored in a session (Poling et al., 1995). The disadvantage of this procedure is that it does not determine whether the two observers scored the same occurrences of behavior (Bijou, Peterson, & Ault, 1968). We do not recommend this index if agreement about specific instances of behavior (as opposed to overall occurrence) is important. However, total reliability can be useful and sufficient to estimate observer accuracy if the primary focus is overall occurrence rather than the distribution of responding in a session (Rolider, Iwata, & Bullock, 2012).

### Interval Agreement

More stringent indices compare scoring in specified, relatively short intervals (e.g., 5–10 seconds) to better evaluate whether the observers are scoring the same behavior at the same time (Bijou et al., 1968; Page & Iwata, 1986). We calculate *interval agreement* by assessing agreement or disagreement for each interval or trial and dividing the number of agreements by the total number of intervals or trials (e.g., Cariveau & Kodak, 2017). This approach is perhaps the most common interobserver agreement calculation method in applied behavior analysis (e.g., Hanley, Iwata, Lindberg, & Conners, 2003; Lannie & Martens, 2004; Thiemann & Goldstein, 2001). We can use it with any collection method involving interval data (e.g., partial- and whole-interval recording or momentary-time sampling; see below) or trial-by-trial data (i.e., correct vs. incorrect responses, compliance with teacher instructions). Each interval or trial typically generates one score—the behavior either occurred or did not—except in the case of block-by-block agreement (see below).

*Exact agreement* is a variant of the interval approach. Intervals in which observers scored the same number of occurrences are exact agreements (e.g., Hagopian, Contrucci Kuhn, Long, & Rush, 2005). The formula for calculating the exact-agreement coefficient is number of intervals with exact agreement divided by the total number of intervals. Although precise, this method may be too stringent for many practical purposes (Page & Iwata, 1986; Rolider et al., 2012).

*Block-by-block agreement* is a slightly less conservative but frequently sufficient method. We calculate total agreement for each interval, calculate the mean of the quotients across the whole session, and convert the ratio to a percentage (Bailey & Burch, 2002; Page & Iwata, 1986; North & Iwata, 2005). Exact and block-by-block agreements are only applicable when observers can score multiple occurrences of behavior in each interval, such as discrete target behaviors.

A less commonly applied variant that is applicable to free-operant data is time-window analysis (Mudford, Martin, Hui, & Taylor, 2009). This approach requires time-stamped data streams for which we can compare the data files of two observers second by second. An example of an agreement for frequency data is when both files contain a scored response in a 1-second window, and an example of an agreement for duration data is if the 1-second window in both data files contains an ongoing occurrence of the behavior. We can modify the stringency of the time window analysis by including a *tolerance interval*. For instance, if we use a tolerance interval of ±2, we would count an agreement if the secondary observer scored a response in a window of 2 seconds before and 2 seconds after a response the primary observer scored. Researchers have not studied time-window analysis extensively. The available data suggest that it may inflate accuracy estimates for high-rate and low-duration behavior, but provide relatively accurate estimates at lower rates and durations (Mudford et al., 2009).

### Occurrence and Nonoccurrence Agreement

Low-rate target behavior produces data streams with many intervals in which the behavior does not occur and few intervals in which the behavior occurs. In this case, the behavior analyst should assess *occurrence agreement* by examining the intervals in which both observers agreed on the occurrence of the behavior (e.g., Lerman et al., 2005). The behavior analyst should assess *nonoccurrence agreement* for high-rate behavior by examining the intervals in which both observers agreed on the nonoccurrence of the behavior. Occurrence and nonoccurrence agreement indices eliminate the risk of inflating interobserver agreement due to disproportionate numbers of intervals in which the target behavior either did or did not occur (Bijou et al., 1968; Page & Iwata, 1986).

### Computerized Data Collection Systems

The use of laptops and handheld computerized devices (e.g., tablets, smartphones) for data collection is common in applied behavior analysis (e.g., Slocum, Grauerholz, Peters, & Vollmer, 2018). Computerized data collection systems operated by human observers have several potential advan-

tages over paper-and-pencil methods, including increased efficiency of data analysis and graphing, and reduced risk of compromised reliability and accuracy due to ambiguity of written records (Dixon, 2003; Jackson & Dixon, 2007; Kahng & Iwata, 1998; Whiting & Dixon, 2013).

In addition, computerized systems that facilitate the coding of video and audio media are available. Such systems allow for the measurement of many simultaneously occurring events, precise detection of response duration, and automatic data analysis and interobserver agreement calculations (e.g., Tapp, 2003; Tapp & Walden, 1993). This approach suffers from the limitation that the observer may need to view each behavioral episode multiple times; therefore, the time expenditure may increase considerably. Behavior analysts should use these kinds of computer programs only if they provide sufficiently important improvements in data collection considering the target behavior and the ultimate goals of data collection.

### Videos and Other Visual Media

We may enhance human data collection by video-recording sessions for later viewing. Video-recorded sessions enable the observer to score many simultaneously occurring responses. Such sessions also are useful for observer training (Miltenberger, Rapp, & Long, 1999). Using videos allows the observer to score duration measures more precisely than live recording (Miltenberger et al., 1999; Tapp & Walden, 1993). Research has suggested that accuracy and reliability generally are not affected adversely by scoring sessions from videos, although low-quality audio recording may affect scoring of vocal responses (Kent, O'Leary, Dietz, & Diament, 1979). However, use of video recordings for data collection is time-consuming; it can create a backlog of media to be scored; and valuable data may be lost if recorded sessions are lost or damaged before they can be viewed. Overall, behavior analysts should weigh these costs against potential benefits when deciding whether to use live recording or to score behavior with the assistance of visual media.

### Mechanical Recording

Much laboratory research in behavior analysis involves measures of target behaviors via mechanical devices (e.g., automatic recording of key strokes or lever presses). Machines are free of many human shortcomings (e.g., expectancy bias, observer drift, illness) and may be less costly (Panos & Freed, 2007). Therefore, behavior analysts may prefer machines over human observers whenever the target behavior lends itself to mechanical recording (Johnston & Pennypacker, 1993). However, many behaviors of interest to applied behavior analysts are not amenable to mechanical recording with current technology. Nevertheless, behavior analysts are using mechanical recording via computer software increasingly in certain areas, especially those that use computer-based instruction. For example, Connell and Witt (2004) used computer-based instruction to teach relations among printed uppercase and lowercase letters, letter names, and letter sounds to kindergartners. The computer software automatically collected data during the study, obviating the need for human observers. Mechanical recording can be useful particularly for dependent variables that may be difficult for human observers to quantify objectively. For example, Wilson, Iwata, and Bloom (2012) used a computerized measurement of wound-surface area to measure the severity of injuries produced by self-injurious behavior. Sigurdsson et al. (2011) used an automated system to measure noise levels in a therapeutic workplace. In these examples, human observers would have had to rely on subjective estimates of injury severity or ambient-sound levels in the absence of mechanical measures.

Mechanical data collection systems have the advantage of completely removing human judgment from the data collection process, thereby eliminating human sources of error and potentially increasing the reliability and accuracy of data collection. We should not, however, automatically trust data gathered through these means. Machines can malfunction, and human designers and programmers can make mistakes that render the systems inaccurate or unreliable. Behavior analysts should conduct calibration tests when using a new data collection system, in which they check output against input of known values. Replication of findings across different laboratories and with different data collection systems is also important.

## INDIRECT VERSUS DIRECT MEASUREMENT

Direct observation requires measuring the target behavior without inferring its occurrence from other events (e.g., products of behavior, verbal recollections), usually by observing the behavior as it occurs in either a natural or contrived set-ting. Direct observation maximizes the validity of measurement, because it decreases the discrepancy between actual behavioral events and sampled behavior (Hersen & Barlow, 1976). Direct observation is preferred whenever possible in behavior analysis; nonetheless, situations may arise in which indirect measures are necessary. For example, the target behavior may occur covertly, so that direct observation is difficult or impossible (e.g., Grace, Thompson, & Fisher, 1996). Furthermore, behavior analysts may want data on past events, in which case the only recourse may be to examine archival information or collect informant reports via interviews, surveys, or questionnaires.

### Indirect Measurement

Indirect measurement involves drawing inferences about the behavior of interest from other behaviors or environmental events. The validity and accuracy of measurement may suffer because we do not observe the target behavior directly, but this approach may be of value to behavior analysts when direct observation is impossible or impractical.

### Permanent-Product Recording

Measuring outcomes of behavior, such as administrative records, completed assignments, or manufactured goods, may supplement or replace direct measurement (Kazdin, 1979). Permanent-product recording involves recording the tangible outcome of a behavior rather than the behavior itself. In some instances, the products may be of primary interest. For example, we might score completed homework for accuracy (Kelly, 1976; Miller & Kelley, 1994). In other cases, permanent products are not of primary interest, but are important indicators of target behavior that is not amenable to direct observation. A study by Grace et al. (1996) illustrated the latter approach. They conducted physical examinations to identify signs of self-injury (e.g., bruises, scratches, swelling, tissue damage). The researchers chose this approach because the participant's self-injury was covert, and observers were unable to observe the behavior directly. Maglieri, DeLeon, Rodriguez-Catter, and Sevin (2000) provided another example: The researchers implemented permanent-product recording to evaluate covert food stealing. Observers recorded the amount of food presented at the start of a session, left the participant alone in the room, and returned later to record the amount of remaining food.

The disadvantage of permanent-product recording lies in its very nature: It measures outcomes rather than the behavior itself. This may be problematic because the outcome may be due to something other than the target behavior, resulting in inaccurate data. For example, measuring performance through examination of worksheets will produce inaccurate measures if someone other than the participant has completed the work (e.g., a parent has done the homework for the child). In addition, the target behavior may not produce the measured outcome (e.g., self-injury may not produce tissue damage; Grace et al., 1996). Therefore, the behavior analyst should exercise caution when implementing product recording. Noting alternative events that may produce the outcome of interest may enhance the accuracy of data collection. For example, if a child falls during outdoor playtime, the resulting bruises and scratches could be difficult to distinguish from injuries produced by self-injurious behavior.

## Self-Monitoring

Self-monitoring or self-recording data is like direct observation, in that the observer records events of interest as they occur. However, the difference is that the client or participant serves as his or her own observer. Self-monitoring is particularly useful in the measurement of private events that only the client can access directly, such as headaches and thinking (Hartmann, 1984; Nelson, 1977). Behavior analysts can use this approach with behavior that is overt and observable by more than one individual, but is not amenable to direct measurement due to practical constraints. For example, adult participants in VanWormer (2004) carried pedometers, which counted the number of steps each participant took, and weighed themselves regularly to produce measures of physical activity and weight loss. Family members and friends served as secondary observers, and the participants periodically e-mailed data to the researcher.

Self-monitoring produces data that otherwise would be unobtainable. Nevertheless, there are at least two major shortcomings of this approach. First, self-recorded data may be less accurate than directly observed data, and the accuracy and reliability of these data are more difficult to verify. Directly training clients to observe their own behavior, and using measurement systems that are convenient and require little effort, are likely to help in this matter. One valuable training strategy is to place contingencies initially on accurate reporting rather than on clinically desirable changes in behavior, so that the behavior analyst rewards data collection that agrees with independent sources, regardless of other outcomes (Hartmann, 1984; Nelson, 1977). Second, observer reactivity (i.e., the effects of observation on the target behavior) is of special concern in self-monitoring. The behavior analyst should attempt to evaluate the effects of intervention via self-monitoring and via less intrusive data collection methods, to ensure that the effects of the independent variable were not due exclusively or primarily to reactivity (Cooper et al., 2020). Although the reactivity inherent in self-monitoring is a threat to effective measurement, the behavior analyst can use it as a treatment protocol. The very act of systematically keeping track of one's own behavior can be an effective tool for self-management and behavior change (Cooper et al., 2020; Critchfield, 1999).

## Interviews, Surveys, and Rating Scales

The behavior analyst can use structured interviews, surveys, or rating scales to collect important information about various aspects of the target behavior, such as topography and environmental correlates (Beaver & Busse, 2000; Merrell, 2000). Depending on the situation, the behavior analyst might gather this information from the client or from significant others in the client's environment (e.g., parents, teachers). Indirect measures of this sort can generate information that may be helpful in the initial stages of assessment (McComas & Mace, 2000; Nay, 1979). Researchers have used behavioral interviews, surveys, and rating scales to generate hypotheses about potential behavioral function (e.g., Applegate, Matson, & Cherry, 1999) and to identify potential reinforcers to use in subsequent treatments (Fisher, Piazza, Bowman, & Amari, 1996; Northup, 2000). Researchers have then used this information to determine what stimuli to include in subsequent preference or reinforcer assessments, and which environmental conditions to include in functional assessments. Importantly, behavior analysts should confirm hypotheses these methods generate through more stringent observation methods, preferably involving direct observation, because informant reports often do not correspond well with the behavior of interest. Direct observation is the gold standard against which to evaluate the accuracy of indirect measures.

## Direct Observation

Direct observation is more consistent with behaviorism's epistemological emphasis on overt behavior, public events, quantification, low levels of inference, and the importance of environmental contingencies (Hartmann & Wood, 1982). Additional advantages of direct observation include an increase in predictive validity as the discrepancy between sampled behavior and predicted behavior decreases, and a close relation between the target behavior and intervention (Hersen & Barlow, 1976). Behavior analysts prefer direct measures to study behavior because of these advantages, and use them widely in numerous contexts (e.g., Alevizos, DeRisi, Liberman, Eckman, & Callahan, 1978; Bijou, Peterson, Harris, Allen, & Johnston, 1969; Cordes, 1994; Doll & Elliott, 1994; Gresham, Gansle, & Noell, 1993; Odom & Ogawa, 1992; Prinz, 1982; Test, Rose, & Corum, 1990; Wasik & Loven, 1980).

Direct measures can be *continuous* or *discontinuous*. Continuous measures record all instances of behavior. Discontinuous measures, also termed *intermittent* measures, sample from all possible occurrences of behavior (Johnston & Pennypacker, 1993). Continuous measures—frequency, duration, latency, and intensity—provide the most complete record of behavior, but may prove expensive and otherwise impractical. Therefore, intermittent or discontinuous methods, such as interval recording and momentary time sampling, are often valuable. However, discontinuous recording produces an incomplete behavior record and consequently raises several questions about the representativeness of the data. As such, discontinuous observational procedures that appropriately sample from all possible occurrences of behavior to yield representative and accurate measures are important.

### Continuous Recording Procedures

Continuous behavior recording is the most rigorous and powerful measurement procedure available to behavior analysts. This approach involves recording behavior based on its occurrence in an uninterrupted, natural time flow (Sanson-Fisher, Poole, Small, & Fleming, 1979; Hartmann & Wood, 1982). We discuss the application of continuous recording to relevant behavioral dimensions in the following paragraphs.

*Frequency.* Frequency recording, also called the *tally method, trial scoring,* and *event recording,* entails continuous recording of separate instances of behavior as they occur (Hartmann & Wood, 1982; Kazdin, 2001; Repp, Roberts, Slack, Repp, & Berkler, 1976). Frequency recording is most appropriate when the number of times a behavior occurs is the response dimension of interest (Hartmann & Wood, 1982; Schinke & Wong, 1977). However, the behavior analyst cannot compare frequencies obtained in different observation sessions meaningfully if observation times are unequal. In those instances, the behavior analyst should convert frequencies to *response rate*, defined as the frequency of behavior per some unit of time (e.g., minute, hour, day; Kazdin, 2001). When behavior is opportunity-bound or trial-based, so that the target responses cannot occur in the absence of specified stimuli (e.g., instructions, stimulus cards), the behavior analyst should convert obtained frequencies to percentages or report the number of responses relative to the number of opportunities for the response to occur. For example, Gutowski and Stromer (2003) measured selection of comparison stimuli that occurred in the presence of specific sample stimuli, and then converted the frequencies into percentages of correct selections.

Frequency recording is best suited for measuring responses that are relatively discrete and have a constant duration. Examples include hitting, throwing objects, pressing buttons or keys, and placing items in containers. In addition, responses that tend to have variable durations can be amenable to frequency recording if the behavior analyst precisely defines their onset and offset. However, the behavior analyst should consider using duration instead of frequency recording given responses with varying durations. Frequency recording can generate much information about behavior (Repp et al., 1976), and observers can use it easily if responding is not excessive. Frequency measures reflect the amount of responding, which is important when the goal is to increase or decrease the number of times the target behavior occurs (Kazdin, 2001).

*Duration.* Duration involves measuring the entire time that the participant performs or engages in the target response (Kazdin, 2001). Duration recording is appropriate when temporal characteristics of a behavior are of interest, and when behaviors vary in the length of time the client engages in them. This approach is best suited to continuous, ongoing behaviors rather than to discrete, short-duration behaviors (Hartmann & Wood, 1982). Observers can measure duration by turning on a stopwatch or a timer at the onset of behavior and turning it off at the offset of behavior. Most computerized data collection systems allow observers to press designated keys at the onset and offset of behavior, and many accommodate multiple, simultaneous duration measures. The behavior analyst can calculate the proportion of session time during which a participant performed the behavior by dividing the total duration of behavior by the total observation time.

Altmann (1974) suggested that duration recording is appropriate for behavioral states versus behavioral events. *Behavioral states* are those behaviors that have appreciable duration. *Behavioral events* are instantaneous occurrences of behavior. Duration recording is useful in measuring *time allocation,* defined as the amount of time spent in certain environmental areas (e.g., sitting in a chair) or engaged in certain response alternatives (e.g., doing homework, practicing a musical instrument; Kazdin, 2001).

As with other continuous measurement procedures, duration recording is appealing because it produces a complete measurement of the response dimension of interest. Like frequency, duration is comprehensible, is socially acceptable, and can be accomplished without complicated observational technology. The reliability of duration measures, however, may be low if the precise onset and offset of behavior are difficult to identify reliably. For instance, observers measuring speech content may have difficulty determining the precise point at which changes in content (e.g., topics) occur, and the reliability of duration measures can suffer. However, observers might agree more easily about whether a conversation topic occurred in an interval. Thus partial-interval recording (see below) may be easier to implement (e.g., Lepper, Devine, & Petursdottir, 2016). Alternatively, behavior analysts could define changes in speech topics by the occurrence of specific keywords, enabling the use of duration measures (e.g., Fisher, Rodriguez, & Owen, 2013). With both approaches, however, there is some risk of failing to capture the entirety of the target behavior. For example, partial-interval recording might overestimate the occurrence of behavior, and keywords may not always correspond with actual changes in content. However, both approaches may produce data that are sufficiently accurate.

In addition, duration recording can be effortful, particularly if we are interested in multiple response topographies, or if observers must measure many individuals' behavior simultaneously. Under these circumstances, the behavior analyst may use appropriate time-sampling techniques (e.g., momentary time sampling; Kazdin, 2001; see below).

*Latency.* Latency refers to the amount of time that elapses between the onset of a specific cue or stimulus and the target behavior (Kazdin, 2001). Like duration, latency can be recorded with the assistance of timing devices or computerized systems that measure duration. Latency recording is appropriate when we are interested in the relation between a certain event and the initiation of a specific response. This includes situations in which the goal is either to reduce or to increase time between antecedent events and target behavior. For example, behavior analysts are frequently interested in reducing the latency between instruction delivery and compliance. Wehby and Hollahan (2000) measured the seconds that passed between the delivery of instructions to engage in academic activities and compliance with the instructions. They used these measures to evaluate the effectiveness of providing a series of high-probability requests (i.e., requests that the participants were likely to engage in immediately) before the delivery of academic instructions. Latency measures have recently been extended to the assessment of challenging behavior (e.g., elopement), which may be beneficial when the target behavior is not continuous or is specific to a particular evocative event (Hansen et al., 2019; Traub & Vollmer, 2019).

Like frequency and duration recording, latency measures consist of complete measurement of the target behavior, and behavior analysts prefer them over discontinuous measures unless practical constraints dictate otherwise. In addition, latency recording is simple, is relatively straightforward, and is likely to be acceptable to consumers and observers. On the other hand, latency recording is only appropriate for measuring a specifically defined relation between antecedent conditions and target responding. As with other continuous measures, practical constraints (e.g., simultaneous measurement of multiple responses or observation of multiple clients) can necessitate the use of discontinuous measures.

*Intensity.* Intensity recording involves measures of magnitude, strength, amplitude, force, or effort of a response. Observers occasionally can record intensity through automated mechanical devices, but degrees of intensity may require judgments that are difficult for observers to make reliably without these devices (Kazdin, 2001). Intensity recording may be appropriate for measuring shouting, throwing an object, hitting, swearing, tantrums, and noise levels. Wilson and Hopkins (1973) recorded intensity while examining the effects of quiet-contingent music on the general noise levels of middle school classrooms. Intensity recording was particularly useful in this situation, because the goal of intervention was to decrease general noise levels in the classrooms.

## Discontinuous Recording Procedures

Continuous measures yield the most accurate behavioral data, but these methods can be impractical, particularly in applied settings where the behavior analyst may have multiple important tasks and limited time to complete them. Therefore, behavior analysts may choose discontinuous measurement procedures, which frequently increase the efficiency of data collection. We discuss the most common varieties of discontinuous recording in the following paragraphs.

*Interval Recording.* The behavior analyst divides the observation session into periods of equal length, such as 10 seconds, and observers score each interval as positive (i.e., occurrence) or negative (i.e., nonoccurrence) according to specific criteria. Varieties include *whole-interval recording,* in which the observer scores a positive interval if the target behavior occurs for the entire observational interval; *partial-interval recording,* in which the observer scores a positive interval if the target behavior occurs at any point during the observational interval; and *predominant-activity sampling,* in which the observer scores a positive interval if the target behavior occurs for more than half the interval (Adams, 1991; Harrop & Daniels, 1986; Poling et al., 1995; Saudargas & Zanolli, 1990; Tyler, 1979). Like other discontinuous measurement procedures, interval recording provides an estimate of behavior rather than a representation of the entire behavioral episode. Therefore, behavior analysts should design interval-recording procedures to minimize error and maximize measurement accuracy.

Researchers have evaluated whether interval recording influences the accuracy of measurement systems when applied to behaviors of different rates and durations (Wirth, Slaven, & Taylor, 2014). Both whole-interval recording and predomi-nant-activity sampling may provide accurate estimates of the time long-duration behavior occurs, but may underestimate instantaneous behavior (Bailey & Burch, 2002; Murphy & Goodall, 1980; Powell, Martindale, & Kulp, 1975). By contrast, partial-interval recording tends to overestimate overall occurrence of long-duration behavior, but tends to underestimate the occurrence of instantaneous, high-rate behavior (Harrop & Daniels, 1993; Murphy & Goodall, 1980; Repp et al., 1976). When overall duration is the response dimension of interest, partial-interval recording almost always provides overestimates (Suen, Ary, & Covalt, 1991), suggesting that the behavior analyst should use whole-interval recording, predominant-activity sampling, or momentary time sampling when duration is the response dimension of interest (but see Harrop & Daniels, 1993, for an alternative interpretation). Behavior analysts can achieve more accurate estimates of frequency with shorter interval lengths (e.g., 10 seconds; Devine, Rapp, Testa, Henrickson, & Schnerch, 2011; Rapp, Colby-Dirksen, Michalski, Carroll, & Lindenberg, 2008). However, shorter interval lengths do not systematically increase the accuracy of estimates of long-duration behavior (Sanson-Fisher, Poole, & Dunn, 1980).

Figures 8.1, 8.2, and 8.3 provide hypothetical demonstrations of the sensitivity of interval-recording conventions with behavioral streams consisting of occurrences of various rates and durations. Figure 8.1 shows that partial-interval recording overestimates and whole-interval recording underestimates frequency and duration of responses of moderate rate and varying duration. Predominant-activity sampling, on the other hand, provides a close estimate. Figure 8.2 shows that partial-interval recording provides a relatively accurate but slightly conservative estimate of the frequency of an instantaneous response of moderate rate, but grossly overestimates its duration. Both predominant-activity sampling and whole-interval recording are unable to detect any responses in a behavioral stream of this sort. Figure 8.3 shows that partial-interval recording somewhat overestimates duration and frequency of long-duration behavior, whereas predominant-activity sampling and whole-interval recording slightly underestimate its duration and overestimate frequency.

Interval measures frequently introduce substantial error into the estimates of behavior, and the amount and type of error depend on the relative rate and duration of behavior and the parameters

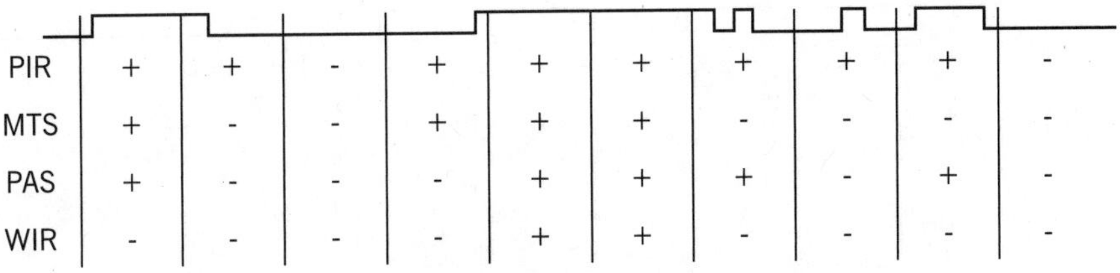

| | Percentage time spent | No. of occurrences |
|---|---|---|
| Actual | 47% | 5 |
| Estimates | | |
| PIR | 80% | 8 |
| MTS | 40% | 4 |
| PAS | 50% | 5 |
| WIR | 20% | 2 |

**FIGURE 8.1.** A demonstration of hypothetical results obtained using different time-sampling conventions by means of an analysis of an event-recorded tape. The width of the figure represents 150 seconds, and the vertical lines represent 15-second intervals. The table presents the results of an analysis of this tape. PIR, partial interval recording; MTS, momentary time sampling; PAS, predominant-activity sampling; WIR, whole-interval recording. Adapted in part from Tyler (1979). Copyright by Elsevier. Adapted by permission.

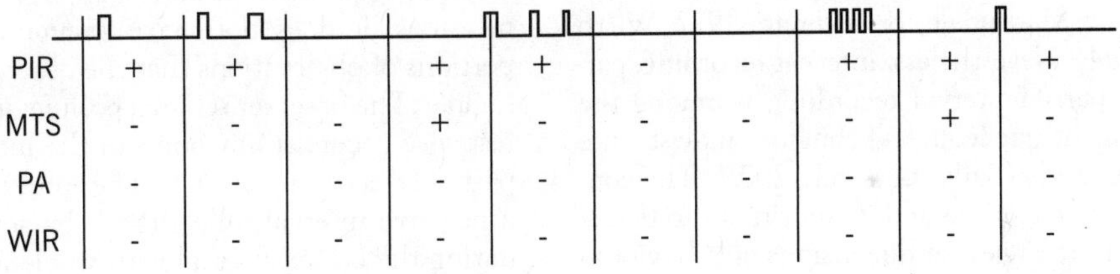

| | Percentage time spent | No. of occurrences |
|---|---|---|
| Actual | 7% | 11 |
| Estimates | | |
| PIT | 70% | 7 |
| MTS | 20% | 2 |
| PAS | 0% | 0 |
| WIR | 0% | 0 |

**FIGURE 8.2.** A demonstration of hypothetical results obtained using different time-sampling conventions by means of an analysis of an event-recorded tape. The width of the figure represents 150 seconds, and the vertical lines represent 15-second intervals. The table presents the results of an analysis of this tape. Abbreviations as in Figure 8.1. Adapted in part from Tyler (1979). Copyright by Elsevier. Adapted by permission.

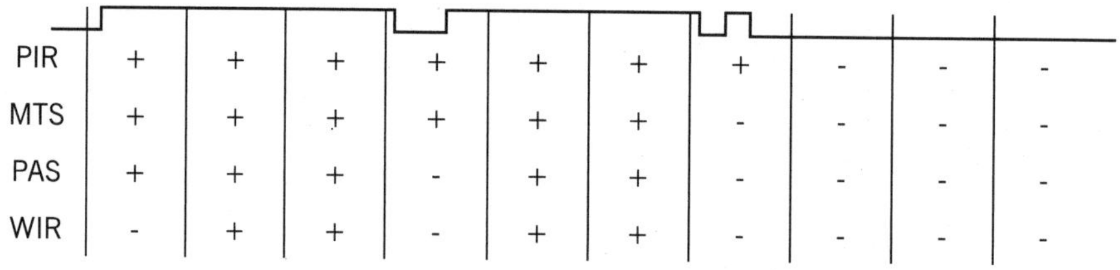

| | | | | | | | | | |
|---|---|---|---|---|---|---|---|---|---|
| PIR | + | + | + | + | + | + | + | - | - | - |
| MTS | + | + | + | + | + | + | - | - | - | - |
| PAS | + | + | + | - | + | + | - | - | - | - |
| WIR | - | + | + | - | + | + | - | - | - | - |

| | Percentage time spent | No. of occurrences |
|---|---|---|
| Actual | 57% | 3 |
| Estimates | | |
| PIT | 70% | 70 |
| MTS | 60% | 6 |
| PAS | 50% | 5 |
| WIR | 40% | 4 |

**FIGURE 8.3.** A demonstration of hypothetical results obtained using different time-sampling conventions by means of an analysis of an event-recorded tape. The width of the figure represents 150 seconds, and the vertical lines represent 15-second intervals. The table presents the results of an analysis of this tape. Abbreviations as in Figure 8.1. Adapted in part from Tyler (1979). Copyright by Elsevier. Adapted by permission.

of the interval-recording system (Powell, Martindale, Kulp, Martindale, & Bauman, 1977; Wirth et al., 2014). Nevertheless, interval recording, particularly partial-interval recording, is among the measurement procedures behavior analysts use most frequently (Bailey & Burch, 2002). The convenience of recording and its sensitivity to detect changes in the relevant dimensions of behavior as a function of intervention are likely reasons for its popularity (Harrop & Daniels, 1986, 1993). For example, partial-interval recording is likely to underestimate the magnitude of change in high-rate, instantaneous behavior and to provide a conservative estimate of behavior change (Harrop & Daniels, 1986; Suen et al., 1991). This is not necessarily a limitation of the procedure, however, because it reduces the probability of Type I errors.

*Momentary Time Sampling.* Momentary time sampling consists of scoring an interval as positive if the target behavior occurs at a predetermined moment (Harrop & Daniels, 1986). A timer set to sound every 10 seconds might prompt observers to assess whether the target behavior occurred. When the timer goes off, the observers look at the client and score whether he or she is performing the target behavior at that precise moment (hence the term *momentary*).

Momentary time sampling is useful in providing estimates of duration of behavior (Harrop &

Daniels, 1986; Suen et al., 1991). Unlike interval measures, it does not make assumptions about portions of observations that the observer did not sample. The observer scores a positive interval if a response occurs at any point in the interval with partial-interval recording. The observer scores a negative interval unless the behavior occurred during the entire interval with whole-interval recording. Momentary time sampling, on the other hand, only makes assumptions about the momentary periods when the observer samples behavior, and the behavior analyst calculates proportional duration estimates by dividing the number of scored occurrences by the total number of intervals, which produces a potentially unbiased estimate of duration (Suen et al., 1991).

Results of research have typically shown that momentary time sampling does not systematically overestimate or underestimate behavior. Errors in estimates tend to be close to random, leading to accurate estimates of the mean (Brookshire, Nicholas, & Krueger, 1978; Green & Alverson, 1978; Harrop & Daniels, 1986; Mudford, Beale, & Singh, 1990; Murphy & Goodall, 1980; Powell et al., 1975, 1977; Repp et al., 1988; Suen et al., 1991; Tyler, 1979). However, Wirth et al. (2014) found that momentary time sampling is biased toward underestimation when cumulative event durations are low and overestimation when cumulative event durations are high. Harrop and Daniels (1993) caution that although momentary time-sampling estimates typically match actual behavior durations, unbiased estimates are not necessarily accurate when based on a single session of observation. Consistent with this notion, researchers have found that increases in the observation period reduce magnitude and variability of error in momentary time sampling (Devine et al., 2011; Wirth et al., 2014). Although definitive guidelines for the use of momentary time sampling do not exist, use of this method may be advisable in some situations over others, such as when high-rate, long-duration behaviors are of interest and when the observation involves multiple responses or organisms (Hanley, Cammilleri, Tiger, & Ingvarsson, 2007; Murphy & Harrop, 1994). We do not recommend momentary time sampling for responses that have a short duration or occur infrequently (Arrington, 1943).

Figures 8.1, 8.2, and 8.3 provide hypothetical demonstrations of the sensitivity of momentary time sampling for behavioral streams with response occurrences of various rates and durations. Figure 8.1 shows that momentary time sampling provides a slight underestimate of behavior of varying duration and moderate rate. Figure 8.2 demonstrates how such sampling may grossly underestimate both frequency and duration of instantaneous responding of moderate rate. However, momentary time sampling is likely to provide a close estimate of the overall duration and an overestimate of the frequency of relatively long-duration behavior that occurs for a large portion of the observation period, as demonstrated in Figure 8.3.

Momentary time sampling has several advantages. Cameron, Crosbie, and Crocker (1988) suggested that it is a good choice because researchers can analyze data with inferential statistics, which can provide a communicative aid when presenting results to psychologists and other professionals subscribing to non-behavior-analytic paradigms. Another key benefit of momentary time sampling is the ease of implementation (Brulle & Repp, 1984; Brookshire et al., 1978). Although momentary time sampling is not an error-free method of observation, Murphy and Goodall (1980) suggested that it may be the best available option when continuous recording is not feasible.

There are several potential limitations of momentary time sampling, including inadequate representation of certain behavioral dimensions and insensitivity to actual duration, frequency, and changes in behavior (Repp et al., 1976). Several authors have reported that momentary time sampling may not be as sensitive to small changes in

actual rates of behavior as partial-interval recording (Harrop & Daniels, 1986; Harrop, Daniels, & Foulkes, 1990). Tyler (1979) discussed the difficulty in using momentary time sampling when the behavior of interest is not amenable to instant recognition. Despite these reservations, several researchers have shown that momentary-time-sampling measures correlate highly with continuous measures (e.g., Brulle & Repp, 1984; Harrop & Daniels, 1986; Powell et al., 1977).

As in interval recording, shorter interval length generally will yield more accurate data in momentary time sampling (Brookshire et al., 1978; Brulle & Repp, 1984; Harrop & Daniels, 1985; Kearns, Edwards, & Tingstrom, 1990; Mansell, 1985; Saudargas & Zanolli, 1990). Brulle and Repp (1984) examined different interval lengths and found that 10-second, 20-second, 30-second, and 60-second intervals provided accurate estimates of the mean duration of the target behavior, but that a 120-second interval was accurate only when the target behavior occurred for more than 10% of the session. The 240-second interval was accurate only when behavior occurred for more than 20% of the session. Harrop and Daniels (1985) cautioned that researchers should only use intervals longer than 30 seconds when the target behavior occurs during 25% or more of the total observation period. Devine et al.'s (2011) results are consistent with the latter recommendation. Thomson, Holmberg, and Baer (1974) examined interval length and the rotation of observation intervals when observing behaviors of multiple organisms. They suggested that the smallest error percentage occurs when behavior is dispersed widely across the observation schedule.

Some research has compared the accuracy of momentary time sampling and interval recording. Green, McCoy, Burns, and Smith (1982) compared whole-interval recording, partial-interval recording, and momentary time sampling; they reported that momentary time sampling provided greater representativeness of the actual behavior and produced fewer observer errors than other interval-recording methods. Wirth et al. (2014) found that momentary time sampling generally resulted in smaller overall absolute magnitude of error when compared to partial-interval recording, but that the variability of error was greater with momentary time sampling (i.e., it sometimes underestimated and sometimes overestimated behavior). As stated previously, overall magnitude of error tends to decrease with increases in the length of observation periods.

## CONCLUSIONS

The purpose of this chapter has been to review observational recording methods, to examine the characteristics of each method, and to provide readers with a method of selecting the optimal observational technique. To aid behavior analysts and researchers in this task, we have developed decision flowcharts (see Figures 8.4 and 8.5). Note that we did not include pathways leading to measures of intensity and latency on the charts, due to the descriptive nature of the measurement labels. The reader should note further that references to interval recording invariably refer to the partial-interval method, but that whole-interval recording and predominant-activity sampling may sometimes be appropriate for responding that is also relatively well captured by momentary time sampling. To simplify the reader's task, we have included separate flowcharts describing recommended decision pathways that are applicable when frequency (Figure 8.4) and duration (Figure 8.5) are the behavioral dimensions of interest.

In deciding which measurement system to use, one must first ask which dimension of behavior—frequency or duration—is of primary interest. We can divide frequency measures of behavior further into three categories, each of which relies on a different form of observation (see Figure 8.4). Permanent products are ideal for instances when behavior results in a tangible product that observers can measure (e.g., number of sentences written). Event recording (i.e., a frequency count) is best suited for instances in which behavior has a clear, definable onset and offset that observers can count (e.g., hitting head with hand). Finally, a partial-interval method is most appropriate for behavior that lacks a delineated onset and offset, or that occurs at such a high rate that observers cannot record it easily and accurately. However, observers may use momentary time sampling if continuous observation is not possible or if responses are of unequal duration. Observers should use duration measures when behavior is discrete (e.g., in-seat behavior), and the observer records a manageable number of response topographies in one individual constantly throughout the entire observation period. Momentary time sampling is best suited for instances in which (1) nondiscrete, ongoing behavior is the target; (2) observations are continuous or discontinuous; (3) when the data collector is observing multiple responses simultaneously, or the same behavior in more than one person; or (4) some combination of these circumstances exists.

However, observers should use interval recording if the behavior is nondiscrete but instantaneous (i.e., responses that do not have a clearly delineated onset or offset but have short durations). Finally, an interval-recording method produces a rough estimate of both frequency and duration.

Because behavior analysts use observational methods widely and matching recording procedures to target behaviors is key, the methods discussed in this chapter are of paramount importance. Correct selection of observation systems is likely to produce more efficient and effective interventions. A comprehensive understanding of measurement methods will help behavior analysts to provide precise information about measurement methods, including their benefits, limitations, and characteristics.

Selecting a system of measurement can be a challenging task, and choices among various measurement systems can have a major impact on the outcome of data collection and subsequent decisions about the data. Behavior analysts must strike a delicate balance between identifying methods to provide the most efficient and representative means of sampling on the one hand, and still considering the behavior's unique characteristics on the other. Therefore, researchers and clinicians should fully understand the nuances among these different recording methods.

## REFERENCES

Adams, R. M. (1991). Momentary and partial interval time sampling: A reply to Harrop, Daniels and Foulkes (1990). *Behavioural Psychotherapy, 19,* 333–336.

Alevizos, P., DeRisi, W., Liberman, R., Eckman, T., & Callahan, E. (1978). The behavior observation instrument: A method of direct observation for program evaluation. *Journal of Applied Behavior Analysis, 11,* 243–257.

Altmann, J. (1974). Observational study of behavior: Sampling methods. *Behaviour, 49,* 227–267.

Applegate, H., Matson, J. L., & Cherry, K. E. (1999). An evaluation of functional variables affecting severe problem behaviors in adults with mental retardation by using the Questions about Behavioral Functions Scale (QABF). *Research in Developmental Disabilities, 20,* 229–237.

Arrington, R. E. (1943). Time-sampling in studies of social behavior: A critical review of techniques and results with research suggestions. *Psychological Bulletin, 40,* 81–124.

Baer, D. M., Wolf, M. M., & Risley, T. R. (1968). Some current dimensions of applied behavior analysis. *Journal of Applied Behavior Analysis, 1,* 91–97.

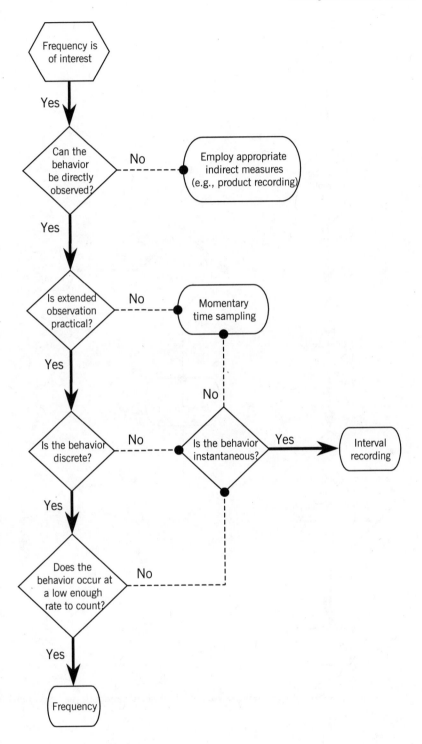

**FIGURE 8.4.** Decision flowchart for selecting an observational method when frequency is the behavioral dimension of interest.

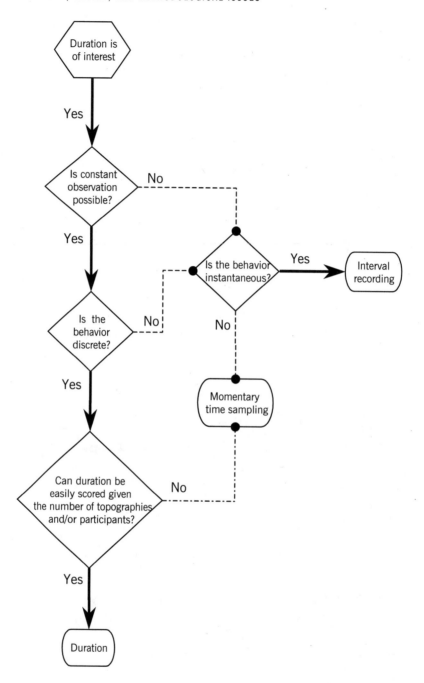

**FIGURE 8.5.** Decision flowchart for selecting an observational method when duration is the behavioral dimension of interest.

Bailey, J. S., & Burch, M. R. (2002). *Research methods in applied behavior analysis.* Thousand Oaks, CA: SAGE.

Bass, R. F. (1987). Computer-assisted observer training. *Journal of Applied Behavior Analysis, 20,* 83–88.

Beaver, B. R., & Busse, R. T. (2000). Informant reports: Conceptual and research bases of interviews with parents and teachers. In E. S. Shapiro & T. R. Kratochwill (Eds.), *Behavioral assessment in schools* (2nd ed., pp. 257–287). New York: Guilford Press.

Bijou, S. W., Peterson, R. F., & Ault, M. H. (1968). A method to integrate descriptive and experimental field studies at the level of data and empirical concepts. *Journal of Applied Behavior Analysis, 1,* 175–191.

Bijou, S. W., Peterson, R. F., Harris, F. R., Allen, K. E., & Johnston, M. S. (1969). Methodology for experimental studies of young children in natural settings. *Psychological Record, 19,* 177–210.

Bowman, L. G., Fisher, W. W., Thompson, R. H., & Piazza, C. C. (1997). On the relation of mands and the function of destructive behavior. *Journal of Applied Behavior Analysis, 30,* 251–265.

Brookshire, R. H., Nicholas, L. S., & Krueger, K. (1978). Sampling of speech pathology treatment activities: An evaluation of momentary and interval time sampling procedures. *Journal of Speech and Hearing Research, 21,* 652–667.

Brulle, A. R., & Repp, A. C. (1984). An investigation of the accuracy of momentary time sampling procedures with time series data. *British Journal of Psychology, 75,* 481–485.

Cameron, D. L., Crosbie, J., & Crocker, A. D. (1988). A fixed interval momentary sampling method for assessing ongoing behaviors induced by dopamine receptor agonists. *Progress in Neuro-Psychopharmacology and Biological Psychiatry, 12,* 595–606.

Cariveau, T., & Kodak, T. (2017). Programming a randomized dependent group contingency and common stimuli to promote durable behavior change. *Journal of Applied Behavior Analysis, 50,* 121–133.

Connell, J. E., & Witt, J. C. (2004). Applications of computer-based instruction: Using specialized software to aid letter-name and letter-sound recognition. *Journal of Applied Behavior Analysis, 37,* 67–71.

Cooper, J. O., Heron, T. E., & Heward, W. L. (2020). *Applied behavior analysis* (3rd ed.). Upper Saddle River, NJ: Pearson.

Cordes, A. K. (1994). The reliability of observational data: I. Theories and methods for speech language pathology. *Journal of Speech and Hearing Research, 37,* 264–278.

Critchfield, T. S. (1999). An unexpected effect of recording frequency in reactive self-monitoring. *Journal of Applied Behavior Analysis, 32,* 389–391.

Dempsey, C. M., Iwata, B. A., Fritz, J. N., & Rolider, N. U. (2012). Observer training revisited: A comparison of *in vivo* and video instruction. *Journal of Applied Behavior Analysis, 45,* 827–832.

Devine, S. L., Rapp, J. T., Testa, J. R., Henrickson, M. L., & Schnerch, G. (2011). Detecting changes in simulated events using partial-interval recording and momentary-time sampling: III. Evaluating sensitivity as a function of session length. *Behavioral Interventions, 26,* 103–124.

Dixon, M. R. (2003). Creating a portable data-collection system with Microsoft® embedded visual tools for the pocket PC. *Journal of Applied Behavior Analysis, 36,* 271–284.

Doll, B., & Elliott, S. N. (1994). Representativeness of observed preschool social behaviors: How many data are enough? *Journal of Early Intervention, 18,* 227–238.

Fisher, W. W., Lindauer, S. E., Alterson, C. J., & Thompson, R. H. (1998). Assessment and treatment of destructive behavior maintained by stereotypic object manipulation. *Journal of Applied Behavior Analysis, 31,* 513–527.

Fisher, W. W., Piazza, C. C., Bowman, L. G., & Amari, A. (1996). Integrating caregiver report with a systematic choice assessment to enhance reinforcer identification. *American Journal on Mental Retardation, 101,* 15–25.

Fisher, W. W., Rodriguez, N. M., & Owen, T. M. (2013). Functional assessment and treatment of perseverative speech about restricted topics in an adolescent with Asperger syndrome. *Journal of Applied Behavior Analysis, 46,* 307–311.

Fritz, J. N., Iwata, B. A., Hammond, J. L., & Bloom, S. E. (2013). Experimental analysis of precursors to severe problem behavior. *Journal of Applied Behavior Analysis, 46,* 101–129.

Fuhrman, A. M., Fisher, W. W., & Greer, B. D. (2016). A preliminary investigation on improving functional communication training by mitigating resurgence of destructive behavior. *Journal of Applied Behavior Analysis, 49,* 884–899.

Grace, N. C., Thompson, R., & Fisher, W. W. (1996). The treatment of covert self-injury through contingencies on response products. *Journal of Applied Behavior Analysis, 29,* 239–242.

Green, S. B., & Alverson, L. G. (1978). A comparison of indirect measures for long-duration behaviors. *Journal of Applied Behavior Analysis, 11,* 530.

Green, S. B., McCoy, J. F., Burns, K. P., & Smith, A. C. (1982). Accuracy of observational data with whole interval, partial interval, and momentary-time-sampling recording techniques. *Journal of Behavioral Assessment, 4,* 103–118.

Gresham, F. M., Gansle, K. A., & Noell, G. H. (1993). Treatment integrity in applied behavior analysis with children. *Journal of Applied Behavior Analysis, 26,* 257–263.

Gutowski, S. J., & Stromer, R. (2003). Delayed matching to two-picture samples by individuals with and without disabilities: An analysis of the role of naming. *Journal of Applied Behavior Analysis, 36,* 487–505.

Hagopian, L. P., Contrucci Kuhn, S. A., Long, E. S., & Rush, K. S. (2005). Schedule thinning following communication training: Using competing stimuli to enhance tolerance to decrements in reinforcer density. *Journal of Applied Behavior Analysis, 38,* 177–193.

Hanley, G. P., Cammilleri, A. P., Tiger, J. H., & Ingvarsson, E. T. (2007). A method for describing preschoolers' activity preferences. *Journal of Applied Behavior Analysis, 40,* 603–618.

Hanley, G. P., Iwata, B. A., Lindberg, J. S., & Conners, J. (2003). Response-restriction analysis: I. Assessment of activity preferences. *Journal of Applied Behavior Analysis, 36,* 47–58.

Hansen, B. D., Sabey, C. V., Rich, M., Marr, D., Robins, N., & Barnett, S. (2019). Latency-based functional analysis in schools: Correspondence and differences across environments. *Behavioral Interventions, 34,* 366–376.

Harrop, A., & Daniels, M. (1985). Momentary time sampling with time series data: A commentary on the paper by Brulle & Repp. *British Journal of Psychology, 76,* 533–537.

Harrop, A., & Daniels, M. (1986). Methods of time sampling: A reappraisal of momentary-time sampling and partial interval recording. *Journal of Applied Behavior Analysis, 19,* 73–77.

Harrop, A., & Daniels, M. (1993). Further reappraisal of momentary-time sampling and partial-interval recording. *Journal of Applied Behavior Analysis, 26,* 277–278.

Harrop, A., Daniels, M., & Foulkes, C. (1990). The use of momentary-time sampling and partial interval recording in behavioral research. *Behavioural Psychotherapy, 18,* 121–127.

Hartmann, D. P. (1984). Assessment strategies. In D. H. Barlow & M. Hersen (Eds.), *Single case experimental designs: Strategies for studying behavior change* (2nd ed., pp. 107–139). New York: Pergamon Press.

Hartmann, D. P., & Wood, D. D. (1982). Observational methods. In A. S. Bellack, M. Hersen, & A. E. Kazdin (Eds.), *International handbook of behavior modification and therapy* (pp. 109–133). New York: Plenum Press.

Hersen, M., & Barlow, D. H. (1976). *Single case experimental designs: Strategies for studying behavior change.* Oxford, UK: Pergamon Press.

Hoch, H., McComas, J. J., Johnson, L., Faranda, N., & Guenther, S. L. (2002). The effects of magnitude and quality of reinforcement on choice responding during play activities. *Journal of Applied Behavior Analysis, 35,* 171–181.

Jackson, J., & Dixon, M. R. (2007). A mobile computing solution for collecting functional analysis data on a Pocket PC. *Journal of Applied Behavior Analysis, 40,* 359–384.

Johnston, J. M., & Pennypacker, H. S. (1993). *Strategies and tactics of behavioral research* (2nd ed.). Hillsdale, NJ: Erlbaum.

Kahng, S., & Iwata, B. A. (1998). Computerized systems for collecting real-time observational data. *Journal of Applied Behavior Analysis, 31,* 253–261.

Kazdin, A. E. (1977). Artifact, bias, and complexity of assessment: The ABC's of reliability. *Journal of Applied Behavior Analysis, 10,* 141–150.

Kazdin, A. E. (1979). Unobtrusive measures in behavioral assessment. *Journal of Applied Behavior Analysis, 12,* 713–724.

Kazdin, A. E. (2001). *Behavior modification in applied settings* (6th ed.). Belmont, CA: Wadsworth/Thomson Learning.

Kearns, K., Edwards, R., & Tingstrom, D. H. (1990). Accuracy of long momentary-time sampling intervals: Implications for classroom data collection. *Journal of Psychoeducational Assessment, 8,* 74–85.

Kelly, M. B. (1976). A review of academic permanent-product data collection and reliability procedures in applied behavior analysis research. *Journal of Applied Behavior Analysis, 9,* 211.

Kent, R. N., Kanowitz, J., O'Leary, K. D., & Cheiken, M. (1977). Observer reliability as a function of circumstances of assessment. *Journal of Applied Behavior Analysis, 10,* 317–324.

Kent, R. N., O'Leary, K. D., Dietz, A., & Diament, C. (1979). Comparison of observational recordings *in vivo,* via mirror, and via television. *Journal of Applied Behavior Analysis, 12,* 517–522.

Lannie, A. L., & Martens, B. K. (2004). Effects of task difficulty and type of contingency on students' allocation of responding to math worksheets. *Journal of Applied Behavior Analysis, 37,* 53–65.

Lepper, T. L., Devine, B., & Petursdottir, A. I. (2016). Application of a lag contingency to reduce perseveration on circumscribed interests: A brief report. *Developmental Neurorehabilitation, 20,* 313–316.

Lerman, D. C., Parten, M., Addison, L. R., Vorndran, C. M., Volkert, V. M., & Kodak, T. (2005). A methodology for assessing the functions of emerging speech in children with developmental disabilities. *Journal of Applied Behavior Analysis, 38,* 303–316.

Maglieri, K. A., DeLeon, I. G., Rodriguez-Catter, V., & Sevin, B. M. (2000). Treatment of covert food stealing in an individual with Prader–Willi syndrome. *Journal of Applied Behavior Analysis, 33,* 615–618.

Mansell, J. (1985). Time sampling and measurement error: the effect of interval length and sampling pattern. *Journal of Behavior Therapy and Experimental Psychiatry, 16,* 245–251.

McComas, J. J., & Mace, F. C. (2000). Theory and practice in conducting functional analysis. In E. S. Shapiro & T. R. Kratochwill (Eds.), *Behavioral assessment in schools* (2nd ed., pp. 78–103). New York: Guilford Press.

Merrell, K. W. (2000). Informant reports: Theory and research in using child behavior rating scales in school settings. In E. S. Shapiro & T. R. Kratochwill (Eds.), *Behavioral assessment in schools* (2nd ed., pp. 233–256). New York: Guilford Press.

Miller, D. L., & Kelley, M. L. (1994). The use of goal

setting and contingency contracting for improving children's homework performance. *Journal of Applied Behavior Analysis, 27,* 73–84.

Miltenberger, R. G., Rapp, J. T., & Long, E. S. (1999). A low-tech method for conducting real-time recording. *Journal of Applied Behavior Analysis, 32,* 119–120.

Mudford, O. C., Beale, I. L., & Singh, N. N. (1990). The representativeness of observational samples of different durations. *Journal of Applied Behavior Analysis, 23,* 323–331.

Mudford, O. C., Martin, N. T., Hui, J. K. Y., & Taylor, S. A. (2009). Assessing observer accuracy in continuous recording of rate and duration: Three algorithms compared. *Journal of Applied Behavior Analysis, 42,* 527–539.

Mudford, O. C., Zeleny, J. R., Fisher, W. W., Klum, M. E., & Owen, T. M. (2011). Calibration of observational measurement of rate of responding. *Journal of Applied Behavior Analysis, 44,* 571–586.

Murphy, G., & Goodall, E. (1980). Case histories and shorter communications: Measurement error in direct observations: A comparison of common recording methods. *Behaviour Research and Therapy, 18,* 147–150.

Murphy, M. J., & Harrop, A. (1994). Observer effort in the use of momentary-time sampling and partial interval recording. *British Journal of Psychology, 85,* 169–180.

Nay, R. N. (1979). *Multimethod clinical assessment.* New York: Gardner Press.

Nelson, R. O. (1977). Methodological issues in assessment via self-monitoring. In J. D. Cone & R. P. Hawkins (Eds.), *Behavioral assessment: New directions in clinical psychology* (pp. 217–240). New York: Brunner/Mazel.

North, S. T., & Iwata, B. A. (2005). Motivational influences on performance maintained by food reinforcement. *Journal of Applied Behavior Analysis, 38,* 317–333.

Northup, J. (2000). Further evaluation of the accuracy of reinforcer surveys: A systematic replication. *Journal of Applied Behavior Analysis, 33,* 335–338.

Odom, S. L., & Ogawa, I. (1992). Direct observation of young children's interactions with peers: A review of methodology. *Behavioral Assessment, 14,* 407–441.

O'Leary, K. D., Kent, R. N., & Kanowitz, J. (1975). Shaping data collection congruent with experimental hypotheses. *Journal of Applied Behavior Analysis, 8,* 43–51.

Page, T. J., & Iwata, B. A. (1986). Interobserver agreement: History, theory, and current practice. In A. Poling & R. W. Fuqua (Eds.), *Research methods in applied behavior analysis: Issues and advances* (pp. 99–126). New York: Plenum Press.

Panos, R., & Freed, T. (2007). The benefits of automatic data collection in the fresh produce supply chain. In *IEEE International Conference on Automation Science and Engineering* (pp. 1034–1038). Piscataway, NJ: Institute of Electrical and Electronics Engineers.

Poling, A., Methot, L. L., & LeSage, M. G. (1995). *Fundamentals of behavior analytic research.* New York: Plenum Press.

Powell, J., Martindale, A., & Kulp, S. (1975). An evaluation of time-sample measures of behavior. *Journal of Applied Behavior Analysis, 8,* 463–469.

Powell, J., Martindale, B., Kulp, S., Martindale, A., & Bauman, R. (1977). Taking a closer look: Time sampling and measurement error. *Journal of Applied Behavior Analysis, 10,* 325–332.

Prinz, R. J. (1982). Observing and recording children's behavior. *Behavioral Assessment, 4,* 120–121.

Rapp, J. T., Colby-Dirksen, A. M., Michalski, D. N., Carroll, R. A., & Lindenberg, A. M. (2008). Detecting changes in simulated events using partial-interval recording and momentary-time-sampling. *Behavioral Interventions, 23,* 237–269.

Repp, A. C., Nieminen, G. S., Olinger, E., & Brusca, R. (1988). Direct observation: Factors affecting the accuracy of observers. *Exceptional Children, 55,* 29–36.

Repp, A. C., Roberts, D. M., Slack, D. J., Repp, C. F., & Berkler, M. S. (1976). A comparison of frequency, interval and time-sampling methods of data collection. *Journal of Applied Behavior Analysis, 9,* 501–508.

Rolider, N. U., Iwata, B. A., & Bullock, C. E. (2012). Influences of response rate and distribution on the calculation of interobserver reliability scores. *Journal of Applied Behavior Analysis, 45,* 753–762.

Sanson-Fisher, R. W., Poole, A. D., & Dunn, J. (1980). An empirical method for determining an appropriate interval length for recording behavior. *Journal of Applied Behavior Analysis, 13,* 493–500.

Sanson-Fisher, R. W., Poole, A. D., Small, G. A., & Fleming, I. R. (1979). Data acquisition in real time: An improved system for naturalistic observations. *Behavior Therapy, 10,* 543–554.

Saudargas, R. A., & Zanolli, K. (1990). Momentary time sampling as an estimate of percentage time: A field validation. *Journal of Applied Behavior Analysis, 23,* 533–537.

Schinke, S. P., & Wong, S. E. (1977). Coding group home behavior with a continuous real-time recording device. *Behavioral Engineering, 4,* 5–9.

Sigurdsson, S. O., Aklin, W., Ring, B. M., Needham, M., Boscoe, J., & Silverman, K. (2011). Automated measurement of noise violations in the therapeutic workplace. *Behavior Analysis in Practice, 4,* 47–53.

Slocum, S. K., Grauerholz-Fisher, E., Peters, K. P., & Vollmer, T. R. (2018). A multicomponent approach to thinning reinforcer delivery during noncontingent reinforcement schedules. *Journal of Applied Behavior Analysis, 51,* 61–69.

Suen, H. K., Ary, D., & Covalt, W. (1991). Reappraisal of momentary-time sampling and partial-interval recording. *Journal of Applied Behavior Analysis, 24,* 803–804.

Tapp, J. (2003). Procoder for digital video: User manual. Retrieved November 23, 2005, from *http://mingus. kc.vanderbilt.edu/pcdv.*

Tapp, J., & Walden, T. (1993). PROCODER: A professional tape control, coding, and analysis system for behavioral research using videotape. *Behavior Research Methods, Instruments, and Computers, 25,* 53–56.

Taravella, C. C., Lerman, D., Contrucci, S. A., & Roane, H. S. (2000). Further evaluation of low-ranked items in stimulus-choice preference assessments. *Journal of Applied Behavior Analysis, 33,* 105–108.

Test, D. W., Rose, T. L., & Corum, L. (1990). Applied behavior analysis with secondary students: A methodological review of research published from 1968 to 1987. *Education and Treatment of Children, 13,* 45–62.

Thiemann, K. S., & Goldstein, H. (2001). Social stories, written text cues, and video feedback: Effects on social communication of children with autism. *Journal of Applied Behavior Analysis, 34,* 425–446.

Thomson, C., Holmberg, M., & Baer, D. M. (1974). A brief report on a comparison of time-sampling procedures. *Journal of Applied Behavior Analysis, 7,* 623–626.

Torres-Viso, M., Strohmeier, C. W., & Zarcone, J. R. (2018). Functional analysis and treatment of problem behavior related to mands for rearrangement. *Journal of Applied Behavior Analysis, 51,* 158–165.

Traub, M. R., & Vollmer, T. R. (2019). Response latency as a measure of behavior in the assessment of elopement. *Journal of Applied Behavior Analysis, 52,* 422–438.

Tyler, S. (1979). Time-sampling: Matter of convention. *Animal Behaviour, 27,* 801–810.

VanWormer, J. J. (2004). Pedometers and brief e-counseling: Increasing physical activity for overweight adults. *Journal of Applied Behavior Analysis, 37,* 421–425.

Wasik, B. H., & Loven, M. D. (1980). Classroom observational data: Sources of inaccuracy and proposed solutions. *Behavioral Assessment, 2,* 211–227.

Wehby, J. H., & Hollahan, M. S. (2000). Effects of high-probability requests on the latency to initiate academic tasks. *Journal of Applied Behavior Analysis, 33,* 259–262.

Whiting, S. W., & Dixon, M. R. (2012). Creating an iPhone application for collecting continuous ABC data. *Journal of Applied Behavior Analysis, 45,* 643–656.

Wilson, C. W., & Hopkins, B. L. (1973). The effects of contingent music on the intensity of noise in junior high home economics classes. *Journal of Applied Behavior Analysis, 6,* 269–275.

Wilson, D. M., Iwata, B. A., & Bloom, S. E. (2012). Computer-assisted measurement of wound size associated with self-injurious behavior. *Journal of Applied Behavior Analysis, 45,* 797–808.

Wirth, O., Slaven, J., & Taylor, M. A. (2014). Interval sampling methods and measurement error: A computer simulation. *Journal of Applied Behavior Analysis, 47,* 83–100.

# CHAPTER 9

# Single-Case Experimental Designs

Nicole M. DeRosa, William E. Sullivan, Henry S. Roane, Andrew R. Craig, and Heather J. Kadey

A primary goal of applied behavior analysis is to understand how specific variables affect socially significant behavior or produce behavior change. Single-case experimental designs are ideal for this type of analysis, because the focus is on the problem, setting, or individual that is the target for evaluation (Kazdin, 2016). Single-case experimental designs involve continuous assessment to measure behavior over time. Thus the use of single-case designs allows a behavior analyst to determine if an independent variable (e.g., intervention) produced the desired change in the target dependent variable (e.g., aggression). These designs also afford the behavior analyst the flexibility to modify the measures and method to suit the problem of interest.

Although well suited for use with individuals, single-case experimental designs in applied behavior analysis do not exclude group designs or statistical analysis (Roane, Ringdahl, Kelley, & Glover, 2011). However, group designs may not allow a behavior analyst to determine individual variations in the effects of an independent variable on the dependent variable of interest for a given individual. In other words, the behavior analyst cannot use a group design to determine the effects (e.g., optimal, minimal, no effect) the independent variable has on behavior change for an individual. Similarly, the use of statistical analysis may obscure behavior change outcomes at the individual's level. For example, suppose an intervention produces a statistically significant reduction in the occurrence of self-injurious behavior; these findings may lack clinical significance if the reduced level of self-injury produces tissue damage. By contrast, single-case experimental designs are appropriate for tracking continuous, moment-to-moment changes in the occurrence of the target behavior that allow the behavior analyst to determine whether behavior change is clinically significant for the individual.

The main goal of single-case experimental design is to demonstrate a *functional relation*—the effects of an independent variable on a dependent variable (Baer, Wolf, & Risley, 1968). An independent variable is one, such as the intervention, that a behavior analyst can manipulate to affect a dependent variable, which is generally the behavior targeted for change. A functional relation exists when changes in the dependent variable occur only during manipulations of the independent variable. Thus the behavior analyst can use a single-case experimental design to systematically identify variables that influence the occurrence of the behavior. In this chapter, we review data collection, visual inspection of data, and specific single-case experimental designs, which we illustrate with hypothetical data and with data from our work and that of others.

## DATA COLLECTION

Effective use of single-case experimental designs depends on accurate and reliable data collection. Important steps in developing an accurate and reliable data collection procedure include defining the target behavior(s), selecting a data collection system, and collecting baseline data (Roane et al., 2011). In addition, we discuss other variables that influence data collection in strategies involving single-case experimental designs. We have focused on how the observation setting and conditions can affect data collection outcomes, as these are variables that behavior analysts often overlook.

Development of an operational definition for the target behavior of interest is an important first step in the data collection process. Operational definitions should be (1) observable, (2) based on an action, and (3) descriptive. Measurement of observable behavior is preferable to measurement of behaviors that are difficult or impossible to observe, such as internal states. Behavior analysts measure observable behavior to avoid making inferences about the cause of behavior, such as "He was angry," and to ensure that the measured behavior is an accurate representation of the behavior of interest as it occurs in the target environment. For example, *hitting* is an observable behavior that has a clear beginning and end, whereas *being angry* is an inferred emotional state. An observer might infer that a person is angry if the person hits someone, but hitting could occur for other reasons.

The behavior analyst should consider the action rather than the outcome of the behavior to develop an operational definition, unless he or she is using a permanent-product measure of behavior, such as number of math problems completed. The observer should record an occurrence of the behavior if it meets the parameters of the definition, regardless of its consequence or perceived intention. For example, the observer should record a head turn during a mealtime observation if the observed behavior matches the operational definition (e.g., the head moving 45 degrees away from the utensil), independently of whether the behavior occurred after the sound of a door opening and someone walking into the room. The operational definition should also include details that differentiate the target behavior from other behaviors, so that two independent observers reliably measure the target behavior. For example, the observer should record appropriate communication if the operational definition is contacting a card with at least one finger on the palm side of the hand, and a child contacts the card with one finger on the palm side of the hand, but not when the child contacts the card with other body parts, such as the arm.

The next step in data collection is to select an appropriate measurement system. There are four categories of behavior measurement: (1) event recording, (2) duration recording, (3) interval recording, and (4) permanent-product recording (Kahng, Ingvarsson, Quigg, Seckinger, & Teichman, 2011; Roane et al., 2011). The operational definition of the target behavior will influence which measurement system is most appropriate. Event recording is often appropriate for discrete responses—behaviors that have a clear beginning and end. The observer typically records each occurrence of the target behavior. The recorded events are typically converted into a rate, such as frequency over unit of time. In some cases, duration recording, in which the observer records the time a behavior occurs, is appropriate for discrete behaviors that occur at high rates. Duration recording is also appropriate for continuous behaviors, such as remaining on task, particularly when the time the behavior occurs is the most important target for change. The observer might report a duration record as a duration of time (e.g., "The child cried for 5 minutes") or as a percentage of time (e.g., "The child cried for 50% of the session"). Interval recording is useful if we want to know whether the behavior occurred or did not occur in a specific interval. The observer would record the occurrence of the behavior if it occurred any time during the interval with partial-interval recording, or if the behavior occurred for the entire interval with whole-interval recording. Interval data are typically reported as percentage of intervals. Permanent-product recording measures the outcome of a behavior, such as number of completed homework sheets.

We have provided a brief overview of operational definitions and behavior measurement in this chapter; the reader can refer to Kahng et al. (Chapter 8, this volume) for a more in-depth review. Below, we discuss how setting and condition variables can affect data collection outcomes.

## SETTING EFFECTS

Careful control of extraneous variables that might affect behavior is necessary to demonstrate a functional relation between the independent and dependent variables. A behavior analyst cannot be sure that observed changes or the absence of observed changes in the dependent variable are a function of manipulating the independent variable in the absence of such control. The setting where the behavior analyst conducts the independent-variable manipulation may affect the dependent variable independently of the manipulation. A simple way to discuss these effects is to consider setting as a dichotomy between natural and contrived settings, although many subtle gradations between the endpoints of this dichotomy exist.

Conducting observations in the natural setting may be advantageous because that is where the target behavior occurs. The disadvantage of the natural setting, however, is that variables in the setting may be more difficult to control. A second and related disadvantage is that variables may be present that may affect the target behavior in an inconsistent way. Clinicians may be more likely to conduct manipulations in the natural setting, particularly if that is the setting in which they work. Clinical researchers, by contrast, often opt to conduct experiments in contrived environments, such as clinics or hospitals, to exert more stringent control over extraneous variables. Control of extraneous variables allows researchers to be more confident about the identified relation between the independent and dependent variables. Use of a contrived setting, however, may reduce confidence in the social validity of the findings. That is, would a researcher identify the same relation between the independent and dependent variables in the natural environment? A second and related disadvantage of the contrived setting is that the setting might exert its own influence on behavior.

Most single-case experimental designs include a measurement of the target behavior in a *baseline* condition. Behavior analysts compare levels or rates of the target behavior in baseline and those after the manipulation, to determine whether the manipulation has produced a change in the level or rate of the target behavior. The behavior analyst can observe behavior in baseline in the presence or absence of planned manipulations of antecedents and consequences. Behavior analysts may use the term *naturalistic observations* to describe observations of the target behavior in the absence of planned manipulations. Measuring the target behavior, such as communication responses, during a regularly scheduled activity is an example of a naturalistic observation, which would provide information about the number of spontaneous communication responses during a free-play activity.

*Contrived observations* involve systematically arranging antecedents, consequences, or both, often with the goal of evoking the target behavior or identifying the effects of antecedents, consequences, or both on the target behavior. In some cases, the target behavior may not occur with sufficient frequency during naturalistic observations for measurement to be practical for the behavior analyst. In these cases, arranging antecedents, consequences, or both may produce a sufficient frequency of the target behavior for practical observation. Contrived observations also help control for potential extraneous variables that would affect target behavior and limit the conclusions the behavior analyst could draw about the effects of the independent variable on the dependent variable. Furthermore, contrived observations may be necessary or advantageous for situations or behaviors that may be difficult or dangerous to observe in naturalistic conditions (e.g., gun play, pica). One disadvantage, however, is that the behavior analyst does not know whether behavior that occurs in a contrived observation is representative of that behavior during a natural observation. Behavior that occurs during the contrived observation may vary to some degree from behavior in more naturalistic conditions (Kazdin, 2011). One way to address this disadvantage might be to conduct initial observations in contrived conditions and subsequent observations in natural conditions, to assess the generality of the observations in the contrived condition.

Lang et al. (2008) implemented functional analyses in two different settings with two participants to assess the potential influence of the observation setting on behavior. One setting was an empty assessment room in the school, and the other was the participant's classroom. Functional-analytic outcomes were the same for both settings for one participant, indicating that the setting did not affect the assessment outcome. Functional-analytic outcomes were different for the settings for the other participant, indicating that the setting did affect the assessment outcome in this case. Results appear in Figure 9.1 for the functional analyses that produced the same result (top) and the functional analyses that produced different re-

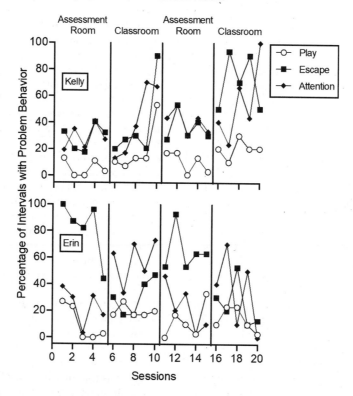

**FIGURE 9.1.** Results from Lang et al. (2008) demonstrating correspondence in behavior function despite differences in setting (top) and variations in behavior function across settings (bottom).

sults (bottom). These results show that functional-analytic outcomes may differ, depending on the setting in which the observation occurs for some individuals.

Developing operational definitions and selecting an appropriate measurement system, observation setting, and observation conditions are integral steps in single-case experimental designs. The primary focus of these designs, however, is demonstration of functional control. Therefore, in the remainder of this chapter, we focus on visual inspection and on variations in single-case experimental designs.

## VISUAL INSPECTION

Visual inspection of graphed data is the primary method of analyzing single-case experimental design data. The goal of visual inspection is to make predictions about the future occurrence of the observed behavior, based on the (1) level, (2) stability, and (3) trend of the data. Other impor-

tant elements to consider during visual inspection of single-case experimental design data include the (1) immediacy of effects; (2) magnitude of effects; and (3) proportion of overlapping data points, which should demonstrate clearly that manipulations of the independent variable produced consistent, meaningful changes in the dependent variable.

The *level* of behavior indicates the extent of the problem. To put this another way, level indicates how frequently the target behavior occurs and whether the graphed data correspond to other observations and records. *Stability* refers to fluctuations in the data over time. Stable levels of behavior are those that occur within a limited range, so that the behavior analyst can predict the future level of the target behavior, given that the independent variable does not change. By contrast, unstable data vary across a wider range from data point to data point, so that the future level of the target behavior is more difficult to predict. *Trend* refers to whether the behavior is improving or worsening over time. An improving trend (e.g., an increase in the number of bites eaten) may suggest a less emergent need for intervention. In other words, why intervene on a behavior that is improving? Improvement in the target behavior before intervention increases the difficulty of determining if further improvements in the target behavior are a function of the intervention or a continuation of the target behavior's trend before intervention. A worsening trend may suggest a more immediate need for intervention. An improvement in a target behavior that was previously worsening increases our confidence that the intervention was the cause of the improved behavior, as the trend of the behavior is different before and after intervention.

Although level, stability, and trend are the fundamental components of visual inspection in single-case experimental designs, a behavior analyst must consider several additional variables when conducting visual inspection. One variable is the *immediacy* of effects, which refers to the latency between the introduction or withdrawal of the independent variable and a change in the dependent variable. Generally, a short latency between independent-variable manipulations and changes in the dependent variable increases our confidence that there is a functional relation (Horner et al., 2005). Figure 9.2 displays hypothetical data of an example (left) and nonexample (right) of immediate effects of the independent-variable manipulation on the rate of the dependent variable.

The *magnitude* of effects across time also contributes to the demonstration of functional control. Changes in the mean and visual inspection of the level, trend, and stability of the data within and across conditions are ways to examine the magnitude of the effect. For example, Figure 9.3,

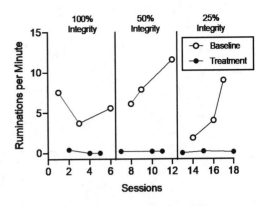

**FIGURE 9.3.** Example from DeRosa, Roane, Bishop, and Stilkowski (2016) of magnitude effects.

which depicts a subset of data from DeRosa, Roane, Bishop, and Silkowski (2016), shows a large, clear differentiation between the baseline and intervention data paths, emphasizing the magnitude of the effects of intervention on the target behavior, rumination. Baseline levels of rumination were elevated and variable (M = 6.5 responses per minute across phases) relative to the intervention condition, which demonstrated near-zero, stable rates of rumination (M = 0.2 response per minute across phases). Finally, the *proportion of overlapping data points* is another factor that influences data interpretation. Smaller and larger proportions of overlapping data support and refute, respectively, a causal relation between independent-variable manipulations and changes in the dependent variable. Figure 9.4 exemplifies overlapping (left) and nonoverlapping (right) data points.

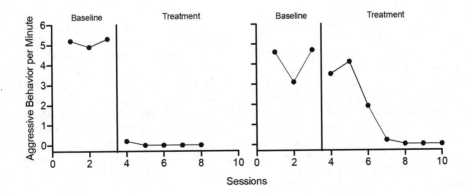

**FIGURE 9.2.** Example of immediate (left) and nonimmediate (right) treatment effects.

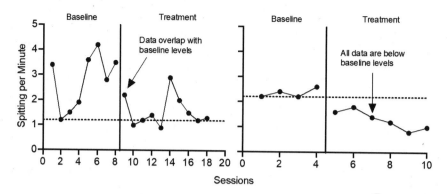

**FIGURE 9.4.** Example of overlapping (left) and nonoverlapping (right) data points across phases.

Visual inspection is the most preferred and most often used method for interpreting graphed data from single-case experimental designs (Horner & Kratochwill, 2012), and accurate interpretation of graphed data is essential for determining the effects of experimental manipulations. One disadvantage is that interpretations during visual inspection of such data may not be reliable among untrained individuals. Thus researchers have developed methods to reduce potential bias and improve agreement during visual inspection of single-case experimental design data. Results of these studies have shown that appropriate training improves interrater agreement to acceptable levels (e.g., Fisher, Kelley, & Lomas, 2003; Kahng et al., 2010; O'Grady, Reeve, Reeve, Vladescu, & Lake, 2018; Stewart, Carr, Brandt, & McHenry, 2007; Wolfe & Slocum, 2015). The generality of these results may be limited, however, because most of the studies used data from sequential designs (Hagopian et al., 1997).

Hagopian et al. (1997) showed that interrater agreement was low (M = .46) when three predoctoral interns used visual inspection to interpret graphed functional-analytic data. Hagopian et al. developed structured criteria for interpretation of such data, based on the consensus of experts in functional analysis. Hagopian et al. used the structured criteria to train the same predoctoral interns to interpret graphed functional-analytic data, and mean interrater agreement increased to .81. One limitation is that Hagopian et al. used functional analyses that included 10 data points per condition; thus behavior analysts could not use the criteria to interpret functional analyses of different lengths.

The results of Study 1 suggested that the interpretation of functional-analytic outcomes was less

reliable in the absence of the modified structured criteria, whereas agreement increased when the criteria were used. During pretraining, in which the reviewers had access to the written modified criteria for visual inspection, the average agreements between the reviewers and the expert judge were .73 and .80, respectively, for the master's-level and postbaccalaureate interns. Following training, interobserver agreement increased for both groups. Specifically, the exact agreement between the master's-level reviewers and the expert judge increased to an average of .98, whereas the average exact agreement between the postbaccalaureate reviewers and the expert judge increased to .95.

Roane, Fisher, Kelley, Mevers, and Bouxsein (2013) modified Hagopian et al.'s (1997) structured criteria to apply them to results of functional analyses with varying lengths. Roane et al. used the criteria to train individuals with different levels of education and clinical experience, which produced high levels of interrater agreement and demonstrated the validity of the modified criteria. Roane et al. then used the criteria to train master's-level and postbaccalaureate participants to interpret graphed functional-analytic data, and agreement between the master's-level and postbaccalaureate participants and an expert judge was .98 and .95, respectively. Finally, Roane et al. applied the criteria to the data from 141 functional analyses and identified the maintaining reinforcement contingency for problem behavior in a similar percentage of cases relative to those reported previously (e.g., Hagopian, Rooker, Jessel, & DeLeon, 2013; Hanley, Iwata, & McCord, 2003). Taken together, these results suggest that behavior analysts can use structured criteria to improve the reliability of visual inspection and interpretation of functional-analytic data. As Hagopian et al., and Roane et al.

note, however, behavior analysts should continue to use visual inspection as the primary method and use structured criteria as an adjunct for interpretation of functional-analytic data.

Researchers and clinicians have recognized the need to evaluate results of single-case experimental designs to expand the pool of scientific evidence available for review for empirically supported interventions (Kratochwill et al., 2010; Pustejovsky & Ferron, 2017). As such, the What Works Clearinghouse drafted standards for single-case experimental designs, based on input from national experts. The information from these standards overlaps with the contents of this chapter, including (1) an overview of single-case experimental designs, (2) the types of questions for which a researcher or clinician might use a single-case experimental design, and (3) a discussion of the internal validity of single-case experimental designs. The panel proposed standards for these designs, which address the internal validity of the designs, and for evidence, which provide guidelines for determining whether the evidence meets the described standards. These guidelines provide another example of the focus on increased objectivity of interpreting single-case experimental design data.

Statistical analysis is a well-accepted method for analyzing group data, but it has not gained widespread acceptance for analysis of single-case experimental design data. One reason for the dearth of statistical analysis in single-case experimental designs is their focus on the individual. Behavior analysts are generally interested in robust intervention effects that have a meaningful impact for the individual. A limitation of statistical analysis for single-case experimental designs is that a statistically significant effect may not be clinically relevant, or a clinically relevant effect may not be statistically significant (Kazdin, 2011). Statistical analysis may be useful in situations in which clinically relevant effects are difficult to determine from visual inspection. Moreover, consensus on and acceptance of statistical analysis to enhance rather than replace visual analysis are growing (Cohen, Feinstein, Masuda, & Vowles, 2014).

Fisher and Lerman (2014) commented that the development of a statistical metric for estimating effect sizes for single-case experimental designs would represent an important advancement in the field. Estimation of effect sizes may increase the likelihood that researchers would use data from single-case experimental-design research in meta-analyses to determine the level of empirical support for behavioral interventions (see Horner & Kratochwill, 2012, for additional discussion). Fisher and Lerman noted that recommendations from researchers who conduct statistical analyses for such data have shifted from a philosophy of statistics as the only method of data analysis to statistics as an adjunct to visual inspection. This shift is likely to become more acceptable, as behavior analysts are not likely to abandon visual inspection completely. One barrier to the addition of statistical analysis to visual inspection is the complexity of statistical-analytic procedures. For example, Shadish, Hedges, and Pustejovsky (2014) used a mean-difference statistic to analyze single-case experimental design data that Fisher and Lerman described as easy to use. By contrast, other researchers (e.g., Shadish, Zuur, & Sullivan, 2014) have evaluated statistical-analytic procedures that require training and skills that behavior analysts in practice might not have (Fisher & Lerman, 2014). Fisher and Lerman concluded that there may be a tradeoff between the appropriateness of statistical methods for single-case experimental design data and the methods' user-friendliness. Additionally, applications of statistical analysis to data from single-case experimental designs are limited, and replications are needed to determine their appropriateness. However, more recent research has identified the use of randomization techniques as possible alternatives to more traditional statistical analyses. Randomization techniques may be more readily appropriate for analyzing single-case experimental design data, due to (1) the lack of assumptions regarding the distribution of outcome variables, (2) the ability to apply the methods to a variety of research designs, and (3) the ability to obtain meaningful outcomes when applied to small-N datasets (Craig & Fisher, 2019). Overall, increased collaboration between statisticians and behavior analysts is encouraged to bridge the gap between the use of visual and statistical analysis for single-case experimental design data (Fisher & Lerman, 2014).

## TYPES OF SINGLE-CASE EXPERIMENTAL DESIGNS

One goal of a single-case experimental design is to show that manipulation of the independent variable is responsible for changes in the dependent variable, which we refer to as internal validity. External validity is the extent to which the results of a study extend beyond the experimental setting.

Behavior analysts must consider and control for threats to internal and external validity during development and execution of the experimental arrangement.

Common threats to internal validity in single-case experimental designs include history, maturation, testing, and instrumentation. These threats could alter, contribute to, or be solely responsible for changes in the dependent variable. *History* in this context refers to events that occur simultaneously with the experimental manipulation (Kratochwill et al., 2010). *Maturation* refers to changes within the experimental participant that occur naturally over time (e.g., aging; Edgington, 1996; Kratochwill et al., 2010). *Testing* refers to the effects of repeated measurement (e.g., a test score improves because the participant took the test multiple times). *Instrumentation* is the way observers measure behaviors, and *observer drift*, which is an example of an instrumentation error, is a change in the way observers record the same target behavior over time.

Threats to external validity may not be apparent until after researchers study and expand on the conditions under which the phenomenon occurred originally (Kazdin, 2011). *External validity* generally refers to whether the results of a study can be applied to other participants, settings, response measures, and behavior change agents (Kazdin, 2011). *Reactivity*, which is another threat to external validity, occurs when a participant changes his or her behavior because of knowledge that he or she is involved in an experimental manipulation or assessment. *Pretest sensitization* occurs when preexperimental measurement (e.g., baseline) produces changes in participant behavior. Finally, *multiple-treatment interference* occurs when the study includes more than one manipulation, and manipulations that occur earlier in the study may affect responding later in the study.

In the remainder of this section, we review the characteristics of the most common single-case experimental designs. We also review advanced applications of single-case experimental designs, such as parametric analysis, component analysis, and combined designs.

## Reversal (ABAB) Design

The most basic experimental design is the *ABAB reversal*, in which one condition (the A phase; e.g., baseline) is followed by another condition (the B phase; e.g., intervention). Demonstration of functional control with the ABAB design depends on (1) relatively stable levels of responding in the A and B phases, or predictably unstable levels of responding; (2) unambiguous differences in the level of responding in the A and B phases; (3) trends in responding in the appropriate direction in the A and B phases; (4) relatively immediate changes in responding during introduction and reversal of A- and B-phase contingencies; (5) a clinically acceptable level of responding if the goal is to increase or decrease target responding; and (6) minimal overlap in the levels of responding in the A and B phases. To put all this another way, responding reliably turns off and on with the introduction and reversal of A- and B-phase contingencies. Additional reversals between the two phases, with corresponding changes in the target response, strengthen the demonstration of a functional relation.

The introduction and reversal of the experimental manipulation are essential but also the most criticized characteristics of the ABAB design. This criticism is most relevant when the behavior analyst withdraws or removes an effective intervention, particularly if the intervention has produced a clinically significant change in a dangerous behavior. Although this is a valid concern in this case, the effects of intervention should be robust, and the clinically significant change in responding should return when the behavior analyst reinstates the intervention. The behavior analyst must balance the advantages of demonstration of functional control over a reemergence of previous levels of responding. Other limitations include responding that does not return to baseline rates during a reversal, and the potential for responding during the reversal to occur at higher rates than during the initial baseline.

## Multiple-Baseline Design

In a concurrent *multiple-baseline design*, the behavior analyst identifies three or four baselines that he or she can use to evaluate the effects of the experimental manipulation (Byiers, Reichle, & Symons, 2010). The baselines could be behaviors, settings, or individuals, and each baseline is referred to as a *leg* of the multiple-baseline design. The behavior analyst implements the experimental manipulation on Leg 1 when the level, stability, and trend of the data are appropriate and continues to implement the baseline contingencies in the other legs. The behavior analyst implements the experimental manipulation in Leg 2 if it produced the targeted effect in Leg 1, and implements the experimental manipulation in Leg 3 if it produced the targeted effect in Leg 2. The behavior analyst implements the experimental manipulation at different times (i.e., staggered) for each leg. The multiple-baseline design demonstrates functional control when changes in responding occur immediately after the introduction of the experimental manipulation for each leg of the multiple baseline. Baseline levels of responding should be maintained for each leg until the behavior analyst implements the experimental manipulation, and this feature controls for the passage of time. That is, the behavior analyst can attribute the changes in responding to the experimental manipulation. Multiple-baseline designs are appropriate when the experimental manipulation targets behavior that is not likely to be reversed (i.e., reading skills) or when a reversal to baseline contingencies may not be desirable (i.e., for dangerous behavior).

One limitation of the multiple-baseline design is that effects of the experimental manipulation may carry over to the baseline(s) of one or more legs of the design. Carry-over effects decrease confidence that the experimental manipulation was responsible for the change in responding. Additionally, the multiple-baseline design may result in prolonged exposure to baseline contingencies for some targets, which may potentially delay behavior change.

## Changing-Criterion Design

The initial baseline of the *changing-criterion design* is like those of other designs. The changing-criterion design differs from other designs in that (1) the experimental manipulation should produce changes in responding that correspond to a criterion that changes over time; (2) levels of responding should change only when the criterion changes; and (3) responding should ultimately correspond to the terminal goal of the manipulation. The other designs we have discussed thus far produce a demonstration of functional control when the level and magnitude of responding after the experimental manipulation are different from those at baseline. By contrast, the changing-criterion design produces a demonstration of functional control when levels of responding correspond to the relatively small incremental changes to the criterion, rather than the large immediate changes we generally expect with other designs. An important component of the changing-criterion design that behavior analysts often overlook is that the participant should have the opportunity to respond

at the level of the terminal goal, independently of the current criterion. For example, if the terminal goal of a training program is to teach an individual to sort 50 knives and 50 forks, the behavior analyst should supply the individual with 50 knives and 50 forks on every trial even if the criterion is to sort 10 knives and 10 forks, 20 knives and 20 forks, 30 knives and 30 forks, or 40 knives and 40 forks.

A limitation of the changing-criterion design is that responding may not correspond to the changes in the criterion, which weakens the demonstration of functional control. This design may be most appropriate for interventions targeting skill acquisition or for manipulations that include fading and shaping. This design may be less desirable when the goal is a large, rapid, or large and rapid change in responding.

## Multielement Design

As the name implies, the *multielement design* involves conducting multiple experimental manipulations that the behavior analyst alternates in rapid succession, such as from session to session. This rapid alternation is equivalent to completing several "mini-reversals." For example, the behavior analyst might evaluate the effects of noncontingent reinforcement in one condition and time out in another condition on rates of disruptive behavior. The design produces a demonstration of functional control when there are differences in responding across the conditions. The ideal demonstration of functional control with a multielement design involves stable, differentiated levels of responding across conditions with no or minimal data overlap. The multielement design is appropriate when the goal is to compare the effects of two or more experimental manipulations while eliminating the sequence effects that are problematic with reversal designs. *Sequence effects* occur when a history with one condition influences responding during a subsequent condition. Behavior analysts may use a multielement design to compare many antecedent and consequent manipulations when the goal is rapid assessment of effects. An advantage of the multielement design is that it does not require a reversal to or a single prolonged baseline phase, given that the behavior analyst can alternate the baseline with the experimental manipulation. Furthermore, implementation of a baseline is not necessarily a requirement of this design. The goal is to evaluate levels of responding during two or more experimental manipulations, rather than to compare levels of responding during the experimental manipulation with those during the baseline.

The multielement design has several limitations that may impede a demonstration of functional control. As with the multiple-baseline design, carry-over effects are a potential limitation of the multielement design. Individuals also may have difficulty discriminating between conditions. Behavior analysts who do not randomize the order of conditions may observe order effects, when the order of the conditions affects responding. Finally, demonstration of functional control may be more difficult with behaviors that change slowly (e.g., reading skills), given the rapid, alternating conditions of the multielement design.

## Combined Designs and Other Design Considerations

Single-case experimental designs are flexible, such that the behavior analyst can combine individual designs to strengthen the demonstration of functional control (Roane et al., 2011). Furthermore, including more than one design in an analysis may mediate several of the disadvantages associated with individual single-case experimental designs. This section provides a case example to demonstrate the flexibility of combined single-case experimental designs. We also discuss design flexibility relative to assessment of the effects of (1) various experimental manipulations and (2) varying levels or intensity of the experimental manipulations.

### Combined Designs

The behavior analyst may need additional design elements when a limitation of a common single-case experimental design impedes the demonstration of a functional relation. Figure 9.5 shows a clinical example in which we evaluated the differential effects of two interventions on inappropriate mealtime behavior across three participants. Our initial plan was to use a multielement design to compare the effects of avoidance and escape extinction on individual participants, which we embedded in a multiple-baseline design to assess intervention effects across participants. Inappropriate mealtime behavior decreased to low levels during the multielement comparison of avoidance and escape extinction. We wondered whether both interventions were equally effective, or whether the simultaneous decrease in rates of inappropriate mealtime behavior for the two interventions was a

result of carry-over effects (a limitation of the multielement design). We then conducted a reversal to baseline, tested the effects of escape extinction, reversed again to baseline, and tested the effects of avoidance. This example illustrates that single-case experimental designs are flexible. When we observed carry-over effects during the multielement comparison of the two interventions, we added a reversal to strengthen the demonstration of functional control.

### Component and Parametric Analyses

Often behavior analysts implement intervention in a package that includes multiple components. For example, consider a child whose disruptive classroom behavior is maintained by adult attention. The classroom teacher implements an intervention in which he or she delivers attention for hand raising and withholds attention when the child engages in disruptive behavior. The teacher can be more confident that the intervention has produced increases in hand raising and decreases in disruptive behavior if the child's responding changes only when the teacher implements the intervention and holds other variables constant. In this section, we discuss how the behavior analyst can use single-case experimental designs to examine the effects of (1) components of a multicomponent intervention and (2) intervention parameters.

*Component Analyses.* Component analyses are useful when an intervention consists of multiple components. Even though a behavior analyst may have demonstrated a functional relation between a multicomponent intervention and levels of responding, he or she may want to conduct a component analysis to evaluate the effects of individual intervention components (Cooper, Heron, & Heward, 2007).

Ward-Horner and Sturmey (2010) have outlined two methods for component analysis. In a *drop-out analysis*, the behavior analyst initially implements the intervention package and then systematically removes one component at a time. In an *add-in analysis*, the behavior analyst implements one component of an intervention and then introduces individual components or combinations of components. A change in responding indicates whether the dropped or added component or components were responsible for changes in responding. Component analyses may be useful when implementation of a package intervention is

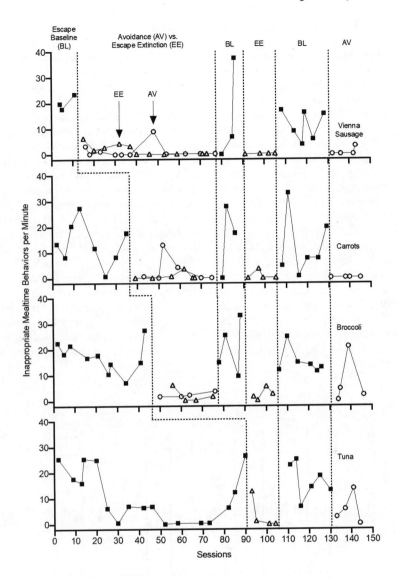

**FIGURE 9.5.** Clinical example for combined designs. The circled data represent examples of potential carry-over effects in baseline, following introduction of treatment in the first leg of the multiple-baseline design.

indicated, but analysis of the effective components is also important.

Cooper et al. (1995) evaluated the components of intervention packages to increase the food acceptance and consumption of four participants with intellectual developmental disorder. We depict the data for one participant in Figure 9.6. The intervention consisted of (1) a choice of food; (2) contingent adult attention for food acceptance; (3) presentation of the food until the feeder could deposit the food into the child's mouth (i.e.,

nonremoval of the spoon); and (4) a warm-up in which the child had access to toys before the feeder presented food. Food acceptance and consumption increased during the multicomponent intervention. The researchers then conducted a component analysis, using a multielement design. Levels of responding did not change when the researchers introduced and withdrew the choice and warm-up components, suggesting that choice and warm-up did not affect responding. By contrast, levels of responding did change when the researchers introduced and withdrew nonremoval of the spoon.

Fisher et al. (1993) used an add-in analysis to evaluate an intervention to reduce the problem behavior of five participants with intellectual developmental disorder. Figure 9.7 depicts responses per minute of disruption (top), aggression (second), and self-injury (third) with one set of demands (Demand 1), and responses per minute of disruption (bottom) during a second set of demands (Demand 2) for one participant. The researchers used reversal and multiple-baseline designs to evaluate rates of problem behavior during (1) baseline, (2) extinction, (3) punishment, (4) functional-communication training (FCT), (5) FCT plus punishment, and (6) FCT plus extinction. For example, Leg 1 shows rates of disruption during a phase of extinction followed by phases of punishment alone, extinction alone, FCT plus punishment, FCT alone, and FCT plus punishment. Rates of disruption were lowest during FCT plus punishment, and the researchers replicated that effect in Leg 2 for aggression and Leg 3 for self-injury.

The researchers compared the effects of FCT plus extinction to FCT plus punishment in Leg 4 for disruption with the second set of demands.

*Parametric Analyses.* Behavior analysts use parametric analyses to evaluate the effects of different parameters of an independent variable, such as magnitude, intensity, and integrity, on the dependent variable. For example, a behavior analyst might use a parametric analysis to assess the effects of 5, 10, 30, or 60 seconds of attention on rates of problem behavior. Parametric analyses allow the behavior analyst to determine the precise level of an experimental manipulation needed to produce and sustain changes in responding (e.g., Athens & Vollmer, 2010; Codding & Lane, 2015; Wilder, Atwell, & Wine, 2006). We provide several clinical examples of parametric analyses below, and we highlight their applied use.

In a four-experiment study, Athens and Vollmer (2010) conducted parametric analyses to examine the effects of duration, quality, and delay to reinforcement on mands and problem behavior.

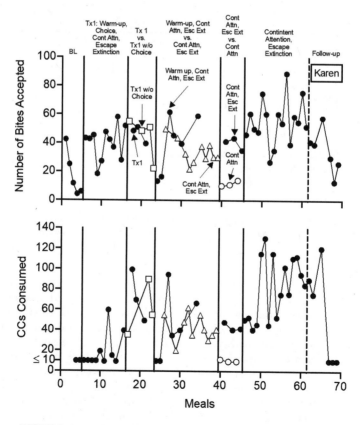

**FIGURE 9.6.** Example of a component analysis from Cooper et al. (1995).

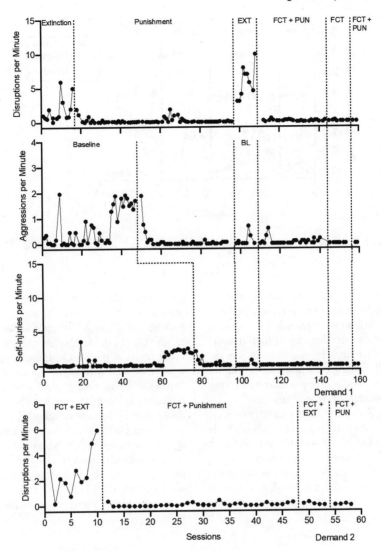

**FIGURE 9.7.** Example of a component analysis from Fisher et al. (1993).

Figure 9.8 shows data for Lana in Experiment 1, in which the researchers used an ABAB design to examine the effects of reinforcement duration. During the A phase, the duration of reinforcement was equal (30 seconds) for mands and problem behavior. Lana accessed reinforcement primarily by engaging in problem behavior when mands and problem behavior produced equal durations of reinforcement. During the B phase, the duration of reinforcement was 30 seconds for mands and 10 seconds for problem behavior. Rates of mands increased and rates of problem behavior decreased, showing that Lana accessed the longer duration of reinforcement by engaging in mands. Athens

and Vollmer replicated the effect in subsequent A and B phases. Figure 9.9 shows data for Clark in Experiment 4, in which the researchers used an ABAB design to examine the effects of reinforcement duration, quality, and delay. During the A phase, mands and problem behavior produced 30 seconds of high-quality reinforcement immediately after the behavior. Clark accessed reinforcement primarily by engaging in problem behavior when mands and problem behavior produced an equal duration of, quality of, and delay to reinforcement. During the B phase, mands produced 30 seconds of high-quality reinforcement immediately, and problem behavior produced 5 seconds of low-qual-

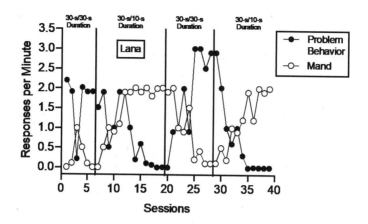

**FIGURE 9.8.** Example of a parametric analysis from Experiment 1 of Athens and Vollmer (2010).

ity reinforcement 10 seconds after the occurrence of problem behavior. Rates of mands increased and rates of problem behavior decreased, showing that Clark accessed the longer duration of high-quality, immediate reinforcement by engaging in mands. In their overall findings, Athens and Vollmer showed that they could bias responding by altering the various parameters of reinforcement.

Kadey, Piazza, Rivas, and Zeleny (2013) provided another example of a parametric analysis in which they evaluated the effects of food texture on *mouth clean,* a product measure of swallowing. Figure 9.10 (top) depicts the percentage of mouth clean during presentation of chopped food, wet ground food, and pureed food. Although levels of mouth clean were highest when the feeder presented the smoothest texture (pureed), mouth clean did not increase to clinically acceptable levels. Kadey et al. identified nine foods that were associated with lower levels of mouth clean and seven foods that were associated with higher levels of it during the texture analysis. Kadey et al. conducted a second texture assessment (Figure 9.10, bottom) in which they compared levels of mouth clean for pureed and Magic Bullet (which is smoother than pureed) textures with the nine foods associated with lower levels of mouth clean in the first texture assessment. The highest levels of mouth clean were associated with the Magic Bullet texture. This parametric analysis allowed the researchers to identify

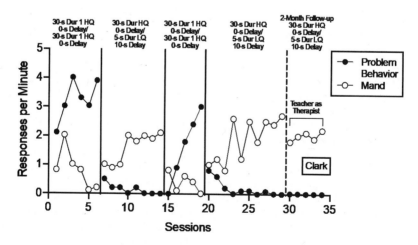

**FIGURE 9.9.** Example of a parametric analysis from Experiment 4 of Athens and Vollmer (2010).

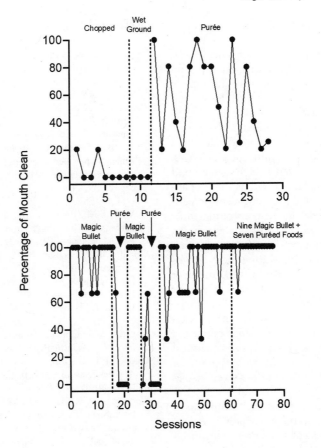

**FIGURE 9.10.** Example of a parametric analysis from Kadey, Piazza, Rivas, and Zeleny (2013).

the level of the independent variable—the pureed texture for seven foods and the Magic Bullet texture for nine foods—that produced the targeted change in the dependent variable (i.e., increases in mouth clean).

As a final example, Carr, Bailey, Ecott, Lucker, and Weil (1998) conducted a parametric analysis to examine the effects of various magnitudes of noncontingent reinforcement (NCR). Figure 9.11 displays the number of chips placed in a cylinder per minute for one participant. During baseline, responses produced preferred edibles on a variable-ratio (VR) 3 or 5 schedule. Next, the researchers delivered high, medium, and low magnitudes of noncontingent edibles, and responses produced no differential consequence. Results suggested that differing magnitudes of NCR produced differential suppression of the response, with the highest magnitudes associated with the lowest levels of responding.

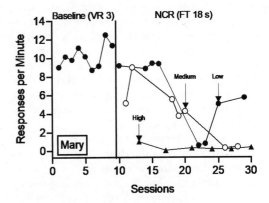

**FIGURE 9.11.** Example of a parametric analysis from Carr, Bailey, Ecott, Lucker, and Weil (1998).

## SUMMARY

The current chapter has provided a general overview of the relevance of single-case experimental designs in applied behavior analysis. This type of experimental arrangement allows for the systematic evaluation of variables to ensure both clinically and socially relevant changes in the behavior of interest at the level of the individual and across a range of socially significant challenges. More specifically, one design or a combination of designs may counterbalance the limitations of another design. The flexibility of single-case experimental designs is ideal for demonstrating functional relations. As such, behavior analysts should incorporate single-case experimental designs into their everyday practice. Integrating these designs into routine clinical practice allows the behavior analyst to provide his or her clients, patients, or students with the highest quality of care. Single-case experimental designs provide information about the efficacy of intervention and provide the clinician with feedback about his or her clinical skills.

A behavior analyst must consider several issues when using single-case experimental designs. Developing clearly defined operational definitions of target behavior and selecting an appropriate measurement system are essential first steps. Historically, visual inspection of data has been the primary way to analyze data from single-case experimental designs; however, critics have questioned the reliability of visual inspection. Research has shown that appropriate training can improve the accuracy and reliability of visual inspection across observers. Statistical analysis may become a viable alternative or complement to visual inspection in the future as these methods improve. However, additional work is needed to establish the role of statistical analysis in interpretation of single-case data. Until then, visual inspection remains the primary means of analysis.

Single-case experimental designs are ideal methods for analyzing the effects of manipulations on responding at the individual level. Thus these design strategies allow the clinician to evaluate whether an intervention has produced a meaningful behavior change. Overall, the flexibility of single-case experimental designs can aid researchers and clinicians in identifying the most effective means for producing socially meaningful changes in behavior.

## REFERENCES

Athens, E. S., & Vollmer, T. R. (2010). An investigation of differential reinforcement of alternative behavior without extinction. *Journal of Applied Behavior Analysis, 43,* 569–589.

Baer, D. M., Wolf, M. M., & Risley, T. R. (1968). Some current dimensions of applied behavior analysis. *Journal of Applied Behavior Analysis, 1,* 91–97.

Byiers, B. J., Reichle, J., & Symons, F. J. (2012). Single-subject experimental design for evidence-based practice. *American Journal of Speech and Language Pathology, 21,* 397–414.

Carr, J. E., Bailey, J. S., Ecott, C. L., Lucker, K. D., & Weil, T. M. (1998). On the effects of non-contingent delivery of differing magnitudes of reinforcement. *Journal of Applied Behavior Analysis, 31,* 313–321.

Codding, R. S., & Lane, K. L. (2015). A spotlight on treatment intensity: An important and often overlooked component of intervention inquiry. *Journal of Behavioral Education, 24,* 1–10.

Cohen, L. L., Feinstein, A., Masuda, A., & Vowles, K. E. (2014). Single-case research design in pediatric psychology: Considerations regarding data analysis. *Journal of Pediatric Psychology, 39,* 124–137.

Cooper, J. O., Heron, T. E., & Heward, W. L. (2007). *Applied behavior analysis* (2nd ed.) Upper Saddle River, NJ: Pearson/Merrill-Prentice Hall.

Cooper, L. L., Wacker, D. P., McComas, J. J., Brown, K., Peck, S. M., Richman, D., et al. (1995). Use of component analyses to identify active variables in treatment packages for children with feeding disorders. *Journal of Applied Behavior Analysis, 28,* 139–153.

Craig, A. R., & Fisher, W. W. (2019). Randomization tests as alternative analysis methods for behavior-analytic data. *Journal of the Experimental Analysis of Behavior, 111,* 309–328.

DeRosa, N. M., Roane, H. S., Bishop, J. R., & Silkowski, E. L. (2016). The combined effects of noncontingent reinforcement and punishment on the reduction of rumination. *Journal of Applied Behavior Analysis, 49,* 680–685.

Edgington, E. S. (1996). Randomized single-subject experimental designs. *Behaviour Research and Therapy, 34,* 567–574.

Fisher, W. W., Kelley, M. E., & Lomas, J. E. (2003). Visual aids and structured criteria for improving visual inspection and interpretation of single-case designs. *Journal of Applied Behavior Analysis, 36,* 387–406.

Fisher, W. W., & Lerman, D. C. (2014). It has been said that, "There are three degrees of falsehoods: Lies, damn lies, and statistics." *Journal of School Psychology, 52,* 243–248.

Fisher, W. W., Piazza, C. C., Cataldo, M. F., Harrell, R., Jefferson, G., & Conner, R. (1993). Functional communication training with and without extinction and punishment. *Journal of Applied Behavior Analysis, 26,* 23–36.

Hagopian, L. P., Fisher, W. W., Thompson, R. H., Owen-DeSchryver, J., Iwata, B. A., & Wacker, D. P. (1997). Toward the development of structured criteria for interpretation of functional analysis data. *Journal of Applied Behavior Analysis, 30,* 313–326.

Hagopian, L. P., Rooker, G. W., Jessel, J., & DeLeon, I. G. (2013). Initial functional analysis outcomes and modifications in pursuit of differentiation: A summary of 176 inpatient cases. *Journal of Applied Behavior Analysis, 46,* 88–100.

Hanley, G. P., Iwata, B. A., & McCord, B. E. (2003). Functional analysis of problem behavior: A review. *Journal of Applied Behavior Analysis, 36,* 147–185.

Horner, R. H., Carr, E. G., Halle, J., McGee, G., Odom, S., & Wolery, M. (2005). Research to identify evidence-base practice in special education. *Exceptional Children, 71,* 165–179.

Horner, R. H., & Kratochwill, T. R. (2012). Synthesizing single-case research to identify evidence-based practices: Some brief reflections. *Journal of Behavioral Education, 21,* 266–272.

Kadey, H. J., Piazza, C. C., Rivas, K. M., & Zeleny, J. (2013). An evaluation of texture manipulations to increase swallowing. *Journal of Applied Behavior Analysis, 46,* 539–543.

Kahng, S. W., Chung, K. M., Gutshall, K., Pitts, S. C., Kao, J., & Girolami, K. (2010). Consistent visual analysis of intra-subject data. *Journal of Applied Behavior Analysis, 43,* 35–45.

Kahng, S., Ingvarsson, E. T., Quigg, A. M., Seckinger, K. E., & Teichman, H. M. (2011). Defining and measuring behavior. In W. W. Fisher, C. C. Piazza, & H. S. Roane (Eds.), *Handbook of applied behavior analysis* (pp. 113–131). New York: Guilford Press.

Kazdin, A. E. (2011). *Single-case research design.* New York: Oxford University Press.

Kazdin, A. E. (2016). Single-case experimental designs. In A. E. Kazdin (Ed.), *Methodological issues and strategies in clinical research* (pp. 459–483). Washington, DC: American Psychological Association.

Kratochwill, T. R., Hitchcock, J., Horner, R. H., Levin, J. R., Odom, S. L., Rindskopf, D. M., et al. (2010). Single-case designs technical documentation. Retrieved from *https://files.eric.ed.gov/fulltext/ED510743.pdf.*

Lang, R., O'Reilly, M., Machalicek, W., Lancioni, G., Rispoli, M., & Chan, J. (2008). A preliminary comparison of functional analysis results when conducted in contrived versus natural settings. *Journal of Applied Behavior Analysis, 41,* 441–445.

O'Grady, A. C., Reeve, S. A., Reeve, K. F., Vladescu, J. C., & Lake, C. M. (2018). Evaluation of computer-based training to teach adults visual analysis skills of baseline-treatment graphs. *Behavior Analysis in Practice, 11,* 254–266.

Pustejovsky, J. E., & Ferron, J. M. (2017). Research synthesis and meta-analysis of single-case designs. In J. M. Kauffman, D. P. Hallahan, & P. C. Pullen (Eds.), *Handbook of special education* (2nd ed., pp. 168–186). New York: Routledge.

Roane, H. S., Fisher, W. W., Kelley, M. E., Mevers, J. L., & Bouxsein, K. J. (2013). Using modified visual-inspection criteria to interpret functional analysis outcomes. *Journal of Applied Behavior Analysis, 46,* 130–146.

Roane, H. S., Ringdahl, J. E., Kelley, M. E., & Glover, A. C. (2011). Single-case experimental designs. In W. W. Fisher, C. C. Piazza, & H. S. Roane (Eds.), *Handbook of applied behavior analysis* (pp. 132–147). New York: Guilford Press.

Shadish, W. R., Hedges, L. V., & Pustejovsky, J. E. (2014). Analysis and meta-analysis of single-case designs with a standardized mean difference statistic: A primer and applications. *Journal of School Psychology, 52,* 15–39.

Shadish, W. R., Zuur, A. F., & Sullivan, K. J. (2014). Using generalized additive (mixed) models to analyze single case designs. *Journal of School Psychology, 52,* 41–70.

Stewart, K. K., Carr, J. E., Brandt, C. W., & McHenry, M. M. (2007). An evaluation of the conservative dual-criterion method for teaching university students to visually inspect AB-design graphs. *Journal of Applied Behavior Analysis, 40,* 713–718.

Ward-Horner, J., & Sturmey, P. (2010). Component analyses using single-subject experimental designs: A review. *Journal of Applied Behavior Analysis, 43,* 685–705.

Wilder, D. A., Atwell, J., & Wine, B. (2006). The effects of varying levels of treatment integrity on child compliance during treatment with a three-step prompting procedure. *Journal of Applied Behavior Analysis, 39,* 369–373.

Wolfe, K., & Slocum, T. A. (2015). A comparison of two approaches to training visual analysis of AB graphs. *Journal of Applied Behavior Analysis, 48,* 472–477.

# PART IV
# BEHAVIORAL ASSESSMENT

In the field of applied behavior analysis, contributions to the assessment of maladaptive behavior have particular societal relevance. Indeed, developments in the functional assessment of maladaptive behavior have resulted in this approach's becoming the recognized standard of care for identifying the determinants of maladaptive behavior. Likewise, behavior-analytic procedures in academic skill development and reinforcer identification have led to countless clinical gains across a range of populations. Part IV of this handbook addresses historical precedents and recent developments in several areas of behavioral assessment.

In Chapter 10, Saini, Retzlaff, Roane, and Piazza have contributed an updated review in the areas of stimulus preference assessment and reinforcer identification. This chapter provides an overview of the basic preference assessment types (e.g., paired-choice assessment, multiple-stimulus assessment) and delves into those factors that might influence preference identification. New to this edition of this chapter is a discussion of procedures that can be used to establish novel reinforcer relations and preference, as well as an overview of research related to reinforcer identification since the publication of the first edition.

In applied behavior analysis, the assessment of a target behavior typically proceeds in one of two manners. Indirect assessments are common in applied settings, and involve data collection across multiple informants through a combination of rating scales, interviews, and the like. By contrast, direct assessments include procedures in which a behavior analyst conducts naturalistic or contrived observations of the client in a setting of interest while recording data on the occurrence of the behavior of interest, among other variables. In both indirect and direct assessments, there have been several new developments since the first edition of this handbook appeared. In Chapter 11, Gadaire, Kelley, and LaRue highlight some of the advances made in indirect assessments, particularly related to new developments in functional-analytic rating scales and structured interviews. Likewise, Thompson and Borrero (Chapter 12) detail some of the advances in direct assessments and direct observation, including updates on descriptive and probability analyses, as well as new recommendations and directions of future research.

Finally, the analogue functional analysis is considered the best practice in the assessment of target behaviors within the field. Thus Part IV concludes with a contribution from Saini, Fisher, Betz, and Piazza on the history and methods of this approach. Though the history of the terminology and core experimental procedures of analogue functional analysis remain unchanged from the first edition of this chapter, the current chapter delves into recent modifications to this methodology. In particular, the current edition provides additional detail on new functional-analytic test conditions, updated procedures for visual inspection, and procedural/design modifications that facilitate the identification of behavior functions.

# CHAPTER 10

# Identifying and Enhancing the Effectiveness of Positive Reinforcement

Valdeep Saini, Billie Retzlaff, Henry S. Roane, and Cathleen C. Piazza

Behavior analysts frequently use positive reinforcement as a key component in programs for increasing appropriate behavior. A common misconception in the lay population is that certain stimuli (e.g., activities, items, food) function as positive reinforcement simply because of the topography of the stimulus. For example, we might hear a parent say, "I used M&Ms as positive reinforcement for my child during potty training." The astute behavior analyst recognizes the potential fallacy in this statement, because our field defines positive reinforcement by its effect on behavior, not by the topographical characteristics of the stimulus. Specifically, we define *positive reinforcement* as delivery of a stimulus contingent on a response that increases the future likelihood of that response (Cooper, Heron, & Heward, 2007). To put this another way, a stimulus presented following a response is a positive reinforcer if the probability of the response increases in the future. A stimulus presented following a response is a not a positive reinforcer if the probability of the response does not increase in the future. Given that we cannot identify positive reinforcement by the topography of a stimulus, an important challenge for the behavior analyst is to identify stimuli that will function as positive reinforcement.

## METHODS TO IDENTIFY PREFERRED STIMULI

Before 1985, researchers either assessed stimulus preference in the absence of assessment of the reinforcing efficacy of the preferred stimuli, or selected potential positive reinforcers somewhat arbitrarily, without using a method to predict whether the stimuli would function as reinforcement. Pace, Ivancic, Edwards, Iwata, and Page (1985) described a procedure to assess the preferences of individuals with intellectual developmental disorder, and tested the extent to which the preferred stimuli functioned as reinforcement. Since the publication of the Pace et al. study, researchers have evaluated many methods for identifying preferred stimuli and have tested whether these assessments predict the efficacy of preferred stimuli as positive reinforcement.

### Single-Stimulus Preference Assessment

Pace et al. (1985) used a single-stimulus preference assessment to assess the preferences of six individuals with intellectual developmental disorder. The therapist presented 16 stimuli, one at a time. Observers scored approach responses (e.g., reaches) as the measure of preference. If the participant approached the stimulus within 5 seconds of presentation, the therapist gave the stimulus to the participant for 5 seconds. If the participant did not approach the stimulus within 5 seconds of presentation, the therapist prompted the participant to touch the stimulus. If the participant did not touch the stimulus within 5 seconds of the prompt, the therapist ended that trial and presented the next stimulus. Pace et al. labeled stimuli approached on at least 80% of presentations *preferred*, and stimuli approached on 50% or less of presentations *nonpreferred*.

Next, Pace et al. (1985) assessed whether assessed stimuli functioned as reinforcement. During baseline, a simple, free-operant response, such as a hand raise, produced no differential consequence. The therapist then delivered either a preferred or a nonpreferred stimulus identified during the preference assessment following the free-operant response. Results indicated that contingent presentation of preferred stimuli increased responding, compared to baseline and presentation of nonpreferred stimuli. That is, stimuli approached more frequently in the preference assessment functioned as reinforcement more often than stimuli approached less frequently.

Although the Pace et al. (1985) single-stimulus preference assessment was one of the first objective methods of identifying preferred stimuli, it has limitations. The most notable is that participants may approach all or most stimuli (Fisher et al., 1992; Mazaleski, Iwata, Vollmer, Zarcone, & Smith, 1993). For example, two of the three participants in Mazaleski et al. (1993) approached most

presented stimuli, raising the question of whether some stimuli identified as highly preferred may not function as effective reinforcers (Paclawskyj & Vollmer, 1995). That is, the single-stimulus assessment may produce *false positives*, or stimuli that appear highly preferred but do not function as reinforcement.

## Paired-Choice Preference Assessment

Fisher et al. (1992) evaluated a variation of the Pace et al. (1985) preference assessment to address its limitations. They used a paired-choice procedure in which they presented stimuli in pairs and prompted each participant, "Pick one." They presented 16 stimuli and paired each stimulus once with every other stimulus. Participant approaches toward one of the two stimuli produced access to that stimulus for approximately 5 seconds. The therapist blocked simultaneous approaches toward both stimuli, removed the stimulus pair, and re-presented it if 5 seconds elapsed with no response. The therapist prompted the participant to sample each stimulus for 5 seconds, re-presented the pair, and then presented the next pair if another 5 seconds elapsed without a response. The choice assessment identified a hierarchy of preferences for participants (see Figure 10.1 for an example).

Fisher et al. (1992) compared the results of the paired-choice assessment with the results of the Pace et al. (1985) single-stimulus assessment. Results showed that both assessments identified certain items as high-preference stimuli. The single-stimulus assessment identified several stimuli as

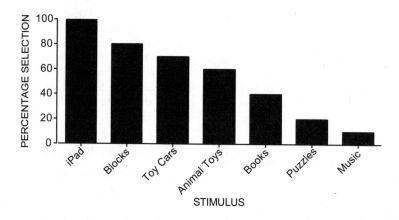

**FIGURE 10.1.** Example of a hierarchy of preferences for one individual, based on the results of a paired-choice preference assessment with the names of the presented stimuli on the *x*-axis and the percentage selection on the *y*-axis.

preferred that the paired-choice assessment did not, as in the findings of Mazaleski et al. (1993). Next, Fisher et al. used a concurrent-operants arrangement to compare the reinforcing effectiveness of stimuli identified as highly preferred on both assessments with that of stimuli identified as highly preferred on the single-stimulus assessment only. Results showed that the stimuli identified as highly preferred on both assessments maintained greater levels of responding than the stimulus identified as highly preferred only on the single-stimulus assessment. Thus the paired-choice assessment produced greater differentiation among stimuli and better predicted which stimuli would function as reinforcers when evaluated in a concurrent-operants arrangement. Researchers have modified the Fisher et al. paired-choice assessment for individuals with visual impairments (Paclawskyj & Vollmer, 1995) and individuals with attention-deficit/hyperactivity disorder (ADHD) (Northup, Fusilier, Swanson, Roane, & Borrero, 1997).

One limitation of the Fisher et al. (1992) paired-choice preference assessment is its administration time (Roane, Vollmer, Ringdahl, & Marcus, 1998; Windsor, Piché, & Lock, 1994). A long administration time may preclude frequent updates of preferences, particularly in settings where participants have competing schedules (e.g., schools) or limited visitation times (e.g., clinics). One way to address this limitation is to decrease the number of presented stimuli. Fisher et al. evaluated 16 stimuli or 120 paired presentations that required about 1 hour to administer, or about 30 seconds per trial. Reducing the number of stimuli to 7, for example, would reduce the number of trials to 21 and the assessment duration to a little over 10 minutes. An alternative method of increasing the efficiency of paired-choice preference assessments is to evaluate a few categories of stimuli (e.g., sweet foods, salty foods) rather than individual stimuli, and to use different stimuli in that category as potential reinforcers (e.g., salty foods; Ciccone, Graff, & Ahearn, 2015).

A second limitation is that presentation and removal of stimuli are inherent components of the paired-choice assessment (Kang et al., 2011; Tung, Donaldson, & Kahng, 2017; Vollmer, Ringdahl, Roane, & Marcus, 1997), which may occasion problem behavior when the therapist withdraws a stimulus. This problem may be more likely in individuals with problem behavior reinforced by access to tangible items.

## Multiple-Stimulus Assessment

Windsor et al. (1994) presented multiple stimuli simultaneously to participants with intellectual developmental disorder, to determine their relative preferences for those stimuli. The therapist presented six stimuli simultaneously to a participant over a series of five sessions, each containing 10 trials. Each trial began with a therapist asking, "Which one do you want?" as he or she presented the stimuli. The therapist waited 20 seconds for participants to emit a selection response (i.e., attempting to grasp an item). The therapist provided the participant brief access to the stimulus if the participant selected one. The trial ended after the participant accessed the stimulus, or after the participant did not respond in 20 seconds. Windsor et al. compared the multiple-stimulus assessment with an extended version of the paired-choice assessment (Fisher et al., 1992). The multiple-stimulus assessment required less time to complete than the extended version of the paired-choice assessment did, but it produced less consistent results across administrations. The paired-choice assessment generally produced a more differentiated preference hierarchy for the assessed stimuli.

## Multiple-Stimulus-without-Replacement Assessment

DeLeon and Iwata (1996) evaluated an extension of the Windsor et al. (1994) procedure, called the *multiple-stimulus-without-replacement* assessment. One limitation of the Windsor et al. procedure was that some participants never selected certain stimuli, perhaps because more highly preferred stimuli were available constantly. DeLeon and Iwata (1996) addressed this limitation by presenting the entire array of stimuli on the first trial and removing selected stimuli on each subsequent trial, resulting in the availability of stimuli the participant had not selected yet on each subsequent trial. Thus this procedure provided opportunities for participants to choose among less preferred alternatives, like the paired-stimulus assessment.

DeLeon and Iwata (1996) compared the multiple-stimulus-without-replacement assessment to paired-choice and multiple-stimulus assessments along three dimensions: (1) rank order of preferred stimuli, (2) time required for administration, and (3) number of potential reinforcers identified. The three assessments identified the same stimulus as the most preferred for four of seven participants.

The researchers found high correlations between the most preferred stimuli in each assessment for the remaining three participants. The multiple-stimulus-with-replacement assessment required the least amount of administration time (M = 16.5 minutes), followed by the multiple-stimulus-without-replacement assessment (M = 21.8 minutes) and the paired-choice assessment (M = 53.3 minutes). Finally, participants selected fewer items in the multiple-stimulus-with-replacement assessment, whereas the multiple-stimulus-without replacement and paired-choice assessments produced better differentiation among the assessed stimuli. Researchers also have used the multiple-stimulus-without-replacement assessment successfully for children in general education classrooms (Daly et al., 2009).

One limitation of both the multiple-stimulus-with-replacement and the multiple-stimulus-without-replacement assessments is that each one requires the participant to discriminate and select from a relatively large array of stimuli. This limits the numbers of stimuli that these assessments can evaluate, because the complexity of the task increases as the array size increases.

## Free-Operant Assessment

Roane et al. (1998) developed a *free-operant* preference assessment, in which participants had continuous access to a stimulus array for 5 minutes. The participants could interact with any stimulus throughout the assessment, because all stimuli remained available. Roane et al. compared the results of the free-operant preference assessment to the Fisher et al. (1992) paired-choice assessment along two dimensions: (1) administration length and (2) occurrence of problem behavior. Results showed that the mean length of the free-operant assessment was shorter than that of the paired-choice assessment (5 minutes vs. 21.7 minutes). Moreover, 85% of the participants displayed significantly higher levels of problem behavior during the paired-choice assessment. Similarly, Kang et al. (2010) showed that the free-operant assessment was associated with less problem behavior than was the multiple-stimulus-without replacement assessment.

One limitation of the free-operant assessment is that it may not produce a preference hierarchy if the participant allocates his or her time to a single stimulus exclusively. A second limitation is that it can be associated with higher levels of problem behavior in individuals who display attention-reinforced problem behavior (Kang et al., 2011).

## Response Restriction

Although single-stimulus, paired-choice, multiple-stimulus-without-replacement, and free-operant assessments appear effective for reinforcement identification, Hanley, Iwata, Lindberg, and Conners (2003) noted that these procedures are associated with limited access to stimuli, and participants often demonstrate exclusive preferences for a few stimuli. Hanley et al. hypothesized that a response restriction method combining free-operant and trial-based assessment procedures might address these limitations. During the response restriction assessment, the therapist provided the participant with a stimulus array and then restricted individual stimuli based on participant interaction with these stimuli. Hanley et al. based their rules for restricting stimuli on the participant's level of interaction with the target stimulus relative to other stimuli. Results showed that the response restriction assessment produced a high degree of consistency for highly ranked items. A comparison of this assessment with an extended free-operant assessment showed that the response restriction assessment produced more differentiated preference and more complete information about engagement across stimuli. The two major limitations of the response restriction assessment are its multiple complex rules for determining when to restrict stimuli, and its lengthy administration time (18 sessions of 5 minutes each to evaluate seven stimuli, considerably longer than most other preference assessments).

## Duration Assessment

DeLeon, Iwata, Conners, and Wallace (1999) suggested that duration of engagement might be an alternative to approach responses as a measure of preference, and described a procedure in which they presented stimuli singly for 2 minutes to adults who engaged in severe problem behavior. They compared results of the duration-based assessment to those of a multiple-stimulus-without-replacement assessment. The duration-based assessment, which measured stimulus engagement, produced a more differentiated preference hierarchy than the multiple-stimulus-without-replacement assessment.

Like DeLeon et al. (1999), Hagopian, Rush, Lewin, and Long (2001) presented stimuli singly and measured participants' level of engagement with each stimulus. Subsequent reinforcement assessments showed that the stimuli identified as highly preferred based on duration of engagement functioned as effective reinforcers. In addition, the researchers compared the results of the duration assessment with those of a paired-choice assessment. Results of the comparison suggested that the duration assessment took less time to administer than the paired-choice assessment, but produced less stable preference rankings across administrations.

## Vocal Report

Vocal report or self-nomination is most appropriate for individuals who can identify preferred stimuli vocally. Many studies have incorporated self-nomination for identifying preferences. For example, Clements and McKee (1968) used a one-page brochure (i.e., the menu of reinforcing events) to identify preferred work activities for 16 inmates. Results showed increases in the amount of daily work completed by the inmates when their work produced access to activities selected on the menu.

Although researchers have used surveys to identify highly preferred stimuli for elementary school students (Fantuzzo, Rohrbeck, Hightower, & Work, 1991) and children (Tourigny Dewhurst & Cautela, 1980) and adults (Fox & DeShaw, 1993) with intellectual developmental disorder, whether the survey results identified stimuli that functioned as reinforcement is not clear. Current research has indicated that self-nominations of preference may be limited in several ways. First, self-nomination of preference may not match observed preferences. For example, Northup, George, Jones, Broussard, and Vollmer (1996) used a survey of common classroom reinforcers to identify differential preferences for four children diagnosed with ADHD and showed that the survey effectively identified differential preferences across participants. However, the results of the survey did not match the results of systematic preference assessments. Thus self-nomination of preferences may not identify preferred stimuli accurately in some cases. In addition, self-nomination may be appropriate only for individuals who possess sufficient expressive and receptive language skills to indicate their preferences vocally (Pace et al., 1985; Rotatori, Fox, & Switzky, 1979; Wehman, 1976).

## Caregiver Nomination

Some researchers have asked caregivers (e.g., staff members, parents) to identify the preferred stimuli of individuals who cannot express their own preferences. In an early comparison of caregiver opinion and observed individual preferences, Favell and Cannon (1976) showed that caregivers did not predict preferences reliably. Other researchers have replicated these findings with different caregivers, such as teachers, and different populations of participants, such as students (Fantuzzo et al., 1991; Green et al., 1988; Parsons & Reid, 1990; Windsor et al., 1994).

Although previous research has shown that caregiver report has not been a consistently effective method of identifying preferences for some individuals, using caregiver input seems like a logical method of identifying preferred stimuli, particularly for individuals who cannot self-report their preferences. To that end, Fisher, Piazza, Bowman, and Amari (1996) developed the Reinforcer Assessment for Individuals with Disabilities (RAISD), a structured interview that prompts caregivers to generate a list of potential reinforcers from the auditory, edible, olfactory, social, tactile, and visual domains. In the Fisher et al. study, caregivers generated a list of potentially preferred stimuli and rank-ordered those stimuli from most to least preferred based on their predictions of child preference. Caregivers also ranked predicted child preferences for a standard list of stimuli that Pace et al. (1985) used. Fisher et al. (1996) conducted paired-choice assessments with caregiver-generated stimuli and with standard stimuli. Caregivers made slightly better predictions of child preference with the stimuli identified via the RAISD than with the standard stimuli. In addition, the most preferred stimuli identified via the RAISD functioned as more effective reinforcers than the most preferred standard stimuli. These results suggest that structured caregiver input can be a useful adjunct to a systematic-choice preference assessment. Cote, Thompson, Hanley, and McKerchar (2007) replicated and extended the Fisher et al. (1996) results with teachers and young children in an early intervention setting. Cote et al. showed that incorporating teacher nomination with a direct assessment, such as the paired-choice assessment, could identify more effective reinforcers for young children in classrooms.

## Pictorial Representations

Pictures are an alternative method of identifying preferred stimuli for individuals who lack a vocal response (Conyers et al., 2002; Daley, 1969; Northup et al., 1996). Daley (1969) presented a picture menu of activities to five children with intellectual developmental disorder. The children showed differential preferences for the pictorially depicted activities. Northup et al. (1996) evaluated the accuracy of a reinforcer survey, a verbal paired-choice questionnaire, and a pictorial paired-choice assessment for preference identification. The verbal and pictorial paired-choice assessments identified high- and low-preference categories for three of the four participants. By contrast, the survey inaccurately identified preferences. One limitation of pictorial representation is that a participant must be able to discriminate that the pictures represent items or activities. For example, Higbee, Carr, and Harrison (1999) found that the picture assessment did not consistently identify stimuli that functioned as reinforcement, and suggested that some individuals may require discrimination training before conducting a pictorial preference assessment.

## Concurrent Chains

Most of the preference assessment procedures described earlier have focused on identification of preferred stimuli that behavior analysts could use as reinforcement in training programs. Researchers also have used preference assessments to measure participants' preferences for positive-reinforcement treatments (Hanley, Piazza, Fisher, Contrucci, & Maglieri, 1997), schedules of reinforcement (Luczynski & Hanley, 2009, 2010, 2014), motivational systems (Heal & Hanley, 2007), punishment and extinction components of interventions (Giles, St. Peter, Pence, & Gibson, 2012; Hanley, Piazza, Fisher, & Maglieri, 2005), and preferences for choice and no-choice arrangements (Fisher, Thompson, Piazza, Crosland, & Gotjen, 1997; Tiger, Hanley, & Hernandez, 2006), among others. For example, Hanley et al. (1997) described a concurrent-chains procedure for evaluating participant preferences for functional-communication training, noncontingent reinforcement, and extinction as treatments for problem behavior. The concurrent-chains procedure consisted of pairing each treatment with a colored card that participants selected to enter a room in which they received their chosen treatment. The results of Hanley et al. showed that the concurrent-chains procedure provided a sensitive measure of participant preferences for treatments for problem behavior.

## Group Arrangement

Most preference assessment studies have focused on shortening administration time for individual participants. By contrast, Layer, Hanley, Heal, and Tiger (2008) assessed the accuracy of preference assessment for multiple children simultaneously. First, the researchers identified a preference hierarchy for each child individually. Next, the researchers evaluated the preferences of three children simultaneously. During the group assessment, each child privately selected a colored card that the experimenters had paired previously with specific food reinforcement. After each child selected a colored card, the researcher placed the three cards in a box. Next, the researcher drew one card from the box, and each child in the group received the food that was associated with that card. Comparisons of individual and group assessment data showed that the two assessments produced similar preference rankings, but that the group assessment identified the preferred stimuli more efficiently. Similarly, Radley, Dart, Battaglia, and Ford (2019) conducted group preference assessments in a classroom of 19 students, with all students responding simultaneously to a prompt (administered via smartphone app) to identify a preferred stimulus. They found that the group procedure was a valid and rapid method of assessing preference within a classroom setting.

Hanley, Cammilleri, Tiger, and Ingvarsson (2007) showed that behavior analysts could use momentary time sampling to assess the activity preferences of 20 children in a preschool classroom. They observed less than a 10% error rate when they evaluated preferences with a 120-second momentary-time-sampling interval. Subsequent analyses showed that observers preferred a 90-second interval relative to other intervals, and that this interval duration accurately identified activity preferences for a classroom of children.

## METHODS FOR EVALUATING REINFORCEMENT EFFECTS

### Correlation between Preference and Reinforcement Efficacy

Researchers have evaluated whether the effectiveness of reinforcement varies positively with the degree of preference (i.e., whether relative preferences demonstrated in preference assessments predict relative reinforcer effectiveness). Piazza, Fisher, Hagopian, Bowman, and Toole (1996) conducted preference assessments with four individuals with severe behavior problems to identify high-, medium-, and low-preference stimuli. Subsequent concurrent-operants reinforcement assessments showed that the results of the preference assessment predicted the reinforcing efficacy of the high-, medium-, and low-preference stimuli. However, DeLeon, Iwata, and Roscoe (1997) and Taravella, Lerman, Contrucci, and Roane (2000) showed that lower-ranked stimuli may function as reinforcement under some circumstances. Graff and Larsen (2011) demonstrated that the reinforcing efficacy of preferred stimuli may be a product of the stimuli used in a preference assessment, independent of the preference hierarchy that is subsequently generated.

Lee, Yu, Martin, and Martin (2010) took a slightly different approach than Piazza et al. (1996) to examine the correspondence between preference and reinforcement effects. Lee et al. identified stimuli that maintained a range of response rates (i.e., high to low) during a reinforcer assessment. Next, they conducted stimulus preference assessments to determine the participants' preferences for those identified reinforcers. They found almost perfect correspondence between the preference and reinforcer assessments for one participant, and partial correspondence for the other participant.

## Simple versus Complex Responses

Most researchers have used simple, free-operant responses (e.g., hand raise, in-chair behavior) to assess the effectiveness of stimuli as reinforcement (e.g., DeLeon & Iwata, 1996; Fisher et al., 1992; Pace et al., 1985; Piazza, Fisher, Hagopian, et al., 1996). Piazza, Fisher, Hagopian, et al. (1996) suggested that the use of a simple, free-operant response during reinforcement assessment has several advantages. The goal of the reinforcement assessment is to evaluate whether the stimulus functions as reinforcement, rather than to teach a specific response. Simple responses are ideal for these types of evaluations, because individuals with varying functional levels can typically discriminate the contingencies rapidly, resulting in a time-efficient assessment. Failure to emit a more complex response during a reinforcement assessment could be due to a skill or a motivational deficit. By contrast, failure to emit a simple response is less likely to be due to a skill deficit. There may be situations, however, in which the use of a more complex response (e.g., on-task behavior) is desirable (Paramore & Higbee, 2005).

## Single versus Concurrent Operants

Fisher et al. (1992) used a concurrent-operants schedule to evaluate the reinforcing efficacy of preferred stimuli. The advantage of a concur-

rent-operants schedule is that the magnitude of responding for each operant is a function of the relative value of each reinforcer, rather than a function of response competition or interference (Catania, 1963; Fisher et al., 1992). The value of reinforcement is a function of its rate, magnitude, and quality, and of the immediacy of delivery and the amount of response effort expended to obtain reinforcement, relative to those of other concurrently available reinforcers (Fisher & Mazur, 1997). Thus the rate of each response is a function of the value of its reinforcer and the value of other concurrently available reinforcers. Assume, for example, that Responses A and B concurrently produce Reinforcers A and B, respectively. Substantially increasing the reinforcement rate for Response A is likely to increase the rate of Response A. The rate of Response B is likely to decrease, even though its reinforcement rate remains unchanged. In most natural environments, multiple sources of reinforcement are available simultaneously, and behavior analysts should assess the value of a given reinforcer relative to other concurrently available reinforcers. Concurrent-operants schedules are ideal for assessing the strength of a reinforcer relative to other available reinforcers.

In some cases, the behavior analyst may want to assess absolute reinforcement effects (e.g., does Stimulus A function as reinforcement for Response A?). For example, Roscoe, Iwata, and Kahng (1999) showed that the most effective reinforcer during a concurrent-operants schedule was the stimulus identified as highly preferred on both single-stimulus and paired-choice assessments. However, stimuli identified as highly preferred only by the single-stimulus assessment functioned as reinforcement during the single-operant schedule. Roscoe et al. suggested that concurrent-schedule procedures are useful for the assessment of relative reinforcement effects (preference for one reinforcer over another), and that single-schedule arrangements may be ideal for assessing the absolute effects of reinforcement.

## Progressive-Ratio Schedules

Roane, Lerman, and Vorndran (2001) used progressive-ratio schedules to assess relative responding for two items identified as similarly preferred during a stimulus preference assessment (Fisher et al., 1992). In a progressive-ratio schedule, the requirement to access reinforcement increases during a single observation (Hodos, 1961). For example, the initial response requirement might be completing one math problem to receive a preferred toy for 20 seconds. After the first reinforcer delivery, the behavior analyst removes the toy and increases the response requirement to two math problems to access 20 seconds of reinforcement. This progression might continue until responding ceases for a specified time. This reinforcer assessment can determine how much work a participant will complete for a given reinforcer before the participant reaches the *breakpoint,* or the schedule requirement at which the participant does not meet the criterion for reinforcement.

Roane et al. (2001) showed that concurrent fixed-ratio (FR) schedules failed to differentiate higher- from lower-preference stimuli, but that increasing the requirements using progressive-ratio schedules enhanced the differences in reinforcer effectiveness. Roane et al. also showed that accurate identification of higher-preference stimuli using progressive-ratio schedules was critical, because the higher-preference stimuli produced greater reductions in problem behavior in reinforcement-based treatments. Moreover, they suggested that the within-session increase in response requirements provided a more expeditious evaluation of relative reinforcer efficacy than did evaluating stimuli across multiple phases of different FR requirements (e.g., DeLeon, Iwata, Goh, & Worsdell, 1997).

Call, Trosclair-Lassare, Findley, Reavis, and Shillingsburg (2012) used progressive-ratio schedules to evaluate the accuracy of the paired-stimulus and multiple-stimulus-without-replacement assessments over time. They administered a paired-choice preference assessment once, followed by daily multiple-stimulus-without-replacement preference assessments and progressive-ratio reinforcer assessments. They evaluated the correspondence between break points and preferences for the two stimulus preference assessments. They found that the highest-ranked stimulus from the paired-choice assessment produced the highest breakpoints for all seven participants, whereas the highest-ranked stimulus from the daily multiple-stimulus-without-replacement assessments corresponded to the highest break point for three of seven participants.

Applied researchers have used progressive-ratio schedules with increased frequency. These applications of progressive-ratio schedules have fallen typically into two categories: bridging basic and applied research, and developing procedures of therapeutic significance (Roane, 2008). Examples of bridging research with progressive-ratio schedules include (1) evaluating the effects of reinforcer assessment under single and concurrent progressive-ratio arrangements (Glover, Roane, Kadey, & Grow, 2008); (2) assessing the relative effects of highly preferred and less preferred stimuli under increasing response requirements (Francisco, Borrero, & Sy, 2008; Penrod, Wallace, & Dyer, 2008); and (3) evaluating whether extra-session access to reinforcement affects rates of academic responding (Roane, Call, & Falcomata, 2005). Applied researchers have used progressive-ratio schedules to evaluate (1) preferences for different staff members in a residential setting (Jerome & Sturmey, 2008); (2) the relative efficacy of different reinforcement durations (Trosclair-Lasserre, Lerman, Call, Addison, & Kodak, 2008); and (3) whether stimuli that function as differentially effective reinforcers under progressive-ratio schedules are also differentially effective when incorporated into reinforcement-based treatments for problem behavior (Roane et al., 2001; Smith, Roane, & Stephenson, 2009). Despite the potential benefits of progressive-ratio schedules, behavior analysts have questioned their utility (e.g., Poling, 2010). Thus researchers should conduct additional studies to evaluate the relative utility of progressive-ratio schedules in applied settings.

## ISSUES RELATED TO SPECIFIC STIMULI AS REINFORCEMENT

### Choice as Reinforcement

Researchers have evaluated whether choice functions as reinforcement. Although initial studies on the effects of choice suggested that the opportunity to make choices functioned as reinforcement (Dunlap et al., 1994; Dyer, Dunlap, & Winterling, 1990; Powell & Nelson, 1997), this work was limited because the choice response produced access to highly preferred stimuli. Thus choice was confounded with the individual's preferences for the chosen items in these investigations.

Fisher et al. (1997) addressed this confound by yoking the choice and no-choice conditions. In Experiment 1, participants could choose from two available preferred stimuli as reinforcement in the choice condition. The researchers yoked the reinforcer they delivered in the no-choice (control) condition to the reinforcer the participant chose in the choice condition. For example, if the participant chose Gummy Bears on the first trial, Skittles on the second trial, and M&Ms on the third trial of the choice condition, then the investigator delivered Gummy Bears on the first trial,

Skittles on the second trial, and M&Ms on the third trial in the no-choice condition. The results of the study showed that higher levels of responding occurred in the choice than in the no-choice condition. In Experiment 2, participants could choose from among lower-preference stimuli in the choice condition or could gain access to higher-preference stimuli in the no-choice condition. Under these arrangements, participants generally allowed the investigator to choose the reinforcer.

One limitation of yoking is that it does not control for momentary fluctuations in preference over time (Tiger et al., 2006). For example, earning Skittles in the previous choice condition may reduce the reinforcing effectiveness of the Skittles in the subsequent no-choice condition. An alternative control for examining the effects of choice is to offer identical options in choice and no-choice conditions (Tiger et al., 2006). For example, Thompson, Fisher, and Contrucci (1998) provided one young boy with autism spectrum disorder (ASD) the opportunity to choose among three identical cups of soda in the choice condition or gain access to one identical cup of soda that the therapist chose in the no-choice condition. Their results showed that the child preferred the choice arrangement. Moreover, the participant continued to select the choice condition even when the reinforcement rate was higher in the no-choice condition. Research has shown that choice functions as reinforcement for children with intellectual developmental disorder and ASD (Fisher et al., 1997; Thompson et al., 1998; Toussaint, Kodak, & Vladescu, 2016), preschool-age children (Ackerlund Brandt, Dozier, Juanico, Laudont, & Mick, 2015; Schmidt, Hanley, & Layer, 2009; Tiger et al., 2006), and individuals with traumatic brain injury (Tasky, Rudrud, Schulze, & Rapp, 2008). Finally, Graff and Libby (1999) showed that participants preferred to make choices during the session as opposed to before it.

## Edible Stimuli

DeLeon, Iwata, and Roscoe (1997) hypothesized that some individuals such as those with intellectual developmental disorder or ASD may be more likely to select food during preference assessments relative to other stimuli. To that end, they assessed whether edible items were more preferred than leisure items and activities during a preference assessment. DeLeon et al. conducted separate multiple-stimulus-without-replacement assessments consisting of food only, leisure items only, and a combination of food and leisure items. The participants displayed a general tendency to select food over nonfood items in the combined preference assessment, even though highly preferred food and highly preferred leisure items from the leisure-only assessment functioned as reinforcement. Similarly, Fahmie, Iwata, and Jann (2015) found that edible items were more preferred than leisure items and resulted in higher rates of responding under maintenance conditions in individuals with and without ASD. Bojak and Carr (1999) found that preference for edible items persisted even after mealtimes. However, adults with dementia did not show a differential preference for edibles over leisure items in a study by Ortega, Iwata, Nogales-González, and Frades (2012). These individuals often have deficits in sensory perception such as smell and taste, which may reduce the value of edible items (Shiffman, 1997). This altered sensory perception might account for Ortega et al.'s finding. Nevertheless, DeLeon et al. suggested that behavior analysts should be cautious about including edibles and leisure items in the same preference assessment.

## Social Stimuli

According to the American Psychiatric Association (2013), deficits in social interaction for children with ASD include but are not limited to a lack of social or emotional reciprocity. This diagnostic feature suggests that social interaction may be less likely to function as reinforcement for children with ASD. However, Nuernberger, Smith, Czapar, and Klatt (2012) demonstrated that children with ASD preferred some social interactions when the researchers presented these stimuli during a multiple-stimulus-without-replacement assessment. These interactions (e.g., chase, tickles, swinging) subsequently functioned as reinforcement. This was true even for interactions that the multiple-stimulus-without-replacement assessment identified as relatively less preferred by the children with ASD. Clay, Samaha, Bloom, Bogoev, and Boyle (2013) found similar results when they evaluated preferences for social interactions and attention in a paired-choice assessment with children with ASD. Morris and Vollmer (2019) found that preferred social interactions could be identified for five children with ASD. These results suggest that social interactions can function as reinforcement for children with ASD, and behavior analysts should include them in preference assessments. This is an important finding, given that one of the primary diagnostic features of ASD is a lack of typical social behavior and social reciprocity.

## Technology as Reinforcement

For some individuals, stimuli that rely on advanced technology (e.g., tablet computers) may have greater preference or reinforcing efficacy than stimuli that do not rely on technology. Hoffmann, Samaha, Bloom, and Boyle (2017) compared the preference and reinforcer efficacy for high- and low-tech stimuli by examining the type and duration of interaction between the two stimuli types. Results suggested that item type and access duration interacted to influence preference and reinforcer efficacy. Participants preferred high-tech items at longer durations of access. However, participants preferred low-tech items at short durations. Moreover, participants engaged in less responding when the high-tech item was provided for short durations and when the low-tech item was provided for long durations. These results suggest that providing longer access to stimuli that rely on technology when arranged during positive reinforcement.

## FACTORS THAT MAY INFLUENCE THE EFFECTIVENESS OF REINFORCEMENT

### Reinforcement Rate, Quality, Delay, and Distribution

Neef and colleagues conducted a series of studies (Mace, Neef, Shade, & Mauro, 1994; Neef, Mace, & Shade, 1993; Neef, Mace, Shea, & Shade, 1992; Neef, Shade, & Miller, 1994) to evaluate how rate, quality, and delay to reinforcement affect responding. Results from these studies suggested that participants preferred schedules of reinforcement associated with higher quality (Neef et al., 1992) and shorter delays to reinforcement (e.g., Neef et al., 1993).

A longer delay to reinforcement will typically reduce the effectiveness of a reinforcer than a shorter delay (Fisher & Mazur, 1997). This is often true even when an individual is given a choice between a delayed larger reinforcer and a smaller but immediate reinforcer (Madden & Bickel, 2010). However, individuals may prefer larger accumulated reinforcement over smaller immediate reinforcement under some circumstances. For example, DeLeon et al. (2014) found that three of four participants preferred accumulating and consuming larger delayed reinforcers (e.g., watch-

ing 5 minutes of a video at the end of a session) over distributed consumption of smaller immediate reinforcers (e.g., watching 30 seconds of the video after each response). These results suggest that accumulated but delayed reinforcement may be as effective as small, immediate reinforcement, and may be even more preferred for some participants and for specific reinforcers (Bukala, Hu, Lee, Ward-Horner, & Fienup, 2015; Fienup, Ahlers, & Pace, 2011). Duration of access to a reinforcer (i.e., accumulated) also may influence preference hierarchies during systematic preference assessments (Steinhilber & Johnson, 2007).

## Stimulus Variation

Stimulus variation is one method that researchers have used to enhance the effectiveness of reinforcement (Bowman, Piazza, Fisher, Hagopian, & Kogan, 1997; Egel, 1980, 1981; Wine & Wilder, 2009). For example, Bowman et al. (1997) found that four of six participants preferred varied versus constant presentation of preferred stimuli; the other two participants preferred constant presentation of preferred stimuli. Wine and Wilder (2009) extended the work of Bowman et al. by examining the effects of varied versus constant reinforcement. Participants could earn access to (1) constant high-preference stimuli; (2) constant medium-preference stimuli; (3) constant low-preference stimuli; or (4) varied stimuli, in which the experimenter randomly selected a high-, medium-, or low-preference stimulus to deliver to the participant on each trial. The greatest increases in work output for both participants occurred in the constant high-preference condition, and the varied-presentation condition resulted in work output comparable to constant delivery of medium-preference stimuli. Moreover, Keyl-Austin, Samaha, Bloom, and Boyle (2012) found that presenting varied medium-preference stimuli produced higher levels and more sustained responding than did presenting those same stimuli singly. However, a single highly preferred stimulus resulted in more total responses and a slower decline in within-session response rate, compared to responding maintained by varied medium-preference stimuli.

## Long-Term Stability of Preferences

Individual preferences for specific stimuli are constantly fluctuating, based on establishing operations and the environmental context in which we deliver them. For example, water may function as reinforcement following consumption of salty pretzels, but may not function as reinforcement in other contexts. Moreover, an individual may prefer candy, and candy may function as reinforcement in most circumstances. The value of candy, however, may wane if an individual has been consuming the same candy every day for a week. Behavior analysts should consider whether preferences change over time and should be reevaluated periodically. Evidence for preference stability across time has been somewhat mixed. For example, the results of several studies have shown that preferences vary over time (e.g., Carr, Nicholson, & Higbee, 2000; Mason, McGee, Farmer-Dougan, & Risley, 1989; Zhou, Iwata, Goff, & Shore, 2001). By, contrast, Hanley, Iwata, and Roscoe (2006) attempted to replicate and extend the literature by evaluating preferences for leisure activities over 3–6 months with 10 adults with intellectual developmental disorder. Unlike previous researchers, Hanley et al. observed relatively stable preferences for 80% of participants. Hanley et al. also showed that naturally occurring changes in establishing operations or conditioning histories disrupted preference stability. Similarly, the results of Kelley, Shillingsburg, and Bowen (2016) were consistent with Hanley et al.'s, in that preferences tended to be relatively stable across time. Subsequent studies have shown that changes in preferences across time does not necessarily affect reinforcer efficacy in practice (Verriden & Roscoe, 2016). DeLeon et al. (2001) showed that when preferences did change over time, behavior analysts could use daily brief preference assessments to monitor and adjust to changes in preferences.

## Satiation versus Deprivation

Limiting access to reinforcement outside training or treatment situations is a commonly recommended strategy to maintain an individual's motivation. Kodak, Lerman, and Call (2007) evaluated whether access to postsession reinforcement influenced responding. Results of the study showed that participants engaged in higher levels of responding when the researchers restricted postsession access to the reinforcer. Hanley, Tiger, Ingvarsson, and Cammilleri (2009) showed that they could alter preschoolers' free-play activity preferences through satiation manipulations. Preschoolers reallocated responding to less preferred but important activities, such as instructional zone, library, and science, when the researchers used a satiation procedure with highly preferred activities. Zhou,

Iwata, and Shore (2002) examined effects of both satiation and deprivation of food as reinforcement on the pre- and postmeal responding of nine adults with intellectual developmental disorder. Less than half the participants had higher premeal than postmeal response rates. The remaining participants had pre- and postmeal response rates that were comparable. Satiation and deprivation effects may be somewhat idiosyncratic, depending on the individual and reinforcement type (e.g., Sy & Borrero, 2009).

## OTHER CONSIDERATIONS IN REINFORCEMENT AND STIMULUS SELECTION

### Teaching New Preferences

Ideally, behavior analysts can identify several highly preferred stimuli to evaluate as reinforcers. However, some individuals may have few items or activities they prefer. In other cases, alternative stimuli may be more appropriate to use as reinforcers in the given environmental context. Researchers have taught individuals to shift their responding to items or activities previously assessed as less preferred by rearranging the environment. Stimulus–stimulus pairing, embedded reinforcement, and manipulation of motivating operations are the most common methods to increase the variety of items or activities an individual prefers or to which the individual allocates his or her responding.

### Pairing Procedures

Stimulus–stimulus pairing involves presenting a highly preferred stimulus and a less preferred stimulus in close temporal proximity, so that the highly preferred stimulus follows the less preferred stimulus after a short delay. The less preferred stimulus often becomes a conditioned reinforcer through repeated pairing. Researchers have used this strategy to condition vocal sounds as reinforcers in children with limited vocal repertoires (e.g., Yoon & Bennett, 2000; Esch, Carr, & Michael, 2005). Researchers have shown that simultaneous presentation of less preferred with highly preferred foods or condiments and highly preferred attention or tangibles, in some cases, increases consumption or selection of the less preferred foods (Ahearn, 2003; Piazza et al., 2002; Solberg, Hanley, Layer, & Ingvarsson, 2007). Furthermore, Hanley, Iwata, Roscoe, Thompson, and Lindberg (2003) presented a highly preferred stimulus on a fixed-time schedule and a less preferred activity continuously, and they found that participant engagement with the less preferred activity increased. However, the increases in consumption of less preferred stimuli produced through stimulus–stimulus pairing may dissipate when the pairings stop. Moreover, stimulus–stimulus pairing procedures have failed to establish stimuli as preferred or as reinforcement in some cases (e.g., Miguel, Carr, & Michael, 2002). Thus researchers should continue to study the behavioral mechanism(s) responsible for shifts in preference (Ahearn, 2003; Hanley, Iwata, Roscoe, et al., 2003; Piazza et al., 2002; Solberg et al., 2007).

### Embedded Reinforcement

Researchers also have provided highly preferred stimuli contingent on engagement with less preferred stimuli, to increase engagement or selection of the less preferred stimuli (Hanley, Iwata, & Lindberg, 1999; Hanley, Iwata, Roscoe, et al., 2003; Hanley et al., 2009). Hanley et al. (2009) provided alternative seating, teacher attention and assistance, tangible items, edibles, or a combination to preschoolers in a classroom who selected activities during free play that they initially engaged with less often during baseline. The embedded-reinforcement condition produced an increase in the percentage of intervals spent in the areas where these activities occurred. Hanley et al. (2002) provided attention, an edible, a highly preferred tangible item, or a combination of these reinforcers for behaviors compatible with engaging in a less preferred activity (e.g., each time the participant strung a bead). The researchers observed increased engagement with the less preferred activity only when they provided reinforcement for engagement with that activity.

### Motivating Operations

Response restriction and satiation of highly preferred stimuli represent antecedent manipulations that may shift response allocation away from highly preferred stimuli and toward less preferred stimuli (Hanley, Iwata, Roscoe, et al., 2003; Hanley et al., 2006, 2009). Restricting access to highly preferred stimuli alone can shift responding to less preferred stimuli for some individuals. The behavior analyst may need to implement a Premack-type contingency for others, which includes presenting the higher preferred activity contingent on engaging in the less preferred activity to shift responding (Hanley, Iwata, Roscoe, et al., 2003).

### Overjustification

The overjustification effect, which is a frequently referenced criticism of reinforcement, is that delivery of extrinsic rewards may decrease intrinsic motivation to engage in the behavior that produced those rewards (Deci, 1971; Greene & Lepper, 1974). For instance, an individual may play the piano because it is a preferred activity. The overjustification hypothesis predicts that piano playing will decrease if the individual receives payment and then payment ceases. However, several meta-analyses and reviews of overjustification have found no detrimental effects of rewards on measures of intrinsic motivation when the researchers defined intrinsic motivation by using observable measures, such as amount of time engaging in an activity (Cameron, Banko, & Pierce, 2001; Cameron & Pierce, 1994; Levy et al., 2017).

### Ecological Validity

Behavior analysts typically use stimulus preference and reinforcer assessments to develop interventions to establish appropriate behaviors, decrease problem behavior, or both. Using reinforcers that have the greatest ecological validity or fit should be a consideration when behavior analysts are designing these interventions (Karsten, Carr, & Lepper, 2011). One way to determine ecological validity is to assess whether a given reinforcer occurs naturally in an individual's environment. Another consideration is whether the reinforcer interferes with ongoing activities or other appropriate behaviors. For instance, giving a child access to toys in an academic setting may be disruptive or distracting to other students in the classroom. Therefore, behavior analysts should select reinforcers that minimally interfere with routine activities whenever possible, such as delivering preferred music through headphones rather than speakers. Other factors that behavior analysts should consider when selecting reinforcers include their cost and any possible untoward side effects, such as weight gain associated with edible reinforcers.

## CONCLUSION

Since 1985, the literature on stimulus preference and reinforcement assessment procedures has advanced markedly. Researchers have identified many effective procedures for assessing preference, and each of these procedures has strengths and weaknesses relative to time efficiency and accuracy. Single-stimulus assessments may be most appropriate for individuals who do not make choices or show approach responses when multiple stimuli are available, although the disadvantage is that some individuals may show high levels of approach responses to all or most stimuli. Paired-choice assessments may produce a more differentiated hierarchy when individuals demonstrate choice-making behavior. The multiple-stimulus-without-replacement, multiple-stimulus-with-replacement, and free-operant procedures have the advantage of time efficiency. Concurrent-chains procedures are useful for evaluating individuals' preferences for procedures such as treatments. Duration assessments may be useful for assessing levels of inappropriate behavior in the presence of specific stimuli (e.g., Piazza, Fisher, Hanley, Hilker, & Derby, 1996; Ringdahl, Vollmer, Marcus, & Roane, 1997). Response restriction combines aspects of both trial- and free-operant-based assessments and may produce well-differentiated preference hierarchies. Vocal assessments may be most appropriate for individuals who can vocalize their preferences, although the correspondence between vocal and observed preferences remains questionable. Pictorial preferences may be an accurate measure for some individuals, but not others. Most research has demonstrated that preference is a relatively good predictor of reinforcement efficacy; however, preference assessments may underestimate the effectiveness of lower-preference stimuli as reinforcement.

The most accurate method of reinforcer identification is to conduct an assessment to test the effectiveness of preferred stimuli as reinforcement. Researchers have used many methods to conduct reinforcer assessments. Single-operant schedules are well suited for evaluating the absolute reinforcing effects of a stimulus. By contrast, concurrent-operants schedules provide information about the relative reinforcing effects of a stimulus. Most studies have used simple, free-operant responses as the target in reinforcement assessments for ease and time efficiency, based on the rationale that if a stimulus does not function as reinforcement for a simple response, then it is not likely to function as reinforcement for a more complex one. Researchers have used progressive-ratio schedules to evaluate relative reinforcer efficacy across many contexts.

Behavior analysts can use several methods to maximize the effectiveness of reinforcement, such as delivering reinforcers immediately after the target response. Stimulus variation may be beneficial under some circumstances. At a minimum, behavior analysts should assess preferences periodically to avoid satiation. They can also minimize satiation by restricting access to reinforcers outside learning or treatment contexts. Furthermore, behavior analysta should assess the quality of potential competing reinforcers in the environment, to ensure that programmed reinforcement is of higher quality than available alternative reinforcements. Finally, research has shown that choice in and of itself may function as reinforcement.

In summary, the existing literature offers many procedures to identify effective positive reinforcers. Some questions that still arise include these:

1. Which procedures are most effective for which individuals?
2. What variables or factors should a behavior analyst consider when choosing a preference assessment?
3. How does a behavior analyst control for various motivational variables when identifying preferred stimuli?
4. What is the best approach for progressing when one or more preference assessments yield inconclusive results?
5. Finally, how does a behavior analyst identify potential negative reinforcers?

Answers to these questions, among others, will further refine our methods for identifying and enhancing positive reinforcers.

## REFERENCES

Ackerlund Brandt, J. A., Dozier, C. L., Juanico, J. F., Laudont, C. L., & Mick, B. R. (2015). The value of choice as a reinforcer for typically developing children. *Journal of Applied Behavior Analysis, 48,* 344–362.

Ahearn, W. H. (2003). Using simultaneous presentation to increase vegetable consumption in a mildly selective child with autism. *Journal of Applied Behavior Analysis, 36,* 361–365.

American Psychiatric Association. (2013). *Diagnostic and statistical manual of mental disorders* (5th ed.). Arlington, VA: Author.

Bojak, S. L., & Carr, J. E. (1999). On the displacement of leisure items by food during multiple-stimulus preference assessments. *Journal of Applied Behavior Analysis, 32,* 515–518.

Bowman, L. G., Piazza, C. C., Fisher, W. W., Hagopian, L. P., & Kogan, J. S. (1997). Assessment of preference for varied versus constant reinforcers. *Journal of Applied Behavior Analysis, 30,* 451–458.

Bukala, M., Hu, M. Y., Lee, R., Ward-Horner, J. C., & Fienup, D. M. (2015). The effects of work-reinforcer schedules on performance and preference in students with autism. *Journal of Applied Behavior Analysis, 48,* 215–220.

Call, N. A., Trosclair-Lasserre, N. M., Findley, A. J., Reavis, A. R., & Shillingsburg, M. A. (2012). Correspondence between single versus daily preference assessment outcomes and reinforcer efficacy under progressive-ratio schedules. *Journal of Applied Behavior Analysis, 45,* 763–777.

Cameron, J., Banko, K. M., & Pierce, W. D. (2001). Pervasive negative effects of rewards on intrinsic motivation: The myth continues. *Behavior Analyst, 24,* 1–44.

Cameron, J., & Pierce, W. D. (1994). Reinforcement, reward, and intrinsic motivation: A meta-analysis. *Review of Educational Research, 64,* 363–423.

Carr, J. E., Nicolson, A. C., & Higbee, T. S. (2000). Evaluation of a brief multiple-stimulus preference assessment in a naturalistic context. *Journal of Applied Behavior Analysis, 33,* 353–357.

Catania, A. C. (1963). Concurrent performances: A baseline for the study of reinforcement magnitude. *Journal of Experimental Animal Behavior, 6,* 299–300.

Ciccone, F. J., Graff, R. B., & Ahearn, W. H. (2015). Increasing the efficiency of paired-stimulus preference assessments by identifying categories of preference. *Journal of Applied Behavior Analysis, 48,* 221–226.

Clay, C. J., Samaha, A. L., Bloom, S. E., Bogoev, B. K., & Boyle, M. A. (2013). Assessing preference for social interactions. *Research in Developmental Disabilities, 34,* 362–371.

Clements, C., & McKee, J. (1968). Programmed instruction for institutionalized offenders: Contingency management and performance contracts. *Psychological Reports, 22,* 957–964.

Conyers, C., Doole, A., Vause, T., Harapiak, S., Yu, D. C. T., & Martin, G. L. (2002). Predicting the relative efficacy of three presentation methods for assessing preferences of persons with developmental disabilities. *Journal of Applied Behavior Analysis, 35,* 49–58.

Cooper, J. O., Heron, T. E., & Heward, W. L. (2007). *Applied behavior analysis* (2nd ed.) Upper Saddle River, NJ: Pearson/Merrill-Prentice Hall.

Cote, C. A., Thompson, R. H., Hanley, G. P., & McKerchar, P. M. (2007). Teacher report and direct assessment of preferences for identifying reinforcers for young children. *Journal of Applied Behavior Analysis, 40,* 157–166.

Daley, M. F. (1969). The "reinforcement menu": Finding effective reinforcers. In J. D. Krumboltz & C. E. Thorsen (Eds.), *Behavioral counseling: Cases and techniques.* New York: Holt, Rinehart & Winston.

Daly, E. J., III, Wells, N. J., Swanger-Gagné, M. S., Carr, J. E., Kunz, G. M., & Taylor, A. M. (2009). Evaluation of the multiple-stimulus without replacement prefer-

ence assessment method using activities as stimuli. *Journal of Applied Behavior Analysis, 42,* 563–574.

Deci, E. L. (1971). Effects of externally mediated rewards on intrinsic motivation. *Journal of Personality and Social Psychology, 18,* 105–115.

DeLeon, I. G., Chase, J. A., Frank-Crawford, M., Carreau-Webster, A., Triggs, M. M., Bullock, C. E., et al. (2014). Distributed and accumulated reinforcement arrangements: Evaluations of efficacy and preference. *Journal of Applied Behavior Analysis, 47,* 293–313.

DeLeon, I. G., Fisher, W. W., Catter, V. R., Maglieri, K., Herman, K., & Marhefka, J. (2001). Examination of relative reinforcement effects of stimuli identified through pretreatment and daily brief preference assessments. *Journal of Applied Behavior Analysis, 34,* 463–473.

DeLeon, I. G., & Iwata, B. A. (1996). Evaluation of a multiple-stimulus presentation format for assessing reinforcer preferences. *Journal of Applied Behavior Analysis, 29,* 519–532.

DeLeon, I. G., Iwata, B. A., Conners, J., & Wallace, M. D. (1999). Examination of ambiguous stimulus preferences with duration-based measures. *Journal of Applied Behavior Analysis, 32,* 111–114.

DeLeon, I. G., Iwata, B. A., Goh, H. L., & Worsdell, A. S. (1997). Emergence of reinforcer preference as a function of schedule requirements and stimulus similarity. *Journal of Applied Behavior Analysis, 30,* 439–449.

DeLeon, I. G., Iwata, B. A., & Roscoe, E. M. (1997). Displacement of leisure reinforcers by food during preference assessments. *Journal of Applied Behavior Analysis, 30,* 475–484.

Dunlap, G., dePerczel, M., Clarke, S., Wilson, D., Wright, S., White, R., & Gomez, A. (1994). Choice making to promote adaptive behavior for students with emotional and behavioral challenges. *Journal of Applied Behavior Analysis, 27,* 505–518.

Dyer, K., Dunlap, G., & Winterling, V. (1990). Effects of choice making on the serious problem behaviors of students with severe handicaps. *Journal of Applied Behavior Analysis, 23,* 515–524.

Egel, A. L. (1980). The effects of constant vs. varied reinforcer presentation on responding by autistic children. *Journal of Experimental Child Psychology, 30,* 455–462.

Egel, A. L. (1981). Reinforcer variation: Implications for motivating developmentally disabled children. *Journal of Applied Behavior Analysis, 14,* 345–350.

Esch, B. E., Carr, J. E., & Michael, J. (2005). Evaluating stimulus-stimulus pairing and direct reinforcement in the establishment of an echoic repertoire of children diagnosed with autism. *Analysis of Verbal Behavior, 21,* 43–58.

Fahmie, T. A., Iwata, B. A., & Jann, K. E. (2015). Comparison of edible and leisure reinforcers. *Journal of Applied Behavior Analysis, 48,* 331–343.

Fantuzzo, J. W., Rohrbeck, C. A., Hightower, A. D., & Work, W. C. (1991). Teachers' use and children's preferences of rewards in elementary school. *Psychology in the Schools, 28*, 175–181.

Favell, J. E., & Cannon, P. R. (1976). Evaluation of entertainment materials for severely retarded persons. *American Journal of Mental Deficiency, 81*, 357–361.

Fienup, D. M., Ahlers, A. A., & Pace, G. (2011). Preference for fluent versus disfluent work schedules. *Journal of Applied Behavior Analysis, 44*, 847–858.

Fisher, W. W., & Mazur, J. E. (1997). Basic and applied research on choice responding. *Journal of Applied Behavior Analysis, 30*, 387–410.

Fisher, W. W., Piazza, C. C., Bowman, L. G., & Amari, A. (1996). Integrating caregiver report with systematic choice assessment to enhance American Journal on Mental Retardation, 101, 15–25.

Fisher, W., Piazza, C. C., Bowman, L. G., Hagopian, L. P., Owens, J. C., & Slevin, I. (1992). A comparison of two approaches for identifying reinforcers for persons with severe and profound disabilities. *Journal of Applied Behavior Analysis, 25*, 491–498.

Fisher, W. W., Thompson, R. H., Piazza, C. C., Crosland, K., & Gotjen, D. (1997). On the relative reinforcing effects of choice and differential consequences. *Journal of Applied Behavior Analysis, 30*, 423–438.

Fox, R. A., & DeShaw, J. M. (1993). Milestone reinforcer survey. *Education and Training in Mental Retardation, 28*, 257–261.

Francisco, M. T., Borrero, J. C., & Sy, J. R. (2008). Evaluation of absolute and relative reinforcer value using progressive-ratio schedules. *Journal of Applied Behavior Analysis, 41*, 189–202.

Giles, A. F., St. Peter, C. C., Pence, S. T., & Gibson, A. B. (2012). Preference for blocking or response redirection during stereotypy treatment. *Research in Developmental Disabilities, 33*, 1691–1700.

Glover, A. C., Roane, H. S., Kadey, H. J., & Grow, L. L. (2008). Preference for reinforcers under progressive- and fixed-ratio schedules: A comparison of single- and concurrent-operant arrangements. *Journal of Applied Behavior Analysis, 41*, 163–176.

Graff, R. B., & Larsen, J. (2011). The relation between obtained preference value and reinforcer potency. *Behavioral Interventions, 26*, 125–133.

Graff, R. B., & Libby, M. E. (1999). A comparison of presession and within-session reinforcement choice. *Journal of Applied Behavior Analysis, 32*, 161–173.

Green, C. W., Reid, D. H., White, L. K., Halford, R. C., Brittain, D. P., & Gardner, S. M. (1988). Identifying reinforcers for persons with profound handicaps: Staff opinion versus systematic assessment of preferences. *Journal of Applied Behavior Analysis, 21*, 31–43.

Greene, D., & Lepper, M. R. (1974). Effects of extrinsic rewards on children's subsequent intrinsic interest. *Child Development, 45*, 1141–1145.

Hagopian, L. P., Rush, K. S., Lewin, A. B., & Long, E. S. (2001). Evaluating the predictive validity of a single stimulus engagement preference assessment. *Journal of Applied Behavior Analysis, 34*, 475–485.

Hanley, G. P., Cammilleri, A. P., Tiger, J. H., & Ingvarsson, E. T. (2007). A method for describing preschoolers' activity preferences. *Journal of Applied Behavior Analysis, 40*, 603–618.

Hanley, G. P., Iwata, B. A., & Lindberg, J. S. (1999). Analysis of activity preferences as a function of differential consequences. *Journal of Applied Behavior Analysis, 32*(4), 419–435.

Hanley, G. P., Iwata, B. A., Lindberg, J. S., & Conners, J. (2003). Response-restriction analysis: I. Assessment of activity preferences. *Journal of Applied Behavior Analysis, 36*, 47–58.

Hanley, G. P., Iwata, B. A., Roscoe, E. M., Thompson, R. H., & Lindberg, J. S. (2003). Response-restriction analysis: II. Alteration of activity preferences. *Journal of Applied Behavior Analysis, 36*, 59–76.

Hanley, G. P., Iwata, B. A., & Roscoe, E. M. (2006). Some determinants of changes in preference over time. *Journal of Applied Behavior Analysis, 39*, 189–202.

Hanley, G. P., Piazza, C. C., Fisher, W. W., Contrucci, S. A., & Maglieri, K. A. (1997). Evaluation of client preference for function-based treatment packages. *Journal of Applied Behavior Analysis, 30*, 459–473.

Hanley, G. P., Piazza, C. C., Fisher, W. W., & Maglieri, K. A. (2005). On the effectiveness of and preference for punishment and extinction components of function-based interventions. *Journal of Applied Behavior Analysis, 38*, 51–65.

Hanley, G. P., Tiger, J. H., Ingvarsson, E. T., & Cammilleri, A. P. (2009). Influencing preschoolers' free-play activity preferences: An evaluation of satiation and embedded reinforcement. *Journal of Applied Behavior Analysis, 42*, 33–41.

Heal, N. A., & Hanley, G. P. (2007). Evaluating preschool children's preferences for motivational systems during instruction. *Journal of Applied Behavior Analysis, 40*, 249–261.

Higbee, T. S., Carr, J. E., & Harrison, C. D. (1999). The effects of pictorial versus tangible stimuli in stimulus-preference assessments. *Research in Developmental Disabilities, 20*, 63–72.

Hodos, W. (1961). Progressive-ratio as a measure of reward strength. *Science, 134*, 943–944.

Hoffmann, A. N., Samaha, A. L., Bloom, S. E., & Boyle, M. A. (2017). Preference and reinforcer efficacy of high- and low-tech items: A comparison of item type and duration of access. *Journal of Applied Behavior Analysis, 50*, 222–237.

Jerome, J., & Sturmey, P. (2008). Reinforcing efficacy of interactions with preferred and non-preferred staff under progressive-ratio schedules. *Journal of Applied Behavior Analysis, 41*, 221–225.

Kang, S., Lang, R. B., O'Reilly, M. F., Davis, T. N., Machalicek, W., Rispoli, M. J., et al. (2010). Problem behavior during preference assessments: An empirical analysis and practical recommendations. *Journal of Applied Behavior Analysis, 43*, 137–141.

Kang, S., O'Reilly, M. F., Fragale, C., Aguilar, J., Rispoli, M., & Lang, R. (2011). Evaluation of the rate of problem behavior maintained by different reinforcers across preference assessments. *Journal of Applied Behavior Analysis, 44,* 835–846.

Karsten, A. M., Carr, J. E., & Lepper, T. L. (2011). Description of practitioner model for identifying preferred stimuli with individuals with autism spectrum disorders. *Behavior Modification, 35,* 347–369.

Kelley, M. E., Shillingsburg, M. A., & Bowen, C. N. (2016). Stability of daily preference across multiple individuals. *Journal of Applied Behavior Analysis, 49,* 394–398.

Keyl-Austin, A. A., Samaha, A. L., Bloom, S. E., & Boyle, M. A. (2012). Effects of preference and reinforcer variation on within-session patterns of responding. *Journal of Applied Behavior Analysis, 45,* 637–641.

Kodak, T., Lerman, D. C., & Call, N. (2007). Evaluating the influence of postsession reinforcement on choice of reinforcers. *Journal of Applied Behavior Analysis, 40,* 515–527.

Layer, S. A., Hanley, G. P., Heal, N. A., & Tiger, J. H. (2008). Determining individual preschoolers' preferences in a group arrangement. *Journal of Applied Behavior Analysis, 41,* 25–37.

Lee, M. S. H., Yu, C. T., Martin, T. L., & Martin, G. L. (2010). On the relation between reinforcer efficacy and preference. *Journal of Applied Behavior Analysis, 43,* 95–100.

Levy, A., DeLeon, I. G., Martinez, C. K., Fernandez, N., Gage, N. A., Sigurdsson, S. Ó., et al. (2017). A quantitative review of overjustification effects in persons with intellectual and developmental disabilities. *Journal of Applied Behavior Analysis, 50,* 206–221.

Luczynski, K. C., & Hanley, G. P. (2009). Do children prefer contingencies?: An evaluation of the efficacy of and preference for contingent versus noncontingent social reinforcement during play. *Journal of Applied Behavior Analysis, 42,* 511–525.

Luczynski, K. C., & Hanley, G. P. (2010). Examining the generality of children's preference for contingent reinforcement via extension to different responses, reinforcers, and schedules. *Journal of Applied Behavior Analysis, 43,* 397–409.

Luczynski, K. C., & Hanley, G. P. (2014). How should periods without social interaction be scheduled?: Children's preference for practical schedules of positive reinforcement. *Journal of Applied Behavior Analysis, 47,* 500–522.

Mace, F. C., Neef, N. A., Shade, D., & Mauro, B. C. (1994). Limited matching on concurrent schedule reinforcement of academic behavior. *Journal of Applied Behavior Analysis, 27,* 585–596.

Madden, G. J., & Bickel, W. K. (2010). *Impulsivity: The behavioral and neurological science of discounting.* Washington, DC: American Psychological Association.

Mason, S. A., McGee, G. G., Farmer-Dougan, V., & Risley, T. R. (1989). A practical strategy for ongoing reinforcer assessment. *Journal of Applied Behavior Analysis, 22,* 171–179.

Mazaleski, J. L., Iwata, B. A., Vollmer, T. R., Zarcone, J. R., & Smith, R. G. (1993). Analysis of the reinforcement and extinction components in DRO contingencies with self-injury. *Journal of Applied Behavior Analysis, 26,* 143–156.

Miguel, C. F., Carr, J. E., & Michael, J. (2002). The effects of a stimulus–stimulus pairing procedure on the vocal behavior of children diagnosed with autism. *Analysis of Verbal Behavior, 18,* 3–13.

Morris, S. L., & Vollmer, T. R. (2019). Assessing preference for types of social interaction. *Journal of Applied Behavior Analysis, 52,* 1064–1075.

Neef, N. A., Mace, F. C., & Shade, D. (1993). Impulsivity in students with serious emotional disturbance: The interactive effects of reinforcer rate, delay, and quality. *Journal of Applied Behavior Analysis, 26,* 37–52.

Neef, N. A., Mace, F. C., Shea, M. C., & Shade, D. (1992). Effects of reinforcer rate and reinforcer quality on time allocation: Extensions of matching theory to educational settings. *Journal of Applied Behavior Analysis, 25,* 691–699.

Neef, N. A., Shade, D., & Miller, M. S. (1994). Assessing influential dimensions of reinforcers on choice in students with serious emotional disturbance. *Journal of Applied Behavior Analysis, 27,* 575–583.

Northup, J., Fusilier, I., Swanson, V., Roane, H., & Borrero, J. (1997). An evaluation of methylphenidate as a potential establishing operation for some common classroom reinforcers. *Journal of Applied Behavior Analysis, 30,* 615–625.

Northup, J., George, T., Jones, K., Broussard, C., & Vollmer, T. R. (1996). A comparison of reinforcer assessment methods: The utility of verbal and pictorial choice procedures. *Journal of Applied Behavior Analysis, 29,* 201–212.

Nuernberger, J. E., Smith, C. A., Czapar, K. N., & Klatt, K. P. (2012). Assessing preference for social interaction in children diagnosed with autism. *Behavioral Interventions, 27,* 33–44.

Ortega, J. V., Iwata, B. A., Nogales-González, C., & Frades, B. (2012). Assessment of preference for edible and leisure items in individuals with dementia. *Journal of Applied Behavior Analysis, 45,* 839–844.

Pace, G. M., Ivancic, M. T., Edwards, G. L., Iwata, B. A., & Page, T. J. (1985). Assessment of stimulus preference and reinforcer value with profoundly retarded individuals. *Journal of Applied Behavior Analysis, 18,* 249–255.

Paclawskyj, T. R., & Vollmer, T. R. (1995). Reinforcer assessment for children with developmental disabilities and visual impairments. *Journal of Applied Behavior Analysis, 28,* 219–224.

Paramore, N. W., & Higbee, T. S. (2005). An evaluation of a brief multiple-stimulus preference assessment with adolescents with emotional–behavioral disorders in an educational setting. *Journal of Applied Behavior Analysis, 38,* 399–403.

Parsons, M. B., & Reid, D. H. (1990). Assessing food preferences among persons with profound mental retardation: Providing opportunities to make choices. *Journal of Applied Behavior Analysis, 23,* 183–195.

Penrod, B., Wallace, M. D., & Dyer, E. J. (2008). Assessing reinforcer potency of high-preference and low-preference reinforcers with respect to response rate and response patterns. *Journal of Applied Behavior Analysis, 41,* 177–188.

Piazza, C. C., Fisher, W. W., Hagopian, L. P., Bowman, L. G., & Toole, L. (1996). Using a choice assessment to predict reinforcer effectiveness. *Journal of Applied Behavior Analysis, 29,* 1–9.

Piazza, C. C., Fisher, W. W., Hanley, G. P., Hilker, K., & Derby, K. M. (1996). A preliminary procedure for predicting the positive and negative effects of reinforcement-based procedures. *Journal of Applied Behavior Analysis, 29,* 137–152.

Piazza, C. C., Patel, M. R., Santana, C. M., Goh, H., Delia, M. D., & Lancaster, B. M. (2002). An evaluation of simultaneous and sequential presentation of preferred and nonpreferred food to treat food selectivity. *Journal of Applied Behavior Analysis, 35,* 259–270.

Poling, A. (2010). Progressive-ratio schedules and applied behavior analysis. *Journal of Applied Behavior Analysis, 43,* 347–349.

Powell, S., & Nelson, B. (1997). Effects of choosing academic assignments on a student with attention deficit hyperactivity disorder. *Journal of Applied Behavior Analysis, 30,* 181–183.

Radley, K. C., Dart, E. H., Battaglia, A. A., & Ford, W. B. (2019). A comparison of two procedures for assessing preference in a classroom setting. *Behavior Analysis in Practice, 12,* 95–104.

Ringdahl, J. E., Vollmer, T. R., Marcus, B. A., & Roane, H. S. (1997). An analogue evaluation of enriched environment: The role of stimulus preference. *Journal of Applied Behavior Analysis, 30,* 203–216.

Roane, H. S. (2008). On the applied use of progressive-ratio schedules of reinforcement. *Journal of Applied Behavior Analysis, 41,* 155–161.

Roane, H. S., Call, N. A., & Falcomata, T. S. (2005). A preliminary analysis of adaptive responding under open and closed economies. *Journal of Applied Behavior Analysis, 38,* 335–348.

Roane, H. S., Lerman, D. C., & Vorndran, C. M. (2001). Assessing reinforcers under progressive schedule requirements. *Journal of Applied Behavior Analysis, 34,* 145–167.

Roane, H. S., Vollmer, T. R., Ringdahl, J. E., & Marcus, B. A. (1998). Evaluation of a brief stimulus preference assessment. *Journal of Applied Behavior Analysis, 31,* 605–620.

Roscoe, E. M., Iwata, B. A., & Kahng, S. (1999). Relative versus absolute reinforcement effects: Implica-

tions for preference assessments. *Journal of Applied Behavior Analysis, 32,* 479–493.

Rotatori, A. F., Fox, B., & Switzky, H. (1979). An indirect technique for establishing preferences for categories of reinforcement for severely and profoundly retarded individuals. *Perceptual and Motor Skills, 48,* 1307–1313.

Schmidt, A. C., Hanley, G. P., & Layer, S. A. (2009). A further analysis of the value of choice: Controlling for illusory discriminative stimuli and evaluating the effects of less preferred items. *Journal of Applied Behavior Analysis, 42,* 711–716.

Shiffman, S. S. (1997). Taste and smell losses in normal aging and disease. *Journal of the American Medical Association, 278,* 1357–1362.

Smith, C. J., Roane, H. S., & Stephenson, K. (2009, May). Evaluation of functional and alternative reinforcers under progressive ratio schedules of reinforcement. In R. G. Smith (Chair), *Advances in preference and choice research across multiple applied contexts.* Symposium conducted at the 35th annual convention of the Association for Behavior Analysis, Phoenix, AZ.

Solberg, K. M., Hanley, G. P., Layer, S. A., & Ingvarsson, E. T. (2007). The effects of reinforcer pairing and fading on preschoolers' snack selection. *Journal of Applied Behavior Analysis, 40,* 633–644.

Steinhilber, J., & Johnson, C. (2007). The effects of brief and extended stimulus availability on preference. *Journal of Applied Behavior Analysis, 40,* 767–772.

Sy, J. R., & Borrero, J. C. (2009). Parametric analysis of presession exposure to edible and nonedible stimuli. *Journal of Applied Behavior Analysis, 42,* 833–837.

Taravella, C. C., Lerman, D. C., Contrucci, S. A., & Roane, H. S. (2000). Further evaluation of low-ranked items in stimulus-choice preference assessments. *Journal of Applied Behavior Analysis, 33,* 105–108.

Tasky, K. K., Rudrud, E. H., Schulze, K. A., & Rapp, J. T. (2008). Using choice to increase on-task behavior in individuals with traumatic brain injury. *Journal of Applied Behavior Analysis, 41,* 261–265.

Thompson, R. H., Fisher, W. W., & Contrucci, S. A. (1998). Evaluating the reinforcing effects of choice in comparison to reinforcement rate. *Research in Developmental Disabilities, 19,* 181–187.

Tiger, J. H., Hanley, G. P., & Hernandez, E. (2006). An evaluation of the value of choice with preschool children. *Journal of Applied Behavior Analysis, 39,* 1–16.

Tourigny Dewhurst, D. L., & Cautela, J. R. (1980). A proposed reinforcement survey schedule for special needs children. *Journal of Behavior Therapy and Experimental Psychiatry, 11,* 109–112.

Toussaint, K. A., Kodak, T., & Vladescu, J. C. (2016). An evaluation of choice on instructional efficacy and individual preferences among children with autism. *Journal of Applied Behavior Analysis, 49,* 170–175.

Trosclair-Lasserre, N. M., Lerman, D. C., Call, N. A., Addison, L. R., & Kodak, T. (2008). Reinforcement magnitude: An evaluation of preference and reinforcer efficacy. *Journal of Applied Behavior Analysis, 41*, 203–220.

Tung, S. B., Donaldson, J. M., & Kahng, S. (2017). The effects of preference assessment type on problem behavior. *Journal of Applied Behavior Analysis, 50*, 861–866.

Verriden, A. L., & Roscoe, E. M. (2016). A comparison of preference-assessment methods. *Journal of Applied Behavior Analysis, 49*, 265–285.

Vollmer, T. R., Ringdahl, J. E., Roane, H. S., & Marcus, B. A. (1997). Negative side effects of noncontingent reinforcement. *Journal of Applied Behavior Analysis, 30*, 161–164.

Wehman, P. (1976). Selection of play materials for the severely handicapped: A continuing dilemma. *Education and Training of the Mentally Retarded, 11*, 46–50.

Windsor, J., Piché, L. M., & Locke, P. A. (1994). Preference testing: A comparison of two presentation methods. *Research in Developmental Disabilities, 15*, 439–455.

Wine, B., & Wilder, D. A. (2009). The effects of varied versus constant high-, medium-, and low-preference stimuli on performance. *Journal of Applied Behavior Analysis, 42*, 321–326.

Yoon, S., & Bennett, G. M. (2000). Effects of a stimulus-stimulus pairing procedure on conditioning vocal sounds as reinforcers. *Analysis of Verbal Behavior, 17*, 75–88.

Zhou, L., Iwata, B. A., Goff, G. A., & Shore, B. A. (2001). Longitudinal analysis of leisure-item preferences. *Journal of Applied Behavior Analysis, 34*, 179–184.

Zhou, L., Iwata, B. A., & Shore, B. A. (2002). Reinforcing efficacy of food on performance during pre- and postmeal sessions. *Journal of Applied Behavior Analysis, 35*, 411–414.

# CHAPTER 11

# Indirect Behavioral Assessments
## *Interviews and Rating Scales*

Dana M. Gadaire, Michael E. Kelley, and Robert H. LaRue

Functional behavioral assessment is an essential part of understanding the variables that affect the occurrence of problem behavior. The Individuals with Disabilities Education Improvement Act of 2004 (IDEA, 2004) guarantees students with disabilities the right to a functional behavioral assessment, thus highlighting its importance. Legislators created and amended the act to ensure free, appropriate public education for students with disabilities. A functional behavioral assessment is part of a comprehensive program used by public school personnel to address a student's specific needs in the least restrictive environment. The law requires that public schools provide necessary learning aids, testing modifications, and other educational accommodations to children with disabilities— accommodations that include a functional behavioral assessment when appropriate.

A *functional behavioral assessment* is a process of gathering information, observing, manipulating environmental variables, or a combination of those activities to develop effective, function-based treatments. There are three general components of a functional behavioral assessment: *indirect assessment, descriptive assessment,* and *experimental functional analysis.* In this chapter, we focus on indirect behavioral assessments, including interviews and rating scales.

## BENEFITS AND LIMITATIONS OF INDIRECT BEHAVIORAL ASSESSMENT

The purpose of indirect functional assessment is to identify antecedent variables (ones that occasion, evoke, or abate target behavior) and consequence variables (ones that affect the future likelihood of the target behavior). An indirect functional assessment usually gathers this information from a rating scale or structured interview (Lloyd & Kennedy, 2014). Indirect methods of functional assessment typically require less intensive training to use and are time efficient to conduct. To illustrate, the time requirement for an indirect functional assessment may range from a few minutes to complete a single rating scale to several hours to compare the results of several scales and to conduct an interview. By contrast, other assessment forms, such as an analogue functional analysis, may take several days, weeks, or even months to complete.

Despite these potential benefits, indirect functional assessment may provide little information about or incorrectly identify the function of target behavior. More concerning is that the assessor may behave as if the information from an indirect assessment is adequate for prescribing treatment in the absence of an analogue functional analysis (Hanley, 2012). For example, indirect functional assessment often does not include direct observation of a client or the target behaviors. Thus the assessor depends on caregiver recollections of the frequency of a target behavior, the settings and conditions in which the target behavior is more and less likely to occur, the consequences that typically follow the target behavior, and so forth. Indirect functional assessment has several other disadvantages. First, investigators have generally not evaluated the psychometric properties of some indirect assessment measures. In fact, results of some studies have shown that some tools for indirect functional assessment lack acceptable levels of *reliability* (the stability of measurement over time or across stimulus parameters), *validity* (whether an assessment measures what investigators designed it to measure), or both. For example, investigators have reported both high and low levels of reliability for the Motivation Assessment Scale (Durand & Crimmins, 1988), depending on how investigators calculated reliability and the topography of the assessed target behavior (Bihm, Kienlen, Ness, & Poindexter, 1991; Iwata, Vollmer, & Zarcone, 1990; Paclawskyj, Matson, Rush, Smalls, & Vollmer, 2001; Sigafoos, Kerr, & Roberts, 1994; Singh et al., 1993). Saini, Ubdegrove, Biran, and Duncan (2019) showed that that both the interrater reliability and concurrent validity of an open-ended functional-analytic interview were relatively low. Therapists typically ask parents and caregivers to provide information about target individuals during indirect assessments. However, Dracobly, Dozier, Briggs, and Juanico (2018) showed that experts were more likely than caregivers to agree with each other (interrater reliability) and to agree with other objective measures (validity). Nevertheless, behavior analysts report frequent use of rating scales and structured interviews to assess the function of problem behavior, probably because they are easy to use (Fryling & Baires, 2016). In the remainder of the chapter, we provide descriptions and analyses of several of the most common rating scales and interviews for indirect behavioral assessment.

## RATING SCALES

Rating scales usually include questions or statements about behavior to which informants respond by using a Likert scale to indicate their level of agreement with the question or statement. Most rating scales include a range of agreement levels. For example, a scale might include this statement:

"My child engages in problem behavior at levels far above that which would be normally accepted in a school." In this hypothetical rating scale, the levels of agreement range from 1 to 5. Thus the informant would indicate his or her level of agreement with this statement as follows: 1—*strongly disagree,* 2—*somewhat disagree,* 3—*neither agree nor disagree,* 4—*somewhat agree,* and 5—*strongly agree.* Rating scales often include methods for summarizing the results, such as adding the scores for each question to produce a total score.

Rating scales are useful because they provide quantifiable information (Hosp, Howell, & Hosp, 2003). Some rating scales assign numerical values to the informant's ratings, and behavior analysts can add those values and analyze the results based on the rating scales' instructions. An advantage is that investigators can assess quantified data for reliability across time, between raters, and within the scale. Investigators also can assess validity by comparing one scale's results to those of scales with known psychometric properties that purport to measure the same construct (*convergent validity*) or a different construct (*discriminant validity*). Second, behavior analysts can compare a rating scale's results across time, raters, or settings to assess changes in the occurrence of target behavior across those dimensions. Third, rating scales may be free of some biases that affect other measures, because a rating scale's quantifiable responses may be less open to interpretation.

Rating scales have some noteworthy disadvantages that warrant consideration (Hanley, 2010, 2012; Iwata, DeLeon, & Roscoe, 2013). Although generating quantifiable outcomes to compare across raters and time may seem appealing, such assessment often produces unreliable results. That is, two independent raters may produce different outcomes when rating the same individual (Newton & Sturmey, 1991; Nicholson, Konstantinidi, & Furniss, 2006; Shogren & Rojahn, 2003; Zarcone, Rodgers, Iwata, Rourke, & Dorsey, 1991). Below, we review some rating scales that behavior analysts often use to aid in identifying the reinforcer(s) for problem behavior.

### Problem Behavior Questionnaire

The Problem Behavior Questionnaire (Lewis, Scott, & Sugai, 1994) has 15 questions about potential antecedent and consequent events for problem behavior designed primarily for classroom teachers. The informant indicates the estimated percentage of time the event is present during a typical episode of problem behavior, using this Likert-scale format: *Never, 10% of the time, 25% of the time, 50% of the time, 75% of the time, 90% of the time,* or *Always.* The questionnaire includes a profile that the interviewer completes, based on the informant's ratings for problem behavior. The profile includes three major categories: peers, adults, and settings. Peers and adults each have two subcategories: attention and escape. Thus the questionnaire identifies five potential functions of problem behavior. Lewis et al. (1994) provide specific scoring criteria for identifying the function of the student's problem behavior. One limitation of the Problem Behavior Questionnaire is that investigators have not assessed its reliability and validity. Thus behavior analysts should not use the Problem Behavior Questionnaire without additional functional assessment.

## Functional Analysis Screening Tool

The Functional Analysis Screening Tool is a rating scale that provides preliminary information about variables that may influence problem behavior (Iwata & DeLeon, 1996). It has several open-ended questions about the informant; his or her relation to the target individual; and the topography, frequency, severity, and context for occurrences and nonoccurrences of problem behavior. Sixteen additional questions assess antecedents and consequences that might affect problem behavior, which the informant answers in a *yes–no* format. For example, one question is "Does the person usually engage in the problem behavior more often when he or she is ill?" The questionnaire assesses antecedents and consequences for social positive and social negative reinforcement and automatic positive and automatic negative reinforcement, and the category with the most *yes* responses indicates a potential reinforcer for problem behavior. Iwata and DeLeon (1996) developed the Functional Analysis Screening Tool to obtain information from caregivers about potential antecedents and consequences for problem behavior that could inform an experimental functional analysis (Iwata et al., 2013).

Iwata et al. (2013) assessed the reliability and validity of the Functional Analysis Screening Tool in a two-study experiment. In Study 1, investigators administered the scale to pairs of raters for 196 problem behaviors. Mean item-to-item agreement was 72% (overall range, 29–100%; range for individual items, 53–85%; M for highest totals = 69%). The agreement coefficients from Iwata et al. were comparable to those from other studies in which investigators assessed agreement for a functional behavior assessment rating scale (Conroy, Fox, Bucklin, & Good, 1996; Duker & Sigafoos, 1998; Sigafoos et al., 1994; Zarcone et al., 1991; see Iwata et al., 2013, for a direct comparison of the agreement scores across studies).

In Study 2, Iwata et al. (2013) evaluated the Functional Analysis Screening Tool's validity by assessing whether its results predicted the condition with the highest rate of problem behavior in each of the analogue functional analyses of 59 individuals. The investigators determined whether the results of the analogue functional analysis matched the results of the Functional Analysis Screening Tool for both informants, one informant, or neither informant. The aggregated results showed the function that one or both informants identified with the scale matched the function the analogue functional analysis identified in 64% of cases. Thus the Functional Analysis Screening Tool lacked predictive validity for functional-analytic outcomes, likely due to its moderate reliability (Iwata et al., 2013).

Although the Functional Analysis Screening Tool was found not to be adequate as a prescriptive tool, the investigators described ways that it might improve the treatment development process. First, it might improve the efficiency and consistency of interviews, because interviewers ask the same questions in every interview. Second, results of the Functional Analysis Screening Tool might provide information about idiosyncratic behaviors or conditions that might not otherwise be apparent. Third, behavior analysts might be able to use rater concordance on the Functional Analysis Screening Tool to rule out reinforcers for problem behavior; this would permit them to conduct fewer conditions in the analogue functional analysis, which could potentially reduce its length. Overall, the results of Iwata et al. (2013) are consistent with the existing literature, which suggests that behavior analysts should use the Functional Analysis Screening Tool as a supplement to experimental functional analyses.

## Motivation Assessment Scale

The Motivation Assessment Scale (Durand & Crimmins, 1988) has 16 questions about potential antecedent and consequent events for problem behavior. Informants rate how often the individual engages in the behavior in response to each question on a Likert scale from 1 (*never*) to 6 (*always*).

The assessor transfers the numerical scores for each question to a scoring guide organized by the motivation types of attention, escape, sensory, and tangible. The highest mean score among the four motivation types indicates the potential reinforcer for problem behavior. Durand and Crimmins (1988, 1992) reported that a reliability assessment produced acceptable interrater reliability (agreement between raters) and test–retest reliability (agreement on separate occasions). The validity assessment compared Motivation Assessment Scale results with direct observation and indicated that the scale predicted situations in which problem behavior was more and less likely to occur.

Studies by other investigators, however, have produced different results (Bihm et al., 1991; Iwata et al., 1990; Paclawskyj, Matson, Rush, Smalls, & Vollmer, 2001; Sigafoos et al., 1994; Singh et al., 1993). For example, Zarcone et al. (1991) evaluated the reliability of the Motivation Assessment Scale with one group of individuals with intellectual developmental disorder in an institution and a second group in a school. Informants for each individual were two staff members who worked with the individual regularly in the institution or school, respectively. Zarcone et al. calculated the reliability coefficients Durand and Crimmins (1988) reported, to directly compare the results from the two studies. The coefficients included (1) a Pearson product–moment correlation that compared the two raters' raw scores across items on the questionnaire, (2) a Pearson product–moment correlation that compared the two raters' mean scores for the four motivation categories, and (3) a Spearman rank-order correlation for each pair of raters on their rank orders for each motivation category. Zarcone et al. also calculated exact agreement (whether the two raters selected the same response on each item of the Motivation Assessment Scale) and agreement for adjacent scores (whether one rater's score for an item was plus or minus 1 from the other rater's score on the item). The five reliability methods produced coefficients of .27, .41, .41, .20, and .40, respectively.

In another study, the reliability coefficients for the Motivation Assessment Scale when aggression was the target behavior were lower (Sigafoos et al., 1994) than those Durand and Crimmins (1988) reported for self-injurious behavior. Finally, Duker and Sigafoos (1998) evaluated the reliability, internal consistency, and construct validity of the Motivation Assessment Scale across three topographies of problem behavior with two calculation methods. Results suggested that the scale had low levels of reliability and ambiguous construct valid-

ity. Overall, results of these studies suggest that the reliability of the Motivation Assessment Scale may not be as high as previously reported. For this reason, behavior analysts should not replace direct observation or experimental manipulation with the Motivation Assessment Scale to determine the function of problem behavior, to develop treatment, or both.

## Questions about Behavioral Function

The Questions about Behavioral Function scale assesses a broader range of potential variables than the rating scales we have reviewed thus far. It includes questions about commonly assessed variables, social attention, escape, tangible reinforcement, and nonsocial reinforcement, as well as underinvestigated variables such as social avoidance and physical discomfort.

Paclawskyj, Matson, Rush, Smalls, and Vollmer (2000) evaluated the test–retest, interrater, and internal-consistency reliability for Questions about Behavioral Function. Results suggested that assessment data were relatively stable over time, that multiple raters produced similar ratings, and that subscales were homogeneous. Simo-Pinatella et al. (2013) assessed the psychometric properties of Questions about Behavioral Function in Spanish and found that it had good test–retest reliability. Matson, Bamburg, Cherry, and Paclawskyj (1999) used Questions about Behavioral Function to identify the function of participants' problem behavior. The scale identified a *clear function*— defined as a minimum score of four of five possible endorsements on a subscale, with no other subscales containing significant endorsements (see Matson & Vollmer, 1995)—for 84% of participants. Next, the investigators assessed whether they could prescribe effective treatment for participants whose Questions about Behavioral Function results identified a function for problem behavior. Treatments based on these results were more effective for decreasing occurrences of problem behavior than those not based on these results. By contrast, Questions about Behavioral Function results matched results of an analogue functional analysis in 56% of cases in Paclawskyj et al. (2001).

Although investigators have evaluated Questions about Behavioral Function more extensively than most other indirect functional behavioral assessments, additional research is warranted. Results thus far are mixed about whether the scale accurately identifies the function of problem behavior and whether behavior analysts can use it to develop effective function-based treatment.

# INTERVIEWS

An interview is likely to be the first step in most assessments. Although interviews may take many forms, we focus on structured interviews in this chapter. In a structured interview, the interviewer gathers information about the prevalence and topography of target behavior, the environments in which the target behavior is more and less likely to occur, and antecedents that precede and consequences that follow the target behavior's occurrence. The behavior analyst usually conducts structured interviews with informants (vs. self-administration of a structured interview), and the structured interview guides the behavior analyst to ask the same questions in the same order with each informant.

Interviews may be useful for gathering anecdotal information about a target behavior from informants with whom the client interacts most often. The interview format is flexible because the behavior analyst can ask follow-up questions to clarify an informant's response. For example, if a caregiver indicates that a client engages in the problem behavior "all day," the behavior analyst might ask a more specific question, such as "Can you think of a time in which Joey does not engage in problem behavior?" These follow-up questions may provide additional detail about antecedents that precede and consequences that follow the target behavior's occurrence.

Interviews have several disadvantages. Bias is one potential problem. That is, the way the interviewer asks the questions and the types of questions that are asked may bias the informant's responses. An informant who does not understand a question, is reluctant to disclose information, or tries to conform to what he or she believes are the interviewer's expectations may provide misleading or erroneous information. In addition, the way the informant answers the questions may bias the interviewer's behavior. For example, an interviewer may prematurely end an interview if an informant provides minimal information that is barely audible, does not make eye contact, and frequently sighs and looks at his or her watch during the interview.

## School-Based Functional Assessment

Steege and Watson (2009) developed a structured interview for functional behavioral assessment, intended to gather information primarily focused in the school. The interview includes several components: the Functional Behavioral Assessment Screening Form, the Behavioral Stream Interview, the Antecedent Variables Assessment Form, the Individual Variables Assessment Form, and the Consequence Variables Assessment Form. We review each of these below.

The Functional Behavioral Assessment Screening Form prompts the interviewer to ask about behavioral strengths, interfering behaviors, potential reinforcers, and current communicative ability. The Behavioral Stream Interview is less structured and is designed to identify how antecedents, behavior, and consequences interact. The interviewer asks informants to describe antecedents, behaviors, and consequences as a sequence of events as they occur in the natural environment. The Antecedent Variables Assessment Form prompts the interviewer to ask questions about the variables that trigger or occasion target behavior. The questions are separated into four domains: environmental variables, such as auditory or visual stimulation; instructional variables, such as task difficulty and instructional pace; social variables, such as specific people or proximity; and transition variables, such as activity initiation or termination or changes in routine. The Individual Variables Assessment Form identifies personal variables that may affect problem behavior, such as communication skills, academic skills, social skills, health issues, sleep issues, and medications. The Consequence Variables Assessment Form identifies events that follow problem behavior, such as social attention from others, access to items or activities, escape from aversive stimulation, or the sensory consequences problem behavior produces. This form also assesses parameters of reinforcement, such as schedule, quality, magnitude, and timing.

## Functional Analysis Interview

The Functional Analysis Interview has 11 sections designed to identify potential reinforcers for problem behavior and takes about 45–90 minutes to complete, depending on the amount of information gathered (O'Neill, Horner, Albin, Storey, & Sprague, 1990). The interviewer prompts the informant to describe (1) the problem behavior, (2) ecological/setting events, (3) antecedents and (4) consequences for problem behavior, (5) the efficiency of problem behavior, (6) functional alternative behavior, (7) primary mode of communicative behavior, (7) things to do and things to avoid, (8) potential preferred stimuli that might function as reinforcement for alternative behavior, and (9) the history of the problem behavior and of previous treatments. The behavior analyst can use the results of the Functional Analysis Interview to inform additional assessment and treatment. We describe each section below.

## Description of Behavior

The interviewer asks the caregiver to identify problem behaviors of concern and to rank the topographies of problem behavior in order of importance. The interviewer uses this section to develop operational definitions for target behavior. Precise operational definitions allow objective observers to measure and agree on occurrences and nonoccurrences of target behavior.

## Ecological/Setting Events

The interviewer asks about events that may affect behavior but do not necessarily occur contiguously with it. For instance, the interviewer might ask about medications, physical problems, routines, sleep patterns, and staffing patterns. Previous research has shown that too little sleep or allergy symptoms (Kennedy & Meyer, 1996), recurrent otitis media (O'Reilly, 1997), or stimulant medication (Kelley, Fisher, Lomas, & Sanders, 2006) may affect the likelihood of target behavior.

## Antecedents

The interviewer asks about environmental events that occur before occurrences of problem behavior to identify antecedents. The literature on establishing operations (Michael, 1993, 2000) suggests that identifying environmental events or conditions that precede the occurrence of a behavior may provide information about the motivation for the behavior, as well as about variables that increase or decrease the effectiveness of the reinforcer for the behavior.

## Consequences

The interviewer asks about events that occur immediately after the occurrence of problem behavior. The purpose of these questions is to identify the reinforcer for problem behavior. Common consequences that function as reinforcement for problem behavior include social positive reinforcement in the form of attention or access to tangibles, social negative reinforcement in the form of escape from demands, and automatic reinforcement that the behavior produces (see Iwata, Dorsey, Slifer, Bauman, & Richman, 1982/1994).

## Efficiency of the Behavior

The interviewer asks about how efficiently problem and alternative behaviors produce reinforcement. Voluminous research suggests that parameters that affect responding include response effort, delay to reinforcement, and reinforcement quality and rate. Response rates tend to be higher when response effort is low, the delay to reinforcement is short, and reinforcement quality and rate are high, relative to the response rate when effort is high, delay to reinforcement is long, and reinforcement quality and rate are low (Fisher & Mazur, 1997; Horner & Day, 1991; Mace, Neef, Shade, & Mauro, 1996; Neef & Lutz, 2001; Neef, Mace, & Shade, 1993; Neef, Shade, & Miller, 1994).

## Functional Alternative Behavior

The interviewer asks about how the target individual recruits reinforcement by using appropriate behavior, such as vocal responses, gestures, signs, or compliance.

## Primary Mode of Communication

The interviewer asks about the target individual's communication skills, to determine whether the individual communicates with gestures, pictures, sign language, vocal language, or a combination.

## Things to Do/Things to Avoid.

The interviewer asks about things that work well and do not work well with the target individual, such as instructional pace and trainer characteristics.

## Potential Reinforcers

The interviewer asks about the target individual's preferred stimuli, such as activities or items, that might function as reinforcers for appropriate behavior (e.g., Fisher et al., 1992; Pace, Ivancic, Edwards, Iwata, & Page, 1985; Roane, Vollmer, Ringdahl, & Marcus, 1998). The interviewer can use this information to inform assessments for stimulus preferences and reinforcers.

## History

The interviewer asks about the problem behavior's history. Questions focus on how long the problem behavior has occurred, as well as effective and ineffective treatments.

## Summary Statements

The interviewer uses the information from the previous sections to develop summary statements that identify the setting events and immediate antecedents for problem behavior, the problem behavior, and the reinforcers for problem behavior.

### Sleep Assessment and Treatment Tool

The Sleep Assessment and Treatment Tool (Jin, Hanley, & Beaulieu, 2013) is an open-ended interview that focuses on sleep problems. The 10-page interview prompts interviewers to obtain demographic information; a history of the sleep problem; information about the caregiver's goals for treatment; a description of specific behavior, such as noncompliance, interfering behavior, problems falling asleep, problems staying asleep, and waking up early; information about the current sleep schedule; a description of the bedtime routine; information about the sleep environment; a description of methods caregivers use to promote sleep, such as giving the child a bottle or rocking the child; and information to help distinguish nighttime and early awakenings, confusional arousals, and nightmares.

Jin et al. (2013) used the Sleep Assessment and Treatment Tool to inform treatments for three children with autism spectrum disorder and sleep problems. The interview-informed treatment included (1) manipulation of establishing operations and discriminative stimuli to weaken sleep-interfering behaviors, (2) adjustment of sleep schedules to decrease the latency to sleep onset (Piazza & Fisher, 1991), and (3) disruption of the putative reinforcers that maintained sleep-interfering behaviors and night wakings. The treatment reduced sleep-onset delay, sleep-interfering behaviors, and night wakings.

## SUMMARY

Some investigators have encouraged behavior analysts to use rating scales and interviews in the context of a comprehensive functional assessment, rather than as the sole methods of assessment. The potential inaccuracy of rating scales and the inadequate psychometric properties of some tools are the likely reasons for this recommendation (Fisher, Piazza, Bowman, & Amari, 1996; Green & Striefel, 1988; Lennox & Miltenberger, 1989; Umbreit, 1996). Most authors who develop and promote indirect methods recommend combining interviews with direct observation or systematic functional analysis (e.g., Durand, 1990; Umbreit, 1996). Ultimately, best practice is likely to include an assessment package that contains a structured interview, at least one rating scale, direct observation, and experimental manipulation of environmental variables. A combination of these assessment methods may produce the most accurate information about the topography of behavior, the conditions under which the behavior is more and less likely to occur, the consequences that typically follow the behavior, and the environmental manipulations that will produce a desirable outcome.

## REFERENCES

Bihm, E. M., Kienlen, T. L., Ness, M. E., & Poindexter, A. R. (1991). Factor structure of the Motivation Assessment Scale for persons with mental retardation. *Psychological Reports, 68,* 1235–1238.

Conroy, M. A., Fox, J. J., Bucklin, A., & Good, W. (1996). An analysis of the reliability and stability of the Motivation Assessment Scale in assessing the challenging behaviors of persons with developmental disabilities. *Education and Training in Mental Retardation and Developmental Disabilities, 31,* 243–250.

Dracobly, J. D., Dozier, C. L., Briggs, A. M., & Juanico, J. F. (2018). Reliability and validity of indirect assessment outcomes: Experts versus caregivers. *Learning and Motivation, 62,* 77–90.

Duker, P. C., & Sigafoos, J. (1998). The Motivation Assessment Scale: Reliability and construct validity across three topographies of behavior. *Research in Developmental Disabilities, 19,* 131–141.

Durand, V. M. (1990). The "aversives" debate is over: And now the work begins. *Journal of the Association for Persons with Severe Handicaps, 15*(3), 140–141.

Durand, V. M., & Crimmins, D. B. (1988). Identifying the variables maintaining self-injurious behavior. *Journal of Autism and Developmental Disorders, 18,* 99–117.

Durand, V. M., & Crimmins, D. B. (1992). *The Motivation Assessment Scale (MAS) administration guide.* Topeka, KS: Monaco & Associates.

Fisher, W. W., & Mazur, J. E. (1997). Basic and applied research on choice responding. *Journal of Applied Behavior Analysis, 30,* 387–410.

Fisher, W. W., Piazza, C. C., Bowman, L. G., & Amari, A. (1996). Integrating caregiver report with systematic choice assessment to enhance reinforcer identification. *American Journal of Mental Retardation, 101,* 15–25.

Fisher, W., Piazza, C. C., Bowman, L. G., Hagopian, L. P., Owens, J. C., & Slevin, I. (1992). A comparison of two approaches for identifying reinforcers for persons with severe and profound disabilities. *Journal of Applied Behavior Analysis, 25,* 491–498.

Fryling, M. J., & Baires, N. A. (2016). The practical importance of the distinction between open and closed-ended indirect assessments. *Behavior Analysis in Practice, 9,* 146–151.

Green, G., & Striefel, S. (1988). Response restriction and substitution with autistic children. *Journal of the Experimental Analysis of Behavior, 50,* 21–32.

Hanley, G. P. (2010). Prevention and treatment of severe problem behavior. In E. Mayville & J. Mulick (Eds.), *Behavioral foundations of autism intervention* (pp. 233–256). New York: Sloman.

Hanley, G. P. (2012). Functional assessment of problem behavior: Dispelling myths, overcoming implementation obstacles, and developing new lore. *Behavior Analysis in Practice, 5,* 54–72.

Horner, R. H., & Day, H. M. (1991). The effects of response efficiency on functionally equivalent competing behaviors. *Journal of Applied Behavior Analysis, 24,* 719–732.

Hosp, J. L., Howell, K. W., & Hosp, M. K. (2003). Characteristics of behavior rating scales: Implications for practice in assessment and behavioral support. *Journal of Positive Behavior Interventions, 5,* 201–208.

Individuals with Disabilities Education Improvement Act of 2004, 20 U.S.C. 1400 et seq. (2004).

Iwata, B. A., & DeLeon, I. G. (1996). *Functional Analysis Screening Tool (FAST).* Gainesville: Florida Center on Self-Injury, University of Florida.

Iwata, B. A., DeLeon, I. G., & Roscoe, E. M. (2013). Reliability and validity of the functional analysis screening tool. *Journal of Applied Behavioral Analysis, 46*(1), 271–284.

Iwata, B. A., Dorsey, M. F., Slifer, K. J., Bauman, K. E., & Richman, G. S. (1994). Toward a functional analysis of self-injury. *Journal of Applied Behavior Analysis, 27,* 197–209. (Reprinted from *Analysis and Intervention in Developmental Disabilities, 2,* 3–20, 1982)

Iwata, B. A., Vollmer, T. R., & Zarcone, J. R. (1990). The experimental (functional) analysis of behavior disorders: Methodology, applications, and limitations. In A. C. Repp & N. N. Singh (Eds.), *Perspectives on the use of nonaversive and aversive interventions for persons with developmental disabilities* (pp. 301–330). Sycamore, IL: Sycamore.

Jin, C. S., Hanley, G. P., & Beaulieu, L. (2013). An individualized and comprehensive approach to treating sleep problems in young children. *Journal of Applied Behavior Analysis, 46,* 161–180.

Kelley, M. E., Fisher, W. W., Lomas, J. E., & Sanders, R. Q. (2006). Some effects of stimulant medication on response allocation: A double-blind analysis. *Journal of Applied Behavior Analysis, 39,* 243–247.

Kennedy, C. H., & Meyer, K. A. (1996). Sleep deprivation, allergy symptoms, and negatively reinforced problem behavior. *Journal of Applied Behavior Analysis, 29,* 133–135.

Lennox, D. B., & Miltenberger, R. G. (1989). Conducting a functional assessment of problem behavior in applied settings. *Journal of the Association for Persons with Severe Handicaps, 14,* 304–311.

Lewis, T. J., Scott, T. M., & Sugai, G. (1994). The Problem Behavior Questionnaire: A teacher-based instrument to develop functional hypotheses of problem behavior in general education classrooms. *Diagnostique, 19,* 103–115.

Lloyd, B. P., & Kennedy, C. H. (2014). Assessment and treatment of challenging behaviour for individuals with intellectual disability: A research review. *Journal of Applied Research in Intellectual Disabilities, 27,* 187–199.

Mace, F. C., Neef, N. A., Shade, D., & Mauro, B. C. (1996). Effects of problem difficulty and reinforcer quality on time allocated to concurrent arithmetic problems. *Journal of Applied Behavior Analysis, 29,* 11–24.

Matson, J. L., Bamburg, J. W., Cherry, K. E., & Paclawskyj, T. R. (1999). A validity study on the Questions about Behavioral Function (QABF) scale: Predicting treatment success for self-injury, aggression, and stereotypies. *Research in Developmental Disabilities, 20,* 142–160.

Matson, J. L., & Vollmer, T. R. (1995). *User's guide: Questions about Behavioral Function (QABF).* Baton Rouge, LA: Scientific.

Michael, J. (1993). Establishing operations. *Behavior Analyst, 16,* 191–206.

Michael, J. (2000). Implications and refinements of the establishing operation concept. *Journal of Applied Behavior Analysis, 33,* 401–410.

Neef, N. A., & Lutz, M. N. (2001). A brief computer-based assessment of reinforcer dimensions affecting choice. *Journal of Applied Behavior Analysis, 34,* 57–60.

Neef, N. A., Mace, F. C., & Shade, D. (1993). Impulsivity in students with serious emotional disturbance: The interactive effects of reinforcer rate, delay, and quality. *Journal of Applied Behavior Analysis, 26,* 37–52.

Neef, N. A., Shade, D., & Miller, M. S. (1994). Assessing influential dimensions of reinforcers on choice in students with serious emotional disturbance. *Journal of Applied Behavior Analysis, 27,* 575–583.

Newton, J. T., & Sturmey, P. (1991). The Motivation Assessment Scale: Inter-rater reliability and internal consistency in a British sample. *Journal of Mental Deficiency Research, 35,* 472–474.

Nicholson, J., Konstantinidi, E., & Furniss, F. (2006). On some psychometric properties of the Questions about Behavioral Function (QABF) scale. *Research in Developmental Disabilities, 27,* 337–352.

O'Neill, R. E., Horner, R. H., Albin, R. W., Sprague, J. R., Storey, K., & Newton, J. (1997). *Functional assessment and program development for problem behavior: A practical handbook.* Pacific Grove, CA: Brooks/Cole.

O'Reilly, M. F. (1997). Functional analysis of episodic self-injury correlated with recurrent otitis media. *Journal of Applied Behavior Analysis, 30,* 165–167.

Pace, G. M., Ivancic, M. T., Edwards, G. L., Iwata, B. A., & Page, T. J. (1985). Assessment of stimulus preference and reinforcer value with profoundly retarded individuals. *Journal of Applied Behavior Analysis, 18,* 249–255.

Paclawskyj, T. R., Matson, J. L., Rush, K. S., Smalls, Y., & Vollmer, T. R. (2000). Questions about Behavioral Function (QABF): A behavioral checklist for functional assessment of aberrant behavior. *Research in Developmental Disabilities, 21,* 223–229.

Paclawskyj, T. R., Matson, J. L., Rush, K. S., Smalls, Y., & Vollmer, T. R. (2001). Assessment of the convergent validity of the Questions about Behavioral Function scale with analogue functional analysis and the Motivation Assessment Scale. *Journal of Intellectual Disability Research, 45,* 484–494.

Piazza, C. C., & Fisher, W. W. (1991). A faded bedtime with response cost protocol for treatment of multiple sleep problems in children. *Journal of Applied Behavior Analysis, 24,* 129–140.

Roane, H. S., Vollmer, T. R., Ringdahl, J. E., & Marcus, B. A. (1998). Evaluation of a brief stimulus preference assessment. *Journal of Applied Behavior Analysis, 31,* 605–620.

Saini, V., Ubdegrove, K., Biran, S., & Duncan, R. (2019). A preliminary evaluation of interrater reliability and concurrent validity of open-ended indirect assessment. *Behavior Analysis in Practice, 13,* 114–125.

Shogren, K. A., & Rojahn, J. (2003). Convergent reliability and validity of the Questions about Behavioral Function and the Motivation Assessment Scale: A replication study. *Journal of Developmental and Physical Disabilities, 15,* 367–375.

Sigafoos, J., Kerr, M., & Roberts, D. (1994). Interrater reliability of the Motivation Assessment Scale: Failure to replicate with aggressive behavior. *Research in Developmental Disabilities, 15,* 333–342.

Simo-Pinatella, D., Alomar-Kurz, E., Font-Roura, J., Gine, C., Matson, J. L., & Cifre, I. (2013). Questions about Behavioral Function (QABF): Adaptation and validation of the Spanish version. *Research in Developmental Disabilities, 34,* 1248–1255.

Singh, N. N., Donatelli, L. S., Best, A., Williams, D. E., Barrera, F. J., Lenz, M. W., et al. (1993). Factor structure of the Motivation Assessment Scale. *Journal of Intellectual Disability Research, 37,* 65–74.

Steege, M. W., & Watson, T. S. (2009). *Conducting school-based functional behavioral assessments* (2nd ed.). New York: Guilford Press.

Umbreit, J. (1996). Functional analysis of disruptive behavior in an inclusive classroom. *Journal of Early Intervention, 20,* 18–29.

Zarcone, J. R., Rodgers, T. A., Iwata, B. A., Rourke, D. A., & Dorsey, M. F. (1991). Reliability analysis of the Motivation Assessment Scale: A failure to replicate. *Research in Developmental Disabilities, 12,* 349–360.

# CHAPTER 12

# Direct Observation

Rachel H. Thompson and John C. Borrero

This chapter focuses on methods of assessment involving the direct observation of behavior. Researchers and behavior analysts typically refer to these as *descriptive* methods, in that the assessments *describe* a series of naturally occurring events, but do not demonstrate a functional relation between those events (i.e., there is no experimental manipulation). As with indirect assessment, the goal of the descriptive analysis[1] is to identify naturally occurring behavior–environment relations. Unlike indirect methods, descriptive analysis involves the measurement of behavior and various environmental events through repeated direct observation.

Researchers have used descriptive-analysis methods widely in the behavioral sciences for decades. In fact, one of the defining features of ethology, a field that grew out of the biological tradition, is direct observation of naturally occurring behavior (Hine, 1982; Tinbergen, 1951). A seminal paper by Bijou, Peterson, and Ault (1968) introduced this approach to the field of applied behavior analysis. This paper highlighted the importance of descriptive studies of behavior, described an ideal interrelation between descriptive and experimental studies, and recommended specific descriptive-analysis procedures to improve the objectivity and ease of interpretation of descriptive data.

Bijou et al. (1968) presented a case study of a young boy in a nursery school setting to illustrate

the key components of a descriptive analysis. They described the classroom, the routine, the number of children and adults present, and precise operational definitions of child and adult behavior. They conducted observations during 3-hour blocks across 28 days during one of several classroom activities such as art or snacktime. They assessed observer reliability and presented data graphically to depict levels of various forms of child and teacher behavior. In short, the researchers developed a model for descriptive analyses and provided a case illustration of the method in application.

Bijou et al. (1968) noted that experimental studies are essential for understanding behavior, in that experimental manipulation uncovers functional relations between behavior and environment. However, as Baer (1973) pointed out, an experimental demonstration that a given variable produces a particular behavior change demonstrates only that the relation is possible. That those same circumstances influence behavior under naturally occurring conditions does not necessarily follow. For example, a behavior analyst might demonstrate language acquisition experimentally, using a shaping procedure (Ghaemmaghami, Hanley, Jessel, & Landa, 2018). These results would indicate only that the behavior analyst *can* shape language, but they do not provide direct evidence that language *is* shaped through typical parent–child interactions. The addition of descriptive data showing that parents provide some potentially reinforcing event following successive approximations to language would support the contention that shaping is responsible for language acquisition outside the laboratory. Thus, as Bijou et al. and Baer point out, descriptive analysis is a vital tool in understanding naturally occurring behavior–environment relations (e.g., Glodowski, Thompson, & Martel, 2019).

## CHOOSING AN APPROPRIATE PROCEDURE

A behavior analyst may consider several factors when selecting a method for a descriptive analysis. Perhaps the most obvious factor is the overall purpose of the descriptive analysis; that is, what is the behavior analyst attempting to accomplish by conducting the analysis? Although behavior analysts conduct descriptive analyses most commonly to develop hypotheses regarding behavioral function, there may be other purposes as well. Such purposes may include (1) identifying common contingencies in naturalistic settings (e.g., Borrero, Woods, Borrero, Masler, & Lesser, 2010; McComas et al., 2009; McKerchar & Thompson, 2004; Rodriguez, Thompson, Stocco, & Schlichenmeyer, 2013; Thompson & Iwata, 2001; Simmons, Akers, & Fisher, 2019); (2) establishing a baseline by which to assess the efficacy of intervention (e.g., Rapp, Vollmer, St. Peter, Dozier, & Cotnoir, 2004); (3) studying basic behavioral processes (e.g., reinforcement, punishment, extinction) under naturally occurring circumstances (Addison & Lerman, 2009; Borrero, Vollmer, Borrero, & Bourret, 2005; Sloman et al., 2005); and (4) studying quantitative models of behavior, such as the matching law (e.g., Borrero & Vollmer, 2002; Cero & Falligant, 2020; Oliver, Hall, & Nixon, 1999) and behavioral momentum (e.g., Strand, Wahler, & Herring, 2000). Even though the focus of this chapter is on applications of descriptive-analysis procedures to develop hypotheses about behavioral function, behavior analysts should recognize that descriptive analysis is a highly flexible and widely used means of studying naturally occurring behavior that they can adapt easily for many purposes.

A second consideration in the selection of descriptive-analysis methods involves available resources. The most sophisticated methods of gathering and analyzing descriptive-analysis data involve (1) direct observation by trained observers who are free from other responsibilities (e.g., patient care) during the observation period; (2) computers to collect, organize, and analyze data; and (3) the availability of a trained professional to interpret and use results to make intervention decisions. When such resources are not available, the only reasonable option may be to implement descriptive-analysis procedures that are relatively easy and inexpensive to carry out. For example, observers might use paper and pencil during brief intervals (e.g., momentary time sampling) to collect data throughout the day. Importantly, behavior analysts should consider how to use the available resources to incorporate descriptive analysis into their everyday clinical practice.

## DEVELOPING HYPOTHESES ABOUT BEHAVIORAL FUNCTION

Behavior analysts often use descriptive analysis in practice to develop hypotheses about the function of behavior. Oliver, Pratt, and Normand (2015) surveyed 682 Board Certified Behavior Analysts and reported that 94% *always* or *almost always* conducted descriptive analyses. Similarly, Roscoe, Phillips, Kelly, Farber and Dube (2015) surveyed 205 behavior analysts in the state of Massachusetts, and 84% of respondents reported using descriptive analysis most frequently. A concerning finding of both studies is that behavior analysts reported frequently using descriptive analyses to generate hypotheses about behavioral function, without using a functional analysis to verify that a functional relation existed. Oliver et al. reported that 63% of behavior analysts reported *never* or *almost never* conducting functional analyses, and the Roscoe et al. survey found that 62% of behavior analysts reported using a descriptive analysis in the absence of a functional analysis.

The practice of prescribing interventions based on the results of a descriptive analysis alone is not empirically supported. Although there are isolated reports of successful intervention based only on descriptive data (e.g., VanDerHeyden, Witt, & Gatti, 2001), there is strong evidence of poor correspondence between descriptive and functional analyses (e.g., Camp, Iwata, Hammond, & Bloom, 2009; Hall, 2005; Mace & Lalli, 1991; Martens et al., 2019; Pence, Roscoe, Bourret, & Ahearn, 2009; Piazza et al., 2003; Thompson & Iwata, 2007). Descriptive analysis may identify events correlated with but not functionally related to the target behavior, or may fail to identify sources of reinforcement that caregivers deliver only intermittently or under circumscribed conditions that the descriptive analysis did not sample (see Lerman & Iwata, 1993, for a discussion). When this occurs, the prescribed intervention may include irrelevant components, may lack essential features, or both. This lack of correspondence between descriptive and functional analyses raises considerable concern about the practice of prescribing interventions based solely on the results of descriptive analyses.

Behavior analysts should use the results of descriptive analyses to generate hypotheses about behavioral function and to inform the development of functional-analysis conditions. Results of the functional analysis are then used to evaluate whether events correlated with problem behavior under natural conditions are functionally related to problem behavior. Hagopian, Rooker, Jessel, and DeLeon (2013) described a clinical model whereby they initially used standard functional-analysis conditions to assess problem behavior, and they modified the functional analysis as necessary to obtain clear results. The standardized analysis yielded an interpretable outcome in only 47% of 176 consecutive clinical cases. The functional analysis ultimately produced clear results in 87% of cases when the researchers modified antecedents, consequences, the experimental design, or a combination of these variables. These results suggest the value of individualizing functional analyses. Hagopian et al. individualized functional analyses only after a standard analysis produced unclear results (see also Roscoe, Schlichenmeyer, & Dube, 2015). An alternative approach is to individualize functional-analysis conditions from the start, rather than waiting for unclear functional-analysis results (see Hanley, 2012, for a discussion). Data from descriptive analyses may be a useful source of information for individualizing functional-analysis conditions (see Schlichenmeyer, Roscoe, Rooker, Wheeler, & Dube, 2015).

The behavior analyst must structure the descriptive analysis to identify idiosyncratic variables for inclusion in a functional analysis. Behavior analysts often structure analyses to identify correlations between problem behavior and the antecedents and consequences described by Iwata, Dorsey, Slifer, Bauman, and Richman (1982/1994). The behavior analyst should expand the descriptive analyses to include more events and to describe specific interactions beyond those that Iwata et al. assessed. For example, Borrero et al. (2010) recorded specific caregiver responses such as coaxing, threats, and statements of concern, rather than simply recording the general category of attention

delivery, to identify potential reinforcers for food refusal. Behavior analysts may refer to Hanley, Iwata, and McCord (2001), Hagopian et al. (2013), and Schlichenmeyer et al. (2015) for guidance on how to identify a broader range of variables to measure during the descriptive analysis. Narrative recording is also a useful starting point for identifying idiosyncratic variables correlated with problem behavior (see Rodriguez et al., 2013).

## VARIATIONS IN MEASUREMENT DURING DIRECT OBSERVATION

Generally, direct observation may involve periodic *sampling* or *continuous recording* of behavior and other environmental events. Considerations for using either sampling or continuous recording include the effort of each method and the amount and quality of the resultant data. Sampling methods involve collecting data at the end of specified intervals. Harding et al. (1999) used a time-sampling procedure to assess child behavior at the end of each 10-second interval, while allocating the remainder of the interval recording to teacher behavior. Sampling procedures require somewhat less effort, depending on how frequently observers collect data, but provide data that are less comprehensive than those of continuous methods. Continuous methods involve collecting data throughout the observation period on each instance of the target response, and in some cases environmental events occurring in close temporal proximity. For example, Moss et al. (2005) used continuous recording to collect data on the self-injurious behavior (SIB) of eight participants diagnosed with Cornelia de Lange syndrome and potential evocative events contiguous with SIB. Continuous methods are more labor-intensive than sampling, but also provide richer samples of behavioral data.

*Event recording* (i.e., recording the number of times a response occurs), and recording the *occurrence* or *nonoccurrence* of behavior in relatively small intervals (e.g., 10–20 seconds), are continuous-observation methods. A study by Anderson and Long (2002) illustrates both methods. Observers recorded each time problem behavior occurred (i.e., event recording) and scored the occurrence or nonoccurrence of potentially evocative environmental events (e.g., periods of low attention) during 5-second intervals.

Partial-interval and whole-interval recording are options for recording the occurrence or nonoccurrence of events. *Partial-interval recording* involves scoring an event if it occurs during any portion of a specified interval, which may overestimate the occurrence of events (Gardenier, MacDonald, & Green, 2004). By contrast, *whole-interval recording* involves scoring an event if it occurs for the duration of the specified interval, which may underestimate the occurrence of events (see Cooper, Heron, & Heward, 2007). Selection of the appropriate measurement procedure will depend in part on whether the response is high- or low-frequency, and whether the response is targeted for increase or decrease.

Below, we describe methods of data collection and analysis that behavior analysts commonly use. We progress from methods that examine behavior–environment relations with relatively low resolution to those with relatively greater resolution. Each method of data collection involves either continuous observation or periodic sampling of behavior. In this section, we highlight methods of summarizing data and make specific recommendations regarding appropriate applications of each method.

## The Scatterplot

The *scatterplot* is a form of descriptive analysis used to identify temporal patterns of a target behavior under naturally occurring conditions. Typically, this form of assessment involves continuous observation of behavior and recording of the target behavior and the time during which the behavior occurred. The scatterplot differs from other forms of descriptive analysis, because the behavior analyst does not record environmental events surrounding the target behavior. In addition, the manner of data depiction is different from that of other methods. In most cases, the behavior analyst uses a code to indicate target behavior frequency on a grid in which each cell indicates a time interval (e.g., 30 minutes), and each column represents a day. For example, an empty cell may indicate that the target behavior did not occur during the interval; a cell with a slash may indicate a low frequency of the target behavior; and a darkened cell may indicate a high frequency of the target behavior (Touchette, MacDonald, & Langer, 1985).

The behavior analyst analyzes data through visual inspection of the grid to identify times associated with zero, low, and high frequencies of problem behavior. If the analyst identifies a temporal pattern of behavior, he or she might use this information to modify features of the environment, such as staffing patterns or activities, that correlate with the problematic times. Further isolating the environmental conditions associated with problem behavior may require additional assessment if multiple variables occur during the problematic times. For example, Arndorfer, Miltenberger, Woster, Rortvedt, and Gaffaney (1994) used a parent-completed scatterplot to identify times during which problem behavior was likely. Observers then recorded antecedents and consequences associated with problem behavior during times identified through the scatterplot.

Touchette et al. (1985) illustrated the use of the scatterplot, presenting data on the temporal patterns of problem behavior displayed by three participants. The scatterplot showed that problem behavior correlated reliably with particular times for two participants, and this information led to environmental modifications aimed at reducing problem behavior. Scatterplot data were uninterpretable for the third participant; problem behavior was not correlated reliably with any particular time. Results of a study by Kahng et al. (1998) suggested that the third case may be more representative. These researchers examined scatterplots depicting the frequency of problem behavior for 15 participants, and found that none of the datasets showed a predictable temporal pattern. However, the researchers identified temporal patterns of behavior for 12 participants, using statistical-control charts of the same data (Pfadt & Wheeler, 1995); these findings suggest that the main limitation of the scatterplot may be the data depiction and analysis rather than the measurement. Nevertheless, the practical utility of the scatterplot is limited severely if the user must construct statistical-control charts for data interpretation.

Behavior analysts report using scatterplots frequently, despite the method's limitations (Ellingson, Miltenberger, & Long, 1999), perhaps because they are easy to use. The published literature describes scatterplot assessment infrequently, but further evaluation of this method may be valuable. For example, the scatterplot may be more useful for temporally organized responses. Ashbaugh and Peck (1998) used a scatterplot to evaluate parent-collected data on disturbed sleep exhibited by a typically developing 2-year-old girl. Data revealed many intervals of sleep during scheduled awake hours, and many intervals awake during scheduled sleep hours. Bedtime fading and response cost modified this pattern. More recently, Maas, Didden, Bouts, Smits, and Curfs (2009) used scatterplot data to assess signs of sleepiness and disruptive behavior for individuals diagnosed with

Prader–Willi syndrome. Conceivably, behavior analysts could use scatterplots to assess temporal patterns of enuresis and feeding among dependent populations (e.g., older adults, infants in child care settings). Results may be useful, for example, in designing interventions (e.g., appropriate timing of scheduled toilet visits) and developing staffing patterns (e.g., allocating more staff members to feeding duties at particular times).

## A-B-C Recording

Unlike the scatterplot, most descriptive analyses involve recording several environmental events, such as antecedents and consequences, surrounding the target behavior. Researchers refer to this type of analysis as *antecedent–behavior–consequence* (A-B-C) recording, because its goal is to capture the familiar three-term contingency. The recorded events are typically those that are contiguous with the target behavior (e.g., Vollmer, Borrero, Wright, Van Camp, & Lalli, 2001), but researchers have made attempts to record more temporally distant events that may occasion or evoke the target behavior (e.g., Carr, Smith, Giacin, Whelan, & Pancari, 2003). This general method may involve either continuous observation and recording of events, or recording antecedent and consequent events only when the target behavior occurs. This section describes several A-B-C recording and analysis procedures.

### Narrative Recording

Narrative recording involves a written account of observed events (Thompson, Symons, & Felce, 2000). The procedure is relatively easy to implement and requires minimal equipment and training. Historically, narrative-recording procedures have included a running description of events without any specific guidelines for recording (e.g., event categories, operational definitions; Bijou, Peterson, Harris, Allen, & Johnston, 1969); however, some forms of narrative recording impose more structure on observations. For example, the Detailed Behavior Report (Groden, 1989; Groden & Lantz, 2001) prompts observers to provide a narrative description of events in specific antecedent (e.g., activity, social, interpersonal) and consequence (e.g., implementation of a behavior-management program) categories.

A potential advantage of narrative recording is the level of detail and amount of qualitative information it captures, relative to other descriptive-analysis methods. In view of these strengths, narrative recording may be useful for developing operational definitions for problem and replacement behavior (Borrero, Vollmer, & Borrero, 2004; Repp & Karsh, 1994; Wahler, Winkel, Peterson, & Morrison, 1965) and may familiarize the observer with scheduled activities and transition periods (Bijou et al., 1969). In addition, narrative-recording procedures may identify idiosyncratic variables associated with problem behavior. For example, narrative recording may be useful in determining qualitative features of naturally occurring antecedent events (e.g., instruction delivery; Borrero et al., 2004) and consequent events (e.g., quality of attention; Richman & Hagopian, 1999; Rodriguez, Thompson, Schlichenmeyer, & Stocco, 2012), which behavior analysts can test in a functional analysis.

A descriptive analysis is unlikely to detect unique features of the behavior or environment when the behavior analyst develops the measurement system a priori, based on common behavior–environment relations. The flexible nature of narrative recording makes it more appropriate than more structured recording methods for these applications. Similarly, narrative-recording procedures may be useful for the evaluation and description of generative or novel behavior (e.g., verbal behavior; Hamo, Blum-Kulka, & Hacohen, 2004; Hart & Risley, 1995) that would be difficult to specify or define before observations.

However, as Bijou et al. (1968) point out, these potential strengths simultaneously present several barriers to analyzing narrative data, which severely limit its usefulness. For example, narrative recording may involve much observer inference, such as when the Detailed Behavior Report prompts observers to describe covert antecedents and affective states (Groden, 1989). This reliance on observer inference is likely to limit both interobserver agreement and the identification of potentially influential and manipulable features of the environment. In addition, narrative recording may lack many quantifiable features of behavior and environment, making it difficult to transform the data into behavioral units (e.g., individual responses, specific antecedents) for analysis. In some respects, the basic components of descriptive analysis described by Bijou et al. represented a response to then-common methods of narrative recording that were lacking in quantifiable dimensions (e.g., Barker & Wright, 1955).

## A-B-C Checklist

The objectivity associated with descriptive analysis is improved greatly when behavior analysts identify and operationally define target events before direct observation, as with an A-B-C checklist. Observers record the occurrence of problem behavior and indicate with a checkmark which of several antecedents and consequences are associated with behavior. Here the term *checklist* refers only to the fact that observers choose from a menu of options when recording antecedents and consequences. Readers should not confuse this approach with indirect forms of assessment (see Gadaire, Kelley, & LaRue, Chapter 11, this volume) that involve caregivers' responding to questionnaires presented in checklist format.

Arndorfer et al. (1994) used this strategy to structure home observations of five children who displayed problem behavior. The researchers based antecedent categories on information gathered during parent interviews, and structured consequence categories based on the common functions of problem behavior (Iwata et al., 1982/1994). Observers checked off the appropriate antecedent and consequence categories when problem behavior occurred during the descriptive analyses. These researchers achieved a high level of interobserver agreement and could relate the results of the descriptive analysis to manipulable features of the environment.

Although there are few examples of this form of direct observation in the literature, behavior analysts report frequently using an A-B-C checklist (Ellingson et al., 1999). Behavior analysts can adopt this method readily because individuals directly responsible for the client (e.g., teachers, direct care staff) can implement it with relatively little training. Lerman, Hovanetz, Strobel, and Tetreault (2009) found that special educators collected data more accurately when they used a structured format to record A-B-C data than when they provided a narrative account of antecedents and consequences. In addition, the A-B-C checklist has the potential to provide more objective information about manipulable features of the environment, compared to the scatterplot or narrative-recording methods. Thus this method may be useful in gathering preliminary data on variables surrounding the target behavior and may be desirable when a trained observer is unavailable.

The A-B-C checklist remains limited in that it provides little information about quantifiable dimensions of behavior and relevant environmental events, although it represents an improvement over narrative recording with respect to objectivity. Typically, A-B-C checklist data simply indicate that a target behavior occurred with unknown frequency and duration, and that some events preceded and followed the behavior without reference to the time between these events and behavior.

## Frequency, Interval, and Time-Sample Recording

A record of the frequency, duration, or occurrence of behavior and environmental events during continuous observation (e.g., Piazza et al., 2003; Vollmer et al., 2001) or time samples (Harding et al., 1999) is most appropriate when the goal is to obtain more detailed information about quantifiable dimensions of naturally occurring events. This method of A-B-C recording is advantageous in that it allows for objective measurement and the analysis of relations between events of quantified dimensions. As a result, this approach to descriptive analysis facilitates integration of descriptive and experimental methods and results, as recommended by Bijou et al. (1968). Therefore, researchers use this method of descriptive analysis commonly in studies involving the integration (e.g., Galiatsatos & Graff, 2003; Roscoe, Schlichenmeyer, & Dube, 2015) or comparison (Camp et al., 2009; Pence et al., 2009) of assessment methods.

Behavior analysts may have more difficulty using this approach than using alternative descriptive-analysis methods when resources are limited. The measurement of the frequency, duration, or occurrence of a target behavior and the surrounding environmental events can involve an elaborate coding system that requires specific training to develop and implement. In addition, trained observers who are free from other duties may be necessary to implement this more detailed form of descriptive analysis.

Although manual (i.e., paper-and-pencil) methods of data collection are appropriate for this type of analysis, computerized data collection may facilitate measurement and data analysis in some cases. For example, computerized systems may be more appropriate when multiple response measures have a negative impact on interobserver agreement, when second-by-second changes in behavior or environmental context are essential to the analysis, or when complex methods of data analysis are desirable.

## METHODS OF DATA ANALYSIS: PROBABILITY ANALYSES

Methods of analysis for direct-observation data range from simple (e.g., tallying the frequency of antecedents, behavior, and consequences) to complex (e.g., computing the Yule's Q statistic; Rahman, Oliver, & Alderman, 2010). Typical methods of data analysis provide gross descriptions of behavior and related environmental events for many of the descriptive-analysis procedures described earlier. However, more complex methods of data analysis provide more fine-grained descriptions. In this section, we focus on two methods that researchers have studied extensively both within and outside applied behavior analysis: comparative-probability analyses and lag-sequential analysis. We can conduct both types of analyses using hand data-collection procedures; however, computerized data collection and analysis programs may facilitate these analyses. Notably, however, comparative-probability and lag-sequential analyses do not represent the end of the complexity continuum. Readers interested in statistics that capture the degree of sequential associations between events may start with Yoder and Symons (2010) and Lloyd, Kennedy, and Yoder (2013).

### Static-Probability Analyses

Many researchers have analyzed descriptive-analysis data by calculating conditional probabilities to determine whether relations exist between behavior and environmental events. *Conditional probabilities* evaluate the likelihood of one event (e.g., attention), *given that* another event occurred (e.g., aggression). Frequently, evaluations of conditional probabilities involve analyses of the target response (e.g., aggression) and a potential reinforcer (e.g., attention). In many cases, researchers calculate and compare the conditional probabilities of various events (e.g., attention, escape, material presentation) to determine the event(s) with the highest conditional probability, given the target behavior (e.g., Reed, Luiselli, Morizio, & Child, 2010). This event or events, then, are considered the likely maintaining variable(s) (e.g., Anderson & Long, 2002; Noell, VanDerHeyden, Gatti, & Whitmarsh, 2001).

One limitation of this approach is that the analysis may identify variables that occur at a high frequency following the target behavior only because the caregiver presents the event at a high frequency, independently of responding. For ex-

ample, it is likely that any observed target behavior will be followed by teacher attention if teacher attention is available (independently of behavior) nearly continuously during an observation. In this case, the conditional probability of attention would be very high, although the target behavior does not increase the probability of attention. To address this weakness, Vollmer et al. (2001) recommend comparing conditional probabilities to unconditional or background probabilities of the same event, to determine whether the probability of an event (e.g., attention) changes due to the target behavior (i.e., to detect a possible contingency) (see also Herscovitch, Roscoe, Libby, Bourret, & Ahearn, 2009). A conceptually similar alternative to comparing the conditional probability of an environmental event, given target behavior, to the unconditional probability of that event is to compare the conditional probability to the probability of the environmental event, given that *no behavior* occurred (e.g., Reed et al., 2010). Though conceptually similar, this approach may prove more challenging, because it requires a somewhat arbitrary determination of what defines a period with no behavior (e.g., Hagopian, Paclawskyj, & Contrucci-Kuhn, 2005).

### Dynamic-Probability Analyses

Closely related to the concept of comparative-probability analysis is the method of lag-sequential analysis (Bakeman & Gottman, 1997). Typically, evaluations of comparative probabilities produce one conditional and one unconditional probability value. For example, observers may record data for 4 hours and report the probability of attention and the probability of attention, given an instance of the target response, for the entire 4-hour observation. This information provides a rather static depiction of what is likely a very dynamic exchange, even though it has proven useful in evaluations of behavior–environment relations. Lag-sequential analysis, on the other hand, can provide a more refined description of exchanges in the natural environment by depicting comparative probabilities before and after an instance of the target response on a second-by-second basis.

The term *lag* conveys that researchers may evaluate behavior–environment relations or behavior–behavior relations several seconds before or after the response occurs (e.g., Emerson, Thompson, Reeves, Henderson, & Robertson, 1995; Samaha et al., 2009). For example, a lag +1 indicates that the probability of an event is calculated 1 unit (e.g., 1 second) after the occurrence of the target response. A lag –1 indicates that the probability of an environmental event is calculated 1 unit (e.g., 1 second) before the occurrence of the target response. Borrero and Borrero (2008) demonstrated the use of lag-sequential analysis. The researchers hypothesized that occurrences of severe problem behavior, such as head hitting, were preceded reliably by less severe forms of problem behavior, such as screaming, for two students with autism spectrum disorder. Borrero and Borrero described the less severe forms of problem behavior as potential *precursors* to more severe forms, to the extent that occurrences of one might be reliable predictors of occurrences of the other. They evaluated the probability of severe problem behavior, given that it was preceded by an instance of less severe problem behavior (i.e., conditional probability), and compared that to the probability of the less severe problem behavior (i.e., the unconditional probability) to quantify this potential relation. The window for the lag-sequential analysis was +50 seconds (i.e., 50 seconds after each instance of problem behavior) and –50 seconds (i.e., 50 seconds before each instance of problem behavior). Results for both students showed a sharp increase in the probability of a potential precursor in the 1-second intervals immediately before an instance of problem behavior.

Vollmer et al. (2001) also conducted comparative-probability analyses and used a variation of the lag-sequential analysis procedure described by Borrero and Borrero (2008). The researchers conducted a descriptive analysis of interactions between participants referred for the assessment and intervention of severe problem behavior and their primary caregivers. Next, the researchers compared the probability of an environmental event to the probability of an environmental event, given problem behavior in the context of various potential establishing operations (e.g., low attention). Researchers evaluated probabilities with lags of +5, +10, +15, and +20, using a variant of the lag-sequential-analysis procedures; that is, the researchers calculated the probability of an event within 5, 10, 15, and 20 seconds of a particular time for the unconditional probability or an instance of the target response for the conditional probability. Even though the procedure does not provide the same level of analysis as the method Borrero and Borrero described, the method does provide four intervals to evaluate probabilistic changes, and Vollmer et al. reported that the method was useful in identifying *potential* contingencies between environmental events and target responses. Furthermore, relative to the method Borrero and Borrero described (which involved analyses of ± 50 seconds), the windows Vollmer et al. evaluated may be more practical for those working in nonresearch settings.

Relative rather than absolute probabilities are important for both static- and dynamic-probability analyses (e.g., Rooker, DeLeon, Borrero, Frank-Crawford, & Roscoe, 2015). For example, a positive contingency between aggression and attention is unlikely if the probability of attention, given problem behavior, is .20. By contrast, problem behavior increases the probability of attention if the probability of attention, given problem behavior, is .10.

Researchers have been the primary users of the data-analysis techniques just described, and they have used them primarily to evaluate descriptive-analysis data for research (e.g., Anderson & Long, 2002; Borrero & Borrero, 2008; Doggett, Edwards, Moore, Tingstrom, & Wilczynski, 2001; Forman, Hall, & Oliver, 2002; Marion, Touchette, & Sandman, 2003; Moss et al., 2005; Noell et al., 2001; Woods, Borrero, Laud, & Borrero, 2010). Perhaps behavior analysts do not use these methods because of their complexity. In addition, although these methods provide a finer-grained analysis of naturally occurring behavior–environment relations than other descriptive-analysis methods produce, they are limited because results suggest correlations between two events (e.g., attention and aggression) but do not identify functional relations (e.g., St. Peter et al., 2005).

## RECOMMENDATIONS

The measurement and analysis of naturally occurring behavior–environment relations are necessary for a complete understanding of behavior. However, the role of descriptive analysis in uncovering potential controlling variables for problem behavior is less clear. The results of two recent surveys show that behavior analysts frequently develop interventions for problem behavior based on the results of descriptive analysis alone. Yet results of several studies showing poor correspondence between descriptive- and experimental-analysis outcomes raise significant concerns about this practice (Camp et al., 2009; Hall, 2005; Mace & Lalli, 1991; Pence et al., 2009; Thompson & Iwata, 2007).

There are inherent limitations to the information that we can gain through descriptive analyses, because this method is limited to correlational and not functional descriptions of naturally occurring behavior–environment relations. Thus we may gain the most complete understanding of these relations by combining descriptive and experimental methods. Descriptive-analysis data provide information regarding the environmental events that are correlated with behavior under naturally occurring conditions, and the experimental analysis identifies those events that are related functionally to the behavior of interest.

We have described several descriptive-analysis methods that vary with respect to the level of detail provided, as well as the level of expertise and amount of resources necessary to conduct the analysis. Of these methods, the scatterplot, narrative recording, and the A-B-C checklist are generally easy to use, and those directly responsible for the participant can implement them with minimal training. A more detailed descriptive analysis involves recording a target behavior and its surrounding events via frequency, interval, or time-sample recording and analyzing relations among the variables. However, this method is resource-intensive and likely to require special training; thus only trained personnel who are dedicated specifically to behavioral assessment are likely to use this type of descriptive analysis. Behavior analysts who allocate resources toward various forms of assessment should remember that even the most sophisticated descriptive analyses yield only correlational data. In many cases, descriptive analyses uncover correlations between problem behavior and events that do not exert control over problem behavior (e.g., Thompson & Iwata, 2007). Therefore, we recommend conducting a brief descriptive analysis to inform the development of functional-analysis conditions in most cases.

## FUTURE RESEARCH

Despite the limitations of descriptive analysis, the apparent ubiquity of its implementation (Oliver et al. 2015; Roscoe, Phillips, et al., 2015) and the importance of understanding the conditions naturally surrounding behavior necessitate additional research. One important use for descriptive analysis is to identify variables for inclusion in a functional analysis. The flexibility of narrative recording is appealing when the behavior analyst's goal is to identify idiosyncratic variables for inclusion in a functional analysis. However, the open-ended nature of this assessment may reduce the accuracy

of recording (Lerman et al., 2009). Mayer and Di-Gennaro Reed (2013) found that narrative data collected by direct care staff did not identify the antecedents of or the consequences for problem behavior accurately. In the same study, researchers demonstrated immediate improvement in accuracy after brief training and the provision of detailed written instructions. Future research should focus on identifying efficient training methods to ensure accuracy of descriptive analyses.

We have focused in this chapter on the use of descriptive analyses to generate hypotheses regarding naturally occurring reinforcers for problem behavior. However, there may be many other uses for descriptive analysis in behavioral assessment. For example, researchers and behavior analysts might use descriptive analysis to identify general practices that appear to promote or interfere with desirable behavior. For example, Austin, Carr, and Agnew (1999) suggested that descriptive analyses might identify the form of instruction that produces the most accurate and efficient performance in organizations. Behavior analysts also might use descriptive analysis to identify socially valid stimuli, responses, or levels of responding to inform social skills training (e.g., Minkin et al., 1976).

## REFERENCES

Addison, L., & Lerman, D. C. (2009). Descriptive analysis of teachers' responses to problem behavior following training. *Journal of Applied Behavior Analysis, 42*, 485–490.

Anderson, C. M., & Long, E. S. (2002). Use of a structured descriptive analysis methodology to identify variables affecting problem behavior. *Journal of Applied Behavior Analysis, 35*, 137–154.

Arndorfer, R. E., Miltenberger, R. G., Woster, S. H., Rortvedt, A. K., & Gaffaney, T. (1994). Home-based descriptive and experimental analysis of problem behaviors in children. *Topics in Early Childhood Special Education, 14*, 64–87.

Ashbaugh, R., & Peck, S. M. (1998). Treatment of sleep problems in a toddler: A replication of the faded bedtime with response cost protocol. *Journal of Applied Behavior Analysis, 31*, 127–129.

Austin, J., Carr, J. E., & Agnew, J. L. (1999). The need for assessment of maintaining variables in OBM. *Journal of Organizational Behavior Management, 19*, 59–87.

Baer, D. M. (1973). The control of the developmental process: Why wait? In J. R. Nesselroade & H. W. Reese (Eds.), *Lifespan developmental psychology: Methodological issues* (pp. 187–193). New York: Academic Press.

Bakeman, R., & Gottman, J. M. (1997). *Observing interaction: An introduction to sequential analyses* (2nd ed.). New York: Cambridge University Press.

Barker, R., & Wright, H. (1955). *Midwest and its children: The psychological ecology of an American town.* Oxford, UK: Peterson.

Bijou, S. W., Peterson, R. F., & Ault, M. H. (1968). A method to integrate descriptive and experimental field studies at the levels of data and empirical concepts. *Journal of Applied Behavior Analysis, 1,* 175–191.

Bijou, S. W., Peterson, R. F., Harris, F. R., Allen, K. E., & Johnston, M. S. (1969). Methodology for experimental studies of young children in natural settings. *Psychological Record, 19,* 177–210.

Borrero, C. S. W., & Borrero, J. C. (2008). Descriptive and experimental analyses of potential precursors to problem behavior. *Journal of Applied Behavior Analysis, 41,* 83–96.

Borrero, C. S. W., Vollmer, T. R., & Borrero, J. C. (2004). Combining descriptive and functional analysis logic to evaluate idiosyncratic variables maintaining aggression. *Behavioral Interventions, 19,* 247–262.

Borrero, C. S. W., Vollmer, T. R., Borrero, J. C., & Bourret, J. (2005). A method of evaluating parameters of reinforcement during parent–child interactions. *Research in Developmental Disabilities, 26,* 577–592.

Borrero, C. S. W., Woods, J. N., Borrero, J. C., Masler, E. A., & Lesser, A. D. (2010). Descriptive analyses of pediatric food refusal and acceptance. *Journal of Applied Behavior Analysis, 43,* 71–88.

Borrero, J. C., & Vollmer, T. R. (2002). An application of the matching law to severe problem behavior. *Journal of Applied Behavior Analysis, 35,* 13–27.

Camp, E. M., Iwata, B. A., Hammond, J. L., & Bloom, S. E. (2009). Antecedent versus consequent events as predictors of problem behavior. *Journal of Applied Behavior Analysis, 42,* 469–483.

Carr, E. G., Smith, C. E., Giacin, T. A., Whelan, B. M., & Pancari, J. (2003). Menstrual discomfort as a biological setting event for severe problem behavior: Assessment and intervention. *American Journal of Mental Retardation, 108,* 117–133.

Cero, I., & Falligant, J. M. (2020). Application of the generalized matching law to chess openings: A gambit analysis. *Journal of Applied Behavior Analysis, 53,* 835–845.

Cooper, J. O., Heron, T. E., & Heward, W. L. (2007). *Applied behavior analysis* (2nd ed.). Upper Saddle River, NJ: Pearson/Merrill-Prentice Hall.

Doggett, R. A., Edwards, R. P., Moore, J. W., Tingstrom, D. H., & Wilczynski, S. M. (2001). An approach to functional assessment in general education classroom settings. *School Psychology Review, 30,* 313–328.

Ellingson, S. A., Miltenberger, R. G., & Long, E. S. (1999). A survey of the use of functional assessment procedures in agencies serving individuals with developmental disabilities. *Behavioral Interventions, 14,* 187–198.

Emerson, E., Thompson, S., Reeves, D., Henderson, D., & Robertson, J. (1995). Descriptive analysis of multiple response topographies of challenging behavior across two settings. *Research in Developmental Disabilities, 16,* 301–329.

Forman, D., Hall, S., & Oliver, C. (2002). Descriptive analysis of self-injurious behavior and self-restraint. *Journal of Applied Research in Intellectual Disabilities, 15,* 1–7.

Galiatsatos, G. T., & Graff, R. B. (2003). Combining descriptive and functional analyses to assess and treat screaming. *Behavioral Interventions, 18,* 123–138.

Gardenier, N. C., MacDonald, R., & Green, G. (2004). Comparison of direct observational methods for measuring stereotypical behavior in children with autism spectrum disorders. *Research in Developmental Disabilities, 25,* 99–118.

Ghaemmaghami, M., Hanley, G. P., Jessel, J., & Landa, R. (2018). Shaping complex functional communication responses. *Journal of Applied Behavior Analysis, 51,* 502–520.

Glodowski, K. R., Thompson, R. H., & Martel. L. (2019). The rooting reflex as an infant feeding cue. *Journal of Applied Behavior Analysis, 52,* 17–27.

Groden, G. (1989). A guide for conducting a comprehensive behavioral analysis of a target behavior. *Journal of Behavior Therapy and Experimental Psychiatry, 20,* 163–170.

Groden, G., & Lantz, S. (2001). The reliability of the Detailed Behavior Report (DBR) in documenting functional assessment observations. *Behavioral Interventions, 16,* 15–25.

Hall, S. S. (2005). Comparing descriptive, experimental and informant-based assessments of problem behaviors. *Research in Developmental Disabilities, 26,* 514–526.

Hagopian, L. P., Paclawskyj, T. R., & Contrucci-Kuhn, S. (2005). The use of conditional probability analysis to identify a response chain leading to the occurrence of eye poking. *Research in Developmental Disabilities, 26,* 393–397.

Hagopian, L. P., Rooker, G. W., Jessel, J., & DeLeon, I. G. (2013). Initial functional analysis outcomes and modifications in pursuit of differentiation: A summary of 176 inpatient cases. *Journal of Applied Behavior Analysis, 46,* 88–100.

Hamo, M., Blum-Kulka, S., & Hacohen, G. (2004). From observation to transcription and back: Theory, practice, and interpretation in the analysis of children's naturally occurring discourse. *Research on Language and Social Interaction, 37,* 71–92.

Hanley, G. P. (2012). Functional assessment of problem behavior: Dispelling myths, overcoming implementation obstacles, and developing new lore. *Behavior Analysis in Practice, 5,* 54–72.

Hanley, G. P., Iwata, B. A., & McCord, B. E. (2001). Functional analysis of problem behavior: A review. *Journal of Applied Behavior Analysis, 36,* 147–185.

Harding, J., Wacker, D. P., Cooper, L. J., Asmus, J., Jensen-Kovalan, P., & Grisolano, L. (1999). Combining descriptive and experimental analyses of young children with behavior problems in preschool settings. *Behavior Modification, 23,* 316–333.

Hart, B., & Risley, T. (1995). *Meaningful differences in the everyday experience of young American children.* Baltimore: Brookes.

Herscovitch, B., Roscoe, E. M., Libby, M. E., Bourret, J. C., & Ahearn, W. H. (2009). A procedure for identifying precursors to problem behavior. *Journal of Applied Behavior Analysis, 42,* 697–702.

Hine, R. A. (1982). *Ethology: Its nature and relations with other sciences.* New York: Oxford University Press.

Iwata, B. A., Dorsey, M. F., Slifer, K. J., Bauman, K. E., & Richman, G. S. (1994). Toward a functional analysis of self-injury. *Journal of Applied Behavior Analysis, 27,* 197–209. (Reprinted from *Analysis and Intervention in Developmental Disabilities, 2,* 3–20, 1982)

Kahng, S. W., Iwata, B. A., Fischer, S. M., Page, T. J., Treadwell, K. R., Williams, D. E., et al. (1998). Temporal distributions of problem behavior based on scatterplot analysis. *Journal of Applied Behavior Analysis, 31,* 593–604.

Lerman, D. C., Hovanetz, A., Strobel, M., & Tetreault, A. (2009). Accuracy of teacher-collected descriptive analysis data: A comparison of narrative and structured recording formats. *Journal of Behavioral Education, 18,* 157–172.

Lerman, D. C., & Iwata, B. A. (1993). Descriptive and experimental analyses of variables maintaining self-injurious behavior. *Journal of Applied Behavior Analysis, 26,* 293–319.

Lloyd, B. P., Kennedy, C. H., & Yoder, P. J. (2013). Quantifying contingent relations from direct observation data: Transitional probability comparisons versus Yule's Q. *Journal of Applied Behavior Analysis, 46,* 479–497.

Maas, A. P. H. M., Didden, R., Bouts, L., Smits, M. G., & Curfs, L. M. G. (2009). Scatterplot analysis of excessive daytime sleepiness and severe disruptive behavior in adults with Prader–Willi syndrome: A pilot study. *Research in Developmental Disabilities, 30,* 529–537.

Mace, F. C., & Lalli, J. S. (1991). Linking descriptive and experimental analyses in the intervention of bizarre speech. *Journal of Applied Behavior Analysis, 24,* 553–562.

Marion, S. D., Touchette, P. E., & Sandman, C. A. (2003). Sequential analysis reveals a unique structure for self-injurious behavior. *American Journal on Mental Retardation, 108,* 301–313.

Martens, B. K., Baxter, E. L., McComas, J. J., Sallade, S. J., Kester, J. S., Caamano, M., et al. (2019). Agreement between structured descriptive assessments and functional analyses conducted over a telehealth system. *Behavior Analysis: Research and Practice, 19,* 343–356.

Mayer, K. L., & DiGennaro Reed, F. D. (2013). Effects of a training package to improve the accuracy of descriptive analysis data recording. *Journal of Organizational Behavior Management, 33,* 226–243.

McComas, J. J., Moore, T., Dahl, N., Hartman, E., Hoch, J., & Symons, F. (2009). Calculating contingencies in natural environments: Issues in the application of sequential analysis. *Journal of Applied Behavior Analysis, 42,* 413–423.

McKerchar, P. M., & Thompson, R. H. (2004). A descriptive analysis of potential reinforcement contingencies in the preschool classroom. *Journal of Applied Behavior Analysis, 37,* 431–444.

Minkin, N., Braukmann, C. J., Minkin, B. L., Timbers, G. D., Timbers, B. J., Fixsen, D. L., et al. (1976). The social validation and training of conversation skills. *Journal of Applied Behavior Analysis, 9,* 127–139.

Moss, J., Oliver, C., Hall, S., Arron, K., Sloneem, J., & Petty, J. (2005). The association between environmental events and self-injurious behaviour in Cornelia de Lange syndrome. *Journal of Intellectual Disability Research, 49,* 269–277.

Noell, G. H., VanDerHeyden, A. M., Gatti, S. L., & Whitmarsh, E. L. (2001). Functional assessment of the effects of escape and attention on students' compliance during instruction. *School Psychology Quarterly, 16,* 253–269.

Oliver, A. C., Pratt, L. A., & Normand, M. P. (2015). A survey of functional behavioral assessment methods used by behavior analysts in practice. *Journal of Applied Behavior Analysis, 48,* 817–829.

Oliver, C., Hall, S., & Nixon, J. (1999). A molecular to molar analysis of communicative and problem behavior. *Research in Developmental Disabilities, 20,* 197–213.

Pence, S. T., Roscoe, E. M., Bourret, J. C., & Ahearn, W. H. (2009). Relative contributions of three descriptive methods: Implications for behavioral assessment. *Journal of Applied Behavior Analysis, 42,* 425–446.

Pfadt, A., & Wheeler, D. J. (1995). Using statistical process control to make data-based clinical decisions. *Journal of Applied Behavior Analysis, 28,* 349–370.

Piazza, C. C., Fisher, W. W., Brown, K. A., Shore, B. A., Patel, M. R., Katz, R. M., et al. (2003). Functional analysis of inappropriate mealtime behaviors. *Journal of Applied Behavior Analysis, 36,* 187–204.

Rahman, B., Oliver, C., & Alderman, N. (2010). Descriptive functional analysis of challenging behaviours shown by adults with acquired brain injury. *Neuropsychological Rehabilitation, 20,* 212–238.

Rapp, J. T., Vollmer, T. R., St. Peter, C., Dozier, C. L., & Cotnoir, N. M. (2004). Analysis of response allocation in individuals with multiple forms of stereotyped behavior. *Journal of Applied Behavior Analysis, 37,* 481–501.

Reed, D. D., Luiselli, J. K., Morizio, L. C., & Child, S. N. (2010). Sequential modification and the identification of instructional components occasioning self-injurious behavior. *Child and Family Behavior Therapy, 32,* 1–16.

Repp, A. C., & Karsh, K. G. (1994). Hypothesis-based interventions for tantrum behaviors of persons with developmental disabilities in school settings. *Journal of Applied Behavior Analysis, 27,* 21–31.

Richman, D. M., & Hagopian, L. P. (1999). On the effects of "quality" of attention in the functional analysis of destructive behavior. *Research in Developmental Disabilities, 20,* 51–62.

Rodriguez, N. M., Thompson, R. H., Schlichenmeyer, K. S., & Stocco, C. S. (2012). Functional analysis of arranging and ordering by individuals with an autism spectrum disorder. *Journal of Applied Behavior Analysis, 45,* 1–22.

Rodriguez, N. M., Thompson, R. H., Stocco, C. S., & Schlichenmeyer, K. S. (2013). Arranging and ordering in autism spectrum disorder: Characteristics, severity, and environmental correlates. *Journal of Intellectual and Developmental Disabilities, 38,* 242–255.

Rooker, G. W., DeLeon, I. G., Borrero, C. S., Frank-Crawford, M. A., & Roscoe, E. M. (2015). Reducing ambiguity in the functional assessment of problem behavior. *Behavioral Interventions, 30,* 1–35.

Roscoe, E. M., Phillips, K. M., Kelly, M. A., Farber, R., & Dube, W. V. (2015). A statewide survey of practitioners' use and perceived utility of functional assessment. *Journal of Applied Behavior Analysis, 48,* 830–844.

Roscoe, E. M., Schlichenmeyer, K. J., & Dube, W. V. (2015). Functional analysis of problem behavior: A systematic approach to identifying idiosyncratic variables. *Journal of Applied Behavior Analysis, 48,* 289–314.

Samaha, A. L., Vollmer, T. R., Borrero, C., Sloman, K., St. Peter Pipkin, C., & Bourret, J. (2009). Analyses of response–stimulus sequences in descriptive observations. *Journal of Applied Behavior Analysis, 42,* 447–468.

Schlichenmeyer, K. J., Roscoe, E. M., Rooker, G. W., Wheeler, E. E., & Dube, W. V. (2013). Idiosyncratic variables affecting functional analysis outcomes: A review (2001–2010). *Journal of Applied Behavior Analysis, 46,* 339–348.

Simmons, C. A., Akers, J. S., & Fisher, W. W. (2019). Functional analysis and treatment of covert food stealing in an outpatient setting. *Behavioral Development, 24,* 42–57.

Sloman, K. N., Vollmer, T. R., Cotnoir, N., Borrero, C. S. W., Borrero, J. C., Samaha, A. L., et al. (2005). Descriptive analyses of parent reprimands. *Journal of Applied Behavior Analysis, 38,* 373–383.

St. Peter, C., Vollmer, T. R., Bourret, J. C., Borrero, C. S. W., Sloman, K. N., & Rapp, J. T. (2005). On the role of attention in naturally occurring matching relations. *Journal of Applied Behavior Analysis, 38,* 429–433.

Strand, P. S., Wahler, R. G., & Herring, M. (2000). Momentum in child compliance and opposition. *Journal of Child and Family Studies, 9,* 363–375.

Thompson, R. H., & Iwata, B. A. (2001). A descriptive analysis of social consequences following problem behavior. *Journal of Applied Behavior Analysis, 34,* 169–178.

Thompson, R. H., & Iwata, B. A. (2007). A comparison of outcomes from descriptive and functional analyses of problem behavior. *Journal of Applied Behavior Analysis, 40,* 333–338.

Thompson, T., Symons, F. J., & Felce, D. (2000). Principles of behavioral observation: Assumptions and strategies. In T. Thompson, D. Felce, & F. J. Symons (Eds.), *Behavioral observation: Technology and applications in developmental disabilities* (pp. 3–16). Baltimore: Brookes.

Tinbergen, N. (1951). *The study of instinct.* Oxford, UK: Clarendon Press.

Touchette, P. E., MacDonald, R. F., & Langer, S. N. (1985). A scatterplot for identifying stimulus control of problem behavior. *Journal of Applied Behavior Analysis, 18,* 343–351.

VanDerHeyden, A. M., Witt, J. C., & Gatti, S. (2001). Descriptive assessment method to reduce overall disruptive behavior in a preschool classroom. *School Psychology Review, 30,* 548–567.

Vollmer, T. R., Borrero, J. C., Wright, C. S., Van Camp, C., & Lalli, J. S. (2001). Identifying possible contingencies during descriptive analyses of severe behavior disorders. *Journal of Applied Behavior Analysis, 34,* 269–287.

Wahler, R. G., Winkel, G. H., Peterson, R. F., & Morrison, D. C. (1965). Mothers as behavior therapists for their own children. *Behaviour Research and Therapy, 3,* 113–124.

Woods, J. N., Borrero, J. C., Laud, R. B., & Borrero, C. S. W. (2010). Descriptive analyses of pediatric food refusal: The structure of parental attention. *Behavior Modification, 34,* 35–36.

Yoder, P., & Symons, F. (2010). *Observational measurement of behavior.* New York: Springer.

# CHAPTER 13

# Functional Analysis
## *History and Methods*

Valdeep Saini, Wayne W. Fisher, Alison M. Betz,
and Cathleen C. Piazza

Traditional methods of classifying behavior disorders (e.g., American Psychiatric Association, 2013) rely primarily on correlations among symptoms. For example, an easily distracted child who often fidgets and squirms while seated might receive a diagnosis of attention-deficit/hyperactivity disorder (ADHD). This approach focuses on the structural characteristics of responses and on the extent to which responses covary. A behavior-analytic alternative to the structural approach is to categorize problem behavior according to environmental variables of which the behavior is a function.

## HISTORY AND CONCEPTUAL FOUNDATION OF FUNCTIONAL ANALYSIS

Skinner (1953) adapted the mathematical term *functional analysis* and introduced it to the field of behavior analysis. According to Skinner, a *functional relation* exists when an independent variable produces an orderly and predictable change in a dependent variable. Among Skinner's primary interests were the effects of environmental events on human behavior, and he used the term *functional analysis* to describe a process to identify independent variables functionally related to human be-

havior. Although Skinner described several procedures for conducting a functional analysis of behavior, we focus in the current chapter on an assessment in which the behavior analyst directly manipulates the consequences hypothesized to reinforce problem behavior. We use the term *functional analysis* to describe this assessment.

### Analyzing Behavioral Function

Researchers in the late 1960s began systematically manipulating environmental variables to study their effects on self-injurious behavior (SIB) and other problem behavior. Lovaas, Freitag, Gold, and Kassorla (1965), for example, observed that the frequency of a participant's SIB increased when the therapist provided attention in the form of sympathetic statements after occurrences of SIB. Similarly, Lovaas and Simmons (1969) established that attention was a reinforcer for one participant's SIB, and that SIB decreased when attention did not follow its occurrence.

Carr and colleagues showed that SIB (Carr, Newsom, & Binkoff, 1976) and aggression (Carr, Newsom, & Binkoff, 1980) occurred more frequently during a condition in which the researcher presented demands than during conditions without demands. These data suggested that escape from demands functioned as negative reinforcement for problem behavior. By contrast, Berkson and Mason (1963, 1964) found that some participants engaged in higher levels of stereotyped movements in a condition in which they removed preferred stimulation, such as leisure items, relative to a condition in which they provided access to those items. These results suggested that the stimulation automatically produced by the stereotyped movements might have functioned as automatic reinforcement, because the movements were maintained in the absence of social consequences.

## Hypotheses about the Motivation of SIB

Results of the studies described above showed that changes in environmental events produced changes in problem behavior, but researchers had not developed a cohesive, systematic explanation for the motivation of problem behavior such as SIB. Carr (1977) reviewed the literature and wrote a seminal paper summarizing the prevailing hypotheses about the motivation of SIB, which indicated that SIB (1) is a learned response reinforced by access to preferred social consequences, such as attention; (2) is a learned response reinforced by the removal of nonpreferred events, such as academic work; (3) is a response reinforced by the sensory stimulation produced by the response; (4) is a response produced by aberrant physiological processes; and (5) is a response that helps to establish ego boundaries or reduce guilt. Carr concluded that several motivational variables either individually or in combination are likely to control SIB, and that those variables may be different for different individuals. Carr recommended that researchers manipulate the antecedents and consequences for SIB, and suggested that these manipulations could serve as tests of the validity of the hypotheses about the motivation of SIB.

## Toward a Functional Analysis of SIB

Iwata, Dorsey, Slifer, Bauman, and Richman (1982/1994) published a landmark study based in part on Carr's (1977) review of the motivational variables for SIB. Iwata et al. described and evaluated a procedure to assess functional relations between environmental variables and SIB and to test the operant hypotheses that Carr described. The functional analysis consisted of test and control conditions that assessed whether (1) attention functioned as positive reinforcement for SIB in the *social disapproval* condition, (2) escape from or avoidance of nonpreferred activities functioned as negative reinforcement for SIB in the *academic demand* condition, (3) the sensory stimulation produced by the response functioned as automatic reinforcement for SIB in the *alone* condition, or (4) a combination of the variables functioned as reinforcement for SIB. Each functional-analysis condition included three components (Iwata, Pace, Cowdery, & Miltenberger, 1994): one or more unique *antecedent stimuli* that signaled the consequence for SIB; a *motivating operation* that altered the effectiveness of the putative reinforcement (Laraway, Snycerski, Michael, & Poling, 2003); and a putative *reinforcing consequence* for SIB.

## Functional-Analysis Conditions

Iwata et al. (1982/1994) used three test conditions (social disapproval, academic demands, and alone) and a control condition (unstructured play) to identify the reinforcers for SIB. We use the general structure Iwata et al. described as the basis for functional analyses in our clinic. However, we also conduct pre-functional-analysis observations to ensure continuity between behavior and events in the natural environment and those in the functional analysis (e.g., Fisher, Ninness, Piazza, & Owen-DeSchryver, et al., 1996; Piazza et al., 2003). During these observations, the caregiver conducts one demand, one attention, and one tangible session, each lasting 5 minutes. We may make modifications to our functional-analysis conditions based on these observations, so that the assessment conditions more closely match what we observe in the natural environment.

## Test for Social Positive Reinforcement, Attention

Iwata et al. (1982/1994) described a *social disapproval* condition that tested whether adult attention functioned as reinforcement for SIB. In this condition, the therapist diverted his or her attention by reading a magazine or book, and provided statements of concern or disapproval and gentle physical contact (e.g., pat on the shoulder) for each occurrence of SIB.

The rationale for the arrangement is that problem behavior maintained by social positive reinforcement often occurs when an adult's attention is diverted, such as when a caregiver is cooking. Problem behavior, such as aggression and SIB, may be particularly effective in interrupting such activities and in producing immediate attention (such as altered facial expressions, physical contact, and reprimands) in the natural environment. Thus the therapist simulates these conditions by diverting his or her attention initially, providing attention following occurrences of problem behavior, and providing no differential consequence for other participant behavior, such as communication. Some behavior analysts include a brief preattention interaction between the therapist and participant, so that the participant samples therapist attention immediately before the session.

Results of several studies have demonstrated that qualitatively different forms of attention may vary in their reinforcing effects on problem behavior (e.g., Fisher et al., 1996; Kodak, Northup, & Kelley, 2007; Piazza et al., 1999). In our clinic, we generally match the type and quality of attention the participant's caregiver provides to our direct observations described above. The therapist will use the same vocal statements, prosody, tone, and volume the caregiver uses to provide attention following problem behavior.

In the Iwata et al. (1982/1994) study, toys were within arm's reach of the participant. Several studies have shown that response-independent availability of preferred items, such as toys, can reduce attention-reinforced problem behavior to near-zero levels (e.g., Fisher, O'Connor, Kurtz, DeLeon, & Gotjen, 2000). The behavior analyst may consider using low-preference items in the attention condition; otherwise, the functional analysis may not identify an attention function that is responsible for the maintenance of problem behavior in the natural environment.

*Divided attention* is a modification of the attention condition in which the therapist provides attention to another child or adult until the participant engages in problem behavior, which then produces the therapist's attention (Fahmie, Iwata, Harper, & Querim, 2013). The rationale for this modification is that an adult providing attention to another child or adult may signal attention availability or increase the value of attention as reinforcement.

### Test for Social Negative Reinforcement, Escape

Iwata et al. (1982/1994) also described an *academic demand* condition, in which the therapist presented demands to complete nonpreferred academic tasks. The therapist used sequential vocal, model, and physical prompts to encourage the individual to complete each task. The therapist provided praise if the participant completed the task after the vocal or model prompt, or physically guided the participant to complete the task if the participant did not complete it after the vocal or model prompt. The therapist removed the task materials, stopped prompting, and turned away from the participant for 30 seconds if the participant engaged in SIB during the prompting sequence.

The rationale for this arrangement is that learning tasks are aversive to some individuals. Problem behavior may postpone, prevent, or remove these aversive events (Iwata, 1987). For example, a caregiver may stop prompting a boy to brush his teeth if the boy becomes aggressive during tooth brushing. Thus the boy may be more likely to engage in aggression again in the future during self-care or other tasks if he learns that it ends the aversive activity. Beavers, Iwata, and Lerman (2013) identified negative reinforcement as the most common reinforcer for problem behavior.

The presentation of learning trials is a defining feature of the demand condition. Iwata et al. (1982/1994) chose tasks the participants were unlikely to complete to increase the participant's motivation to escape. We select tasks based on our pre-functional-analysis observations, caregiver or teacher reports of tasks that correlate with problem behavior, or a combination of these methods (Fisher, Adelinis, Thompson, Worsdell, & Zarcone, 1998; McComas, Hoch, Paone, & El-Roy, 2000). The tasks that evoke problem behavior may differ for individual participants, depending on variables such as amount of movement required, difficulty level, and presentation rate (McCord, Thompson, & Iwata, 2001; Smith, Iwata, Goh, & Shore, 1995). Thus selection and use of tasks that evoke problem behavior in the natural environment may increase the probability of accurate functional-analysis results.

### Test for Automatic Reinforcement

Iwata et al. (1982/1994) described an *alone* condition, in which the participant was alone in a room with no toys or materials that would function as external stimulation. The rationale for this arrangement is that some problem behaviors occur in the absence of social reinforcement—reinforcement that another person mediates or controls. Rather, the stimulation that the problem behavior automatically produces reinforces problem behavior. The absence of stimulation in the alone condition increases the probability that no other reinforcement is available that would compete with the automatic reinforcement the problem behavior produces.

The risk of harm for some participants may outweigh the benefits of an alone condition. An *ignore* condition is an alternative in which a therapist in the room blocks the participant's problem behavior to reduce injury risk, but provides no additional programmed consequence for problem behavior. An ignore condition also may be appropriate if the therapist suspects that automatic reinforcement maintains problem behavior, such as aggression or property destruction. These cases require the therapist in the room for the participant to exhibit aggression or materials in the room for the participant to exhibit property destruction.

Another variation is a *baited environment*, which provides the participant with the materials to engage in the problem behavior. Piazza et al. (1998) described a procedure for a baited environment to assess pica (consumption of unsafe items such as lead paint chips). The researchers identified each participant's pica items and bought or made items that would serve as proxies. For example, Piazza et al. made simulated paint chips from flour and water for participants who consumed paint chips (Finney, Russo, & Cataldo, 1982). This preparation allowed Piazza et al. to observe and measure proxies of pica without exposing these participants to the risks associated with consumption of the pica materials in the natural environment (e.g., paint chips containing lead).

Querim et al. (2013) used the alone condition as a screening tool to predict whether automatic or social reinforcement would maintain problem behavior. After conducting a series of consecutive 5-minute sessions, they hypothesized that automatic reinforcement likely maintained problem behavior that persisted across sessions, and that social reinforcement likely maintained problem behavior that extinguished across sessions. This screening tool predicted whether automatic or social reinforcement maintained problem behavior in 28 of 30 cases.

Withdrawing and reinstating reinforcement consequences constitute another method for confirming the reinforcer for problem behavior. This method is more difficult when problem behavior produces automatic reinforcement. For example, a therapist may not be able to block or prevent SIB if a participant has multiple topographies that occur simultaneously at a high rate. In addition, the behavior analyst may not be able to control the onset or offset of automatic reinforcement. One exception in the literature was a study by Rincover (1978). He hypothesized that auditory stimulation was the automatic reinforcement for a participant's stereotypical object flipping and spinning. He assessed this hypothesis by placing a carpet on the table to attenuate the sound of the objects while flipping and spinning. Decreases and increases in flipping and spinning occurred with the introduction and withdrawal of the carpet, respectively.

### Control Condition

Iwata et al. (1982/1994) used an *unstructured play* condition as the control condition of the functional analysis. The participant had toys; the therapist interacted with the participant about once every 30 seconds in the absence of SIB, but provided no differential consequence after occurrences of SIB. The rationale for this arrangement is that noncontingent attention, the absence of demands, the presence of toys, and the absence of a contingency for problem behavior should decrease the participant's motivation to engage in problem behavior to access attention, escape, or automatic reinforcement, respectively.

### Test for Social Positive Reinforcement, Tangible

Children may engage in problem behavior to access a preferred item or activity, such as when Child B hits Child A to get the truck with which Child A is playing. Researchers have systematically tested whether access to *tangible* items functions as reinforcement for problem behavior (cf. Fisher et al., 1993), which is an addition to the original Iwata et al. (1982/1994) procedure. The therapist gives the participant the tangible item briefly before the session, starts the session by removing the tangible item, and then provides the tangible item for about 30 seconds after occurrences of problem behavior. The rationale for this arrangement is that removal of the tangible item should increase the participant's motivation to engage in problem behavior to access the item if the item functions as reinforcement for problem behavior.

We select the tangible item based on our direct observations of participant behavior or caregiver report. We conduct a stimulus preference assessment (Fisher et al., 1992) and use the most preferred item(s) from the assessment if the caregiver reports that the participant engages in problem behavior to access several tangible items.

We only conduct a tangible condition if we observe or a caregiver reports a relationship between a problem behavior and a tangible item, because of the risk of teaching the participant a response–reinforcement relation that does not exist currently in the individual's natural environment (Rooker, Iwata, Harper, Fahmie, & Camp, 2011; Shirley, Iwata, & Kahng, 1999). For example, Shirley et al. (1999) showed that occurrences of automatically reinforced hand mouthing increased when the participant received a tangible item after occurrences of hand mouthing. Shirley et al. concluded that the tangible item *became* a reinforcer for hand mouthing, because the researchers provided it after occurrences of hand mouthing.

## MITIGATING THE RISKS OF CONDUCTING A FUNCTIONAL ANALYSIS

The occurrence of problem behavior during a functional analysis is necessary to identify response–reinforcement relations. The possibility exists, therefore, that the functional analysis will increase the risk of harm to the participant, the caregiver or therapist, or the environment, due to occurrences of problem behavior. Iwata et al. (1982/1994) implemented safeguards to minimize risks to participants in their study. First, each participant received a medical examination and appropriate diagnostic consultations to assess the participant's physical status and to rule out organic causes for the participant's SIB, such as headaches. Second, the participants' physician recommended criteria for terminating functional-analysis sessions based on degree of injury or level of responding, and intermittently observed sessions and modified termination criteria if needed. Third, the therapist stopped the session if a participant met the termination criterion, and a physician or nurse examined the participant and determined whether sessions could continue. Fourth, a nurse examined participants after every four sessions and noted any issues from SIB. Iwata et al. concluded that the risk of study participation was no greater than the risk the participants experienced from occurrences of SIB in the natural environment, due to their study's safeguards.

Standard functional-analysis practice should include safeguards to minimize risk to participants (Weeden, Mahoney, & Poling, 2010). These might include interviewing the caregiver(s) to determine how often, when, and where problem behavior has produced harm to the participant, others, or the environment. The behavior analyst should have a plan to block or prevent SIB that might cause significant damage, such as using arm splints to prevent eye gouging or a helmet if head banging might cause a concussion (e.g., Fisher, Piazza, Bowman, Hanley, & Adelinis, 1997). Therapists who conduct functional analyses should also wear protective equipment, such as arm guards, if problem behavior (e.g., biting) might cause injury to them. Functional analyses should have session termination criteria when problem behavior causes or has the potential to cause injury, as well as criteria for resuming sessions, such as when the injuries heal or after consulting with a medical care provider. In general, behavior analysts should consider the risks carefully and only conduct a functional analysis when the benefits clearly outweigh the risks.

Kahng et al. (2015) evaluated whether participation in a functional analysis increased injury risk relative to when the participants were not in the functional analysis, based on records from 99 patients with SIB treated in an inpatient hospital. The frequency of injury was comparable during and outside of the functional analyses. Injury rate adjusted for time tended to be higher during the functional analysis, but the injuries that occurred were relatively infrequent and of low severity.

## INTERPRETING FUNCTIONAL-ANALYSIS DATA

The goal of a functional analysis is to identify the reinforcer(s) for problem behavior. Observers collect data on the target problem behavior via direct observation during the test and control conditions. The behavior analyst converts the data to a measure that is comparable across conditions, such as responses per minute; plots the data on a line graph; and visually inspects the line graph to determine whether levels of problem behavior are higher in one or more test conditions than in the control condition. Generally, when levels of problem behavior are higher in one or more test conditions than in the control condition, the behavior analyst concludes that the functional analysis has identified the reinforcer(s) for problem behavior, or says that the analysis is *differentiated*. Iwata et al. (1982/1994) found that higher levels of SIB occurred in specific test conditions for six of the nine participants. The researchers concluded that the "data provide information regarding the specific conditions that may affect self-injury" (p. 203).

Visual inspection is a reasonable method of data analysis when functional-analysis results are relatively clear, but it may not be the most reliable method of interpreting such results (Hagopian et al., 1997). Researchers have developed and used structured criteria to interpret functional-analysis data, to address the problem of visual inspection's poor interrater reliability.

## Structured Visual-Inspection Criteria

Fisher and colleagues (Hagopian et al., 1997; Roane, Fisher, Kelley, Mevers, & Bouxsein, 2013; Saini, Fisher, & Retzlaff, 2018; Saini, Fisher, Retzlaff, & Keevey, 2020) developed and evaluated structured criteria, using consensus interpretations of functional-analysis data by an expert panel as the criterion variable. The first version of their structured visual-inspection procedure included drawing criterion lines on the functional-analysis graph that indicated the range and variance for the levels of responding in the control condition (Hagopian et al., 1997). The interpreter drew the upper criterion line (UCL) about one standard deviation above the mean for the control condition, and the lower criterion line (LCL) about one standard deviation below the mean for the control condition. The visual inspector counted the number of data points for each test condition that were above the UCL and the number of data points that were below the LCL, and subtracted the latter number from the former ($X_{UCL} - X_{LCL}$). If the difference was larger than or equal to one-half the total number of data points for that test condition (e.g., $X_{UCL} - X_{LCL} \geq 5$, with 10 data points per condition), the interpreter concluded that the test condition was differentiated from the control condition, and that the tested consequence functioned as reinforcement for problem behavior. Other components of the structured criteria included specific rules for (1) functions of automatic reinforcement, (2) trends in the data, (3) magnitude of effects, (4) low-level responding, and (5) multiply controlled responding. The reliability of functional-analysis interpretations increased from a mean of 54% correct in baseline to a mean of 90% correct after training when participants used the structured criteria. A limitation was that the procedure only applied to functional analyses with 10 points per condition.

Roane et al. (2013) modified Hagopian et al. (1997)'s visual-inspection criteria by using percentage rather than number of data points to calculate differences in responding between the test and control conditions. They concluded that responding was differentiated when 50% or more of the data points for the test condition were above the UCL than were below the LCL. These modified criteria increased the agreement between expert reviewers from a mean of 62% in baseline to 92% after training, and increased agreement between nonexperts and experts from a mean of 73% in baseline to 95% after training. The Roane et al. procedure provided more flexibility than the Hagopian et al. procedure, because it was applied to functional analyses with varying numbers of data points.

One limitation of both the Hagopian et al. (1997) and Roane et al. (2013) criteria is that they applied the criteria post hoc (i.e., after they completed the functional analysis). Saini et al. (2018) extended the Roane et al. study by providing rules for *ongoing visual inspection*. That is, Saini et al. applied the criteria while conducting the functional analysis. They also added a criterion for objectively determining when to end the functional analysis. When Saini et al. applied the criteria for ongoing visual inspection to published functional analyses, they produced highly convergent interpretations with the Roane et al. criteria. Recall that Roane et al. applied their criteria to the entire functional-analysis dataset, and their exact agreement on identified functions was 92%. Ongoing visual inspection decreased the mean length of the functional analyses by more than 40%. Thus, ongoing visual inspection using structured criteria can produce reliable and valid interpretations of functional analyses more efficiently (Saini et al., 2020).

### Single-Function Problem Behavior

When levels of problem behavior are higher in one test condition than in other test conditions or the control condition, we conclude that problem behavior has a *single* function. That is, the consequence in the test condition with the highest levels of problem behavior functions as reinforcement for problem behavior. We conclude that (1) attention functions as social positive reinforcement if levels of problem behavior are highest in the attention condition; (2) escape functions as social negative reinforcement if levels of problem behavior are highest in the demand condition; and (3) automatic reinforcement is the reinforcer if levels of problem behavior are highest in the alone or ignore condition. The functional analysis in Figure 13.1 shows that rates of problem behavior for Mike are clearly and consistently higher in the attention condition than in the other test and control conditions. These data suggest that attention functions as social positive reinforcement for Mike's problem behavior. Figure 13.2 shows high levels of problem behavior across multiple conditions, but highest in the ignore condition for Hank. This pattern of responding suggests that the consequence produced by problem behavior functions as automatic reinforcement.

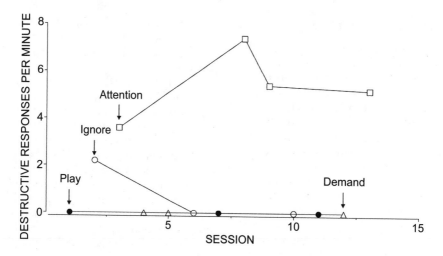

**FIGURE 13.1.** An example of a functional analysis in which contingent attention functions as social positive reinforcement for Mike's problem behavior.

### Multiply Controlled Problem Behavior

When more than one reinforcer maintains problem behavior, behavior analysts use the term *multiply controlled* to describe the behavior. In other words, levels of multiply controlled problem behavior are higher in more than one test condition of a functional analysis relative to the control condition. The functional analysis in Figure 13.3 shows that rates of Willie's problem behavior are highest in the tangible condition relative to the other test and control conditions, and that rates of problem behavior are higher in the attention condition than in the control condition. These data suggest that the tangible item and attention function as social positive reinforcement for problem behavior.

### Undifferentiated Functional Analysis

Interpretation of functional-analysis data may be more difficult when problem behavior occurs at

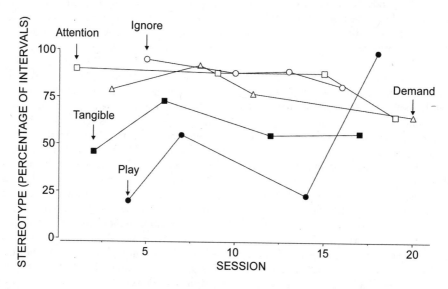

**FIGURE 13.2.** An example of a functional analysis in which automatic reinforcement likely maintains Hank's problem behavior.

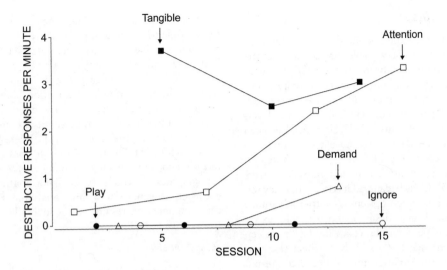

**FIGURE 13.3.** An example of a functional analysis in which multiple consequences function as reinforcement for Willie's problem behavior.

relatively equivalent rates across conditions, rates of problem behavior are variable across conditions, or problem behavior seldom or never occurs during the functional analysis. In this case, the behavior analyst might conclude that problem behavior is *undifferentiated*; that is, the functional analysis did not identify the reinforcer for problem behavior. Figure 13.4 depicts undifferentiated responding, in which rates of Lynn's problem behavior are low and variable across conditions.

## Variables That May Affect Interpretation

Although we expect the programmed antecedents and consequences of a functional analysis to control responding, research has shown that other procedural components of the functional analysis may affect the results. We review these issues below. We then review procedures for clarifying data on undifferentiated problem behavior in the subsequent section.

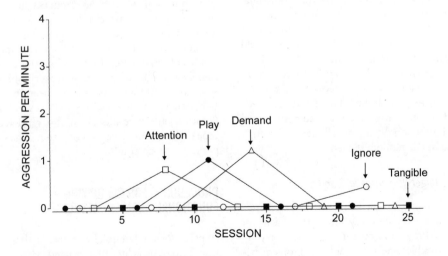

**FIGURE 13.4.** An example of an undifferentiated, inconclusive functional analysis for Lynn.

## Experimental Design

The single-case experimental design for the functional analysis is one variable that could affect the clarity of the results. Iwata et al. (1982/1994) used a multielement design in which the therapist conducted repeated series of four sessions (one of each condition), presented in a random order until levels of SIB were stable, unstable levels of SIB persisted for 5 days, or 12 days of sessions elapsed. Functional-analysis research published in the literature also has favored the multielement design (81%; Beavers et al., 2013), likely because of its time efficiency relative to other design options. Another advantage of the multielement design is that variables external to the experimental preparation (such as sleep deprivation) may be less likely to affect the clarity of functional-analysis results, because external variables should affect each condition equally, due to the rapid alternation of conditions.

One disadvantage of the multielement design is that carry-over effects or multiple-treatment interference, in which the programmed antecedents or consequences in one condition affect responding in another condition, may affect the clarity of the results. A second disadvantage is that the participant may not discriminate between conditions, due to their rapid alternation.

## Session Order

Hammond, Iwata, Rooker, Fritz, and Bloom (2013) examined the effects of a fixed functional-analysis condition sequence (ignore, attention, play, and demand) versus a random condition sequence. The purpose was to evaluate whether individual conditions in the fixed sequence would function as motivating operations for the reinforcement in the subsequent condition. For example, would the attention deprivation in the ignore condition increase a participant's motivation to engage in problem behavior to access attention in a subsequent attention condition? The fixed sequence produced more clearly differentiated results and increased functional-analysis efficiency by 57% compared to the random sequence.

## Number of Target Responses Included

The number of problem behaviors targeted in a functional analysis can also affect the clarity of the results. Programming contingencies for only the most troublesome topography of problem behavior generally leads to clearer functional-anal-ysis results relative to programming contingencies for multiple topographies, particularly when these topographies have different reinforcers (Asmus, Franzese, Conroy, & Dozier, 2003; Derby et al., 1994, 2000). Graphing each response topography individually may provide information about the reinforcers for individual response topographies that is not evident in a single graph of combined response topographies (Derby et al., 1994, 2000). Nevertheless, Hanley, Iwata, and McCord (2003) recommended minimizing the number of response topographies for which the behavior analyst programs contingencies in a functional analysis, because inconclusive results may be more likely.

## Session Duration

Cooper, Wacker, Sasso, Reimers, and Donn (1990) described a method for conducting a brief functional analysis of problem behavior that produced interpretable results for most cases during a 90-minute outpatient visit (Derby et al., 1992). The therapist conducted one session of each test condition and one session of the control condition initially. The therapist identified the reinforcer that produced the highest levels of problem behavior in the initial series of sessions, provided that reinforcer for appropriate behavior and placed problem behavior on extinction in the next session, and provided reinforcement only for problem behavior in the final session.

Wallace and Iwata (1999) analyzed data from 46 functional analyses of SIB in which session duration was 15 minutes. They created and interpreted 138 graphs: 46 with data from the first 5 minutes of each session, 46 with data from the first 10 minutes of each session, and 46 with data from the 15-minute session. Results from the 5-minute sample were the same as those from the 15-minute sessions for 94% of cases. Results from the 10-minute sample were the same as those from the 15-minute sessions for 100% of cases. Our current practice is to conduct 5-minute sessions and to extend session duration only if results are undifferentiated after repeated exposure to each condition (e.g., four exposures to each condition).

## PROCEDURES FOR CLARIFYING FUNCTIONAL-ANALYSIS RESULTS

A behavior analyst might conclude that a functional analysis is undifferentiated when problem behavior occurs at relatively equivalent rates across conditions, rates of problem behavior are variable across conditions, or problem behavior seldom or never occurs during the functional analysis. However, an alternative conclusion is that some other variable(s)—such as carry-over effects, multiple-treatment interference, or a participant's failure to discriminate the condition contingencies—have contributed to the unclear results. In these cases, researchers have described and tested several procedures to clarify the results. Hagopian, Rooker, Jessel, and DeLeon (2013) modified the functional analysis for 176 cases with initially undifferentiated results. The modifications included (1) conducting sessions in a different location, (2) implementing extinction for certain problem behaviors, or (3) increasing session duration. These manipulations identified the function of problem behavior in 153 of 176 cases. Below, we review specific procedures researchers have used to clarify undifferentiated functional-analysis results.

## Providing Extended Alone Sessions

Vollmer, Marcus, Ringdahl, and Roane (1995) suggested conducting consecutive or extended alone or ignore sessions when problem behavior occurs during a functional analysis, but the results are undifferentiated (Querim et al., 2013; Vollmer et al., 1995). Automatic reinforcement is the likely function of problem behavior that persists during extended alone sessions, because no other conditions are present to cause multiple-treatment interference, and alternative sources of reinforcement are not available in the alone condition. Figure 13.5

shows data from an undifferentiated functional analysis followed by extended alone sessions in the final phase. Problem behavior was maintained during extended alone sessions, suggesting automatic reinforcement as the function.

## Re-Presenting Social-Reinforcement Test Conditions

When problem behavior does not persist during extended alone or ignore sessions, re-presenting the social-reinforcement conditions of the functional analysis in a reversal design may clarify results. Figure 13.6 shows that problem behavior did not persist during an extended ignore condition. The behavior analyst then conducted a reversal between a contingent-escape condition and an ignore condition. Rates of behavior were higher in the contingent-escape conditions, suggesting that escape functioned as negative reinforcement for problem behavior. A potentially more time-efficient alternative is to conduct a pairwise comparison of one test condition and the control condition (Iwata, Duncan, Zarcone, Lerman, & Shore, 1994).

## Including Additional Discriminative Stimuli

Some functional analyses may produce undifferentiated results because the discriminative stimuli associated with the conditions do not control the participant's problem behavior. Adding different, salient discriminative stimuli in each condition may address this problem (Conners et al., 2000). For example, a therapist might wear a red shirt

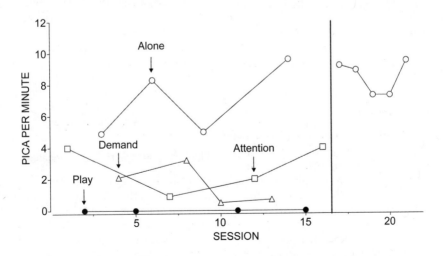

**FIGURE 13.5.** An example of a functional analysis with an extended alone condition.

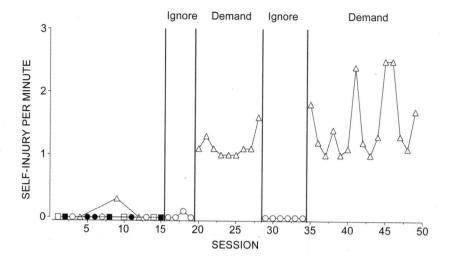

**FIGURE 13.6.** An example of an extended analysis with a reversal design.

during the attention condition, a purple shirt during the demand condition, and a yellow shirt during the control condition.

## Altering Motivating Operations, Reinforcement Contingencies, or Both

Another reason for undifferentiated functional-analysis results is that the motivating operation for problem behavior may not be present in the functional analysis. Altering one or several of the motivating operations may produce more differentiated or conclusive results. Finally, a functional analysis may produce undifferentiated or inconclusive results because the consequences that maintain problem behavior may not be present in the functional analysis. Therefore, adding or altering the consequences for problem behavior may produce more differentiated or conclusive results (Hagopian et al., 2013).

## Extending Session Duration

Extending the duration of sessions for a functional analysis may add clarity to the results. For example, the participant in Kahng, Abt, and Schonbachler (2001) never displayed aggression during the 10-minute functional-analysis sessions. Conducting one condition per day from 9:00 A.M. to 4:00 P.M. produced data suggesting that attention functioned as positive reinforcement for problem behavior, and a treatment analysis validated this conclusion.

## Analyzing Within-Session Response Patterns

Vollmer, Iwata, Zarcone, Smith, and Mazaleski (1993) analyzed within-session data for a participant whose rates of SIB were high in the alone and control conditions. The analysis showed that extinction bursts occurred at the beginning of alone and control sessions that immediately followed an attention session. These results supported the conclusion that attention reinforced SIB.

Roane, Lerman, Kelley, and Van Camp (1999) suggested analyzing within-session data to determine the effects of momentary changes in the establishing operation on problem behavior. Roane et al. used within-session data to determine whether problem behavior occurred when the condition's motivating operation was present versus absent. Results of the within-session analysis generally agreed with the results of the multielement functional analysis: Problem behavior tended to occur when the motivating operation for problem behavior identified by the functional analysis was present versus when it was absent.

## Identifying Idiosyncratic Consequences

Still another possible explanation for undifferentiated results is that the reinforcer for problem behavior is not present in the functional analysis. For example, Van Camp et al. (2000) observed a correlation between the occurrence of problem behavior and the presence of a Bumble Ball® during an undifferentiated functional analysis. Researchers evaluated this relationship in conditions in which (1) the participant had the ball, and the therapist removed the ball for 20 seconds after occurrences of problem behavior; (2) the therapist gave the ball to the participant for 20 seconds after occurrences of problem behavior; and (3) the participant had access to toys but not social interaction. Results suggested that rates of problem behavior were higher when the ball was present, but that automatic reinforcement maintained problem behavior. Schlichenmeyer, Roscoe, Rooker, Wheeler and Dube (2013) identified more than 30 idiosyncratic variables that influenced problem behavior during functional analyses published between 2001 and 2010. Thus behavior analysts should assess whether idiosyncratic consequences reinforce problem behavior.

Our research group has used informal descriptive assessments to generate hypotheses about idiosyncratic reinforcers for problem behavior, and these hypotheses inform our subsequent test and control conditions (Bowman, Fisher, Thompson, & Piazza, 1997; Fisher, Adelinis, et al., 1998; Fisher, Lindauer, Alterson, & Thompson, 1998; Thompson, Fisher, Piazza, & Kuhn, 1998). For example, Bowman et al. (1997) conducted informal observations of participants with undifferentiated functional analyses and their caregivers. Each caregiver frequently acquiesced to the participant's requests or mands, even ones that were unreasonable, such as telling the adult to hop on one foot while playing a card game. Bowman et al. hypothesized that a precurrent relation had developed in which the precurrent response (problem behavior) increased the probability of reinforcement of the current response (the mand). In this case, because problem behavior occurred when the caregiver did not acquiesce to the participant's mand, the caregiver was likely to deliver reinforcement for the mand to avoid the occurrence of problem behavior.

Bowman et al. (1997) conducted a mand analysis in which the therapist complied with the participant's mands for 1–2 minutes before the test session started. The therapist stopped complying with the participant's mands when the session started, and occurrences of problem behavior produced 30 seconds of therapist compliance with the mand. The therapist complied with the participant's mands in the control condition, and problem behavior produced no differential consequence. Problem behavior occurred at high rates in the test condition and at near-zero rates in the control condition. The mand analysis informed a treatment that reduced problem behavior to near-zero levels.

Currently, we use the following steps to identify idiosyncratic reinforcers for problem behavior. First, we interview caregivers to establish (1) the participant's daily routine, (2) the times when problem behavior is most likely to occur during the routine, and (3) which activities correlate with the occurrence of problem behavior. Next, we ask caregivers to collect descriptive antecedent–behavior–consequence data (Sulzer-Azaroff & Mayer, 1977), and therapists conduct observations based on caregiver interview and descriptive data to identify the antecedents that evoke or occasion problem behavior and the consequences that reinforce it. A therapist then conducts several 1- to 2-minute sessions in which he or she presents the identified antecedents and consequences to *recreate the scene* (see Van Houten & Rolider, 1988). We develop hypotheses and test and control conditions if problem behavior reliably occurs when we re-create the scene (e.g., Bowman et al., 1997).

Roscoe, Schlichenmeyer, and Dube (2015) developed a systematic method to generate and test hypotheses about idiosyncratic functions of problem behavior when initial functional-analysis results were undifferentiated. They first administered questionnaires to two informants familiar with each participant, to identify potential idiosyncratic antecedents and consequences of problem behavior. Next, Roscoe et al. video-recorded and observed participants when problem behavior reportedly occurred. This method identified the reinforcer(s) for problem behavior for five of six participants.

## VARIATIONS OF FUNCTIONAL-ANALYSIS PROCEDURES

### Trial-Based Functional Analysis

A trial-based functional analysis capitalizes on naturally occurring events, but also allows the behavior analyst to manipulate variables that potentially reinforce participant problem behavior in a discrete-trial format (Bloom, Iwata, Fritz, Roscoe, & Carreau, 2011; Sigafoos & Saggers, 1995). Each trial consists of presentation and removal of the motivating operation for the putative reinforcer. For example, the attention condition of a trial-based functional analysis in a classroom might consist of sequential 2-minute intervals in which the teacher presents attention in one interval and removes it in the next interval. Conceptually, the presentation and removal of teacher attention are the test and control conditions, respectively. Observers collect data on the occurrence of problem behavior per trial, and the behavior analyst converts occurrences to a percentage of trials. Figure 13.7 shows the results of a trial-based functional analysis for David, which suggests that attention functions as positive reinforcement for aggression.

Conducting the assessment in the environment where the behavior occurs is an advantage of the trial-based functional analysis. Researchers have conducted trial-based functional analyses in classrooms for typically developing children (Austin, Groves, Raynish, & Francis, 2015) and children with autism spectrum disorder (Kodak, Fisher, Paden, & Dickes, 2013). Moreover, classroom teachers and residential staff working with adults with developmental disabilities have implemented trial-based functional analyses with good procedural integrity (Bloom, Lambert, Dayton, & Samaha, 2013; Lambert, Bloom, Kunnavatana, Collins, & Clay, 2013).

Trial duration may be one limitation of trial-based functional analyses. Exposure to the motivating operation is short and may be insufficient to evoke problem behavior for some participants. Research thus far, however, has shown that trial-based functional analysis is a relatively simple, efficient, and effective method for identifying the function of problem behavior in natural environments.

### Functional Analysis in the Natural Environment

The trial-based method is not the only procedure for conducting a functional analysis in the natural environment (e.g., Broussard & Northup, 1995; Ringdahl & Sellers, 2000; Sigafoos & Saggers, 1995; Umbreit, 1996). Thomason-Sassi, Iwata, and Fritz (2013) directly compared the results of analogue functional analyses and functional analyses conducted in natural environments, such as in the home with the caregiver as therapist. Results of the two types of functional analyses corresponded for four of five participants. Additional research is needed to assess the correspondence of analogue and naturalistic functional analyses (Hanley et al., 2003).

### Latency-Based Functional Analysis

The occurrence of problem behavior may be necessary for a functional analysis to identify the reinforcer for problem behavior. Some participants, however, exhibit problem behavior that is a danger to themselves, caregivers and staff, property, or a combination of these. Measuring latency to the occurrence of problem behavior is one way to minimize the risk of problem behavior. As in other functional-analysis procedures, the behavior analyst presents the motivating operation in test condition sessions; however, the session ends when the participant engages in problem behavior. Shorter latencies to the occurrence of problem behavior in a test condition relative to the control condition suggest that the tested consequence functions as reinforcement for problem behavior.

Thomason-Sassi, Iwata, Neidert, and Roscoe (2011) examined response rate and response latency in 38 functional analyses, and found that rate and latency identified the same reinforcer for problem behavior in 33 of 38 cases. Latency-based functional analysis may be time-efficient if problem behavior occurs reliably and lawfully because the session ends after the first occurrence of problem behavior or after a specific time has elapsed. Figure 13.8 shows the results of a latency-based functional analysis for Brian. The short latencies

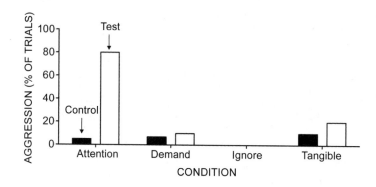

**FIGURE 13.7.** An example of a trial-based functional analysis.

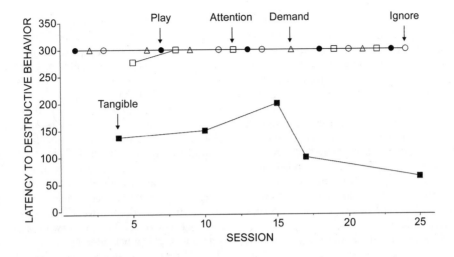

**FIGURE 13.8.** An example of a latency-based functional analysis.

to problem behavior in the tangible condition suggest that access to tangible items reinforces problem behavior.

## Precursor Functional Analysis

The risk of harm from some forms of problem behavior significantly outweighs the benefits of observing the behavior in a functional analysis, such as when a few occurrences of eye poking could cause blindness. One strategy that researchers have used to address this problem is *precursor functional analysis*. A precursor is a behavior that occurs reliably before the participant engages in problem behavior. A precursor functional analysis is one in which the behavior analyst arranges contingencies for the precursor(s) to problem behavior rather than for the problem behavior. If a precursor behavior is in the same functional response class as the problem behavior, identifying the reinforcer for the precursor behavior will identify the reinforcer for problem behavior.

Researchers have used descriptive assessments, lag-sequential analyses, and conditional-probability analyses to identify precursors to problem behavior (Dracobly & Smith, 2012; Fritz, Iwata, Hammond, & Bloom, 2013). Fritz et al. (2013) identified precursors to the problem behavior for eight participants, and conducted a functional analysis of precursor behavior and another one of problem behavior. The outcomes of these two types of functional analyses identified the same reinforcer(s) for seven of the eight participants. Developing an intervention based on the function of precur-

sor behavior is a reasonable approach, particularly when the risks outweigh the benefits of conducting a functional analysis of problem behavior.

## Synthesized Conditions

Hanley, Jin, Vanselow, and Hanratty (2014) described a procedure for a synthesized assessment informed by open-ended interviews with relevant stakeholders, such as caregivers and teachers, and followed by a brief, structured observation of the individual. Hanley and colleagues later referred to this assessment as the *interview-informed synthesized contingency analysis* (IISCA; Ghaemmaghami, Hanley, Jin, & Vanselow, 2016). The test condition included the simultaneous presentation of multiple potential motivating operations (e.g., presentation of demands and deprivation from tangible items) and multiple putative reinforcers following problem behavior (e.g., escape plus access to tangible items). Researchers compared the test condition with a control condition that included continuous, noncontingent presentation of the putative reinforcers from the test condition (e.g., no demands plus access to tangible items). Hanley et al. suggested that the IISCA method is highly efficient because it includes one test and one control condition (Jessel, Hanley, & Ghaemmaghami, 2016).

Although the IISCA efficiently verifies that one or more of the synthesized contingencies reinforces problem behavior, it cannot determine whether one, some, or all the individual contingencies are necessary or sufficient for reinforcement of problem behavior. For example, in a synthesized contingency of contingent escape and access to toys, the behavior analyst cannot determine whether problem behavior is maintained by (1) negative reinforcement as an individual contingency, (2) positive reinforcement as an individual contingency, or (3) the combination of negative and positive reinforcers as a synthesized contingency. Moreover, researchers use an open-ended interview and informal observations to identify the contingencies they include in an IISCA. The open-ended interview is of unknown reliability, and informal observations often identify events that correlate with but do not reinforce the target behavior (Thompson & Borrero, 2011).

Fisher, Greer, Romani, Zangrillo, and Owen (2016) conducted within-participant comparisons of the results of an IISCA and a traditional functional analysis. An IISCA is based on the assumption that the multiple, synthesized contingencies interact to reinforce problem behavior, rather than operating on the behavior independently, but it tests neither the interactive nor the independent effects of those contingencies. By contrast, a traditional functional analysis assumes that the putative reinforcement contingencies (e.g., attention, escape) operate independently on problem behavior, and it tests this assumption by testing each contingency in isolation. Fisher et al. found that both the IISCA and the functional analysis produced clear and differentiated results for four of five participants. In each of these four cases, results supported the assumption of a traditional functional analysis that the tested contingencies operated in isolation, but not the assumption that the putative reinforcers included in the IISCA interacted to produce a differential effect on problem behavior. In addition, 6 (55%) of the 11 contingencies the IISCA included across these four participants appeared to be irrelevant, in that they did not increase problem behavior relative to the individual contingency identified by the traditional functional analysis. Greer, Mitteer, Briggs, Fisher, and Sodawasser (2020) replicated and extended the findings of Fisher et al. with a larger cohort and produced equivalent findings.

One limitation of studies that compare functional-analysis procedures, such as an IISCA and a traditional functional analysis, is that the behavior analyst cannot determine the *true* function of problem behavior in the participant's natural environment before he or she conducts the analyses. Retzlaff, Fisher, Akers, and Greer (2020) conducted a translational investigation to address this

limitation, in which they trained a function (e.g., escape) for a surrogate problem response (e.g., hitting a cushioned pad) that had no prior history of reinforcement. They then conducted a traditional functional analysis, followed by a synthesized contingency analysis based on the IISCA, and then another traditional functional analysis for this newly established response. The traditional functional analysis only identified the trained function of the surrogate problem behavior for all six cases, thus providing support for the validity of the traditional functional analysis. By contrast, after the surrogate problem behavior was exposed to the synthesized contingency analysis, three of the six participants showed a new function of the surrogate problem behavior during the second traditional functional analysis. These results suggest that synthesizing contingencies in a manner such as that of the IISCA has the potential to produce new functions of problem behavior. Behavior analysts should consider this potential side effect of an IISCA before using such synthesized analyses.

## CONCLUSION

Functional analysis has emerged as the predominant method of prescribing effective behavioral treatments for persons with intellectual developmental disorder who display problem behavior (Repp, 1994). Several investigations have compared behavioral interventions that are and are not based on a functional analysis, and the results have favored the function-based approach consistently (Kuhn, DeLeon, Fisher, & Wilke, 1999; Smith, Iwata, Vollmer, & Zarcone, 1992). In addition, the results across studies included in large-scale meta-analyses have indicated that behavioral interventions tend to be more effective than pharmacological interventions, and that function-based behavioral interventions tend to be more effective than non-function-based interventions (Didden, Duker, & Korzilius, 1997; Iwata, Pace, Dorsey, et al., 1994). Although Iwata et al. (1982/1994) originally developed their procedure to assess the SIB of individuals with intellectual developmental disorder, researchers have adapted this procedure and applied it to ADHD (Northup et al., 1997), autism spectrum disorder (Fisher, Piazza, Alterson, & Kuhn, 1999), breath holding (Kern, Mauk, Marder, & Mace, 1995), bruxism (Armstrong, Knapp, & McAdam, 2014; Lang et al., 2013), disruptive behavior (Asmus et al., 1999), drug ingestion (Chapman, Fisher, Piazza, & Kurtz,

1993), elopement (Lang et al., 2010; Lehardy, Lerman, Evans, O'Connor, & LeSage, 2013; Piazza et al., 1997), feeding problems (Piazza et al., 2003), behavior in nonhuman animals (Dorey, Rosales-Ruiz, Smith, & Lovelace, 2009; Martin, Bloomsmith, Kelley, Marr, & Maple, 2011), noncompliance (Wilder, Harris, Reagan, & Rasey, 2007), pica and coprophagia (Ing, Roane, & Veenstra, 2011; Piazza et al., 1998), physical exercise (Larson, Normand, Morley, & Miller, 2013), psychotic speech (Fisher, Piazza, & Page, 1989), rumination (Woods, Luiselli, & Tomassone, 2013), and tantrums (Repp & Karsh, 1994). Researchers also have modified functional-analysis procedures to improve their accuracy (e.g., Vollmer et al., 1995), applicability to different populations (e.g., Cooper et al., 1992), applicability to telehealth (e.g., Wacker et al., 2013), efficiency (e.g., Derby et al., 1992; Kahng & Iwata, 1999; Wallace & Iwata, 1999), generality to natural environments (e.g., Mace & Lalli, 1991; Thomason-Sassi, Iwata, & Fritz, 2013), and use for identifying idiosyncratic reinforcers (e.g., Fisher, Lindauer, et al., 1998; Roscoe et al., 2015; Saini, Greer, & Fisher, 2015).

In summary, the functional-analysis procedure Iwata et al. (1982/1994) developed arguably represents the most important advance in applied behavior analysis in the last half century. It is a prescriptive assessment, in that its results directly inform intervention. Functional analysis generally leads to more effective intervention (Didden et al., 1997; Iwata, Pace, Dorsey, et al., 1994). Functional analysis has led to the development of many innovative interventions (Bowman et al., 1997; Iwata, Pace, Cowdery, et al., 1994). Finally, functional analysis provides a controlled method for conducting large-scale epidemiological investigations to study environmental influences on problem behavior (Iwata, Pace, Dorsey, et al., 1994).

# REFERENCES

American Psychiatric Association. (2013). *Diagnostic and statistical manual of mental disorders* (5th ed.). Arlington, VA: Author.

Armstrong, A., Knapp, V. M., & McAdam, D. B. (2014). Functional analysis and treatment of the diurnal bruxism of a 16-year-old girl with autism. *Journal of Applied Behavior Analysis, 47,* 415–419.

Asmus, J. M., Franzese, J. C., Conroy, M. A., & Dozier, C. L. (2003). Clarifying functional analysis outcomes for disruptive behaviors by controlling consequence delivery for stereotypy. *School Psychology Review, 32,* 624–630.

Asmus, J. M., Wacker, D. P., Harding, J., Berg, W. K., Derby, K. M., & Kocis, E. (1999). Evaluation of antecedent stimulus parameters for the treatment of escape-maintained aberrant behavior. *Journal of Applied Behavior Analysis, 32,* 495–513.

Austin, J. L., Groves, E. A., Reynish, L. C., & Francis, L. L. (2015). Validating trial-based functional analyses in mainstream primary school classrooms. *Journal of Applied Behavior Analysis, 48,* 274–288.

Beavers, G. A., Iwata, B. A., & Lerman, D. C. (2013). Thirty years of research on the functional analysis of problem behavior. *Journal of Applied Behavior Analysis, 46,* 1–21.

Berkson, G., & Mason, W. A. (1963). Stereotyped movements of mental defectives: III. Situation effects. *American Journal of Mental Deficiency, 68,* 409–412.

Berkson, G., & Mason, W. A. (1964). Stereotyped movements of mental defectives: IV. The effects of toys and the character of the acts. *American Journal of Mental Deficiency, 68,* 511–524.

Bloom, S. E., Iwata, B. A., Fritz, J. N., Roscoe, E. M., & Carreau, A. B. (2011). Classroom application of trial-based functional analysis. *Journal of Applied Behavior Analysis, 44,* 19–31.

Bloom, S. E., Lambert, J. M., Dayton, E., & Samaha, A. L. (2013). Teacher-conducted trial-based functional analyses as the basis for intervention. *Journal of Applied Behavior Analysis, 46,* 208–218.

Bowman, L. G., Fisher, W. W., Thompson, R. H., & Piazza, C. C. (1997). On the relation of mands and the function of problem behavior. *Journal of Applied Behavior Analysis, 30,* 251–265.

Broussard, C. D., & Northup, J. (1995). An approach to functional assessment and analysis of disruptive behavior in regular education classrooms. *School Psychology Quarterly, 10,* 151–164.

Carr, E. G. (1977). The motivation of self-injurious behavior: A review of some hypotheses. *Psychological Bulletin, 84,* 800–816.

Carr, E. G., Newsom, C. D., & Binkoff, J. A. (1976). Stimulus control of self-destructive behavior in a psychotic child. *Journal of Abnormal Child Psychology, 4,* 139–153.

Carr, E. G., Newsom, C. D., & Binkoff, J. A. (1980). Escape as a factor in the aggressive behavior of two retarded children. *Journal of Applied Behavior Analysis, 13,* 101–117.

Chapman, S., Fisher, W. W., Piazza, C. C., & Kurtz, P. F. (1993). Functional assessment and treatment of life-threatening drug ingestion in a dually diagnosed youth. *Journal of Applied Behavior Analysis, 26,* 255–256.

Conners, J., Iwata, B. A., Kahng, S., Hanley, G. P., Worsdell, A. S., & Thompson, R. H. (2000). Differential responding in the presence and absence of discriminative stimuli during multielement functional analyses. *Journal of Applied Behavior Analysis, 33,* 299–308.

Cooper, L. J., Wacker, D. P., Sasso, G. M., Reimers, T. M., & Donn, L. K. (1990). Using parents as therapists to evaluate appropriate behavior of their children: Application to a tertiary diagnostic clinic. *Journal of Applied Behavior Analysis, 23,* 285–296.

Cooper, L. J., Wacker, D. P., Thursby, D., Plagmann, L. A., Harding, J., Millard, T., et al. (1992). Analysis of the effects of task preferences, task demands, and adult attention on child behavior in outpatient and classroom settings. *Journal of Applied Behavior Analysis, 25,* 823–840.

Derby, K. M., Hagopian, L., Fisher, W. W., Richman, D., Augustine, M., Fahs, A., et al. (2000). Functional analysis of aberrant behavior through measurement of separate response topographies. *Journal of Applied Behavior Analysis, 33,* 113–117.

Derby, K. M., Wacker, D. P., Peck, S., Sasso, G., DeRaad, A., Berg, W., et al. (1994). Functional analysis of separate topographies of aberrant behavior. *Journal of Applied Behavior Analysis, 27,* 267–278.

Derby, K. M., Wacker, D. P., Sasso, G., Steege, M., Northup, J., Sigrand, K., et al. (1992). Brief functional assessment techniques to evaluate aberrant behavior in an outpatient setting: A summary of 79 cases. *Journal of Applied Behavior Analysis, 25,* 713–721.

Didden, R., Duker, P. C., & Korzilius, H. (1997). Meta-analytic study on treatment effectiveness for problem behaviors with individuals who have mental retardation. *American Journal on Mental Retardation, 101,* 387–399.

Dorey, N. R., Rosales-Ruiz, J., Smith, R., & Lovelace, B. (2009). Functional analysis and treatment of self-injury in a captive olive baboon. *Journal of Applied Behavior Analysis, 42,* 785–794.

Dracobly, J. D., & Smith, R. G. (2012). Progressing from identification and functional analysis of precursor behavior to treatment of self-injurious behavior. *Journal of Applied Behavior Analysis, 45,* 361–374.

Fahmie, T. A., Iwata, B. A., Harper, J. M., & Querim, A. C. (2013). Evaluation of the divided attention condition during functional analyses. *Journal of Applied Behavior Analysis, 46,* 71–78.

Finney, J. W., Russo, D. C., & Cataldo, M. F. (1982). Reduction of pica in young children with lead poisoning. *Journal of Pediatric Psychology, 7,* 197–207.

Fisher, W. W., Adelinis, J. D., Thompson, R. H., Worsdell, A. S., & Zarcone, J. R. (1998). Functional analysis and treatment of problem behavior maintained by termination of "don't" (and symmetrical "do") requests. *Journal of Applied Behavior Analysis, 31,* 339–356.

Fisher, W. W., Greer, B. D., Romani, P. W., Zangrillo, A. N., & Owen, T. M. (2016). Comparisons of synthesized- and individual-reinforcement contingencies during functional analysis. *Journal of Applied Behavior Analysis, 49,* 596–616.

Fisher, W. W., Lindauer, S. E., Alterson, C. J., & Thompson, R. H. (1998). Assessment and treatment of problem behavior maintained by stereotypic object manipulation. *Journal of Applied Behavior Analysis, 31,* 513–527.

Fisher, W. W., Ninness, H. A. C., Piazza, C. C., & Owen-DeSchryver, J. S. (1996). On the reinforcing effects of the content of verbal attention. *Journal of Applied Behavior Analysis, 29,* 235–238.

Fisher, W. W., O'Connor, J. T., Kurtz, P. F., DeLeon, I. G., & Gotjen, D. L. (2000). The effects of noncontingent delivery of high- and low-preference stimuli on attention-maintained problem behavior. *Journal of Applied Behavior Analysis, 33,* 79–83.

Fisher, W. W., Piazza, C. C., Alterson, C. J., & Kuhn, D. E. (1999). Interresponse relations among aberrant behaviors displayed by persons with autism and developmental disabilities. In P. M. Ghezzi, W. L. Williams, & J. E. Carr (Eds.), *Autism: Behavior-analytic perspectives* (pp. 113–135). Reno, NV: Context Press.

Fisher, W., Piazza, C. C., Bowman, L. G., Hagopian, L. P., Owens, J. C., & Slevin, I. (1992). A comparison of two approaches for identifying reinforcers for persons with severe and profound disabilities. *Journal of Applied Behavior Analysis, 25,* 491–498.

Fisher, W. W., Piazza, C. C., Bowman, L. G., Hanley, G. P., & Adelinis, J. D. (1997). Direct and collateral effects of restraints and restraint fading. *Journal of Applied Behavior Analysis, 30,* 105–120.

Fisher, W. W., Piazza, C. C., Cataldo, M., Harrell, R., Jefferson, G., & Conner, R. (1993). Functional communication training with and without extinction and punishment. *Journal of Applied Behavior Analysis, 26,* 23–36.

Fisher, W. W., Piazza, C. C., & Page, T. J. (1989). Assessing independent and interactive effects of behavioral and pharmacologic interventions for a client with dual diagnoses. *Journal of Behavior Therapy and Experimental Psychiatry, 20,* 241–250.

Fritz, J. N., Iwata, B. A., Hammond, J. L., & Bloom, S. E. (2013). Experimental analysis of precursors to severe problem behavior. *Journal of Applied Behavior Analysis, 46,* 101–129.

Ghaemmaghami, M., Hanley, G. P., Jin, S. C., & Vanselow, N. R. (2016). Affirming control by multiple reinforcers via progressive treatment analysis. *Behavioral Interventions, 31,* 70–86.

Greer, B. D., Mitteer, D. R., Briggs, A. M., Fisher, W. W., & Sodawasser, A. J. (2020). Comparisons of standardized and interview-informed synthesized reinforcement contingencies relative to functional analysis. *Journal of Applied Behavior Analysis, 53,* 82–101.

Hammond, J. L., Iwata, B. A., Rooker, G. W., Fritz, J. N., & Bloom, S. E. (2013). Effects of fixed versus random condition sequencing during multielement functional analyses. *Journal of Applied Behavior Analysis, 46,* 22–30.

Hanley, G. P., Iwata, B. A., & McCord, B. E. (2003). Functional analysis of problem behavior: A review. *Journal of Applied Behavior Analysis, 36,* 147–185.

Hanley, G. P., Jin, C. S., Vanselow, N. R., & Hanratty, L. A. (2014). Producing meaningful improvements in problem behavior of children with autism via synthesized analyses and treatments. *Journal of Applied Behavior Analysis, 47,* 16–36.

Hagopian, L. P., Fisher, W. W., Thompson, R. H., Owen-DeSchryver, J., Iwata, B. A., & Wacker, D. P. (1997). Toward the development of structured criteria for interpretation of functional analysis data. *Journal of Applied Behavior Analysis, 30,* 313–326.

Hagopian, L. P., Rooker, G. W., Jessel, J., & DeLeon, I. G. (2013). Initial functional analysis outcomes and modifications in pursuit of differentiation: A summary of 176 inpatient cases. *Journal of Applied Behavior Analysis, 46,* 88–100.

Ing, A. D., Roane, H. S., & Veenstra, R. A. (2011). Functional analysis and treatment of coprophagia. *Journal of Applied Behavior Analysis, 44,* 151–155.

Iwata, B. A. (1987). Negative reinforcement in applied behavior analysis: An emerging technology. *Journal of Applied Behavior Analysis, 20,* 361–378.

Iwata, B. A., Dorsey, M. F., Slifer, K. J., Bauman, K. E., & Richmand, G. S. (1994). Toward a functional analysis of self-injury. *Journal of Applied Behavior Analysis, 27,* 197–209. (Reprinted from *Analysis and Intervention in Developmental Disabilities, 2,* 3–20, 1982)

Iwata, B. A., Duncan, B. A., Zarcone, J. R., Lerman, D. C., & Shore, B. A. (1994). A sequential, test-control methodology for conducting functional analyses of self-injurious behavior. *Behavior Modification, 18,* 289–306.

Iwata, B. A., Pace, G. M., Cowdery, G. E., & Miltenberger, R. G. (1994). What makes extinction work: An analysis of procedural form and function. *Journal of Applied Behavior Analysis, 27,* 131–144.

Iwata, B. A., Pace, G. M., Dorsey, M. F., Zarcone, J. R., Vollmer, T. R., Smith, R. G., et al. (1994). The functions of self-injurious behavior: An experimental–epidemiological analysis. *Journal of Applied Behavior Analysis, 27,* 215–240.

Jessel, J., Hanley, G. P., & Ghaemmaghami, M. (2016). Interview-informed synthesized contingency analyses: Thirty replications and reanalysis. *Journal of Applied Behavior Analysis, 49,* 576–595.

Kahng, S., Abt, K. A., & Schonbachler, H. E. (2001). Assessment and treatment of low-rate high intensity problem behavior. *Journal of Applied Behavior Analysis, 34,* 225–228.

Kahng, S., Hausman, N. L., Fisher, A. B., Donaldson, J. M., Cox, J. R., Lugo, M., et al. (2015). The safety of functional analyses of self-injurious behavior. *Journal of Applied Behavior Analysis, 48,* 107–114.

Kahng, S., & Iwata, B. A. (1999). Correspondence between outcomes of brief and extended functional analyses. *Journal of Applied Behavior Analysis, 32,* 149–159.

Kern, L., Mauk, J. E., Marder, T. J., & Mace, F. C. (1995). Functional analysis and intervention for breath-holding. *Journal of Applied Behavior Analysis, 28,* 339–340.

Kodak, T., Fisher, W. W., Paden, A., & Dickes, N. (2013). Evaluation of the utility of a discrete-trial functional analysis in early intervention classrooms. *Journal of Applied Behavior Analysis, 46,* 301–306.

Kodak, T., Northup, J., & Kelley, M. E. (2007). An evaluation of the types of attention that maintain problem behavior. *Journal of Applied Behavior Analysis, 40,* 167–171.

Kuhn, D. E., DeLeon, I. G., Fisher, W. W., & Wilke, A. E. (1999). Clarifying an ambiguous functional analysis with matched and mismatched extinction procedures. *Journal of Applied Behavior Analysis, 32,* 99–102.

Lambert, J. M., Bloom, S. E., Kunnavatana, S. S., Collins, S. D., & Clay, C. J. (2013). Training residential staff to conduct trial-based functional analyses. *Journal of Applied Behavior Analysis, 46,* 296–300.

Lang, R., Davenport, K., Britt, C., Ninci, J., Garner, J., & Moore, M. (2013). Functional analysis and treatment of diurnal bruxism. *Journal of Applied Behavior Analysis, 46,* 322–327.

Lang, R., Davis, T., O'Reilly, M., Machalicek, W., Rispoli, M., Sigafoos, J., et al. (2010). Functional analysis and treatment of elopement across two school settings. *Journal of Applied Behavior Analysis, 43,* 113–118.

Laraway, S., Snycerski, S., Michael, J., & Poling, A. (2003). Motivating operations and terms to describe them: Some further refinements. *Journal of Applied Behavior Analysis, 36,* 407–414.

Larson, T. A., Normand, M. P., Morley, A. J., & Miller, B. G. (2013). A functional analysis of moderate-to-vigorous physical activity in young children. *Journal of Applied Behavior Analysis, 46,* 199–207.

Lehardy, R. K., Lerman, D. C., Evans, L. M., O'Connor, A., & LeSage, D. L. (2013). A simplified methodology for identifying the function of elopement. *Journal of Applied Behavior Analysis, 46,* 256–270.

Lovaas, O. I., Freitag, G., Gold, V. J., & Kassorla, I. C. (1965). Experimental studies in childhood schizophrenia: Analysis of self-destructive behavior. *Journal of Experimental Child Psychology, 2,* 67–84.

Lovaas, O. I., & Simmons, J. Q. (1969). Manipulation of self-destruction in three retarded children. *Journal of Applied Behavior Analysis, 2,* 143–157.

Mace, F. C., & Lalli, J. S. (1991). Linking descriptive and experimental analyses in the treatment of bizarre speech. *Journal of Applied Behavior Analysis, 24,* 553–562.

Martin, A. L., Bloomsmith, M. A., Kelley, M. E., Marr, M. J., & Maple, T. L. (2011). Functional analysis and treatment of human-directed undesirable behavior exhibited by a captive chimpanzee. *Journal of Applied Behavior Analysis, 44,* 139–143.

McComas, J., Hoch, H., Paone, D., & El-Roy, D. (2000). Escape behavior during academic tasks: A preliminary analysis of idiosyncratic establishing operations. *Journal of Applied Behavior Analysis, 33,* 479–493.

Northup, J., Jones, K., Broussard, C., DiGiovanni, G., Herring, M., Fusilier, I., et al. (1997). A preliminary analysis of interactive effects between common class-room contingencies and methylphenidate. *Journal of Applied Behavior Analysis, 30,* 121–125.

Piazza, C. C., Bowman, L. G., Contrucci, S. A., Delia, M. D., Adelinis, J. D., & Goh, H. (1999). An evaluation of the properties of attention as reinforcement for problem and appropriate behavior. *Journal of Applied Behavior Analysis, 32,* 437–449.

Piazza, C. C., Fisher, W. W., Brown, K. A., Shore, B. A., Patel, M. R., Katz, R. M., et al. (2003). Functional analysis of inappropriate mealtime behaviors. *Journal of Applied Behavior Analysis, 36,* 187–204.

Piazza, C. C., Fisher, W. W., Hanley, G. P., LeBlanc, L. A., Worsdell, A. S., Lindauer, S. E., et al. (1998). Treatment of pica through multiple analyses of its reinforcing functions. *Journal of Applied Behavior Analysis, 31,* 165–189.

Piazza, C. C., Hanley, G. P., Bowman, L. G., Ruyter, J. M., Lindauer, S. E., & Saiontz, D. M. (1997). Functional analysis and treatment of elopement. *Journal of Applied Behavior Analysis, 30,* 653–672.

Querim, A. C., Iwata, B. A., Roscoe, E. M., Schlichenmeyer, K. J., Ortega, J. V., & Hurl, K. E. (2013). Functional analysis screening for problem behavior maintained by automatic reinforcement. *Journal of Applied Behavior Analysis, 46,* 47–60.

Repp, A. (1994). Comments on functional analysis procedures for school-based behavior problems. *Journal of Applied Behavior Analysis, 27,* 409–411.

Repp, A. C., & Karsh, K. G. (1994). Hypothesis-based interventions for tantrum behaviors of persons with developmental disabilities in school settings. *Journal of Applied Behavior Analysis, 27,* 21–31.

Retzlaff, B. J., Fisher, W. W., Akers, J. S., & Greer, B. D. (2020). A translational evaluation of potential iatrogenic effects of single and combined contingencies during functional analysis of target responses. *Journal of Applied Behavior Analysis, 53,* 67–81.

Rincover, A. (1978). Sensory extinction: A procedure for eliminating self-stimulatory behavior in developmentally disabled children. *Journal of Abnormal Child Psychology, 6,* 299–310.

Ringdahl, J. E., & Sellers, J. A. (2000). The effects of different adults as therapists during functional analyses. *Journal of Applied Behavior Analysis, 33,* 247–250.

Roane, H. S., Fisher, W. W., Kelley, M. E., Mevers, J. L., & Bouxsein, K. J. (2013). Using modified visual-inspection criteria to interpret functional analysis outcomes. *Journal of Applied Behavior Analysis, 46,* 130–146.

Roane, H. S., Lerman, D. C., Kelley, M. E., & Van Camp, C. M. (1999). Within-session patterns of responding during functional analyses: The role of establishing operations in clarifying behavioral function. *Research in Developmental Disabilities, 20,* 73–89.

Rooker, G. W., Iwata, B. A., Harper, J. M., Fahmie, T. A., & Camp, E. M. (2011). False-positive tangible outcomes of functional analyses. *Journal of Applied Behavior Analysis, 44,* 737–745.

Roscoe, E. M., Schlichenmeyer, K. J., & Dube, W. V. (2015). Functional analysis of problem behavior: A systematic approach for identifying idiosyncratic variables. *Journal of Applied Behavior Analysis, 48,* 289–314.

Saini, V., Fisher, W. W., & Retzlaff, B. J. (2018). Predictive validity and efficiency of ongoing visual-inspection criteria for interpreting functional analyses. *Journal of Applied Behavior Analysis, 51,* 303–320.

Saini, V., Fisher, W. W., Retzlaff, B. J., & Keevy, M. D. (2020). Efficiency in functional analysis of problem behavior: A quantitative and qualitative review. *Journal of Applied Behavior Analysis, 53,* 44–66.

Saini, V., Greer, B. D., & Fisher, W. W. (2015). Clarifying inconclusive functional analysis results: Assessment and treatment of automatically reinforced aggression. *Journal of Applied Behavior Analysis, 48,* 315–330.

Schlichenmeyer, K. J., Roscoe, E. M., Rooker, G. W., Wheeler, E. E., & Dube, W. V. (2013). Idiosyncratic variables that affect functional analysis outcomes: A review (2001–2010). *Journal of Applied Behavior Analysis, 46,* 339–348.

Shirley, M. J., Iwata, B. A., & Kahng, S. (1999). False-positive maintenance of self-injurious behavior by access to tangible reinforcers. *Journal of Applied Behavior Analysis, 32,* 201–204.

Sigafoos, J., & Saggers, E. A. (1995). Discrete-trial approach to the functional analysis of aggressive behaviour in two boys with autism. *Australian and New Zealand Journal of Developmental Disabilities, 20,* 287–297.

Skinner, B. F. (1953). *Science and human behavior.* New York: Free Press.

Smith, R. G., Iwata, B. A., Goh, H. L., & Shore, B. A. (1995). Analysis of establishing operations for self-injury maintained by escape. *Journal of Applied Behavior Analysis, 28,* 515–535.

Smith, R. G., Iwata, B. A., Vollmer, T. R., & Zarcone, J. R. (1992). Experimental analysis and treatment of multiply controlled self-injury. *Journal of Applied Behavior Analysis, 26,* 183–196.

Sulzer-Azaroff, B., & Mayer, G. (1977). *Applying behavior analysis procedures with children and youth.* Austin, TX: Holt, Rinehart & Winston.

Thomason-Sassi, J. L., Iwata, B. A., & Fritz, J. N. (2013). Therapist and setting influences on functional analysis outcomes. *Journal of Applied Behavior Analysis, 46,* 79–87.

Thomason-Sassi, J. L., Iwata, B. A., Neidert, P. L., & Roscoe, E. M. (2011). Response latency as an index of response strength during functional analyses of problem behavior. *Journal of Applied Behavior Analysis, 44,* 51–67.

Thompson, R. H., & Borrero, J. C. (2011). Direct observation. In W. W. Fisher, C. C. Piazza, & H. S. Roane (Eds.), *Handbook of applied behavior analysis* (pp. 191–205). New York: Guilford Press.

Thompson, R. H., Fisher, W. W., Piazza, C. C., & Kuhn,

D. E. (1998). The evaluation and treatment of aggression maintained by attention and automatic reinforcement. *Journal of Applied Behavior Analysis, 31,* 103–116.

Thompson, R. J., & Iwata, B. A. (2001). Functional analysis and treatment of self-injury associated with transitions. *Journal of Applied Behavior Analysis, 34,* 195–210.

Umbreit, J. (1996). Functional analysis of disruptive behavior in an inclusive classroom. *Journal of Early Intervention, 20,* 18–29.

Van Camp, C. M., Lerman, D. C., Kelley, M. E., Roane, H. S., Contrucci, S. A., & Vorndran, C. M. (2000). Further analysis of idiosyncratic antecedent influences during the assessment and treatment of problem behavior. *Journal of Applied Behavior Analysis, 33,* 207–221.

Van Houten, R., & Rolider, A. (1988). Recreating the scene: An effective way to provide delayed punishment for inappropriate motor behavior. *Journal of Applied Behavior Analysis, 21,* 187–192.

Vollmer, T. R., Iwata, B. A., Zarcone, J. R., Smith, R. G., & Mazaleski, J. L. (1993). Within-session patterns of self-injury as indicators of behavioral function. *Research in Developmental Disabilities, 14,* 479–492.

Vollmer, T. R., Marcus, B. A., Ringdahl, J. E., & Roane, H. S. (1995). Progressing from brief assessments to extended experimental analyses in the evaluation of aberrant behavior. *Journal of Applied Behavior Analysis, 28,* 561–576.

Wacker, D. P., Lee, J. F., Dalmau, Y. C. P., Kopelman, T. G., Lindgren, S. D., Kuhle, J., et al. (2013). Conducting functional analyses of problem behavior via telehealth. *Journal of Applied Behavior Analysis, 46,* 31–46.

Wallace, M. D., & Iwata, B. A. (1999). Effects of session duration on functional analysis outcomes. *Journal of Applied Behavior Analysis, 32,* 175–183.

Weeden, M., Mahoney, A., & Poling, A. (2010). Self-injurious behavior and functional analysis: Where are the descriptions of participant protections? *Research in Developmental Disabilities, 31,* 299–303.

Wilder, D. A., Harris, C., Reagan, R., & Rasey, A. (2007). Functional analysis and treatment of noncompliance by preschool children. *Journal of Applied Behavior Analysis, 40,* 173–177.

Woods, K. E., Luiselli, J. K., & Tomassone, S. (2013). Functional analysis and intervention for chronic rumination. *Journal of Applied Behavior Analysis, 46,* 328–332.

# PART V

# INTERVENTIONS FOR INCREASING DESIRABLE BEHAVIOR

Applied behavior analysis has a rich history and an array of procedures to promote skill development and increase desirable behavior across a broad range of learners. The topics covered in Part V reflect the breadth of these procedures and progress from teaching alternatives to problem behavior, to teaching novel verbal behavior, to teaching complex, multistep behavior repertoires, to providing staff training.

In Chapter 14, Tiger and Hanley discuss the topic of differential reinforcement and the many ways in which differential-reinforcement paradigms may be used to promote desirable behavior and decrease maladaptive behavior. Attention is given to the subtypes of differential-reinforcement procedures, their various applications, and the conditions under which some procedures might be warranted. For their current chapter, the authors have expanded their discussion in the first edition to summarize recent research on differential reinforcement and describe tools to facilitate programming for maintenance and increasing delays to reinforcement.

It is common for behavior analysts to focus on promoting extended behavioral sequences or chains (e.g., assembling a bicycle). In Chapter 15, Noell, Call, Ardoin, and Miller have updated their first-edition chapter on building complex behaviors through stimulus control, chaining, and strategic behavior. New for this edition is an increased focus on the conceptualization of complex behavior repertoires, as well as new information on promoting maintenance, generalization, self-management, and response variability.

Since the first edition of this handbook appeared, there have been several advances in the area of verbal behavior. Chapter 16, by Tincani, Miguel, Bondy, and Crozier, summarizes much of this recent research. The chapter begins by reviewing Skinner's formulation of verbal behavior before reviewing applications for developing verbal behavior repertoires. It then provides a summary of recent developments related to procedures and considerations for teaching various components of verbal behavior.

The final chapter in this section addresses staff training. This is an area of critical importance for promoting the efficacy of behavior change programs. In Chapter 17, Reid, O'Kane, and Macurik highlight the many considerations and data-based procedures associated with staff training. Of note, these authors highlight recent advances in the application of functional assessment and preference assessment to staff training, and highlight steps that behavior analysts might take to promote generalization beyond training environments. Finally, this chapter includes considerations for applying procedures developed under controlled settings with children to adults living in more naturalistic settings.

# CHAPTER 14

# Differential-Reinforcement Procedures

Jeffrey H. Tiger and Gregory P. Hanley

The term *reinforcement* describes the process in which a behavior strengthens when its occurrence is followed by some improvement in the environment. By *strengthened*, we mean that the behavior is more likely to occur in the future in similar environmental conditions. The process of reinforcement is fundamental to the way people interact with and learn from their environment. For instance, children repeat phrases that made their parents laugh; teenagers wear the same clothes that made their friends take notice; and adults swing a golf club with a particular form when doing so has produced long and accurate drives.

We can understand much of early human learning by acknowledging the regular, natural, and often accidental reinforcement and punishment contingencies that infants experience (Bijou, 1996; Schlinger, 1995). For example, an infant girl may experience reinforcers for grasping her food only when she applies the appropriate amount of grip strength. Grasping too hard will squash the food or cause it to slip from her hands. Grasping too softly will not capture the food. Such gradual and natural reinforcement processes may at least partially account for learning to reach, grasp, and then chew, and other important behaviors such as babbling, standing, and walking.

Although natural contingencies may account for much of human learning, alone they may change behavior in a slow and inefficient man-

ner, particularly when reinforcers for engaging in important behavior are delayed or intermittent, or when a chain of behavior is necessary to produce reinforcement. Imagine trying to learn to drive a manual-transmission car based solely on the natural consequences of that behavior. Two distinguishing capacities of humans are the abilities to relay personal learning histories to other people through verbal behavior, such as speech and writing, and to arrange contingencies to develop and refine important behaviors in others. Thus we can increase the speed at which important behavior develops and eventually contacts natural reinforcement contingencies. In this regard, *differential reinforcement* is applicable as a *procedural* term to describe the act of increasing the occurrence of a desirable behavior in others by arranging for improvements to follow such behavior.

By arranging for reinforcers to occur more often following one behavior than following another, differential reinforcement has two effects: It strengthens the target behavior and weakens other behavior that is functionally similar. Given this latter effect, investigators have used differential reinforcement to reduce problem behavior (see Vollmer, Athens, & Fernand, Chapter 19, this volume). By many accounts, differential-reinforcement procedures have revolutionized the educational and care practices for young children, especially children with intellectual developmental disorder and severe problem behaviors (Risley, 2005). However, the accelerative effects of differential reinforcement are also valuable for designing teaching and habilitative environments, and our chapter focuses primarily on the use of differential reinforcement to develop and refine new behavior and to maintain this behavior in many settings.

Differential reinforcement as a procedure is deceptively simple: Identify a behavior you would like to occur more often, arrange reinforcers to follow the occurrence of the behavior or features of the behavior, and do not present these same reinforcers following occurrences of other behaviors. Socially important behavior change, however, is often not that simple. Behavior analysts have developed a comprehensive technology for increasing desirable behavior through differential reinforcement and have used this technology since the inception of the field in the early 1960s. We review those technological developments in this chapter. Specifically, we provide descriptions and examples of features of behavior that behavior analysts may strengthen through differential reinforcement and highlight considerations for analysts designing differential-reinforcement-based interventions. In addition, we highlight the diverse array of applications with differential reinforcement at their core.

## FEATURES OF BEHAVIOR TO TARGET WITH DIFFERENTIAL REINFORCEMENT

In this section, we define features of behavior that are sensitive to differential reinforcement and provide illustrative examples of how differential reinforcement has modified these features.

### Topography

Common uses of differential reinforcement involve reinforcement of appropriate behavior in lieu of problem behavior. We often refer to this procedure as *differential reinforcement of alternative behavior* (DRA). Pinkston, Reese, LeBlanc, and Baer (1973) provided an example of DRA for appropriate peer interactions in lieu of aggression. In baseline, teachers typically responded to instances of peer aggression with reprimands (e.g., "You can't do that here!") and responded infrequently to appropriate social interaction, resulting in relatively high rates of aggression. The investigators then taught the teachers to withhold attention following aggression and to provide attention when the children engaged in desirable peer interactions.

This simple manipulation produced increased appropriate peer interactions and decreased occurrences of aggression.

In *differential reinforcement of other behavior* (DRO), by contrast, reinforcement is arranged for periods in which target behavior does not occur, and this may produce shifts from one topography to another. For instance, Protopopova, Kisten, and Wynne (2016) delivered food remotely to dogs that historically engaged in high rates of nuisance barking after periods in which no barking occurred. This DRO schedule eliminated nuisance barking for four of five dogs. DRO is not as precise as DRA for strengthening target behavior, and response topographies that the omission contingency did not target may emerge and be strengthened (Jessel, Borrero, & Becraft, 2015; Jessel & Ingvarsson, 2016).

### Rate

*Rate* is the number of responses emitted in a certain period. Some responses must occur repeatedly in a period to be useful or functional (e.g., typing speed, answering math facts). Much differential-reinforcement research focuses on increasing the rate of various socially important behaviors. In a recent creative example, Stasolla et al. (2017) used automated differential reinforcement to increase the ambulation rate of two girls with multiple disabilities. When optic sensors detected a forward step, the automated device provided brief access to music, lights, or tactile vibration, and this arrangement produced large increases in ambulation rate. Furthermore, these girls showed higher indices of happiness when ambulation produced reinforcement than when the same reinforcers were available noncontingently. These findings are like those of studies in which children demonstrated a preference for differential over noncontingent reinforcement during concurrent-chain schedules (Hanley, Piazza, Fisher, Contrucci, & Maglieri, 1997; Luczynski & Hanley, 2009, 2010).

When the base rate of a behavior is insufficient, *differential reinforcement of high-rate behavior* (DRH) can produce acceleration in the behavior's base rate. A DRH schedule arranges reinforcement delivery if the participant emits a minimum number of responses before the end of a specified interval. Ingham and Andrews (1973) used a procedure to treat stuttering that we can conceptualize as a DRH schedule. The investigators treated participants for stuttering with auditory feedback in which a tone sounded when the participant stuttered. This treatment produced stutter-free speech, but the speech was slow and unnatural, according to the investigators. Ingham and Andrews then delivered token reinforcement for progressively higher rates of spoken words. This DRH maintained stutter-free speech and increased the rate and naturalness of the spoken words.

In other cases, certain behaviors are socially acceptable only when they occur at moderate to low rates. For instance, recruiting teacher attention is a common and desirable behavior of young children and is a common target for children who do not demonstrate this skill (e.g., Stokes, Fowler, & Baer, 1978). However, children who make frequent bids for attention can be disruptive to typical classroom environments. In *differential reinforcement of low-rate behavior* (DRL), reinforcement is arranged when a behavior occurs below a certain threshold. Investigators have used DRL schedules to maintain moderate or low rates of behavior, frequently as an initial treatment for problem behavior. For instance, Austin and Bevan (2011) described what they called a full-session DRL procedure with three elementary school students. The classroom teacher set a maximum-response criterion for each student, such as nine responses in a 20-minute session, and each student who made fewer requests than their individualized maximum received a point that he or she could use in the classroom behavior management system. This procedure reduced requesting behavior to levels more appropriate for the classroom. Unlike forms of differential reinforcement that target zero or near-zero levels of a behavior, DRL schedules may maintain behavior at low rates, but see Jessel and Borrero (2014) and Becraft, Borrero, Davis, Mendres-Smith, and Castillo (2018) for laboratory-based studies including variations of DRL schedules that produced response maintenance relative to response suppression.

## Duration

*Duration* is the amount of time a participant performs a behavior. For behaviors such as completing homework, exercising, or reading, the number of instances of behavior is less informative than the amount of time a participant performs the behavior. For instance, knowing that a student studied for 3 hours in the past week is likely more informative than knowing that the student studied on three occasions, particularly if the three occasions lasted only 30 seconds each. Thus response duration may be a more important target than response frequency in these cases.

Our previous examples of differential reinforcement target increased frequency or speed of behaviors, but behavior analysts can also use differential reinforcement to sustain responding. Miller and Kelley (1994) taught parents to use differential reinforcement to sustain the homework engagement of four school-age children. After the parent and child set a goal for such engagement, the parent provided access to preferred activities when the child met or exceeded the goal. Investigators also have used DRO schedules to increase the duration of other important behavior. For instance, Cox, Virues-Ortega, Julio, and Martin (2017) arranged DRO schedules to reduce the excessive motion of children with autism spectrum disorder during magnetic resonance imaging (MRI). The DRO schedule arranged reinforcement for movement-free intervals, and participants learned to lie still up to 5 minutes during mock MRI sessions. These findings are important because excessive movement produces unusable MRI results, with the subsequent need to repeat this expensive procedure to obtain usable results.

## Intensity

*Intensity* is the physical force or magnitude of the target response. For instance, the volume at which an individual emits speech is integral to a conversation partner's ability to respond. An individual who speaks too softly may not be heard, and excessively loud speech may be aversive to the listener. Fleece et al. (1981) demonstrated the use of differential reinforcement of response intensity to increase the speech volume of two preschool children with intellectual developmental disorder. Investigators used a sound-sensitive apparatus that they calibrated to respond to participant vocalizations that exceeded a minimum threshold by producing red- and green-colored lights in the shape of a Christmas tree, which was a presumed reinforcer. The investigators increased the minimum threshold for reinforcement as the children successfully activated the device. The speech volume of the participants increased but did not exceed the speech volume of their peers.

## Latency

*Latency* is the amount of time that passes between the occurrence of some event and the completion of behavior. For instance, we might define latency to awakening as the time between an alarm clock's sounding and a person's getting out of bed. Tiger, Bouxsein, and Fisher (2007) used differential reinforcement of response latencies with an adult with Asperger syndrome who displayed delayed responding to questions. The investigators asked the participant for information, such as his siblings' names and their addresses, during baseline. The participant responded accurately, but mean response latency was 24 seconds. The investigators then arranged a differential-reinforcement contingency in which the participant earned tokens exchangeable for access to a movie for each question he answered within an identified latency. By the third differential-reinforcement session, the participant's mean latency to respond was 5 seconds.

## Interresponse Time

*Interresponse time* is the time between two instances of a response. Differential reinforcement of short interresponse times produces rapid responding (i.e., short pausing between similar responses) and differential reinforcement of longer interresponse times produces slow responding (i.e., greater pausing between similar responses). For instance, Lennox, Miltenberger, and Donnelly (1987) reduced the rapid eating of three adults with profound intellectual developmental disorder by differentially reinforcing long interresponse times between consumption of bites of food. The investigators used baseline data to set a target interresponse time of 15 seconds. They blocked participants' attempts to place food in the mouth more often than once every 15 seconds. Lennox et al. also prompted the participant to engage in an incompatible response during the 15-second interval, and participants' rate of bite consumption decreased.

## CONSIDERATIONS FOR DIFFERENTIAL-REINFORCEMENT PROCEDURES

Behavior analysts can implement differential reinforcement in many ways. Several parameters of the response–reinforcer relation affect the likelihood of differential reinforcement's effectiveness. These include the effort of the target response and the immediacy, schedule, magnitude, type, and quality of reinforcement. We discuss each of these parameters below.

## Response Effort

The *response effort* is likely to affect the rate at which an individual learns a response. Individuals acquire responses with lower effort more quickly than those with higher effort, and simple responses more quickly than complex responses. Horner,

Sprague, O'Brien, and Heathfield (1990) showed the importance of response effort when teaching alternative communicative responses to two participants who engaged in socially mediated problem behavior. Acquisition was slow and incomplete, and problem behavior persisted when the investigators required participants to type a full sentence on an augmentative-communication device to access reinforcement. Participants learned and maintained a less effortful alternative (pressing a key to generate the same sentence) more quickly, and problem behavior decreased and remained low. When speed of acquisition is critical, decreasing response effort is an important tactic to consider. The behavior analyst may still teach more effortful and complex responses by first arranging differential-reinforcement contingencies for less effortful or more simple responses, and then gradually increasing the response effort and response complexity required to access reinforcement (see Hernandez, Hanley, Ingvarsson, & Tiger, 2007, for an example of this strategy).

## Immediacy of Reinforcers

*Reinforcer immediacy* or *reinforcer contiguity* is the time between an instance of behavior and reinforcement delivery (Vollmer & Hackenberg, 2001). Individuals may acquire responses when considerable time expires between the response and a reinforcing event (i.e., acquisition under delayed-reinforcement conditions; Gleeson & Lattal, 1987), and short delays may sometimes increase response persistence for primary reinforcers (Leon, Borrero, & DeLeon, 2016). The acquisition process is usually substantially longer or incomplete, however, even with brief delays (Carroll, Kodak, & Adolf, 2016; Gleeson & Lattal, 1987). The contingency-weakening effects of delayed reinforcement are well documented (Fisher, Thompson, Hagopian, Bowman, & Krug, 2000; Hanley, Iwata, & Thompson, 2001), and sometimes a single instance of immediate reinforcement will strengthen a response (Skinner, 1948). Thus ensuring the immediate delivery of reinforcement following a target behavior is critical for rapidly increasing the behavior through differential reinforcement (Hanley et al., 2001).

Delays to social and tangible reinforcement are inevitable outside of highly resourced teaching conditions, however. Differential reinforcement is still essential for generating and maintaining important behavior under these conditions. In an early example, Lalli, Casey, and Kates (1995) used differential reinforcement of progressively increasing chains of responses to strengthen task completion and maintain functional communication, despite consistent delay to reinforcement. Ghaemmaghami, Hanley, and Jessel (2016) extended this work by showing that socially important behavior such as functional communication, tolerance, and compliance with instructions maintained despite long delays to reinforcement by (1) providing immediate reinforcement for each behavior type at least intermittently, and (2) progressively strengthening chains of appropriate behavior with the contingent termination of the delay versus time-based termination of the delay. This process strengthens initial behaviors in the response chain, even though initial behaviors do not contact much immediate reinforcement. The process also mitigates resurgence of problem behavior during delays by strengthening appropriate behavior during the delay. Thus the appropriate behavior that occurs during the delay is available for reinforcement when the delay ends. Investigators also have shown that procedures that develop behavior chains mitigate the untoward effects of delays to automatic reinforcement. For instance, Slaton and Hanley (2016) showed that chained schedules produced more consistent item engagement and lower levels of stereotypy.

## Reinforcement Schedules

Reinforcement schedules specify the number and type of responses required to produce reinforcement or the time that must elapse before reinforcement is available. The reinforcement schedule specifies the rules for reinforcement delivery. Because Mace, Pritchard, and Penney (Chapter 4, this volume) describe reinforcement schedules more fully, we only briefly review them here.

### Ratio Schedules

*Ratio* schedules arrange reinforcement delivery based on number of responses, which may be constant, variable, or progressive. In a *fixed-ratio* (FR) schedule, the number of responses required to produce reinforcement remains constant. For instance, every response produces a reinforcer in an FR 1 schedule; every fifth response produces a reinforcer in an FR 5 schedule. Behavior analysts use FR 1 schedules commonly to establish and strengthen behavior. FR schedules may produce a pause-and-run pattern in which responding occurs at consistent high rates until reinforcement delivery; the organism then pauses for a period before high-rate responding resumes (Ferster & Skinner, 1957; Orlando & Bijou, 1960).

*Variable-ratio* (VR) schedules arrange reinforcement delivery around a mean number of responses that changes from trial to trial. For instance, reinforcement delivery would occur after a mean of five responses in a VR 5 schedule. Thus, reinforcement delivery might occur after one, three, five, seven, or nine responses. VR schedules tend to produce high response rates without postreinforcement pauses, and behavior analysts often use them for response maintenance (Ferster & Skinner, 1957; Schlinger, Derenne, & Baron, 2008).

*Progressive-ratio* schedules arrange reinforcement delivery on a schedule that changes across reinforcer deliveries. These schedules progress either by the addition of a fixed number of responses (arithmetic increases) or by multiplying each progressive-schedule value by a constant (geometric increases). For instance, an investigator might use a geometric progressive-ratio schedule in which the number of responses required to produce reinforcement doubles after each reinforcer delivery. Investigators use progressive-ratio schedules to compare the strength of two or more stimuli as reinforcers (see DeLeon et al., Chapter 7, this volume). For instance, Roane, Lerman, and Vorndran (2001) demonstrated that progressive-ratio schedules were more sensitive to differences in the reinforcing efficacy of stimuli than traditional preference assessments.

### Interval Schedules

*Interval* schedules arrange for reinforcement delivery for the first response occurring after a specified interval and may be either fixed or variable. In a *fixed-interval* (FI) schedule, reinforcement delivery occurs for the first response that occurs after interval lengths that remain constant. For instance, the first response after 60 seconds will produce a reinforcer in an FI 60-second schedule. FI schedules may generate high rates of responding, especially with low-effort responses and relatively small schedule values (e.g., Hanley et al., 2001). These schedules tend to produce a scalloped behavior pattern in which little responding occurs early in the interval, but responding gradually accelerates as the interval progresses (Ferster & Skinner, 1957; Weiner, 1969).

A *variable-interval* (VI) schedule arranges reinforcement for the first response occurring after a specified interval that varies around a defined mean. For instance, reinforcement delivery might occur for the first response after 10, 30, 80, or 90 seconds in a VI 60-second schedule. VI schedules tend to produce steady response rates with little pausing (Orlando & Bijou, 1960).

## Reinforcer Magnitude

*Reinforcer magnitude* is the amount or duration of a reinforcer. Social or practical constraints often influence a reinforcer's magnitude, such as when a teacher is available only for 5 minutes, or when someone wants to limit the amount of candy a child consumes. These constraints, however, may influence the efficacy of differential-reinforcement procedures. For instance, Trosclair-Lasserre, Lerman, Call, Addison, and Kodak (2008) showed that larger amounts of attention and toys maintained responding at higher schedule values than did smaller amounts for three children diagnosed with autism spectrum disorder. Like most functional relations, there are relevant boundary conditions. For instance, delivering copious amounts of reinforcement may produce reinforcer satiation and limit the effectiveness of the differential-reinforcement procedure. Therefore, behavior analysts should base their selection of reinforcement amount or magnitude on practicality, social acceptability, and effectiveness.

## Types of Reinforcers

Behavior analysts generally distinguish between *positive* and *negative* reinforcement and *social* and *nonsocial* reinforcement. A positive reinforcer is one that a behavior analyst presents contingent on a response, which increases the future probability of the response. A negative reinforcer is one the behavior analyst removes contingent on a response, which increases the future probability of a response. Social reinforcers are ones that we can control, such as saying, "Nice work!" or giving a child a cookie. By contrast, nonsocial or automatic reinforcers are events that occur as a direct result of the behavior (e.g., obtaining a cookie from a vending machine; Vaughan & Michael, 1982).

### Positive versus Negative Reinforcers

Most reported applied-behavior-analytic studies of differential reinforcement have used positive reinforcers, such as vocal and physical attention, edible items, or leisure activities. Although investigators use differential negative reinforcement

less often (Iwata, 1987), examples include studies by Piazza et al. (1997) and Lalli et al. (1999). They provided negative reinforcement in the form of a break when the participant complied with a task demand.

Error correction is a common differential-negative-reinforcement procedure that behavior analysts incorporate into teaching programs. Error correction involves prompting additional responding when a learner makes an error. For instance, the teacher might point to the correct picture, say, "That is the elephant," and then prompt the child to "Point to the elephant" in an error correction trial for receptive identification. Research has shown that learners will acquire novel skills to avoid these additional prompts (Kodak et al., 2016; McGhan & Lerman, 2013; Rodgers & Iwata, 1991).

### Automatic Reinforcers

Most studies of differential reinforcement in the literature have used social reinforcers. Nevertheless, programming nonsocial or automatic reinforcers following the occurrence of target behavior is possible and may be useful. For instance, Linscheid, Iwata, Ricketts, Williams, and Griffin (1990) described a device to treat severe self-injurious behavior that could detect occurrences of head banging and deliver a preferred event, such as music or visual stimulation, when head banging did not occur for a specified period.

Behavior analysts also can arrange differential automatic negative reinforcement for target responses. For instance, Azrin, Ruben, O'Brien, Ayllon, and Roll (1968) engineered a device that emitted a quiet tone, followed in 3 seconds by a loud tone when participants engaged in slouching. Participants could correct their posture after the quiet tone and avoid the loud tone, or could remain erect and avoid both tones.

Investigators have shown that providing access to automatically reinforced stereotypical behavior can function as reinforcement for other target responses, such as academic discriminations and play skills (Charlop-Christy & Haymes, 1996; Charlop, Kurtz, & Casey, 1990; Wolery, Kirk, & Gast, 1985). For instance, Hanley, Iwata, Thompson, and Lindberg (2000) showed that participants' stereotypic behavior persisted in the absence of social consequences during an experimental functional analysis, suggesting that the consequences produced by the behavior functioned as automatic reinforcement. Hanley et al. provided access to stereotypic behaviors contingent on play with leisure materials, which increased participants' play with leisure materials. Potter, Hanley, Augustine, Clay, and Phelps (2013) used a similar arrangement to teach complex, multistep play to adolescents with autism spectrum disorder. The participants could engage in stereotypy by completing progressively complicated play routines. Slaton and Hanley (2016) taught participants to inhibit stereotypy and engage appropriately with items, using access to stereotypy as reinforcement. A chained schedule of reinforcement produced higher levels of item engagement and stimulus control of stereotypy than a schedule in which access to stereotypy was time-based.

Using automatic reinforcers in differential-reinforcement contingencies may be desirable for several additional reasons. First, the delivery of social reinforcers commonly requires a caregiver to continuously monitor and document participant behavior. The procedures described by Linscheid et al. (1990) and Azrin et al. (1968) require neither, which may increase their utility. Second, automated delivery of reinforcers is likely to be more precise and immediate than delivery of reinforcers by humans if the device functions properly. Third, individuals may acquire skills more readily when the consequence of responding results directly from the behavior (Thompson & Iwata, 2000).

### Reinforcer Quality

*Reinforcer quality* is a participant's subjective valuation of a reinforcing stimulus. Results of multiple studies have shown that attention to quality improves the efficacy of reinforcement programs (e.g., Johnson, Vladescu, Kodak, & Sidener, 2017; Mace, Neef, Shade, & Mauro, 1996) and their acceptability to the participants (e.g., Johnson et al., 2017). Presumably, effective procedures rely on reinforcers of sufficient quality, and reinforcer value is idiosyncratic and may change over time.

## STRATEGIES TO INCREASE OR MAINTAIN THE EFFECTIVENESS OF REINFORCERS

### Motivating Operations

A *motivating operation* is an event that alters the effectiveness of a stimulus as reinforcement. There are two broad categories of motivating operations (Laraway, Snycerski, Michael, & Poling, 2003): those that temporarily increase the value of a reinforcer, called *establishing operations*, and those

that temporarily diminish the value of a reinforcer, called *abolishing operations*. The most common establishing operation is deprivation, and the most common abolishing operation is satiation. Control and manipulation of establishing operations can increase the effectiveness of differential-reinforcement procedures. For instance, Goh, Iwata, and DeLeon (2000) showed that no participants acquired a novel mand when the reinforcer for the mand was available on a dense schedule of noncontingent reinforcement (NCR). When the investigators made the NCR schedule progressively leaner, participants acquired the novel mand, presumably because the relevant establishing operation increased with decreases in time-based reinforcer deliveries.

Satiation is a serious challenge when a behavior analyst is arranging reinforcement contingencies, because each reinforcer delivery serves as an abolishing operation for the reinforcer that subsequent responses produce. For instance, each sip of water decreases the establishing operation for subsequent sips of water over the near term. Using the smallest amount of reinforcement necessary to maintain responding is one way to mitigate satiation. Another is to restrict the reinforcer to the environment for the contingency arrangement. For instance, Roane, Call, and Falcomata (2005) demonstrated that responding persisted more when they restricted the reinforcer to the progressive-ratio-schedule arrangement than when the reinforcer was available outside the progressive-ratio-schedule arrangement.

In some cases, a behavior analyst cannot ethically or legally restrict a potential reinforcer. In these cases, the behavior analyst can schedule training in ways that maximize the effectiveness of reinforcers. For instance, the analyst might schedule a training session before the participant's regularly scheduled lunch and use food as a reinforcer (e.g., North & Iwata, 2005; Vollmer & Iwata, 1991).

### Reinforcer Variation

Varying reinforcers for responding may delay satiation and prolong the effectiveness of differential reinforcement (Bowman, Piazza, Fisher, Hagopian, & Kogan, 1997; Egel, 1981; Koehler, Iwata, Roscoe, Rolider, & O'Steen, 2005). For instance, Bowman et al. (1997) showed that five of seven participants preferred varied delivery of three lesser preferred items to constant delivery of a more preferred item, and Egel (1981) showed that varying reinforcers produced more stable levels of correct responding and on-task behavior for several children diagnosed with autism spectrum disorder.

## Reinforcer Choice

Providing a choice of reinforcers may be a simple yet highly effective means of improving the efficacy of differential-reinforcement procedures (Ackerlund Brandt, Dozier, Juanico, Laudont, & Mick, 2015; Dunlap et al., 1994; Dyer, Dunlap, & Winterling, 1990; Fisher, Thompson, Piazza, Crosland, & Gotjen, 1997; Sellers et al., 2013; Thompson, Fisher, & Contrucci, 1998; Tiger, Hanley, & Hernandez, 2006; Toussaint, Kodak, & Vladescu, 2016). Choice making may be effective because it produces reinforcer variation, which minimizes satiation secondary to the repeated delivery of the same reinforcer. In addition, choice making capitalizes on establishing operations that produce momentary fluctuations in the value of reinforcers, because the participant can choose the reinforcer he or she prefers at that moment.

There also is evidence that the opportunity to choose adds value to differential reinforcement beyond the value of obtaining the most preferred item. For instance, we (Tiger & Hanley, 2006) showed that six of seven preschoolers preferred to engage in academic seatwork when they could choose a single edible from an identical edible array for correct responding, rather than when the teacher provided the same amount and type of edible from the same type of array for correct responding. Note that reinforcer amount, quality, and type were identical in the two conditions; the only difference was the choice component. We also showed that children engaged in 12 to 16 times more academic work in the choice condition. These data show that programming opportunities to make choices may enhance the efficacy of differential reinforcement.

## Token Reinforcement Systems

Using conditioned reinforcers that an individual can trade later for preferred items, known as *backup reinforcers*, is another strategy to decrease satiation. Token economies, for instance, involve providing arbitrary items, such as tickets, tokens, stickers, or points, following the occurrence of target behaviors. Later the individual can exchange the tokens for preferred items (see Reitman, Boerke, & Vassilopoulos, Chapter 22, this volume, or reviews by Hackenberg, 2018; Kazdin, 1982; Kazdin & Bootzin, 1972). Token systems allow caregivers to deliver multiple reinforcers contingent on desirable behavior without adversely affecting the value of the primary or backup reinforcers, and without interrupting learning tasks or complex behaviors for reinforcer consumption. For instance, Krentz, Miltenberger, and Valbuena (2016) used token reinforcement to increase the distance walked by overweight and obese adults with intellectual developmental disorder at an adult day training center.

## COMPLEMENTARY PROCEDURES TO DEVELOP NEW BEHAVIOR

Although differential reinforcement alone can produce new behavior, combining it with other procedures when teaching new behavior is often more effective. This section describes procedures to complement differential reinforcement to develop new behavior.

### Prompting

Behavior analysts often pair prompting with differential reinforcement to teach new behavior. The general sequence involves prompting the individual to engage in a response, providing reinforcement for the prompted response, and gradually eliminating the prompt over time. The behavior analyst can provide prompts in many forms (such as vocal, visual, or physical-response prompts; within-stimulus prompts; or extrastimulus prompts) and can choose the prompt based on the modality of the target behavior and the individual's capabilities. For instance, Thompson, McKerchar, and Dancho (2004) used delayed physical prompts and differential reinforcement to teach three infants to emit the manual signs *Please* and *More* with food as the reinforcer.

By contrast, behavior analysts cannot prompt nonmotor target behavior, such as vocalizations; therefore, they must pair alternative prompting procedures with differential reinforcement. Bourret, Vollmer, and Rapp (2004) used vocal and model prompts to teach vocalizations to two children with autism spectrum disorder. The therapist vocally prompted the participant to emit the target vocalization (e.g., "Say *tunes*"). Correct vocalizations produced access to music. If the participant did not emit the target vocalization, the therapist modeled progressively shorter vocalizations (e.g., changing "Say *tunes*" to "Say *tuh*"). As the participant successfully emitted the modeled vocalization, the therapist required the participant to emit a vocalization that more closely approximated the target vocalization before receiving reinforcement.

One disadvantage is that prompting may produce prompt dependence. The behavior analyst can pair differential reinforcement with various tactics to fade and to eliminate prompts eventually (see Halle, 1987, for a discussion of spontaneity). Thompson et al. (2004) and Bourret et al. (2004) eliminated prompts by increasing the delay between the presentation of the evocative event (such as placing a toy in a participant's reach) and the prompts, so that reinforcement was more immediate for independent responses. Other tactics include withholding reinforcement for prompted responses (Touchette & Howard, 1984) or decreasing the physical intensity of the prompts (see Wolery & Gast, 1984).

## Shaping and Percentile Schedules

When prompting is not appropriate to increase responding, we recommend shaping as an alternative tool. *Shaping* involves differential reinforcement of successive approximations of a behavior. To initiate a shaping procedure, a behavior analyst must (1) identify a behavior the individual currently emits that approximates the target behavior; (2) provide reinforcement for that behavior; and (3) require closer approximations to the terminal behavior, such as more complex forms or different rates or durations of behavior, for reinforcer delivery. Investigators have used shaping to teach many complex behaviors, including eye contact in children with autism spectrum disorder (e.g., McConnell, 1967), vocal speech in mute adults diagnosed with psychosis (Sherman, 1965), and limb use in patients after strokes (Taub et al., 1994). Although shaping is among behavior analysts' oldest and most celebrated tools, there are few formalized rules for shaping.

Galbicka (1994) described a formalized shaping system using *percentile schedules*, and investigators have published studies in which percentile schedules are the cornerstones of their behavior change procedures (Athens, Vollmer, & St. Peter Pipkin, 2007; Lamb, Kirby, Morral, Galbicka, & Iguchi, 2004; Lamb, Morral, Kirby, Iguchi, & Galbicka, 2004). Percentile schedules dictate rules for the timing of reinforcement delivery, and these rules can be adjusted based on recent or local rates, durations, or types of responding. The behavior analyst rank-orders responses from the simplest to the most complex to arrange percentile schedules for complex behavior. The behavior analyst keeps a running stream of the temporal order and form of the behavior, with a focus on the most recent responses. The behavior analyst delivers a reinforcer for a response if it exceeds the formal qualities of the most recent subset of responses.

Behavior analysts may use percentile schedules to shape higher rates or durations of responding. For instance, Athens et al. (2007) used percentile schedules to increase the academic-task engagement of four students with intellectual developmental disorder. The investigators measured the duration of task engagement for each participant. During the percentile-schedule phase, engagement produced a token exchangeable for food if engagement duration exceeded the median duration of the previous 5, 10, or 20 engagement durations, depending on the experimental condition. Thus the reinforcement criterion constantly shifted, given the participant's recent engagement duration. The percentile schedule produced increased engagement durations, with the biggest increases in conditions in which the participant's previous behavior determined the momentary criterion for reinforcement. For instance, Athens et al. observed higher engagement durations when they used the previous 20 versus the previous 5 engagement durations to determine the reinforcement criterion.

## Response Chaining and Task Analysis

Commonly taught behaviors are often not single, unitary responses; instead, they include a series of topographically distinct behaviors that a participant must complete in sequence. Behavior analysts often refer to these behaviors as *response chains* and to each component behavior as a *link* in the chain. Providing reinforcement for a single response in a chain or for the entire response chain may not be an efficient or effective way to shape behavior. Therefore, behavior analysts typically use prompting and differential reinforcement or shaping to establish individual links of the response chain, then differentially reinforce sequences of links until a participant produces an entire response chain. Behavior analysts use one of two general procedures, called *forward chaining* and *backward chaining*, to teach response chains. Forward chaining involves teaching the response chain in the same order in which the participant will ultimately perform it. That is, the behavior analyst differentially reinforces emission of the first behavior in the chain, then the first and second behaviors, and so forth. By contrast, the behavior analyst provides differential reinforcement for the last behavior in the chain and adds behaviors of the chain to the differential-reinforcement contingency in reverse order, in backward chaining.

*Task analysis,* or identifying individual behaviors in the response chain, is necessary before teaching a complex behavior. For instance, Neef, Parrish, Hannigan, Page, and Iwata (1989) demonstrated the importance of task analysis. They taught self-catheterization skills to two young girls with spina bifida by identifying each step of self-catheterization and then partitioning the task into 6–11 component steps. They taught each step to each participant, using prompting and differential reinforcement, until the two girls could independently self-catheterize (see also Noell, Call, Ardoin, & Miller, Chapter 15, this volume).

## RESPONSE MAINTENANCE AND SCHEDULE THINNING

Although immediate, dense schedules of reinforcement are important for establishing responses, caregivers may have difficulty implementing such schedules with high integrity over the long term. Therefore, thinning of a reinforcement schedule is an important part of response maintenance.

One method of reinforcement schedule thinning is to deliver reinforcement intermittently by progressively increasing response requirements for reinforcement. For instance, Van Houten and Nau (1980) used FR- and VR-like reinforcement schedules to increase the attending behaviors of elementary school students. The fixed schedule arranged reinforcement for every eight intervals with attending behavior. Children could reach into a grab bag with a one-eighth probability of payoff after 5 minutes of continuous attending behavior in the VR schedule. Procedures like these may allow caregivers to miss a few instances of an important behavior without inadvertently weakening the behavior.

A second technique for making differential reinforcement more practical is to include delays to reinforcement, which allows extra time for caregivers to provide the reinforcer. However, delays to reinforcement often result in extinction of newly acquired behaviors (Fisher et al., 2000; Hanley et al., 2001), and exposure to extinction may produce resurgence (i.e., the reemergence of previously reinforced behavior) and increase the likelihood of problem behavior returning (Fuhrman, Fisher,

& Greer, 2016). Other methods for introducing delays successfully include introducing brief delays that gradually increase (Schweitzer & Sulzer-Azaroff, 1988), providing a signal when the delay begins (Vollmer, Borrero, Lalli, & Daniel, 1999), and providing alternative activities during the delay (Austin & Tiger, 2015; Fisher et al., 2000; Hagopian, Contrucci Kuhn, Long, & Rush, 2005).

A *multiple schedule* is another effective method for thinning reinforcement schedules (Hanley et al., 2001; Tiger & Hanley, 2004). During a multiple schedule, the behavior analyst correlates reinforcement and extinction periods with distinct discriminative signals. Hanley et al. (2001) showed that multiple schedules maintained newly acquired social manding, even though reinforcement was available only one-fifth of the time. In addition, we (Tiger & Hanley, 2006) showed that children preferred conditions with signaled reinforcement and extinction versus ones without signals. Luczynski and Hanley (2009) showed that children preferred multiple schedules to briefly signaled delays.

Slaton and Hanley (2016) showed that students preferred chained schedules of reinforcement in which the reinforcement component included differential versus noncontingent reinforcement. Ghaemmaghami et al. (2016) used intermittent and unpredictable reinforcement of several alternative responses to thin the reinforcement schedule. Ghaemmaghami et al. suggested that the schedule they used was more like those in natural environments, where reinforcement contingencies are often ambiguous.

## DIFFERENTIAL REINFORCEMENT OF DIVERSE RESPONDING

Behavior analysts use differential reinforcement to increase the occurrence of a target behavior and to increase the diversity of behavior. For instance, Goetz and Baer (1973) provided descriptive praise (e.g., "Wow, a tower; that is new") to preschoolers for creating a block structure that they had not built that day, and new forms of building increased. Investigators have used similar procedures to increase diverse verbal responses to questions (Lee, McComas, & Jawor, 2002), activity selections during free-play periods (Cammilleri & Hanley, 2005), and martial-arts performances (Harding, Wacker, Berg, Rick, & Lee, 2004). A renewed emphasis on using differential-reinforcement schedules to promote diverse verbal behavior also is apparent in the applied literature. Investigators have used lag-differential-reinforcement schedules to increase preschoolers' diversity of selections during free-play periods (Cammilleri & Hanley, 2005), mand variability in young children with autism spectrum disorder (Brodhead, Higbee, Gerencser, & Akers, 2016), varied intraverbal responses of children with autism spectrum disorder (Contreras & Betz, 2016), and varied item naming of typically developing children (Wiskow & Donaldson, 2016).

## GROUP CONTINGENCIES

When the behavior of many individuals is the target of intervention, dependent- or interdependent-group contingencies may be useful. The consequences for the group depend on the behavior of one or some members of the group with a *dependent-group contingency*. For instance, an entire classroom may earn extra recess time if one child scores well on an exam (Litow & Pumroy, 1975). Dependent contingencies may motivate students to aid each other, such as helping each other prepare for an exam (Speltz, Shimamura, & McReynolds, 1982) or to help one child behave more appropriately. Poorly designed group contingencies may cause unwelcome peer pressure, however, and some children may not prefer reinforcement contingencies that depend on someone else's behavior (e.g., Speltz et al., 1982). One way to mitigate the negative effects of a dependent-group contingency is to randomly select the student on whose behavior the contingencies will depend (Cariveau & Kodak, 2017).

In an *interdependent-group contingency*, the group's behavior determines whether the group receives reinforcement (Litow & Pumroy, 1975). For instance, the group receives reinforcement if the students score above 80% on an exam. Hirsch, Healy, Judge, and Lloyd (2016) used an interdependent-group contingency to increase second-grade students' engagement in physical education activities; the students rated this group contingency favorably. Interdependent-group contingencies may involve competition between two or more groups, with the highest-scoring group receiving the reinforcer, such as the Good Behavior Game for students in classrooms (Barrish, Saunders, & Wolf, 1969) or the Good Productivity Game for staff members in hospitals (Lutzker & White-Blackburn, 1979). Groves and Austin (2017) recently found both independent- and interdependent-group contingencies to be effective in reducing students' verbal disruptions, inappropriate sitting, and off-task behaviors during the Good Behavior Game, but students preferred the interdependent-group contingency.

## LOTTERY CONTINGENCIES

*Lottery* contingencies are useful for increasing the time- and cost-effectiveness of differential reinforcement. For instance, Petry et al. (1998) used a lottery-type reinforcement procedure to decrease inappropriate verbal behavior in a heroin treatment center. Patients earned stickers for engaging in desirable verbal behavior. Investigators entered the names of sticker recipients into a lottery and drew one name from the lottery at the end of each week. The winner received $25. This procedure produced increased compliments and pleasantries, and decreased profanity and discussion of evading the police.

## CONCLUSION

Differential reinforcement is one of the most well-researched procedures available to behavior analysts. A mature understanding of differential reinforcement involves knowledge of (1) the range and complexity of behavior it affects, (2) the parameters that are responsible for or increase its effectiveness, and (3) the procedures that may complement it to produce significant and lasting changes in socially important behavior. This sort of understanding, combined with supervised and dedicated practice in implementing differential reinforcement, is critical to the development of an effective behavior analyst.

## REFERENCES

Ackerlund Brandt, J. A., Dozier, C. L., Juanico, J. F., Laudont, C. L., & Mick, B. R. (2015). The value of choice as a reinforcer for typically developing children. *Journal of Applied Behavior Analysis, 48,* 344–362.

Athens, E. S., Vollmer, T. R., & St. Peter Pipkin, C. C. (2007). Shaping academic task engagement with percentile schedules. *Journal of Applied Behavior Analysis, 40,* 475–488.

Austin, J. E., & Tiger, J. H. (2015). Providing alternative reinforcers to facilitate tolerance to delayed reinforcement following functional communication training. *Journal of Applied Behavior Analysis, 48,* 663–668.

Austin, J. L., & Bevan, D. (2011). Using differential reinforcement of low rates to reduce children's requests for teacher attention. *Journal of Applied Behavior Analysis, 44,* 451–461.

Azrin, N., Rubin, H., O'Brien, F., Ayllon, T., & Roll, D. (1968). Behavioral engineering: Postural control by a portable operant apparatus. *Journal of Applied Behavior Analysis, 1,* 99–108.

Barrish, H. H., Saunders, M., & Wolf, M. M. (1969). Good Behavior Game: Effects of individual contingencies for group consequences on disruptive behavior in a classroom. *Journal of Applied Behavior Analysis, 2,* 119–124.

Becraft, J. L., Borrero, J. C., Davis, B. J., Mendres-Smith, A. E., & Castillo, M. I. (2018). The role of signals in two variations of differential-reinforcement-of-low-rate procedures. *Journal of Applied Behavior Analysis, 51,* 3–24.

Bijou, S. W. (1996). *New directions in behavior development.* Reno, NV: Context Press.

Bourret, J., Vollmer, T. R., & Rapp, J. T. (2004). Evaluation of a vocal mand assessment and vocal mand training procedures. *Journal of Applied Behavior Analysis, 37,* 129–144.

Bowman, L. G., Piazza, C. C., Fisher, W. W., Hagopian, L. P., & Kogan, J. S. (1997). Assessment of preference for varied versus constant reinforcers. *Journal of Applied Behavior Analysis, 30,* 451–458.

Brodhead, M. T., Higbee, T. S., Gerencser, K. R., & Akers, J. S. (2016). The use of a discrimination-training procedure to teach mand variability to children with autism. *Journal of Applied Behavior Analysis, 49,* 34–48.

Cammilleri, A. P., & Hanley, G. P. (2005). Use of a lag differential reinforcement contingency to increase varied selections of classroom activities. *Journal of Applied Behavior Analysis, 38,* 111–115.

Cariveau, T., & Kodak, T. (2017). Programming a randomized dependent group contingency and common stimuli to promote durable behavior change. *Journal of Applied Behavior Analysis, 50,* 121–133.

Carroll, R. A., Kodak, T., & Adolf, K. J. (2016). Effect of delayed reinforcement on skill acquisition during discrete-trial instruction: Implications for treatment-integrity errors in academic settings. *Journal of Applied Behavior Analysis, 49,* 176–181.

Charlop, M. H., Kurtz, P. F., & Casey, F. G. (1990). Using aberrant behaviors as reinforcers for autistic children. *Journal of Applied Behavior Analysis, 23,* 163–181.

Charlop-Christy, M. H., & Haymes, L. K. (1996). Using obsessions as reinforcers with and without mild reductive procedures to decrease inappropriate behaviors of children with autism. *Journal of Autism and Developmental Disorders, 26,* 527–546.

Contreras, B. P., & Betz, A. M. (2016). Using lag schedules to strengthen the intraverbal repertoires of chil-

dren with autism. *Journal of Applied Behavior Analysis, 49,* 3–16.

Cox, A. D., Virues-Ortega, J., Julio, F., & Martin, T. L. (2017). Establishing motion control in children with autism and intellectual disability: Applications for anatomical and functional MRI. *Journal of Applied Behavior Analysis, 50,* 8–26.

Dunlap, G., dePerczel, M., Clarke, S., Wilson, D., Wright, S., White, R., et al. (1994). Choice making to promote adaptive behavior for students with emotional and behavioral challenges. *Journal of Applied Behavior Analysis, 27,* 505–518.

Dyer, K., Dunlap, G., & Winterling, V. (1990). Effects of choice making on the serious problem behaviors of students with severe handicaps. *Journal of Applied Behavior Analysis, 23,* 515–524.

Egel, A. L. (1981). Reinforcer variation: Implications for motivating developmentally disabled children. *Journal of Applied Behavior Analysis, 14,* 345–350.

Ferster, C. B., & Skinner, B. F. (1957). *Schedules of reinforcement.* New York: Appleton-Century-Crofts.

Fisher, W. W., Thompson, R. H., Hagopian, L. P., Bowman, L. G., & Krug, A. (2000). Facilitating tolerance to delayed reinforcement during functional communication training. *Behavior Modification, 24,* 3–29.

Fisher, W. W., Thompson, R. H., Piazza, C. C., Crosland, K., & Gotjen, D. (1997). On the relative reinforcing effects of choice and differential consequences. *Journal of Applied Behavior Analysis, 30,* 423–438.

Fleece, L., Gross, A., O'Brien, T., Kistner, J., Rothblum, E., & Drabman, R. (1981). Elevation of voice volume in young developmentally delayed children via an operant shaping procedure. *Journal of Applied Behavior Analysis, 14,* 351–355.

Fuhrman, A. M., Fisher, W. W., & Greer, B. D. (2016). A preliminary investigation on improving functional communication training by mitigating resurgence of destructive behavior. *Journal of Applied Behavior Analysis, 49,* 884–899.

Galbicka, G. (1994). Shaping in the 21st century: Moving percentile schedules into applied settings. *Journal of Applied Behavior Analysis, 27,* 739–760.

Ghaemmaghami, M., Hanley, G. P., & Jessel, J. (2016). Contingencies promote delay tolerance. *Journal of Applied Behavior Analysis, 49,* 548–575.

Gleeson, S., & Lattal, K. A. (1987). Response–reinforcer relations and the maintenance of behavior. *Journal of the Experimental Analysis of Behavior, 48,* 383–393.

Goetz, E. M., & Baer, D. M. (1973). Social control of form diversity and the emergence of new forms in children's block building. *Journal of Applied Behavior Analysis, 6,* 209–217.

Goh, H., Iwata, B. A., & DeLeon, I. G. (2000). Competition between noncontingent and contingent reinforcement schedules during response acquisition. *Journal of Applied Behavior Analysis, 33,* 195–205.

Groves, E. A., & Austin, J. L. (2017). An evaluation of interdependent and independent group contingencies during the Good Behavior Game. *Journal of Applied Behavior Analysis, 50*, 552–566.

Hackenberg, T. D. (2018). Token reinforcement: Translational research and application. *Journal of Applied Behavior Analysis, 51*, 393–435.

Hagopian, L. P., Contrucci Kuhn, S. A., Long, E. S., & Rush, K. S. (2005). Schedule thinning following communication training: Using competing stimuli to enhance tolerance to decrements in reinforcer density. *Journal of Applied Behavior Analysis, 38*, 177–193.

Halle, J. W. (1987). Teaching language in the natural environment: An analysis of spontaneity. *Journal of the Association for Persons with Severe Handicaps, 12*, 28–37.

Hanley, G. P., Iwata, B. A., & Thompson, R. H. (2001). Reinforcement schedule thinning following treatment with functional communication training. *Journal of Applied Behavior Analysis, 34*, 17–38.

Hanley, G. P., Iwata, B. A., Thompson, R. H., & Lindberg, J. S. (2000). A component analysis of "stereotypy as reinforcement" for alternative behavior. *Journal of Applied Behavior Analysis, 33*, 285–297.

Hanley, G. P., Piazza, C. C., Fisher, W. W., Contrucci, S. A., & Maglieri, K. A. (1997). Evaluation of client preference for function-based treatments. *Journal of Applied Behavior Analysis, 30*, 459–473.

Harding, J. W., Wacker, D. P., Berg, W. K., Rick, G., & Lee, J. F. (2004). Promoting response variability and stimulus generalization in martial arts training. *Journal of Applied Behavior Analysis, 37*, 185–195.

Hernandez, E., Hanley, G. P., Ingvarsson, E. T., & Tiger, J. H. (2007). An evaluation of the emergence of novel mand forms. *Journal of Applied Behavior Analysis, 40*, 137–156.

Hirsch, S. E., Healy, S., Judge, J. P., & Lloyd, J. W. (2016). Effects of an interdependent group contingency on engagement in physical education. *Journal of Applied Behavior Analysis, 49*, 975–979.

Horner, R. H., Sprague, J. R., O'Brien, M., & Heathfield, L. T. (1990). The role of response efficiency in the reduction of problem behaviors through functional equivalence training: A case study. *Journal of the Association for Persons with Severe Handicaps, 15*, 91–97.

Ingham, R. J., & Andrews, G. (1973). An analysis of a token economy in stuttering therapy. *Journal of Applied Behavior Analysis, 6*, 219–229.

Iwata, B. A. (1987). Negative reinforcement in applied behavior analysis: An emerging technology. *Journal of Applied Behavior Analysis, 20*, 361–378.

Jessel, J., & Borrero, J. C. (2014). A laboratory comparison of two variations of differential-reinforcement-of-low-rate procedures. *Journal of Applied Behavior Analysis, 47*, 314–324.

Jessel, J., Borrero, J. C., & Becraft, J. L. (2015). Differential reinforcement of other behavior increases untargeted behavior. *Journal of Applied Behavior Analysis, 48*, 402–416.

Jessel, J., & Ingvarsson, E. T. (2016). Recent advances in applied research on DRO procedures. *Journal of Applied Behavior Analysis, 49*, 991–995.

Johnson, K. A., Vladescu, J. C., Kodak, T., & Sidener, T. M. (2017). An assessment of differential reinforcement procedures for learners with autism spectrum disorder. *Journal of Applied Behavior Analysis, 50*, 290–303.

Kazdin, A. E. (1982). The token economy: A decade later. *Journal of Applied Behavior Analysis, 15*, 431–445.

Kazdin, A. E., & Bootzin, R. R. (1972). The token economy: An evaluative review. *Journal of Applied Behavior Analysis, 5*, 343–372.

Kodak, T., Campbell, V., Bergmann, S., LeBlanc, B., Kurtz-Nelson, E., Cariveau, T., et al. (2016). Examination of efficacious, efficient, and socially valid error-correction procedures to teach sight words and prepositions to children with autism spectrum disorder. *Journal of Applied Behavior Analysis, 49*, 532–547.

Koehler, L. J., Iwata, B. A., Roscoe, E. M., Rolider, N. U., & O'Steen, L. E. (2005). Effects of stimulus variation on the reinforcing capability of nonpreferred stimuli. *Journal of Applied Behavior Analysis, 38*, 469–484.

Krentz, H., Miltenberger, R., & Valbuena, D. (2016). Using token reinforcement to increase walking for adults with intellectual disabilities. *Journal of Applied Behavior Analysis, 49*, 745–750.

Lalli, J. S., Casey, S., & Kates, K. (1995). Reducing escape behavior and increasing task completion with functional communication training, extinction, and response chaining. *Journal of Applied Behavior Analysis, 28*, 261–268.

Lalli, J. S., Vollmer, T. R., Progar, P. R., Wright, C., Borrero, J., Daniel, D., et al. (1999). Competition between positive and negative reinforcement in the treatment of escape behavior. *Journal of Applied Behavior Analysis, 32*, 285–296.

Lamb, R. J., Kirby, K. C., Morral, A. R., Galbicka, G., & Iguchi, M. Y. (2004). Improving contingency management programs for addiction. *Addictive Behaviors, 29*, 507–523.

Lamb, R. J., Morral, A. R., Kirby, K. C., Iguchi, M. Y., & Galbicka, G. (2004). Shaping smoking cessation using percentile schedules. *Drug and Alcohol Dependence, 76*, 247–259.

Laraway, S., Snycerski, S., Michael, J., & Poling, A. (2003). Motivating operations and terms to describe them: Some further refinements. *Journal of Applied Behavior Analysis, 36*, 407–414.

Lee, R., McComas, J. J., & Jawor, J. (2002). The effects of differential and lag reinforcement schedules on varied verbal responding by individuals with autism. *Journal of Applied Behavior Analysis, 35*, 391–402.

Lennox, D. B., Miltenberger, R. G., & Donnelly, D. R. (1987). Response interruption and DRL for the reduction of rapid eating. *Journal of Applied Behavior Analysis, 20*, 279–284.

Leon, Y., Borrero, J. C., & DeLeon, I. G. (2016). Parametric analysis of delayed primary and conditioned reinforcers. *Journal of Applied Behavior Analysis, 49,* 639–655.

Linscheid, T. R., Iwata, B. A., Ricketts, R. W., Williams, D. E., & Griffin, J. C. (1990). Clinical evaluation of the self-injurious behavior inhibiting system. *Journal of Applied Behavior Analysis, 23,* 53–78.

Litow, L., & Pumroy, D. K. (1975). Brief technical report: A brief review of classroom group-oriented contingencies. *Journal of Applied Behavior Analysis, 8,* 341–347.

Luczynski, K. C., & Hanley, G. P. (2009). Do children prefer contingencies?: An evaluation of the efficacy of and preference for contingent versus noncontingent social reinforcement during play. *Journal of Applied Behavior Analysis, 42,* 511–525.

Luczynski, K. C., & Hanley, G. P. (2010). Examining the generality of children's preference for contingent reinforcement via extension to different responses, reinforcers, and schedules. *Journal of Applied Behavior Analysis, 43,* 397–409.

Lutzker, J. R., & White-Blackburn, G. (1979). The Good Productivity Game: Increasing work performance in a rehabilitation setting. *Journal of Applied Behavior Analysis, 12,* 488.

Mace, F. C., Neef, N. A., Shade, D., & Mauro, B. C. (1996). Effects of problem difficulty and reinforcer quality on time allocated to concurrent arithmetic problems. *Journal of Applied Behavior Analysis, 29,* 11–24.

McConnell, O. L. (1967). Control of eye contact in an autistic child. *Journal of Child Psychology and Psychiatry, 8,* 249–255.

McGhan, A. C., & Lerman, D. C. (2013). An assessment of error-correction procedures for learners with autism. *Journal of Applied Behavior Analysis, 46,* 626–639.

Miller, D. L., & Kelley, M. L. (1994). The use of goal setting and contingency contracting for improving children's homework performance. *Journal of Applied Behavior Analysis, 27,* 73–84.

Neef, N. A., Parrish, J. M., Hannigan, K. F., Page, T. J., & Iwata, B. A. (1989). Teaching self-catheterization skills to children with neurogenic bladder complications. *Journal of Applied Behavior Analysis, 22,* 237–243.

North, S. T., & Iwata, B. A. (2005). Motivational influences on performance maintained by food reinforcement. *Journal of Applied Behavior Analysis, 38,* 317–333.

Orlando, R., & Bijou, S. W. (1960). Single and multiple schedules of reinforcement in developmentally retarded children. *Journal of the Experimental Analysis of Behavior, 3,* 339–348.

Petry, N. M., Bickel, W. K., Tzanis, E., Taylor, R., Kubik, E., Foster, M., et al. (1998). A behavioral intervention for improving verbal behaviors of heroin addicts in a treatment clinic. *Journal of Applied Behavior Analysis, 31,* 291–297.

Piazza, C. C., Fisher, W. W., Hanley, G. P., Remick, M. A., Contrucci, S. A., & Aitken, T. (1997). The use of positive and negative reinforcement in the treatment of escape-maintained destructive behavior. *Journal of Applied Behavior Analysis, 30,* 279–297.

Pinkston, E. M., Reese, N. M., LeBlanc, J. M., & Baer, D. M. (1973). Independent control of a preschool child's aggression and peer interaction by contingent teacher attention. *Journal of Applied Behavior Analysis, 6,* 115–124.

Potter, J. N., Hanley, G. P., Augustine, M., Clay, C. J., & Phelps, M. C. (2013). Treating stereotypy in adolescents diagnosed with autism by refining the tactic of "using stereotypy as reinforcement." *Journal of Applied Behavior Analysis, 46,* 407–423.

Protopopova, A., Kisten, D., & Wynne, C. (2016). Evaluating a humane alternative to the bark collar: Automated differential reinforcement of not barking in a home-alone setting. *Journal of Applied Behavior Analysis, 49,* 735–744.

Risley, T. R. (2005). Montrose M. Wolf (1935–2004). *Journal of Applied Behavior Analysis, 38,* 279–287.

Roane, H. S., Call, N. A., & Falcomata, T. S. (2005). A preliminary analysis of adaptive responding under open and closed economies. *Journal of Applied Behavior Analysis, 38,* 335–348.

Roane, H. S., Lerman, D. C., & Vorndran, C. M. (2001). Assessing reinforcers under progressive schedule requirements. *Journal of Applied Behavior Analysis, 34,* 145–167.

Rodgers, T. A., & Iwata, B. A. (1991). An analysis of error-correction procedures during discrimination training. *Journal of Applied Behavior Analysis, 24,* 775–781.

Schlinger, H. D. (1995). *A behavior analytic view of child development.* New York: Plenum Press.

Schlinger, H. D., Derenne, A., & Baron, A. (2008). What 50 years of research tell us about pausing under ratio schedules of reinforcement. *Behavior Analyst, 31,* 39–60.

Schweitzer, J. B., & Sulzer-Azaroff, B. (1988). Self-control: Teaching tolerance for delay in impulsive children. *Journal of the Experimental Analysis of Behavior, 50,* 173–186.

Sellers, T. P., Bloom, S. E., Samaha, A. L., Dayton, E., Lambert, J. M., & Keyl-Austin, A. A. (2013). Evaluation of some components of choice making. *Journal of Applied Behavior Analysis, 46,* 455–464.

Sherman, J. A. (1965). Use of reinforcement and imitation to reinstate verbal behavior in mute psychotics. *Journal of Abnormal Psychology, 70,* 155–164.

Skinner, B. F. (1948). "Superstition" in the pigeon. *Journal of Experimental Psychology, 38,* 168–272.

Slaton, J., & Hanley, G. P. (2016). Effects of multiple versus chained schedules on stereotypy and functional engagement. *Journal of Applied Behavior Analysis, 49,* 927–946.

Speltz, M. L., Shimamura, J. W., & McReynolds, W. T. (1982). Procedural variations in group contingencies:

Effects on children's academic and social behaviors. *Journal of Applied Behavior Analysis, 15,* 533–544.

Stasolla, F., Caffò, A. O., Perilli, V., Boccasini, A., Stella, A., Damiani, R., et al. (2017). A microswitch-based program for promoting initial ambulation responses: An evaluation with two girls with multiple disabilities. *Journal of Applied Behavior Analysis, 50,* 345–356.

Stokes, T. F., Fowler, S. A., & Baer, D. M. (1978). Training preschool children to recruit natural communities of reinforcement. *Journal of Applied Behavior Analysis, 11,* 285–303.

Taub, E., Crago, J. E., Burgio, L. D., Groomes, T. E., Cook, E. W., DeLuca, S. C., et al. (1994). An operant approach to rehabilitation medicine: Overcoming learned nonuse by shaping. *Journal of the Experimental Analysis of Behavior, 61,* 281–293.

Thompson, R. H., Fisher, W. W., & Contrucci, S. A. (1998). Evaluating the reinforcing effects of choice in comparison to reinforcement rate. *Research in Developmental Disabilities, 19,* 181–187.

Thompson, R. H., & Iwata, B. A. (2000). Response acquisition under direct and indirect contingencies of reinforcement. *Journal of Applied Behavior Analysis, 33,* 1–11.

Thompson, R. H., McKerchar, P. M., & Dancho, K. A. (2004). The effects of delayed physical prompts and reinforcement on infant sign language acquisition. *Journal of Applied Behavior Analysis, 37,* 379–383.

Tiger, J. H., Bouxsein, K. J., & Fisher, W. W. (2007). Treating excessively slow responding of a young man with Asperger syndrome using differential reinforcement of short response latencies. *Journal of Applied Behavior Analysis, 40,* 559–563.

Tiger, J. H., & Hanley, G. P. (2004). Developing stimulus control of preschooler mands: An analysis of schedule-correlated and contingency-specifying stimuli. *Journal of Applied Behavior Analysis, 37,* 517–521.

Tiger, J. H., & Hanley, G. P. (2006). The effectiveness of and preschoolers' preferences for variations of multiple-schedule arrangements. *Journal of Applied Behavior Analysis, 39,* 475–488.

Tiger, J. H., Hanley, G. P., & Hernandez, E. (2006). A further evaluation of the reinforcing value of choice. *Journal of Applied Behavior Analysis, 39,* 1–16.

Touchette, P. E., & Howard, J. S. (1984). Errorless learning: Reinforcement contingencies and stimulus control transfer in delayed prompting. *Journal of Applied Behavior Analysis, 17,* 175–188.

Toussaint, K. A., Kodak, T., & Vladescu, J. (2016). An evaluation of choice on instruction efficacy and individual preference for children with autism. *Journal of Applied Behavior Analysis, 40,* 170–175.

Trosclair-Lasserre, N. M., Lerman, D. C., Call, N. A., Addison, L. R., & Kodak, T. (2008). Reinforcement magnitude: An evaluation of preference and reinforcer efficacy. *Journal of Applied Behavior Analysis, 41,* 203–220.

Van Houten, R., & Nau, P. A. (1980). A comparison of the effects of fixed and variable ratio schedules of reinforcement on the behavior of deaf children. *Journal of Applied Behavior Analysis, 13,* 13–21.

Vaughan, M. E., & Michael, J. L. (1982). Automatic reinforcement: An important but ignored concept. *Behaviorism, 10,* 101–112.

Vollmer, T. R., Borrero, J. C., Lalli, J. S., & Daniel, D. (1999). Evaluating self-control and impulsivity in children with severe behavior disorders. *Journal of Applied Behavior Analysis, 32,* 451–466.

Vollmer, T. R., & Hackenberg, T. D. (2001). Reinforcement contingencies and social reinforcement: Some reciprocal relations between basic and applied research. *Journal of Applied Behavior Analysis, 34,* 241–253.

Vollmer, T. R., & Iwata, B. A. (1991). Establishing operations and reinforcement effects. *Journal of Applied Behavior Analysis, 24,* 279–291.

Weiner, H. (1969). Controlling human fixed-interval performance. *Journal of the Experimental Analysis of Behavior, 12,* 349–373.

Wiskow, K. M., & Donaldson, J. M. (2016). Evaluation of a lag schedule of reinforcement in a group contingency to promote varied naming of categories items with children. *Journal of Applied Behavior Analysis, 49,* 472–484.

Wolery, M., & Gast, D. L. (1984). Effective and efficient procedures for the transfer of stimulus control. *Topics in Early Childhood Special Education, 4,* 52–77.

Wolery, M., Kirk, K., & Gast, D. L. (1985). Stereotypic behavior as a reinforcer: Effects and side-effects. *Journal of Autism and Developmental Disorders, 15,* 149–161.

# CHAPTER 15

# Building Complex Repertoires from Discrete Behaviors

*Establishing Stimulus Control, Behavioral Chains, and Strategic Behavior*

George H. Noell, Nathan A. Call, Scott P. Ardoin, and Sarah J. Miller

Complexity is a cardinal feature of human behavior. Humans routinely exhibit behavior that is varied; is subtly discriminated; requires long-term planning; is maintained by delayed, ambiguous contingencies; is initiated by verbal rules; and is recursive. Human behavior's complexity, subtle capacity of adaptation, and incorporation of rich language largely accounts for our evolutionary dominance over the earth (Ehrlich & Ehrlich, 2008). This wondrous capacity has also created enormous challenges for individual human beings, as societies have developed increasingly complex behavioral requirements for successful adaptation. As the complexity of behavioral expectations increases, the demand for efficient teaching increases.

Cognitive-constructivist approaches to teaching have achieved dominance in many areas, because they explicitly emphasize the complex, varied nature of the target material and its accompanying behavior (e.g., Haywood, 2004; Martens & Daly, 1999; Richardson, 2003). This approach to teaching makes sense to many consumers and is sufficient for many learners. By contrast, behavior-analytic teaching procedures have commonly emphasized an elemental approach, in which the be-

havior analyst reduces complex behavior to small teachable units. For some consumers, this approach initially appears reductive and far removed from the goal of teaching subtle, complex, and adaptive behavior. When behavior analysts have sought to establish more complex behavior, they have typically achieved it by combining simpler behaviors to form a more complex chain, or by elaborating on a simpler behavior to produce a more complex behavior (e.g., Sauttfr, LeBlanc, Jay, Goldsmith, & Carr, 2011). Due to different conceptual bases and emphasis on different outcomes (e.g., understanding vs. behaving), cognitivist and behavior-analytic approaches are commonly viewed as conflicting or competing approaches, but the two approaches have much in common. For example, they both identify some of the same procedures as effective, such as practice with feedback, but provide different explanations for how and why the procedures are effective (Carroll, Kodak, & Adolf, 2016, vs. Trapman, van Gelderen, van Steensel, van Schooten, & Hulstijn, 2014). Both approaches seek to help individuals develop complex behavioral repertoires that include flexible and generalized responding to diverse stimuli.

A strength of the systematic, elemental building approach that behavior-analytic teaching adopts is that simplified behaviors can be taught to individuals who have difficulty acquiring new or complex behavior (Luiselli & Hurley, 2005). By contrast, some have criticized behavior-analytic approaches for failing to capture the symbolic meaning or underlying structure of complex behaviors and for fostering dependence on instructors (Hickey, Moore, & Pellegrino, 2001; Kroesbergen, Van Luit, & Maas, 2004). This criticism of behavior-analytic teaching appears quite reasonable when we examine studies for which the goal was to establish a specific response (e.g., Swain, Lane, & Gast, 2015). It appears less tenable in the context of broader and more systematic behavior-analytic approaches to teaching, such as direct instruction, that clearly emphasize meaning, structure, and behaviors that represent understanding (Liem & Martin, 2013).

## COMPLEXITY: FLEXIBLE, DIVERSE BEHAVIOR

Behavioral complexity is difficult to define, because it exists as a relative comparison of behaviors within and across individuals. Driving to the corner market to buy a gallon of milk can be insurmountably complex for some individuals or quite simple for others. Behaviors also vary in complexity. For example, talking to a friend who is present is less complex than e-mailing the friend. Behaviors that were complex will become simple as an individual develops greater skill in a domain. Decoding a single word can be a complex process that includes many discriminations (Snow, Burns, & Griffin, 1998). Later in the process of becoming literate, reading that same word can become a simple behavior in which the reader perceives the word as a single stimulus. A common goal of teaching is to help learners master simple behaviors that will become elements of more complex behaviors.

Complexity emerges in all parts of the antecedent–behavior–consequence (A-B-C) chain. For example, a behavior is more complex when its antecedent is ambiguous (Harding, Wacker, Cooper, Millard, & Jensen-Kovalan, 1994); when a delay occurs between the onset of the discriminative stimulus and the target behavior; or when the same stimulus is discriminative for different behavioral repertoires, depending on the context (Hughes & Barnes-Holmes, 2014). Complex stimuli whose functional properties change across contexts are common aspects of social interactions, academic activities, and vocational activities.

Behaviors themselves are the most intuitive source of complexity. No generally accepted definition of behavioral complexity exists in the behavior-analytic literature. We suggest that the following five dimensions are important to consider in establishing new behavior: (1) subordinate and superordinate skills, (2) sequencing, (3) promoting variability in responding, (4) ambiguity in natural criteria, and (5) establishing self-management skills. Most complex behaviors include or require several subordinate or prerequisite skills. For example, fluent decoding skills are precursors to text search and reading comprehension skills (National Reading Panel, 2000).

Another considerable challenge is identifying the required proficiency level for prerequisite behaviors before teaching the target skill. That a student must be able to complete addition and subtraction operations correctly before learning to balance a checkbook may be obvious. However, defining which operations and what accuracy and fluency levels to require before teaching the target skill may pose a considerable challenge (see Kelley, Reitman, & Noell, 2002, for a discussion of accuracy and fluency criteria in subordinate skills).

A second source of complexity arises from *behavioral chains*, a series of behaviors that occur sequentially and produce a consistent end state (Cooper, Heron, & Heward, 2007). Sequences of a different order of behaviors or variations within the chain may produce the same end state. For example, many successful variations of the handwashing chain are possible, dependent on personal preferences and environmental context. Each behavior in an established chain produces the conditioned reinforcer that serves as the discriminative stimulus for the next behavior in the chain (Cooper et al., 2007).

The requirement that competence includes varied behavior, which is necessary for response generalization, creates a third source of complexity. For example, initiating play with peers requires variety across occasions and available materials (Ledbetter-Cho et al., 2015). Variable behavior that maintains contact with reinforcement is a common feature of social, vocational, and academic behaviors. For example, the person who tells the same joke over and over is not likely to receive continued reinforcement for joke telling, even if the joke initially occasioned laughter. Response generalization and behavioral flexibility are very challenging for some learners. Individuals who require many trials with carefully controlled antecedent and consequent stimuli to learn also have difficulty learning to respond to variability in natural contexts, and this is one of the central features of some developmental disabilities (Reitzel et al., 2013).

A fourth source of complexity is evident for behaviors that are so varied that correct and incorrect responses are difficult to define. These behaviors are so common in human interaction that we might describe them as normative. For example, a response to a simple greeting may have a nearly infinite number of acceptable responses.

A fifth source of complexity arises when behavior requires substantial planning, progress monitoring, and plan revision, also known as *executive control* (Mahy, Moses, & Kliegel, 2014) or *self-management* (Gureasko-Moore, DuPaul, & White, 2006). Executive control or self-management in this context refers to organizing and evaluating responses necessary to complete complex behaviors. Although the term *executive control* typically describes internal unobservable processes, planning, progress monitoring, and plan revision can be observable behaviors.

The consequences of behavior can create an additional source of complexity in establishing and maintaining behaviors. Delayed consequences, thin reinforcement schedules, and small-magnitude, cumulative consequences are extraordinarily common in human endeavor (Malott, 1989) and are frequently problematic in establishing and sustaining behavior. Natural consequences can be sufficiently delayed, on such thin schedules, and so ambiguous in their presentation that they are insufficient to teach behavior or maintain existing behavior (Malott, 1989).

Behavior-analytic teaching often focuses on specific responses, using tightly controlled procedures that can produce inflexible, tightly controlled responding. We should conceptualize this outcome, however, as a beginning rather than an end. This approach arose in part from demonstrations that individuals regarded as "unteachable" or "disabled" could learn far more and far faster than anyone thought was possible. The striking success in using principles of applied behavior analysis (ABA) led to ABA's successful application to typically developing individuals (Daly, Persampieri, McCurdy, & Gortmaker, 2005; Koscinski & Hoy, 1993). Moving from discrete teachable behaviors to elaborate flexible repertoires is a fundamental goal of teaching represented in the ABA literature (e.g., Reid, Lienemann, & Hagaman, 2013). In the balance of this chapter, we focus on critical issues for establishing new behaviors and the elaboration of those behaviors to produce more flexible, adaptive repertoires. We first discuss selected issues in the assessment of behaviors and individuals before teaching begins. We then discuss many specific procedures behavior analysts might use to establish new behavior. We present the procedures as they might arise in practice as an analyst moves from establishing an initial response, to elaborating on that response, to creating a more complex repertoire. Thus these sections progress from shaping and prompting, to chaining, to strategy instruction, and finally to generalization.

## ASSESSING BEHAVIORS AND INDIVIDUALS

Any program to establish new behavior should begin with an assessment of the individual's current skills, behaviors, goals, and preferences. We can conceptualize establishing new behavior as the answers to three questions. First, what do we expect the learner to do? Second, what does the learner know how to do? Third, what procedures can we use to build on what the learner does now, so that he or she can meet the new expectations? Although these questions are intuitive, complexity arises in the details. For example, most individuals will need to learn many new behaviors that likely overlap in function and topography. We often must prioritize the behaviors that we will teach. Space limitations preclude an extensive consideration of prioritizing strategies in this chapter. Generally, we should target those behaviors that have the broadest possible adaptive importance and those that are prerequisites of these broad and important behaviors. Researchers have used the term *behavioral cusps* to describe behaviors that make broad contributions to an individual's adaptive success (Rosales-Ruiz & Baer, 1997). Obvious examples include spoken language in social contexts, and reading in educational and vocational contexts.

Instructional planning should begin by identifying criteria for competence that indicate when we should terminate instruction or shift to new targets. The end point might be age-appropriate oral-language skills or reading text and correctly answering comprehension questions with an intermediate stage to prepare the student to learn additional material. For example, teaching a child with autism spectrum disorder (ASD) to articulate targeted words in response to appropriate antecedent stimuli is less likely to be an end than a stage in the process of building oral-language skills.

Once we identify the immediate goal of instruction, we can identify the behavior's critical components. We often identify relevant approximations or create a task analysis of the behavior. Relevant *approximations* are behaviors that are topographically like the target behavior, and that we can potentially shape through differential reinforcement to produce the target behavior (Isaacs, Thomas, & Goldiamond, 1960). For example, a student may already read grade-level words, but with insufficient fluency to be competent. In this case, we may be able to use reading slowly to shape fluent reading (e.g., Noell et al., 1998).

A *task analysis* is the process of breaking down a complex behavior into a series of discrete, measurable, and teachable components. For example, students must read numbers and operation signs, identify correct answers, and write the correct answers to complete multiplication problems. The three strategies researchers most commonly recommend for completing task analyses are as follow. First, we can watch the performance and record the steps that competent individuals use to complete the task. Second, we can consult an expert (an individual with specialized content expertise or a specialized published resource). Third is simply to complete the target behavior ourselves and record the steps that were necessary to complete the task.

Once we identify the component steps of the target task, assessment will shift to the learner. We will ask the learner to complete the task and record which steps the learner completes independently. We will compare the learner's performance to a performance standard to identify which steps the learner preformed competently and which we need to teach, including instructional targets. Unfortunately, evidence-based standards are not available for many tasks, but we can apply rational and local, normative standards for some tasks. Adequate standards typically require attention to quality, accuracy, and fluency (see Kelley et al., 2002). For example, the assessment may show that the student's reading fluency is too low for him or her to answer comprehension questions accurately. Assessment of reading performance may suggest that the student has sufficient fundamental skills but needs fluency building, that some critical sight words are missing, that phonics/decoding skills are insufficient for reading novel words, or a combination. Each of these outcomes suggests a different initial focus for instruction.

One of the central tenets of ABA is that the environment changes behavior. This fact is as important to behavior assessment as it is to behavior treatment. A standardized assessment may suggest that a learner lacks a skill, when in fact the assessment environment simply lacked the supports necessary to elicit the learner's performance. The absence of contingencies for competent responding and reinforcement for competing responses or distractions can yield negatively biased assessments (Noell, Freeland, Witt, & Gansle, 2001). Behavior analysts should assess behavior under varied conditions that test consequences.

The next stage is to identify an instructional procedure that is appropriate for establishing or refining the target behavior. We describe specific ABA teaching procedures below. Behavior analysts should note that the assessment–treatment or assessment–teaching process is recursive and continuous. Once teaching begins, ongoing assessment data should guide decisions that will change the instructional plan as necessary.

## SHAPING

*Shaping* is an instructional approach that is particularly important for learners who have a low probability of exhibiting the target behavior even with prompting, but engage in some related behavior that we can use to begin instruction. Shaping involves increasing the probability of a behavior's occurrence through the gradual transformation of some property of responding. Differential reinforcement of successive approximations of a targeted operant class produces this transformation. *Shaping across topographies* modifies the topography of a response, and researchers have demonstrated it in several classic studies (Horner, 1971; Isaacs et al., 1960; Skinner, 1938). For example, Isaacs et al. (1960) shaped the eye movements of an individual diagnosed with comatose schizophrenia into lip movements, then speech sounds, and eventually recognizable words. *Shaping within topography* modifies the rate, magnitude, or some other property of the target operant. Researchers have used this type of shaping to increase the arm extension of an athlete during a critical step in pole vaulting (Rea & Williams, 2002) and to increase the duration individuals held their breath before measuring exhaled carbon monoxide levels during treatment for smoking cessation (Scott, Scott, & Goldwater, 1997).

Learners typically emit a distribution of behaviors relevant to the targeted response dimension. Shaping uses extinction and reinforcement to shift this distribution, so that the proportion of responses that contain the desired response property increases (Galbicka, 1994). Continued differential reinforcement of responses above a criterion value produces differentiation in which an increasing proportion of behavior is at or nearer to the target behavior. Factors affecting the probability of successful shaping include properties of the initial response and the way we establish the criterion for reinforcement. The response targeted early in the process must occur at a sufficient level or rate to permit initial reinforcement. It must also approximate the target behavior, so that we can differentially reinforce the relevant response dimension. Finally, the initial response must have enough variability that we can provide differential reinforcement for responses that exceed an established criterion, thus shaping the response toward the target. Note that increased variability is a predictable side effect of both reinforcement (Skinner, 1938) and extinction (Lerman & Iwata, 1996), so initial responses that seem relatively invariant may be amenable to shaping.

Determining which responses to reinforce and which responses to extinguish can be challenging. If the criterion for reinforcement is too low, we will reinforce a large proportion of responses and shaping will proceed slowly. By contrast, if the criterion is too high, we will reinforce a small proportion of responses, and responding may be extinguished. Galbicka (1994) recommended that instructors use percentile schedules to empirically determine the criterion for reinforcement during shaping. All responses that exceed a preestablished rank-ordered response from a sample of the previous responses produce reinforcement (e.g., the third highest from the last 10). Researchers have successfully used this approach to shape behaviors such as eye contact (Hall, Maynes, & Reiss, 2009) and academic-task engagement (Athens, Vollmer, & St. Peter Pipkin, 2007; Clark, Schmidt, Mezhoudi, & Kahng, 2016).

The advantage of a percentile schedule is that it constantly updates the distribution of responses it uses to establish the criterion for reinforcement as responding varies, which keeps the proportion of reinforced responses constant. To date, researchers have conducted few studies to determine the optimal rank order and number of responses to sample to establish a percentile schedule. In a notable exception, Athens et al. (2007) found that percentile schedule procedures were more effective when they based the criterion for reinforcement on a larger number of observations. However, using more observations has the potential to decrease efficiency, because we must postpone reinforcement until the learner has emitted a sufficiently large number of responses to establish the criterion.

## PROMPTING

When a response is not in a learner's repertoire or is not under appropriate stimulus control, prompting may be necessary to evoke the response so that we can reinforce it. *Prompts* are antecedent stimuli that increase the probability of a desired response. Prompting can help a stimulus become discriminative by increasing opportunities to provide differential reinforcement in its presence (Alberto & Troutman, 1986; Cooper et al., 2007; Demchak, 1990; Miltenberger, 2001). Researchers have used prompts to teach communication (Matson, Sevin, Fridley, & Love, 1990; Williams, Donley, & Keller, 2000), academic skills (Noell, Connell, & Duhon, 2006; Stevens, Blackhurst, & Slaton, 1991), leisure skills (DiCarlo, Reid, & Stricklin, 2003; Schleien, Wehman, & Kiernan, 1981; Oppenheim-Leaf, Leaf, & Call, 2012), social skills (Krantz & McClannahan, 1993; Garcia-Albea, Reeve, Brothers, & Reeve, 2014), self-help skills (Pierce & Schreibman, 1994; Taylor, Hughes, Richard, Hoch, & Coello, 2004), and vocational skills (Bennett, Ramasamy, & Honsberger, 2013).

Behavior analysts have categorized prompts as stimulus and response prompts (Schoen, 1986; Wolery & Gast, 1984). *Stimulus prompts* are those in which we alter or present some property of the criterion stimulus (Etzel & LeBlanc, 1979). For example, a teacher uses a stimulus prompt when he or she places two pictures in front of the learner, and the correct picture is larger than the incorrect one. By contrast, *response prompts* involve teacher behavior to evoke the desired learner behavior. For example, a teacher uses a response prompt when he or she points to the correct picture after the learner did not respond when the teacher said, "Point to [correct picture]."

A *script* is a stimulus prompt that we can use to facilitate complex behavior, especially conversational skills. Subtlety is a distinct advantage of prompting social behaviors such as conversations with a script, because more contrived prompts (such as vocal instructions) might be off-putting to conversational partners. We can fade the script length from a complete text to a single word or a symbol (e.g., Krantz & McClannahan, 1993), or eliminate the script entirely (e.g., Garcia-Albea et al., 2014). Researchers have used scripts as a caregiver-mediated intervention for children with ASD to promote verbal interactions during play (Reagon & Higbee, 2009). However, scripts are limited to learners who can read, and script fading can be lengthy with some learners.

Response prompts exist along a continuum of intrusiveness in the amount of assistance required to evoke the desired behavior from the least intrusive verbal prompts, to the moderately intrusive gestural or model prompts, to the more intrusive physical prompts (Cooper et al., 2007; Miltenberger, 2001). We can deliver most prompts at different intrusiveness levels, such as a partial verbal prompt instead of a complete instruction or a physical prompt, to guide the learner to perform the first portion instead of the entire behavior.

*Modeling,* in which the antecedent stimulus is topographically identical to the target behavior, is a prompt that can be especially effective for teaching complex behaviors (Bandura, Ross, & Ross, 1963). Video modeling and prompting are methods to demonstrate target behavior without requiring an instructor to model the behavior each time the learner receives the prompt. The prompt in video modeling is a video of an individual completing the behavior, which provides the learner with a visual overview of the steps in the behavior sequence. The prompt in video prompting is a clip of an individual completing one step of a behavior sequence and a video clip of the next step after the learner completes the previous step (Domire & Wolfe, 2014). Researchers have used both methods to teach complex chains of behavior, including social skills and daily living tasks (Ayres & Langone, 2005). There is some evidence that video prompting may facilitate acquisition of chained responses more effectively than video modeling (Cannella-Malone et al., 2006).

Several factors can influence the effectiveness of modeling, such as the learner's observing the modeled behavior produce reinforcement, as well as the similarity between the model and the learner or between discriminative stimuli presented to the model and the learner (Bandura et al., 1963). Video self-modeling, in which the learner is also the model in the video, is one way to maximize similarity between model and learner (Buggey & Ogle, 2012). Although modeling is effective, two of its limitations are that the learner must have generalized imitation skills and attend to the model during instruction. Further research is needed to identify the components that influence the effectiveness of video modeling and video

prompting, such as evaluating the effects of model type and of recording perspective (e.g., Domire & Wolfe, 2014).

## PROMPT FADING

*Prompt dependence* occurs when the prompt overshadows the criterion stimulus to such an extent that it never takes on discriminative properties in the absence of the prompt. Thus we must transfer stimulus control from the prompt to the criterion stimulus. *Fading* is a method of gradually removing a prompt so that the behavior eventually comes under control of the criterion stimulus in the absence of prompts. For example, Wichnick-Gillis, Vener, and Poulson (2019) used textual prompts embedded within instructional stimuli (i.e., scripts) to teach three children with ASD to engage in social interactions. During generalization, the scripts were gradually faded by removing one word at a time from the end of a given script until all words were faded.

### Fading Stimulus Prompts

There are two primary methods of fading stimulus prompts: stimulus shaping and stimulus fading. In *stimulus shaping,* we alter the property of the criterion stimulus that is critical to the intended discrimination, so that the learner can initially make the discrimination. For example, when a chef is teaching a sous-chef to make subtle discriminations of saltiness, initial training may include samples with very distinct differences in salt content. Once the learner is reliably making the discrimination, we gradually diminish the altered stimulus property until the stimulus is representative of the criterion stimulus (Etzel & LeBlanc, 1979). Thus the difference in the amount of salt in the two samples during stimulus shaping may become smaller until the sous-chef can detect even subtle differences.

In *stimulus fading,* we alter a property of the criterion stimulus other than the dimension critical for the discrimination (Etzel & LeBlanc, 1979; Wichnick-Gillis et al., 2019). For example, we can alter position prompts or the size of a target letter when teaching letter identification. In this case, neither position nor size is the critical dimension for discriminating the target letter from other letters. Rather, the form of the letter is the critical property. During stimulus fading, we bring the size or position of the target letter closer to the position or size of the alternative letter until the learner can discriminate the letter by its form.

A review of studies comparing stimulus shaping and stimulus fading found that both were effective instructional approaches (Ault, Wolery, Doyle, & Gast, 1989). However, stimulus shaping appears to be more effective than stimulus fading, perhaps because stimulus fading requires the learner to shift the discrimination from an irrelevant stimulus dimension to the relevant dimension. Making such a shift may be difficult for some learners—especially those who selectively attend to certain dimensions of stimuli, such as some individuals with ASD (Wolery & Gast, 1984).

## Fading Response Prompts

The five main fading procedures researchers have studied for transferring stimulus control from a response prompt to a criterion stimulus are least-to-most, graduated guidance, most-to-least, time-delay, and simultaneous prompting. *Least-to-most prompting*, or the system of least prompts, is adaptable to teaching behavior chains such as a series of motor responses (e.g., folding laundry) and discrete behavior such as object labeling. During least-to-most prompting, the instructor presents the criterion stimulus so the learner can emit the correct response independently. If the learner does not emit the correct response, the instructor presents increasingly intrusive prompts until the learner emits the target behavior. For example, an instructor may use least-to-most prompting to teach a learner to correctly identify sight words by first presenting the criterion stimulus, a flash card. The instructor provide a more intrusive prompt, such as the first syllable, if the learner does not make the target response before an interval expired (e.g., 5 seconds), and an even more intrusive prompt, the word, if the learner does not make the target response after the previous prompt. Wolery and Gast (1984) suggested that as instructors, we should present the criterion stimulus at each prompt level and use a constant response interval after each prompt. We should also consider whether successive prompts increase the probability of the target behavior. If not, we should use the least intrusive prompt that is likely to occasion the behavior.

An advantage of least-to-most prompt fading is that the learner can emit the correct behavior without prompts. It also may be easier to implement than other strategies, because more intrusive prompts become unnecessary as the individual learns to emit the target behavior independently (Billingsley & Romer, 1983).

During *graduated guidance*, the instructor gradually eliminates the controlling prompt by only presenting the level of prompt necessary to evoke the target behavior. A *controlling prompt* is one that consistently results in the learner's exhibiting the target behavior (Wolery et al., 1992). We can use least-to-most prompting to identify controlling prompts, which often include physical guidance. For example, parents taught yoga poses to their children by gradually fading the amount of physical guidance from a firm hold to shadowing their children (Gruber & Poulson, 2015). We can use graduated guidance to fade physical guidance and to transfer stimulus control to other types of controlling prompts, such as verbal prompts (Schoen, 1986).

An advantage of graduated guidance is that the learner can be as independent as possible, because the instructor only provides the minimum amount of guidance necessary. A disadvantage is that fading is not systematic. Fading relies on subjective judgments about the required prompting level (Wolery & Gast, 1984), which the instructor must make rapidly, based on the learner's responses. This can affect implementation integrity and can be difficult to evaluate in the absence of systematic research.

*Most-to-least fading* begins with the delivery of a controlling prompt, and the amount of assistance necessary for the individual to complete the behavior correctly varies across trials instead of within a trial. The intrusiveness of the prompt decreases or increases on subsequent trials, based on whether the learner meets a mastery or failure criterion, respectively, for the current prompt level. Note that if the first prompting level is a controlling prompt, the learner should always meet the mastery criterion, because the response should always occur following this most intrusive prompt. Graduated guidance and most-to-least prompt fading are well suited for teaching chained motor responses and for learners who require many response–reinforcer pairings to achieve independence (Wolery & Gast, 1984).

Libby, Weiss, Bancroft, and Ahearn (2008) modified most-to-least prompt fading by inserting a delay between controlling prompts to allow learners an opportunity for independence. This *time-delay fading* procedure produced mastery almost as rapidly as least-to-most prompting, but with fewer errors. The two types of time-delay fading, constant and progressive (O'Neill, McDowell,

& Leslie, 2018; Snell & Gast, 1981), begin with 0-second-delay trials in which the criterion stimulus and prompt occur simultaneously. We typically use more 0-second-delay trials for difficult tasks or lower-functioning learners. In *progressive time-delay fading*, the time between the criterion stimulus presentation and the prompt gradually increases after each trial, several trials, or each instructional session (Heckaman, Alber, Hooper, & Heward, 1998). With *constant time-delay fading*, the instructor delays the prompt for a specified time after presentation of the criterion stimulus, and this latency remains fixed during instructional sessions (Snell & Gast, 1981).

Some advantages of time-delay fading include its low error rate and its simplicity. Constant time-delay fading is especially simple to use, which may produce better treatment integrity (Wolery et al., 1992). Simplicity may be especially important when caregivers or supervisees implement interventions. For example, DiPipi-Hoy and Jitendra (2004) showed that parents could implement constant time-delay procedures with good fidelity.

During *simultaneous prompting*, the instructor delivers the controlling prompt immediately after presenting the demand (Morse & Schuster, 2004). That is, trials have a 0-second delay, and the instructor does not introduce a delay. The instructor conducts an assessment before instructional sessions to determine whether the learner can emit the target response without the prompt. Researchers have used simultaneous prompting to teach discrete behaviors (Tekin-Iftar, Acar, & Kurt, 2003), chained tasks (Parrott, Schuster, Collins, & Gassaway, 2000), and vocational tasks (Fetko, Schuster, Harley, & Collins, 1999). The advantages of simultaneous prompting are low error rate and simplicity, but it may be less sensitive to detecting the moment at which mastery occurs. However, instructors can conduct more trials per time than they can with prompt-delay procedures, and simultaneous prompting produces more rapid mastery than other prompting strategies do (Akmanoglu, Kurt, & Kapan, 2015; Schuster, Griffen, & Wolery, 1992; Swain et al., 2015).

Studies comparing prompt-fading methods have produced conflicting results. Limitations of these comparative studies is that most participants displayed generalized imitation, attended well, waited for teacher assistance, and demonstrated clear preferences for potential reinforcers. Wolery and Gast (1984) suggested that constant time-delay may be more efficient for students who exhibit these behaviors, but that other prompt-fading strategies may be more appropriate for individuals who lack these skills. In general, research has shown that the prompt-fading methods described above can effectively transfer stimulus control to a criterion stimulus for at least some tasks and participants. We cannot draw further conclusions about prompt fading beyond the idiosyncratic variables evaluated, such as participant characteristics, tasks, and prompting variations.

## CHAINING

Each step or component of a behavior chain has its own conditioned reinforcers and discriminative stimuli (Kelleher, 1966; Skinner, 1938). That is, the consequence following completion of each component of the behavior chain may function as both a conditioned reinforcer for the previous behavior and a discriminative stimulus for the next one. We typically complete a task analysis for the chain of target behaviors and teach the chain by using forward chaining, backward chaining, or total-task presentation.

During *backward chaining* and *forward chaining*, the instructor teaches one component of the behavior chain at a time. The instructor teaches each additional component as the learner meets the mastery criterion for the previous components. The difference is that in backward chaining, the instructor teaches the behavior chain in reverse order, starting with the last component; in forward chaining, behaviors are taught in the order they occur in the chain, starting with the first component. In total- or whole-task chaining, the learner performs the entire behavior chain on every instructional trial.

During *reverse chaining*, the instructor physically guides the learner to perform the behavior chain's components until the last one, which the learner performs independently (Sternberg & Adams, 1982). The instructor teaches components in reverse order by physically guiding progressively fewer components (e.g., last two, last three) as the learner masters each component. In *backward chaining with leap ahead* (Spooner, Spooner, & Ulicny, 1986), the instructor does not teach every component directly, to increase time efficiency. Rather, the instructor conducts ongoing assessment to determine whether the learner can perform some components without training.

A potential advantage of backward chaining is that the learner produces natural reinforcement by completing each component of the behavior chain, whereas completing initial components during forward-chaining produces conditioned reinforcement (Spooner et al., 1986). However, the natural consequences produced in backward chaining may not function as reinforcement for some individuals. The advantage of total-task presentation is that the learner has increased opportunities for conditioned reinforcement by practicing every component in the behavior chain on every trial. However, total-task presentation may be less time-efficient. Forward chaining may be easiest to use, because the instructor teaches components in the order in which they occur in the chain, and this may produce the best long-term performance (Watters, 1992).

Smith (1999) showed that fewer errors occurred at the beginning of the chain during forward chaining and at the end of the chain during backward chaining. Thus an instructor should use forward chaining if a learner is unlikely to complete the chain after an error. Direct comparisons of the different chaining methods have shown mixed results (Ash & Holding, 1990; Hur & Osborne, 1993; Slocum & Tiger, 2011; Spooner & Spooner, 1984; Spooner, Weber, & Spooner, 1983; Watters, 1992; Wightman & Sistrunk, 1987). As with other methods described in this chapter, acquisition of skills via different chaining methods is likely to be idiosyncratic across populations and highly influenced by the target skill.

## PROMOTING RESPONSE GENERALIZATION AND VARIETY

We direct readers to Chapters 5 (Spradlin, Simon, & Fisher) and 6 (Podlesnik, Jimenez-Gomez, & Kelley) of this volume for discussions of generalization and methods useful for its facilitation, including descriptions of stimulus control, equivalence classes, and recombinative generalization. We review some issues about generalization relevant to establishing complex behaviors. For example, *multiple-exemplar training*, in which the instructor prompts and reinforces responding to several members of a stimulus class, can produce generalization and promote spontaneous or varied responding (Stokes & Baer, 1977). For example, Krantz and McClannahan (1993) used scripts with varied content that prompted comments about activities to teach children with ASD to initiate social interactions. Scripted comments increased, and spontaneous, unscripted comments also increased for several participants. Such vari-

ability in responding can be important, because it often determines whether a response will produce natural reinforcers. For example, peers may perceive a student who always asks for help using a single phrase in the same tone of voice as odd, and may ignore or shun the student. McClannahan and Krantz (2005) used scripts to teach several mand frames (i.e., *I want, I need,* or *I would like*) to participants and observed increases in spontaneous, novel mand frames. Similarly, Betz, Higbee, Kelley, Sellers, and Pollard (2011) taught varied responses to individuals with ASD by using stimulus prompts, each associated with a unique color. They faded the stimulus prompts and used the color prompts, and faded the color prompts for two of three participants who continued to emit the varied responses.

We can promote response variability by manipulating the consequences of responding. Extinction-induced variability is one example in which extinction of a previously reinforced response increases the likelihood that various other responses will occur (Goetz & Baer, 1973; Sullivan et al., 2020). Extinction-induced variability has the unique benefit of eliminating instructional time for behaviors that are in the learner's repertoire but occur infrequently. For example, Valentino, Shillingsburg, Call, Burton, and Bowen (2011) implemented extinction for the signed mands of children with limited vocalizations, and observed increases in vocalizations. The chances for extinction of the original target behavior and emergence of problem behavior are disadvantages of extinction-induced variability.

Another method to produce response variability is a lag schedule of reinforcement. The instructor reinforces a response in a lag schedule if it differs from a designated number of previously emitted responses (Falcomata et al., 2018; Page & Neuringer, 1985). For example, if an individual had previously emitted the response *hi* followed by *hello*, neither of these greetings would be eligible for reinforcement as the third response on a Lag 2 schedule. Only a novel greeting (e.g., *good morning*) would produce reinforcement, but a novel response or *hi* for the fourth greeting would produce reinforcement, because neither was one of the previous two responses. Researchers have used lag schedules to establish variety for verbal behavior (Esch, Esch, & Love, 2009; Falcomata et al., 2018; Lee, McComas, & Jawor, 2002; Silbaugh, Falcomata, & Ferguson, 2018; Wiskow, Matter, & Donaldson, 2018) and building block structures (Napolitano, Smith, Zarcone, Goodkin, & McAdam, 2010), and to maintain variable responding after discontinuation of the lag schedule (Heldt & Schlinger, 2012). A disadvantage is that patterned responding may emerge. Using variable-lag schedules may mitigate this problem (Lee et al., 2002).

## STRATEGIC INSTRUCTION

*Strategies* are more complex sequences of behavior that include assessment, planning, execution, and evaluation of a course of action. Importantly, a strategy is a behavioral process by which an individual chooses, orders, and evaluates behavior toward solving diverse problems, rather than a fixed behavioral sequence. We can distinguish skills and strategies by the unique roles that they play in learning and achievement. Alexander and Murphy (1999) describe *skills* as procedural knowledge that students develop, which enables them to perform tasks effectively with speed and accuracy. Students who achieve automaticity or fluency of skills can attend to more complex task dimensions (e.g., comprehending text after mastering decoding and sight words). For example, Wagner et al. (2011) reported that fluency in writing individual letters contributed to the quality and complexity of first- and fourth-grade students' writing. One critical goal of effective education is to provide students with sufficient opportunities to practice fundamental skills (e.g., decoding, computing basic math facts), so that they can develop adequate fluency to use those basic skills in a strategic manner (Ardoin & Daly, 2007).

As they do with basic skills, students learn and perform strategies better when we teach these explicitly, when the environment supports effective skill use, and when the environment naturally rewards strategy use (Duffy, Roehler, Sivan, & Rackliffe, 1987; Manset-Williamson & Nelson, 2005). An extensive literature exists describing models of strategy instruction in reading, writing, and mathematics for students with and without learning difficulties (Alexander, Graham, & Harris, 1998; Reid et al., 2013).

Instructors who use effective strategy instruction ensure that students have the prerequisite background skills, explain the strategy to them, model the strategy, and explain why they should use the strategy. For example, Self-Regulated Strategy Development, an empirically validated curriculum for teaching writing strategies, involves explaining to students how good writers might use a strategy (e.g., planning, listing main ideas) and the benefits of using the strategy. Teachers then model the strategy for students by writing essays while asking themselves questions aloud, followed by modeling self-instruction procedures (e.g., self-evaluation and self-reinforcement). A second common component of strategy instruction is providing students with opportunities to practice problems in a programmed sequence from simpler to more complex problems. Teachers provide students with corrective feedback, reinforcement, and many models, allowing the students to practice skills collaboratively. Collaborative practice, when possible, enables teachers to support students while gradually providing them with greater independence. Teachers provide students with mnemonics for remembering the strategy's steps and teach them to use self-monitoring, prompt cards, or a combination to foster independence and generalization. The students practice these steps verbally until they memorize the strategy's steps. Providing students with opportunities to practice newly learned strategies across multiple exemplars promotes generalization and adaptation of strategies (Alber-Morgan, Hessler, & Konrad, 2007). For example, teachers should provide students with opportunities to practice reading and writing strategies and continued support across a variety of text types and writing tasks, so that the students effectively use these strategies.

Teaching students to use self-regulatory strategies, such as self-monitoring, self-recording, self-assessing, and self-reinforcing, will promote strategy use (Alexander et al., 1998; Reid et al., 2013). Teachers meet with students individually, review students' work to establish a baseline, explain the benefits of each self-regulatory behavior, help students to establish self-monitoring goals, and verbally model the strategy. Research has shown that teaching students self-regulatory behaviors increases their understanding of their academic abilities, which enables them to connect strategy use and successful performance. Students who have been taught explicitly to use self-regulatory behaviors experience greater acquisition, maintenance, and generalization of self-regulatory strategy development (De La Paz, 1999; Pressley & Levin, 1987).

## DIRECT INSTRUCTION

*Direct instruction* focuses on teaching skills and strategies to a level of mastery via explicit teacher-directed instruction (Grossen, 2004). A guiding principle of direct instruction is that students can learn, and failure to learn is viewed as the function of inappropriate teaching, curriculum, or both rather than as a student characteristic. Siegfried Englemann and Carl Bereiter developed direct instruction in the 1960s to enable students who many believed could not learn to read to learn at a pace that would allow them to catch up to their nondisabled peers. Over 30 years of research suggests that the Corrective Reading Program (Englemann, 1999) improves reading skills at two to three times the typical rate if implemented consistently and with integrity, allowing struggling students to catch up to their peers (see Grossen, 1998, for a review of the research). Researchers have broadened direct instruction's application to include critical reading (Darch & Kame'enui, 1987), chemistry (Carnine, 1989), earth science (BFA Educational Media, 1991), expressive writing (Walker, Shippen, Alberto, Houchins, & Cihak, 2005), U.S. history (Carnine, Crawford, Harniss, & Hollenbeck, 1994), and problem solving (BFA Educational Media, 1991).

Direct-instruction curricula share several common characteristics to ensure that students with various needs will succeed. For example, assessment of a student's instructional needs drives placement in a direct-instruction curriculum. Ongoing assessment provides information about the student's skill development and teacher effectiveness. Students are commonly placed in homogeneous skill groups to ensure that students in a group need the same level of instruction and guidance. It also decreases the probability that some students either have mastered the targeted skills or do not have the prerequisite skills to benefit from instruction. Groupings are temporary, however, because teachers use ongoing individualized performance assessment to alter group membership appropriately.

Direct-instruction materials streamline lessons when this is practical. Engelmann recommends not teaching information students do not need, so that struggling students can catch up (Engelmann & Becker, 1978). Direct-instruction lessons are organized as logical developmental sequences, so that students know the rules, concepts, operations, and strategies necessary to learn the target skill (Kim & Axelrod, 2005; Kozloff, LaNuiziata, Cowardin, & Bessellieu, 2000). For example, teachers only teach letter sounds, not names, to students learning to sound out words, because the letter names are not needed to sound out words. The teacher teaches generalizable skills, concepts, and strategies, so that students can apply what

they learn to the trained examples and to the widest array of new items and situations. Engelmann and Becker (1978) referred to this as *general-case programming*. Teachers show students examples and nonexamples in a specific sequence that allows students to easily recognize differences and generalize what they have learned (Watkins & Slocum, 2004).

A misperception is that direct instruction focuses only on rote learning and promotes passive learning (Adams & Engelmann, 1996; Leontovich, 1999). Results of studies suggest that direct instruction promotes more generalization than alternative programs supported by constructivists, who commonly argue that teachers should only guide students as the students discover rules and strategies on their own. To examine this issue, Klahr and Nigam (2004) assigned 112 third- and fourth-grade students to a direct-instruction or a discovery-learning condition to teach the control-of-variables strategy, an elementary science objective. Teachers provided students in the direct-instruction condition with information on how and why control of variables works, showed examples and nonexamples of the strategy, and explained the differences between the examples. In the discovery-learning condition, teachers provided students with identical materials, and students developed their own experiments. Researchers conducted acquisition assessments in which students developed four of their own experiments, and a generalization assessment in which students evaluated two science fair projects. Results replicated previous studies indicating that acquisition of the control-of-variables strategy was greater for students in the direct-instruction condition (Chen & Klahr, 1999). In addition, results extended the literature by showing that students in the direct-instruction condition demonstrated more generalization, based on their science fair evaluations, than students in the discovery-learning condition did. Results of a meta-analytic study showed that explicit instructions produced a mean effect size of $d = -0.38$, suggesting that explicit instruction produced greater learning than unassisted discovery instruction (Alfieri, Brooks, Aldrich, & Tenenbaum, 2011).

Teachers teach direct-instruction lessons at a brisk pace, to provide students with more learning and response opportunities and to maintain active student engagement. Teachers and students use consistent language to define concepts, state rules, and employ strategies, which prevents confusion from variations in language. Teachers also use consistent verbal signals, nonverbal signals, or both for frequent group unison responding. Students write their answers on dry-erase boards; this facilitates academic engagement and practice, as well as assessment of student performance (Watkins & Slocum, 2004). Haydon and Hunter (2011) reported that unison responding decreased teachers' redirective statements and increased their praise statements, and that it increased students' on-task behavior, correct responses, and test scores.

Teachers consistently use a model–lead–test–delayed-test procedure in which teachers first model the target content, and then the teachers and students work through skills and operations together (Kozloff et al., 2000). As students become more proficient, teachers provide less information, decrease their prompts, and fade their corrective feedback from immediate to delayed. Problems increase in complexity. These shifts ensure initial and ongoing student success, thus maintaining their motivation to learn, to master skills, and to become more independent. Teaching skills to mastery increases the likelihood that students will maintain their learning and will generalize and adapt it to new situations (Binder, 1996). After modeling, teachers test students' acquisition through unison responding and provide immediate corrective feedback for mistakes. Teachers conduct group and individual delayed tests later in the same lesson and during subsequent lessons, to ensure maintenance and to promote generalization (Kozloff et al., 2000).

Adhering to the precise sequence of teaching skills and strategies, and maintaining the clarity and consistency of instructions, are the keys to the effectiveness of direct instruction. Teachers use lesson scripts to increase the integrity and planfulness of instruction (Watkins & Slocum, 2004). A direct-instruction approach or curriculum is a relatively comprehensive instructional method that incorporates explicit strategy instruction into teaching basic skills and more complex behavioral chains. Direct instruction includes ongoing assessment of student progress and needs, with recursive plan revision, shaping, prompting, chaining, and strategy instruction.

## GENERALIZATION OF COMPLEX SKILLS

Both strategy instruction and direct instruction devote considerable attention to generalization from the outset of teaching. Typically, the goal of teaching is for the student to demonstrate the new behaviors in the teaching context and across contexts, persons, and times, and to exhibit a range of related behaviors that were never explicitly instructed. The likelihood of students' retaining and generalizing learning increases substantially when generalization is part of the curriculum rather than an afterthought (Daly, Martens, Barnett, Witt, & Olson, 2007).

One technique to promote generalization is to provide students with numerous opportunities to practice skills and strategies to promote mastery. Evidence exists that teaching students to a high level of fluency, rather than just accuracy, promotes maintenance, generalization, and adaptation (Binder, 1996). There are also data suggesting that *overlearning* further increases retention and generalization. Overlearning is achieved by bringing students to levels of mastery and then providing additional practice opportunities (Driskell, Copper, & Willis, 1992). For example, Ardoin, Williams, Klubnik, and McCall (2009) found that overlearning through increased opportunities to respond enhanced maintenance effects, but did not substantially increase students' initial reading fluency.

Frequent reinforcement for accurate and fluent responding also promotes generalization. Teacher assistance in the form of modeling and performance feedback ensures success. Teachers should graduate their assistance such that students experience success, but they should also require students to apply the skills and strategies independently across tasks that systematically increase in difficulty. Teachers should systematically plan what academic responses to reinforce, which will increase the probability of skill generalization and allow for natural contingencies to serve eventually as reinforcers (Daly et al., 2007).

Teachers should model and provide practice opportunities, using various examples of when students should use the target skill or strategy (Troia, 2002), and should provide students with examples and nonexamples. In a study by Hicks, Bethune, Wood, Cooke, and Mims (2011), teachers taught correct preposition use to students with intellectual disabilities. For example, the teacher first placed a ball on a box and said, "This is on" (example), and then placed the ball at least 0.3 meters from the box and said, "This is not on" (nonexample). The teacher next decreased the distance between the ball and the box. After this, the teacher replaced the ball with common classroom objects to demonstrate examples and nonexamples of *on*. Finally, students participated in a scavenger hunt to find examples of the recently learned prepositions. The researchers gradually increased the complexity of the tasks and used multiple exemplars, while assisting students to discriminate between when to use and not use their recently learned skill. Such purposeful sequencing teaches students that skills and strategies build upon one another and are important to remember (Watkins & Slocum, 2004).

## SELF-MANAGEMENT

Teaching new complex skills by no means ensures that students will use those skills outside of training. In fact, students with learning disabilities may have the necessary skills to perform tasks at the levels of their peers, but simply do not use those skills (Reid et al., 2013). Perhaps high response effort or an inadequate reinforcement history contributes to the absence of skill use. Nguyen, Binder, Nemier, and Ardoin (2014) reported that 22% of second-grade students in their study did not read passages for comprehension. The researchers observed that several highly skilled readers engaged in behavior that was inconsistent with reading for comprehension. Strategy instruction and direct instruction teach students to use self-regulatory skills with the goal that natural contingencies will eventually maintain these skills, and that students will use skills, strategies, and behaviors independently across settings and times (Brooks, Todd, Tofflemoyer, & Horner, 2003).

Research has shown that self-monitoring modifies the behavior and improves the academic performance of children and adults with and without developmental disabilities (Delano, 2007; Gureasko-Moore et al., 2006; Plavnick, Ferreri, & Maupin, 2010; Silla-Zaleski & Vesloski, 2010). To teach self-management, a teacher first evaluates a student's performance and shows/explains the evaluation to the student. The teacher provides the student with examples of how he or she would rate the student's behavior; then the student and teacher evaluate the student's behavior, compare the ratings, and discuss the differences. The teacher provides reinforcement for accurate evaluations (i.e., performance feedback) and gradually fades assistance as the student becomes an accurate self-evaluator (Briesch & Chafouleas, 2009). Ideally, students use these self-regulatory skills across settings, thus helping them to evaluate problems, choose an appropriate strategy to use, evaluate the outcome of strategy use, and reinforce appropriate responding (Pressley & Levin, 1987; Troia, 2002).

## CONCLUSION

Behavior-analytic approaches to establishing new behaviors have achieved their most striking successes in permitting individuals whose learning capacity was perceived as substantially limited to learn more than had previously been thought possible. The success of ABA-derived teaching procedures for learners with disabilities led to the use of behavior-analytic teaching to permit faster and more precise learning for typically developing persons. Findings with more typically developing learners have paralleled the positive results from populations of students with disabilities. Research has demonstrated that typically developing students learn material more quickly and with greater precision when teaching includes a systematic, graduated approach of direct instruction with carefully sequenced targets, reinforcement of responding, and explicit instruction for complex behaviors (Grossen, 1998).

Interestingly, the development of behavior-analytic approaches to teaching parallels the development of individual instructional programs. The literature is oldest and most well developed at the beginning of instruction: the establishment of discrete behaviors. The work on procedures such as prompting, shaping, and chaining is well established. The research literature on teaching complex behavioral repertoires is better developed than one might initially assume, given the mass of the more basic discrete-instruction literature, but to some degree it is fragmented. Although some of the literature related to establishing strategic behavior appears in traditional behavior-analytic outlets (e.g., Ledbetter-Cho et al., 2015), some of this literature appears in research outlets that we would describe as more broadly educational than behavior-analytic, and there is simply less volume than in the literature on discrete responses.

Behavior analysts who are engaged in the establishment of new behaviors should keep the long view in mind. The long-term goal of teaching is not to bring individual operants under stimulus control, but to help learners develop complex, flexible repertoires that are adaptive, will remain in contact with reinforcement, will confer adaptive advantage, and will endure. Developing these complex behavioral repertoires requires a complex array of analyst behavior that will progress from procedures designed to teach discrete behaviors to those that explicitly support the development of the generalized and strategic behaviors that form effective flexible response classes.

# REFERENCES

Adams, G., & Engelmann, S. (1996). *Research on direct instruction: 25 years beyond DISTAR*. Seattle, WA: Educational Achievement System.

Akmanoglu, N., Kurt, O., & Kapan, A. (2015). Comparison of simultaneous prompting and constant time delay procedures in teaching children with autism the response to questions about personal information. *Educational Sciences: Theory and Practice, 15*(3), 723–737.

Alber-Morgan, S. R., Hessler, T., & Konrad, M. (2007). Teaching writing for keeps. *Education and Treatment of Children, 30*(3), 107–128.

Alberto, P. A., & Troutman, A. C. (1986). *Applied behavior analysis for teachers*. Columbus, OH: Merrill.

Alexander, P. A., Graham, S., & Harris, K. R. (1998). A perspective on strategy research: Progress and prospects. *Educational Psychology Review, 10*, 129–154.

Alexander, P. A., & Murphy, P. K. (1999). What cognitive psychology has to say to school psychology: Shifting perspectives and shared purposes. In C. R. Reynolds & T. B. Gutkin (Eds.), *The handbook of school psychology* (3rd ed., pp. 167–193). New York: Wiley.

Alfieri, L., Brooks, P. J., Aldrich, N. J., & Tenenbaum, H. R. (2011). Does discovery-based instruction enhance learning? *Journal of Educational Psychology, 103*(1), 1–18.

Ardoin, S. P., & Daly, E. J., III. (2007). Introduction to the special series: Close encounters of the instructional kind—How the instructional hierarchy is shaping instructional research 30 years later. *Journal of Behavioral Education, 16*, 1–6.

Ardoin, S. P., Williams, J. C., Klubnik, C., & McCall, M. (2009). Three versus six rereadings of practice passages. *Journal of Applied Behavior Analysis, 42*, 375–380.

Ash, D. W., & Holding, D. H. (1990). Backward versus forward chaining in the acquisition of a keyboard skill. *Human Factors, 32*, 139–146.

Athens, E. S., Vollmer, T. R., & St. Peter Pipkin, C. C. (2007). Shaping academic task engagement with percentile schedules. *Journal of Applied Behavior Analysis, 40*, 475–488.

Ault, M. J., Wolery, M., Doyle, P. M., & Gast, D. L. (1989). Review of comparative studies in the instruction of students with moderate and severe handicaps. *Exceptional Children, 55*(4), 346–356.

Ayres, K. M., & Langone, J. (2005). Intervention and instruction with video for students with autism: A review of the literature. *Education and Training in Developmental Disabilities, 40*(2), 183–196.

Bandura, A., Ross, D., & Ross, S. A. (1963). Vicarious reinforcement and imitative learning. *Journal of Abnormal and Social Psychology, 67*(6), 601–607.

Bennett, K. D., Ramasamy, R., & Honsberger, T. (2013). The effects of covert audio coaching on teaching clerical skills to adolescents with autism spectrum disorder. *Journal of Autism and Developmental Disorders, 43*(3), 585–593.

Betz, A. M., Higbee, T. S., Kelley, K. N., Sellers, T. P., & Pollard, J. S. (2011). Increasing response variability of mand frames with script training and extinction. *Journal of Applied Behavior Analysis, 44*, 357–362.

BFA Educational Media. (1991). *Problem solving with tables, graphs, and statistics*. St. Louis, MO: Author.

Billingsley, F. F., & Romer, L. T. (1983). Response prompting and the transfer of stimulus control: Methods, research, and a conceptual framework. *Journal of the Association for the Severely Handicapped, 8*(2), 3–12.

Binder, C. (1996). Behavioral fluency: Evolution of a new paradigm. *Behavior Analyst, 19*, 163–197.

Briesch, A. M., & Chafouleas, S. M. (2009). Review and analysis of literature on self-management interventions to promote appropriate classroom behaviors (1988–2008). *School Psychology Quarterly, 24*(2), 106–118.

Brooks, A., Todd, A. W., Tofflemoyer, S., & Horner, R. H. (2003). Use of functional assessment and a self-management system to increase academic engagement and work completion. *Journal of Positive Behavior Interventions, 5*, 144–152.

Buggey, T., & Ogle, L. (2012). Video self-modeling. *Psychology in the Schools, 49*(1), 57–70.

Cannella-Malone, H., Sigafoos, J., O'Reilly, M., de la Cruz, B., Edrisinha, C., & Lancioni, G. E. (2006). Comparing video prompting to video modeling for teaching daily living skills to six adults with developmental disabilities. *Education and Training in Developmental Disabilities, 41*(4), 344–356.

Carnine, D. (1989). Teaching complex content to learning disabled students: The role of technology. *Exceptional Children, 55*, 524–533.

Carnine, D., Crawford, D., Harniss, M., & Hollenbeck, K. (1994). *Understanding U.S. history* (Vols. 1–2). Eugene, OR: Considerate.

Carroll, R. A., Kodak, T., & Adolf, K. J. (2016). Effect of delayed reinforcement on skill acquisition during discrete-trial instruction: Implications for treatment-integrity errors in academic settings. *Journal of Applied Behavior Analysis, 49*, 1–6.

Chen, Z., & Klahr, D. (1999). All other things being equal: Acquisition and transfer of the control of variables strategy. *Child Development, 70*, 1098–1120.

Clark, A. M., Schmidt, J. D., Mezhoudi, N., & Kahng, S. W. (2016). Using percentile schedules to increase academic fluency. *Behavioral Interventions, 31*, 283–290.

Cooper, J. O., Heron, T. E., & Heward, W. L. (2007). *Applied behavior analysis* (2nd ed.). Upper Saddle River, NJ: Pearson/Merrill-Prentice Hall.

Daly, E. J., III, Martens, B. K., Barnett, D., Witt, J. C., & Olson, S. C. (2007). Varying intervention delivery in response to intervention: Confronting and resolving challenges with measurement, instruction, and intensity. *School Psychology Review, 36*(4), 562–581.

Daly, E. J., III, Persampieri, M., McCurdy, M., & Gort-maker, V. (2005). Generating reading interventions through experimental analysis of academic skills: Demonstration and empirical evaluation. *School Psychology Review, 34*(3), 395–414.

Darch, C. B., & Kame'enui, E. J. (1987). Teaching LD students critical reading skills: A systematic replication. *Learning Disability Quarterly, 10,* 82–91.

De La Paz, S. (1999). Self-regulated strategy instruction in regular education settings: Improving outcomes for students with and without learning disabilities. *Learning Disabilities Research and Practice, 14,* 92–106.

Delano, M. E. (2007). Improving written language performance of adolescents with Asperger syndrome. *Journal of Applied Behavior Analysis, 40,* 345–351.

Demchak, M. (1990). Response prompting and fading methods: A review. *American Journal on Mental Retardation, 94,* 603–615.

DiCarlo, C. F., Reid, D. H., & Stricklin, S. B. (2003). Increasing toy play among toddlers with multiple disabilities in an inclusive classroom: A more-to-less, child-directed intervention continuum. *Research in Developmental Disabilities, 24,* 195–209.

DiPipi-Hoy, C., & Jitendra, A. (2004). A parent-delivered intervention to teach purchasing skills to young adults with disabilities. *Journal of Special Education, 38*(3), 144–157.

Domire, S. C., & Wolfe, P. (2014). Effects of video prompting techniques on teaching daily living skills to children with autism spectrum disorder: A review. *Research and Practice for Persons with Severe Disabilities, 39*(3), 211–226.

Driskell, J. E., Copper, C., & Willis, R. P. (1992). Effect of overlearning on retention. *Journal of Applied Psychology, 77,* 615–622.

Duffy, G. G., Roehler, L. R., Sivan, E., & Rackliffe, G. (1987). Effects of explaining the reasoning associated with using reading strategies. *Reading Research Quarterly, 22*(3), 347–368.

Ehrlich, P. R., & Ehrlich, A. H. (2008). *The dominant animal.* Washington, DC: Island Press.

Englemann, S. (1999). *Corrective reading program.* Blacklick, OH: Science Research Associates.

Englemann, S., & Becker, W. S. (1978). Systems for basic instruction: Theory and applications. In A. C. Catania & T. A. Bringham (Eds.), *Handbook of applied behavior analysis* (pp. 325–377). New York: Irvington.

Esch, J. W., Esch, B. E., & Love, J. R. (2009). Increasing vocal variability in children with autism using a lag schedule of reinforcement. *Analysis of Verbal Behavior, 25*(1), 73–78.

Etzel, B. C., & LeBlanc, J. M. (1979). The simplest treatment alternative: Appropriate instructional control and errorless learning procedures for the difficult-to-teach child. *Journal of Autism and Developmental Disorders, 9,* 361–382.

Falcomata, T. S., Muething, C. S., Silbaugh, B. C.,

Adami, S. Hoffman, K., Shpall, C., et al. (2018). Lag schedules and functional communication training: Persistence of mands and relapse of problem behavior. *Behavior Modification, 42,* 314–334.

Fetko, K. S., Schuster, J. W., Harley, D. A., & Collins, B. C. (1999). Using simultaneous prompting to teach a chained vocational task to young adults with severe intellectual disabilities. *Education and Training in Mental Retardation and Developmental Disabilities, 34,* 318–329.

Galbicka, G. (1994). Shaping in the 21st century: Moving percentile schedules into applied settings. *Journal of Applied Behavior Analysis, 27,* 739–760.

Garcia-Albea, E., Reeve, S. A., Brothers, K. J., & Reeve, K. F. (2014). Using audio script fading and multiple-exemplar training to increase vocal interactions in children with autism. *Journal of Applied Behavior Analysis, 47,* 325–343.

Goetz, E. M., & Baer, D. M. (1973). Social control of form diversity and the emergence of new forms in children's blockbuilding. *Journal of Applied Behavior Analysis, 62,* 209–217.

Grossen, B. (1998). *The research base for Corrective Reading.* Blacklick, OH: Science Research Associates.

Grossen, B. (2004). Success of a direct instruction model at a secondary level school with high risk students. *Reading and Writing Quarterly, 20,* 161–178.

Gruber, D. J., & Poulson, C. L. (2015). Graduated guidance delivered by parents to teach yoga to children with developmental delays. *Journal of Applied Behavior Analysis, 49,* 1–6.

Gureasko-Moore, S., DuPaul, G. J., & White, G. P. (2006). The effects of self-management in general education classrooms on the organizational skills of adolescents with ADHD. *Behavior Modification, 30,* 159–183.

Hall, S. S., Maynes, N. P., & Reiss, A. L. (2009). Using percentile schedules to increase eye contact in children with fragile X syndrome. *Journal of Applied Behavior Analysis, 42,* 171–176.

Harding, J., Wacker, D. P., Cooper, L. J., Millard, T., & Jensen-Kovalan, P. (1994). Brief hierarchical assessment of potential treatment components with children in an outpatient clinic. *Journal of Applied Behavior Analysis, 27,* 291–300.

Haydon, T., & Hunter, W. (2011). The effects of two types of teacher questioning on teacher behavior and student performance: A case study. *Education and Treatment of Children, 34*(2), 229–245.

Haywood, H. C. (2004). Thinking in, around, and about the curriculum: The role of cognitive education. *International Journal of Disability, Development and Education, 51,* 231–252.

Heckaman, K. A., Alber, S., Hooper, S., & Heward, W. L. (1998). A comparison of least-to-most prompts and progressive time delay on the disruptive behavior of students with autism. *Journal of Behavioral Education, 8*(2), 171–201.

Heldt, J., & Schlinger, H. D. (2012). Increased variability in tacting under a lag 3 schedule of reinforcement. *Analysis of Verbal Behavior, 28*(1), 131–136.

Hickey, D. T., Moore, A. L., & Pellegrino, J. W. (2001). The motivational and academic consequences of elementary mathematics environments: Do constructivist innovations and reforms make a difference? *American Educational Research Journal, 38*, 611–652.

Hicks, S. C., Bethune, K. S., Wood, C. L., Cooke, N. L., & Mims, P. J. (2011). Effects of direct instruction on the acquisition of prepositions by students with intellectual disabilities. *Journal of Applied Behavior Analysis, 44*, 675–679.

Horner, R. D. (1971). Establishing use of crutches by a mentally retarded spina bifida child. *Journal of Applied Behavior Analysis, 4*, 183–189.

Hughes, S., & Barnes-Holmes, D. (2014). Associative concept learning, stimulus equivalence, and relational frame theory: Working out the similarities and differences between human and nonhuman behavior. *Journal of the Experimental Analysis of Behavior, 101*(1), 156–160.

Hur, J., & Osborne, S. (1993). A comparison of forward and backward chaining methods used in teaching corsage making skills to mentally retarded adults. *British Journal of Developmental Disabilities, 39*(77), 108–117.

Isaacs, W., Thomas, J., & Goldiamond, I. (1960). Application of operant conditioning to reinstate verbal behavior in psychotics. *Journal of Speech and Hearing Disorders, 25*, 8–12.

Kelleher, R. T. (1966). Chaining and conditioned reinforcement. In W. K. Honig (Ed.), *Operant behavior: Areas of research and application* (pp. 160–212). Englewood Cliffs, NJ: Prentice-Hall.

Kelley, M. L., Reitman, D., & Noell, G. H. (2002). *Practitioner's guide to empirically based measures of school behavior.* New York: Kluwer Academic/Plenum.

Kim, T., & Axelrod, S. (2005). Direct instruction: An educators' guide and a plea for action. *Behavior Analyst Today, 6*(2), 111–120.

Klahr, D., & Nigam, M. (2004). The equivalence of learning paths in early science instruction: Effects of direct instruction and discovery learning. *Psychological Science, 15*, 661–667.

Koscinski, S. T., & Hoy, C. (1993). Teaching multiplication facts to students with learning disabilities: The promise of constant time delay procedures. *Learning Disabilities Research and Practice, 8*(4), 260–263.

Kozloff, M. A., LaNuiziata, L., Cowardin, J., & Bessellieu, F. B. (2000). Direct instruction: Its contributions to high school achievement. *High School Journal, 84*, 54–77.

Krantz, P. J., & McClannahan, L. E. (1993). Teaching children with autism to initiate to peers: Effects of a script-fading procedure. *Journal of Applied Behavior Analysis, 26*, 121–132.

Kroesbergen, E. H., Van Luit, J. E. H., & Maas, C. J. M. (2004). Effectiveness of explicit and constructivist mathematics instruction for low-achieving students in the Netherlands. *Elementary School Journal, 104*, 233–251.

Ledbetter-Cho, K., Lang, R., Davenport, K., Moore, M., Lee, A., Howell, A., et al. (2015). Effects of script training on the peer-to-peer communication of children with autism spectrum disorder. *Journal of Applied Behavior Analysis, 48*, 785–799.

Lee, R., McComas, J. J., & Jawor, J. (2002). The effects of differential and lag reinforcement schedules on varied verbal responding by individuals with autism. *Journal of Applied Behavior Analysis, 35*, 391–402.

Leontovich, M. (1999, August). Direct controversial: Direct instruction makes enemies, converts. *Title I Report.* Retrieved July 2004, from *www.ncld.org/summit99/keys99-nichd.htm.*

Lerman, D. C., & Iwata, B. A. (1996). Developing a technology for the use of operant extinction in clinical settings: An examination of basic and applied research. *Journal of Applied Behavior Analysis, 29*, 345–382.

Libby, M. E., Weiss, J. S., Bancroft, S., & Ahearn, W. H. (2008). A comparison of most-to-least and least-to-most prompting on the acquisition of solitary play skills. *Behavior Analysis in Practice, 1*(1), 37–43.

Liem, G. D., & Martin, A. J. (2013). Direct instruction. In J. Hattie & E. M. Anderman (Eds.), *International guide to student achievement* (pp. 366–368). New York: Routledge.

Luiselli, J. K., & Hurley, A. D. (2005). The significance of applied behavior analysis in the treatment of individuals with autism spectrum disorders (ASD). *Mental Health Aspects of Developmental Disabilities, 8*, 128–130.

Mahy, C. V., Moses, L. J., & Kliegel, M. (2014). The development of prospective memory in children: An executive framework. *Developmental Review, 34*(4), 305–326.

Malott, R. W. (1989). The achievement of evasive goals. In S. C. Hayes (Ed.), *Rule-governed behavior: Cognition, contingencies, and instructional control* (pp. 269–322). New York: Plenum Press.

Manset-Williamson, G., & Nelson, J. M. (2005). Balanced, strategic reading instruction for upper-elementary and middle school students with reading disabilities: A comparative study of two approaches. *Learning Disability Quarterly, 28*, 59–74.

Martens, B. K., & Daly, E. J. (1999). Discovering the alphabetic principle: A lost opportunity for educational reform. *Journal of Educational Psychology, 9*, 35–43.

Matson, J. L., Sevin, J. A., Fridley, D., & Love, S. R. (1990). Increasing spontaneous language in three autistic children. *Journal of Applied Behavior Analysis, 23*, 227–233.

McClannahan, L. E., & Krantz, P. J. (2005). *Teaching conversation to children with autism: Scripts and script fading.* Bethesda, MD: Woodbine House.

Miltenberger, R. G. (2001). *Behavior modification: Principles and procedures* (2nd ed.). Belmont, CA: Wadsworth/Thomson Learning.

Morse, T. E., & Schuster, J. W. (2004). Simultaneous prompting: A review of the literature. *Education and Training in Developmental Disabilities, 39*(2), 153–168.

Napolitano, D. A., Smith, T., Zarcone, J. R., Goodkin, K., & McAdam, D. B. (2010). Increasing response diversity in children with autism. *Journal of Applied Behavior Analysis, 43,* 265–271.

National Reading Panel. (2000). *Report of the National Reading Panel. Teaching children to read: An evidence-based assessment of the scientific research literature on reading and its implications for reading instruction* (NIH Publication No. 00-4769). Washington, DC: National Institute of Child Health and Human Development.

Nguyen, K.-V., Binder, K. S., Nemier, C., & Ardoin, S. P. (2014). Gotcha!: Catching kids during mindless reading. *Scientific Studies of Reading, 18*(4), 274–290.

Noell, G. H., Connell, J. M., & Duhon, G. J. (2006). Spontaneous response generalization during whole word instruction: Reading to spell and spelling to read. *Journal of Behavioral Education, 15*(3), 121–130.

Noell, G. H., Freeland, J. T., Witt, J. C., & Gansle, K. A. (2001). Using brief assessments to identify effective interventions for individual students. *Journal of School Psychology, 39*(4), 335–355.

Noell, G. H., Gansle, K. A., Witt, J. C., Whitmarsh, E. L., Freeland, J. T., LaFleur, L. H., et al. (1998). Effects of contingent reward and instruction on oral reading performance at differing levels of passage difficulty. *Journal of Applied Behavior Analysis, 31,* 659–664.

O'Neill, S. J., McDowell, C., & Leslie, J. (2018). A comparison of prompt delays with trial-and-error instruction in conditional discrimination training. *Behavior Analysis in Practice, 11,* 370–380.

Oppenheim-Leaf, M. L., Leaf, J. B., & Call, N. A. (2012). Teaching board games to two children with autism spectrum disorder. *Journal of Developmental and Physical Disabilities, 24*(4), 347–358.

Page, S., & Neuringer, A. (1985). Variability is an operant. *Journal of Experimental Psychology: Animal Behavior Processes, 11*(3), 429–452.

Parrott, K. A., Schuster, J. W., Collins, B. C., & Gassaway, L. J. (2000). Simultaneous prompting and instructive feedback when teaching chained tasks. *Journal of Behavioral Education, 10*(1), 3–19.

Pierce, K. L., & Schreibman, L. (1994). Teaching daily living skills to children with autism in unsupervised settings through pictorial self-management. *Journal of Applied Behavior Analysis, 27,* 471–481.

Plavnick, J. B., Ferreri, S. J., & Maupin, A. N. (2010). The effects of self-monitoring on the procedural integrity of a behavioral intervention for young children with developmental disabilities. *Journal of Applied Behavior Analysis, 43,* 315–320.

Pressley, M., & Levin, J. R. (1987). Elaborative learning strategies for the inefficient learner. In S. J. Ceci (Ed.), *Handbook of cognitive, social, and neuropsychological aspects of learning disabilities* (pp. 175–212). Hillsdale, NJ: Erlbaum.

Rea, J., & Williams, D. (2002). Shaping exhale durations for breath CO detection for men with mild mental retardation. *Journal of Applied Behavior Analysis, 35,* 415–418.

Reagon, K. A., & Higbee, T. S. (2009). Parent-implemented script fading to promote play-based verbal initiations in children with autism. *Journal of Applied Behavior Analysis, 42,* 659–664.

Reid, R., Lienemann, T. O., & Hagaman, J. L. (2013). *Strategy instruction for students with learning disabilities* (2nd ed.). New York: Guilford Press.

Reitzel, J., Summers, J., Lorv, B., Szatmari, P., Zwaigenbaum, L., Georgiades, S., et al. (2013). Pilot randomized controlled trial of a functional behavior skills training program for young children with autism spectrum disorder who have significant early learning skill impairments and their families. *Research in Autism Spectrum Disorders, 7*(11), 1418–1432.

Richardson, V. (2003). Constructivist pedagogy. *Teachers College Record, 105*(9), 1623–1640.

Rosales-Ruiz, J., & Baer, D. M. (1997). Behavioral cusps: A developmental and pragmatic concept for behavior analysis. *Journal of Applied Behavior Analysis, 30,* 533–544.

Sauttfr, R. A., LeBlanc, L. A., Jay, A. A., Goldsmith, T. R., & Carr, J. E. (2011). The role of problem solving in complex intraverbal repertoires. *Journal of Applied Behavior Analysis, 44,* 227–244.

Schleien, S. J., Wehman, P., & Kiernan, J. (1981). Teaching leisure skills to severely handicapped adults: An age-appropriate darts game. *Journal of Applied Behavior Analysis, 14,* 513–519.

Schoen, S. F. (1986). Assistance procedures to facilitate the transfer of stimulus control: Review and analysis. *Education and Training of the Mentally Retarded, 21*(1), 62–74.

Schuster, J. W., Griffin, A. K., & Wolery, M. (1992). Comparisons of simultaneous prompting and constant time delay procedures in teaching sight words to elementary students with moderate mental retardation. *Journal of Behavioral Education, 2*(3), 302–325.

Scott, D., Scott, L. M., & Goldwater, B. (1997). A performance improvement program for an international-level track and field athlete. *Journal of Applied Behavior Analysis, 30,* 573–575.

Silbaugh, B. C., Falcomata, T. S., & Ferguson, R. H. (2018). Effects of a lag schedule of reinforcement with progressive time delay on topographical mand variability in children with autism. *Developmental Neurorehabilitation, 21,* 166–177.

Silla-Zaleski, V. A., & Vesloski, M. J. (2010). Using DRO, behavioral momentum, and self-regulation to reduce scripting by an adolescent with autism. *Journal of Speech and Language Pathology–Applied Behavior Analysis, 5*(1), 80–87.

Skinner, B. F. (1938). *The behavior of organisms: An experimental analysis.* New York: Appleton-Century-Crofts.

Slocum, S. K., & Tiger, J. H. (2011). An assessment of the efficiency of and child preference for forward and backward chaining. *Journal of Applied Behavior Analysis, 44,* 793–805.

Smith, G. J. (1999). Teaching a long sequence of a behavior using whole task training, forward chaining, and backward chaining. *Perceptual and Motor Skills, 89,* 951–965.

Snell, M. E., & Gast, D. L. (1981). Applying time delay procedure to the instruction of the severely handicapped. *Journal of the Association for the Severely Handicapped, 6*(3), 3–14.

Snow, C. E., Burns, M. S., & Griffin, P. (1998). *Preventing reading difficulties in young children.* Washington, DC: National Academy Press.

Spooner, F., & Spooner, D. (1984). A review of chaining techniques: Implications for future research and practice. *Education and Training of the Mentally Retarded, 19,* 114–124.

Spooner, F., Spooner, D., & Ulicny, G. (1986). Comparisons of modified backward chaining: Backward chaining with leap-aheads and reverse chaining with leap-aheads. *Education and Treatment of Children, 9*(2), 122–134.

Spooner, F., Weber, L. H., & Spooner, D. (1983). The effects of backward chaining and total task presentation on the acquisition of complex tasks by severely retarded adolescents and adults. *Education and Treatment of Children, 6,* 401–420.

Sternberg, L., & Adams, G. L. (1982). *Educating severely and profoundly handicapped students.* Rockville MD: Aspen Systems.

Stevens, K. B., Blackhurst, A. E., & Slaton, D. B. (1991). Teaching memorized spelling with a microcomputer: Time delay and computer-assisted instruction. *Journal of Applied Behavior Analysis, 24,* 153–160.

Stokes, T. F., & Baer, D. M. (1977). An implicit technology of generalization. *Journal of Applied Behavior Analysis, 10,* 349–367.

Sullivan, W. E., Saini, V., DeRosa, N. M., Craig, A. R., Ringdahl, J. E., & Roane, H. S. (2020). Measurement of nontargeted problem behavior during investigations of resurgence. *Journal of Applied Behavior Analysis, 53,* 249–264.

Swain, R., Lane, J. D., & Gast, D. L. (2015). Comparison of constant time delay and simultaneous prompting procedures: Teaching functional sight words to students with intellectual disabilities and autism spectrum disorder. *Journal of Behavioral Education, 24*(2), 210–229.

Taylor, B. A., Hughes, C. E., Richard, E., Hoch, H., & Coello, A. R. (2004). Teaching teenagers with autism to seek assistance when lost. *Journal of Applied Behavior Analysis, 37,* 79–82.

Tekin-Iftar, E., Acar, G., & Kurt, O. (2003). The effects of simultaneous prompting on teaching expressive identification of objects: An instructive feedback study. *International Journal of Disability, Development, and Education, 50*(2), 149–167.

Trapman, M., van Gelderen, A., van Steensel, R., van Schooten, E., & Hulstijn, J. (2014). Linguistic knowledge, fluency and meta-cognitive knowledge as components of reading comprehension in adolescent low achievers: Differences between monolinguals and bilinguals. *Journal of Research in Reading, 37,* S3–S21.

Troia, G. A. (2002). Teaching writing strategies to children with disabilities: Setting generalization as the goal. *Exceptionality, 10,* 249–269.

Valentino, A. L., Shillingsburg, M. A., Call, N. A., Burton, B., & Bowen, C. N. (2011). An investigation of extinction-induced vocalizations. *Behavior Modification, 35*(3), 284–298.

Wagner, R. K., Puranik, C. S., Foorman, B., Foster, E., Wilson, L. G., Tschinkel, E., et al. (2011). Modeling the development of written language. *Reading and Writing, 24,* 203–220.

Walker, B., Shippen, M. E., Alberto, P., Houchins, D. E., & Cihak, D. F. (2005). Using the expressive writing program to improve the writing skills of high school students with learning disabilities. *Learning Disabilities Research and Practice, 20,* 175–183.

Watkins, C. L., & Slocum, T. A. (2004). The components of direct instruction. In N. E. Marchand-Martella, T. A. Slocum, & R. C. Martella (Eds.), *Introduction to direct instruction* (pp. 28–65). Boston: Allyn & Bacon.

Watters, J. K. (1992). Retention of human sequenced behavior following forward chaining, backward chaining, and whole task training procedures. *Journal of Human Movement Studies, 22*(3), 117–129.

Wichnick-Gillis, A. M., Vener, S. M., & Poulson, C. L. (2019). Script fading for children with autism: Generalization of social initiation skills from school to home. *Journal of Applied Behavior Analysis, 52,* 451–466.

Wightman, D. C., & Sistrunk, F. (1987). Part-task training strategies in simulated carrier landing final-approach training. *Human Factors, 29*(3), 245–254.

Williams, G., Donley, C. R., & Keller, J. W. (2000). Teaching children with autism to ask questions about hidden objects. *Journal of Applied Behavior Analysis, 33,* 627–630.

Wiskow, K. M., Matter, A. L., & Donaldson, J. M. (2018). An evaluation of log schedules and prompting methods to increase variability of naming category items in children with autism spectrum disorder. *Analysis of Verbal Behavior, 34,* 100–123.

Wolery, M., & Gast, D. L. (1984). Effective and efficient procedures for the transfer of stimulus control. *Topics in Early Childhood Special Education, 4*(3), 52–77.

Wolery, M., Holcombe, A., Cybriwsky, C., Doyle, P. M., Schuster, J. W., Ault, M. J., et al. (1992). Constant time delay with discrete responses: A review of effectiveness and demographic, procedural, and methodological parameters. *Research in Developmental Disabilities, 13*(3), 239–266.

# CHAPTER 16

# Teaching Verbal Behavior

Matt Tincani, Caio Miguel, Andy Bondy, and Shannon Crozier

Lori is eating popcorn in a classroom while she prepares a lesson for her preschool students, who are on the playground. Lily walks into the classroom, approaches Lori, and says, "Popcorn!" Lori smiles and gives Lily popcorn. Jack walks into the classroom and sees the popcorn. He grabs for the bag without saying anything. Lori looks at him and says, "What do you want?" Jack says, "Popcorn!" Lori smiles and gives Jack popcorn. Char walks into the classroom, sees the popcorn, and grabs for the bag while remaining silent. Lori says, "What do you want?", but Char continues to grab for the bag while remaining silent. Lori then says, "Say *popcorn.*" Char immediately says, "Popcorn!" Lori smiles and gives Char popcorn.

If Lori were to complete a checklist based on these interactions that included the question "Can each child say *popcorn*?", the correct answer would be *yes*. However, if we were to ask Lori, "Does each child do the same thing?", the correct answer would be *no*. Although the form of the response *popcorn* is the same, each example involves a different controlling relation. The difference in perspective between the first and second questions is at the heart of a functional analysis of verbal behavior. Although knowing the *form* of verbal behavior is useful, understanding its *functional control* is more important. This chapter reviews how a functional analysis of verbal behavior can provide guidance about the complex issues associated with teaching communication and language to those with limited or no verbal repertoire.

## SKINNER'S ANALYSIS OF VERBAL BEHAVIOR

In his seminal book *Verbal Behavior*, Skinner (1957) showed how we can analyze language by using the principles of operant and respondent conditioning. Skinner chose the term *verbal behavior* rather than *speech*, because he did not want to restrict his analysis to vocal behavior. Additionally, traditionalists had already used the term *language* to refer to an ability or system in the organism responsible for generating speech. The source of control for language or verbal behavior, respectively, was a major difference between the traditional approach and Skinner's approach. According to the traditionalists, control for language originates within the organism. According to Skinner, by contrast, control for verbal behavior originates from contingencies of reinforcement acting upon the organism's behavior. Skinner's terminology emphasized that verbal behavior is like any other operant behavior. The term *verbal behavior*, which at that time was "relatively unfamiliar in traditional modes of explanation" (Skinner, 1957, p. 1), set the stage for a departure from traditional explanations of language.

Skinner (1957) defined *verbal behavior* as "behavior reinforced through the mediation of other persons" (p. 2). In other words, a *speaker's* behavior is reinforced through or mediated by the behavior of a *listener*.[1] The topography of the speaker's behavior, such as vocal, gestural, or visual, is irrelevant within this definition. Skinner stated his unique orientation to verbal behavior explicitly: "In defining verbal behavior as behavior reinforced through the mediation of other persons, we do not, and cannot, specify any one form, mode, or medium" (p. 14). Sometimes our behavior influences the environment in direct ways. For example, a little boy ties his own shoelaces and can run around immediately. At other times, our behavior influences other people whose actions lead to reinforcement. For example, the boy asks his brother to tie his shoes and runs around after his brother does so. Although the first example does not meet the definition of verbal behavior, the second one does.

The verbal community selects specific forms of verbal behavior to function in certain ways. The behavior forms may be vocal, such as spoken words; graphic lines, such as writing; or hand postures and movements, such as sign language. These behavior forms produce an effect on the environment. Skinner added an important refinement to the definition of verbal behavior when he wrote, "The listener must be responding in ways that have been conditioned *precisely to reinforce the behavior of the speaker*" (p. 225, emphasis in original). An individual learns listening behavior as a member of a verbal community. Thus the listener learns to react to the speaker's verbal behavior, and this is a requirement for behavior to be verbal. In the example above, when the little boy asks his brother, "Will you tie my shoes?", the auditory product of this behavior, the sound pattern, serves as a stimulus that evokes his brother's shoe tying. But notice that the brother can react appropriately as a listener by performing the task only if he has learned how to respond to this request previously. In lay terms, the listener must understand the speaker.[2]

We contrast the behavioral approach Skinner (1957) advocated with the traditional approach to language development and intervention of Chomsky (1965), Brown (1973), and Piaget (1951), who conceptualized language by the form or topography of the learner's verbal repertoire (i.e., vocabulary, grammar, syntax), with little regard for function. From the traditional perspective, language development is the function of hypothesized innate developmental, neurological, and cognitive structures. We use the term *language deficit* or *delay* when a learner's verbal repertoire is deficient in comparison to the verbal repertoire of a same-age, typically developing learner. Proponents of a traditional-language approach often relate language deficits to genetic or neurological abnormalities (Lord, Cook, Leventhal, & Amaral, 2000). Intervention tends to focus on the acquisition of forms, from sounds to words to larger structures, with less attention to the behavioral function of such forms (American Speech–Language–Hearing Association, 2016).

By contrast, the behavioral approach focuses on contingency or functional analysis of language or verbal behavior. Specific environment–behavior relations or contingencies of reinforcement are responsible for language development, according to the behavioral approach. Although Skinner (1957) did not review language deficits extensively in his book, researchers have applied his analysis to teaching language to children and adults with language difficulties (Barbera & Rasmussen, 2007; Carr & Miguel, 2013; Frost & Bondy, 2002; LaFrance & Miguel, 2014; Sundberg, 2008; Sundberg & Partington, 1998). However, some behaviorally oriented language training programs (e.g., Lovaas, 2003; Maurice, Green, & Luce, 1996) have not used Skinner's analysis as a framework for teaching verbal behavior. In our view, Skinner's analysis is essential to developing successful programs for training verbal behavior. In the sections that follow, we illustrate the basic tenets of Skinner's approach to verbal behavior and illustrate how we may apply it in specific training protocols.

## PRIMARY VERBAL OPERANTS

Skinner (1957) identified and named six types of functional relations between controlling variables and verbal responses. These consist of the *mand, tact, intraverbal, textual, echoic,* and *audience relations.* He named two more in the section on transcription: *copying a text* and *taking dictation.* Skin-

---

[1] Even though we commonly use the terms *speaker* and *listener* to refer to vocal behavior (i.e., speech), in Skinner's terms, the speaker is the one behaving (e.g., talking, signing, using pictures), and the listener is the one being affected by the response products of the speaker's behavior.

[2] During any given verbal episode, we behave as both speakers and listeners, as when we make a request or fulfill one, respectively. Additionally, we can react as listeners to our own verbal behavior, in that we can understand and react to the things we say (Miguel, 2016).

ner referred to these relations as *verbal operants,* because he classified them by the antecedents and consequences that control their form (i.e., operant behavior).

A *mand* is a verbal operant that a characteristic consequence reinforces, and the relevant conditions of deprivation or aversive stimulation control the response. Deprivation or aversive stimulation are *motivating operations,* or events that alter the value of a reinforcer. *Establishing operations* increase the value of a stimulus as a reinforcer. *Abolishing operations* decrease the value of a stimulus as a reinforcer[3] (Michael & Miguel, 2020; Michael, 1993). For example, behavior that produces water, such as touching a communication card that signals the therapist to deliver water, is likely to increase after consumption of salty snacks, which is the motivating operation in this example. The learner is likely to emit behavior that has produced water in the past under these conditions. Newborn babies and crying provide another example. Although newborns cry reflexively, they learn to cry when hungry when crying produces food. In this example, food deprivation is the motivating operation, which will control crying if crying produces food. These examples show that mands develop when specific response forms, such as touching a communication card or crying, produce specific consequences, such as water or food, respectively.

Mands are unique among verbal operants, because mands are controlled by relevant motiving operations. By contrast, discriminative stimuli control other verbal operants, such as tacts and intraverbals. Another difference between mands and other verbal operants is that specific stimulus forms reinforce mands. By contrast, nonspecific, generalized stimuli reinforce other verbal operants.

The *tact* is a verbal operant in which a response of a given form, such as vocal, sign, or writing, is controlled by a nonverbal stimulus or "a particular object or event or property of an object or event" (Skinner, 1957, p. 82). The presence of a car, for example, increases the likelihood of the learner's emitting the vocal, signed, or written response *car.* The object evokes the response because the English-speaking verbal community reinforced this specific verbalization in the presence of this object. An object may serve as a discriminative stimulus for various response forms. A toy car can evoke not only the response *car,* but also other

tacts such as *vehicle, red,* and *fast.* Environmental stimuli are likely to control many verbal responses, and we discuss this issue more fully below.

Skinner (1957) also illustrated that tacts can occur in the presence of novel objects or events to which the speaker has not been exposed previously if the novel object shares physical properties with the original stimulus. For example, a child may give the verbal response *car* in the presence of a novel exemplar because it shares common physical properties with the stimulus that was present when the child learned to say, sign, or write *car.* In his book, Skinner referred to this type of stimulus generalization as *generic tact extension.* Other types of extensions include *metaphorical* and *metonymic extensions.* A metaphoric extension occurs when the novel stimulus shares some, but not all, characteristics with the original stimulus. The word *surfing* when referring to the Internet is an example. A metonymical extension occurs when the novel stimulus does not share any physical similarity with the original one. Rather, they just happened to appear together during the acquisition of the tact. For example, the sentence *The White House released a statement* is equivalent to *The President released a statement,* because the President and the White House usually appear together.

Skinner (1957) identified other verbal operants whose forms, such as what a learner says or writes, are all evoked by *verbal discriminative stimuli* (i.e., the products of someone else's verbal behavior). The *echoic relation* is one of these operants in which the speaker's behavior is controlled by the auditory stimulus arising from someone else's vocal behavior. In the case of the echoic, the response bears formal similarity to the stimulus. For instance, a girl says, "Ball," after her teacher says, "Ball," when there is no ball in view. *Copying a text* is like the echoic in that the response form also bears formal similarity with the stimulus, and reinforcement may also depend on close correspondence between the stimulus and response. For instance, a girl writes the word *ball* after seeing the printed word *ball. Taking dictation* is writing what someone says. Writing *ball* when hearing someone say, "Ball," is an example. There is still correspondence between the stimulus and response, because specific sound patterns control specific hand movements. There is no physical similarity between them, however, because the stimulus is auditory, and the response produces a printed word or visual stimulus. Like taking dictation, *the textual relation* consists of reading printed words.

---

[3]Motivating operations may also modulate the effectiveness of consequences as punishers.

The *intraverbal* relation is a response form evoked by a verbal discriminative stimulus. The stimulus and response are different words and do not resemble each other. For example, a parent asks, "What day is it today?", and the child responds, "Thursday." Or the teacher says, "Two, four, six . . . ," and the student responds, "Eight." In these cases, there are no parts or subdivisions of the stimulus controlling parts or subdivisions of the response.

Even though all verbal operants except the mand are maintained by generalized conditioned reinforcement, Skinner suggested that "the action that a listener takes with respect to a verbal response is often more important to the speaker than generalized reinforcement" (p. 151). In other words, verbal behavior is sensitive to listener behavior, such as a listener's nodding as a speaker provides directions to a restaurant. This observation suggests that if we want to establish an effective speaker repertoire, we must establish listener reactions as effective forms of reinforcement (e.g., Maffei, Singer-Dudek, & Keohane, 2014).

## THE LISTENER

Emphasizing the role of the listener in these primary verbal relations, including the sources of control for the listener's behavior, is important. According to Skinner (1957), an analysis of both speaker and listener behavior is necessary to understand the "total verbal episode" (p. 36). The mand primarily benefits the speaker, such as when a girl requests and receives water. By contrast, other primary verbal operants, such as the tact, largely benefit the listener. For example, if a speaker says, "It's going to rain," in response to a dark sky, the listener may contact reinforcement that he or she would not have contacted otherwise. The stimulus may evoke listener behavior such as carrying an umbrella or delaying a walk outside. The reinforcer for the listener is avoidance of an aversive stimulus: getting wet. Thus competent speakers extend a listener's contact with the stimulating environment, and this effect on the listener may serve as an important yet subtle source of reinforcement for the speaker's verbal behavior.

Additionally, effective programs for training language must explicitly teach the speaker to engage the listener. For example, after beginning speakers learn to make requests to attentive listeners, they may need to learn to recruit atten-tion from inattentive listeners. In applied settings, increasing the consistency of the communicative partner's attention and responses to the speaker's communicative attempts is an important intervention goal (Goldstein, Kaczmarek, Pennington, & Shafer, 1992). This is necessary to support the efforts of the speaker in his or her communicative attempts.

Importantly, effective communicators can act as both speakers and listeners, which allows them to understand (i.e., react to) their own verbal behavior. Unfortunately, young children or those with developmental disabilities may not speak readily after learning to react to words as listeners, or vice versa (Petursdottir & Carr, 2011). This suggests that when attempting to establish functional verbal skills, we must teach speaker and listener behavior simultaneously (e.g., Fiorile & Greer, 2007).

## MULTIPLE CONTROL

The verbal operants discussed thus far involve control by a single variable, such as a motivating operation or a verbal or nonverbal stimulus. However, most verbal behavior involves different topographies under control of multiple variables (Michael, Palmer, & Sundberg, 2011). *Multiple control* occurs when a single response is controlled by more than one variable, or a single variable controls more than one response (Bondy, Tincani, & Frost, 2004; Skinner, 1957). The first type of multiple control, *convergent* control, occurs when the verbal community arranges reinforcement for a response form in the presence of more than one stimulus. For example, a girl receives reinforcement for saying, "Ball," in response to the printed word *ball*, a picture of a ball, and the question "What do you throw?" The second type of multiple control, *divergent* control, occurs when a given variable strengthens multiple responses. An example is when liquid deprivation strengthens verbal responses such as *Water please*, *May I have a drink?*, and *I'm thirsty*.

Multiple control that produces *impure* verbal operants, (i.e., those that more than one variable strengthens simultaneously) may be present when teaching verbal responses (Skinner, 1957, p. 151). For example, a boy who is liquid-deprived is more likely to say, "Juice, please," if we present him with a cup of juice than when deprivation or the cup of juice is presented alone. The motivating operation and nonverbal stimulus have a combined effect, producing an impure verbal operant, which is the mand–tact. Several variables may combine to produce a response. When a mother asks, "Would you like some juice?" with a cup of juice present, and her daughter says, "Yes, please," we may call the girl's response a mand–tact–intraverbal if it is multiply controlled by a motivating operation (deprivation), nonverbal stimulus (cup of juice), and verbal stimulus (mother's question). In this manner, we can identify the potential sources of control and establish multiply controlled operants.

The relation among the different verbal operants is important in teaching verbal skills. For example, does acquisition of a response form under one set of variables lead to emission of the same response form under a different set of variables? There is considerable evidence that verbal operants are functionally independent under certain conditions (Kelley, Shillingsburg, Castro, Addison, & LaRue, 2007; LaFrance, Wilder, Normand, & Squires, 2009; LaMarre & Holland, 1985; Petursdottir, Carr, & Michael, 2005; Twyman, 1996). That is, a response topography (i.e., word) learned with one set of controlling variables will not necessarily occur in the presence of different variables unless it is explicitly taught. A response topography taught as a mand, therefore, will not occur automatically as a tact, or vice versa. For example, a boy who is taught to say, sign, or write *tree* in response to the question "What is it?" and a picture of a tree may not reply with *tree* in the presence of the picture of the tree by itself (tact), because the learned response involves a different controlling relation—the picture of the tree plus the question.

The analysis of multiply controlled verbal operants becomes particularly relevant in the design of communication training programs. Even though many behaviorally oriented language training programs seek to establish complex verbal operants (e.g., Leaf & McEachin, 1999; Lovaas, 2003; Maurice et al., 1996), they do not describe procedures to transfer control from the question plus object to the object itself. Without explicit procedures for transfer of stimulus control, the learner is likely to develop a highly selective repertoire in which tacts will occur only in the presence of objects accompanied by questions. By contrast, a more functional tacting repertoire involves response topographies that occur in several stimulus combinations, including presentation of the object alone.

Intraverbals are usually under the control of multiple verbal stimuli. For example, the response *toast* in the presence of the question "What do you eat for breakfast?" must be under control of both the verbal stimuli *eat* and *breakfast*. Although the stimulus *eat* may evoke several responses (divergent control), including, *pasta, pizza, toast,* and *broccoli,* the addition of the stimulus *breakfast* will serve to strengthen the response *toast* (convergent control). In the absence of specific instructions to distinguish between both features of this compound verbal stimulus, *eat* and *breakfast,* a learner may attend to only one component (i.e., *eat*) and continue to respond with *toast* to any question that includes the stimulus *eat* (e.g., Q: "What do rabbits eat?" A: *toast*). Behavior analysts can prevent this kind of failure, or *rote responding,* by teaching learners to respond to both features of the complex verbal stimulus at the onset of instruction (Axe, 2008; DeSouza, Fisher, & Rodriguez, 2019; Sundberg & Sundberg, 2011)

The determination of controlling variables helps direct teaching protocols for several relevant situations. For example, a seemingly simple verbal skill, such as Martin's learning to say, "Swing," may have many possible sources of control:

1. Martin learns an echoic. He says, "Swing," when the teacher says, "Swing," and the teacher provides praise.

2. Martin learns an echoic–mand. When his teacher says, "Swing," he says, "Swing," and his teacher puts him on the swing.

3. Martin learns a mand. Martin says, "Swing," to his teacher, and his teacher puts him on the swing.

4. Martin learns a mand–tact. Martin sees a swing and says, "Swing," to his teacher. His teacher puts him on the swing.

5. Martin learns an intraverbal–mand. His teacher asks, "What do you want to do?", without a swing in sight. Martin says, "Swing," and his teacher puts him on the swing.

6. Martin learns a pure tact. Martin sees a swing, and he says, "Swing." The teacher says, "Yes, I see it too," but does not put him on the swing.

7. Martin learns an intraverbal–tact. When his teacher points to a swing and asks, "What is that?", Martin says, "Swing." He teacher provides praise, but does not put him on the swing.

8. Martin learns an intraverbal–mand–tact. Martin sees a swing, and his teacher asks, "What do you want to do?" Martin says, "Swing," and his teacher puts him on the swing.

Martin's teacher must determine which variables are relevant and explicitly arrange each variation to teach Martin to say, "Swing."

## SELECTING A RESPONSE MODALITY

Skinner (1957) wrote that modality is not a determinant of whether a behavior can function as a verbal operant. Therefore, gestures, sign language, picture-based communication, and digitally based modalities of communication may all function as verbal behavior (Tincani & Zawacki, 2012). There is little reason to suggest that one modality of communication is inherently better than other ones (Bondy et al., 2004; Tincani, 2004). Rather, some learners may demonstrate higher rates of acquisition with one modality, and others with a different modality (Lorah et al., 2013). Of course, the most common modality of verbal behavior is speech. In typical development, infants acquire nonvocal mands, such as pointing or gesturing to an object while looking back and forth between the object and parent, before developing specific spoken words (Mundy, 1995). Speech arises out of babbling sounds that appear to be species and not culturally specific. That is, young children around the world tend to produce similar sounds, some of which produce direct or automatic reinforcement in particular language groups (Miguel, Carr, & Michael, 2002; Werker & Tees, 1999).

Many issues may interfere with typical language development, from structural problems associated with oral functioning to difficulties in acquiring imitative repertoires (Fey, 1986). When learners do not speak, most interventionists try to promote speech first (Mirenda, 2003). When learners do not acquire speech via the typical pattern, researchers have identified several promising strategies to promote verbal behavior, though none is universally effective (Wankoff, 2005). Broadly speaking, such strategies encourage speech production, often without regard to function. The therapist engages the learner in various playful and reinforcing activities to increase the learner's production of sound. If sounds occur, the therapist attempts to reinforce their frequency. Next, the therapist teaches an echoic repertoire. The therapist makes a sound and provides reinforcement if the learner makes the same sound. The therapist then teaches the learner to blend sounds together in increasingly complex patterns, forming words and then short phrases (e.g., "Want cookie").

Several factors may make speech a difficult modality to acquire for many young learners, particularly those with intellectual or developmental disorders. Speech production requires refined coordination of many actions, including breath and oral–motor movements. A generalized imitative repertoire is particularly critical to speech development (Garcia, Baer, & Firestone, 1971; Young, Krantz, McClannahan, & Poulson, 1994). Teaching a learner an echoic repertoire is difficult until the learner displays generalized imitative responding. If the learner does not display generalized imitative responding, he or she is not likely to acquire a comprehensive vocal repertoire. The onset of speech via babbling appears to be relatively time-restricted and may not be available when some learners with disabilities begin communication training (Werker & Tees, 2005).

We should consider training verbal behavior via other modalities if speech is a low-probability option. Most speakers use body language and gestures, which Skinner (1957) called *autoclitics*, to modify the meaning of their statements. We can shape these behaviors into sign language, either conforming to the grammar of a specific language or involving unique grammatical rules. One potential advantage of this approach is that sign language involves topographically different movements of the hands, thus requiring no external support (Sundberg & Partington, 1998). Modalities that use visual icons can include pictures, symbols, or print media. Some systems are low-tech, such as the Picture Exchange Communication System (PECS; Frost & Bondy, 2002); others are high-tech or digital, such as speech-generating devices (Alzrayer, Banda, & Koul, 2014; Tincani & Boutot, 2005). Learners can acquire writing skills with either a keyboard or a writing implement without prior use of speech (Lovaas & Lovaas, 1999).

A behavior analyst should consider the ease of and the necessary prompts for response acquisition and the role of the verbal community's responses to a learner when selecting a communication modality (Mirenda, 2003). Although we currently have little empirical evidence to guide modality selection (cf. McLay et al., 2017), the behavior analyst should consider the following issues. First, a learner who does not have a generalized vocal imitation repertoire may not learn speech readily. In such instances, the behavior analyst should consider an augmentative and alternative communication system. Sign language also may be a viable alternative for learners who lack a vocal imitative repertoire. However, a learner must have a generalized motor imitation repertoire to acquire a functional sign-language vocabulary because of its topography-based nature. The behavior analyst should consider an aided or device-based alternative and augmentative communication system if the learner does not display vocal and motor imitation skills. Aided systems include picture-based systems, such as PECS (Frost & Bondy, 2002), and speech-generating devices (Lorah, Parnell, Whitby, & Hantula, 2015). Relevant factors for selecting an aided system may include (1) the availability of a device or system; (2) the ease of use for the primary listeners, such as parents, siblings, or teachers; (3) the potential for the device or system to accommodate several communication symbols and vocabulary; and (4) the capability of the device or system to produce a repertoire of independent, functional verbal behavior for the listener (Tincani, 2007; Tincani & Boutot, 2005).

## TEACHING THE MAND

The mand directly benefits the speaker; thus assessment of the people, items, and events that function as reinforcers for the learner is critical before teaching the mand. Researchers have developed systematic strategies to assess learners' preferences for reinforcers, though a detailed description of these is beyond the scope of this chapter (see Saini, Retzlaff, Roane, & Piazza, Chapter 10, this volume). Extensive research has focused on teaching the mand as a component of functional-communication training (Durand & Merges, 2001; Greer, Fisher, Saini, Owen, & Jones, 2016; Mancil, 2006; Saini, Miller, & Fisher, 2016). The primary purpose of functional-communication training is to reduce challenging behavior by teaching alternative responses (i.e., mands) that produce the same reinforcing consequences as challenging behavior (see Fisher, Greer, & Bouxsein, Chapter 20, this volume). Other researchers have evaluated procedures to establish independent or spontaneous mand repertoires for learners who do not engage in challenging behavior. Several studies have established the efficacy of time-delay prompting procedures for teaching mand repertoires to learners with developmental disabilities (e.g., Halle, Baer, & Spradlin, 1981; Halle, Marshall, & Spradlin, 1979; Kratzer, Spooner, & Test, 1993; Landa, Hansen, & Shillingsburg, 2017; Shillingsburg, Marya, Bartlett, & Thompson, 2019). For instance, Halle et al. (1981) used a 5-second time-delay prompting procedure to teach learners with intellectual developmental disorder and language delays to mand in a naturalistic setting. The teacher arranged a cue likely to evoke a mand, such as approaching the learner with a cup of juice. The teacher waited 5 seconds for the learner to perform the mand before delivering a prompt.

*Progressive time-delay prompting* or *errorless teaching* (Karsten & Carr, 2009; Touchette & Howard, 1984) is a variation of the time-delay procedure, in which the teacher presents the cue simultaneously with the prompt and gradually increases the duration between the cue and prompt as the learner makes independent responses. Such time-delay procedures use establishing operations (Michael, 1993) to promote mand acquisition. The *interrupted-chain* procedure (Hall & Sundberg, 1997) also uses establishing operations, in which the teacher prevents the learner from completing a behavior chain until the learner performs an appropriate mand. For example, a teacher might hide a step stool from a learner who typically uses the stool to access a game on a shelf. The teacher would use this situation to teach the learner to request help in locating the missing stool. A common feature of these procedures is a systematic manipulation of the learner's environment to promote a functional manding repertoire (Carnett et al., 2017; Ingvarsson & Hollobaugh, 2013; Landa et al., 2017; Lechago, Carr, Grow, Love, & Almason, 2010; Shillingsburg, Bowen, Valentino, & Pierce, 2014; Shillingsburg et al., 2019).

Three basic response forms that beginning communicators need to learn are asking for a break, asking for help, and saying (or otherwise communicating) *no* to an offered item or activity. These simple skills are important, because they allow the learner to exert control over his or her environment and bring the learner into contact with contingencies that will be critical for developing other skills (Hixson, 2004). Asking for a break or assistance and communicating *no* are under functional control of aversive events such as demands, uncompleted or difficult tasks, or unwanted items. Communicating *no* allows the learner to escape or avoid an unwanted item or activity. It functions as a qualifying autoclitic in a mand function (see Skinner, 1957, p. 322). When a learner requests an alternative item or activity in the context of an escape or avoidance situation, the request can also function as a form of rejection maintained in part by negative reinforcement. Such choice-making responses may have the collateral effect of reducing challenging behavior associated with escape or avoidance contingencies.

Researchers have validated several strategies for teaching requesting and rejecting behaviors. Best practice integrates instruction of communicative responses into daily routines by systematically identifying all potential opportunities for a learner to engage in target behaviors and embedding instruction into naturally occurring events (Carnett et al., 2017; Sigafoos, Kerr, Roberts, & Couzens, 1994; Ylvisaker & Feeney, 1994). Strategies for creating opportunities for verbal behavior focus on teaching communication in real-life activities. These strategies include (1) delaying access to an item or activity that is present until the learner makes a request (Halle et al., 1981); (2) withholding an item necessary to complete a preferred activity (Cipani, 1988; Lechago et al., 2010); (3) blocking a response or interrupting an activity to create the need for a request (Carnett, Bravo, & Waddington, 2019; Shafer, 1995; Sigafoos et al., 1994); (4) providing only part of what the learner has requested to create a new need (Duker, Kraaykamp, & Visser, 1994); (5) intentionally giving the learner the incorrect item (Choi, O'Reilly, Sigafoos, & Lancioni, 2010; Sigafoos et al., 1994); or (6) delaying offers of assistance until the learner makes a request for help (Rodriguez, Levesque, Cohrs, & Niemeier, 2017; Sigafoos & Roberts-Pennell, 1999).

The learner escapes or avoids nonpreferred items or activities in a socially acceptable manner if he or she can make a rejection response. Learners who do not communicate this need may adopt an idiosyncratic behavior that is difficult to interpret (Iacono, Carter, & Hook, 1998), or may learn to escape or avoid activities through challenging behavior (Carr, 1994). The learner is more likely to acquire socially appropriate escape or avoidance communication in situations where he or she is motivated to escape or avoid an item or activity. The behavior analyst can create a context for teaching the learner to reject an offer appropriately if the analyst can identify items or activities the learner is motivated to escape or avoid (Chezan, Drasgow, Martin, & Halle, 2016; Sigafoos & Roberts-Pennell, 1999).

There are several techniques for teaching rejection or refusal behavior. First, the behavior analyst can strengthen an existing appropriate behavior to make it more effective, specific, or consistent (Warren, Yoder, Gazdag, Kim, & Jones, 1993). Second, the behavior analyst can teach new communicative behaviors by chaining the new response to an existing, inefficient behavior (Keen, Sigafoos, & Woodyatt, 2001) or by prompting (Drasgow, Halle, Ostrosky, & Harbers, 1996). Third, the behavior analyst can replace socially unacceptable communicative behaviors with acceptable, functionally equivalent behaviors. For example, the behavior analyst could teach a learner to point to the word *stop* on a communication board to end a task instead of throwing a tantrum (Carr,

1994). Fourth, the behavior analyst must teach the learner that escape or avoidance will not always be possible even when the learner has requested it appropriately (Sigafoos, 1998). Even though we are suggesting that we should initially teach communicating *no* as a mand, more advanced learners will benefit from acquiring *no* and *yes* as tacts and intraverbals. For example, we should teach a learner who can speak to say, "No," if the teacher asks, "Is this a giraffe?" when she presents a picture of a cow (tact), and to say, "Yes," when the teacher asks, "Does a cow says moo?" (intraverbal; see Shillingsburg, Kelley, Roane, Kisamore, & Brown, 2009).

## TEACHING OTHER VERBAL OPERANTS

Although much research has focused on the acquisition of mands, research also has shown that the tact repertoire is foundational for the development of other verbal and nonverbal behaviors, such as mands, intraverbals, stimulus categorization, and analogical reasoning (e.g., Finn, Miguel, & Ahearn, 2012; Greer & Du, 2010; Miguel et al., 2015; Miguel & Kobari-Wright, 2013; Miguel, Petursdottir, & Carr, 2005; Sprinkle & Miguel, 2012). Additionally, tacts may not readily emerge after receptive-discrimination instruction (Contreras, Cooper, & Kahng, 2020; Petursdottir & Carr, 2011), especially if a child lacks a generalized echoic repertoire (Horne & Lowe, 1996). For this reason, a behavior analyst should prioritize tacts when attempting to expand a learner's vocal repertoire (e.g., Greer & Du, 2010). Tact training should focus initially on preferred, familiar, and functional three-dimensional stimuli readily found in the learner's environment; it should then move toward two-dimensional complex stimuli, including functions, features, relations, and private events (LeBlanc, Dillon, & Sautter, 2009).

Behavior analysts should teach echoics early in programming when teaching vocal tacts, because therapists then can use echoic prompts for other verbal operants (e.g., Kodak & Clements, 2009). Although researchers have studied generalized vocal imitation (e.g., Kymissis & Poulson, 1990), more recent investigations have focused on procedures to establish vocalizations in learners who are otherwise nonvocal. One of these procedures, called *stimulus–stimulus pairing,* establishes vocalizations as conditioned reinforcers. Thus the response-produced auditory stimulus may function as reinforcement for the vocalizations that produced them (Lepper & Petursdottir, 2017; Shillingsburg, Hollander, Yosick, Bowen, & Muskat, 2015). Other more naturalistic procedures evoke vocalizations by capturing the learner's interest while modeling vocal sounds (Charlop-Christy, LeBlanc, & Carpenter, 1999).

Behavior analysts can teach simple intraverbals in the form of fill-in-the-blanks at the same time they are teaching simple mands and tacts. By contrast, the behavior analyst should teach more complex intraverbals after the learner can respond to the same topography or word as a listener (i.e., receptive discrimination) and speaker (i.e., tact). For example, before the analyst teaches a learner to say, "Carrot," when the learner hears, "What does a rabbit eat?", he or she should first learn to tact *carrot* and *eat* and respond as a listener when hearing these words (Petursdottir, Ólafsdóttir, & Aradóttir, 2008). As with other verbal operants, the behavior analyst can teach intraverbals by using time-delay procedures with either vocal or visual prompts, although the learner's prior experience with prompts seems to determine which will be more effective (Coon & Miguel, 2012; Roncati, Souza, & Miguel, 2019).

Behavior analysts should assess learners' current repertoires before teaching these verbal operants and use assessment results to guide programming. Unfortunately, many language assessments focus on the form rather than function of verbal responses (Esch, LaLonde, & Esch, 2010), so they do not measure the strength and breadth of a learner's verbal repertoire (Carr & Miguel, 2013). Thus a behavior analyst might use criterion-referenced assessments like the Assessment of Basic Language and Learning Skills—Revised (ABLLS-R; Partington, 2006) and the Verbal Behavior Milestones Assessment and Placement Program (VB-MAPP; Sundberg, 2008) to evaluate a learner's repertoire, suggest goals for intervention, and track progress. Although many behavior analysts often use these assessments, research has not evaluated their psychometric properties and interobserver reliability (Carr & Miguel, 2013), so analysts should not rely on them solely when making clinical decisions.

## OTHER ISSUES

Learner characteristics may influence how we teach verbal skills and which ones we teach. Some of these variables may be learner-specific. For example, a behavior analyst should use a learner's most potent reinforcers identified via a formal preference assessment when initiating mand training (DeLeon & Iwata, 1996; Fisher et al., 1992; Frost & Bondy, 2002). Other factors that may be important in selecting verbal responses to teach relate to the learner's behavioral development. For example, learners tact items and events that are part of the public environment before they can tact private events (see Skinner, 1957, p. 131). In other words, learners name common items, such as toys, furniture, and important people, before they learn to comment about things happening within them, such as pain, pleasure, or other emotional changes. Therefore, we must ensure that a learner can comment about items or events in his or her environment before teaching comments about a possibly painful knee.

Strategies for teaching verbal behavior such as incidental teaching and pivotal-response training (Koegel & Koegel, 2005) depend on a teacher's awareness of the learner's current repertoire; that is, these strategies seek to expand upon current skill sets in small steps. Each lesson depends more on what the learner is doing than on what the teacher wants the learner to do. Thus, if a learner has demonstrated a clear preference for a large as opposed to a small ball and can ask for a ball, teaching the learner to request the *large ball* represents a viable target response. For learners who either do not like balls or cannot request a ball in any modality, trying to teach *large* in this way is not likely to be effective.

Response production issues also may influence which skills behavior analysts teach. Importantly, behavior analysts must determine how production issues may interfere with learning. For example, learners who display some vocal responses may have difficulty in sound production or blending; similarly, learners who sign may have difficulty forming or stringing signs together. Some learners may select letters on a keyboard more easily than they can produce them with a writing implement. Research on fluency (Johnson & Layng, 1992) suggests that when core response production rates (such as the rate of producing individual sounds, writing individual letters, or selecting specific pictures) are very low, acquisition of more complex skills (such as stringing together letters to spell words or speaking in increasingly complex sentences) will be difficult.

Attributing characteristics to an individual learner based on a general characteristic of the population to which he or she belongs is often risky. Nevertheless, a behavior analyst may consider such characteristics on a probabilistic basis.

For example, learners with autism spectrum disorder (ASD) tend to be less sensitive than typically developing learners to social reinforcers, especially when they first enter treatment programs. As such, praise, smiles, and words of encouragement are usually not highly motivating for learners with ASD. Skills that produce social consequences, such as tacts, intraverbals, and most autoclitics, will be difficult for these learners to acquire (Fisher et al., 2019). If a teacher replaces social consequences with more concrete but powerful reinforcers, such as food or toys, a learner with ASD may acquire a verbal operant that may remain partially controlled by the item rather than an operant controlled by generalized conditioned reinforcers. Simply substituting one reinforcer for another can have a significant impact on the acquisition of verbal operants. In this case, the limited availability of reinforcers may affect the behavior analyst's selection of target skills. If social consequences do not function as reinforcement, then teaching mands for items and activities may be more effective than teaching verbal operants with social reinforcers.

Learners may have difficulty acquiring sophisticated language skills if social consequences do not function as reinforcers at all or function only as weak reinforcers (Greer & Keohane, 2006). For example, learners with Asperger syndrome or other mild forms of ASD typically develop global language skills on par with their typically developing peers. However, some of these learners may have difficulty acquiring communication skills that relate to social effectiveness—from using and understanding puns and other word play, to more general skills associated with successful dating and romantic involvement. Thus a learner may tell a joke, but may not discriminate why it is funny.

Skinner (1957) pointed out the critical role of social reinforcement in the development of language and self-knowledge: "As we have noted, it is *social reinforcement* which leads the individual to know himself. It is only through the gradual growth of a verbal community that the individual becomes 'conscious.' He comes to see himself only as others see him, or at least only as others insist that he see himself" (p. 140, emphasis added). Learners who show limited responsivity to social consequences are likely to show concomitant limits in language development.

For other populations, such as children with Down syndrome, social consequences may be particularly powerful reinforcers. In such cases, lessons associated with tacting, such as naming animals, identifying sounds, and describing items, may be reinforcing and acquired readily. A learner's diagnostic or educational classification does not set or fix educational goals, but it may suggest consequences that do and do not function as reinforcers.

Behavior analysts should use many reinforcers when teaching manding. Although manipulating access to concrete rewards such as food, drink, and toys may be relatively easy, lessons should extend to activities and social events with many potential communicative partners. Specifically, we should teach learners to request items from peers (Schwartz, Garfinkle, & Bauer, 1998) and from adults; to talk about and play games and related activities with siblings (Taylor, Levin, & Jasper, 1999); and to seek information (Williams, Pérez-González, & Vogt, 2003). Thus two general training aims are to broaden the array of reinforcers associated with manding and to increase potential mediators for various reinforcers.

Finally, much of this chapter has focused on acquisition of verbal behavior and related interventions in childhood; however, certain developmental disabilities, such as ASD, produce deficits in verbal behavior that may persist across the lifespan (Shattuck et al., 2007). These learners are likely to need empirically supported interventions to increase and maintain functional verbal behavior well into adulthood. The demonstrated continuity in principles of behavior across the lifespan suggests that Skinner's (1957) analysis is just as relevant to teaching verbal behavior skills to adults as it is to children. Nonetheless, research on strategies to teach such skills to adults with developmental disabilities is far less abundant than research with children (e.g., Bishop-Fitzpatrick, Minshew, & Eack, 2014). Preliminary evidence suggests that the conceptual approach and teaching strategies based in Skinner's analysis that produce functional verbal behavior in children also produce functional verbal behavior in adults with similar impairments (Bracken & Rohrer, 2014; Nepo, Tincani, Axelrod, & Meszaros, 2015). Nevertheless, researchers should focus on the specific nature of developmentally compatible and effective strategies for improving verbal behavior in adults.

## SUMMARY

Skinner's (1957) work provides a platform on which behavior analysts can develop effective targets and strategies to help children and adults acquire or improve verbal repertoires. Considering the relevant motivational and stimulus conditions is essential in teaching verbal responses. Behavior analysts can provide critical guidance regarding the importance of reinforcement and how context affects the function of new responses when designing lessons. Our emphasis on the function rather than the form of verbal behavior also suggests that behavior analysts should be adept at helping learners develop verbal repertoires in several modalities, even while recognizing the societal importance of speech. Indeed, the techniques for teaching verbal responses described in this chapter accommodate several response modalities, including speech, sign language, picture-based systems, and other augmentative devices.

# REFERENCES

Alzrayer, N., Banda, D. R., & Koul, R. K. (2014). Use of iPad/iPods with individuals with autism and other developmental disabilities: A meta-analysis of communication interventions. *Review Journal of Autism and Developmental Disorders, 1,* 179–191.

American Speech–Language–Hearing Association. (2016). Scope of practice in speech–language pathology. Retrieved from *www.asha.org/policy/SP2016-00343.*

Axe, J. B. (2008). Conditional discrimination in the intraverbal relation: A review and recommendations for future research. *Analysis of Verbal Behavior, 24,* 159–174.

Barbera, M. L., & Rasmussen, T. (2007). *The verbal behavior approach: How to teach children with autism and related disorders.* London: Jessica Kingsley.

Bishop-Fitzpatrick, L., Minshew, N. J., & Eack, S. M. (2014). A systematic review of psychosocial interventions for adults with autism spectrum disorders. In F. R. Volkmar, B. Reichow, & J. McPartland (Eds.), *Adolescents and adults with autism spectrum disorders* (pp. 315–327). New York: Springer.

Bondy, A., Tincani, M., & Frost, L. (2004). Multiply controlled verbal operants: An analysis and extension to the Picture Exchange Communication System. *Behavior Analyst, 27,* 247–261.

Bracken, M., & Rohrer, N. (2014). Using an adapted form of the Picture Exchange Communication System to increase independent requesting in deafblind adults with learning disabilities. *Research in Developmental Disabilities, 35,* 269–277.

Brown, R. (1973). *A first language.* Cambridge, MA: Harvard University Press.

Carnett, A., Bravo, A., & Waddington, H. (2019). Teaching mands for actions to children with autism spectrum disorder using systematic instruction, behavior chain interruption, and a speech-generating device. *International Journal of Developmental Disabilities, 65,* 98–107.

Carnett, A., Waddington, H., Hansen, S., Bravo, A., Sigafoos, J., & Lang, R. (2017). Teaching mands to children with autism spectrum disorder using behavior chain interruption strategies: A systematic review. *Advances in Neurodevelopmental Disorders, 1,* 203–220.

Carr, E. G. (1994). Emerging themes in the functional analysis of problem behavior. *Journal of Applied Behavior Analysis, 27,* 393–399.

Carr, J. E., & Miguel, C. F. (2013). The analysis of verbal behavior and its therapeutic applications. In G. J. Madden (Ed.), *APA handbook of behavior analysis: Vol. 2. Translating principles into practice* (pp. 329–352). Washington, DC: American Psychological Association.

Charlop-Christy, M. H., LeBlanc L. A., & Carpenter, M. H. (1999). Naturalistic teaching strategies (NaTS) to teach speech to children with autism: Historical perspective, development, and current practice. *California School Psychologist, 4,* 30–46.

Chezan, L. C., Drasgow, E., Martin, C. A., & Halle, J. W. (2016). Negatively-reinforced mands: An examination of resurgence to existing mands in two children with autism and language delays. *Behavior Modification, 40,* 922–953.

Choi, H., O'Reilly, M., Sigafoos, J., & Lancioni, G. (2010). Teaching requesting and rejecting sequences to four children with developmental disabilities using augmentative and alternative communication. *Research in Developmental Disabilities, 31,* 560–567.

Chomsky, N. (1965). *Aspects of a theory of syntax.* Cambridge, MA: MIT Press.

Cipani, E. (1988). The missing item format. *Teaching Exceptional Children, 21,* 25–27.

Contreras, B. P., Cooper, A. J., & Kahng, S. (2020). Recent research on the relative efficiency of speaker and listener instruction for children with autism spectrum disorder. *Journal of Applied Behavior Analysis, 53,* 584–589.

Coon, J. T., & Miguel, C. F. (2012). The role of increased exposure to transfer of stimulus control procedures on the acquisition of intraverbal behavior. *Journal of Applied Behavior Analysis, 45,* 657–666.

DeLeon, I. G., & Iwata, B. A. (1996). Evaluation of a multiple-stimulus presentation format for assessing reinforcer preferences. *Journal of Applied Behavior Analysis, 29,* 519–532.

DeSouza, A. A., Fisher, W. W., & Rodriguez, N. M. (2019). Facilitating the emergence of convergent intraverbals in children with autism. *Journal of Applied Behavior Analysis, 52,* 28–49.

Drasgow, E., Halle, J. W., Ostrosky, M. M., & Harbers, H. M. (1996). Using behavioral indication and functional communication training to establish initial sign repertoire with a young child with severe disabilities. *Topics in Early Childhood Special Education, 16,* 500–521.

Duker, P. C., Kraaykamp, M., & Visser, E. (1994). A stimulus control procedure to increase requesting with individuals who are severely/profoundly intellectually disabled. *Journal of Intellectual Disability Research, 38,* 177–186.

Durand, V. M., & Merges, E. (2001). Functional communication training: A contemporary behavior analytic intervention for problem behavior. *Focus on Autism and Other Developmental Disabilities, 16,* 110–119.

Esch, B. E., LaLonde, K. B., & Esch, J. W. (2010). Speech and language assessment: A verbal behavior analysis. *Journal of Speech–Language Pathology–Applied Behavior Analysis, 5,* 166–191.

Fey, M. (1986). *Language intervention with young children.* Boston: College Hill Press.

Finn, H. E., Miguel, C. F., & Ahearn, W. H. (2012). The emergence of untrained mands and tacts in children with autism. *Journal of Applied Behavior Analysis, 45*(2), 265–280.

Fiorile, C. A., & Greer, R. D. (2007). The induction of naming in children with no prior tact responses as a function of multiple exemplar histories of instruction. *Analysis of Verbal Behavior, 23,* 71–87.

Fisher, W., Piazza, C. C., Bowman, L. G., Hagopian, L. P., Owens, J. C., & Slevin, I. (1992). A comparison of two approaches for identifying reinforcers for persons with severe and profound disabilities. *Journal of Applied Behavior Analysis, 25,* 491–498.

Fisher, W. W., Retzlaff, B. J., Akers, J. S., DeSouza, A. A., Kaminski, A. J., & Machado, M. A. (2019). Establishing initial auditory–visual conditional discriminations and emergence of initial tacts in young children with autism spectrum disorder. *Journal of Applied Behavior Analysis, 52,* 1089–1106.

Frost, L., & Bondy, A. (2002). *The Picture Exchange Communication System (PECS) training manual* (2nd ed.). Newark, DE: Pyramid Products.

Garcia, E. E., Baer, D. M., & Firestone, I. (1971). The development of generalized imitation in topographically determined boundaries. *Journal of Applied Behavior Analysis, 4,* 101–113.

Goldstein, H., Kaczmarek, L., Pennington, R., & Shafer, K. (1992). Peer-mediated intervention: Attending to, commenting on, and acknowledging the behavior of preschoolers with autism. *Journal of Applied Behavior Analysis, 25,* 289–305.

Greer, B. D., Fisher, W. W., Saini, V., Owen, T. M., & Jones, J. K. (2016). Functional communication training during reinforcement schedule thinning: An analysis of 25 applications. *Journal of Applied Behavior Analysis, 49,* 105–121.

Greer, R. D., & Du, L. (2010). Generic instruction versus intensive tact instruction and the emission of spontaneous speech. *Journal of Speech–Language Pathology–Applied Behavior Analysis, 5,* 1–19.

Greer, R. D., & Keohane, D.-D. (2006). The evolution of verbal behavior in children. *Journal of Speech and Language Pathology–Applied Behavior Analysis, 1,* 111–140.

Hall, G., & Sundberg, M. L. (1987). Teaching mands by manipulating conditioned establishing operations. *Analysis of Verbal Behavior, 5,* 41–53.

Halle, J. W., Baer, D., & Spradlin, J. (1981). Teachers' generalized use of delay as a stimulus control procedure to increase language use in handicapped children. *Journal of Applied Behavior Analysis, 14,* 389–409.

Halle, J. W., Marshall, A. M., & Spradlin, J. E. (1979). Time delay: A technique to increase language use and generalization in retarded children. *Journal of Applied Behavior Analysis, 12,* 431–439.

Hixson, M. (2004). Behavioral cusps, basic behavioral repertoires, and cumulative-hierarchical learning. *Psychological Record, 54,* 387–403.

Horne, P. J., & Lowe, C. F. (1996). On the origins of naming and other symbolic behavior. *Journal of the Experimental Analysis of Behavior, 65,* 185–241.

Iacono, T., Carter, M., & Hook, J. (1998). Identification of intentional communication in students with severe and multiple disabilities. *Augmentative and Alternative Communication, 14,* 417–431.

Ingvarsson, E. T., & Hollobaugh, T. (2010). Acquisition of intraverbal behavior: Teaching children with autism to mand for answers to questions. *Journal of Applied Behavior Analysis, 43,* 1–17.

Johnson, K. R., & Layng, T. J. (1992). Breaking the structuralist barrier: Literacy and numeracy with fluency. *American Psychologist, 47,* 1475–1490.

Karsten, A. M., & Carr, J. E. (2009). The effects of differential reinforcement of unprompted responding on the skill acquisition of children with autism. *Journal of Applied Behavior Analysis, 42,* 327–334.

Keen, D., Sigafoos, J., & Woodyatt, G. (2001). Replacing prelinguistic behaviors with functional communication. *Journal of Autism and Developmental Disorders, 31,* 385–398.

Kelley, M. E., Shillingsburg, M. A., Castro, M. J., Addison, L. R., & LaRue, R. H., Jr. (2007). Further evaluation of emerging speech in children with developmental disabilities: Training verbal behavior. *Journal of Applied Behavior Analysis, 40,* 431–445.

Kodak, T., & Clements, A. (2009). Acquisition of mands and tacts with concurrent echoic training. *Journal of Applied Behavior Analysis, 42,* 839–843.

Koegel, R. L., & Koegel, L. K. (2005). *Pivotal response treatments for autism: Communication, social, and academic development.* Baltimore: Brookes.

Kratzer, D. A., Spooner, F., & Test, D. W. (1993). Extending the application of constant time delay: Teaching a requesting skill to students with severe multiple disabilities. *Education and Treatment of Children, 16,* 235–253.

Kymissis, E., & Poulson, C. L. (1990). The history of imitation in learning theory: The language acquisition process. *Journal of the Experimental Analysis of Behavior, 54,* 113–127.

LaFrance, D. L., & Miguel, C. F. (2014). Teaching language to children with autism spectrum disorder. In J. Tarbox, D. R. Dixon, P. Sturmey, & J. L. Matson

(Eds.), *Handbook of early intervention for autism spectrum disorders: Research, practice, and policy* (pp. 403–436). New York: Springer.

LaFrance, D. L., Wilder, D. A., Normand, M. P., & Squires, J. L. (2009). Extending the assessment of functions of vocalizations in children with limited verbal repertoires. *Analysis of Verbal Behavior, 25,* 19–32.

LaMarre, J., & Holland, J. G. (1985). The functional independence of mands and tacts. *Journal of the Experimental Analysis of Behavior, 43,* 5–19.

Landa, R. K., Hansen, B., & Shillingsburg, M. A. (2017). Teaching mands for information using 'when' to children with autism. *Journal of Applied Behavior Analysis, 50,* 538–551.

Leaf, R., & McEachin, J. (1999). *A work in progress: Behavior management strategies and a curriculum for intensive behavior treatment of autism.* New York: DRL Books.

LeBlanc, L. A., Dillon, C. M., & Sautter, R. A. (2009). Establishing mand and tact repertoires. In R. A. Rehfeldt & Y. Barnes-Holmes (Eds.), *Derived relational responding: Applications for learners with autism and other developmental disabilities* (pp. 79–108). Oakland, CA: New Harbinger.

Lechago, S. A., Carr, J. E., Grow, L. L., Love, J. R., & Almason, S. M. (2010). Mands for information generalize across establishing operations. *Journal of Applied Behavior Analysis, 43,* 381–395.

Lepper, T. L., & Petursdottir, A. I. (2017). Effects of response-contingent stimulus pairing on vocalizations of nonverbal children with autism. *Journal of Applied Behavior Analysis, 50,* 756–774.

Lorah, E. R., Parnell, A., Whitby, P. S., & Hantula, D. (2015). A systematic review of tablet computers and portable media players as speech generating devices for individuals with autism spectrum disorder. *Journal of Autism and Developmental Disorders, 45,* 3792–3804.

Lorah, E. R., Tincani, M., Dodge, J., Gilroy, S., Hickey, A., & Hantula, D. (2013). Evaluating picture exchange and the iPad™ as a speech generating device to teach communication to young children with autism. *Journal of Developmental and Physical Disabilities, 25,* 637–649.

Lord, C., Cook, E. H., Leventhal, B. L., & Amaral, D. G. (2000). Autism spectrum disorders. *Neuron, 28,* 355–363.

Lovaas, O. I. (2003). *Teaching individuals with developmental delays.* Austin, TX: PRO-ED.

Lovaas, N. W., & Lovaas, E. E. (1999). *The Reading and Writing Program: An alternative form of communication.* Austin, TX: PRO-ED.

Maffei, J., Singer-Dudek, S., & Keohone, D. (2014). The effects of the establishment of adult faces and/or voices as conditioned reinforcers for children with ASD and related disorders. *Acta de Investigacion Psicologia, 4,* 1621–1641.

Mancil, G. (2006). Functional communication training: A review of the literature related to children with autism. *Education and Training in Developmental Disabilities, 41,* 213–224.

Maurice, C., Green, G., & Luce, S. C. (1996). *Behavioral intervention for young children with autism: A manual for parents and professionals.* Austin, TX: PRO-ED.

McLay, L., Schäfer, M. C., van der Meer, L., Couper, L., McKenzie, E., O'Reilly, M. F., et al. (2017). Acquisition, preference and follow-up comparison across three AAC modalities taught to two children with autism spectrum disorder. *International Journal of Disability, Development and Education, 64,* 117–130.

Michael, J. (1993). Establishing operations. *Behavior Analyst, 16,* 191–206.

Michael, J., & Miguel, C. F. (2020). Motivating operations. In J. O. Cooper, T. E. Heron, & W. L. Heward (Eds.), *Applied behavior analysis* (3rd ed., pp. 372–394). Hoboken, NJ: Pearson.

Michael, J., Palmer, D. C., & Sundberg, M. L. (2011). The multiple control of verbal behavior. *Analysis of Verbal Behavior, 27,* 3–22.

Miguel, C. F. (2016). Common and intraverbal bidirectional naming. *Analysis of Verbal Behavior, 32,* 125–138.

Miguel, C. F., Carr, J. E., & Michael, J. (2002). The effects of a stimulus–stimulus pairing procedure on the vocal behavior of children diagnosed with autism. *Analysis of Verbal Behavior, 18,* 3–13.

Miguel, C. F., Frampton, S. E., Lantaya, C. A., LaFrance, D. L., Quah, K., Meyer, C. S., et al. (2015). The effects of tact training on the development of analogical reasoning. *Journal of the Experimental Analysis of Behavior, 104,* 96–118.

Miguel, C. F., & Kobari-Wright, V. V. (2013). The effects of tact training on the emergence of categorization and listener behavior in children with autism. *Journal of Applied Behavior Analysis, 46,* 669–673.

Miguel, C. F., Petursdottir, A. I., & Carr, J. E. (2005). The effects of multiple-tact and receptive-discrimination training on the acquisition of intraverbal behavior. *Analysis of Verbal Behavior, 21,* 27–41.

Mirenda, P. (2003). Toward functional augmentative and alternative communication for students with autism: Manual signs, graphic symbols, and voice output communication aids. *Language, Speech, and Hearing Services in Schools, 34,* 203–216.

Mundy, P. (1995). Joint attention and social–emotional approach behavior in children with autism. *Development and Psychopathology, 7,* 63–82.

Nepo, K., Tincani, M., Axelrod, S., & Meszaros, L. (2015). iPod Touch® to increase functional communication of adults with autism spectrum disorder and significant intellectual disability. *Focus on Autism and Other Developmental Disabilities, 32*(3), 209–217.

Partington, J. W. (2006). *The Assessment of Basic Language and Learning Skills—Revised (The ABLLS-R).* Pleasant Hill, CA: Partington Behavior Analysts.

Petursdottir, A. I., & Carr, J. E. (2011). A review of recommendations for sequencing receptive and expressive language instruction. *Journal of Applied Behavior Analysis, 44,* 859–876.

Petursdottir, A. I., Carr, J. E., & Michael, J. (2005). Emergence of mands and tacts of novel objects among preschool children. *Analysis of Verbal Behavior, 21,* 59–74.

Petursdottir, A. I., Ólafsdóttir, A. R., & Aradóttir, B. (2008). The effects of tact and listener training on the emergence of bidirectional intraverbal relations. *Journal of Applied Behavior Analysis, 41,* 411–415.

Piaget, J. (1951). *The psychology of intelligence.* London: Routledge & Kegan Paul.

Rodriguez, N. M., Levesque, M. A., Cohrs, V. L., & Niemeier, J. J. (2017). Teaching children with autism to request help with difficult tasks. *Journal of Applied Behavior Analysis, 50,* 717–732.

Roncati, A. L., Souza, A. C., & Miguel, C. F. (2019), Exposure to a specific prompt topography predicts its relative efficiency when teaching intraverbal behavior to children with autism spectrum disorder. *Journal of Applied Behavior Analysis, 52,* 739–745.

Saini, V., Miller, S. A., & Fisher, W. W. (2016). Multiple schedules in practical application: Research trends and implications for future investigation. *Journal of Applied Behavior Analysis, 49,* 421–444.

Schwartz, I. S., Garfinkle, A. N., & Bauer, J. (1998). Communicative outcomes for young children with disabilities. *Topics in Early Childhood Special Education, 18,* 144–159.

Shafer, E. (1995). A review of interventions to teach a mand repertoire. *Analysis of Verbal Behavior, 12,* 53–66.

Shattuck, P. T., Seltzer, M. M., Greenberg, J. S., Orsmond, G. I., Bolt, D., Kring, S., et al. (2007). Change in autism symptoms and maladaptive behaviors in adolescents and adults with an autism spectrum disorder. *Journal of Autism and Developmental Disorders, 37*(9), 1735–1747.

Shillingsburg, M. A., Bowen, C. N., Valentino, A. L., & Pierce, L. E. (2014). Mands for information using "who?" and "which?" in the presence of establishing and abolishing operations. *Journal of Applied Behavior Analysis, 47,* 136–150.

Shillingsburg, M. A., Hollander, D. L., Yosick, R. N., Bowen, C., & Muskat, L. R. (2015). Stimulus–stimulus pairing to increase vocalizations in children with language delays: A review. *Analysis of Verbal Behavior, 31,* 215–235.

Shillingsburg, M. A., Kelley, M. E., Roane, H. S., Kisamore, A., & Brown, M. R. (2009). Evaluation and training of yes–no responding across verbal operants. *Journal of Applied Behavior Analysis, 42,* 209–223.

Shillingsburg, M. A., Marya, V., Bartlett, B. L., & Thompson, T. M. (2019). Teaching mands for information using speech generating devices: A replication and extension. *Journal of Applied Behavior Analysis, 52,* 756–771.

Sigafoos, J. (1998). Assessing conditional use of graphic mode requesting in a young boy with autism. *Journal of Developmental and Physical Disabilities, 10,* 133–151.

Sigafoos, J., Kerr, M., Roberts, D., & Couzens, D. (1994). Increasing opportunities for requesting in classrooms serving children with developmental disabilities. *Journal of Autism and Developmental Disorders, 24,* 631–645.

Sigafoos, J., & Roberts-Pennell, D. (1999). Wrong-item format: A promising intervention for teaching socially appropriate forms of rejecting to children with developmental disabilities? *Augmentative and Alternative Communication, 15,* 135–140.

Skinner, B. F. (1957). *Verbal behavior.* Englewood Cliffs, NJ: Prentice-Hall.

Sprinkle, E. C., & Miguel, C. F. (2012). The effects of listener and speaker training on emergent relations in children with autism. *Analysis of Verbal Behavior, 28,* 111–117.

Sundberg, M. L. (2008). *Verbal Behavior Milestones Assessment and Placement Program (VB-MAPP): A language and social skills assessment program for children with autism or other developmental disabilities.* Concord, CA: AVB Press.

Sundberg, M. L., & Partington, J. W. (1998). *Teaching language to children with autism or other developmental disabilities.* Danville, CA: Behavior Analysts.

Sundberg, M. L., & Sundberg, C. A. (2011). Intraverbal behavior and verbal conditional discriminations in typically developing children and children with autism. *Analysis of Verbal Behavior, 27,* 23–43.

Taylor, B. A., Levin, L., & Jasper, S. (1999). Increasing play-related statements in children with autism toward their siblings: Effects of video modeling. *Journal of Developmental and Physical Disabilities, 11,* 253–264.

Tincani, M. (2004). Comparing sign language and picture exchange training for students with autism and multiple disabilities. *Focus on Autism and Other Developmental Disabilities, 19,* 162–173.

Tincani, M. (2007). Beyond consumer advocacy: Autism spectrum disorders, effective instruction, and public schooling. *Intervention in School and Clinic, 43,* 47–51.

Tincani, M. J., & Boutot, E. A. (2005). Autism and technology: Current practices and future directions. In D. L. Edyburn, K. Higgins, & R. Boone (Eds.), *The handbook of special education technology research and practice* (pp. 413–421). Whitefish Bay, WI: Knowledge by Design.

Tincani, M., & Zawacki, J. (2012). Evidence based practice for communication skill acquisition. In E. E. Barton & B. A. Harn (Eds.), *Educating young children with autism spectrum disorder* (pp. 171–189). Thousand Oaks, CA: Corwin Press.

Touchette, P. E., & Howard, J. S. (1984). Errorless learning: Reinforcement contingencies and stimulus control transfer in delayed prompting. *Journal of Applied Behavior Analysis, 17,* 175–188.

Twyman, J. (1996). The functional independence of impure mands and tacts of abstract stimulus properties. *Analysis of Verbal Behavior, 13*, 1–19.

Wankoff, L. S. (2005). *Innovative methods in language intervention.* Austin, TX: PRO-ED.

Warren, S. F., Yoder, P. J., Gazdag, G. E., Kim, K., & Jones, H. A. (1993). Facilitating prelinguistic communication skills in young children with developmental delay. *Journal of Speech and Hearing Research, 36*, 83–97.

Werker, J. F., & Tees, R. C. (1999). Influences on infant speech processing: Toward a new synthesis. *Annual Review of Psychology, 50*, 509–535.

Werker, J. F., & Tees, R. C. (2005). Speech perception as a window for understanding plasticity and commit-ment in language systems of the brain. *Developmental Psychobiology, 46*, 233–251.

Williams, G., Pérez-González, L. A., & Vogt, K. (2003). The role of specific consequences in the maintenance of three types of questions. *Journal of Applied Behavior Analysis, 36*, 285–296.

Ylvisaker, M., & Feeney, T. J. (1994). Communication and behavior: Collaboration between speech–language pathologists and behavioral psychologists. *Topics in Language Disorders, 15*(1), 37–54.

Young, J. M., Krantz, P. J., McClannahan, L. E., & Poulson, C. L. (1994). Generalized imitation and response-class formation in children with autism. *Journal of Applied Behavior Analysis, 27*, 685–697.

# CHAPTER 17

# Staff Training and Management

Dennis H. Reid, Niamh P. O'Kane, and Kenneth M. Macurik

Staff training and management represent a long-standing area of focus in applied behavior analysis. Soon after initial demonstrations of the efficacy of behavior analysis for improving the behavior of people with special needs in the 1960s, behavior analysis directed its attention to disseminating the emerging technology among human-service staff. Concern first centered on training staff in basic behavioral procedures to use with people with developmental and related disabilities (e.g., Gardner, 1972). Shortly thereafter, behavior analysts recognized that the same principles underlying behavior change procedures for people with developmental disabilities were applicable with staff members' work performance (Hollander, Plutchik, & Horner, 1973; Quilitch, 1975; Welsch, Ludwig, Radiker, & Krapfl, 1973).

Interest in training human-service staff to use behavioral procedures and applying behavioral strategies to manage staff performance continues today. Such interest is due to several factors, including recognition that many services for people with disabilities warrant improvement (Reid, Parsons, & Green, 2012, Ch. 1). A related factor is the continuing gap between evidence-based procedures for promoting desirable behavior among people with special needs and caregivers' provision of day-to-day services to those people (Lerman, 2009; Neef, 1995). We consider staff training and management as one way to disseminate behavior

analysis and bridge that gap (Babcock, Fleming, & Oliver, 1998; Parsons, Rollyson, & Reid, 2012).

Staff training and management have constituted a consistent but not a large area of focus in applied behavior analysis since the field's inception. Investigations on staff performance in human-service settings represent a small percentage of published research in behavior analysis. Nonetheless, when we consider that investigators have been addressing staff performance for over 40 years, behavior analysts have conducted a substantial amount of research. Such research has produced highly relevant information for improving staff performance. The purpose of this chapter is to summarize the existing knowledge base from behavior-analytic research on staff training and management. An additional purpose is to describe gaps in the current knowledge and suggest areas for future research.

## FOCUS OF CHAPTER

A specialty area of applied behavior analysis, *organizational behavior management*, has conducted the behavioral research on staff training and management. Although the primary emphasis in organizational behavior management more recently has been business and industry rather than human-service settings, behavioral research has continued in the latter settings. The focus of the current chapter is on staff training and management specifically in human-service settings. (For fuller discussion of organizational behavior management in general, see Wilder & Gravina, Chapter 32, this volume.) The principles of behavior change and many of the applications are the same in the two settings, but significant differences in business and industry versus typical human-service settings exist (e.g., variations in outcomes reflecting successful operations; personnel policies; potential performance incentives and reinforcers).

As with investigations in behavior analysis in general, most staff research has targeted settings for people with intellectual and other developmental disabilities. Such settings are likewise the focus of this chapter. However, we include research on improving staff performance in other settings, particularly schools, where relevant.

## FORMAT OF CHAPTER

The chapter consists of two primary sections. The first section summarizes the technology of staff training and management from behavior-analytic research to date. The second section describes current gaps in the technology and areas in need of investigation, based on the noted gaps and emerging trends in human-service settings.

## EXISTING TECHNOLOGY OF STAFF TRAINING AND MANAGEMENT

We can categorize behavior-analytic research on staff performance in the human services generally in three areas: (1) training staff in work performance, (2) improving ongoing work performance, and (3) maintaining proficient work performance. Although these three areas are closely related and often overlap, they represent a useful means of organizing and describing investigations of staff work performance.

### Behavioral Procedures to Train Human-Service Staff

The first investigations using behavioral procedures to train staff members typically involved teaching basic behavior modification skills to human-service staff for use with people with developmental disabilities (e.g., Gardner, 1972; Koegel, Russo, & Rincover, 1977; Watson & Uzzell, 1980). Two major findings resulted from the early staff-

training research. First, investigators demonstrated that behavior analysts could teach professionals and paraprofessionals to use behavioral procedures to change the behavior of individuals with significant disabilities. Although this research outcome is not surprising now, it was noteworthy at the time. The research demonstrated that behavior analysts could apply behavioral procedures in existing service settings to teach important skills to people with severe and profound cognitive disabilities who previously were considered unteachable (Whitman, Hantula, & Spence, 1990). Successful teaching demonstrations played an important role in major changes in residential, vocational, and educational opportunities subsequently offered to people with developmental disabilities across the United States as part of the movements toward deinstitutionalization, rights to education, and community inclusion.

A second major outcome of initial studies on training staff to use behavioral procedures pertained to what constituted effective training. Research demonstrated that typical training approaches relying on verbal procedures (i.e., lectures and written material) were useful for training knowledge about job skills, but rarely were effective for training staff how to perform the skills (Gardner, 1972). More performance-oriented training procedures were necessary, such as modeling and practice, to teach staff the skills necessary to perform job duties (for summaries, see Jahr, 1998; Reid, 2004; Reid, Parsons, & Green, 1989, Ch. 3).

Implications of findings from early behavioral research regarding effective staff-training procedures have proven especially noteworthy. The findings highlight a primary reason for many problems with nonproficient staff performance in the human services: In many cases, staffers may not have not been trained effectively to perform the skills supervisors expected. Human-service settings usually provide staff training, but the training frequently relies on verbal approaches that research has shown are insufficient for training performance skills.

Early training research established the foundation for the development of a highly effective training technology for human-service staff to perform work skills. The development and evaluation of that technology have been described in several reviews (Adkins, 1996; Demchak, 1987; Gravina et al., 2018; Jahr, 1998; Parsons et al., 2012; Reid, 2004), and we generally refer to it as *behavioral skills training*. The technology represents a rather straightforward approach for training many work skills, such as discrete-trial teaching (Clayton & Headley, 2019; Sarokoff & Sturmey, 2004), safety-related performance (Nabeyama & Sturmey, 2010), systematic preference assessments (Lavie & Sturmey, 2002), school-based behavior plans (Hogan, Knez, & Kahng, 2015), and courteous service (Johnson & Fawcett, 1994).

We provide a prototypical illustration of a behavioral approach to staff training below. The illustration includes two critical features of effective staff-training programs: *competency-based* and *performance-based* training components (Reid, Rotholz, et al., 2003). *Competency-based* refers to specifying the component behaviors of the target skills clearly, establishing a criterion for adequately performing the behaviors, and continuing training until each trainee achieves the criterion (see Reid, 2017, for a review). *Performance-based* refers to a trainer demonstrating the skills as part of the training and requiring trainees to perform the target skills.

## Prototypical Staff-Training Approach

The prototypical staff-training approach is as follows:

1. Specify target skills.
2. Verbally describe the target skills and the rationale for their importance.
3. Provide a written summary of the target skills.
4. Demonstrate performance of the target skills.
5. Support staff members in practicing the target skills.
6. Provide positive and corrective feedback based on staff proficiency in performing the target skills.
7. Repeat Steps 4–6 until staffers proficiently perform the target skills.

Although ample research has validated the efficacy of the behavioral technology of staff training, investigations also have demonstrated that training alone will not necessarily result in staff members' appropriately applying their newly acquired skills (Alavosius & Sulzer-Azaroff, 1990; Greene, Willis, Levy, & Bailey, 1978; Mozingo, Smith, Riordan, Reiss, & Bailey, 2006; Smith, Parker, Taubman, & Lovaas, 1992). In short, staff training is often necessary for enhancing staff job performance, but is rarely sufficient. To ensure that staff members proficiently apply skills acquired through staff-training programs, follow-up management procedures usually are needed during staff members' regular job performance.

## Behavioral Procedures to Improve Ongoing Staff Work Performance

The second major area of behavior-analytic research with human-service staff is the use of behavioral procedures to improve day-to-day work performance. This area pertains to situations in which staffers have the requisite skills to perform their jobs, but they do not use those skills during daily job performance. Investigations designed to improve ongoing work performance represent the largest area of behavior-analytic research involving human-service staff.

Researchers have used behavior analysts' traditional *antecedent–behavior–consequence* (A-B-C) model to improve ongoing staff performance. Staff performance is the behavior. Researchers then use antecedent interventions to prompt or set the occasion for the behavior, consequence interventions to reinforce the target behavior or punish competing or undesirable behavior, or a combination. Another category of interventions is self-control procedures to assist staffers in controlling their own behavior to improve work performance. A fourth category is multicomponent interventions, in which behavior analysts combine antecedent, consequence, and self-control procedures.

Several reviews have summarized research on antecedent, consequence, self-control, and multicomponent interventions to improve staff performance (Alvero, Bucklin, & Austin, 2001; Phillips, 1998; Reid, 2004; Reid et al., 1989, 2012), and we do not repeat these reviews here. Rather, we summarize key points regarding the existing technology for improving ongoing staff performance with various procedures.

### Antecedent Interventions for Improving Staff Performance

The most commonly investigated antecedent approach for improving work performance is staff training. Other antecedent interventions, which investigators have often implemented after initial training, have included instructions to staff to perform a work duty (Fielding, Errickson, & Bettin, 1971); having a supervisor or similar individual model target skills at the work site (Gladstone & Spencer, 1977; Wallace, Davis, Liberman, & Baker, 1973); and prompts or cues to perform a work task, such as duty cards (Sneed & Bible, 1979). These interventions are attractive because, except for modeling, they typically require relatively little time and effort. However, antecedent interventions are inconsistently effective for improving staff performance (for reviews, see Phillips, 1998; Reid & Whitman, 1983).

Research demonstrating the inconsistent effectiveness of antecedent interventions has important implications. Antecedent interventions, such as a supervisor's providing vocal or written instructions, represent the most commonly used training method for improving staff performance in human-service settings. Consequently, supervisors often attempt to improve staff performance by using procedures that research has shown are not effective consistently (cf. Sturmey, 1998).

The continued use of antecedent procedures, despite their inconsistent effectiveness, prompts the question of why supervisors employ such strategies so frequently. One likely answer is a pervasive problem in the human services: lack of supervisor training in evidence-based procedures for improving staff performance (Reid, Parsons, Lattimore, Towery, & Reade, 2005; Sturmey, 1998). Lacking knowledge and skills of evidence-based procedures, supervisors may well resort to familiar strategies, such as simply telling staffers what they should do. Another likely reason is that intermittent changes in staff work behavior after supervisor instructions episodically reinforces supervisors' instructional behavior.

Clearly, some staff members respond to supervisory instructions by altering their work behavior in some situations. Increased research is warranted to determine conditions in which instructions and other antecedent interventions are likely to be effective (cf. Graff & Karsten, 2012). For example, staff behavior may be more likely to change following an instruction if the targeted behavior involves minimal response effort or represents a one-time, discrete event, as opposed to involving more considerable effort or requiring repeated activity. Staffers may be more responsive to supervisory instructions if supervisors have a history of following staff (non)compliance with feedback or other consequences. If investigations could identify conditions in which antecedents are more and less effective, then we could describe the efficacious procedures trainers should use routinely.

### Consequence Interventions for Improving Staff Performance

Behavior-analytic research on consequence-based training procedures has focused on reinforcing desired staff performance. Investigators have directed relatively little attention to punishing undesired behavior. Early investigations often employed tangible consequences as potential reinforcers, such as money (Katz, Johnson, & Gelfand, 1972), trading stamps (Bricker, Morgan, & Grabowski, 1972), and free meals (Shoemaker & Reid, 1980). Due in large part to practical considerations with tangible consequences, such as cost to an agency and lack of supervisory control necessary to provide money frequently and contingently, recent investigations have targeted more readily available consequences. The most frequently investigated consequence has been performance feedback.

Investigators have provided feedback contingent on target staff behavior in many formats, including spoken (Realon, Lewallen, & Wheeler, 1983), written (Kneringer & Page, 1999), graphic (Miles & Wilder, 2009), privately presented to individual staff members (Shoemaker & Reid, 1980), publicly presented to groups of staffers (Cotnoir-Bichelman, Thompson, McKerchar, & Haremza, 2006), and a combination of formats (Casey & McWilliam, 2011; Luck, Lerman, Wu, Dupuis, & Hussein, 2018). Although each type of feedback has relative advantages and disadvantages, each generally has been effective in increasing targeted staff behavior over time (for reviews, see Alvero et al., 2001; Balcazar, Hopkins, & Suarez, 1986; Ford, 1980). The most commonly investigated type of feedback is positive comments (e.g., praise) regarding target staff behavior. Some debate exists regarding the mechanism underlying contingent feedback as a behavior change intervention with staff (Alvero et al., 2001). Nonetheless, ample evidence demonstrates feedback can improve staff performance.

Despite the frequently demonstrated efficacy of feedback with staff performance in the research literature, systematic use of feedback has not been common practice in many human-service settings (Harchik, Sherman, Hopkins, Strouse, & Sheldon, 1989; Reid, 2004). Two likely reasons exist for this. One reason is that supervisors may not receive appropriate training in the skills they need to provide effective feedback to staff (Reid et al., 2005; Sturmey, 1998). A second reason is that providing systematic feedback requires consistent supervisor effort. Consequently, effective supervisor feedback to staff is likely to require training and feedback to the supervisor from upper management.

Little research exists on consequences to punish inadequate staff performance. Available research has shown that punishment is not an effective way to change staff behavior consistently (e.g., Gardner, 1970; Repp & Deitz, 1979). Nonetheless, supervisors often attempt to use punishment to change staff behavior. One early survey indicated that over 90% of supervisors in settings serving people with developmental disabilities relied on punishment procedures for managing staff performance problems (Mayhew, Enyart, & Cone, 1979). Such results are disconcerting, because research suggests that such approaches are not effective and may even be detrimental to an agency's staff (Sturmey, 1998).

## Self-Control Interventions for Improving Staff Performance

A small but relatively persistent area of research on improving staff performance has been the evaluation of self-control procedures involving staffers' use of goal setting, self-recording, and (to a lesser extent) self-reinforcement. Researchers have used each procedure with one or more other self-control strategies. A primary rationale for evaluating self-control procedures from a management perspective is that the procedures have been effective behavior change interventions in areas other than staff management. Logically, we might expect them to promote behavior change among human-service staff. Additionally, self-control procedures can require less time and effort for supervisors, because staff members are implementing the procedures to enhance their own performance in contrast to requiring implementation by a supervisor (Williams, Vittorio, & Hausherr, 2002).

Investigations on self-control interventions with human-service staff have reported mixed results. In some cases, self-control procedures produced significant improvements in staff performance (e.g., Burgio, Whitman, & Reid, 1983; Plavnick, Ferreri, & Maupin, 2010), whereas the improvements were inconsistent or temporary across staff members in others (Doerner, Miltenberger, & Bakken, 1989; Petscher & Bailey, 2006; Richman, Riordan, Reiss, Pyles, & Bailey, 1988; Suda & Miltenberger, 1993). Even in the former research, separating effects of self-control procedures from effects of supervisor behavior that was occurring simultaneously was often difficult. Another concern is that supervisory behavior may be necessary to promote staff use of self-control procedures (Adkins, 1996), which reduces the time-efficiency advantage of the procedures. A potential advantage of self-control procedures may be to maintain improvements in staff performance that initially accompanied supervisory interventions (Brackett, Reid, & Green, 2007; Kissel, Whitman, & Reid, 1983). Nonetheless, the overall research on self-control procedures to improve staff performance suggests that such approaches can be effective, but the conditions under which they are effective are unclear and warrant continued research.

## Multicomponent Interventions for Improving Staff Performance

Most interventions for improving staff performance have been multicomponent. Typically, the researcher conducts an initial training or instructional procedure, followed by application of performance consequences and self-control procedures, to a lesser degree. The primary purpose of research with multicomponent interventions has been to demonstrate a reliable means of improving a designated area of staff performance. The rationale generally has been that combining various procedures enhances the likelihood of success of the intervention relative to reliance on only one procedure.

Although different strategies comprise multicomponent interventions, an underlying conceptual basis for the interventions remains the basic A-B-C model noted earlier. Behavior analysts have attempted to streamline and provide more systemization to multicomponent interventions by employing a rather generic model of *behavioral supervision* (Hawkins, Burgio, Langford, & Engel, 1992; Reid & Shoemaker, 1984). Coinciding with a popular movement to provide consumer-centered services (Ivancic & Helsel, 1998), Reid and Parsons (2002) developed *behavioral outcome management*, which is an update of behavioral supervision. Outcome management, which has demonstrated efficacy in several human-service settings (Parsons, Rollyson, & Reid, 2004; Reid, Green, & Parsons, 2003; Reid et al., 2005), identifies desired outcomes for agency consumers to attain and specifies respective staff performances necessary to assist consumers in attaining the outcomes. We summarize the outcome management approach to working with staff below.

## Basic Steps of Behavioral Outcome Management

The basic steps of behavioral outcome management are as follows:

1. Specify a target consumer outcome.
2. Specify the staff performance necessary to assist consumers in attaining target outcome.
3. Train staff members in targeted behavior using performance- and competency-based training procedures.

4. Monitor staffers' job performance.
5. Provide supportive feedback for proficient staff performance.
6. Provide corrective feedback for nonproficient staff performance.

Multicomponent programs have improved staff performance in many situations. However, because of the reliance on multiple intervention components, these approaches require certain supervisory skills plus consistent time and effort. The latter features likely represent one reason why systematic, multicomponent behavioral approaches to staff training and management are more prevalent in the research literature than in routine practice.

## Behavioral Procedures to Maintain Staff Performance

The third major area of behavioral research on staff performance is maintenance of behavior change after training and management interventions. Behavior analysts often consider maintenance a subcategory of training or management research, rather than a specific category itself. However, we address maintenance as its own category for two reasons. First, maintaining improvements in staff performance is critical for demonstrating the social significance of behavioral research on staff training. Second, maintaining target staff performance has proven difficult.

Behavior analysts have long recognized the difficulty of maintaining improved staff performance after staff training and management interventions. Liberman (1983), for example, acknowledged that effects of behavioral interventions on staff performance often ended as soon as investigators completed their study in one human-service setting. Subsequently, investigators have recognized the need to promote maintenance of initial improvements in staff performance after behavioral interventions (Carr, Wilder, Majdalany, Mathisen, & Strain, 2013; Phillips, 1998).

Although behavior analysts recognize the importance of maintaining staff performance change and difficulties in this regard, they have conducted much less research in this area than on training and management interventions to improve staff performance initially (Downs, Downs, & Rau, 2008; van Oorsouw, Embregts, Bosman, & Jahoda, 2009). One likely reason for the relative lack of maintenance research is the time involved in this research. Investigators must work with agency personnel to initially implement and evaluate a training or management program and continue reliable observations for extended maintenance periods. Furthermore, experimental manipulations must occur after the initial intervention, and observations must continue to evaluate variables *functionally affecting* maintenance.

Despite these difficulties in conducting maintenance research, the available data are encouraging regarding use of behavioral procedures to maintain effects of training and management interventions. Investigators have published several demonstrations that staff behavior change can be maintained for up to several years (e.g., Harchik, Sherman, Sheldon, & Strouse, 1992; Parsons, Schepis, Reid, McCarn, & Green, 1987; Pollack, Fleming, & Sulzer-Azaroff, 1994; Richman et al., 1988) and even across a 30-year period (Reid, Parsons, & Jensen, 2017). These data suggest that behavioral management interventions are accompanied by sustained improvements in staff performance if some components of the initial interventions remain in place. However, sustaining supervisor procedures to maintain changes in staff behavior can be problematic.

One way to maintain the effects of staff performance interventions is to incorporate behavioral procedures, like supervisory feedback, in an agency's routine management system. Although some research has demonstrated positive effects of institutionalizing such procedures in an agency's operation (Christian, 1983; Fielding & Blasé, 1993) those positive findings have not been consistent (Green, Rollyson, Passante, & Reid, 2002). More specifically, contingencies seem necessary to ensure that supervisors carry out the maintenance systems. In short, we have much to learn about incorporating effective maintenance procedures in an agency's routine operation.

## GAPS IN STAFF-TRAINING AND MANAGEMENT TECHNOLOGY, AND FUTURE RESEARCH AREAS

We have gained considerable knowledge from behavior-analytic research on staff training and management. Research has identified effective training programs, and we have an effective technology for teaching performance skills to human-service staff. Behavior analysts have used the A-B-C model as a conceptual basis for developing many procedures, particularly in consequence and multicomponent interventions. Findings have been promising for producing long-term performance improvements with the behavioral procedures researchers have investigated.

The knowledge base and technology for training and managing staff performance remain incomplete, however. This section provides a synthesis of significant gaps in the existing technology and corresponding areas warranting future research. We can view the applied-behavior-analytic research needs on staff training and management from two perspectives. The first perspective is research on expanding the technology for training staff members and managing their performance. The second is how to disseminate and incorporate the technology more effectively in the routine operation of human-service settings.

## Expanding the Technology of Staff Training and Management

Like its parent discipline of applied behavior analysis, organizational behavior management and related areas of behavioral staff training and management are continually evolving. The evolution occurs as research enhances behavior analysts' understanding of human behavior and their ability to promote socially valued behavior in different contexts. The evolution also occurs as behavioral researchers target new or previously unaddressed problem areas. Knowledge and technology derived from research represents the evidence-based foundation that separates behavioral staff training and management from almost every other approach to supervision in human services (Reid & Parsons, 2002). As such, we anticipate and desire that researchers will continue to expand and refine the behavioral technology of staff training and management.

### Training and Managing Staff in the Use of New Behavioral Technologies

In one way, research on staff training and management in human-service settings follows research on changing the behavior of people with special needs. As research in behavior analysis demonstrates new or better means of teaching individuals and overcoming challenging behavior, for example, behavior analysts conduct staff training and management research to disseminate those means to human-service staff.

Research on the functional assessment of challenging behavior among people with developmental disabilities provides an illustration of how research on staff performance follows other

behavior-analytic research. Behavior analysts have conducted much research over the last three decades on assessing the function of challenging behavior and developing function-based interventions. Subsequently, research has addressed how to train staff in functional-assessment procedures (Chok, Shlesinger, Studer, & Bird, 2012; Moore et al., 2002; Schnell, Sidener, DeBar, Vladescu, & Kahng, 2018; Wallace, Doney, Mintz-Resudek, & Tarbox, 2004). Similar developments have occurred in other areas, such as training staff to identify the preferences of people with disabilities (Ausenhus & Higgins, 2019; Lavie & Sturmey, 2002; Roscoe, Fisher, Glover, & Volkert, 2006). Training and managing staff in the use of new technologies from behavior-analytic research represent an area of continuing importance.

### Expanding Staff-Training and Management Research to Other Problematic Performance Areas

Although behavioral research has addressed numerous types of staff behavior in the human services, several important performance areas remain frequently problematic but have not been examined thoroughly. One notable example is staff turnover. High rates of staff turnover represent one of the most troublesome issues facing many human-service settings, yet turnover has received infrequent attention from behavioral researchers (Strouse, Carroll-Hernandez, Sherman, & Sheldon, 2003).

Another area of concern that has received relatively little attention pertains to agencies that provide support for adults with autism spectrum disorder (ASD). Behavior-analytic research and application involving children with ASD has grown tremendously in the last two decades, with a corresponding increase (albeit to a lesser degree) in training staff to work in this area (e.g., Catania, Almeida, Liu-Constant, & DiGennaro Reed, 2009; DiGennaro Reed, Codding, Catania, & Maguire, 2010; Graff & Karsten, 2012). However, many children with ASD who have received intensive behavioral services have grown up and entered service systems for adults, which do not provide the same degree of behavioral support. Adults with disabilities such as ASD also have needs that go beyond children's, and these needs require support staff with special skills (Reid, 2016). To illustrate, many adults with ASD and other severe disabilities spend much of their time in center-based settings (Wehman, 2011). A longstanding concern with these settings is a lack of meaningful activity involvement among participating consumers, exemplified by frequent occurrences of consumers' putting the same puzzle together day after day, coloring in children's coloring books, and being involved in activities with no apparent purpose other than to keep them busy (Reid et al., 2017). Research on staff training and performance identified this problem relatively early and reported ways of working with staffers to promote more meaningful activity involvement (Dyer, Schwartz, & Luce, 1984; Parsons et al., 1987; Reid et al., 1985). However, recent observational studies indicate that a lack of meaningful activity involvement among adults with ASD and other severe disabilities continues to be prevalent across the United States (Reid et al., 2017).

### Training and Managing Staff's Use of Behavioral Technologies in New Venues

Just as behavior analysis is continually evolving as a professional discipline, the human-service field tends to evolve over time. If behavior analysts intend to practice in new and altered venues, such as in clients' homes with caregivers, then behavioral technologies must be amenable to those venues. Successfully applying behavior analysis in new venues represents another area for future research.

The change from institutional to community living for people with disabilities in the United States is an example of how we need research on behavioral staff training and management in new venues. Much early staff-training research occurred in institutional settings. As the community-living trend became more widespread, a need arose for demonstrations of how to improve staff performance in community settings (Harchik & Campbell, 1998). For example, much early research on institutional staffers' performance involved the frequent presence of a supervisor for intervention implementation. Community-living arrangements do not often include frequent supervisor involvement with staff. Consequently, a need has arisen for research on ways to improve staff performance without frequent supervisory presence. A similar situation exists in many home-based behavior-analytic early intervention programs for children with ASD (e.g., Ausenhu & Higgins, 2019).

### Use of New Information Technology in Staff Training and Management

Technology has revolutionized information dissemination in recent years. Internet access, training videos and DVDs, and interactive software, for example, are now readily available to many human-service settings (Severtson & Carr, 2012). Correspondingly, researchers have directed significant attention to evaluating and demonstrating the effectiveness of these approaches to training (e.g., Catania et al., 2009; Moore & Fisher, 2007; Rosales, Gongola, & Homlitas, 2015; Scott, Lerman, & Luck, 2018; Weldy, Rapp, & Capocasa, 2014).

New information technologies offer many attractive features for training important work behavior to human-service staff. To illustrate, training DVDs and videos in other formats may represent a means of providing relevant information and procedural demonstrations that require minimal trainer time relative to more traditional training procedures (Macurik, O'Kane, Malanga, & Reid, 2008). Continued research evaluating these approaches to staff training seems warranted. However, caution also is warranted. Information technologies still rely heavily on dissemination of verbal information, with the addition of performance-based modeling in many cases, and previous research has produced inconsistent effects for training mastery-level performance. This may explain the inconsistencies regarding the effectiveness of this type of training technology (e.g., DiGennaro Reed et al., 2010; Neef, Trachtenberg, Loeb, & Sterner, 1991). Research to determine ways to incorporate performance-based training with new information technologies is warranted.

## Expanding Adoption of Behavioral Training and Management

We have noted the lack of widespread adoption of the behavioral technology of staff training and management in human-service settings, as have others (Babcock et al., 1998; LeBlanc, Raetz, & Feliciano, 2011; Reid, 2004). The social significance of the evidence-based approach for staff training and management will remain limited until the human services use it consistently. The following sections suggest areas for research to aid wider use of the existing technology.

### Developing Personnel Preparation Programs in Staff Training and Management

One means of incorporating the staff-training and management technology in human-service settings is to ensure that professionals entering those settings are knowledgeable about the technology and skilled in its application. Traditionally, professionals have received little or no training in this area (Schell, 1998). Indications exist that personnel preparation programs are directing more attention to behavioral staff training and management. For example, some university programs for training behavior analysts are including courses with content on staff training and management, partly because behavior-analyst certification requires knowledge of these areas (Moore & Shook, 2001). Nonetheless, only a few university programs currently focus on organizational behavior management, and their emphasis is often on business and industry in contrast to human-service settings.

### Training Supervisors in Behavioral Staff Training and Management

We cannot expect supervisors in the human services to be proficient in behavioral staff training and management unless they have had training in these areas. Few investigations have addressed training supervisors in behavioral applications with staff (e.g., Clark et al., 1985; Fleming, Oliver, & Bolton, 1996; Methot, Williams, Cummings, & Bradshaw, 1996; Parsons & Reid, 1995; Reid et al., 2005). Evidence-based curricula for training supervisors are likely to aid expansion of supervisor training. The American Association on Intellectual and Developmental Disabilities has developed one such curriculum (Reid, Parsons, & Green, 2009).

In research on supervisor training, attention to the results of staff training research as summarized earlier is warranted. Results of staff-training research suggest that supervisor training is not likely to affect supervisor behavior unless upper management prompts and reinforces the supervisors' performance of the trained skills. With few exceptions (e.g., Gillat & Sulzer-Azaroff, 1994; Methot et al., 1996), research addressing the behavior of senior managers or executives in human-service settings is lacking.

### Maintaining Human-Service Staff Performance

The need for research on maintaining improvements in staff performance after training and management interventions is related closely to the need for research with supervisors and senior managers. Research to date suggests that improved staff performance is likely to be maintained only if supervisors implement some relevant components of the initial interventions. In turn, senior man-

agement needs to promote supervisors' continued use of intervention components.

The acceptability of behavioral management procedures is another research area relevant to maintaining supervisor performance. Behavior analysts have recognized the importance of management procedures that are acceptable to supervisors for potentially promoting continued use of supervisory skills (Reid & Whitman, 1983). Correspondingly, several investigators have attempted to evaluate acceptable components of supervisory procedures (see Parsons, 1998, for a review). However, as the Parsons (1998) review indicated (see also Parsons et al., 2012), researchers have concerns regarding the validity of typical measures of supervisory acceptance (i.e., questionnaire responses). We need continued research on improving the acceptability of management procedures to supervisors and identifying valid measures of acceptability.

Functional assessment of staff performance is another way of potentially promoting maintenance of appropriate staff behavior. Human-service staff members have many tasks to perform and many contingencies on their work performance. Investigations on improving staffers' performance often impose new contingencies without apparent regard for existing contingencies. As a result, staff members resume responding to the more common contingencies when investigators discontinue the research contingencies. One way of avoiding this obstacle is to identify when supervisors could introduce new contingencies that would not compete with existing contingencies (Green, Reid, Perkins, & Gardner, 1991). For example, Green et al. (1991) conducted a structural analysis of staffers' work performance to identify periods of nonwork behavior. The researchers then increased performance of selected duties during those nonwork periods. Targeting periods of nonwork allowed staffers to increase their performance of selected duties without competing with their other duties.

The Green et al. (1991) investigation also highlights staff performance problems due to an apparent lack of contingencies on certain work duties. Several investigations have addressed reducing staff time spent in nonwork activities (Brown, Willis, & Reid, 1981; Green et al., 1991; Iwata, Bailey, Brown, Foshee, & Alpern, 1976). This research assumed that staff spent time in such activities due to a lack of supervisor contingencies on such behavior or a lack of contingencies on more desired performance.

More detailed analysis of contingencies or lack of contingencies on staff behavior in human-service settings may produce information relevant for promoting sustained improvements in staff performance. Investigators have noted the significance of conducting functional assessments with staff performance (Austin, 2000; Sturmey, 1998), and research in this area appears promising. Particularly, investigators have used the Performance Diagnostic Checklist—Human Services to design interventions to improve problematic staff performance, based on systematically assessed variables related to the lack of desired performance (Carr et al., 2013; Ditzian, Wilder, King, & Tanz, 2015). We support the continuation of this line of research and offer it as an important means of furthering the contribution of applied behavior analysis to promoting high-quality staff performance.

## REFERENCES

Adkins, V. K. (1996). Discussion: Behavioral procedures for training direct care staff in facilities serving dependent populations. *Behavioral Interventions, 11,* 95–100.

Alavosius, M. P., & Sulzer-Azaroff, B. (1990). Acquisition and maintenance of health-care routines as a function of feedback density. *Journal of Applied Behavior Analysis, 23,* 151–162.

Alvero, A. M., Bucklin, B. R., & Austin, J. (2001). An objective review of the effectiveness and essential characteristics of performance feedback in organizational settings. *Journal of Organizational Behavior Management, 21*(1), 3–29.

Ausenhus, J. A., & Higgins, W. J. (2019). An evaluation of real-time feedback delivered via telemedicine: Training staff to conduct preference assessments. *Behavior Analysis in Practice, 12,* 643–648.

Austin, J. (2000). Some thoughts on the field of organizational behavior management. *Journal of Organizational Behavior Management, 20*(3–4), 191–202.

Babcock, R. A., Fleming, R. K., & Oliver, J. R. (1998). OBM and quality improvement systems. *Journal of Organizational Behavior Management, 21*(1), 33–59.

Balcazar, F., Hopkins, B. L., & Suarez, Y. (1986). A critical, objective review of performance feedback. *Journal of Organizational Behavior Management, 7*(3–4), 65–89.

Brackett, L., Reid, D. H., & Green, C. W. (2007). Effects of reactivity to observations on staff performance. *Journal of Applied Behavior Analysis, 40,* 191–195.

Bricker, W. A., Morgan, D. G., & Grabowski, J. G. (1972). Development and maintenance of a behavior modification repertoire of cottage attendants through TV feedback. *American Journal of Mental Deficiency, 77,* 128–136.

Brown, K. M., Willis, B. S., & Reid, D. H. (1981). Differential effects of supervisor verbal feedback and feedback plus approval on institutional staff performance. *Journal of Organizational Behavior Management, 3*(1), 57–68.

Burgio, L. D., Whitman, T. L., & Reid, D. H. (1983). A participative management approach for improving direct-care staff performance in an institutional setting. *Journal of Applied Behavior Analysis, 16,* 37–53.

Carr, J. E., Wilder, D. A., Majdalany, L., Mathisen, D., & Strain, L. A. (2013). An assessment-based solution to a human-service employee performance problem: An evaluation of the Performance Diagnostic Checklist—Human Services. *Behavior Analysis in Practice, 6,* 16–32.

Casey, A. M., & McWilliam, R. A. (2011). The impact of checklist-based training on teachers' use of the zone defense schedule. *Journal of Applied Behavior Analysis, 44,* 397–401.

Catania, C. N., Almeida, D., Liu-Constant, B., & DiGennaro Reed, F. D. (2009). Video modeling to train staff to implement discrete-trial instruction. *Journal of Applied Behavior Analysis, 42,* 387–392.

Chok, J. T., Shlesinger, A., Studer, L., & Bird, F. L. (2012). Description of a practitioner training program on functional analysis and treatment development. *Behavior Analysis in Practice, 5,* 25–36.

Christian, W. P. (1983). A case study in the programming and maintenance of institutional change. *Journal of Organizational Behavior Management, 5*(3–4), 99–153.

Clark, H. B., Wood, R., Kuehnel, T., Flanagan, S., Mosk, M., & Northup, J. T. (1985). Preliminary validation and training of supervisory interaction skills. *Journal of Organizational Behavior Management, 7*(1–2), 95–115.

Clayton, M., & Headley, A. (2019). The use of behavioral skills training to improve staff performance of discrete trial training. *Behavioral Intervention, 34,* 136–143.

Cotnoir-Bichelman, N. M., Thompson, R. H., McKerchar, P. M., & Haremza, J. L. (2006). Training student teachers to reposition infants frequently. *Journal of Applied Behavior Analysis, 39,* 489–494.

Demchak, M. A. (1987). A review of behavioral staff training in special education settings. *Education and Training in Mental Retardation, 22,* 205–217.

DiGennaro Reed, F. D., Codding, R., Catania, C. N., & Maguire, H. (2010). Effects of video modeling on treatment integrity of behavioral interventions. *Journal of Applied Behavior Analysis, 43,* 291–295.

Ditzian, K., Wilder, D. A., King, A., & Tanz, J. (2015). An evaluation of the Performance Diagnostic Checklist—Human Services to assess an employee performance problem in a center-based autism treatment facility. *Journal of Applied Behavior Analysis, 48,* 199–203.

Doerner, M., Miltenberger, R. G., & Bakken, J. (1989). The effects of staff self-management on positive social interactions in a group home setting. *Behavioral Residential Treatment, 4,* 313–330.

Downs, A., Downs, R. C., & Rau, K. (2008). Effects of training and feedback on discrete trial teaching skills and student performance. *Research in Developmental Disabilities, 29,* 235–246.

Dyer, K., Schwartz, I. S., & Luce, S. C. (1984). A supervision program for increasing functional activities for severely handicapped students in a residential setting. *Journal of Applied Behavior Analysis, 17,* 249–259.

Fielding, D. L., & Blasé, K. A. (1993). Creating new realities: Program development and dissemination. *Journal of Applied Behavior Analysis, 26,* 597–613.

Fielding, L. T., Errickson, E., & Bettin, B. (1971). Modification of staff behavior: A brief note. *Behavior Therapy, 2,* 550–553.

Fleming, R. K., Oliver, J. R., & Bolton, D. (1996). Training supervisors to train staff: A case study in a human service organization. *Journal of Organizational Behavior Management, 16*(1), 3–25.

Ford, J. E. (1980). A classification system for feedback procedures. *Journal of Organizational Behavior Management, 2*(3), 183–191.

Gardner, J. M. (1970). Effects of reinforcement conditions on lateness and absence among institutional personnel. *Ohio Research Quarterly, 3,* 315–316.

Gardner, J. M. (1972). Teaching behavior modification to nonprofessionals. *Journal of Applied Behavior Analysis, 5,* 517–521.

Gillat, A., & Sulzer-Azaroff, B. (1994). Promoting principals' managerial involvement in instructional improvement. *Journal of Applied Behavior Analysis, 27,* 115–129.

Gladstone, B. W., & Spencer, C. J. (1977). The effects of modeling on the contingent praise of mental retardation counselors. *Journal of Applied Behavior Analysis, 10,* 75–84.

Graff, R. B., & Karsten, A. M. (2012). Evaluation of a self-instruction package for conducting stimulus preference assessments. *Journal of Applied Behavior Analysis, 45,* 69–82.

Gravina, N., Villacorta, J., Albert, K., Clark, R., Curry, S., & Wilder, D. (2018). A literature review of organizational behavior management interventions in human service settings from 1990 to 2016. *Journal of Organizational Behavior Management, 38,* 191–224.

Green, C. W., Reid, D. H., Perkins, L. I., & Gardner, S. M. (1991). Increasing habilitative services for persons with profound handicaps: An application of structural analysis to staff management. *Journal of Applied Behavior Analysis, 24,* 459–471.

Green, C. W., Rollyson, J. H., Passante, S. C., & Reid, D. H. (2002). Maintaining proficient supervisor performance with direct support personnel: An analysis of two management approaches. *Journal of Applied Behavior Analysis, 35,* 205–208.

Greene, B. F., Willis, B. S., Levy, R., & Bailey, J. S. (1978). Measuring client gains from staff-implemented programs. *Journal of Applied Behavior Analysis, 11,* 395–412.

Harchik, A. E., & Campbell, A. R. (1998). Supporting people with developmental disabilities in their homes in the community: The role of organizational behavior management. *Journal of Organizational Behavior Management, 18*(2–3), 83–101.

Harchik, A. E., Sherman, J. A., Hopkins, B. L., Strouse, M. C., & Sheldon, J. B. (1989). Use of behavioral techniques by paraprofessional staff: A review and proposal. *Behavioral Residential Treatment, 4,* 331–357.

Harchik, A. E., Sherman, J. A., Sheldon, J. B., & Strouse, M. C. (1992). Ongoing consultation as a method of improving performance of staff members in a group home. *Journal of Applied Behavior Analysis, 25,* 599–610.

Hawkins, A. M., Burgio, L. D., Langford, A., & Engel, B. T. (1992). The effects of verbal and written supervisory feedback on staff compliance with assigned prompted voiding in a nursing home. *Journal of Organizational Behavior Management, 13*(1), 137–150.

Hogan, A., Knez, N., & Kahng, S. (2015). Evaluating the use of behavioral skills training to improve school staffs' implementation of behavior intervention plans. *Journal of Behavioral Education, 24,* 242–254.

Hollander, M., Plutchik, R., & Horner, V. (1973). Interaction of patient and attendant reinforcement programs: The "piggyback" effect. *Journal of Consulting and Clinical Psychology, 41,* 43–47.

Ivancic, M. T., & Helsel, W. J. (1998). Organizational behavior management in large residential organizations: Moving from institutional to client-centered care. *Journal of Organizational Behavior Management, 18*(2–3), 61–82.

Iwata, B. A., Bailey, J. S., Brown, K. M., Foshee, T. J., & Alpern, M. (1976). A performance-based lottery to improve residential care and training by institutional staff. *Journal of Applied Behavior Analysis, 9,* 417–431.

Jahr, E. (1998). Current issues in staff training. *Research in Developmental Disabilities, 19,* 73–87.

Johnson, M. D., & Fawcett, S. B. (1994). Courteous service: Its assessment and modification in a human service organization. *Journal of Applied Behavior Analysis, 27,* 145–152.

Katz, R. C., Johnson, C. A., & Gelfand, S. (1972). Modifying the dispensing of reinforcers: Some implications for behavior modification with hospitalized patients. *Behavior Therapy, 3,* 579–588.

Kissel, R. C., Whitman, T. L., & Reid, D. H. (1983). An institutional staff training and self-management program for developing multiple self-care skills in severely/profoundly retarded individuals. *Journal of Applied Behavior Analysis, 16,* 395–415.

Kneringer, M., & Page, T. J. (1999). Improving staff nutritional practices in community-based group homes: Evaluation, training, and management. *Journal of Applied Behavior Analysis, 32,* 221–224.

Koegel, R. L., Russo, D. C., & Rincover, A. (1977). Assessing and training teachers in the generalized use of behavior modification with autistic children. *Journal of Applied Behavior Analysis, 10,* 197–205.

Lavie, T., & Sturmey, P. (2002). Training staff to conduct a paired-stimulus preference assessment. *Journal of Applied Behavior Analysis, 35,* 209–211.

LeBlanc, L. A., Raetz, P. B., & Feliciano, L. (2011). Behavioral gerontology. In W. W. Fisher, C. C. Piazza, & H. S. Roane (Eds.), *Handbook of applied behavior analysis* (pp. 472–486). New York: Guilford Press.

Lerman, D. C. (2009). An introduction to the Volume 2, Number 2 of Behavior Analysis in Practice (BAP). *Behavior Analysis in Practice, 2,* 2–3.

Liberman, R. P. (1983). Guest editor's preface. *Analysis and Intervention in Developmental Disabilities, 3,* iii–iv.

Luck, K. M., Lerman, D. C., Wu, W. L., Dupuis, D. L., & Hussein, L. A. (2018). A comparison of written, vocal, and video feedback when training teachers. *Journal of Behavioral Education, 27,* 124–144.

Macurik, K. M., O'Kane, N. P., Malanga, P., & Reid, D. H. (2008). Video training of support staff in intervention plans for challenging behavior: Comparison with live training. *Behavioral Interventions, 23,* 143–163.

Mayhew, G. L., Enyart, P., & Cone, J. D. (1979). Approaches to employee management: Policies and preferences. *Journal of Organizational Behavior Management, 2*(2), 103–111.

Methot, L. L., Williams, W. L., Cummings, A., & Bradshaw, B. (1996). Measuring the effects of a manager–supervisor training program through the generalized performance of managers, supervisors, front-line staff, and clients in a human service setting. *Journal of Organizational Behavior Management, 16*(2), 3–34.

Miles, N. I., & Wilder, D. A. (2009). The effects of behavioral skills training on caregiver implementation of guided compliance. *Journal of Applied Behavior Analysis, 42,* 405–410.

Moore, J. W., Edwards, R. P., Sterling-Turner, H. E., Riley, J., DuBard, M., & McGeorge, A. (2002). Teacher acquisition of functional analysis methodology. *Journal of Applied Behavior Analysis, 35,* 73–77.

Moore, J. W., & Fisher, W. W. (2007). The effects of videotape modeling on staff acquisition of functional analysis methodology. *Journal of Applied Behavior Analysis, 40,* 197–202.

Moore, J., & Shook, G. L. (2001). Certification, accreditation, and quality control in behavior analysis. *Behavior Analyst, 24,* 45–55.

Mozingo, D. B., Smith, T., Riordan, M. R., Reiss, M. L., & Bailey, J. S. (2006). Enhancing frequency recording by developmental disabilities treatment staff. *Journal of Applied Behavior Analysis, 39,* 253–256.

Nabeyama, B., & Sturmey, P. (2010). Using behavioral skills training to promote safe and correct staff guarding and ambulation distance of students with multiple physical disabilities. *Journal of Applied Behavior Analysis, 43,* 341–345.

Neef, N. A. (1995). Research on training trainers in program implementation: An introduction and future directions. *Journal of Applied Behavior Analysis, 28,* 297–299.

Neef, N. A., Trachtenberg, S., Loeb, J., & Sterner, K. (1991). Video-based training of respite care providers: An interactional analysis of presentation format. *Journal of Applied Behavior Analysis, 24,* 473–486.

Parsons, M. B. (1998). A review of procedural acceptability in organizational behavior management. *Journal of Organizational Behavior Management, 18*(2–3), 173–190.

Parsons, M. B., & Reid, D. H. (1995). Training residential supervisors to provide feedback for maintaining staff teaching skills with people who have severe disabilities. *Journal of Applied Behavior Analysis, 28,* 317–322.

Parsons, M. B., Rollyson, J. H., & Reid, D. H. (2004). Improving day-treatment services for adults with severe disabilities: A norm-referenced application of outcome management. *Journal of Applied Behavior Analysis, 37,* 365–377.

Parsons, M. B., Rollyson, J. H., & Reid, D. H. (2012). Evidence-based staff training: A guide for practitioners. *Behavior Analysis in Practice, 5,* 2–11.

Parsons, M. B., Schepis, M. M., Reid, D. H., McCarn, J. E., & Green, C. W. (1987). Expanding the impact of behavioral staff management: A large-scale, long term application in schools serving severely handicapped students. *Journal of Applied Behavior Analysis, 20,* 139–150.

Petscher, E. S., & Bailey, J. S. (2006). Effects of training, prompting, and self-monitoring on staff behavior in a classroom for students with disabilities. *Journal of Applied Behavior Analysis, 39,* 215–226.

Phillips, J. F. (1998). Applications and contributions of organizational behavior management in schools and day treatment settings. *Journal of Organizational Behavior Management, 18*(2–3), 103–129.

Plavnick, J. B., Ferreri, S. J., & Maupin, A. N. (2010). The effects of self-monitoring on the procedural integrity of a behavioral intervention for young children with developmental disabilities. *Journal of Applied Behavior Analysis, 43,* 315–320.

Pollack, M. J., Fleming, R. K., & Sulzer-Azaroff, B. (1994). Enhancing professional performance through organizational change. *Behavioral Interventions, 9,* 27–42.

Quilitch, H. R. (1975). A comparison of three staff-management procedures. *Journal of Applied Behavior Analysis, 8,* 59–66.

Realon, R. E., Lewallen, J. D., & Wheeler, A. J. (1983). Verbal feedback vs. verbal feedback plus praise: The effects on direct care staff's training behaviors. *Mental Retardation, 21,* 209–212.

Reid, D. H. (2004). Training and supervising direct support personnel to carry out behavioral procedures. In J. L. Matson, R. B. Laud, & M. L. Matson (Eds.), *Behavior modification for persons with developmental disabilities: Treatments and supports* (pp. 73–99). Kingston, NY: NADD Press.

Reid, D. H. (2016). *Promoting happiness among adults with autism and other severe disabilities: Evidence-based strategies.* Morganton, NC: Habilitative Management Consultants.

Reid, D. H. (2017). Competency-based staff training. In J. K. Luiselli (Ed.), *Applied behavior analysis advanced guidebook: A manual for professional practice* (pp. 21–40). San Diego, CA: Elsevier/Academic Press.

Reid, D. H., Green, C. W., & Parsons, M. B. (2003). An outcome management program for extending advances in choice research into choice opportunities for supported workers with severe multiple disabilities. *Journal of Applied Behavior Analysis, 36,* 575–578.

Reid, D. H., & Parsons, M. B. (2002). *Working with staff to overcome challenging behavior among people who have severe disabilities: A guide for getting support plans carried out.* Morganton, NC: Habilitative Management Consultants.

Reid, D. H., Parsons, M. B., & Green, C. W. (1989). *Staff management in human services: Behavioral research and application.* Springfield, IL: Charles C Thomas.

Reid, D. H., Parsons, M. B., & Green, C. W. (2009). *The supervisor training curriculum: Evidence-based ways to promote work quality and enjoyment among support staff.* Washington, DC: American Association on Intellectual and Developmental Disabilities.

Reid, D. H., Parsons, M. B., & Green, C. W. (2012). *The supervisor's guidebook: Evidence-based strategies for promoting work quality and enjoyment among human service staff.* Morganton, NC: Habilitative Management Consultants.

Reid, D. H., Parsons, M. B., & Jensen, J. M. (2017). Maintaining staff performance following a training intervention: Suggestions from a 30-year case example. *Behavior Analysis in Practice, 10,* 12–21.

Reid, D. H., Parsons, M. B., Lattimore, L. P., Towery, D. L., & Reade, K. K. (2005). Improving staff performance through clinician application of outcome management. *Research in Developmental Disabilities, 26,* 101–116.

Reid, D. H., Parsons, M. B., McCarn, J. M., Green, C. W., Phillips, J. F., & Schepis, M. M. (1985). Providing a more appropriate education for severely handicapped persons: Increasing and validating functional classroom tasks. *Journal of Applied Behavior Analysis, 18,* 289–301.

Reid, D. H., Rotholz, D. A., Parsons, M. B., Morris, L., Braswell, B. A., Green, C. W., et al. (2003). Training human service supervisors in aspects of PBS: Evaluation of a statewide, performance-based program. *Journal of Positive Behavior Interventions, 5,* 35–46.

Reid, D. H., & Shoemaker, J. (1984). Behavioral supervision: Methods of improving institutional staff performance. In W. P. Christian, G. T. Hannah, & T. J. Glahn (Eds.), *Programming effective human services: Strategies for institutional change and client transition* (pp. 39–61). New York: Plenum Press.

Reid, D. H., & Whitman, T. L. (1983). Behavioral staff management in institutions: A critical review of effectiveness and acceptability. *Analysis and Intervention in Developmental Disabilities, 3,* 131–149.

Repp, A. C., & Deitz, D. E. D. (1979). Improving administrative-related staff behaviors at a state institution. *Mental Retardation, 17,* 185–192.

Richman, G. S., Riordan, M. R., Reiss, M. L., Pyles, D. A., & Bailey, J. S. (1988). The effects of self-monitoring and supervisor feedback on staff performance in a residential setting. *Journal of Applied Behavior Analysis, 21,* 401–409.

Rosales, R., Gongola, L., & Homlitas, C. (2015). An evaluation of video modeling with embedded instructions to teach implementation of stimulus preference assessments. *Journal of Applied Behavior Analysis, 48,* 209–214.

Roscoe, E. M., Fisher, W. W., Glover, A. C., & Volkert, V. M. (2006). Evaluating the relative effects of feedback and contingent money for staff training of stimulus preference assessments. *Journal of Applied Behavior Analysis, 39,* 63–77.

Sarokoff, R. A., & Sturmey, P. (2004). The effects of behavioral skills training on staff implementation of discrete-trial teaching. *Journal of Applied Behavior Analysis, 37,* 535–538.

Schell, R. M. (1998). Organizational behavior management: Applications with professional staff. *Journal of Organizational Behavior Management, 18(2–3),* 157–171.

Schnell, L. K., Sidener, T. M., DeBar, R. M., Vladescu, J. C., & Kahng, S. (2018). Effects of computer-based training on procedural modifications to standard functional analyses. *Journal of Applied Behavior Analysis, 51,* 87–98.

Scott, J., Lerman, D. C., & Luck, K. (2018). Computer-based training to detect antecedents and consequences of problem behavior. *Journal of Applied Behavior Analysis, 51,* 784–801.

Severtson, J. M., & Carr, J. E. (2012). Training novice instructors to implement errorless discrete-trial teaching: A sequential analysis. *Behavior Analysis in Practice, 5,* 13–23.

Shoemaker, J., & Reid, D. H. (1980). Decreasing chronic absenteeism among institutional staff: Effects of a low-cost attendance program. *Journal of Organizational Behavior Management, 2(4),* 317–328.

Smith, T., Parker, T., Taubman, M., & Lovaas, O. I. (1992). Transfer of staff training from workshops to group homes: A failure to generalize across settings. *Research in Developmental Disabilities, 13,* 57–71.

Sneed, T. J., & Bible, G. H. (1979). An administrative procedure for improving staff performance in an institutional setting for retarded persons. *Mental Retardation, 17,* 92–94.

Strouse, M. C., Carroll-Hernandez, T. A., Sherman, J. A., & Sheldon, J. B. (2003). Turning over turnover: The evaluation of a staff scheduling system in a community-based program for adults with developmental disabilities. *Journal of Organizational Behavior Management, 23*(2–3), 45–63.

Sturmey, P. (1998). History and contribution of organizational behavior management to services for persons with developmental disabilities. *Journal of Organizational Behavior Management, 18*(2–3), 7–32.

Suda, K. T., & Miltenberger, R. G. (1993). Evaluation of staff management strategies to increase positive interactions in a vocational setting. *Behavioral Residential Treatment, 8*, 69–88.

van Oorsouw, W. M., Embregts, P. J., Bosman, A. M., & Jahoda, A. (2009). Training staff serving clients with intellectual disabilities: A meta-analysis of aspects determining effectiveness. *Research in Developmental Disabilities, 30*, 503–511.

Wallace, C. J., Davis, J. R., Liberman, R. P., & Baker, V. (1973). Modeling and staff behavior. *Journal of Consulting and Clinical Psychology, 41*, 422–425.

Wallace, M. D., Doney, J. K., Mintz-Resudek, C. M., & Tarbox, R. S. F. (2004). Training educators to implement functional analyses. *Journal of Applied Behavior Analysis, 37*, 89–92.

Watson, L. S., & Uzzell, R. (1980). A program for teaching behavior modification skills to institutional staff. *Applied Research in Mental Retardation, 1*, 41–53.

Wehman, P. (2011). Employment for persons with disabilities: Where are we now and where do we need to go? *Journal of Vocational Rehabilitation, 35*, 145–151.

Weldy, C. R., Rapp, J. T., & Capocasa, K. (2014). Training staff to implement brief stimulus preference assessments. *Journal of Applied Behavior Analysis, 47*, 214–218.

Welsch, W. V., Ludwig, C., Radiker, J. E., & Krapfl, J. E. (1973). Effects of feedback on daily completion of behavior modification projects. *Mental Retardation, 11*, 24–26.

Whitman, T. L., Hantula, D. A., & Spence, B. H. (1990). Current issues in behavior modification with mentally retarded persons. In J. L. Matson (Ed.), *Handbook of behavior modification with the mentally retarded* (pp. 9–50). New York: Plenum Press.

Williams, W. L., Vittorio, T. D., & Hausherr, L. (2002). A description and extension of a human services management model. *Journal of Organizational Behavior Management, 22*(1), 47–71.

# INTERVENTIONS FOR DECREASING PROBLEM BEHAVIOR

The chapters and their order in Part VI remain the same in this edition of the handbook as in the first edition. In Chapter 18, Smith introduces the reader to the term *antecedent stimuli* and describes the many ways these stimuli affect behavior, their role in functional analysis, and the mechanisms by which they change behavior. The effects of motivating operations, which are one type of antecedent stimuli, constitute a recurring theme in the subsequent chapters of Part VI; thus Smith's chapter sets the stage for new research that the authors of subsequent chapters discuss. An exciting addition to Chapter 18 in this edition is a review of novel research on the effects of environmental enrichment on the brain and on human behavior. In Chapter 19, Vollmer, Athens, and Fernand use the procedure that Iwata et al. described in their classic study on functional analysis as the framework for their discussion of function-based extinction procedures. The chapter includes reviews of classic and more recent studies that have incorporated extinction as treatment for problem behavior. The latter half of the chapter is a review of the response patterns associated with extinction and of why a sound understanding of these patterns is important in clinical practice.

Fisher, Greer, and Bouxsein have updated Chapter 20 on developing function-based positive reinforcement procedures with a focus on new research on functional-communication training. They review studies on the effects of the duration of exposure to the establishing operation and on the effects of multiple schedules on reinforcement schedule thinning, transfer of treatment effects, and relapse. Lerman and Toole note in Chapter 21 that the advent of function analysis has improved the effectiveness of treatments for problem behavior. Thus research on punishment has not grown substantially in recent years outside of that on response interruption and redirection, which Lerman and Toole review. As with punishment, investigators conducted the bulk of research on the token economy in the 1960s and 1970s. Reitman, Boerke, and Vassilopoulos review that research in Chapter 22. They also introduce the reader to studies in which researchers have combined tokens with medication for children with attention-deficit/hyperactivity disorder, and have evaluated children's preference for programs in which children earn versus lose tokens. In sum, readers will find a plethora of useful information in Part VI that they can apply in clinical practice.

# CHAPTER 18

# Developing Antecedent Interventions for Problem Behavior

## Richard G. Smith

Behavioral interventions to treat problem behavior typically involve the manipulation or management of some environmental event or condition, with the intended result to eliminate or reduce problem behavior. We use the term *antecedent intervention* when we manipulate the events or conditions that occur before the behavior.

We can broadly classify antecedent interventions into two categories. *Default* interventions do not depend on identification of the variables that set the occasion for and maintain the problem behavior. Default interventions can be effective for problem behaviors maintained by a range of reinforcers. Examples are antecedent exercise, environmental enrichment, protective equipment, and restraint. By contrast, *function-based* interventions involve identifying the antecedents and consequences that maintain problem behavior, and then directly manipulating at least one component of that operant contingency. We use the term *functional reinforcer* for the consequence that maintains problem behavior (Saini, Fisher, Retzlaff, & Keevy, 2020). For example, *noncontingent reinforcement* (NCR; Vollmer, 1999) is a function-based intervention in which the behavior analyst schedules delivery of the *functional reinforcer* on a time-based, response-independent schedule.

We can further classify antecedent interventions according to the mechanism by which they decrease behavior. Some interventions affect mo-tivating operations for problem behavior (Fisher et al., 2018; Laraway, Snycerski, Michael, & Poling, 2003), whereas others may alter discriminative functions. *Motivating operations* temporarily alter the effectiveness of consequences and the momentary probability of behavior that has produced those consequences in the past (Laraway et al., 2003). For example, NCR involves repeated, response-independent presentation of functional reinforcers; therefore, NCR may decrease problem behavior by abolishing the reinforcing effectiveness of those consequences via satiation or habituation (Murphy, McSweeney, Smith, & McComas, 2003). Thus we would classify NCR as a motivating-operation-based procedure. Other antecedent interventions may manage conditions or stimuli associated with differential consequences for problem behavior, thus altering discriminative control over the behavior. For example, problem behavior will decrease in contexts in which it fails to produce functional reinforcers, and the context will become an *S-delta*.[1] Finally, some interventions

---

[1] Interventions based on discriminative control require manipulation of both antecedent and consequent events to establish and maintain their effectiveness; thus we do not properly characterize them as exclusively antecedent interventions (i.e., the behavior analyst must actively control consequences to maintain the effectiveness of the antecedent stimulus).

arrange the environment so that problem behavior is difficult or impossible to emit. Examples include protective equipment and mechanical restraint.

In the following sections, I describe antecedent behavioral interventions designed to reduce or eliminate behavior. I present a brief review of the literature for each intervention and discuss procedural variations, functional properties (i.e., the behavioral principles that describe their effects), and strengths and limitations, starting with default interventions and following with function-based interventions.

## DEFAULT INTERVENTIONS

Some antecedent procedures will decrease behavior, regardless of the operant function of problem behavior. That is, identification of the functional reinforcer is not necessary when using these interventions. As a result, we may not understand the precise mechanisms associated with these procedures' effects, compared to our understanding of procedures that correspond with a reinforcement contingency. Although prescribing intervention without requiring a prior functional analysis seems clinically expedient, default procedures have significant limitations and produce side effects.

We use the term *default interventions* for interventions whose effects do not depend on the operant function of problem behavior. The term *default* does not mean that problem behavior or the intervention effects are not operant. Like function-based interventions, some default interventions may alter discriminative stimuli ($S^d$s) or motivating operations for problem behavior. However, identifying the contingency maintaining problem behavior is not a necessary component of a potentially effective default intervention.

### Antecedent Exercise

Research has shown that *antecedent exercise* can decrease problem behavior (e.g., Allison, Basile, & MacDonald, 1991; Bachman & Fuqua, 1983; Baumeister & MacLean, 1984; Celiberti, Bobo, Kelly, Harris, & Handleman, 1997; Kern, Koegel, & Dunlap, 1984; Lochbaum & Crews, 2003; McGimsey & Favell, 1988; Powers, Thibadeau, & Rose, 1992). Antecedent exercise engages participants in a program of effortful activities such as aerobic exercise (e.g., jogging, walking, dancing, roller skating) or strength training (e.g., weight lifting). The behavior analyst typically conducts observations during or within a few minutes after exercise completion. Researchers have used antecedent exercise to decrease self-injurious behavior (SIB; Baumeister & MacLean, 1984), aggression (McGimsey & Favell, 1988; Powers et al., 1992), inappropriate vocalizations (Bachman & Fuqua, 1983; Powers et al., 1992), off-task behavior (Bachman & Fuqua, 1983), out-of-seat behavior (Celiberti et al., 1997), and stereotypy (Celiberti et al., 1997; Kern et al., 1984; Powers et al., 1992) exhibited by persons with developmental disabilities. Researchers have also used antecedent exercise to treat depression, with varying degrees of reported success (Doyne, Chambless, & Beutler, 1983); panic disorder (Broocks et al., 1998); and pain disorder (Turner & Clancy, 1988) in persons without developmental disabilities.

Antecedent exercise differs from other interventions involving effortful activity such as overcorrection (Foxx & Azrin, 1972, 1973) because participants engage in it independently of occurrences of the problem behavior, typically before observation sessions. By contrast, overcorrection prescribes effortful activities contingent on problem behavior. Unlike overcorrection, the process of punishment cannot account for the effectiveness of antecedent exercise in decreasing problem behavior, because we do not present it as a consequence for problem behavior.

### Mechanisms Underlying the Effects of Antecedent Exercise

Although the production of a general state of fatigue is an intuitively appealing account of the effects of antecedent exercise, research outcomes seem inconsistent with this interpretation. For example, increases in on-task behavior (Powers et al., 1992), increases in appropriate responding (Kern, Koegel, Dyer, Blew, & Fenton, 1982), and the absence of overt signs of fatigue (Baumeister & MacLean, 1984) after bouts of exercise indicate that the response-decreasing effects of this intervention are at least somewhat specific to problem behavior. In fact, researchers have reported *increases* in several forms of appropriate behavior after antecedent exercise in several studies (e.g., Baumeister & MacLean, 1984; Celiberti et al., 1997; Kern et al., 1982; Powers et al., 1992). These outcomes are somewhat paradoxical. This specificity of action appears to correlate most clearly with the social acceptability of the classes of behavior affected: Problematic behavior decreases and socially acceptable behavior increases after exercise.

Antecedent exercise may alter the reinforcing effectiveness of the consequences that maintain problem behavior (i.e., a motivating-operations effect) (Smith & Iwata, 1997). Some researchers have suggested that antecedent exercise may function as *matched stimulation*, in which exercise produces free access to stimulation like that produced by problem behavior, presumably functioning as an abolishing operation for the maintaining reinforcer. For example, Morrison, Roscoe, and Atwell (2011) observed decreases in automatically reinforced problem behavior both during and after antecedent exercise for three of four participants, suggesting that exercise *devalued* the automatically reinforcing consequences of problem behavior. However, few studies have directly investigated the mechanisms underlying the effects of antecedent exercise. Behavior analysts tend to embrace an abolishing-operation account due to conceptual inconsistencies associated with a stimulus control (or discrimination) account of this effect. However, we should consider a motivating-operations account tentative until more definitive evidence about the behavioral mechanisms underlying the effectiveness of antecedent exercise becomes available.

### Strengths and Limitations of Antecedent Exercise

Strengths of antecedent exercise are that it decreases problem behavior, increases appropriate behavior, and improves both physical and psychological health. Exercise programs have obvious physiological and medical benefits, including improved cardiovascular fitness, muscle tone, and adaptive skills. Results of some studies suggest that antecedent exercise may decrease depression and anxiety and improve measures of general psychological health (Lochbaum & Crews, 2003).

A limitation of antecedent exercise is that its effects appear to be temporary, limited to a brief period immediately following the exercise. Most studies have analyzed only the short-term effects of exercise, often during or just after bouts of exercise; however, the results of more temporally extended analyses suggest that the effects of exercise on problem behavior may be transient (Bachman & Fuqua, 1983; Mays, 2013). For example, two of four participants in one study showed large and immediate decreases in problem behavior after vigorous exercise; however, these results waned across 15-minute observation sessions immediately, 1 hour, and 2 hours after exercise periods (Bachman & Fuqua, 1983). By contrast, a recent study tracked problem behavior over entire school days and showed that the effects of antecedent exercise can persist for several hours (Cannella-Malone, Tullis, & Kazee, 2011). These inconsistent results indicate that we need additional research to determine what alters the durability of the effects of antecedent exercise on problem behavior. Another potential limitation of antecedent exercise is that it may be inconvenient or impossible to implement in some situations (e.g., during academic instruction).

### Enriched Environment

Another way of arranging antecedent conditions to decrease problem behavior is to provide a stimulus-enriched environment. Environmental enrichment involves making preferred items, toys, educational materials, leisure and recreation items, activities, social interaction, or a combination available on a continuous, response-independent schedule. Several studies have demonstrated that environmental enrichment can be an effective intervention for SIB and stereotypic problem behavior (Berkson & Davenport, 1962; Berkson & Mason, 1963, 1965; Cuvo, May, & Post, 2001; Horner, 1980; Rapp, 2006; Ringdahl, Vollmer, Marcus, & Roane, 1997; Saini et al., 2016). Although environmental enrichment may reduce problem behavior maintained by social reinforcement, much of the literature about it has focused on stereotypic problem behavior, suggesting that it may be most appropriate to treat automatically reinforced behavior.

### Mechanisms Underlying the Effects of Environmental Enrichment

At least two reasonable accounts exist for the reductive effects of environmental enrichment. First, environmental enrichment may involve competition between behavior allocated toward the enriching stimuli and problem behavior. That is, environmental enrichment may reduce problem behavior indirectly by providing alternative, competing sources of reinforcement. Results of studies indicate that environmental enrichment is more effective when researchers use highly preferred versus less preferred stimuli (e.g., Vollmer, Marcus, & LeBlanc, 1994). This finding is consistent with the notion that highly preferred stimuli compete effectively with the consequences maintaining problem behavior. One study showed that rotating sets of noncontingently available stimuli produced more durable decreases in problem behavior than did continuous availability of one set of stimuli (DeLeon, Anders, Rodriguez-Catter, & Neidert, 2000). These results suggest that the participant engaged in problem behavior to produce automatic reinforcement when the effectiveness of alternative reinforcement sources waned, due to repeated or extended contact with the single-stimulus set. Rotating alternative stimuli apparently maintained the relative effectiveness of those stimuli and more effectively decreased problem behavior.

On the other hand, environmental enrichment may function as an abolishing operation and may reduce problem behavior if its consequences and those of the environment-enriching materials are similar. In this case, we would consider environmental enrichment a function-based intervention, because its effectiveness would depend on a functional *match* or a relation of *substitutability* between the reinforcers that environmental enrichment produces and those that maintain problem behavior. The effectiveness of the reinforcer for problem behavior may be reduced temporarily or abolished through satiation or habituation, because environmental enrichment produces the same or similar reinforcement (Murphy et al., 2003). Research indicating that antecedent availability of stimuli such as those suspected of maintaining problem behavior (matched stimuli) more effectively suppresses problem behavior than availability of unmatched stimuli (e.g., Favell, McGimsey, & Schell, 1982; Piazza et al., 1998) is consistent with this account. Indeed, Piazza, Adelinis, Hanley, Goh, and Delia (2000) demonstrated that matched stimuli were more effective in decreasing problem behavior than stimuli that participants indicated were more preferred during a preintervention preference assessment. These results indicate that mere competition among reinforcing options may not completely account for the effects of environmental enrichment, and that environmental enrichment may qualify as a function-based intervention in some cases.

A substantial body of research suggests that environmental enrichment can have direct and beneficial effects on the brain, such as increased plasticity in the cerebral cortex and increases in synaptic density (Alwis & Rajan, 2014). Moreover, research results have shown that environmental enrichment can produce improved learning and memory, and that it may be useful to treat a range of neurological disorders, such as Alzheimer's disease and autism spectrum disorder. Thus the effects of environmental enrichment as an intervention for problem behavior may involve both operant conditioning and basic neurological mechanisms; however, direct evidence for the contributions of neurological changes for these effects does not currently exist.

## Strengths and Limitations of Environmental Enrichment

There are several clear benefits to the use of environmental enrichment in practice. First, environmental enrichment is simple, straightforward, easily implemented, and cost-effective. It appears to be especially effective to decrease stereotypic and automatically reinforced behavior, as it provides either a source of competing reinforcement or an alternative means to access reinforcement similar to that maintaining problem behavior. Providing a wide array of alternative forms of stimulation makes sense when the operant function of problem behavior is unclear or difficult to assess directly. In such cases, the probability that a stimulus will function to compete effectively with or replace the reinforcer that problem behavior produces can be increased simply by providing many alternatives. We can further increase the probability of finding an effective alternative stimulus by matching the sensory properties of those stimuli with those associated with the problem behavior. Although environmental enrichment does not teach new or alternative behavior directly, the availability of alternative activities and items appears to be associated with improvements in appropriate object-directed behavior (Horner, 1980).

## Restraint, Protective Equipment, and Other Forms of Response Restriction

Researchers have evaluated the effects of restraint, protective equipment, and other means to mitigate or prevent injury from occurrences of problem behavior (DeRosa, Roane, Wilson, Novak, & Silkowski, 2015; Fisher, Piazza, Bowman, Hanley, & Adelinis, 1997). These interventions physically impede the occurrence or completion of problem behavior. Although these interventions are unquestionably effective in decreasing or eliminating problem behavior, most consider them a highly intrusive, undesirable, and inadequate approach that behavior analysts should only use in emergency situations, such as when problem behavior poses immediate and serious risk to the participant or others or will produce substantial property damage.

We typically categorize procedures for physically restricting problem behavior by their form. *Personal restraint* involves caregivers' physically securing and holding body parts so that problem behavior cannot occur, and caregivers often use it after an episode of problem behavior has begun (i.e., as a consequence-based intervention). However, they can also use personal restraint as an antecedent intervention in situations where problem behavior is highly likely to occur. For example, caregivers may physically restrain a child during dental visits if that child has engaged in problem behavior during previous dental exams and procedures. Mechanical restraint involves securing limbs and body parts with devices designed for this purpose, such as four-point restraints, arm splints, and straightjackets. Caregivers most frequently use mechanical restraint, such as personal restraint, to stop ongoing episodes of problem behavior, but they can also use it as a proactive, antecedent intervention when they anticipate severe problem behavior. Finally, protective equipment is like restraint in that mechanical devices are used; however, protective equipment typically permits the wearer to engage in unrestricted motion but prevents problem behavior from producing damage (e.g., a padded helmet to prevent trauma from head banging). Protective equipment is usually less confining than restraints and may include the use of devices such as safety goggles, helmets, and lap or wheelchair belts. Caregivers can use restraint devices to prevent the occurrence of a range of problem behaviors (e.g., aggression, property destruction, SIB), but protective equipment is used primarily for SIB, as the devices generally protect the wearer from injury.

## Strengths and Limitations of Restraint and Protective Equipment

Restraint and protective equipment eliminate problem behavior effectively when they are used. They are designed specifically to restrict occurrences of problem behavior. Thus no targeted problem behavior typically occurs during restraint periods. However, restraints and protective equipment have serious limitations and side effects. First, many restraint procedures are intrusive, in that they disrupt ongoing activities and often prevent the occurrence of appropriate alternative behavior. That is, the use of restraint may limit many activities, including participation in learning opportunities and appropriate social interactions. Thus restrictive restraint procedures (e.g.,

four-point restraints, straightjackets) are nonconstructive because they do not teach or encourage alternative, replacement behavior; in fact, they may actively impede acquisition of alternative behavior if they restrict appropriate behavior. Second, restraint appears to have aversive properties for some people. For example, some research has indicated that contingent application of restraint can suppress behavior that produces it (e.g., Lerman, Iwata, Shore, & DeLeon, 1997), which is a defining effect of aversive stimulation. Therefore, it is important to consider issues associated with aversive intervention before using restraint. For example, attempts to apply antecedent restraint may and often do occasion avoidance or escape behaviors such as running away or aggression. Additionally, a caregiver may threaten to use contingent restraint if it appears aversive (e.g., "If you do that again, I'll put you in a straightjacket!") or use it as punishment.

Another limitation of restraint is that some individuals who engage in SIB also actively seek opportunities to be placed into restraints or *self-restrain* (e.g., Baroff & Tate, 1969). In extreme cases, individuals may engage in problem behavior to produce access to restraint (Smith, Lerman, & Iwata, 1996; Vollmer & Vorndran, 1998). Some individuals engage in self-restraint almost continuously, interfering with active engagement in habilitative or other desirable behavior. Finally, restricting an individual's ability to engage in a behavior may increase his or her motivation to engage in that behavior. For example, research outcomes have shown that limiting access to leisure activities can produce subsequent increases in engagement in such activities, presumably due to deprivation of their reinforcing aspects (Klatt, Sherman, & Sheldon, 2000). Similarly, restricted access to problem behavior such as SIB may increase subsequent levels of the behavior for some individuals (Blevins, 2003; Rapp, 2006). Thus restraint may merely postpone and ultimately exacerbate the very behavior it is intended to reduce in some cases.

## FUNCTION-BASED INTERVENTIONS

If we know the operant function of problem behavior (i.e., if we can identify the functional reinforcer), we can develop a function-based intervention. Function-based interventions correspond specifically to a maintaining contingency of reinforcement. As such, intervention procedures vary according to the contingency identified to maintain problem behavior. Function-based antecedent interventions manipulate motivating operations, discriminative stimuli, or both. Below, I describe function-based antecedent interventions and their procedural variations. After introducing each general strategy, I describe specific tactical variations associated with those strategies as they relate to different types of maintaining contingencies for problem behavior.

## Noncontingent Reinforcement

NCR involves presentation of the reinforcing consequence for problem behavior on a time-based, or response-independent, schedule (Kettering, Fisher, Kelley, & LaRue, 2018). The behavior analyst often withholds the functional reinforcer when the participant engages in problem behavior (i.e., the problem behavior is placed on extinction). Initial NCR schedules are often dense, in that the behavior analyst provides the functional reinforcer frequently (Hagopian, Fisher, & Legacy, 1994). Subsequently, the behavior analyst may thin the NCR schedule systematically, usually based on low rates of problem behavior (e.g., Vollmer, Iwata, Zarcone, Smith, & Mazaleski, 1993). The goal is to reach a schedule that is manageable in natural environments, or the effective parameters of NCR become apparent as further schedule thinning produces unacceptable increases in problem behavior. Research has shown that NCR is an effective intervention for SIB (Vollmer et al., 1993), aggression (Lalli, Casey, & Kates, 1997), disruption (Fisher, Ninness, Piazza, & Owen-DeSchryver, 1996), food refusal (Cooper et al., 1995), inappropriate vocalizations (Falcomata, Roane, Hovanetz, Kettering, & Keeney, 2004), pica (Goh, Iwata, & Kahng, 1999), and pseudoseizures (DeLeon, Uy, & Gutshall, 2005). See Carr and LeBlanc (2006) for a detailed and comprehensive review of NCR.

Some behavior analysts have criticized the term *noncontingent reinforcement* as technically inaccurate, because (1) reinforcement involves a contingency by definition (i.e., the process of reinforcement is defined in part by a contingency between a response and a consequence), and (2) the target of reinforcement in NCR is unclear (Poling & Normand, 1999). Other behavior analysts have acknowledged the validity of these criticisms (Vollmer, 1999), and many researchers now use more technically correct descriptors, referring to time-based delivery of stimuli or events (e.g., fixed time [FT] 1-minute attention). However, many re-searchers continue to use the term NCR and have established its utility as shorthand for a general class of interventions involving response-independent delivery of stimuli and events (Vollmer, 1999). Therefore, I use the term NCR in the following discussion to describe general procedures, but more descriptively accurate labels for procedural details.

### NCR with Problem Behavior Maintained by Social Positive Reinforcement

As with all function-based interventions, NCR procedures vary according to the functional properties of the problem behavior. For example, if caregiver attention functions as positive reinforcement for problem behavior, then NCR would consist of presenting attention on a time-based schedule and withholding attention following problem behavior. In an early and influential application of NCR, Vollmer et al. (1993) showed that providing no differential consequence following their participants' attention-maintained SIB and providing attention on a time-based schedule produced immediate and substantial decreases in SIB. Initially, the therapist provided continuous attention; however, the therapist subsequently faded the reinforcement schedule to one brief presentation of attention every 5 minutes. Researchers have used NCR to treat a range of problem behaviors maintained by positive reinforcement, including SIB (Vollmer et al., 1993), destructive behavior (Hagopian et al., 1994), and bizarre speech (Mace & Lalli, 1991). Although most NCR procedures schedule time-based stimulus deliveries and withhold functional reinforcement for problem behavior (i.e., extinction), several studies have shown that stimulus presentation alone – *without extinction* – can be sufficient to produce substantial decreases in problem behavior (e.g., Fisher et al., 1999; Lalli et al., 1997).

A few studies have investigated NCR arrangements in which the researchers presented stimuli other than the functional reinforcer for problem behavior (i.e., arbitrary stimuli; Fischer, Iwata, & Mazaleski, 1997; Fisher, DeLeon, Rodriguez-Catter, & Keeney, 2004; Fisher, O'Connor, Kurtz, DeLeon, & Gotjen; 2000; Hanley, Piazza, & Fisher, 1997). For example, Hanley et al. (1997) showed that time-based presentation of a stimulus identified as preferred via formal preference assessment was as effective as presentation of attention (the functional reinforcer for problem behavior) to decrease two participants' problem behavior. Fischer et al. (1997) extended these findings, showing that continuous access to preferred stimuli decreased the positively reinforced problem behavior of two participants, even when the behavior continued to produce the functional reinforcer.

Researchers have used results of preference assessments to select the stimuli for arbitrary NCR arrangements. Fisher et al. (2000) showed that stimuli identified as highly preferred via paired-choice preference assessment (Fisher et al., 1992) more effectively decreased problem behavior than did less preferred stimuli. Researchers have used competing-stimulus assessments to empirically identify preferred stimuli that occasion low levels of problem behavior and high levels of stimulus engagement (Fisher et al., 2000; Fisher et al., 2004). For example, Piazza et al. (1998) used a paired-choice preference assessment to identify a pool of preferred stimuli. Subsequently, therapists provided each stimulus to participants while problem behavior continued to produce the identified maintaining reinforcer. Effective competing stimuli were those stimuli that occasioned low levels of problem behavior and high levels of stimulus engagement during the assessment.

Noncontingent presentation of arbitrary stimuli represents a promising alternative, because it potentially increases the number of available stimuli and may decrease the need for extensive preintervention functional assessment. However, the empirical support for the use of arbitrary stimuli in NCR is currently limited, and several questions remain about the conditions under which arbitrary stimuli will or will not decrease problem behavior, how to best select and present stimuli, and the mechanisms underlying the effects of this procedure.

## NCR with Problem Behavior Maintained by Social Negative Reinforcement

NCR for behavior maintained by escape from aversive stimuli or activities consists of providing time-based breaks from those events. For example, following functional analyses indicating that the SIB of two adult participants with developmental disabilities was maintained by escape from aversive training activities, Vollmer, Marcus, and Ringdahl (1995) implemented NCR interventions in which they presented breaks from these activities independently of the participants' problem behavior. Initially, reinforcement schedules were very dense, with one participant receiving no training tasks, and the second receiving only 15 seconds of training before each 20-second break. However, the researchers systematically decreased the schedule of breaks based on low levels of problem behavior during previous sessions until one participant received a 30-second break once every 10 minutes, and the second participant received a 20-second break every 2.5 minutes. Although only a few studies have evaluated the use of noncontingent escape as intervention, researchers have produced similar outcomes with disruptive behavior during speech therapy (Coleman & Holmes, 1998), problem behavior of children with disabilities during instruction (Kodak, Miltenberger, & Romaniuk, 2003), and disruptive behavior of children without disabilities during dental routines (O'Callaghan, Allen, Powell, & Salama, 2006).

Some researchers have found that providing access to positive reinforcers on time-based schedules can produce decreases in problem behavior maintained by negative reinforcement. For example, several studies have investigated the effectiveness of NCR schedules using positive reinforcers as intervention for negatively reinforced food refusal (e.g., Cooper et al., 1995; Piazza, Patel, Gulotta, Sevin, & Layer, 2003; Reed et al., 2004; Wilder, Normand, & Atwell, 2005). The outcomes of these studies have been mixed. Whereas positive NCR has decreased problem behavior and increased food acceptance for some participants (Wilder et al., 2005), other intervention components such as extinction were necessary to produce clinically acceptable effects for other participants (Piazza et al., 2003; Reed et al., 2004). Ingvarsson, Hanley, and Welter (2009) compared the effectiveness of contingent reinforcement versus NCR, using arbitrary reinforcers to treat escape-maintained disruptive behavior. When both reinforcement schedules were implemented without extinction, results showed that NCR produced a clinically significant decrease in disruptive behavior for one participant; however, extinction was ultimately necessary for a second participant, and additional procedures were necessary for the third participant. These results illustrate the need for further research into the effectiveness of positive NCR to treat problem behavior maintained by negative reinforcement.

## NCR with Problem Behavior Maintained by Automatic Reinforcement

NCR for automatically reinforced behavior typically involves an attempt to identify the automatically produced reinforcer for the behavior, followed by provision of that event on a time-based schedule. In a groundbreaking study, Favell et al. (1982) provided noncontingent access to stimuli that corresponded to the SIB topographies of six participants. For example, the researchers provided toys and items with striking visual properties (e.g., brightly colored toys, lights) to two participants who engaged in eye poking. The researchers provided toys participants could mouth or small food items to participants who engaged in hand mouthing or pica. Results suggested that providing noncontingent access to items that appeared to match the hypothesized functional properties of automatically reinforced problem behavior produced substantial decreases in problem behavior for some participants.

Subsequent research has further investigated the importance of providing stimuli that match the functional properties of automatically reinforced problem behavior in NCR arrangements. For example, Piazza et al. (1998) conducted a series of analyses to identify the specific functional reinforcers for the pica of three participants, and to evaluate the effects of interventions that corresponded to the outcomes. Results indicated that the participants' pica was maintained at least in part by automatic reinforcement. An assessment of the effects of matched (e.g., food) versus unmatched stimuli (e.g., light-up wand) showed that matched stimuli more effectively reduced pica for two participants. Subsequently, the researchers conducted analyses of specific characteristics of matched stimuli, such as taste and texture. Results indicated that food with a firmer texture more effectively decreased pica than less firm food items.

Piazza et al. (2000) extended this approach to other topographies of problem behavior. These investigators compared the effects of providing access to matched versus unmatched stimuli to treat diverse topographies of automatically reinforced behavior (e.g., climbing on furniture, jumping out of windows, aggression, saliva play, hand mouthing) exhibited by three children with developmental disabilities. Researchers compared conditions in which available stimuli matched the hypothesized functional properties of automatically reinforced problem behavior; stimuli did not match the hypothesized functional properties of automatically reinforced problem behavior; or no toys or leisure items were available. Matched stimuli nearly eliminated problem behavior for all three participants, although unmatched stimuli also reduced problem behavior.

Although these outcomes highlight the importance of selecting items that appear to produce stimulation like that suspected of maintaining problem behavior in NCR arrangements, other findings suggest that a match may not always be necessary. Several researchers have used assessments to identify competing stimuli for NCR arrangements with automatically reinforced problem behavior (e.g., Piazza, Fisher, Hanley, Hilker, & Derby, 1996; Ringdahl et al., 1997; Shore, Iwata, DeLeon, Kahng, & Smith, 1997). Researchers have provided participants with access to individual stimuli to identify those that are associated with high levels of engagement and low levels of problem behavior. Using competing-stimulus assessments to select arbitrary stimuli for NCR arrangements seems a promising approach, given the potential difficulty of identifying the hypothesized functional properties of automatically reinforced problem behavior.

## Mechanisms Underlying the Effects of NCR

The behavioral principles that describe the effects of NCR have received considerable attention in the literature. One explanation is that frequent, repeated contact with the functional reinforcer for problem behavior during NCR schedules acts as an abolishing operation, which temporarily decreases the effectiveness of the functional reinforcer and decreases the occurrence of the class of behavior maintained by that reinforcer (Laraway et al., 2003). Although most researchers refer to satiation to explain this decrease in reinforcer effectiveness, some suggest that habituation may better account for these effects (Murphy et al., 2003). Habituation is a decrease in responsiveness to stimuli after repeated presentation of those stimuli (Thompson & Spencer, 1966) and is typically associated with respondent rather than operant behavior. However, Murphy et al. (2003) reviewed research findings that appear to support a habituation account for many operant phenomena, including NCR.

The two accounts have different implications for intervention. For example, habituation is facilitated by fixed rather than variable schedules of stimulus presentation (e.g., Broster & Rankin, 1994); therefore, a habituation account predicts that FT schedules should more effectively abolish the effectiveness of the functional reinforcer than variable-time (VT) schedules. However, some basic research outcomes suggest that VT schedules more effectively suppress responding (e.g., Lattal, 1972; Neuringer, 1973; Ono, 1987), and the results of one applied investigation showed slightly more rapid decreases in VT than in FT conditions (Van

Camp, Lerman, Kelley, Contrucci, & Vorndran, 2000). Another characteristic of habituated behavior is *stimulus specificity*, in which unpredictable changes in the presented stimulus disrupt habituation. Therefore, ensuring a minimum of variation in type, magnitude, and mode of stimulus presentation should enhance NCR effects. Although outcomes in basic research are consistent with this account (e.g., Swithers & Hall, 1994; Whitlow, 1975), no applied research has investigated the effects of stimulus specificity by using time-based schedules.

Regardless of whether the effects of repeated stimulus exposure represent satiation or habituation, both accounts are consistent with the notion that NCR schedules decrease problem behavior due to an abolishing-operation effect, in which the procedure produces a decrease in the value of the functional reinforcer and decreases in responses that have produced that reinforcer in the past. Alternatively, NCR may decrease behavior due to a disruption of the reinforcement contingency. Most NCR procedures contain an extinction component, in that the researcher does not present the functional reinforcer contingent on problem behavior. The response-independent presentation of the functional reinforcer further disrupts the problem behavior–reinforcer contingency. Therefore, decreases in problem behavior may be a function of extinction, at least in part.

Several studies have investigated the relative contributions of extinction and abolishing operations to NCR's reductive effects. For example, some researchers have shown that when they combined NCR schedules with concurrent schedules of response-contingent access to the same reinforcer, responding that produced contingent reinforcement was typically low during dense NCR schedules but increased as NCR schedules were thinned (e.g., Goh, Iwata, & DeLeon, 2000; Marcus & Vollmer, 1996). Others have observed that problem behavior occurred during NCR schedules without extinction (e.g., Kahng, Iwata, Thompson, & Hanley, 2000), or as the researchers thinned the NCR schedule (e.g., Kahng et al., 2000; Simmons, Smith, & Kliethermes, 2003).

Abruptly discontinuing NCR should produce immediate increases in problem behavior according to an extinction account for NCR's behavior-reducing effects. By contrast, in NCR functions as an abolishing operation, problem behavior initially occurs at low levels, followed by an increase as deprivation from the functional reinforcer occurs. Outcomes of investigations have shown both

effects: Problem behavior occurs at relatively low levels following dense NCR schedules, but increases almost immediately following leaner NCR schedules. Thus it seems possible that the effects of NCR reflect a combination of extinction and motivational processes.

Wallace, Iwata, Hanley, Thompson, and Roscoe (2012) directly examined the relative contributions of abolishing operations and extinction during NCR with three participants. In Study 1, lean and dense schedules of NCR with extinction were equally effective in producing large and immediate reductions in problem behavior. In Study 2, the researchers implemented NCR with and without extinction in a multielement design. The procedures were equally effective initially for two participants at dense NCR schedules. Noncontingent reinforcement without extinction was ineffective for the third participant. Problem behavior increased during NCR without extinction as the researchers thinned the NCR schedule. These outcomes, combined with previously reported differences in the persistence of NCR's effects (e.g., Simmons et al., 2003), and the effects of dense and lean NCR schedules on responding in concurrent contingent-reinforcement schedules (e.g., Goh et al., 2000)— suggest that abolishing-operation and extinction processes may combine to produce NCR effects, but that the dynamics that influence their relative contributions (e.g., differences in NCR schedules, amounts, etc.) await further research.

An alternative account of the effects of NCR is that time-based reinforcement delivery produces adventitious reinforcement of alternative behaviors that compete with problem behavior. Using an inventive laboratory preparation to model NCR procedures, Ecott and Critchfield (2004) investigated the effects of NCR on classes of targeted and alternative behaviors. These researchers used college students as participants and designed an experimental environment in which they could (1) measure multiple behaviors and (2) constrain the range of alternative behavior to capture changes in alternative behavior as a function of NCR. Results indicated that behavior previously maintained by contingent reinforcement decreased and alternative behavior increased during NCR, suggesting that alternative behavior was adventitiously reinforced during NCR. The patterns of response reallocation in this experiment were consistent with an account based on *matching law* (e.g., McDowell, 1989), which holds that relative rates of responding among response options corresponds to relative rates of reinforcement for those options. These outcomes may be particularly relevant for arbitrary NCR arrangements, which seem inconsistent with abolishing operation or extinction accounts. A matching law interpretation suggests that NCR may reinforce alternative behavior, thus tipping the scales toward behavior maintained by alternative reinforcement rather than problem behavior. Because we do not typically identify behavior that could be adventitiously reinforced during NCR schedules, behavior analysts using them should closely monitor participants' behavior to assure that NCR does not produce adventitious reinforcement of nontargeted, undesirable behavior.

### Strengths and Limitations of NCR

A large and growing body of research indicates that NCR can be effective to decrease or eliminate problem behavior. Its effects are rapid, and it can mitigate some of the negative side effects of extinction, such as response bursts, aggression, and escape or avoidance of the intervention context (Vollmer et al., 1993). NCR does not produce deprivation when researchers use functional reinforcers. Thus problem behavior may not reemerge as rapidly if events occasionally disrupt the intervention procedures and the reinforcement schedule temporarily thins or stops (Simmons et al., 2003). Researchers have characterized NCR as benign, socially acceptable, and relatively easy to apply (Vollmer et al., 1993).

Despite its apparent strengths, NCR has limitations: It does not directly establish appropriate alternative behavior, and it may limit the effectiveness of training due to potential abolishing-operation effects. For example, Goh et al. (2000) showed that although NCR successfully decreased problem behavior, alternative mands did not increase until substantial decreases in the density of the NCR schedule occurred, which produced an increase in problem behavior for one participant. Another potential limitation is that NCR may produce adventitious reinforcement of unspecified behavior, which may include target or other problem behavior. Indeed, researchers have reported apparent adventitious reinforcement of target problem behavior (e.g., Hagopian, Crockett, van Stone, DeLeon, & Bowman, 2000; Vollmer, Ringdahl, Roane, & Marcus, 1997). Researchers have recommended using differential-reinforcement schedules to overcome this limitation (e.g., Vollmer et al., 1997).

## Stimulus Control Strategies

Schaefer (1970) showed that SIB could be established in rhesus monkeys by presenting food following the response. Furthermore, the monkeys engaged in higher levels of SIB when a control stimulus that had been correlated with the contingent food procedure was present than when it was absent. These results and similar observations suggest that we can bring problem behavior under *stimulus control* through differential reinforcement. Stimulus control develops when an antecedent event, stimulus, or condition regulates behavior because of a history of differential consequences when it is present versus when it is absent (Michael, 2004). These stimuli become *discriminative* because they predict or signal changes in contingencies, and behavior changes correspondingly in their presence.

Although we generally consider stimulus control an antecedent behavioral process, it involves both antecedent and consequent manipulations. The differential consequences that produce discriminative control are ultimately responsible for the effectiveness of discriminative stimuli. Therefore, we should consider stimulus control strategies relative to the characteristics and effects of the consequences with which they are associated. For example, antecedent stimuli that have been correlated with punishment for target behavior may also produce negative side effects, such as aggression and attempts to escape the stimulus.

Researchers have used many different stimulus control procedures to treat problem behavior. For example, researchers have used discrimination training to treat behavior that is only problematic when it occurs in certain circumstances. For example, removing and consuming food from a refrigerator are not inappropriate; however, removing and consuming food that belongs to another person (i.e., food stealing) are. Maglieri, DeLeon, Rodriguez-Catter, and Sevin (2000) paired mild reprimands and placed a warning sticker on prohibited foods to decrease the food stealing of a girl with moderate intellectual developmental disorder and Prader–Willi syndrome. Subsequently, the girl consumed only foods without a warning sticker, even when the researchers delayed contingent reprimands, administered them intermittently, or both.

Researchers have also used stimulus control procedures to promote generalization of intervention effects in contexts and at times when intervention procedures cannot be conducted. For example, Piazza, Hanley, and Fisher (1996) implemented a response interruption procedure for pica in the presence of a signal card. Subsequently, pica decreased when the card was present, even when they did not implement the response interruption procedure. Similarly, McKenzie, Smith, Simmons, and Soderlund (2008) delivered reprimands contingent on eye poking when their participant was wearing wristbands, but not when the wristbands were absent. Eye poking decreased when the participant wore the wristbands, both in the intervention environment and at times when and in places where the researchers did not and had never delivered reprimands.

Researchers have also used discrimination-training procedures to signal changes in contingencies during reinforcement-based interventions for problem behavior. For example, in some situations it may not be possible to deliver functional reinforcers for appropriate communication (such as when a child with attention-maintained SIB requests attention when his or her caregiver is changing an infant sibling's diaper), or the alternative response may occur excessively (such as when a child requests attention continuously). The communication response may be extinguished and problem behavior may increase if the caregiver does not deliver reinforcement for communication responses immediately and consistently (e.g., Briggs, Fisher, Greer, & Kimball, 2018; Hagopian, Fisher, Sullivan, Acquisto, & LeBlanc, 1998). Therefore, procedures to mitigate these effects would be useful. Fisher, Kuhn, and Thompson (1998) taught two participants to mand for functional and alternative reinforcers, and subsequently correlated specific stimuli with the functional and alternative reinforcers. Results showed that problem behavior decreased when either functional or alternative reinforcers were available, and that participants manded appropriately for functional and alternative reinforcers in the presence of the relevant discriminative stimuli (i.e., the mand for the functional reinforcer but not the mand for the alternative reinforcer occurred in the presence of the stimulus correlated with the functional reinforcer's availability, and vice versa). Thus the stimulus control procedure managed problem behavior when delivery of the functional reinforcer for the communication response was not possible. Subsequent studies have used stimulus-control training, typically with condition-correlated stimuli, to manage the rates

of and establish contextual control over communicative responses (e.g., Fisher, Greer, Fuhrman, & Querim, 2015; Hanley, Iwata, & Thompson, 2001; Tiger & Hanley, 2004).

A strength of stimulus control procedures is that they can bring behavior under the control of consequence-based contingencies without necessitating frequent or prolonged contact with those contingencies. Specifically, a behavior analyst can decrease use of aversive consequences by presenting antecedent stimuli that he or she has correlated with those consequences previously. Consider the effects of visible patrol cars on highway speeding. Drivers are more likely to observe speed limits in the presence of patrol cars, which are correlated with an increased probability of receiving a speeding ticket. Frequent punishment of speeding is not necessary to have this effect; police only need to present a stimulus that signals a higher probability of punishment. All *warning* stimuli operate on the same principle: Unwanted behavior decreases *in the moment* not because it is punished, but because a signal has been presented warning that punishment is likely to follow that behavior.

## Antecedent Interventions Designed Specifically to Treat Escape Behavior

Researchers have developed several distinct antecedent interventions to decrease problem behavior maintained by negative reinforcement in the form of escape from or avoidance of aversive events. These strategies are particularly important for several reasons. First, the outcomes of comprehensive reviews indicate that escape from task demands maintains escape behavior for approximately 32% of individuals exhibiting severe problem behavior; a proportion that is greater than any other contingency (Beavers, Iwata, & Lerman, 2013). Second, the antecedents that occasion escape and avoidance are often more obvious and available to immediate manipulation than those that occasion positively reinforced behavior. For example, escape behavior typically is motivated by the presence of some obvious source of aversive stimulation, whereas positive reinforcement is more often motivated by less-apparent operations, such as deprivation. Third, caregivers and therapists often control those sources of aversive stimulation, such as task demands or requests to participate in activities such as educational, dental, medical, or other therapeutic routines. Thus antecedent approaches to the management of potentially aversive situations in ways that might prevent occurrences of problematic escape behavior is, in a sense, "low hanging fruit," in that the antecedent conditions that set the occasion for problem behavior are relatively obvious and available to the caregiver. Below, I describe several antecedent strategies tailored specifically to escape behavior. See Miltenberger (2006) for a comprehensive discussion of antecedent interventions for negatively reinforced behavior.

### Elimination of Aversive Stimulation

Perhaps the most straightforward antecedent intervention for escape behavior is to remove the aversive event that motivates the behavior. By definition, escape behavior occurs in the presence of an aversive stimulus; therefore, removal of that stimulus should eliminate escape behavior, and a large body of literature indicates that it does. The functional-analytic literature is replete with examples in which problem behavior occurs in the presence but not the absence of task demands (e.g., Carr, Newsom, & Binkoff, 1980; Iwata, Dorsey, Slifer, Bauman, & Richman, 1982/1994; Iwata et al., 1994). Although the removal of task demands or other aversive antecedent stimuli is undeniably effective in reducing problem behavior maintained by escape, it is an impractical and unrealistic approach for all but the most serious cases. Eliminating all potentially aversive responsibilities and requirements is simply not possible for most people. Withholding as many of these events as possible on an emergency basis may be necessary in extreme cases when the presentation of task demands or other stressful events sets the occasion for severe and dangerous behavior. A behavior analyst can reintroduce the antecedents of problem behavior systematically when the behavior has decreased to acceptable levels.

A notable exception in which removal of aversive stimulation is the first-choice intervention is when pain or discomfort associated with illness, injury, or other biological factors occasions problem behavior. Several researchers have suggested that conditions such as allergies (Kennedy & Meyer, 1996), constipation (Carr & Smith, 1995), menstrual discomfort (Carr, Smith, Giacin, Whelan, & Pancari, 2003; Taylor, Rush, Hetrick, & Sandman, 1993), otitis media (Carr & Smith, 1995; Cataldo & Harris, 1982; O'Reilly, 1995), and sleep deprivation (Kennedy & Meyer, 1996) may be associated with escape-maintained problem behavior. Caregivers should arrange immediate

treatment for any medical or biological condition that they suspect contributes to the motivation of SIB. They may consider additional interventions if SIB persists after medical intervention.

### Fading in Aversive Stimuli

One way to return aversive events to the environment following their elimination is through stimulus fading (e.g., Pace, Ivancic, & Jefferson, 1994; Pace, Iwata, Cowdery, Andree, & McIntyre, 1993; Zarcone, Iwata, Smith, Mazaleski, & Lerman, 1994; Zarcone et al., 1993). Fading is the gradual and systematic reintroduction of stimuli that occasion escape behavior. Zarcone et al. (1993) compared fading plus extinction with extinction alone to reduce the escape-maintained SIB of three participants. During fading, the researchers eliminated task demands that occasioned SIB. Subsequently, they reintroduced task demands slowly and systematically while providing no differential consequence for SIB (i.e., extinction). Extinction alone produced more rapid decreases in SIB, but also resulted in initial extinction bursts that were not observed during fading. Attempts to use fading procedures without extinction have met with mixed results. Some researchers have produced encouraging outcomes (e.g., Pace et al., 1994), and others have failed to maintain initial decreases in problem behavior without extinction (e.g., Zarcone, Iwata, Smith, et al., 1994).

The behavioral processes underlying the effectiveness of fading procedures are not well understood. Fading with extinction may permit behavior to contact extinction contingencies in the presence of a relatively weak establishing operation. That is, extinction may proceed more smoothly if the antecedent stimuli that motivate escape are altered to decrease their aversiveness (Greer, Fisher, Saini, Owen, & Jones, 2016). Slow but repeated exposure may reduce the overall aversiveness of stimuli when fading is effective without extinction. Indeed, desensitization, or graduated exposure to stimuli that occasion escape or avoidance, is a widely used procedure to treat phobias (e.g., Shabani & Fisher, 2006). The precise mechanism responsible for this effect is not understood, although habituation offers a potentially viable account (Murphy et al., 2003).

### High-Probability Sequence/Behavioral Momentum

Like fading, high-probability (high-p) sequences can be used to facilitate reintroduction of aversive stimuli to the environment. A behavior analyst delivers several high-*p* requests (ones with a high probability of compliance and that do not occasion escape behavior) before delivering a *low-probability* (low-*p*) request (one that has a low probability of compliance, occasions problematic escape behavior, or both). Researchers have used high-*p* sequences to increase compliance with low-*p* requests (e.g., Mace et al., 1988) and to treat escape-maintained problem behavior (e.g., Mace & Belfiore, 1990). Researchers have used the metaphor of *behavioral momentum* to describe these effects. According to this account, a high density of reinforcement for high-*p* requests increases mass and creates velocity in compliance, which makes this class of behavior resistant to change (Nevin, 1996). Thus compliance persists and problematic escape behavior is unlikely to occur when the behavior analyst presents a low-*p* request. Researchers have used high-*p* sequences successfully to treat noncompliance to *do* and *don't* commands (Mace et al., 1988), academic tasks (Belfiore, Lee, Vargas, & Skinner, 1997; Wehby & Hollahan, 2000), and medical routines (McComas, Wacker, & Cooper, 1998). However, results of research suggest that extinction may be necessary to treat active escape behavior such as SIB and aggression. In some cases, using the high-*p* sequence without extinction may exacerbate escape behavior (e.g., Zarcone, Iwata, Mazaleski, & Smith, 1994).

Recent research on high-*p* sequences to treat food refusal or selectivity illustrates both the promise and some apparent limitations of such interventions. McComas, Wacker, et al. (2000) showed that adding a high-*p* sequence to escape extinction for bite refusal improved the effectiveness of extinction. Subsequently, Dawson et al. (2003) observed increases in acceptance and decreases in problem behavior only during high-*p* sequences plus escape extinction, and not during high-*p* sequences alone. However, other researchers have shown that a high-*p* sequence without extinction can be sufficient to increase bite acceptance for some participants (e.g., Ewry & Fryling, 2015; Meier, Fryling, & Wallace, 2012; Patel et al., 2006). Interestingly, studies reporting successful outcomes of high-*p* sequences without extinction used high-*p* requests that were topographically like the behavior targeted for increase. For example, Meier et al. (2012) used acceptance of highly preferred food as the high-*p* response that preceded low-*p* requests to accept bites of nonpreferred food. Given that the nature of high-*p* requests appears to have influenced the effectiveness of such request sequences, the mechanism(s) responsible for intervention effects in these studies are unclear. Specifically, topographical features of the high- and low-*p* responses should not be relevant for a behavioral-momentum-based account of the effects of high-*p* sequences. Thus additional investigations will be necessary to clearly identify the conditions under which high-*p* sequences are most efficacious, and the behavioral mechanisms that produce their effects.

## Altering the Aversive Stimulus

Altering the features of the aversive stimulus or event that sets the occasion for escape behavior to reduce its evocative effect is a possible intervention. For example, Cameron, Ainsleigh, and Bird (1992) showed that the escape SIB of one participant was more likely to occur during washing routines with bar rather than liquid soap. Thus researchers simply altered the task and presented liquid rather than bar soap during washing routines. Similarly, researchers have shown that changes such as using a computer instead of pencil and paper for writing (Ervin, DuPaul, Kern, & Friman, 1998), or using checkers or a calculator as counting aids during math tasks (McComas, Hoch, Paone, & El-Roy, 2000), can function as abolishing operations, effectively decreasing the aversiveness of tasks so that they no longer evoke escape behavior. Despite these encouraging results, altering aversive events to make them more benign may not always be possible (e.g., when liquid soap, computers, checkers, or calculators are unavailable). Thus problem behavior will likely return to preintervention levels when avoiding contact with aversive events is not possible.

## Altering the Aversive Context

Another way to reduce the aversiveness of antecedent stimuli is to alter features of the context in which a behavior analyst presents those stimuli. With contextual interventions, the analyst changes the surrounding environment to reduce the aversiveness of antecedent stimuli. Thus contextual interventions do not involve direct manipulation of the aversive stimulus or event per se; rather, the behavior analyst alters other aspects of the environment, which then decrease the evocative function (aversiveness) of the stimulus or event. Researchers have shown that many contextual variables alter the occurrence of problematic escape behavior and have manipulated them as interventions. For example, results of studies have shown that embedding task demands in pleasant stories (Carr, Newsom, & Binkoff, 1976) or in preferred activities (Carr & Carlson, 1993) decreases escape behavior. Similarly, Dunlap, Kern-Dunlap, Clarke, and Robbins (1991) increased on-task behavior and decreased problem behavior for one participant by altering session length, type of motor activity, and the functional nature of presented tasks.

Several researchers have shown that offering a choice among putatively aversive activities can decrease escape behavior (e.g., Dunlap et al., 1994; Dyer, Dunlap, & Winterling, 1990; Vaughn & Horner, 1997). Some outcomes suggest that this effect will occur even if the researchers' choices are yoked to those of participants' (Dyer et al., 1990), or if participants choose from low-preference tasks that have evoked high levels of escape behavior previously (Vaughn & Horner, 1997).

Research outcomes have shown that temporally distant routines and events can sometimes set the occasion for later occurrences of problem behavior. Some use the term *setting events*, but see Smith and Iwata (1997) for a discussion of issues with that term. For example, Kennedy and Itkonen (1993) showed that one participant's problem behavior at school was more likely to occur on days when she awakened late. A second participant's problem behavior correlated with the number of stops on her ride to school. Each participant's problem behavior decreased when researchers eliminated these situations from their routines. When behavior analysts cannot eliminate events that set the occasion for problem behavior, they may be able to neutralize their influence. For example, Horner, Day, and Day (1997) found that prior postponements or delays in planned activities exacerbated the escape-maintained problem behavior of two participants during subsequent instructional routines. The researchers conducted *neutralizing* routines (the opportunity to draw and write for one participant, and the opportunity to reschedule the event and look at a yearbook for the other participant) on days when the conditions correlated with problem behavior were present before instructional sessions. Problem behavior decreased substantially on the days when researchers conducted neutralizing routines.

Some other contextually based interventions include altering the timing of requests to avoid interrupting preferred activities (e.g., Fritz, DeLeon, & Lazarchick, 2004), presenting stimuli associated with a positive mood (e.g., Carr, Magito McLaugh-lin, Giacobbe-Grieco, & Smith, 2003), and the presentation of corrective feedback before (as antecedent prompts) rather than after task trials (Ebanks & Fisher, 2003), among others. The effects of most contextual strategies appear to be due to abolishing-operation effects, in which changing an apparently unrelated condition alters the motivational properties of aversive events; that is, they decrease the aversiveness of the events that motivate escape. Additional research will be necessary to identify the specific mechanisms associated with the effectiveness of various contextual strategies.

## SUMMARY

Researchers have used an array of antecedent interventions to decrease problem behavior. Some strategies decrease the motivation to engage in the behavior; others signal differential consequences for the behavior; and still others physically impede the occurrence of behavior in some way. Although each intervention has unique benefits and limitations, all share the characteristic that they are implemented before the occurrence of problem behavior. Thus a shared strength among antecedent strategies is that they do not require the occurrence of problem behavior for their effectiveness (certain discrimination-based interventions constitute a possible exception, as previously discussed). In some cases, problem behavior may not occur at all after the first implementation of intervention.

Antecedent interventions may also complement or accelerate the effects of consequence-based interventions. Researchers have paired antecedent strategies with extinction procedures to decrease negative side effects associated with extinction (e.g., Zarcone, Iwata, Smith, et al., 1994). Researchers also have incorporated antecedent strategies into packages including differential reinforcement (e.g., Kodak et al., 2003; Marcus & Vollmer, 1996; Shabani & Fisher, 2006), punishment (e.g., Thompson, Iwata, Conners, & Roscoe, 1999), and pharmacological interventions (e.g., Allison et al., 1991).

A shared limitation of antecedent strategies is that they do not build or encourage new, alternative forms of behavior (i.e., they are not constructive), because the establishment of new behavior or maintenance of alternative behavior requires that we manage reinforcing consequences. Certainly behavior analysts incorporate antecedent manipulations such as prompts and instructions into repertoire-building interventions. But because the analysts also must manage the consequences that are ultimately responsible for the effectiveness of these strategies (i.e., reinforcement), these are not considered antecedent strategies. Also, some antecedent strategies, such as NCR, may interfere with acquisition of alternative behavior due to habituation or satiation effects. When combining NCR with procedures to increase appropriate behavior, behavior analysts should closely monitor the outcomes and use alternative reinforcers or varied consequences to ensure adequate progress. Thus antecedent strategies—alone—do not systematically establish or maintain positive alternatives to problem behavior.

Although researchers have shown that antecedent procedures are effective in treating problem behavior, a behavior analyst should implement them as components in a comprehensive intervention package that includes both antecedent and consequence strategies. Antecedents alone can produce behavior and consequences alone can affect behavior that produces it; however, combining both can enhance the effects of each, improving the ability of antecedents to evoke or suppress behavior and providing more opportunities to contact more effective consequences. Thus behavior analysts should carefully match antecedents and consequences in behavior intervention programs to maximize the potential effectiveness of each strategy. As shown in this chapter, a wide range of proven antecedent strategies is available for integration in comprehensive intervention packages to treat problem behaviors and help establish appropriate alternative repertoires.

## REFERENCES

Allison, D. B., Basile, V. C., & MacDonald, R. B. (1991). Brief report: Comparative effects of antecedent exercise and lorazepam on aggressive behavior of an autistic man. *Journal of Autism and Developmental Disorders, 21,* 89–94.

Alwis, D. S., & Rajan, R. (2014). Environmental enrichment and the sensory brain: The role of enrichment in remediating brain injury. *Frontiers in Systems Neuroscience, 8,* 156.

Bachman, J. E., & Fuqua, R. W. (1983). Management of inappropriate behaviors of trainable mentally impaired students using antecedent exercise. *Journal of Applied Behavior Analysis, 16,* 477–484.

Baroff, G. S., & Tate, B. G. (1968). The use of aversive stimulation in the treatment of chronic self-injurious

behavior. *Journal of the American Academy of Child Psychiatry, 7,* 454–470.

Baumeister, A. A., & MacLean, W, E., Jr. (1984). Deceleration of self-injurious and stereotypic responding by exercise. *Applied Research in Mental Retardation, 5,* 385–393.

Beavers, G. A., Iwata, B. A., & Lerman, D. C. (2013). Thirty years of research on the functional analysis of problem behavior. *Journal of Applied Behavior Analysis, 46,* 1–21.

Belfiore, P. J., Lee, D. L., Vargas, A. U., & Skinner, C. H. (1997). Effects of high-preference single-digit mathematics problem completion on multiple-digit mathematics problem performance. *Journal of Applied Behavior Analysis, 30,* 327–330.

Berkson, G., & Davenport, R. K. (1962). Stereotyped movements of mental defectives. *American Journal of Mental Deficiency, 66,* 849–852.

Berkson, G., & Mason, W. A. (1963). Stereotyped movements of mental defectives: III. Situation effects. *American Journal of Mental Deficiency, 68,* 409–412.

Blevins, T. (2003). *The effects of response restriction on non-socially maintained self-injury.* Unpublished master's thesis, University of North Texas, Denton, TX.

Briggs, A. M., Fisher, W. W., Greer, B. D., & Kimball, R. T. (2018). Prevalence of resurgence of destructive behavior when thinning reinforcement schedules during functional communication training. *Journal of Applied Behavior Analysis, 51,* 620–633.

Broocks, A., Bandelow, B., Pekrun, G., George, A., Meyer, T., Bartmann, U., et al. (1998). Comparison of aerobic exercise, chlomipramine, and placebo in the treatment of panic disorder. *American Journal of Psychiatry, 155,* 603–609.

Broster, B. S., & Rankin, C. H. (1994). Effects of changing interstimulus interval during habituation in *Caenorhabditis elegans. Behavioral Neuroscience, 108,* 1019–1029.

Cameron, M. J., Ainsleigh, S. A., & Bird, F. L. (1992). The acquisition of stimulus control of compliance and participation during an ADL routine. *Behavioral Residential Treatment, 7,* 327–340.

Cannella-Malone, H. I., Tullis, C. A., & Kazee, A. R. (2011). Using antecedent exercise to decrease challenging behavior in boys with developmental disabilities and an emotional disorder. *Journal of Positive Behavior Interventions, 13,* 230–239.

Carr, E. G., & Carlson, J. I. (1993). Reduction of severe behavior problems in the community using a multicomponent treatment approach. *Journal of Applied Behavior Analysis, 26,* 157–172.

Carr, E. G., Magito McLaughlin, D., Giacobbe-Grieco, T., & Smith, C. E. (2003). Using mood ratings and mood induction in assessment and intervention for severe problem behavior. *American Journal on Mental Retardation, 108,* 32–55.

Carr, E. G., Newsom, C. D., & Binkoff, J. A. (1976). Stimulus control of self-destructive behavior in a psychotic child. *Journal of Abnormal Child Psychology,* 4, 139–153.

Carr, E. G., Newsom, C. D., & Binkoff, J. A. (1980). Escape as a factor in the aggressive behavior of two retarded children. *Journal of Applied Behavior Analysis,* 13, 101–117.

Carr, E. G., & Smith, C. E. (1995). Biological setting events for self-injury. *Mental Retardation and Developmental Disabilities Research Reviews,* 1, 94–98.

Carr, E. G., Smith, C. E., Giacin, T. A., Whelan, B. M., & Pancari, J. (2003). Menstrual discomfort as a biological setting event for severe problem behavior: Assessment and intervention. *American Journal on Mental Retardation,* 108, 117–133.

Carr, J. E., & LeBlanc, L. A. (2006). Noncontingent reinforcement as antecedent behavior support. In J. Luiselli (Ed.), *Antecedent assessment and intervention: Supporting children and adults with developmental disabilities in community settings* (pp. 147–164). Baltimore: Brookes.

Cataldo, M. F., & Harris, J. (1982). The biological basis of self-injury in the mentally retarded. *Analysis and Intervention in Developmental Disabilities,* 7, 21–39.

Celiberti, D. A., Bobo, H. E., Kelly, K. S., Harris, S. L., & Handleman, J. S. (1997). The differential and temporal effects of antecedent exercise on the self-stimulatory behavior of a child with autism. *Research in Developmental Disabilities,* 18, 139–150.

Coleman, C., & Holmes, P. (1998). The use of noncontingent escape to reduce disruptive behaviors in children with speech delays. *Journal of Applied Behavior Analysis,* 31, 687–690.

Cooper, L. J., Wacker, D. P., McComas, J., Brown, K., Peck, S. M., Richman, D., et al. (1995). Use of component analysis to identify active variables in treatment packages for children with feeding disorders. *Journal of Applied Behavior Analysis,* 28, 139–153.

Cuvo, A. J., May, M. E., & Post, T. M. (2001). Effects of living room, Snoezelen room, and outdoor activities on stereotypic behavior and engagement by adults with profound mental retardation. *Research in Developmental Disabilities,* 22, 183–204.

Dawson, J. E., Piazza, C. C., Sevin, B. M., Gulotta, C. S., Lerman, D., & Kelly, M. L. (2003). Use of the high-probability instructional sequence and escape extinction in a child with food refusal. *Journal of Applied Behavior Analysis,* 36, 105–108.

DeLeon, I. G., Anders, B. M., Rodriguez-Catter, V., & Neidert, P. L. (2000). The effects of noncontingent access to single-versus multiple-stimulus sets on self-injurious behavior. *Journal of Applied Behavior Analysis,* 33, 623–626.

DeLeon, I. G., Uy, M., & Gutshall, K. (2005). Noncontingent reinforcement and competing stimuli in the treatment of pseudoseizures and destructive behaviors. *Behavioral Interventions,* 20, 203–217.

DeRosa, N. M., Roane, H. S., Wilson, J. L., Novak, M. D., & Silkowski, E. L. (2015). Effects of arm-splint rigidity on self-injury and adaptive behavior. *Journal of Applied Behavior Analysis,* 48, 860–864.

Doyne, E. J., Chambless, D. L., & Beutler, L. E. (1983). Aerobic exercise as a treatment for depression in women. *Behavior Therapy,* 14, 434–440.

Dunlap, G., dePerczel, M., Clarke, S., Wilson, D., Wright, S., White, R., et al. (1994). Choice making to promote adaptive behavior for students with emotional and behavioral challenges. *Journal of Applied Behavior Analysis,* 27, 505–518.

Dunlap, G., Kern-Dunlap, L., Clarke, S., & Robbins, F. R. (1991). Functional assessment, curricular revision, and severe behavior problems. *Journal of Applied Behavior Analysis,* 24, 387–397.

Dyer, K., Dunlap, G., & Winterling, V. (1990). Effects of choice making on the serious problem behaviors of students with severe handicaps. *Journal of Applied Behavior Analysis,* 23, 515–524.

Ebanks, M. E., & Fisher, W. W. (2003). Altering the timing of academic prompts to treat destructive behavior maintained by escape. *Journal of Applied Behavior Analysis,* 36, 355–359.

Ecott, C. L., & Critchfield, T. S. (2004). Noncontingent reinforcement, alternative reinforcement, and the matching law: A laboratory demonstration. *Journal of Applied Behavior Analysis,* 37, 249–265.

Ervin, R. A., DuPaul, G. J., Kern, L., & Friman, P. C. (1998). Classroom-based functional and adjunctive assessments: Proactive approaches to intervention selection for adolescents with attention deficit hyperactivity disorder. *Journal of Applied Behavior Analysis,* 31, 65–78.

Ewry, D. M., & Fryling, M. J. (2015). Evaluating the high-probability instructional sequence to increase the acceptance of foods with an adolescent with autism. *Behavior Analysis in Practice,* 8, 1–4.

Falcomata, T. S., Roane, H. S., Hovanetz, A. N., Kettering, T. L., & Keeney, K. M. (2004). An evaluation of response cost in the treatment of inappropriate vocalizations maintained by automatic reinforcement. *Journal of Applied Behavior Analysis,* 37, 83–87.

Favell, J. E., McGimsey, J. F., & Schell, R. M. (1982). Treatment of self-injury by providing alternate sensory activities. *Analysis and Intervention in Developmental Disabilities,* 2, 83–104.

Fischer, S. M., Iwata, B. A., & Mazaleski, J. L. (1997). Noncontingent delivery of arbitrary reinforcers as treatment for self-injurious behavior. *Journal of Applied Behavior Analysis,* 30, 239–249.

Fisher, W. W., DeLeon, I. G., Rodriguez-Catter, V., & Keeney, K. M. (2004). Enhancing the effects of extinction on attention-maintained behavior through noncontingent delivery of attention or stimuli identified via a competing stimulus assessment. *Journal of Applied Behavior Analysis,* 37, 171–184.

Fisher, W. W., Greer, B. D., Fuhrman, A. M., & Querim, A. C. (2015). Using multiple schedules during functional communication training to promote rapid transfer of treatment effects. *Journal of Applied Behavior Analysis, 48,* 713–733.

Fisher, W. W., Greer, B. D., Mitteer, D. R., Fuhrman, A. M., Romani, P. W., & Zangrillo, A. N. (2018). Further evaluation of differential exposure to establishing operations during functional communication training. *Journal of Applied Behavior Analysis, 51,* 360–373.

Fisher, W. W., Kuhn, D. E., & Thompson, R. H. (1998). Establishing discriminative control of responding using functional and alternative reinforcers during functional communication training. *Journal of Applied Behavior Analysis, 31,* 543–560.

Fisher, W. W., Ninness, H. A. C., Piazza, C. C., & Owen-DeSchryver, J. S. (1996). On the reinforcing effects of the content of verbal attention. *Journal of Applied Behavior Analysis, 29,* 235–238.

Fisher, W. W., O'Connor, J. T., Kurtz, P. F., DeLeon, I. G., & Gotjen, D. L. (2000). The effects of noncontingent delivery of high- and low-preference stimuli on attention-maintained destructive behavior. *Journal of Applied Behavior Analysis, 33,* 79–83.

Fisher, W., Piazza, C. C., Bowman, L. G., Hagopian, L. P., Owens, J. C., & Slevin, I. (1992). A comparison of two approaches for identifying reinforcers for persons with severe and profound disabilities. *Journal of Applied Behavior Analysis, 25,* 491–498.

Fisher, W. W., Piazza, C. C., Bowman, L. G., Hanley, G. P., & Adelinis, J. D. (1997). Direct and collateral effects of restraints and restraint fading. *Journal of Applied Behavior Analysis, 30,* 105–120.

Fisher, W. W., Thompson, R. H., DeLeon, I. G., Piazza, C. C., Kuhn, D. E., Rodriquez-Catter, V., et al. (1999). Noncontingent reinforcement: Effects of satiation versus choice responding. *Research in Developmental Disabilities, 20,* 411–427.

Foxx, R. M., & Azrin, N. H. (1972). Restitution: A method of eliminating aggressive disruptive behavior of retarded and brain damaged patients. *Behaviour Research and Therapy, 10,* 15–27.

Foxx, R. M., & Azrin, N. H. (1973). The elimination of autistic self-stimulatory behavior by overcorrection. *Journal of Applied Behavior Analysis, 6,* 1–14.

Fritz, J., DeLeon, I. G., & Lazarchick, W. (2004). Separating the influence of escape and access to preferred activities on problem behavior occurring in instructional contexts. *Behavioral Interventions, 19,* 159–171.

Goh, H., Iwata, B. A., & DeLeon, I. G. (2000). Competition between noncontingent and contingent reinforcement schedules during response acquisition. *Journal of Applied Behavior Analysis, 33,* 195–205.

Goh, H., Iwata, B. A., & Kahng, S. (1999). Multicomponent assessment and treatment of cigarette pica. *Journal of Applied Behavior Analysis, 32,* 297–316.

Greer, B. D., Fisher, W. W., Saini, V., Owen, T. M., & Jones, J. K. (2016). Functional communication training during reinforcement schedule thinning: An analysis of 25 applications. *Journal of Applied Behavior Analysis, 49,* 105–121.

Hagopian, L. P., Crockett, J. L., van Stone, M., DeLeon, I. G., & Bowman, L. G. (2000). Effects of noncontingent reinforcement on problem behavior and stimulus engagement: The role of satiation, extinction, and alternative reinforcement. *Journal of Applied Behavior Analysis, 33,* 433–449.

Hagopian, L. P., Fisher, W. W., & Legacy, S. M. (1994). Schedule effects of noncontingent reinforcement on attention-maintained destructive behavior in identical quadruplets. *Journal of Applied Behavior Analysis, 27,* 317–325.

Hagopian, L. P., Fisher, W. W., Sullivan, M. T., Acquisto, J., & LeBlanc, L. A. (1998). Effectiveness of functional communication training with and without extinction and punishment: A summary of 21 inpatient cases. *Journal of Applied Behavior Analysis, 31,* 211–235.

Hanley, G. P., Iwata, B. A., & Thompson, R. H. (2001). Reinforcement schedule thinning following treatment with functional communication training. *Journal of Applied Behavior Analysis, 34,* 17–38.

Hanley, G. P., Piazza, C. C., & Fisher, W. W. (1997). Noncontingent presentation of attention and alternative stimuli in the treatment of attention maintained destructive behavior. *Journal of Applied Behavior Analysis, 30,* 229–237.

Horner, R. D. (1980). The effects of an environmental enrichment program on the behavior of institutionalized profoundly retarded children. *Journal of Applied Behavior Analysis, 13,* 473–491.

Horner, R. H., Day, H. M., & Day, J. R. (1997). Using neutralizing routines to reduce problem behaviors. *Journal of Applied Behavior Analysis, 30,* 601–614.

Ingvarsson, E. T., Hanley, G. P., & Welter, K. M. (2009). Treatment of escape-maintained behavior with positive reinforcement: The role of reinforcement contingency and density. *Education and Treatment of Children, 32,* 371–401.

Iwata, B. A., Dorsey, M. F., Slifer, K. J., Bauman, K. E., & Richman, G. S. (1994). Toward a functional analysis of self-injury. *Journal of Applied Behavior Analysis, 27,* 197–209. (Reprinted from *Analysis and Intervention in Developmental Disabilities, 2,* 3–20, 1982)

Iwata, B. A., Pace, G. M., Dorsey, M. F., Zarcone, J. R., Vollmer, T. R., Smith, R. G., et al. (1994). The functions of self-injurious behavior: An experimental-epidemiological analysis. *Journal of Applied Behavior Analysis, 27,* 215–240.

Kahng, S., Iwata, B. A., Thompson, R. H., & Hanley, G. P. (2000). A method for identifying satiation versus extinction effects under noncontingent reinforcement schedules. *Journal of Applied Behavior Analysis, 33,* 419–432.

Kennedy, C. H., & Itkonen, T. (1993). Effects of setting events on the problem behavior of students with severe disabilities. *Journal of Applied Behavior Analysis, 26,* 321–328.

Kennedy, C. H., & Meyer, K. A. (1996). Sleep deprivation, allergy symptoms, and negatively reinforced problem behavior. *Journal of Applied Behavior Analysis, 29,* 133–135.

Kern, L., Koegel, R. L., & Dunlap, G. (1984). The influence of vigorous versus mild exercise on autistic stereotyped behaviors. *Journal of Autism and Developmental Disorders, 14,* 57–67.

Kern, L., Koegel, R. L., Dyer, K., Blew, P. A., & Fenton, L. R. (1982). The effects of physical exercise on self-stimulatory and appropriate responding in autistic children. *Journal of Autism and Developmental Disabilities, 12,* 399–419.

Kettering, T. L., Fisher, W. W., Kelley, M. E., & LaRue, R. H. (2018). Sound attenuation and preferred music in the treatment of problem behavior maintained by escape from noise. *Journal of Applied Behavior Analysis, 51,* 687–693.

Klatt, K. P., Sherman, J. A., & Sheldon, J. B. (2000). Effects of deprivation on engagement in preferred activities by persons with developmental disabilities. *Journal of Applied Behavior Analysis, 33,* 495–506.

Kodak, T., Miltenberger, R. G., & Romaniuk, C. (2003). The effects of differential negative reinforcement of other behavior and noncontingent escape on compliance. *Journal of Applied Behavior Analysis, 36,* 379–382.

Lalli, J. S., Casey, S. D., & Kates, K. (1997). Noncontingent reinforcement as treatment for severe problem behavior: Some procedural variations. *Journal of Applied Behavior Analysis, 30,* 127–137.

Laraway, S., Snycerski, S., Michael, J., & Poling, A. (2003). Motivating operations and terms to describe them: Some further refinements. *Journal of Applied Behavior Analysis, 36,* 407–414.

Lattal, K. A. (1972). Response–reinforcer independence and conventional extinction after fixed-interval and variable-interval schedules. *Journal of the Experimental Analysis of Behavior, 18,* 133–140.

Lerman, D. C., Iwata, B. A., Shore, B. A., & DeLeon, I. G. (1997). Effects of intermittent punishment on self-injurious behavior: An evaluation of schedule thinning. *Journal of Applied Behavior Analysis, 30,* 187–201.

Lochbaum, M. R., & Crews, D. J. (2003). Viability of cardiorespiratory and muscular strength programs for the adolescent with autism. *Complementary Health Practice Review, 8,* 225–233.

Mace, F. C., & Belfiore, P. (1990). Behavioral momentum in the treatment of escape-motivated stereotypy. *Journal of Applied Behavior Analysis, 23,* 507–514.

Mace, F. C., Hock, M. L., Lalli, J. S., West, B. J., Belfiore, P., Pinter, E., et al. (1988). Behavioral momentum in the treatment of noncompliance. *Journal of Applied Behavior Analysis, 21,* 123–141.

Mace, F. C., & Lalli, J. S. (1991). Linking descriptive and experimental analysis in the treatment of bizarre speech. *Journal of Applied Behavior Analysis, 24,* 553–562.

Maglieri, K. A., DeLeon, I. G., Rodriguez-Catter, V., & Sevin, B. (2000). Treatment of covert food stealing in an individual with Prader–Willi syndrome. *Journal of Applied Behavior Analysis, 33,* 615–618.

Marcus, B. A., & Vollmer, T. R. (1996). Combining noncontingent reinforcement and differential reinforcement schedules as treatment for aberrant behavior. *Journal of Applied Behavior Analysis, 29,* 43–51.

Mays, M. N. (2013). *Using antecedent aerobic exercise to decrease stereotypic behavior in children with autism.* Unpublished doctoral dissertation, Georgia State University, Atlanta, GA.

McComas, J., Hoch, H., Paone, D., & El-Roy, D. (2000). Escape behavior during academic tasks: A preliminary analysis of idiosyncratic establishing operations. *Journal of Applied Behavior Analysis, 33,* 479–493.

McComas, J. J., Wacker, D. P., & Cooper, L. J. (1998). Increasing compliance with medical procedures: Application of the high-probability request procedure to a toddler. *Journal of Applied Behavior Analysis, 31,* 287–290.

McComas, J. J., Wacker, D. P., Cooper, L. J., Peck, S., Golonka, Z., Millard, T., et al. (2000). Effects of the high-probability request procedure: Patterns of responding to low-probability requests. *Journal of Developmental and Physical Disabilities, 12,* 157–171.

McDowell, J. J. (1989). Matching theory in natural human environments. *Behavior Analyst, 11,* 95–108.

McGimsey, J. F., & Favell, J. E. (1988). The effects of increased physical exercise on disruptive behavior in retarded persons. *Journal of Autism and Developmental Disabilities, 18,* 167–179.

McKenzie, S. D., Smith, R. G., Simmons, J. N., & Soderlund, M. J. (2008). Suppressive effects of a stimulus correlated with reprimands for automatically maintained eye poking. *Journal of Applied Behavior Analysis, 41,* 255–259.

Meier, A. E., Fryling, M. J., & Wallace, M. D. (2012). Using high-probability foods to increase the acceptance of low-probability foods. *Journal of Applied Behavior Analysis, 45,* 149–153.

Michael, J. L. (2004). *Concepts and principles of behavior analysis.* Kalamazoo: Western Michigan University, Association for Behavior Analysis International.

Miltenberger, R. G. (2006). Antecedent intervention for challenging behavior maintained by escape from instructional activities. In J. Luiselli (Ed.), *Antecedent assessment and intervention: Supporting children and adults with developmental disabilities in community settings* (pp. 101–124). Baltimore: Brookes.

Morrison, H., Roscoe, E. M., & Atwell, A. (2011). An evaluation of antecedent exercise on behavior maintained by automatic reinforcement using a three-component multiple schedule. *Journal of Applied Behavior Analysis, 44,* 523–541.

Murphy, E. S., McSweeney, F. K., Smith, R. G., & McComas, J. J. (2003). Dynamic changes in reinforcer effectiveness: Theoretical, methodological, and practical implications for applied research. *Journal of Applied Behavior Analysis, 36,* 421–438.

Neuringer, A. (1973). Pigeons respond to produce periods in which rewards are independent of responding. *Journal of the Experimental Analysis of Behavior, 19,* 39–54.

Nevin, J. A. (1996). The momentum of compliance. *Journal of Applied Behavior Analysis, 29,* 535–547.

O'Callaghan, P. M., Allen, K. D., Powell, S., & Salama, F. (2006). The efficacy of noncontingent escape for decreasing children's disruptive behavior during restorative dental treatment. *Journal of Applied Behavior Analysis, 39,* 161–171.

O'Reilly, M. F. (1995). Functional analysis and treatment of escape-maintained aggression correlated with sleep deprivation. *Journal of Applied Behavior Analysis, 28,* 225–226.

Ono, K. (1987). Superstitious behavior in humans. *Journal of the Experimental Analysis of Behavior, 47,* 261–271.

Pace, G. M., Ivancic, M. T., & Jefferson, G. (1994). Stimulus fading as treatment for obscenity in a brain-injured adult. *Journal of Applied Behavior Analysis, 27,* 301–305.

Pace, G. M., Iwata, B. A., Cowdery, G. E., Andree, P. J., & McIntyre, T. (1993). Stimulus (instructional) fading during extinction of self-injurious escape behavior. *Journal of Applied Behavior Analysis, 26,* 205–212.

Patel, M. R., Reed, G. K., Piazza, C. C., Bachmeyer, M. H., Layer, S. A., & Pabico, R. S. (2006). An evaluation of a high-probability instructional sequence to increase acceptance of food and decrease inappropriate behavior in children with pediatric feeding disorders. *Research in Developmental Disabilities, 27,* 430–442.

Piazza, C. C., Adelinis, J. D., Hanley, G., P., Goh, H., & Delia, M. D. (2000). An evaluation of the effects of matched stimuli on behaviors maintained by automatic reinforcement. *Journal of Applied Behavior Analysis, 33,* 13–27.

Piazza, C. C., Fisher, W. W., Hanley, G. P., Hilker, K., & Derby, K. M. (1996). A preliminary procedure for predicting the positive and negative effects of reinforcement-based procedures. *Journal of Applied Behavior Analysis, 29,* 137–152.

Piazza, C. C., Fisher, W. W., Hanley, G. P., LeBlanc, L. A., Worsdell, A. S., Lindauer, S. E., et al. (1998). Treatment of pica through multiple analyses of its reinforcing functions. *Journal of Applied Behavior Analysis, 31,* 165–189.

Piazza, C. C., Hanley, G. P., & Fisher, W. W. (1996). Functional analysis and treatment of cigarette pica. *Journal of Applied Behavior Analysis, 29,* 437–450.

Piazza, C. C., Patel, M. R., Gulotta, C. S., Sevin, B. M., & Layer, S. A. (2003). On the relative contributions of positive reinforcement and escape extinction in the treatment of food refusal. *Journal of Applied Behavior Analysis, 36,* 309–324.

Poling, A., & Normand, M. (1999). Noncontingent reinforcement: An inappropriate description of time-based schedules that reduce behavior. *Journal of Applied Behavior Analysis, 32,* 237–238.

Powers, S., Thibadeau, S., & Rose, K. (1992). Antecedent exercise and its effects on self-stimulation. *Behavioral Residential Treatment, 7,* 15–22.

Rapp, J. T. (2006). Toward an empirical method for identifying matched stimulation for automatically reinforced behavior: A preliminary investigation. *Journal of Applied Behavior Analysis, 39,* 137–140.

Reed, G. K., Piazza, C. C., Patel, M. R., Layer, S. A., Bachmeyer, M. H., & Bethke, S. D. (2004). On the relative contributions of noncontingent reinforcement and escape extinction in the treatment of food refusal. *Journal of Applied Behavior Analysis, 37,* 27–42.

Ringdahl, J. E., Vollmer, T. R., Marcus, B. A., & Roane, H. S. (1997). An analogue evaluation of environmental enrichment: The role of stimulus preference. *Journal of Applied Behavior Analysis, 30,* 203–216.

Saini, V., Fisher, W. W., Retzlaff, B. J., & Keevy, M. (2020). Efficiency in functional analysis of problem behavior: A quantitative and qualitative review. *Journal of Applied Behavior Analysis, 53,* 44–66.

Saini, V., Greer, B. D., Fisher, W. W., Lichtblau, K. R., DeSouza, A. A., & Mitteer, D. R. (2016). Individual and combined effects of noncontingent reinforcement and response blocking on automatically reinforced problem behavior. *Journal of Applied Behavior Analysis, 49,* 693–698.

Schaefer, H. H. (1970). Self-injurious behavior: Shaping head-banging in monkeys. *Journal of Applied Behavior Analysis, 3,* 111–116.

Shabani, D. B., & Fisher, W. W. (2006). Stimulus fading and differential reinforcement for the treatment of needle phobia in a youth with autism. *Journal of Applied Behavior Analysis, 39,* 449–452.

Shore, B. A., Iwata, B. A., DeLeon, I. G., Kahng, S., & Smith, R. G. (1997). An analysis of reinforcer substitutability using object manipulation and self-injury as competing responses. *Journal of Applied Behavior Analysis, 30,* 21–40.

Simmons, J. N., Smith, R. G., & Kliethermes, L. (2003). A multiple-schedule evaluation of immediate and subsequent effects of fixed-time food presentation on automatically maintained mouthing. *Journal of Applied Behavior Analysis, 36,* 541–544.

Smith, R. G., & Iwata, B. A. (1997). Antecedent influences of behavior disorders. *Journal of Applied Behavior Analysis, 30,* 343–375.

Smith, R. G., Lerman, D. C., & Iwata, B. A. (1996). Self-restraint as positive reinforcement for self-injurious behavior. *Journal of Applied Behavior Analysis, 29,* 99–102.

Swithers, S. E., & Hall, W. G. (1994). Does oral experience terminate ingestion? *Appetite, 23,* 113–138.

Taylor, D. V., Rush, D., Hetrick, W. P., & Sandman, C. A.

(1993). Self-injurious behavior within the menstrual cycle of developmentally delayed women. *American Journal on Mental Retardation, 97,* 659–664.

Thompson, R. F., & Spencer, W. A. (1966). Habituation: A model phenomenon for the study of neuronal substrates of behavior. *Psychological Review, 73,* 16–43.

Thompson, R. H., Iwata, B. A., Conners, J., & Roscoe, E. M. (1999). Effects of reinforcement for alternative behavior during punishment of self-injury. *Journal of Applied Behavior Analysis, 32,* 317–328.

Tiger, J. H., & Hanley, G. P. (2004). Developing stimulus control of preschooler mands: An analysis of schedule-correlated and contingency-specifying stimuli. *Journal of Applied Behavior Analysis, 37,* 517–521.

Turner, J. A., & Clancy, S. (1988). Comparison of operant behavioral and cognitive-behavioral group treatment for chronic low back pain. *Journal of Consulting and Clinical Psychology, 56,* 261–266.

Van Camp, C. M., Lerman, D. C., Kelley, M. E., Contrucci, S. A., & Vorndran, C. M. (2000). Variable-time reinforcement schedules in the treatment of socially maintained problem behavior. *Journal of Applied Behavior Analysis, 33,* 545–557.

Vaughn, B. J., & Horner, R. H. (1997). Identifying instructional tasks that occasion problem behaviors and assessing the effects of student versus teacher choice among these tasks. *Journal of Applied Behavior Analysis, 30,* 299–312.

Vollmer, T. R. (1999). Noncontingent reinforcement: Some additional comments. *Journal of Applied Behavior Analysis, 32,* 239–240.

Vollmer, T. R., Iwata, B. A., Zarcone, J. R., Smith, R. G., & Mazaleski, J. L. (1993). The role of attention in the treatment of attention-maintained self-injurious behavior: Noncontingent reinforcement and differential reinforcement of other behavior. *Journal of Applied Behavior Analysis, 26,* 9–21.

Vollmer, T. R., Marcus, B. A., & LeBlanc, L. (1994). Treatment of self-injury and hand mouthing following inconclusive functional analyses. *Journal of Applied Behavior Analysis, 27,* 331–344.

Vollmer, T. R., Marcus, B. A., & Ringdahl, J. E. (1995). Noncontingent escape as treatment for self-injurious behavior maintained by negative reinforcement. *Journal of Applied Behavior Analysis, 28,* 15–26.

Vollmer, T. R., Ringdahl, J. E., Roane, H. S., & Marcus, B. A. (1997). Negative side effects of noncontingent reinforcement. *Journal of Applied Behavior Analysis, 30,* 161–164.

Vollmer, T. R., & Vorndran, C. M. (1998). Assessment of self-injurious behavior maintained by access to self-restraint materials. *Journal of Applied Behavior Analysis, 31,* 647–650.

Wallace, M. D., Iwata, B. A., Hanley, G. P., Thompson, R. H., & Roscoe, E. M. (2012). Noncontingent reinforcement: A further examination of schedule effects during treatment. *Journal of Applied Behavior Analysis, 45,* 709–719.

Wehby, J. H., & Hollahan, M. S. (2000). Effects of high-probability requests on the latency to initiate academic tasks. *Journal of Applied Behavior Analysis, 33,* 259–262.

Whitlow, J. W. (1975). Short-term memory in habituation and dishabituation. *Journal of Experimental Psychology: Animal Behavior Processes, 1,* 196–209.

Wilder, D. A., Normand, M., & Atwell, J. (2005). Noncontingent reinforcement as treatment for food refusal and associated self-injury. *Journal of Applied Behavior Analysis, 38,* 549–553.

Zarcone, J. R., Iwata, B. A., Mazaleski, J. L., & Smith, R. G. (1994). Momentum and extinction effects on self-injurious escape behavior and noncompliance. *Journal of Applied Behavior Analysis, 27,* 649–658.

Zarcone, J. R., Iwata, B. A., Smith, R. G., Mazaleski, J. L., & Lerman, D. C. (1994). Reemergence and extinction of self-injurious escape behavior during stimulus (instructional) fading. *Journal of Applied Behavior Analysis, 27,* 307–316.

Zarcone, J. R., Iwata, B. A., Vollmer, T. R., Jagtiani, S., Smith, R. G., & Mazaleski, J. L. (1993). Extinction of self-injurious escape behavior with and without instructional fading. *Journal of Applied Behavior Analysis, 26,* 353–360.

# CHAPTER 19

# Developing Function-Based Extinction Procedures for Problem Behavior

Timothy R. Vollmer, Elizabeth Athens, and Jonathan K. Fernand

*Extinction* is the operation of discontinuing response-contingent reinforcement, and the effect of extinction is the reduction in responding that follows this operation (Catania, 2007). Identification of the reinforcer that maintains problem behavior is the critical first step in the development of an extinction treatment. In fact, implementing extinction with any degree of certainty without identifying the reinforcer for problem behavior is not possible.

Iwata, Dorsey, Slifer, Bauman, and Richman (1982/1994) described a functional-analytic procedure that improved the efficiency and specificity with which investigators could identify the reinforcer(s) for problem behavior. Iwata et al. used functional analyses to assesses the sensitivity of self-injurious behavior (SIB) of participants with developmental disabilities to (1) socially mediated positive reinforcement, (2) socially mediated negative reinforcement, and (3) automatic reinforcement. Subsequently, investigators have conducted functional analyses across many target behaviors (e.g., aggression, property destruction, elopement, tantrums) and populations (e.g., individuals with autism spectrum disorder, with dementia, with traumatic brain injury, and without disabilities; see Beavers & Iwata, 2013, for a comprehensive review).

Pretreatment functional analyses have improved the efficacy of extinction treatments, because the procedures that define extinction for problem behavior dictate its functional properties (Iwata, Pace, Cowdery, & Miltenberger, 1994). Iwata, Pace, Cowdery, et al. (1994), for example, examined the effects of extinction based on and not based on the function of problem behavior. We explain the results for one participant to illustrate their findings. Results of a functional analysis showed that attention functioned as social positive reinforcement for head banging. The investigators tested the effect of two types of putative extinction: attention extinction, in which the investigator no longer delivered attention when the participant engaged in head banging; and extinction of automatic reinforcement, in which the investigator used a helmet to attenuate the sensory consequences produced by head banging. Attention extinction but not extinction of automatic reinforcement decreased head banging. These findings showed that (1) the functional analysis identified the reinforcer that maintained head banging, (2) head banging decreased when the investigator discontinued delivery of the functional reinforcer for head banging, and (3) head banging did not decrease when the investigator discontinued delivery of a stimulus that was not a functional reinforcer. Thus the functional analysis was useful for prescribing the correct form and function of the extinction treatment.

In this chapter, we discuss the three functional variations of extinction for problem behavior described by Iwata, Pace, Cowdery, et al. (1994): extinction of problem behavior maintained by (1) socially mediated positive reinforcement, (2) socially mediated negative reinforcement, and (3) automatic reinforcement. In addition, we discuss response patterns associated with extinction, factors influencing the efficacy of extinction, and other practical considerations.

## FUNCTIONAL VARIATIONS OF EXTINCTION

### Extinction of Problem Behavior Maintained by Socially Mediated Positive Reinforcement

*Positive reinforcement* is both the operation of presenting a stimulus (i.e., a positive reinforcer) contingent on the occurrence of a behavior, and the resulting increase in responding that produced the reinforcer (Catania, 2007). *Socially mediated reinforcement* is that which another individual delivers (Iwata, Pace, Dorsey, et al., 1994). Extinction is a logical approach for decreasing problem behavior maintained by social positive reinforcement, because the source of reinforcement is delivered by other people (hence the term *social*). If individuals can deliver reinforcement, then we should be able to teach them to withhold reinforcement. For example, if access to tangible items functions as positive reinforcement for problem behavior (e.g., a caregiver provides a toy when a child hits themself), extinction would consist of discontinuing delivery of the tangible item when problem behavior occurs. Similarly, if access to adult attention functions as positive reinforcement for problem behavior (e.g., a caregiver says, "Stop," when the child has a tantrum), extinction would consist of discontinuing attention when problem behavior occurs.

Before the publication of studies on functional analysis, investigators appeared to presume that positive reinforcement maintained problem behavior in many studies. Williams (1959), for example, used extinction in the form of social isolation for a child who displayed tantrums at bedtime. The caregiver placed the child into bed at bedtime, left the room, and did not reenter. Tantrums decreased to zero rates in eight sessions, suggesting that adult attention maintained the tantrums. Wolf, Risley, and Mees (1964) used social isolation for one child's tantrums. The investigators immediately placed the child in his hospital room and left him alone until the tantrum ceased; tantrums

decreased to near-zero rates. The results of Wolf et al. are difficult to interpret, however, because the procedure was structurally similar to time out. That is, Wolf et al. placed the child in social isolation (time out), which also resulted in discontinuing attention delivery (extinction). Thus, whether the discontinuation of attention, placement into social isolation, or both was responsible for the effects is not clear.

Lovaas and Simmons (1969) hypothesized that social consequences reinforced the problem behavior of two children. Lovaas and Simmons isolated each child in a room noncontingently, which resulted in relatively high rates of problem behavior initially, followed by a gradual decrease in rates of problem behavior over time. These results supported the presumption that social positive reinforcement maintained problem behavior and the efficacy of extinction as treatment.

Mazaleski, Iwata, Vollmer, Zarcone, and Smith (1993) evaluated the effects of differential reinforcement of other behavior (DRO) and extinction on SIB emitted by three women living in a state residential facility for individuals with disabilities. The pretreatment functional analysis indicated that socially mediated positive reinforcement (e.g., attention) maintained each woman's SIB. The investigators demonstrated that SIB persisted when they delivered preferred stimuli (e.g., music) for short intervals in which the women refrained from SIB (i.e., DRO). However, SIB decreased when the necessary extinction component was in place (i.e., the investigators withheld attention). These results suggested that extinction was necessary to decrease problem behavior maintained by attention and might be the critical component of DRO schedules.

### Extinction of Problem Behavior Maintained by Socially Mediated Negative Reinforcement

Negative reinforcement, just like positive reinforcement, is both an operation and a process. *Negative reinforcement* is the removal of an aversive stimulus contingent on the occurrence of a behavior and the resulting increase in responding that produced the removal of that stimulus (Catania, 2007). Furthermore, negative reinforcement is socially mediated when another individual delivers reinforcement (Iwata, Pace, Dorsey, et al., 1994). The functional-analytic approach has demonstrated that a high proportion of problem behavior is sensitive to negative reinforcement, such as escape from bite presentations (e.g., Bachmeyer, Kirkwood,

Criscito, Mauzy, & Berth, 2019), environmental changes (Fisher, Felber, et al., 2019), instructional activities (Iwata, Pace, Kalsher, Cowdery, & Cataldo, 1990), self-care activities (Dowdy, Tincani, Nipe, & Weiss, 2018; Steege, Wacker, Cigrand, & Berg, 1990), and social proximity (Vollmer et al., 1998), among others. In fact, large-scale summaries of functional-analytic outcomes have shown that about 33–48% of problem behavior is sensitive to negative reinforcement (Derby et al., 1992; Iwata, Pace, Cowdery, et al., 1994).

The finding that a substantial proportion of problem behavior is sensitive to negative reinforcement is important for extinction interventions. As Iwata, Pace, Cowdery, et al. (1994) illustrated, the functional properties of reinforcement dictate the form and function of extinction. For example, discontinuation of social attention may reinforce problem behavior maintained by negative reinforcement. Discontinuation of negative reinforcement requires an entirely different approach to extinction than investigators previously considered in the literature on applied behavior analysis. Investigators appeared to presume in the early literature that problem behavior was maintained only by attention as many putative extinction procedures included time out or planned ignoring (Fyffe, Kahng, Fittro, & Russell, 2004; Pinkston, Reese, LeBlanc, & Baer, 1973; Wolf et al., 1964). These procedures were like extinction of positively reinforced problem behavior structurally, in that the investigators discontinued attention. A decrease in problem behavior under those contingency arrangements would have provided support for the assumption that attention reinforced problem behavior. Of course, publication practices are such that journals mainly publish positive rather than negative results, so it is impossible to say how many failed attempts at extinction of negatively reinforced problem behavior may have occurred due to a faulty assumption that attention reinforced problem behavior.

Extinction for negatively reinforced problem behavior requires no change of the aversive stimulation as a function of problem behavior and discontinuation of the escape or avoidance contingency. Hineline (1977) pointed out that early conceptualizations of extinction of negatively reinforced behavior were incorrect. For example, some investigators believed that extinction involved eliminating the aversive stimulation that produced the escape or avoidance behavior. Simply removing instructional demands to eliminate escape behavior, however, is not extinction, because it does not involve discontinuation of a response–reinforcer relation (Smith & Iwata, 1997). In the laboratory, extinction of negatively reinforced behavior involves continued presentation of aversive stimulation, despite the occurrence of behavior previously reinforced by escape or avoidance.

Early applications of extinction of negatively reinforced behavior alone are difficult to find because most such studies had at least one confounding variable. For example, in a study by Heidorn and Jensen (1984), a participant's SIB correlated with demands, suggesting that it was escape behavior. The treatment included physical guidance to complete the requested task when SIB occurred. Conceptually, continuation of task demands was an extinction procedure, as SIB no longer produced escape. However, the physical-guidance component resembled punishment in that the investigators presented putative aversive stimulation contingent on SIB. The treatment also included other components, such as praise, food reinforcement, and session termination contingent on compliance. Nevertheless, Heidorn and Jensen's approach was innovative with respect to the escape extinction component, continuation of task demands.

Iwata et al. (1990) were the first to apply escape extinction explicitly as a treatment for problem behavior based on the results of a functional analysis. Functional analyses showed that participants displayed escape-maintained SIB. The investigators used a three-step prompting sequence to present task demands during baseline and treatment. During baseline, SIB produced escape from the task demands. During treatment, SIB no longer produced escape, and an investigator guided each participant to complete the task if they engaged in SIB. In five of six cases, extinction plus physical guidance decreased SIB. In the sixth case, the investigators added response blocking. An additional case involved different procedures that were not relevant to this discussion, and we do not include a description of this here. As with the Heidorn and Jensen (1984) study, an interpretive limitation of Iwata et al.'s approach was that physical guidance possibly functioned as punishment. An extinction procedure would have continued three-step prompting when SIB occurred rather than physically guiding task completion. Thus the possibility exists that both extinction and punishment contributed to decreases in SIB. From a practical standpoint, however, contingent physical guidance is more likely to ensure that no escape follows occurrences of problem behavior.

Food refusal is a good example of a clinical disorder that investigators have treated effectively by using escape extinction as one component of an intervention. In most studies, reinforcement is available for alternative behavior as part of a treatment package, and investigators have not identified the function of the behavior (Cooper et al., 1995; Hoch, Babbitt, Coe, Krell, & Hackbert, 1994; Piazza, Patel, Gulotta, Sevin, & Layer, 2003). For example, Patel, Piazza, Martinez, Volkert, and Santana (2002) compared the effects of delivering reinforcement for acceptance or for *mouth clean*, which is a product measure of swallowing. The investigators found that differential reinforcement without escape extinction was ineffective in increasing acceptance or mouth clean or decreasing inappropriate mealtime behavior. Second, they added escape extinction in the form of nonremoval of the spoon or cup to the reinforcement procedures, such that inappropriate mealtime behavior no longer produced escape. A feeder held the spoon or cup touching or near a child's lips until the child opened their mouth and allowed the feeder to deposit the bite or drink. The feeder re-presented expelled food or drink. Acceptance and mouth clean increased for the three participants, independently of the target of differential reinforcement, after the feeder implemented the escape extinction procedure.

In a similar study, Piazza, Patel, et al. (2003) compared the individual effects of positive reinforcement alone, escape extinction alone, and the combined effect of positive reinforcement with escape extinction on food and liquid refusal exhibited by four children with total food refusal. Results indicated that positive reinforcement alone did not increase acceptance or decrease inappropriate mealtime behavior, whereas escape extinction alone increased acceptance. However, the investigators showed that the addition of positive reinforcement to escape extinction produced lower levels of inappropriate mealtime behavior relative to escape extinction alone for some participants in some phases.

Other investigators have conducted functional analyses of inappropriate mealtime behavior and used the results to develop a function-based treatment (e.g., Bachmeyer et al., 2009; Berth et al., 2019; Girolami & Scotti, 2001; Piazza, Fisher, et al., 2003). Bachmeyer et al. (2009) treated four children whose inappropriate mealtime behavior was sensitive to both social positive and social negative reinforcement identified by a pretreatment functional analysis. The investigators

validated the results of the functional analysis by matching treatment to one (i.e., attention extinction with escape and escape extinction with attention) or both (i.e., attention and escape extinction) functions of inappropriate mealtime behavior. They determined that attention extinction alone did not decrease inappropriate mealtime behavior or increase bite acceptance. In comparison, escape extinction alone effectively decreased inappropriate mealtime behavior and increased bite acceptance, even though inappropriate mealtime behavior produced delivery of attention. However, the combined attention and escape extinction procedure decreased inappropriate mealtime behavior to near-zero levels and increased bite acceptance to 100% of trials. These pediatric feeding studies show that escape extinction may be a necessary component in the treatment of food refusal; they also emphasize the importance of identifying functional relations to inform the successful treatment of inappropriate mealtime behavior.

There is no definitive study on the effects of escape extinction, because early studies on extinction of negatively reinforced behavior generally confounded it with other treatment components (e.g., punishment, reinforcement), and more recent approaches have used extinction in combination with procedures derived from a functional analysis (e.g., differential negative reinforcement). A pure application of escape extinction would involve a continuation of the aversive stimulation without the introduction of some other variable (e.g., physical guidance). Therefore, from a conceptual standpoint, future investigators should isolate the effects of continuation of aversive stimulation and physical guidance.

## Extinction of Problem Behavior Maintained by Automatic Reinforcement

The defining characteristic of automatic reinforcement is that reinforcement is not mediated socially; rather, the problem behavior produces reinforcement (Vaughan & Michael, 1982). Note that automatic reinforcement can be positive or negative (Hagopian, Rooker, & Zarcone, 2015: Hagopian, Rooker, Zarcone, Bonner, & Arevalo, 2017). For example, head hitting can be reinforced by endorphin release (positive reinforcement; Sandman & Hetrick, 1995), or self-scratching may attenuate an itching sensation (negative reinforcement). Investigators have referred to automatically reinforced problem behavior as *self-stimulation* (e.g., Lovaas, Newsom, & Hickman, 1987) or *sen-*

sory-reinforced behavior (e.g., Rincover, 1978). The term *automatically reinforced problem behavior* is preferred, because it best describes behavior that is not maintained socially and may be a positive- or negative-reinforcement contingency. On the other hand, the terms *self-stimulation* and *sensory-reinforced behavior* leave out the possibility that the behavior may serve a negative-reinforcement function.

Extinction of automatically reinforced problem behavior is likely to be more challenging than extinction of socially reinforced problem behavior. The social environment controls socially mediated reinforcement (Vollmer, 1994); therefore, investigators can rearrange the environment to discontinue reinforcement. By contrast, problem behavior rather than the social environment produces automatic reinforcement; thus automatically reinforced problem behavior is more difficult to control via changes in the environment.

One approach to extinction of automatically reinforced behavior is called *sensory extinction* (Rincover, Cook, Peoples, & Packard, 1979). The term is a misnomer, because the problem behavior producing reinforcement is extinguished, rather than the sensory reinforcement. Nonetheless, the term has gained widespread usage, so we use it here for consistency. During sensory extinction, the investigator terminates or blocks the putative source of automatic reinforcement. For example, Rincover (1978) reduced stereotypical object spinning by blocking the auditory feedback produced by the object. Rincover put carpet on the table where the participant spun the object, thereby eliminating the sound the object produced.

Investigators have used sensory-extinction-like approaches as treatments for SIB. For example, Dorsey, Iwata, Reid, and Davis (1982) used a helmet to block the sensory products of head hitting. There are difficulties, however, in interpreting the results of some sensory-extinction studies. The source or sources of reinforcement that protective equipment altered are unclear, because investigators implemented treatment in the absence of a functional analysis. For example, Rincover and Devany (1982) used a helmet with one participant and noted decreases in head banging, presumably as a function of extinction of automatic reinforcement. An alternative explanation is that teacher attention maintained head banging, and the teacher ignored head banging when the child wore a helmet, but not when he did not wear a helmet (Vollmer, 1994). Another interpretation is that application of protective equipment functions as punishment. For example, hitting a hard helmet might cause pain to an individual's hand.

Mazaleski, Iwata, and Rodgers (1994) conducted a functional analysis showing that hand mouthing was automatically reinforced, and that noncontingent and contingent application of oven mitts decreased hand mouthing. Mazaleski et al. proposed that the effects of noncontingent and contingent mitts may have been a function of (1) the aversive properties of wearing mitts (e.g., mitts were uncomfortable) or (2) time out from the opportunity to obtain automatic reinforcement from hand mouthing. Another possibility was that sensory extinction accounted for the effect of noncontingent mitts, and that punishment or time out accounted for the effect of contingent mitts (Mazaleski et al., 1994).

Response blocking is another procedure investigators have conceptualized as extinction for automatically reinforced problem behavior (Saini et al., 2016). Presumably, blocking prevents the automatic reinforcement produced by the response; however, extinction may not explain the effects of response blocking in all cases. Lerman and Iwata (1996a) varied the number of blocked SIB responses systematically to distinguish between extinction and punishment effects. They hypothesized that intermittent response blocking would produce effects like an intermittent schedule of reinforcement if response blocking functioned as extinction. If so, intermittent response blocking would maintain or increase the frequency of SIB. Alternatively, the same intermittent schedule of response blocking would produce effects like an intermittent schedule of punishment if response blocking functioned as punishment. If so, intermittent response blocking would decrease the frequency of SIB. Lerman and Iwata (1996a) found that response blocking functioned as punishment for an adult female engaging in chronic hand mouthing, because rates of hand mouthing were near zero with intermittent and continuous response blocking. Alternatively, Smith, Russo, and Le (1999) examined the function of response blocking on the eye-poking behavior of an adult female. Levels of eye poking increased relative to baseline during intermittent blocking, like the effect of an intermittent schedule of reinforcement. By contrast, levels of eye poking decreased during continuous blocking, consistent with an extinction schedule.

Taken together, these results indicate that response blocking can function as extinction in some cases and as punishment in others. Response blocking would be contraindicated, then, if the investigator could not implement it with near-perfect integrity if response blocking functioned as extinction. By contrast, intermittent response blocking still might be effective if response blocking functioned as punishment. Thus a distinction between the extinction and punishment effects of response blocking is of clinical significance.

## RESPONSE PATTERNS ASSOCIATED WITH EXTINCTION

Skinner (1938) demonstrated in the animal laboratory that operant behavior decreases in frequency, duration, and intensity when the investigator terminates the delivery of reinforcement. Investigators have observed these patterns with SIB (Roscoe, Iwata, & Goh, 1998), nighttime sleep disruptions (Blampied & France, 1993), and bizarre vocalizations (Wilder, Masuda, O'Connor, & Baham, 2001), to name a few. In addition, investigators have observed other response patterns associated with extinction—some of which are undesirable, such as the extinction or response burst, response variation, aggression, emotional behavior, and spontaneous recovery. We discuss these five extinction-associated response patterns because of their clinical relevance. Behavior analysts should recognize and anticipate these response patterns and prepare for them accordingly (e.g., provide caregivers with protective equipment in case of extinction-induced aggression).

### Extinction Burst

The *extinction burst* is the temporary increase in the frequency, intensity, or duration of a target response that can occur with the onset of extinction (Cooper, Heron, & Heward, 1987). Extinction bursts can be detrimental for at least two reasons. First, a temporary increase in the frequency, intensity, or duration of problem behavior may produce greater injury or destruction if the problem behavior is dangerous (e.g., aggression). Second, caregivers may be less inclined to follow through with treatment if it produces a worsening of behavior, even if that worsening is temporary (Sloman et al., 2005).

Although textbooks frequently present the extinction burst as a common side effect, published data suggest that extinction bursts may not be as prevalent as once believed (e.g., Lerman & Iwata, 1995; Lerman, Iwata, & Wallace, 1999; Woods & Borrero, 2019). Lerman and Iwata (1995) reported

that extinction bursts occurred in 36% of 113 published and unpublished cases when investigators used extinction in isolation. By contrast, extinction bursts occurred in only 12% of cases when investigators combined extinction with other procedures (e.g., differential reinforcement). Lerman, Iwata, and Wallace (1999) found that extinction bursts occurred in 62% of cases when investigators used extinction in isolation, and in 39% of cases when investigators used extinction with other procedures. The Lerman et al. data are especially important, because investigators implemented treatment in a highly controlled environment where extinction was only in effect during data collection for the study. Thus these data presumably measured levels of responding at the onset of extinction, which is the only time extinction bursts can occur. Lerman and Iwata, by contrast, conducted their study on an inpatient unit where clinicians might have been implementing extinction throughout the day. Lerman and Iwata collected data during short sessions; thus those data might not have measured levels of responding at the onset of extinction. This difference in the implementation of extinction across the two studies could account for the larger percentage of cases of extinction bursts in Lerman et al. More generally, investigators have found that extinction bursts are more likely with extinction in isolation and less likely with extinction combined with other procedures.

### Extinction-Induced Response Variation

Another commonly reported response pattern associated with extinction is *response variation*, which is an increased tendency for novel or diverse behavior to occur during extinction. For example, if an adult denies a child access to reinforcement after the child asks politely for reinforcement, the child may engage in an alternative behavior (e.g., whining) to access reinforcement. At times, extinction-induced response variation is desirable. For example, response variation may produce successive approximations of behavior that an investigator can differentially reinforce to shape new and desired response forms (Grow, Kelley, Roane, & Shillingsburg, 2008). Response variation can be desirable during treatment of problem behavior if appropriate behavior emerges. On the other hand, response variation is undesirable if other forms of problem behavior emerge.

To date, no studies have examined response variation explicitly during implementation of extinction for problem behavior. Nonetheless, basic research has reported response variation for decades (e.g., Antonitis, 1951). Some applied research has reported response variation when the investigators implemented extinction, although response variation was not the focus of the study. For example, Lerman, Kelley, Vorndran, and Van Camp (2003) blocked a participant's head and tooth tapping, and hand wringing increased. Similarly, Lerman, Kelley, Van Camp, and Roane (1999) implemented extinction for screaming, and hand clapping increased. Lerman, Kelley, et al. (1999) then provided reinforcement for hand clapping as an alternative response. One explanation of these results is that the newly emerged responses were results of extinction-induced response variation. An alternative explanation is that the newly emerged responses were members of the same functional response class. That is, the newly emerged responses historically produced the same reinforcement as the response on extinction. More research is needed to determine whether extinction-induced response variation occurs in applied settings.

## Extinction-Induced Aggression

Basic research has shown that aggression can emerge as a result of withholding previously presented contingent or noncontingent reinforcement (e.g., Azrin, Hutchinson, & Hake, 1966). The evidence for extinction-induced aggression in humans is fairly clear (e.g., Frederiksen & Peterson, 1974; Kelly & Hake, 1970; Todd, Morris, & Fenza, 1989). For example, Kelly and Hake (1970) examined the effect of extinction on a punching response in laboratory participants. Participants exhibited few punches when button pressing was effective as an avoidance response. Punching increased for seven of nine participants when button pressing was on extinction.

An alternative explanation of extinction-induced aggression is that the emergent aggressive behavior is a member of the same functional response class as the behavior on extinction. If so, aggression may emerge when other problem behavior no longer produces reinforcement. For example, Vollmer, Iwata, Zarcone, Smith, and Mazaleski (1993) reported that noncontingent reinforcement and extinction as treatment for SIB resulted in a burst of one participant's aggression. One possibility is that aggression and SIB were in the same functional response class; that is, the same reinforcer (social attention in Vollmer et al.) maintained aggression and SIB. This explanation is speculative, as Vollmer et al. did not conduct a functional analysis of aggression.

Research on response hierarchies provides additional evidence for a functional-response-class interpretation of extinction-induced aggression. For example, Richman, Wacker, Asmus, Casey, and Andelman (1999) conducted functional analyses in which the reinforcement contingency for mild (e.g., screaming, disruption) and severe (e.g., aggression) forms of problem behavior was the same, and they only observed mild problem behavior. Severe problem behavior emerged when Richman et al. implemented extinction for mild problem behavior but continued to deliver reinforcement for severe problem behavior. They found that the same reinforcer maintained mild and severe problem behavior. Two of the three participants had a response pattern indicative of a response class hierarchy in which mild problem behavior typically occurred before severe problem behavior. These data suggest that when severe forms of problem behavior continue to produce reinforcement, such as when a caregiver cannot withhold reinforcement, terminating the reinforcement contingency for less severe forms is likely to produce a concomitant increase in more severe forms of problem behavior. This increased likelihood of aggression and much more severe problem behavior when other problem behavior is placed on extinction highlights the importance of protecting not only the client, but therapists, caregivers, and other individuals who might be affected by implementing an extinction procedure.

## Extinction-Induced Emotional Behavior

*Extinction-induced emotional behavior* is another pattern of responding associated with extinction (Lerman & Iwata, 1996b). Such behavior in humans can include crying, attempting to escape, protesting, acting upset, and other forms of agitation (e.g., Baumeister & Forehand, 1971; Rovee-Collier & Capatides, 1979; Sullivan, Lewis, & Alessandri, 1992). For example, Sullivan et al. examined the emotional responding of 4-month-old infants during baseline, reinforcement, and extinction phases, in which the baseline and extinction phases were procedurally identical except that baseline preceded and extinction followed the learning history provided in the reinforcement phase. They concluded that positive reinforcement correlated with positive emotional expressions (e.g., facial expressions) and physiological measures (e.g., heart rate) when compared to baseline measures. By contrast, extinction correlated with negative emotional responding and physiological measures. Extinction-induced emotional behavior in basic research may include whisker cleaning in rats, sniffing, and ambulating (Gallup & Altomari, 1969; Lerman & Iwata, 1996b). Whether emotional behavior in humans (e.g., crying) parallels responding exhibited by nonhuman animals (e.g., whisker cleaning) is not clear. Crying and protesting in humans may be members of the same functional response class as problem behavior on extinction, rather than induced by the extinction procedure itself.

Whatever the functional properties of emotional behavior may be, its occurrence in clinical contexts is important to note. Caregivers might interpret emotional behavior as a sign of discomfort (Blampied & France, 1993; France & Hudson, 1990), and its occurrence could decrease the acceptability of extinction and negatively affect the integrity with which caregivers implement extinction. Furthermore, extinction-induced emotional behavior could be indicative that the stimulus context is aversive and might increase the likelihood of escape or avoidance behavior. Such behavior could have a negative impact if the context is a learning environment or if the individual consistently attempts to escape or avoid a caregiver.

## Spontaneous Recovery

*Spontaneous recovery* refers to the reemergence of previously extinguished behavior after a period away from the context in which the investigator implemented extinction (Skinner, 1938). Evidence for spontaneous recovery is ample in basic research (e.g., Hatton, 1965; Lewis, 1956; Miller & Stevenson, 1936; Youtz, 1938), and there are some reports of it in applied research (Lerman, Kelley, et al., 1999). Skinner (1938) showed that exposing a previously reinforced response to extinction decreased responding to pretraining levels by the end of the first exposure. When Skinner exposed the subject to extinction a second time, responding reappeared at the beginning of the session, with a gradual decrease to pretraining levels by the end of the session. The subject repeated this pattern during subsequent exposures to extinction, with gradually decreasing response curves.

Spontaneous recovery is likely an important phenomenon to consider in application. For example, suppose a parent enters a child's bedroom contingent on disruptive behavior at bedtime, and parent attention functions as reinforcement. France and Hudson (1990) taught caregivers to implement extinction that consisted of eliminating attention for bedtime disruptive behavior by

not entering the room, unless a child had a medical problem. The investigators observed the expected extinction effect (i.e., eventual decrease of nighttime disruptive behavior). However, brief increases in nighttime disruptive behavior occurred periodically across nights, which might have been due to the time between extinction trials.

There are practical reasons to be aware of spontaneous recovery. First, if the recovery occurs unexpectedly, caregivers may infer that the intervention does not work, and they may not continue implementing it. Clinicians should inform caregivers to expect spontaneous recovery, but also note that the recovery should be lower in magnitude and easier to eliminate each time it occurs. Second, clinicians can anticipate spontaneous recovery and arrange the environment accordingly. For example, clinicians can implement safety precautions for severe aggression or SIB, even though prior extinction trials have produced low or eventually even zero rates of problem behavior.

## FACTORS THAT INFLUENCE THE EFFICACY OF EXTINCTION

Several factors influence the efficacy of extinction. Although the list of potential variables influencing extinction is long, some key variables highlighted in this section include schedule of and parameters of reinforcement during baseline; the availability of alternative sources of reinforcement during treatment; and stimulus control, including rules.

### Baseline Schedule of Reinforcement

*Resistance to extinction*, which is persistence in responding during extinction, is one measure investigators use to evaluate the effects of extinction. Catania (2007) defines resistance to extinction as the responses emitted, time elapsed, or number of trials until responding reaches a predetermined extinction criterion, such as the number of responses emitted before 2 minutes elapses without the occurrence of a response. Behavior maintained on an intermittent-reinforcement schedule generally is more resistant to extinction than behavior maintained on a continuous-reinforcement schedule (Ferster & Skinner, 1957). The more intermittent the schedule, the more resistant the behavior is to extinction (Lerman & Iwata, 1996b). The influence of intermittent reinforcement is known as the *partial-reinforcement extinction effect*. Reviews discussing the partial-reinforcement extinction effect suggest that the phenomenon is quite complex (e.g., Lerman & Iwata, 1996b; Lewis, 1960; Mackintosh, 1974).

Research on the partial-reinforcement extinction effect highlights this complexity. For example, some investigators have used total number of responses that occur during extinction to evaluate the partial-reinforcement extinction effect (Lerman & Iwata, 1996b). However, Nevin (1988) has argued that proportion of response rate during baseline is a more appropriate measure of this effect. The proportional decrease in responding when extinction follows an intermittent-reinforcement schedule could be greater than the proportional decrease in responding when extinction follows a continuous-reinforcement schedule. MacDonald, Ahearn, Parry-Cruwys, Bancroft, and Dube (2013) found that mean proportional rates of problem behavior were higher when extinction followed a continuous-reinforcement schedule than when extinction followed an intermittent-reinforcement schedule. Although most research shows that problem behavior decreases more quickly when extinction follows a continuous-reinforcement schedule, findings are sometimes mixed (Lerman, Kelley, Vorndran, Kuhn, & LaRue, 2002). Results of some studies have shown that problem behavior decreases more quickly when extinction follows an intermittent-reinforcement schedule (e.g., Siqueland, 1968). Future investigators might examine the conditions under which this occurs.

## Baseline Parameters of Reinforcement

Lerman and Iwata (1996b) outlined several other baseline parameters of reinforcement that appear to influence responding during extinction. These parameters include but are not limited to the number of reinforcers delivered, the delay to reinforcement, and the magnitude of reinforcement.

### Number of Reinforcers

Basic behavioral research has shown generally that the longer the acquisition period (i.e., history of reinforcement) or the greater the density of reinforcer delivery (even if response independent) before extinction is implemented, the more resistant the behavior is to extinction (e.g., Fisher, Saini, et al., 2019; Nevin, Tota, Torquato, & Shull, 1990). Nevertheless, basic research also has shown

that the effects of number of reinforcers reach an asymptote after which resistance to extinction does not increase further, sometimes after as few as 100 reinforcers (Lerman & Iwata, 1996b). We do not know if the asymptotic effect of reinforcement number on resistance to extinction during baseline applies to humans in complex environments. If so, resistance to extinction should reach its highest point quickly if problem behavior has occurred at a high rate in baseline.

### Delay to Reinforcement

Basic research has shown that the delay to reinforcement before implementation of extinction influences its effects. According to Lerman and Iwata (1996b), the literature suggests that problem behavior is more resistant to extinction in conditions where delays to reinforcement are unpredictable and variable than in conditions with no reinforcement delay. Conversely, resistance to extinction is less pronounced (i.e., responding does not persist as much) if the reinforcer delay is constant and predictable. Findings related to delay have powerful implications for extinction-based treatments. The consequences for problem behavior are often delayed, and the length of the delay is often variable (e.g., Borrero, Vollmer, Borrero, & Bourret, 2005)—conditions that would decrease the efficacy of extinction. Delivery of immediate reinforcement on a continuous schedule at a constant delay might reduce the deleterious effects of reinforcement delay.

### Magnitude of Reinforcement

Basic research shows that if we define reinforcement magnitude by amount, then smaller reinforcement magnitudes during baseline produce more resistance to extinction. If we define reinforcement magnitude by intensity, then larger reinforcement magnitudes during baseline produce more resistance to extinction. The clinical implication of these findings is that the magnitude or intensity of baseline reinforcement, depending on the function of problem behavior, should influence resistance to extinction. For example, problem behavior maintained by food might be more resistant to extinction if reinforced during baseline with a small snack relative to a large meal. Conversely, problem behavior maintained by attention might be more resistant to extinction if reinforced during baseline with high-intensity attention relative to low-intensity attention. Some applied research is beginning to evaluate qualitative differences in attention as reinforcement. The issue of reinforcer intensity as it relates to social attention could be like the issue of higher-quality attention (e.g., Fisher, Ninness, Piazza, & Owen-DeSchryver, 1996; Piazza et al., 1999). However, investigators have not evaluated the effects of reinforcer quality on resistance to extinction in the context of behavioral treatments.

## Extinction Combined with Reinforcement

Extinction is more effective in reducing problem behavior when it is combined with differential or noncontingent reinforcement (Lalli, Casey, & Kates, 1997; Reed et al., 2004; Vollmer et al., 1998). We emphasize two of the possible reasons for this finding.

First, the availability of reinforcement for alternative behavior should decrease problem behavior and increase alternative behavior, in accordance with the principles of the *matching law* (Herrnstein, 1974). The matching law posits that the relative rate of a response will match the relative rate of reinforcement for that response. For example, if twice as many reinforcers are available for problem behaviors than for other behaviors, the individual will engage in twice as many problem behaviors as other behaviors (Borrero & Vollmer, 2002; Martens & Houk, 1989; McDowell, 1988). Borrero and Vollmer (2002) conducted descriptive observations in which they observed the problem behavior emitted by four children with developmental disabilities and the environmental events that followed them (e.g., potential reinforcers). After the naturalistic observations, the investigators identified the functional reinforcer maintaining each child's problem behavior by conducting a functional analysis. Subsequently, they calculated the relative rate of responding from the naturalistic observation and showed that it matched the relative rate of reinforcement, as predicted by the matching law. In addition to this study, Borrero et al. (2010) experimentally manipulated reinforcement rates to show that response rates to problem behavior adjusted accordingly. Therefore, extinction of problem behavior should produce a shift in responding from problem behavior to behavior that produces reinforcement. For example, extinction of problem behavior maintained by attention and delivery of attention for a communication response should produce a decrease in problem behavior and an increase in the communication response (Carr & Durand, 1985).

Second, treatment integrity failures during extinction alone are likely to have a detrimental effect on treatment, because these failures would be equivalent to an intermittent-reinforcement schedule for problem behavior. By contrast, such failures may not be as detrimental when we combine extinction with reinforcement if the schedule of reinforcement is sufficiently dense. That is, an individual is not likely to shift responding to problem behavior after occasional reinforcement of problem behavior if reinforcement is available differentially for alternative behavior or noncontingently.

Although extinction combined with reinforcement is more effective than extinction alone, resurgence can occur if the newly acquired and reinforced alternative behavior (e.g., compliance, communication) undergoes extinction (Epstein, 1983). *Resurgence* is the reemergence of an extinguished behavior (e.g., problem behavior). The schedule of reinforcement for appropriate behavior in a reinforcement plus extinction intervention will affect whether resurgence occurs.

## Stimulus Control

*Stimulus control* is the change in the probability of a response due to the presence, absence, or change in an antecedent stimulus event (Pierce & Cheney, 2013). One way that stimulus control is relevant to extinction is during multiple schedules. *Multiple schedules* are compound schedules in which different correlated stimuli signal two or more alternating component schedules of reinforcement, extinction, or punishment (Ferster & Skinner, 1957). Basic research has shown that signaled-extinction schedules yield more immediate suppression of and stimulus control over responding than do unsignaled-extinction schedules (e.g., mixed schedules of reinforcement). The findings from applied studies have confirmed those from basic research (e.g., Cammilleri, Tiger, & Hanley, 2008; Fisher, Greer, Fuhrman, Saini, & Simmons, 2018; Fuhrman, Fisher, & Greer, 2016; Hanley, Iwata, & Thompson, 2001). For example, Hanley et al. (2001) used signaled-reinforcement and signaled-extinction components during functional-communication training and then thinned the reinforcement schedules. Results generally showed that extinction was more effective if the investigators signaled it. That is, SIB was much more likely in the unsignaled-extinction component (i.e., mixed schedule) than in the signaled-extinction component (i.e., multiple schedule). In addition, signals were effective in keeping SIB below baseline levels as the investigators thinned reinforcement, and periods of extinction increased. The schedule-thinning procedure (in which periods of extinction increased), plus schedule-correlated stimuli that are common in research on multiple schedules, likely served to mitigate the negative side effects of extinction. However, further research on multiple schedules is necessary to measure the various side effects described earlier. Finally, research also suggests that individuals may prefer interventions with signaled-extinction and reinforcement schedules over interventions with unsignaled-extinction and reinforcement schedules (Tiger, Hanley, & Heal, 2006).

One specific form of stimulus control is instructional control. Investigators have shown that the effects of extinction are more rapid when verbal instructions signal an extinction schedule than when there are no verbal instructions (Notterman, Schoenfeld, & Bersh, 1952; Weiner, 1970). The effects of brief verbal instructions on extinction are comparable to the effects of signals that are present during the duration of the scheduled component (i.e., continuously signaled; Tiger, Hanley, & Larsen, 2008). An example of verbal instructions as a signal for extinction might be "Beginning today, I will not give you a toy when you scream." This approach makes intuitive sense when one considers common daily occurrences, such as when a friend or colleague suggests, "Do not put your money in the soda machine; it is broken today." Under such conditions, one is far less likely to engage in a response such as placing money into the machine. Presumably, the rule plus an extinction trial would yield a more rapid effect than an extinction trial presented in isolation of rules if one were to test the contingencies. For example, Tiger et al. (2008) evaluated the effect of providing brief verbal instructions (e.g., saying, "It is your time," or "It is my time") during reinforcement and extinction components of a multiple schedule, compared to when they did not provide those instructions (i.e., a mixed schedule). They found that all children engaged in discriminated responding when investigators provided brief signals (i.e., the verbal instructions) during the reinforcement and extinction components. Furthermore, three of four children engaged in near-zero levels of responding during the extinction component when the investigators provided verbal instructions at the beginning of the reinforcement and extinction components, or when they only signaled the reinforcement component.

## PRACTICAL CONSIDERATIONS

In this section, we discuss three considerations in the practical implementation of extinction: (1) use of extinction as one component of a treatment package, (2) alternative strategies when extinction is impossible or impractical, and (3) the relation between extinction and establishing operations.

### Treatment Packages

In practical applications, clinicians are likely to combine extinction with other procedures, such as differential reinforcement (McCord, Iwata, Galensky, Ellingson, & Thomson, 2001; McCord, Thomson, & Iwata, 2001; Piazza, Moes, & Fisher, 1996) or noncontingent reinforcement (Hagopian, Wilson, & Wilder, 2001; Hanley, Piazza, Fisher, Contrucci, & Maglieri, 1997). For example, Fyffe et al. (2004) used functional-communication training and extinction to treat one participant's problem behavior (i.e., touching others inappropriately). A functional analysis showed that attention was the reinforcer for problem behavior. Fyffe et al. taught the participant to request attention by using an attention card. During extinction, investigators blocked and provided no other differential consequences for problem behavior. Problem behavior decreased relative to baseline. Similar studies have shown the efficacy of extinction combined with differential reinforcement of alternative behavior (Rehfeldt & Chambers, 2003; Wilder et al., 2001), functional-communication training (Fyffe et al., 2004; Hanley, Piazza, Fisher, & Maglieri, 2005), and noncontingent reinforcement (Vollmer et al., 1993).

Investigators have shown that antecedent components (e.g., rules), modification of establishing operations (e.g., demand fading), or the use of consequent events other than reinforcement (i.e., punishment) influence the efficacy of extinction (e.g., decrease responding rapidly compared to extinction alone; Cote, Thompson, & McKerchar, 2005; Lerman et al., 2003; Zarcone, Iwata, Smith, Mazaleski, & Lerman, 1994). For example, Cote et al. evaluated a 2-minute warning or access to a toy during transitions between activities on compliance to transitioning and problem behavior. The two interventions were ineffective when implemented alone. However, adding one of the intervention components enhanced the effects of extinction for two of three participants. That is, compliance for these participants increased rapidly and was more consistent in the treatment package relative to extinction alone.

## Modification of Extinction

There are circumstances in which researchers, clinicians, or caregivers cannot implement extinction with high integrity. Examples include the difficulty of physical guidance with a large, strong individual; the danger of providing no differential consequences to life-threatening SIB; or the difficulty of eliminating the automatic reinforcement produced by a behavior. In these cases, a general approach might be to minimize reinforcement for problem behavior and maximize reinforcement for appropriate behavior (Vollmer, Peters, Kronfli, Lloveras, & Ibañez, 2020). For example, Athens and Vollmer (2010) investigated parameters of the functional reinforcer maintaining problem behavior, including duration, quality, delay, and a combination of these parameters. Results indicated that altering each of the parameters of reinforcement to favor the alternative response (e.g., increased duration) relative to problem behavior (e.g., decreased duration) produced a decrease in problem behavior, even though extinction was not in effect. Furthermore, the most marked decreases in problem behavior occurred when the investigators altered all reinforcement parameters to favor the alternative response, and these findings were consistent across behavior maintained by different sources of socially mediated reinforcement (i.e., attention, tangible, escape).

## Motivating Operations

A *motivating operation* is any environmental event that alters the reinforcing effectiveness of other events (e.g., reinforcement) and the likelihood of a response class that has historically produced those events (Michael, 1993). Identifying the variables that alter the effectiveness of escape, attention, and automatic reinforcement may establish the appropriateness of extinction as treatment (Fisher, Greer, Mitteer, et al., 2018). For example, extinction may be inappropriate for escape-maintained problem behavior in an instructional context if the tasks are not appropriate for the individual's abilities, or for automatic or attention-maintained problem behavior in a sterile environment. Several investigators have demonstrated methods for reducing problem behavior in the absence of extinction (e.g., Lalli et al., 1999; Fritz, Jackson, Stiefler, Wimberly, & Richardson, 2017; Slocum & Vollmer, 2015; Vollmer, Marcus, & Ringdahl, 1995). Lalli et al. (1999) demonstrated that compliance increased and problem behavior decreased when they provided positive reinforcement (edible

items) for compliance in the absence of extinction. Clinicians should alter motivating operations directly if they are aberrant (e.g., excessively harsh demands, sterile environment) before considering extinction as a treatment.

## CONCLUSION

Extinction is one of the most basic behavioral principles in our field and is the operation of discontinuing reinforcement of a response. If an investigator can identify the reinforcement for problem behavior, and that reinforcement is in the investigator's control, then they can discontinue the response–reinforcer relation. Extinction takes different forms, depending on the source of reinforcement.

Basic and applied research has shown that extinction is effective for decreasing problem behavior. In addition, some studies have reported patterns of responding associated with extinction, such as the extinction burst, response variation, emotional behavior, aggression, and spontaneous recovery. Reviews of the literature suggest that these response patterns may not be as common as once believed, and that investigators can attenuate them by combining extinction with other procedures, such as reinforcement.

Several factors influence the efficacy of extinction, including (1) identification of the operant function of problem behavior, (2) the baseline schedule of reinforcement, (3) the baseline parameters of reinforcement, (4) use of other procedures (e.g., reinforcement), and (5) the discriminative properties of the environment. Recognition of these variables is likely to improve the efficacy of extinction-based interventions for problem behavior. Investigators should consider alternatives if caregivers cannot implement extinction with high integrity or if motivating operations are aberrant.

## REFERENCES

Antonitis, J. J. (1951). Response variability in the white rat during conditioning, extinction, and reconditioning. *Journal of Experimental Psychology, 42,* 273–281.

Athens, E. S., & Vollmer, T. R. (2010). Investigation of differential reinforcement of alternative behavior without extinction. *Journal of Applied Behavior Analysis, 43,* 569–589.

Azrin, N. H., Hutchinson, R. R., & Hake, D. F. (1966). Extinction-induced aggression. *Journal of the Experimental Analysis of Behavior, 9,* 191–204.

Bachmeyer, M. H., Kirkwood, C. A., Criscito, A. B., Mauzy, C. R., & Berth, D. P. (2019). A comparison of functional analysis methods of inappropriate mealtime behavior. *Journal of Applied Behavior Analysis, 52,* 603–621.

Bachmeyer, M. H., Piazza, C. C., Fredrick, L. D., Reed, G. K., Rivas, K. D., & Kadey, H. J. (2009). Functional analysis and treatment of multiply controlled inappropriate mealtime behavior. *Journal of Applied Behavior Analysis, 42,* 641–658.

Baumeister, A. A., & Forehand, R. (1971). Effects of extinction of an instrumental response on stereotyped body rocking in severe retardates. *Psychological Record, 21,* 235–240.

Beavers, G. A., & Iwata, B. A. (2013). Thirty years of research on the functional analysis of problem behavior. *Journal of Applied Behavior Analysis, 46,* 1–21.

Berth, D. P., Bachmeyer, M. H., Kirkwood, C. A., Mauzy, C. R., Retzlaff, B. J., & Gibson, A. L. (2019). Noncontingent and differential reinforcement in the treatment of pediatric feeding problems. *Journal of Applied Behavior Analysis, 52,* 622–641.

Blampied, N. M., & France, K. G. (1993). A behavioral model of infant sleep disturbance. *Journal of Applied Behavior Analysis, 26,* 477–492.

Borrero, C. S. W., Vollmer, T. R., Borrero, J. C., & Bourret, J. (2005). A method for evaluating parameters of reinforcement during parent–child interactions. *Research in Developmental Disabilities, 26,* 577–592.

Borrero, C. S. W., Vollmer, T. R., Borrero, J. C., Bourret, J. C., Sloman, K. N., Samaha, A. L., et al. (2010). Concurrent reinforcement schedules for problem behavior and appropriate behavior: Experimental applications of the matching law. *Journal of the Experimental Analysis of Behavior, 93,* 455–469.

Borrero, J. C., & Vollmer, T. R. (2002). An application of the matching law to severe problem behavior. *Journal of Applied Behavior Analysis, 35,* 13–27.

Cammilleri, A. P., Tiger, J. H., & Hanley, G. P. (2008). Developing stimulus control of young children's requests to teachers: Classwide applications of multiple schedules. *Journal of Applied Behavior Analysis, 41,* 299–303.

Carr, E. G., & Durand, V. M. (1985). Reducing behavior problems through functional communication training. *Journal of Applied Behavior Analysis, 18,* 111–126.

Catania, A. C. (2007). *Learning* (4th ed.). Cornwall-on-Hudson, NY: Sloan.

Cooper, J. O., Heron, T. E., & Heward, W. L. (1987). *Applied behavior analysis.* Columbus, OH: Merrill.

Cooper, L. J., Wacker, D. P., McComas, J. J., Brown, K., Peck, S. M., Richman, D., et al. (1995). Use of component analyses to identify active variables in treatment packages for children with feeding disorders. *Journal of Applied Behavior Analysis, 28,* 139–153.

Cote, C. A., Thompson, R. H., & McKerchar, P. M. (2005). The effects of antecedent interventions and extinction on toddlers' compliance during transitions. *Journal of Applied Behavior Analysis, 38,* 235–238.

Derby, K. M., Wacker, D. P., Sasso, G., Steege, M., Northup, J., Cigrand, K., et al. (1992). Brief functional assessment techniques to evaluate aberrant behavior in an outpatient setting: A summary of 79 cases. *Journal of Applied Behavior Analysis, 25,* 713–721.

Dorsey, M. F., Iwata, B. A., Reid, D. H., & Davis, P. A. (1982). Protective equipment: Continuous and contingent application in the treatment of self-injurious behavior. *Journal of Applied Behavior Analysis, 15,* 217–230.

Dowdy, A., Tincani, M., Nipe, T., & Weise, M. J. (2018). Effects of reinforcement without extinction on increasing compliance with nail cutting: A systematic replication. *Journal of Applied Behavior Analysis, 51,* 924–930.

Epstein, R. (1983). Resurgence of previously reinforced behavior during extinction. *Behaviour Analysis Letters, 3,* 391–397.

Ferster, C. B., & Skinner, B. F. (1957). *Schedules of reinforcement.* New York: Appleton-Century-Crofts.

Fisher, W. W., Felber, J. M., Phillips, L. A., Craig, A. R., Paden, A. R., & Niemeier, J. J. (2019). Treatment of resistance to change in children with autism. *Journal of Applied Behavior Analysis, 52,* 974–993.

Fisher, W. W., Greer, B. D., Fuhrman, A. M., Saini, V., & Simmons, C. A. (2018). Minimizing resurgence of destructive behavior using behavioral momentum theory. *Journal of Applied Behavior Analysis, 51,* 831–853.

Fisher, W. W., Greer, B. D., Mitteer, D. R., Fuhrman, A. A., Romani, P. W., & Zangrillo, A. N. (2018). Further evaluation of differential exposure to establishing operations during functional communication training. *Journal of Applied Behavior Analysis, 51,* 360–373.

Fisher, W. W., Ninness, H. A. C., Piazza, C. C., & Owen-DeSchryver, J. S. (1996). On the reinforcing effects of the content of verbal attention. *Journal of Applied Behavior Analysis, 29,* 235–238.

Fisher, W. W., Saini, V., Greer, B. D., Sullivan, W. E., Roane, H. S., Fuhrman, A. M., et al. (2019). Baseline reinforcement rate and resurgence of destructive behavior. *Journal of the Experimental Analysis of Behavior, 111,* 75–93.

France, K. G., & Hudson, S. M. (1990). Behavior management of infant sleep disturbance. *Journal of Applied Behavior Analysis, 23,* 91–98.

Frederiksen, L. W., & Peterson, G. L. (1974). Schedule-induced aggression in nursery school children. *Psychological Record, 24,* 343–351.

Fritz, J. N., Jackson, L. M., Stiefler, N. A., Wimberly, B. S., & Richardson, A. R. (2017). Noncontingent reinforcement without extinction plus differential reinforcement of alternative behavior during treatment of problem behavior. *Journal of Applied Behavior Analysis, 50,* 590–599.

Fuhrman, A. M., Fisher, W. W., & Greer, B. D. (2016). A preliminary investigation on improving functional communication training by mitigating resurgence of destructive behavior. *Journal of Applied Behavior Analysis. 49,* 884–889.

Fyffe, C. E., Kahng, S., Fittro, E., & Russell, D. (2004). Functional analysis and treatment of inappropriate sexual behavior. *Journal of Applied Behavior Analysis, 37,* 401–404.

Gallup, G. G., & Altomari, T. S. (1969). Activity as a postsituation measure of frustrative nonreward. *Journal of Comparative and Physiological Psychology, 68,* 382–384.

Girolami, P. A., & Scotti, J. R. (2001). Use of analog functional analysis in assessing the function of mealtime behavior problems. *Education and Training in Mental Retardation and Developmental Disabilities, 36,* 207–223.

Grow, L. L., Kelley, M. E., Roane, H. S., & Shillingsburg, M. A. (2008). Utility of extinction-induced response variability for the selection of mands. *Journal of Applied Behavior Analysis, 41,* 15–24.

Hagopian, L. P., Rooker, G. W., & Zarcone, J. R. (2015). Delineating subtypes of self-injurious behavior maintained by automatic reinforcement. *Journal of Applied Behavior Analysis, 48,* 523–543.

Hagopian, L. P., Rooker, G. W., Zarcone, J. R., Bonner, A. C., & Arevalo, A. R. (2017). Further analysis of subtypes of automatically reinforced SIB: A replication and quantitative analysis of published datasets. *Journal of Applied Behavior Analysis, 50,* 48–66.

Hagopian, L. P., Wilson, D. M., & Wilder, D. A. (2001). Assessment and treatment of problem behavior maintained by escape from attention and access to tangible items. *Journal of Applied Behavior Analysis, 34,* 229–232.

Hanley, G. P., Iwata, B. A., & Thompson, R. H. (2001). Reinforcement schedule thinning following treatment with functional communication training. *Journal of Applied Behavior Analysis, 34,* 17–38.

Hanley, G. P., Piazza, C. C., Fisher, W. W., Contrucci, S. A., & Maglieri, K. A. (1997). Evaluation of client preference for function-based treatment packages. *Journal of Applied Behavior Analysis, 30,* 459–473.

Hanley, G. P., Piazza, C. C., Fisher, W. W., & Maglieri, K. A. (2005). On the effectiveness of and preference for punishment and extinction components of function-based interventions. *Journal of Applied Behavior Analysis, 38,* 51–65.

Hatton, G. I. (1965). Drive shifts during extinction: Effects on extinction and spontaneous recovery of bar-pressing behavior. *Journal of Comparative and Physiological Psychology, 59,* 385–391.

Heidorn, S. D., & Jensen, C. C. (1984). Generalization and maintenance of the reduction of self-injurious behavior maintained by two types of reinforcement. *Behaviour Research and Therapy, 22,* 581–586.

Herrnstein, R. J. (1974). Formal properties of the matching law. *Journal of the Experimental Analysis of Behavior, 21,* 159–164.

Hineline, P. N. (1977). Negative reinforcement and avoidance. In W. K. Honig & J. E. R. Staddon (Eds.), *Handbook of operant behavior* (pp. 364–414). Englewood Cliffs, NJ: Prentice-Hall.

Hoch, T. A., Babbitt, R. L., Coe, D. A., Krell, D. M., & Hackbert, L. (1994). Contingency contacting: Combining positive reinforcement and escape extinction procedures to treat persistent food refusal. *Behavior Modification, 18,* 106–128.

Iwata, B. A., Dorsey, M. F., Slifer, K. J., Bauman, K. E., & Richman, G. S. (1994). Toward a functional analysis of self-injury. *Journal of Applied Behavior Analysis, 27,* 197–209. (Reprinted from *Analysis and Intervention in Developmental Disabilities, 2,* 3–20, 1982)

Iwata, B. A., Pace, G. M., Cowdery, G. E., & Miltenberger, R. G. (1994). What makes extinction work: An analysis of procedural form and function. *Journal of Applied Behavior Analysis, 27,* 131–144.

Iwata, B. A., Pace, G. M., Dorsey, M. F., Zarcone, J. R., Vollmer, T. R., Smith, R. G., et al. (1994). The functions of self-injurious behavior: An experimental–epidemiological analysis. *Journal of Applied Behavior Analysis, 27,* 215–240.

Iwata, B. A., Pace, G. M., Kalsher, M. J., Cowdery, G. E., & Cataldo, M. F. (1990). Experimental analysis and extinction of self-injurious escape behavior. *Journal of Applied Behavior Analysis, 23,* 11–27.

Kelly, J. F., & Hake, D. F. (1970). An extinction induced increase in an aggressive response with humans. *Journal of the Experimental Analysis of Behavior, 14,* 153–164.

Lalli, J. S., Casey, S. D., & Kates, K. (1997). Noncontingent reinforcement as treatment for severe problem behavior: Some procedural variations. *Journal of Applied Behavior Analysis, 30,* 127–137.

Lalli, J. S., Vollmer, T. R., Progar, P. R., Wright, C., Borrero, J., Daniel, D., et al. (1999). Competition between positive and negative reinforcement in the treatment of escape behavior. *Journal of Applied Behavior Analysis, 32,* 285–296.

Lerman, D. C., & Iwata, B. A. (1995). Prevalence of the extinction burst and its attenuation during treatment. *Journal of Applied Behavior Analysis, 28,* 93–94.

Lerman, D. C., & Iwata, B. A. (1996a). A methodology for distinguishing between extinction and punishment effects associated with response blocking. *Journal of Applied Behavior Analysis, 29,* 231–233.

Lerman, D. C., & Iwata, B. A. (1996b). Developing a technology for the use of operant extinction in clinical settings: An examination of the basic and applied research. *Journal of Applied Behavior Analysis, 29,* 345–382.

Lerman, D. C., Iwata, B. A., & Wallace, M. D. (1999). Side effects of extinction: Prevalence of bursting and aggression during the treatment of self-injurious behavior. *Journal of Applied Behavior Analysis, 32,* 1–8.

Lerman, D. C., Kelley, M. E., Van Camp, C. M., & Roane, H. S. (1999). Effects of reinforcement magnitude on spontaneous recovery. *Journal of Applied Behavior Analysis, 32,* 197–200.

Lerman, D. C., Kelley, M. E., Vorndran, C. M., Kuhn, S. A. C., & LaRue, R. H., Jr. (2002). Reinforcement magnitude and responding during treatment with differential reinforcement. *Journal of Applied Behavior Analysis, 35,* 29–48.

Lerman, D. C., Kelley, M. E., Vorndran, C. M., & Van Camp, C. M. (2003). Collateral effects of response blocking during the treatment of stereotypic behavior. *Journal of Applied Behavior Analysis, 36,* 119–123.

Lewis, D. J. (1956). Acquisition, extinction, and spontaneous recovery as a function of percentage of reinforcement and intertrial intervals. *Journal of Experimental Psychology, 51,* 45–53.

Lewis, D. J. (1960). Partial reinforcement: A selective review of the literature since 1950. *Psychological Bulletin, 57,* 1–28.

Lovaas, I., Newsom, C., & Hickman, C. (1987). Self-stimulatory behavior and perceptual reinforcement. *Journal of Applied Behavior Analysis, 20,* 45–68.

Lovaas, O. I., & Simmons, J. Q. (1969). Manipulation of self-destruction in three retarded children. *Journal of Applied Behavior Analysis, 2,* 143–157.

MacDonald, J. M., Ahearn, W. H., Parry-Cruwys, D., Bancroft, S., & Dube, W. V. (2013). Persistence during extinction: Examining the effects of continuous and intermittent reinforcement on problem behavior. *Journal of Applied Behavior Analysis, 46,* 333–338.

Mackintosh, N. J. (1974). *The psychology of animal learning.* New York: Academic Press.

Martens, B. K., & Houk, J. L. (1989). The application of Herrnstein's law of effect to disruptive and on-task behavior of a retarded adolescent girl. *Journal of the Experimental Analysis of Behavior, 51,* 17–27.

Mazaleski, J. L., Iwata, B. A., & Rodgers, T. A. (1994). Protective equipment as treatment for stereotypic hand mouthing: Sensory extinction or punishment. *Journal of Applied Behavior Analysis, 27,* 345–355.

Mazaleski, J. L., Iwata, B. A., Vollmer, T. R., Zarcone, J. R., & Smith, R. G. (1993). Analysis of the reinforcement and extinction components in DRO contingencies with self-injury. *Journal of Applied Behavior Analysis, 26,* 143–156.

McCord, B. E., Iwata, B. A., Galensky, T. L., Ellingson, S. A., & Thomson, R. J. (2001). Functional analysis and treatment of problem behavior evoked by noise. *Journal of Applied Behavior Analysis, 34,* 447–462.

McCord, B. E., Thomson, R. J., & Iwata, B. A. (2001). Functional analysis and treatment of self-injury associated with transitions. *Journal of Applied Behavior Analysis, 34,* 195–210.

McDowell, J. J. (1988). Matching theory in natural human environments. *Behavior Analyst, 11,* 95–108.

Michael, J. (1993). Establishing operations. *Behavior Analyst, 16,* 191–206.

Miller, N. E., & Stevenson, S. S. (1936). Agitated behavior of rats during experimental extinction and a curve of spontaneous recovery. *Journal of Comparative Psychology, 21,* 205–231.

Nevin, J. A. (1988). Behavioral momentum and the practical reinforcement effect. *Psychological Bulletin, 103,* 44–56.

Nevin, J. A., Tota, M. E., Torquato, R. D., & Shull, R. L. (1990). Alternative reinforcement increases resistance to change: Pavlovian or operant contingencies? *Journal of the Experimental Analysis of Behavior, 53,* 359–379.

Notterman, J. M., Schoenfeld, W. N., & Bersh, P. J. (1952). A comparison of three extinction procedures following heart rate conditioning. *Journal of Abnormal and Social Psychology, 47,* 674–677.

Patel, M. R., Piazza, C. C., Martinez, C. J., Volkert, V. M., & Santana, C. M. (2002). An evaluation of two differential reinforcement procedures with escape extinction to treat food refusal. *Journal of Applied Behavior Analysis, 35,* 363–374.

Piazza, C. C., Bowman, L. G., Contrucci, S. A., Delia, M. D., Adelinis, J. D., & Goh, H. (1999). An evaluation of the properties of attention as reinforcement for destructive and appropriate behavior. *Journal of Applied Behavior Analysis, 32,* 437–449.

Piazza, C. C., Fisher, W. W., Brown, K. A., Shore, B. A., Patel, M. R., Katz, R. M., et al. (2003). Functional analysis of inappropriate mealtime behavior. *Journal of Applied Behavior Analysis, 36,* 187–204.

Piazza, C. C., Moes, D. R., & Fisher, W. W. (1996). Differential reinforcement of alternative behavior and demand fading in the treatment of escape-maintained destructive behavior. *Journal of Applied Behavior Analysis, 29,* 569–572.

Piazza, C. C., Patel, M. R., Gulotta, C. S., Sevin, B. M., & Layer, S. A. (2003). On the relative contributions of positive reinforcement and escape extinction in the treatment of food refusal. *Journal of Applied Behavior Analysis, 36,* 309–324.

Pierce, W. D., & Cheney, C. D. (2013). *Behavior analysis and learning* (5th ed.). New York: Psychology Press.

Pinkston, E. M., Reese, N. M., LeBlanc, J. M., & Baer, D. M. (1973). Independent control of a preschool child's aggression and peer interaction by contingent teacher attention. *Journal of Applied Behavior Analysis, 6,* 115–124.

Reed, G. K., Piazza, C. C., Patel, M. R., Layer, S. A., Bachmeyer, M. H., Bethke, S. D., et al. (2004). On the relative contributions of noncontingent reinforcement and escape extinction in the treatment of food refusal. *Journal of Applied Behavior Analysis, 37,* 27–41.

Rehfeldt, R. A., & Chambers, M. R. (2003). Functional analysis and treatment of verbal perseverations displayed by an adult with autism. *Journal of Applied Behavior Analysis, 36,* 259–261.

Richman, D. M., Wacker, D. P., Asmus, J. M., Casey, S. D., & Andelman, M. (1999). Further analysis of problem behavior in response class hierarchies. *Journal of Applied Behavior Analysis, 32,* 269–283.

Rincover, A. (1978). Sensory extinction: A procedure for eliminating self-stimulatory behavior in developmentally disabled children. *Journal of Abnormal Child Psychology, 6,* 299–310.

Rincover, A., Cook, R., Peoples, A., & Packard, D. (1979). Sensory extinction and sensory reinforcement principles for programming multiple adaptive behavior change. *Journal of Applied Behavior Analysis, 12,* 221–233.

Rincover, A., & Devany, J. (1982). The application of sensory extinction procedures to self-injury. *Journal of Applied Behavior Analysis, 2,* 67–81.

Roscoe, E. M., Iwata, B. A., & Goh, H. (1998). A comparison of noncontingent reinforcement and sensory extinction as treatments for self-injurious behavior. *Journal of Applied Behavior Analysis, 31,* 635–646.

Rovee-Collier, C. K., & Capatides, J. B. (1979). Positive behavioral contrast in 3-month-old infants on multiple conjugate reinforcement schedules. *Journal of the Experimental Analysis of Behavior, 32,* 15–27.

Saini, V., Greer, B. D., Fisher, W. W., Lichtblau, K. R., DeSouza, A. A., & Mitteer, D. R. (2016). Individual and combined effects of noncontingent reinforcement and response blocking on automatically reinforced problem behavior. *Journal of Applied Behavior Analysis, 49,* 693–698.

Sandman, C. A., & Hetrick, W. P. (1995). Opiate mechanisms in self-injury. *Mental Retardation and Developmental Disabilities Research Reviews, 1,* 130–136.

Siqueland, E. R. (1968). Reinforcement patterns and extinction in human newborns. *Journal of Experimental Child Psychology, 6,* 431–432.

Skinner, B. F. (1938). *The behavior of organisms: An experimental analysis.* Englewood Cliffs, NJ: Prentice-Hall.

Slocum, S. K., & Vollmer, T. R. (2015). A comparison of positive and negative reinforcement for compliance to treat problem behavior maintained by escape. *Journal of Applied Behavior Analysis, 48,* 563–574.

Sloman, K. N., Vollmer, T. R., Cotnoir, N. M., Borrero, C. S. W., Borrero, J. C., Samaha, A. L., et al. (2005). Descriptive analyses of caregiver reprimands. *Journal of Applied Behavior Analysis, 38,* 373–383.

Smith, R. G., & Iwata, B. A. (1997). Antecedent influences on behavior disorders. *Journal of Applied Behavior Analysis, 30,* 343–375.

Smith, R. G., Russo, L., & Le, D. D. (1999). Distinguishing between extinction and punishment effects of response blocking: A replication. *Journal of Applied Behavior Analysis, 32,* 367–370.

Steege, M. W., Wacker, D. P., Cigrand, K. C., & Berg, W. K. (1990). Use of negative reinforcement in the treatment of self-injurious behavior. *Journal of Applied Behavior Analysis, 23,* 459–467.

Sullivan, M. W., Lewis, M., & Alessandri, S. M. (1992). Cross-age stability in emotional expressions during learning and extinction. *Developmental Psychology, 28,* 58–63.

Tiger, J. H., Hanley, G. P., & Heal, N. A. (2006). The effectiveness of and preschoolers' preference for variations of multiple-schedule arrangements. *Journal of Applied Behavior Analysis, 41,* 475–488.

Tiger, J. H., Hanley, G. P., & Larsen, K. M. (2008). A practical variation of a multiple-schedule procedure: Brief schedule-correlated stimuli. *Journal of Applied Behavior Analysis, 41,* 125–130.

Todd, J. T., Morris, E. K., & Fenza, K. M. (1989). Temporal organization of extinction-induced responding in preschool children. *Psychological Record, 39,* 117–130.

Vaughan, M. E., & Michael, J. L. (1982). Automatic reinforcement: An important but ignored concept. *Behaviorism, 10,* 217–227.

Vollmer, T. R. (1994). The concept of automatic reinforcement: Implications for behavioral research in developmental disabilities. *Research in Developmental Disabilities, 15,* 187–207.

Vollmer, T. R., Iwata, B. A., Zarcone, J. R., Smith, R. G., & Mazaleski, J. L. (1993). The role of attention in the treatment of attention-maintained self-injurious behavior: Noncontingent reinforcement and differential reinforcement of other behavior. *Journal of Applied Behavior Analysis, 26,* 9–21.

Vollmer, T. R., Marcus, B. A., & Ringdahl, J. E. (1995). Noncontingent escape as treatment for self-injurious behavior maintained by negative reinforcement. *Journal of Applied Behavior Analysis, 28,* 15–26.

Vollmer, T. R., Peters, K. P., Kronfli, F. R., Lloveras, L. A., & Ibañez, V. F. (2020). On the definition of differential reinforcement of alternative behavior. *Journal of Applied Behavior Analysis, 53,* 1299–1303.

Vollmer, T. R., Progar, P. R., Lalli, J. S., Van Camp, C. M., Sierp, B. J., Wright, C. S., et al. (1998). Fixed-time schedules attenuate extinction-induced phenomena in the treatment of severe aberrant behavior. *Journal of Applied Behavior Analysis, 31,* 529–542.

Weiner, H. (1970). Instructional control of human operant responding during extinction following fixed-ratio conditioning. *Journal of the Experimental Analysis of Behavior, 13,* 391–394.

Wilder, D. A., Masuda, A., O'Connor, C., & Baham, M. (2001). Brief functional analysis and treatment of bizarre vocalizations in an adult with schizophrenia. *Journal of Applied Behavior Analysis, 34,* 65–68.

Williams, C. D. (1959). The elimination of tantrum behavior by extinction procedures. *Journal of Abnormal and Social Psychology, 59,* 269.

Wolf, M., Risley, T., & Mees, H. (1964). Application of operant conditioning procedures to the behavior problems of an autistic child. *Behaviour Research and Therapy, 1,* 305–312.

Woods, J. N., & Borrero, C. S. W. (2019). Examining extinction bursts in the treatment of pediatric food refusal. *Behavioral Interventions, 34,* 307–322.

Youtz, R. E. P. (1938). Reinforcement, extinction, and spontaneous recovery in a non-Pavlovian reaction. *Journal of Experimental Psychology, 22,* 305–318.

Zarcone, J. R., Iwata, B. A., Smith, R. G., Mazaleski, J. L., & Lerman, D. C. (1994). Reemergence and extinction of self-injurious escape behavior during stimulus (instructional) fading. *Journal of Applied Behavior Analysis, 27,* 307–316.

## CHAPTER 20

# Developing Function-Based Reinforcement Procedures for Problem Behavior

Wayne W. Fisher, Brian D. Greer, and Kelly J. Bouxsein

When a functional analysis shows that social consequences reinforce an individual's problem behavior, a behavior analyst can alter those consequences in ways that decrease the problem behavior and increase appropriate alternative behavior (Carr & Durand, 1985; Fisher et al., 1993; Horner & Day, 1991; Lalli, Casey, & Kates, 1995; Wacker et al., 1990). For example, the behavior analyst can teach an individual whose problem behavior is reinforced by adult attention to obtain that attention through an appropriate communication response—a differential-reinforcement treatment called *functional communication training* (FCT; Carr & Durand, 1985). Even when a functional analysis determines that the consequences automatically produced by problem behavior functions as reinforcement (Piazza et al., 1998), the behavior analyst can arrange alternative reinforcement procedures in ways that decrease the problem behavior, though it continues to produce its reinforcer automatically (e.g., Piazza et al., 1998; Vollmer, Marcus, & LeBlanc, 1994). In this chapter, we first discuss the operant mechanisms responsible for the effectiveness of function-based reinforcement procedures. We then review the possible outcomes of functional analyses and show how behavior analysts can use those results to develop effective reinforcement-based treatments for problem behavior.

## OPERANT MECHANISMS IN FUNCTION-BASED TREATMENTS

Iwata and colleagues (Iwata, Pace, Cowdery, & Miltenberger, 1994; Iwata, Dorsey, Slifer, Bauman, & Richman, 1982/1994) described three operant mechanisms related to the function of problem behavior that behavior analysts should incorporate into a functional analysis. The first component of a functional-analysis condition is its *discriminative stimulus*. Each functional-analysis condition has one or more unique antecedent stimuli that correlate with and signal the specific reinforcer for problem behavior in that condition. For example, the therapist sits in a chair reading a magazine only in the attention condition; the participant is alone in a room only in the alone condition; the therapist presents demands only in the demand condition; and the therapist plays with the participant only in the toy play condition. Research by Conners et al. (2000) showed that correlating functional-analysis conditions with additional salient, discriminative stimuli, such as unique therapists and different-colored rooms, can improve the efficiency, clarity, or both of a functional analysis with some participants. Their results also suggested that correlating baseline and treatment conditions with unique and salient discriminative stimuli may lead to more rapid treatment effects.

The second functional component of a functional-analysis condition is its *motivating operation* (Laraway, Snycerski, Michael, & Poling, 2003), an environmental event that has two effects. One effect of a motivating operation is to increase or to decrease motivation for a reinforcer (e.g., skipping lunch increases motivation for an afternoon snack; eating a big lunch decreases it). The other effect of a motivating operation is to increase or decrease the probability of responses that have produced that reinforcer in the past (e.g., walking to the snack room is more probable after skipping lunch and less probable after a big lunch). *Establishing operations* are motivating operations that increase motivation for a given reinforcer (Peterson, Lerman, & Nissen, 2016), and *abolishing operations* are those that decrease motivation (Laraway et al., 2003).

Each test condition of a functional analysis has a specific establishing operation to increase motivation for the reinforcer associated with that condition. Attention deprivation in the attention condition and demands in the demand condition increase the effectiveness of attention and escape from demands, respectively, as reinforcement and serve to evoke problem behavior. Similarly, no stimulation is available except for stimulation automatically produced by problem behavior in the alone condition. By contrast, we eliminate the previously mentioned establishing operations from the toy-play condition, which is the control condition, to decrease the probability of problem behavior.

Hammond, Iwata, Rooker, Fritz, and Bloom (2013) extended this logic by examining whether a specific sequence of functional-analysis conditions could strengthen the establishing operations in each test condition further. Participants experienced two functional analyses that differed only by condition order. Therapists conducted the functional analysis in the fixed order of ignore, attention, toy play, and demand in the fixed-sequence functional analysis. Therapists implemented those same conditions in a quasi-random order in the other functional analysis. Only the fixed sequence produced a clear function for problem behavior for three of the participants.

Understanding how establishing operations influence the probability of problem behavior during a functional analysis is important not only for assessing the function of problem behavior but also for developing an effective treatment. That is, behavior analysts can manipulate establishing operations that increase the probability of problem behavior during a functional analysis in ways that decrease its probability during treatment. For example, time-based delivery of highly preferred items (e.g., edibles) can reduce negatively reinforced problem behavior to near-zero levels by abolishing the effectiveness of escape as reinforcement (Lomas, Fisher, & Kelley, 2010; Mevers, Fisher, Kelley, & Fredrick, 2014).

The third functional component of a functional-analysis condition is its *reinforcing consequence*. A behavior analyst delivers a specific consequence following problem behavior in each test condition of a functional analysis and does so according to a dense schedule, usually a fixed-ratio (FR) 1 schedule. One advantage of delivering the putative reinforcer following problem behavior on a dense schedule and not delivering that consequence in the absence of problem behavior is that the contingency should be strong and salient (Vollmer, Borrero, Wright, Van Camp, & Lalli, 2001). Strong and salient differential contingencies in the functional-analysis conditions should lead to clearer results. A second potential advantage is that response rates are generally much lower under FR 1 schedules than under intermittent schedules, which may reduce the risks associated with severe self-injurious behavior (SIB) or aggressive behavior. A third potential advantage of delivering the putative reinforcer on an FR 1 schedule is that decreases in problem behavior may occur more rapidly if extinction is a treatment component (Lerman, Iwata, Shore, & Kahng, 1996).

## TREATMENTS FOR RESPONSES REINFORCED BY SOCIAL POSITIVE REINFORCEMENT

Functional-analysis research has shown that social positive reinforcement maintains many problem behaviors, such as aggression, SIB, pica, and property destruction (Beavers, Iwata, & Lerman, 2013; Hanley, Iwata, & McCord, 2003). For example, Iwata, Pace, Dorsey, et al. (1994) found that social positive reinforcement maintained the SIB of 40 of their 152 participants (26%). Social reactions to problem behavior that may inadvertently function as positive reinforcement in the natural environment include delivery of preferred stimuli such as attention, food, toys, music, or TV.

Function-based treatment for problem behavior maintained by social positive reinforcement generally manipulates one or more of the three functional components of a functional analysis described earlier (i.e., the discriminative stimulus that signals reinforcement for problem behavior, the motivating operation that establishes the effectiveness of a consequence as reinforcement for problem behavior, and the consequence for problem behavior). Thus one reasonable way to begin the process of developing a function-based treatment after a functional analysis has identified the reinforcer(s) for problem behavior is to ask questions related to these three functional components:

1. How can we arrange discriminative stimuli to signal (a) the availability of reinforcement for the alternative behavior at appropriate times, and (b) the unavailability of reinforcement for problem behavior?
2. How can we alter the relevant motivating operations to reduce the probability of problem behavior and increase the probability of appropriate behavior?
3. How can we alter the reinforcement contingency to reduce problem behavior and to increase appropriate behavior?

We now discuss how we can use these questions to guide development of two commonly prescribed treatments for problem behavior reinforced by social positive reinforcement: FCT and *noncontingent reinforcement* (NCR).

## Functional-Communication Training

FCT typically manipulates the consequence for problem behavior in two important ways: (1) A behavior analyst delivers the consequence the functional analysis identified as the reinforcer for problem behavior contingent on an appropriate communication response (i.e., a form of differential reinforcement of alternative behavior), and (2) the behavior analyst no longer delivers that consequence contingent on problem behavior (i.e., operant extinction). For example, if the functional analysis indicates that contingent attention reinforces problem behavior, then the behavior analyst teaches the participant (1) to obtain attention via an appropriate communication response and (2) that problem behavior no longer produces attention. The first component, delivering the functional reinforcer contingent on a communication response, is important because the participant can receive frequent reinforcement via the communication response. Providing reinforcement for the communication response minimizes periods of deprivation from attention that may act

as an establishing operation that evokes problem behavior (Lerman & Iwata, 1995). The second component is important because problem behavior becomes less probable if the behavior analyst implements extinction, so that problem behavior no longer produces attention. Behavior analysts often use FCT to treat problem behavior that is reinforced by social consequences (e.g., access to attention or tangibles, escape from demands) because FCT typically involves withholding the reinforcer following problem behavior and delivering it following an appropriate communication response. Researchers have used FCT infrequently for problem behavior maintained by automatic reinforcement because withholding reinforcers that are an automatic consequence of the behavior is often difficult (Rapp & Lanovaz, 2014).

### Selecting and Teaching the FCT Response

Investigators have rarely described how they selected the FCT response (for notable exceptions, see Grow, Kelley, Roane, & Shillingsburg, 2008; Horner & Day, 1991), although FCT is one of the most researched operant treatments (Tiger, Hanley, & Bruzek, 2008). In addition, few studies have provided clear and replicable details on how the researchers trained the FCT response (e.g., Fisher et al., 1993; Shirley, Iwata, Kahng, Mazaleski, & Lerman, 1997; Wacker et al., 1990). Horner and Day (1991) studied three components of the FCT response that have direct implications for selecting an appropriate response. In the first study of the investigation, they showed that a simple and less effortful response was more effective as an FCT response than a more complex and effortful one was. That is, problem behavior decreased more when the FCT response was signing a single word (i.e., "Break") versus a complete sentence (i.e., "I want to go, please"). In the second study, Horner and Day showed that the response was more effective when reinforced on a dense schedule (i.e., FR 1) versus a leaner schedule (i.e., FR 3). Finally, in the third study, they showed that the FCT response was more effective when it produced reinforcement almost immediately (after a 1-second delay) than when it produced the same reinforcer after a longer delay (20 seconds).

DeRosa, Fisher, and Steege (2015) extended the research by Horner and Day (1991) by showing that another important factor in predicting the effectiveness of FCT is whether the therapist can control the establishing operation for problem behavior. First, they compared two forms of FCT that differed according to the type of response targeted. Therapists modeled the vocal FCT response at prescribed times throughout the session in the vocal FCT condition. Therapists in the card FCT condition physically guided a card-touch FCT response on the same schedule they used to model the vocal response. Thus, the difference between the conditions was whether the therapist could (card FCT condition) or could not (vocal FCT condition) physically guide the FCT response. Physical guidance in the card FCT condition resulted in less exposure to the establishing operation for problem behavior for both participants. Decreased establishing-operation exposure in the card FCT condition corresponded to lower rates of problem behavior than in the vocal FCT condition. In a follow-up study, Fisher et al. (2018) directly manipulated exposure to the establishing operation during initial stages of FCT and showed that establishing-operation exposures in the range of 5–20 seconds evoked extinction bursts in five of six applications, whereas shorter exposures to the establishing operation produced rapid reductions in problem behavior without extinction bursts.

We have developed the following guidelines for selecting and training the FCT response, based on studies by Horner and Day (1991), DeRosa et al. (2015), and Tiger et al. (2008). The response should be simple for the participant to emit and easily recognized by other individuals. A response that is already in the participant's response repertoire is preferable to one that is not. A short request is an appropriate FCT response (e.g., "Play with me, please") for participants who speak in complete sentences if the participant reliably imitates a model of the vocal FCT response. We usually teach participants who do not speak and participants who speak but do not imitate a model of a vocal FCT response readily to touch a picture card that depicts the functional reinforcer (e.g., touching a picture card that shows the participant and adult playing together). We use physical guidance to help participants who do not perform the FCT response independently, then deliver the reinforcer. We reduce exposure to the establishing operation by delivering reinforcement even if we guide the participant to complete the response initially, which helps to decrease the probability of evoking problem behavior while we are training the FCT response. Over time, we fade the physical prompts until the participant emits the response independently during 90% of training trials for two consecutive sessions. Finally, we deliver the reinforcer identified during the functional analysis

immediately (i.e., a 0-second delay) and following each FCT response (i.e., an FR 1 schedule). In summary, the critical components are to (1) select an FCT response that is simple for the participant, and one we can prompt and reinforce reliably; (2) reinforce the response on a dense schedule; and (3) deliver the reinforcer as immediately as possible following the response.

## Time-Based Delivery of the Reinforcer for Problem Behavior

Another reinforcement-based approach for the treatment of problem behavior is to deliver the functional reinforcer on a time-based schedule (e.g., Fisher, DeLeon, Rodriguez-Catter, & Keeney, 2004; Vollmer, Iwata, Zarcone, Smith, & Mazaleski, 1993). Some researchers have referred to this approach as *noncontingent reinforcement* (NCR), but other researchers have criticized the label because the intended and generally observed effect is a reduction in and weakening of problem behavior. By contrast, we define *reinforcement* as an increase in responding due to the contingent presentation of a positive or negative reinforcer (Poling & Normand, 1999). Poling and Normand (1999) suggested the term *fixed-time (FT) schedules*. This label, however, does not acknowledge the prior functional relation between problem behavior and the stimulus delivered on a time-based schedule during treatment or the fact that the results of a functional analysis are used to prescribe treatment. We use the term *NCR* in this chapter to be consistent with the relevant applied literature, while acknowledging the inconsistency in referring to a treatment to reduce problem behavior as reinforcement.

We typically deliver the stimulus that previously reinforced problem behavior on a dense schedule when we initiate NCR schedules. For example, Vollmer et al. (1993) introduced NCR as a treatment for SIB reinforced by attention. The baseline was identical to the attention condition of the functional analysis, in which the therapist delivered 10 seconds of statements of concern or disapproval contingent on SIB. The researchers discontinued the contingency between SIB and attention (i.e., extinction), and they delivered praise and general conversation independently of SIB during NCR.

The delivery of attention on a dense, time-based schedule removes or lessens the establishing operation for problem behavior, which often results in immediate and large reductions in responding. For example, Hagopian, Fisher, and Legacy (1994) compared dense (FT 10-second) and lean (FT 5-minute) schedules of NCR and found that the dense schedule produced large and immediate reductions in problem behavior, whereas the lean schedule produced smaller and less consistent reductions. Researchers have observed similar differences with larger and smaller magnitudes of reinforcement on time-based schedules, even when they implemented NCR without extinction (Roscoe, Iwata, & Rand, 2003). Finally, Fisher et al. (2004) showed that NCR with extinction resulted in larger and more immediate reductions in problem behavior than implementation of extinction alone. Behavior analysts can avoid contiguous pairing of problem behavior and time-based reinforcement delivery by using a changeover delay, in which the occurrence of problem behavior at the scheduled reinforcement interval delays reinforcement delivery (Herrnstein, 1961).

## Choosing between FCT and NCR

Given that research has shown that FCT and NCR are effective treatments for problem behavior, especially when combined with extinction or mild punishment (Hagopian, Fisher, Sullivan, Acquisto, & LeBlanc, 1998), how should a behavior analyst decide which one to use and when? Perhaps the first consideration should be whether problem behavior is dangerous and likely to produce imminent harm to the participant or others. NCR may be the treatment of choice if the risk of harm is high, because FCT generally requires an initial training period, and NCR does not. NCR also has the advantage of requiring less monitoring of the participant's ongoing behavior than FCT. That is, the caregiver delivers reinforcement on a time-based schedule during NCR. By contrast, the caregiver must monitor and respond to the participant's FCT response during FCT, although most participants learn to find the caregiver and recruit reinforcement with the FCT response.

Another important consideration in choosing between FCT and NCR is whether establishing a communication response in and of itself is an important treatment goal. In such cases, FCT is the obvious choice. FCT also may have an advantage over NCR when the amount of reinforcement necessary to reduce or eliminate the establishing operation for problem behavior is unclear. For example, extended exposure to attention deprivation, such as when the caregiver is on the telephone, establishes the effectiveness of attention as a reinforcer

and evokes problem behavior that has produced attention previously. Exposure to the establishing operation may be more likely to evoke the FCT response during FCT because of its recent history of reinforcement with attention (cf. Hoffman & Falcomata, 2014).

## TREATMENTS FOR RESPONSES REINFORCED BY SOCIAL NEGATIVE REINFORCEMENT

In 1987, Iwata described negative reinforcement as an emerging technology in the field of applied behavior analysis. Research on the unique role of negative reinforcement in the development, maintenance, and treatment of problem behavior has grown exponentially since that time, despite criticisms that the distinction between positive and negative reinforcement is ambiguous, is without functional significance, and should be abandoned (Baron & Galizio, 2005; Michael, 1975).

The field has defined *negative reinforcement* as an increase in responding due to the response-contingent removal of a stimulus. However, Baron and Galizio (2005) and Michael (1975) argued that we should view reinforcement as an increase in responding due to a response-contingent environmental change from one stimulus condition to another. Their argument is based in part on the fact that a behavior analyst may have difficulty determining whether an individual is responding to terminate one event or to gain access to the opposite event in some circumstances. For example, does a person turn up the thermostat to escape from cold air or to gain access to warm air? Other behavior analysts have argued that the distinction between positive and negative reinforcement is useful and sufficiently engrained among behavior analysts that abandoning the distinction may be unwarranted; it certainly is unlikely (Iwata, 2006; Lattal & Lattal, 2006; Sidman, 2006).

Our purpose in discussing this issue is twofold. First, applied behavior analysts should recognize that there is disagreement in the field on whether the distinction between positive and negative reinforcement is meaningful. More importantly, behavior analysts on both sides of this argument would agree that considering, describing, and analyzing the stimulus conditions in effect before and after the target response are important, regardless of whether the analysts use the adjectives *positive* or *negative* to modify the term *reinforcement*. We highlight both sides of the stimulus change by (1) describing and analyzing the relevant establishing operations and discriminative stimuli present before the target response, and (2) retaining the terms *positive* and *negative reinforcement* to describe whether the stimulus change involved the introduction (positive reinforcement) or withdrawal (negative reinforcement) of a stimulus following problem behavior.

Functional-analysis research has shown that termination of demands often reinforces problem behavior. In fact, Iwata, Pace, Dorsey, et al. (1994) found that 38% of their 152 participants displayed SIB maintained by social negative reinforcement, which was a higher percentage than for any other behavioral function. Recent reviews of the functional-analysis literature also have found that a high percentage of problem behavior is negatively reinforced (Beavers et al., 2013; Hanley et al., 2003). Other forms of negatively reinforced problem behavior include escape from noise (Kettering, Fisher, Kelley, & LaRue, 2018; McCord, Iwata, Galensky, Ellingson, & Thomson, 2001) and from social interaction (Hall, DeBernardis, & Reiss, 2006).

### Choosing between FCT and NCR

FCT and NCR are both reasonable and effective treatments for problem behavior reinforced by escape from demands or other aversive events, and the issues and considerations discussed earlier, such as selecting the FCT response, are applicable to negatively reinforced problem behavior. We teach individuals whose problem behavior is reinforced by escape to request breaks with an FCT response (e.g., saying "Break, please"; touching a picture card showing the child leaving the worktable; Hagopian et al., 1998) when we use FCT. We deliver escape on a dense, time-based schedule (Vollmer, Marcus, & Ringdahl, 1995) when we use NCR. In most cases, we generally combine FCT or NCR with escape extinction (discussed further by Vollmer, Athens, & Fernand, Chapter 19, this volume).

One limitation common to FCT and NCR is that a participant with negatively reinforced problem behavior frequently escapes all or most instructional demands during initial treatment. Thus, the participant does not benefit from instruction or learn new skills (Fisher et al., 1993). Demand or instructional fading, in which a behavior analyst increases the number of presented demands gradually, is one approach to address this problem. We discuss this approach later as we describe procedures that increase treatment practicality. Presenting instructions and delivering differential reinforcement for compliance rather than for communication (Marcus & Vollmer, 1995) is another approach behavior analysts use to reduce problem behavior.

Selecting compliance as the alternative response in differential reinforcement of alternative behavior has several potential advantages. First, the individual continues to receive instructions and is more likely to learn skills that will produce alternative sources of reinforcement. Second, the continued exposure to instructions may produce habituation and make their subsequent presentation less aversive. Third, differential reinforcement of compliance can add to the effectiveness of escape extinction in unique and important ways. For example, Cataldo and colleagues showed that reinforcement of compliance can both increase that response and concomitantly decrease problem behavior, even when the consequences for problem behavior remain unchanged (Parrish, Cataldo, Kolko, Neef, & Egel, 1986; Russo, Cataldo, & Cushing, 1981). Conversely, treatments that directly target problem behavior, such as extinction, can decrease problem behavior and simultaneously increase compliance, even though the consequences for compliance remain unchanged. Parrish et al. (1986) and Russo et al. (1981) have hypothesized that compliance and problem behavior are inverse members of an overarching response class called *instruction following*, which may include these two topographically distinct responses in environmental contexts in which compliance historically has produced reinforcement and problem behavior historically has produced punishment or extinction (Parrish et al., 1986).

Selecting potent reinforcement is important in targeting problem behavior through differential reinforcement of compliance. Differential negative reinforcement of compliance is one approach to treat problem behavior maintained by negative reinforcement. The therapist delivers escape from instructions and provides no differential consequence for problem behavior (i.e., escape extinction). For example, Vollmer et al. (1995) delivered escape in the form of breaks from work on a dense FT schedule that produced immediate and large reductions in SIB. They subsequently thinned the schedule of time-based breaks from work to 10 minutes for one participant and 2.5 minutes for the other, using an instruction-fading procedure such as the one we describe below.

## Additional Considerations

Another approach to treat negatively reinforced problem behavior is to deliver positive reinforcement for compliance. For example, Lalli et al. (1999) showed that reinforcement of compliance with a preferred food increased compliance and decreased negatively reinforced problem behavior, even though problem behavior continued to produce escape. Several researchers have replicated this finding (e.g., DeLeon, Neidert, Anders, & Rodriguez-Catter, 2001; Kodak, Lerman, Volkert, & Trosclair, 2007; Slocum & Vollmer, 2015). Payne and Dozier (2013) discussed these findings in a brief review. Differential reinforcement of compliance is particularly useful when escape extinction is difficult or impossible to implement (e.g., when the participant is larger and stronger than the therapist).

Lalli et al. (1999) suggested two possible operant mechanisms for the effectiveness of differential positive reinforcement of compliance as treatment for negatively reinforced problem behavior. One possibility is that the participant prefers positive relative to negative reinforcement. The other possibility is that the presence of highly preferred positive reinforcement during instructions acts as an abolishing operation that lessens the effectiveness of escape as reinforcement for problem behavior. DeLeon et al. (2001) showed that one participant consistently chose positive reinforcement over escape when given a choice between these two reinforcers following compliance. Conversely, Lomas et al. (2010) reduced escape-reinforced problem behavior to near-zero levels with the variable-time-based delivery of preferred food and praise, showing that a highly preferred stimulus in the demand context acted as an abolishing operation and lessened the effectiveness of escape as negative reinforcement for problem behavior. These results collectively indicate that one or both of the operant mechanisms Lalli et al. described may be responsible for reductions in escape-reinforced problem behavior for a given individual.

Finally, there are additional ways of manipulating motivating operations to treat problem behavior reinforced by escape. For example, Smith, Iwata, Goh, and Shore (1995) found that escape-reinforced SIB was more probable when they presented novel tasks, when the instructional-session duration was longer, and when they presented demands at a higher rate. Other variables that establish the effectiveness of escape as reinforcement for problem behavior include difficult tasks (Weeks & Gaylord-Ross, 1981), less preferred tasks (Dunlap, Kern-Dunlap, Clarke, & Robbins, 1991), cancellation of a planned and preferred activity before the instructional session (Horner, Day, & Day, 1997), and sleep deprivation (O'Reilly, 1995). Conversely, we can reverse these establishing operations to abolish or lessen the effectiveness of escape as negative reinforcement for problem behavior, such as interspersing less aversive tasks (Ebanks & Fisher, 2003; Horner, Day, Sprague, O'Brien, & Heathfield, 1991), gradually increasing the rate or aversiveness of tasks (Pace, Ivancic, & Jefferson, 1994; Pace, Iwata, Cowdery, Andree, & McIntyre, 1993), and providing choices among tasks (Romaniuk et al., 2002.)

## TREATMENTS FOR AUTOMATICALLY REINFORCED RESPONSES

In the preceding sections, we have discussed problem behavior reinforced by consequences that individuals in the environment deliver (i.e., socially mediated reinforcement). However, some problem behavior persists at high rates in the absence of social consequences, such as when the participant is alone, and consequences that the problem behavior automatically or intrinsically produces may reinforce the response. We use the term *automatic reinforcement* to refer to a response that produces a favorable consequence automatically, and this automatic consequence increases the future probability of the response (Skinner, 1953; Vaughan & Michael, 1982; Vollmer, 1994). An everyday example is loosening a tie, which is reinforced by the discomfort it relieves. Potential examples among individuals with autism spectrum disorder or other developmental disabilities include rocking, which may produce favorable kinesthetic sensations; repeatedly dropping colorful objects in front of the eyes, which may produce favorable visual sensations; lining up objects, which may bring order to an otherwise confusing environment; and hand flapping, which may occur during physiological excitation because it mitigates arousal and reduces muscle tension.

Problem behavior reinforced by consequences that are automatically produced by the response pose a challenge because behavior analysts may not be able to control or even observe these consequences. For example, eye poking is more likely in participants who have visual impairments but intact visual sensory–neural pathways (Hyman, Fisher, Mercugliano, & Cataldo, 1990). A reasonable hypothesis regarding the function of this unique form of SIB is that it occurs because the response produces a visual-like sensation that functions as reinforcement for the response in someone who is deprived of such stimulation. However, testing whether this hypothesized automatic consequence is the functional reinforcer for SIB is difficult if not impossible, because it cannot be manipulated during a functional analysis or during treatment (for a notable exception, see Rincover, 1978).

One treatment approach is to provide the individual with alternative forms of appropriate stimulation that compete with the automatic reinforcer for problem behavior (Piazza et al., 1998; Wilder, Draper, Williams, & Higbee, 1997). Horner (1980) implemented one of the first applications of this approach, although he did not base it on a functional analysis. Horner added manipulables (such as puzzles, pull and push toys, and a rocking horse) to an otherwise austere institutional environment and called the treatment an *enriched environment*. This simple treatment increased adaptive behavior with the manipulables and reduced SIB and stereotypical behavior.

Vollmer et al. (1994) refined and extended this treatment approach by (1) prescribing the enriched-environment treatment based on the results of a functional analysis in which problem behavior persisted in the absence of social contingencies and (2) selecting the stimuli for environmental enrichment based on the results of a preference assessment (Fisher et al., 1992). Piazza et al. (1998) further refined this approach by developing a preference assessment, called the *competing-stimulus assessment,* specifically designed to identify preferred stimuli associated with high levels of interaction and low levels of problem behavior. The competing-stimulus assessment is particularly well suited for identifying preferred stimuli for reinforcement-based treatments for problem behavior maintained by automatic reinforcement and for problem behavior maintained by social positive reinforcement (e.g., Fisher, O'Connor, Kurtz, DeLeon, & Gotjen, 2000).

The competing-stimulus assessment is simple and involves a series of short sessions (e.g., 2 minutes each). The behavior analyst presents a single competing stimulus in each session, and the participant can interact with the competing stimulus, display the automatically reinforced problem behavior, or both. Observers record stimulus interaction and problem behavior to identify one or more stimuli associated with high levels of interaction and low levels of problem behavior. The behavior analyst uses the identified stimulus or stimuli by presenting them to the participant on a time-based schedule when the automatically reinforced problem behavior is most likely to occur, such as "down times" and times when alternative stimulation is unavailable.

## IMPROVING THE PRACTICALITY OF REINFORCEMENT-BASED TREATMENTS

A common criticism of behavioral treatments is that they are often labor-intensive relative to drug or milieu treatments and frequently require caregivers to (1) continuously monitor the behavior and (2) accurately deliver various prompts and consequences. Thus, behavior analysts have worked to develop and validate treatment components that make behavioral treatments easier and more practical to implement.

### Alternative Reinforcement

One approach to increasing the practicality of reinforcement-based treatments is to identify alternative reinforcers (e.g., toys) to deliver when a caregiver would have difficulty delivering the consequence that previously reinforced problem behavior (Austin & Tiger, 2015; Hagopian, Contrucci Kuhn, Long, & Rush, 2005; Hanley, Piazza, & Fisher, 1997; Rooker, Jessel, Kurtz, & Hagopian, 2013). This approach is especially useful for problem behavior reinforced by attention because caregivers are not available to deliver attention constantly (e.g., when a caregiver is in the bathtub). Delivering highly preferred toys noncontingently can decrease the probability that attention-reinforced problem behavior will reemerge when a caregiver is busy.

Several researchers have shown that providing alternative reinforcers with the functional reinforcer (e.g., a break with preferred toys) can produce more robust decreases in problem behavior than delivering the functional reinforcer alone (Rooker et al., 2013; Zangrillo, Fisher, Greer, Owen, & DeSouza, 2016). For example, therapists in Zangrillo et al. (2016) delivered escape (i.e., the functional reinforcer for problem behavior) following an FCT response in one condition and escape plus preferred toys in the other. Rates of problem behavior were lower and levels of compliance were higher for the two participants when the escape interval included preferred toys. Researchers have reported similar findings when delivering multiple, functional reinforcers instead of a single functional reinforcer (Piazza et al., 1997; Piazza, Moes, & Fisher, 1996; Rooker et al., 2013).

Selecting effective reinforcement is important regardless of whether a behavior analyst delivers functional reinforcement or alternative reinforcement when functional reinforcement is unavailable. Fisher et al. (2000) described an adaptation of the competing-stimulus assessment (Piazza et al., 1998) for problem behavior reinforced by social contingencies. Fisher et al. presented stimuli individually; problem behavior produced the functional reinforcer, which was attention, and they measured stimulus interaction and problem behavior. Stimuli associated with high levels of interaction and low levels of problem behavior effectively reduced problem behavior when the researchers delivered them on a time-based schedule, and problem behavior produced attention (Fisher et al., 2000).

Another approach to identifying effective alternative stimuli involves a behavior analyst's carefully observing the consequences produced automatically by the problem behavior. The purpose of these observations is to generate hypotheses about the nature of the stimulation produced by the behavior, which the behavior analyst uses to identify stimuli that produce the same or similar stimulation in the absence of problem behavior. Researchers have called these *matched stimuli* because they match the type of stimulation produced by problem behavior (Piazza, Adelinis, Hanley, Goh, & Delia, 2000). Behavior analysts can conduct a competing-stimulus assessment to identify one or more matched stimuli associated with high levels of interaction and low levels of problem behavior after they identify a preliminary set of matched stimuli. Matched stimuli sometimes produce greater reductions in automatically reinforced problem behavior than alternative stimuli do (Piazza et al., 1998, 2000), perhaps because they more effectively reduce the establishing operation for problem behavior.

## Thinning the Reinforcement Schedule

FCT is an effective treatment for problem behavior that behavior analysts use frequently. Initial implementation is often labor-intensive, however, because it involves providing reinforcement for the FCT response on a dense schedule, to maximize the likelihood that problem behavior will

decrease rapidly to near-zero levels. Caregivers may be unable to maintain such a dense schedule in the natural environment (Fisher et al., 1993). Thus, researchers have developed procedures to thin the reinforcement schedule effectively and efficiently during FCT while (1) maintaining low levels of problem behavior; (2) decreasing the FCT response rate, to make treatment easier and more practical to implement; and (3) bringing the FCT response under stimulus control, so that it occurs at appropriate times but does not weaken because reinforcement is periodically unavailable (Fisher, Kuhn, & Thompson, 1998; Fyffe, Kahng, Fittro, & Russell, 2004; Hanley, Iwata, & Thompson, 2001; Saini, Miller, & Fisher, 2016).

A practical approach to thinning the reinforcement schedule is to restrict access to the picture card immediately following reinforcement delivery when the FCT response is a picture exchange (Fisher, Greer, Querim, & DeRosa, 2014; Greer, Fisher, Saini, Owen, & Jones, 2016; Roane, Fisher, Sgro, Falcomata, & Pabico, 2004). The absence of the FCT response card serves as a discriminative stimulus for the unavailability of reinforcement and prevents the occurrence of the response when it is not likely to produce reinforcement. For example, a child cannot request a caregiver's attention if the card is unavailable while the caregiver is changing a sibling's diaper. The picture card should be available continuously during initial treatment. The caregiver initiates schedule thinning after several sessions with high levels of the FCT response and low levels of problem behavior by restricting access to the card (e.g., by placing it out of sight) for a few seconds after the reinforcement interval. Over time, the caregiver progressively increases the duration of the picture card's unavailability. For example, the caregiver might double the duration of the picture card's unavailability after every two sessions in which levels of problem behavior remain low until reaching a practical schedule. A reasonable schedule-thinning goal would be to present the FCT card once every 10–15 minutes and to provide functional reinforcement for 1–3 minutes. Terminal reinforcement schedules are likely to vary across participants and situations. However, reinforcement density should remain sufficiently high throughout and after schedule thinning, such that the participant does not experience long periods without access to the functional reinforcer (Roane, Falcomata, & Fisher, 2007).

We generally use separate discriminative stimuli to signal reinforcement availability when the FCT response is a vocal operant (e.g., "Play, please"; "Break, please"). For example, we might hang a large square of green or red paper alternately on the wall to signal the availability or unavailability of reinforcement, respectively, according to the current reinforcement schedule (e.g., Fisher et al., 1998). The green paper serves as the $S^D$ (pronounced "ess-dee") because it signals the availability of reinforcement, and the red paper serves as the $S^\Delta$ (pronounced "ess-delta") because it signals the unavailability of reinforcement.

We typically conduct training trials to expose the participant to the contingencies correlated with each discriminative stimulus, such as a green $S^D$ to signal reinforcement and a red $S^\Delta$ to signal extinction. We thin the reinforcement schedule over time by increasing the duration the $S^\Delta$ is present, decreasing the duration the $S^D$ is present, or both (Hanley et al., 2001). We continue thinning the schedule when levels of problem behavior remain low.

Reinforcement schedule thinning for problem behavior reinforced by escape from instructions typically involves increasing the number of instructions or trials the participant must complete before escape is available (e.g., a chain schedule of reinforcement), which researchers refer to as *instructional* or *demand fading* (Pace et al., 1993; Zarcone et al., 1993). Instructional fading can be used alone (Pace et al., 1994) or with other treatments, such as escape extinction (Zarcone et al., 1993) or FCT (Hagopian et al., 1998). The therapist arranges the treatment with instructional materials present when instructional fading begins, but the therapist delivers no instructions initially (i.e., continuous noncontingent escape). When problem behavior remains low in the absence of instruction delivery, the therapist introduces a single instruction (e.g., "Point to red") about halfway through the session. The therapist subsequently increases the number of instructions per session gradually (e.g., by adding one instruction after each session in which problem behavior is at least 90% below the baseline mean; Pace et al., 1993) until reaching a criterion, such as a 10-minute instructional period.

We generally do not reduce the number of instructions per session when we implement instructional fading with FCT. Rather, we introduce a chained schedule in which the participant must complete one instruction first, and then we present a discriminative stimulus to signal reinforcement availability (i.e., escape) for the FCT response. In subsequent sessions, we gradually in-

crease the number of instructions that we require the participant to complete before we present the discriminative stimulus and provide escape for the FCT response. We only increase the response requirement (i.e., the number of instructions) if the rate of problem behavior remains below a criterion (e.g., 90% below the baseline mean; Hagopian et al., 1998).

Similarly, several procedures are available for increasing the practicality and ease of NCR schedules after we achieve initial reductions in problem behavior with a dense NCR schedule. For example, Hagopian et al. (1994) gradually thinned the dense (FT 10-second) schedule to a lean (FT 5-minute) schedule and obtained near-zero rates of problem behavior. Importantly, treatment effects transferred from the clinic to the classroom and were maintained at a 2-month follow-up.

## Discriminative Stimuli

Developing stimulus control over the FCT response so that it occurs reliably, but only during programmed availability of functional reinforcement, is important for reinforcement schedule thinning. A behavior analyst often presents a unique discriminative stimulus (e.g., green card, green bracelet) continuously while reinforcement is available. The behavior analyst uses a different stimulus (e.g., red card, red bracelet) to signal that reinforcement is not available (i.e., extinction). Incorporating discriminative stimuli during reinforcement schedule thinning for the FCT response can improve the efficiency and efficacy of FCT.

A study by Betz, Fisher, Roane, Mintz, and Owen (2013) compared the effects of multiple- and mixed-reinforcement schedules for four participants who engaged in problem behavior. The multiple schedule included discriminative stimuli that signaled the availability of reinforcement, but the mixed schedule did not. Therapists during the mixed-reinforcement schedule alternated quasi-randomly between 60-second unsignaled periods in which functional reinforcement for the FCT response was available or unavailable. The procedure was identical during the multiple-reinforcement schedule, with the addition of discriminative stimuli such as a colored bracelet, vest, or card to signal the availability and unavailability of functional reinforcement for the FCT response. The participants showed high rates of the FCT response during the extinction component of the mixed schedule, but relatively few responses during the extinction component of the multiple schedule, indicating that the stimuli facilitated discrimination between the FCT components. Next, the researchers evaluated whether they could thin the reinforcement schedule rapidly with a multiple schedule. The participants showed near-perfect discrimination between the components during rapid thinning of the schedule when discriminative stimuli signaled the availability and unavailability of reinforcement.

The Betz et al. (2013) results are important because they show that behavior analysts can forgo lengthy schedule thinning under some conditions and arrive more quickly at terminal FCT schedules if they establish discriminative control first. Fisher, Greer, Fuhrman, and Querim (2015) recently extended the Betz et al. findings. They showed that other individuals could implement treatment in other contexts with little loss of treatment effects after participants readily discriminated between the multiple-reinforcement-schedule components during FCT. That is, the FCT treatment proved portable and easily transferred to other individuals and other settings. Greer et al. (2019) replicated and extended these findings by showing that the use of discriminative stimuli facilitated the rapid transfer of treatment effects from behavior therapists to the participants' caregivers.

Greer et al. (2016) described other potential advantages of establishing stimulus control initially during FCT. The researchers summarized 25 consecutive applications of FCT in which they used discriminative stimuli to thin the reinforcement schedule. Results indicated a 96% reduction in levels of problem behavior from baseline, relatively few FCT responses (8%) during extinction, and only one (4%) application of punishment.

Perhaps some of the most fascinating data on discriminative stimuli during FCT show that such stimuli can reduce the probability of treatment relapse. Fuhrman, Fisher, and Greer (2016) exposed two participants who engaged in problem behavior to two sequences of phases in which they implemented FCT with or without discriminative stimuli. After rates of problem behavior decreased with each FCT type, researchers then conducted extinction sessions in which FCT responses never produced reinforcement. Researchers used the same discriminative stimulus that they used during FCT (i.e., the $S^\Delta$) during the extinction sessions that followed FCT, to determine whether using the discriminative stimulus to signal extinction during some phases (i.e., $S^\Delta$ present) but not others (i.e., $S^\Delta$ absent) would reduce the re-emergence of problem behavior. Both participants emitted considerably fewer problem behaviors in the condition in which the researchers signaled extinction (i.e., $S^\Delta$ present) relative to the condition in which they did not (i.e., $S^\Delta$ absent). Fisher, Fuhrman, Greer, Mitteer, and Piazza (2020) replicated and extended these findings with four additional participants by isolating the effects of the discriminative stimuli and applying those stimuli in a new context. These studies are important because they show that behavior analysts can use discriminative stimuli to mitigate or even prevent treatment relapse when the functional reinforcer is unavailable for extended periods.

## ADDRESSING COMMON PROBLEMS IN REINFORCEMENT-BASED TREATMENTS

Hagopian et al. (1998) reviewed 21 cases in which they implemented FCT-based treatments and found that FCT was effective in most when combined with extinction. However, FCT plus extinction lost its effectiveness in about one-half of the cases when they thinned the reinforcement schedule. Similarly, Volkert, Lerman, Call, and Trosclair-Lasserre (2009) observed resurgence of problem behavior in most cases when they placed the FCT response on extinction or rapidly decreased the frequency of reinforcement for the response from an FR 1 to an FR 12 schedule. As previously mentioned, signaling extended periods in which reinforcement will be unavailable can help to mitigate resurgence (e.g., Fuhrman et al., 2016). In addition, providing substitute reinforcers may also prevent occurrences of problem behavior when the functional reinforcer is unavailable (e.g., Fisher et al., 2000; Rooker et al., 2013). However, adding a function-based punishment component may be warranted when these reinforcement-based treatments are ineffective (Hagopian et al., 1998; see Lerman & Toole, Chapter 21, this volume, for a detailed discussion of this issue).

## CONCLUDING COMMENTS

Functional-reinforcement-based treatments are likely to be efficient and effective, because results of the functional analysis provide specific information that directs treatment development to relevant antecedents and consequences. That is, the functional-analysis results allow a behavior analyst to focus the treatment on the contexts (e.g., demand contexts when escape is the reinforcer, low-attention contexts when attention is the reinforcer), rather than implementing a treatment across environmental contexts. Focusing on one or a few specific contexts allows for easier treatment implementation in the natural environment. The functional analysis also specifies a relatively small number of procedures to reduce problem behavior (e.g., eliminate the contingency between problem behavior and its reinforcer) and increase appropriate alternative behavior (e.g., provide access to the functional reinforcer following an appropriate communication response). This leads to more efficient treatment development, in that results of the functional analysis prescribe a specific treatment and avoid a trial-and-error approach to selecting treatments.

In conclusion, accurate functional-analysis results promote quicker development of effective treatments; easier implementation of the treatment in the natural environment, by specifying the contexts in which the treatment is relevant; and generalization and maintenance of treatment effects, by using the functional reinforcer to maintain an appropriate alternative behavior in the natural environment (Durand, Berotti, & Weiner, 1993).

## REFERENCES

Austin, J. E., & Tiger, J. H. (2015). Providing alternative reinforcers to facilitate tolerance to delayed reinforcement following functional communication training. *Journal of Applied Behavior Analysis, 48,* 663–668.

Baron, A., & Galizio, M. (2005). Positive and negative reinforcement: Should the distinction be preserved? *Behavior Analyst, 28,* 85–98.

Beavers, G. A., Iwata, B. A., & Lerman, D. C. (2013). Thirty years of research on the functional analysis of problem behavior. *Journal of Applied Behavior Analysis, 46,* 1–21.

Betz, A. M., Fisher, W. W., Roane, H. S., Mintz, J. C., & Owen, T. M. (2013). A component analysis of schedule thinning during functional communication training. *Journal of Applied Behavior Analysis, 46,* 219–241.

Carr, E. G., & Durand, V. M. (1985). Reducing behavior problems through functional communication training. *Journal of Applied Behavior Analysis, 18,* 111–126.

Conners, J., Iwata, B. A., Kahng, S. W., Hanley, G. P., Worsdell, A. S., & Thompson, R. H. (2000). Differential responding in the presence and absence of discriminative stimuli during multielement functional analyses. *Journal of Applied Behavior Analysis, 33,* 299–308.

DeLeon, I. G., Neidert, P. L., Anders, B. M., & Rodriguez-Catter, V. (2001). Choices between positive and negative reinforcement during treatment for escape-maintained behavior. *Journal of Applied Behavior Analysis, 34,* 521–525.

DeRosa, N. M., Fisher, W. W., & Steege, M. W. (2015). An evaluation of time in establishing operation on the effectiveness of functional communication training. *Journal of Applied Behavior Analysis, 48,* 115–130.

Dunlap, G., Kern-Dunlap, L., Clarke, S., & Robbins, F. R. (1991). Functional assessment, curricular revision, and severe behavior problems. *Journal of Applied Behavior Analysis, 24,* 387–397.

Durand, V. M., Berotti, D., & Weiner, J. (1993). Functional communication training: Factors affecting effectiveness, generalization, and maintenance. In J. Reichle & D. P. Wacker (Eds.), *Communicative alternatives to challenging behavior: Integrating functional assessment and treatment strategies* (pp. 317–340). Baltimore: Brookes.

Ebanks, M. E., & Fisher, W. W. (2003). Altering the timing of academic prompts to treat destructive behavior maintained by escape. *Journal of Applied Behavior Analysis, 36,* 355–359.

Fisher, W. W., DeLeon, I. G., Rodriguez-Catter, V., & Keeney, K. M. (2004). Enhancing the effects of extinction on attention-maintained behavior through noncontingent delivery of attention or stimuli identified via a competing stimulus assessment. *Journal of Applied Behavior Analysis, 37,* 171–184.

Fisher, W. W., Fuhrman, A. M., Greer, B. D., Mitteer, D. R., & Piazza, C. C. (2020). Mitigating resurgence of destructive behavior using the discriminative stimuli of a multiple schedule. *Journal of the Experimental Analysis of Behavior, 113,* 263–277.

Fisher, W. W., Greer, B. D., Fuhrman, A. M., & Querim, A. C. (2015). Using multiple schedules during functional communication training to promote rapid transfer of treatment effects. *Journal of Applied Behavior Analysis, 48,* 713–733.

Fisher, W. W., Greer, B. D., Mitteer, D. R., Fuhrman, A. M., Romani, P. W., & Zangrillo, A. N. (2018). Further evaluation of differential exposure to establishing operations during functional communication training. *Journal of Applied Behavior Analysis, 51,* 360–373.

Fisher, W. W., Greer, B. D., Querim, A. C., & DeRosa, N. (2014). Decreasing excessive functional communication responses while treating destructive behavior using response restriction. *Research in Developmental Disabilities, 35,* 2614–2623.

Fisher, W. W., Kuhn, D. E., & Thompson, R. H. (1998). Establishing discriminative control of responding using functional and alternative reinforcers during functional communication training. *Journal of Applied Behavior Analysis, 31,* 543–560.

Fisher, W. W., O'Connor, J. T., Kurtz, P. F., DeLeon, I. G., & Gotjen, D. L. (2000). The effects of noncontingent delivery of high- and low-preference stimuli on attention-maintained destructive behavior. *Journal of Applied Behavior Analysis, 33,* 79–83.

Fisher, W., Piazza, C. C., Bowman, L. G., Hagopian, L. P., Owens, J. C., & Slevin, I. (1992). A comparison of two approaches for identifying reinforcers for persons with severe and profound disabilities. *Journal of Applied Behavior Analysis, 25,* 491–498.

Fisher, W., Piazza, C., Cataldo, M., Harrell, R., Jefferson, G., & Conner, R. (1993). Functional communication training with and without extinction and punishment. *Journal of Applied Behavior Analysis, 26,* 23–36.

Fuhrman, A. M., Fisher, W. W., & Greer, B. D. (2016). A preliminary investigation on improving functional communication training by mitigating resurgence of destructive behavior. *Journal of Applied Behavior Analysis, 49,* 884–899.

Fyffe, C. E., Kahng, S. W., Frittro, E., & Russell, D. (2004). Functional analysis and treatment of inappropriate sexual behaviors. *Journal of Applied Behavior Analysis, 37,* 401–404.

Greer, B. D., Fisher, W. W., Briggs, A. M., Lichtblau, K. R., Phillips, L. A., & Mitteer, D. R. (2019). Using schedule-correlated stimuli during functional communication training to promote the rapid transfer of treatment effects. *Behavioral Development, 24,* 100–119.

Greer, B. D., Fisher, W. W., Saini, V., Owen, T. M., & Jones, J. K. (2016). Functional communication training during reinforcement schedule thinning: An analysis of 25 applications. *Journal of Applied Behavior Analysis, 49,* 105–121.

Grow, L. L., Kelley, M. E., Roane, H. S., & Shillingsburg, M. A. (2008). Utility of extinction-induced response variability for the selection of mands. *Journal of Applied Behavior Analysis, 41,* 15–24.

Hagopian, L. P., Contrucci Kuhn, S. A., Long, E. S., & Rush, K. S. (2005). Schedule thinning following communication training: Using competing stimuli to enhance tolerance to decrements in reinforcer density. *Journal of Applied Behavior Analysis, 38,* 177–193.

Hagopian, L. P., Fisher, W. W., & Legacy, S. M. (1994). Schedule effects of noncontingent reinforcement on attention-maintained destructive behavior in identical quadruplets. *Journal of Applied Behavior Analysis, 27,* 317–325.

Hagopian, L. P., Fisher, W. W., Sullivan, M. T., Acquisto, J., & LeBlanc, L. A. (1998). Effectiveness of functional communication training with and without extinction and punishment: A summary of 21 inpatient cases. *Journal of Applied Behavior Analysis, 31,* 211–235.

Hall, S., DeBernardis, M., & Reiss, A. (2006). Social escape behaviors in children with fragile X syndrome. *Journal of Autism and Developmental Disorders, 36,* 935–947.

Hammond, J. L., Iwata, B. A., Rooker, G. W., Fritz, J. N., & Bloom, S. E. (2013). Effects of fixed versus random condition sequencing during multielement functional analyses. *Journal of Applied Behavior Analysis, 46,* 22–30.

Hanley, G. P., Iwata, B. A., & McCord, B. E. (2003). Functional analysis of problem behavior: A review. *Journal of Applied Behavior Analysis, 36,* 147–185.

Hanley, G. P., Iwata, B. A., & Thompson, R. H. (2001). Reinforcement schedule thinning following treatment with functional communication training. *Journal of Applied Behavior Analysis, 34,* 17–38.

Hanley, G. P., Piazza, C. C., & Fisher, W. W. (1997). Noncontingent presentation of attention and alternative stimuli in the treatment of attention-maintained destructive behavior. *Journal of Applied Behavior Analysis, 30,* 229–237.

Herrnstein, R. J. (1961). Relative and absolute strength of response as a function of frequency of reinforcement. *Journal of the Experimental Analysis of Behavior, 4,* 267–272.

Hoffman, K., & Falcomata, T. S. (2014). An evaluation of resurgence of appropriate communication in individuals with autism who exhibit severe problem behavior. *Journal of Applied Behavior Analysis, 47,* 651–656.

Horner, R. D. (1980). The effects of an environmental "enrichment" program on the behavior of institutionalized profoundly retarded children. *Journal of Applied Behavior Analysis, 13,* 473–491.

Horner, R. H., & Day, H. M. (1991). The effects of response efficiency on functionally equivalent competing behaviors. *Journal of Applied Behavior Analysis, 24,* 719–732.

Horner, R. H., Day, H. M., & Day, J. R. (1997). Using neutralizing routines to reduce problem behaviors. *Journal of Applied Behavior Analysis, 30,* 601–614.

Horner, R. H., Day, H. M., Sprague, J. R., O'Brien, M., & Heathfield, L. T. (1991). Interspersed requests: A nonaversive procedure for reducing aggression and self-injury during instruction. *Journal of Applied Behavior Analysis, 24,* 265–278.

Hyman, S. L., Fisher, W., Mercugliano, M., & Cataldo, M. F. (1990). Children with self-injurious behavior. *Pediatrics, 85,* 437–441.

Iwata, B. A. (1987). Negative reinforcement in applied behavior analysis: An emerging technology. *Journal of Applied Behavior Analysis, 20,* 361–378.

Iwata, B. A. (2006). On the distinction between positive and negative reinforcement. *Behavior Analyst, 29,* 121–123.

Iwata, B. A., Dorsey, M. F., Slifer, K. J., Bauman, K. E., & Richman, G. S. (1994). Toward a functional analysis of self-injury. *Journal of Applied Behavior Analysis, 27,* 197–209. (Reprinted from *Analysis and Intervention in Developmental Disabilities, 2,* 3–20, 1982)

Iwata, B. A., Pace, G. M., Cowdery, G. E., & Miltenberger, R. G. (1994). What makes extinction work: An analysis of procedural form and function. *Journal of Applied Behavior Analysis, 27,* 131–144.

Iwata, B. A., Pace, G. M., Dorsey, M. F., Zarcone, J. R., Vollmer, T. R., Smith, R. G., et al. (1994). The functions of self-injurious behavior: An experimental-epidemiological analysis. *Journal of Applied Behavior Analysis, 27,* 215–240.

Kettering, T. L., Fisher, W. W., Kelley, M. E., & LaRue, R. H. (2018). Sound attenuation and preferred music in the treatment of problem behavior maintained by escape from noise. *Journal of Applied Behavior Analysis, 51,* 687–693.

Kodak, T., Lerman, D. C., Volkert, V. M., & Trosclair, N. (2007). Further examination of factors that influence preference for positive versus negative reinforcement. *Journal of Applied Behavior Analysis, 40,* 25–44.

Lalli, J. S., Casey, S., & Kates, K. (1995). Reducing escape behavior and increasing task completion with functional communication training, extinction, and response chaining. *Journal of Applied Behavior Analysis, 28,* 261–268.

Lalli, J. S., Vollmer, T. R., Progar, P. R., Wright, C., Borrero, J., Daniel, D., et al. (1999). Competition between positive and negative reinforcement in the treatment of escape behavior. *Journal of Applied Behavior Analysis, 32,* 285–296.

Laraway, S., Snycerski, S., Michael, J., & Poling, A. (2003). Motivating operations and terms to describe them: Some further refinements. *Journal of Applied Behavior Analysis, 36,* 407–414.

Lattal, K. A., & Lattal, A. D. (2006). And yet . . . : Further comments on distinguishing positive and negative reinforcement. *Behavior Analyst, 29,* 129–134.

Lerman, D. C., & Iwata, B. A. (1995). Prevalence of the extinction burst and its attenuation during treatment. *Journal of Applied Behavior Analysis, 28,* 93–94.

Lerman, D. C., Iwata, B. A., Shore, B. A., & Kahng, S. W. (1996). Responding maintained by intermittent reinforcement: Implications for the use of extinction with problem behavior in clinical settings. *Journal of Applied Behavior Analysis, 29,* 153–171.

Lomas, J. E., Fisher, W. W., & Kelley, M. E. (2010). The effects of variable-time delivery of food items and praise on problem behavior reinforced by escape. *Journal of Applied Behavior Analysis, 43,* 425–435.

Marcus, B. A., & Vollmer, T. R. (1995). Effects of differential negative reinforcement on disruption and compliance. *Journal of Applied Behavior Analysis, 28,* 229–230.

McCord, B. E., Iwata, B. A., Galensky, T. L., Ellingson, S. A., & Thomson, R. J. (2001). Functional analysis and treatment of problem behavior evoked by noise. *Journal of Applied Behavior Analysis, 34,* 447–462.

Mevers, J. E. L., Fisher, W. W., Kelley, M. E., & Fredrick, L. D. (2014). The effects of variable-time versus contingent reinforcement delivery on problem behavior maintained by escape. *Journal of Applied Behavior Analysis, 47,* 277–292.

Michael, J. (1975). Positive and negative reinforcement, a distinction that is no longer necessary: Or better ways to talk about bad things. *Behaviorism, 3,* 33–45.

O'Reilly, M. F. (1995). Functional analysis and treatment of escape-maintained aggression correlated with sleep deprivation. *Journal of Applied Behavior Analysis, 28,* 225–226.

Pace, G. M., Ivancic, M. T., & Jefferson, G. (1994). Stimulus fading as treatment for obscenity in a brain-injured adult. *Journal of Applied Behavior Analysis, 27,* 301–305.

Pace, G. M., Iwata, B. A., Cowdery, G. E., Andree, P. J., & McIntyre, T. (1993). Stimulus (instructional) fading during extinction of self-injurious escape behavior. *Journal of Applied Behavior Analysis, 26,* 205–212.

Parrish, J. M., Cataldo, M. F., Kolko, D. J., Neef, N. A., & Egel, A. L. (1986). Experimental analysis of response covariation among compliant and inappropriate behaviors. *Journal of Applied Behavior Analysis, 19,* 241–254.

Payne, S. W., & Dozier, C. L. (2013). Positive reinforcement as treatment for problem behavior maintained by negative reinforcement. *Journal of Applied Behavior Analysis, 46,* 699–703.

Peterson, C., Lerman, D. C., & Nissen, M. A. (2016). Reinforcer choice as an antecedent versus consequence. *Journal of Applied Behavior Analysis, 49,* 286–293.

Piazza, C. C., Adelinis, J. D., Hanley, G. P., Goh, H. L., & Delia, M. D. (2000). An evaluation of the effects of matched stimuli on behaviors maintained by automatic reinforcement. *Journal of Applied Behavior Analysis, 33,* 13–27.

Piazza, C. C., Fisher, W. W., Hanley, G. P., LeBlanc, L. A., Worsdell, A. S., Lindauer, S. E., et al. (1998). Treatment of pica through multiple analyses of its reinforcing functions. *Journal of Applied Behavior Analysis, 31,* 165–189.

Piazza, C. C., Fisher, W. W., Hanley, G. P., Remick, M. L., Contrucci, S. A., & Aitken, T. L. (1997). The use of positive and negative reinforcement in the treatment of escape-maintained destructive behavior. *Journal of Applied Behavior Analysis, 30,* 279–298.

Piazza, C. C., Moes, D. R., & Fisher, W. W. (1996). Differential reinforcement of alternative behavior and demand fading in the treatment of escape-maintained destructive behavior. *Journal of Applied Behavior Analysis, 29,* 569–572.

Poling, A., & Normand, M. (1999). Noncontingent reinforcement: An inappropriate description of time-based schedules that reduce behavior. *Journal of Applied Behavior Analysis, 32,* 237–238.

Rapp, J. T., & Lanovaz, M. J. (2014). Introduction to the special issue on assessment and treatment of stereotypy. *Behavior Modification, 38,* 339–343.

Rincover, A. (1978). Sensory extinction: A procedure form eliminating self-stimulatory behavior in developmentally disabled children. *Journal of Abnormal Child Psychology, 6,* 299–310.

Roane, H. S., Falcomata, T. S., & Fisher, W. W. (2007). Applying the behavioral economics principle of unit price to DRO schedule thinning. *Journal of Applied Behavior Analysis, 40,* 529–534.

Roane, H. S., Fisher, W. W., Sgro, G. M., Falcomata, T. S., & Pabico, R. R. (2004). An alternative method of thinning reinforcer delivery during differential reinforcement. *Journal of Applied Behavior Analysis, 37,* 213–218.

Romaniuk, C., Miltenberger, R., Conyers, C., Jenner, N., Jurgens, M., & Ringenberg, C. (2002). The influence of activity choice on problem behaviors maintained by escape versus attention. *Journal of Applied Behavior Analysis, 35,* 349–362.

Rooker, G. W., Jessel, J., Kurtz, P. F., & Hagopian, L. P. (2013). Functional communication training with and without alternative reinforcement and punishment: An analysis of 58 applications. *Journal of Applied Behavior Analysis, 46,* 708–722.

Roscoe, E. M., Iwata, B. A., & Rand, M. S. (2003). Effects of reinforcer consumption and magnitude on response rates during noncontingent reinforcement. *Journal of Applied Behavior Analysis, 36,* 525–539.

Russo, D. C., Cataldo, M. F., & Cushing, P. J. (1981). Compliance training and behavioral covariation in the treatment of multiple behavior problems. *Journal of Applied Behavior Analysis, 14,* 209–222.

Saini, V., Miller, S. A., & Fisher, W. W. (2016). Multiple schedules in practical application: Research trends and implications for future investigation. *Journal of Applied Behavior Analysis, 49,* 421–444.

Shirley, M. J., Iwata, B. A., Kahng, S., Mazaleski, J. L., & Lerman, D. C. (1997). Does functional communication training compete with ongoing contingencies of reinforcement?: An analysis during response acquisition and maintenance. *Journal of Applied Behavior Analysis, 30,* 93–104.

Sidman, M. (2006). The distinction between positive and negative reinforcement: Some additional considerations. *Behavior Analyst, 29,* 135–139.

Skinner, B. F. (1953). *Science and human behavior.* New York: Free Press.

Slocum, S. K., & Vollmer, T. R. (2015). A comparison of positive and negative reinforcement for compliance to treat problem behavior maintained by escape. *Journal of Applied Behavior Analysis, 48,* 563–574.

Smith, R. G., Iwata, B. A., Goh, H., & Shore, B. A. (1995). Analysis of establishing operations for self-injury maintained by escape. *Journal of Applied Behavior Analysis, 28,* 515–535.

Tiger, J. H., Hanley, G. P., & Bruzek, J. (2008). Functional communication training: A review and practical guide. *Behavior Analysis in Practice, 1,* 16–23.

Vaughan, M. E., & Michael, J. L. (1982). Automatic reinforcement: An important but ignored concept. *Behaviorism, 10,* 217–228.

Volkert, V. M., Lerman, D. C., Call, N. A., & Trosclair-Lasserre, N. (2009). An evaluation of resurgence during treatment with functional communication training. *Journal of Applied Behavior Analysis, 42,* 145–160.

Vollmer, T. R. (1994). The concept of automatic reinforcement: Implications for behavioral research in developmental disabilities. *Research in Developmental Disabilities, 15,* 187–207.

Vollmer, T. R., Borrero, J. C., Wright, C. S., Van Camp, C., & Lalli, J. S. (2001). Identifying possible contingencies during descriptive analyses of severe behavior disorders. *Journal of Applied Behavior Analysis, 34,* 269–287.

Vollmer, T. R., Iwata, B. A., Zarcone, J. R., Smith, R. G., & Mazaleski, J. L. (1993). The role of attention in the treatment of attention-maintained self-injurious behavior: Noncontingent reinforcement and differential reinforcement of other behavior. *Journal of Applied Behavior Analysis, 26,* 9–21.

Vollmer, T. R., Marcus, B. A., & LeBlanc, L. (1994). Treatment of self-injury and hand mouthing following inconclusive functional analyses. *Journal of Applied Behavior Analysis, 27,* 331–344.

Vollmer, T. R., Marcus, B. A., & Ringdahl, J. E. (1995). Noncontingent escape as treatment for self-injurious behavior maintained by negative reinforcement. *Journal of Applied Behavior Analysis, 28,* 15–26.

Wacker, D. P., Steege, M. W., Northup, J., Sasso, G., Berg, W., Reimers, T., et al. (1990). A component analysis of functional communication training across three topographies of severe behavior problems. *Journal of Applied Behavior Analysis, 23,* 417–429.

Weeks, M., & Gaylord-Ross, R. (1981). Task difficulty and aberrant behavior in severely handicapped students. *Journal of Applied Behavior Analysis, 14,* 449–463.

Wilder, D. A., Draper, R., Williams, W. L., & Higbee, T. S. (1997). A comparison of noncontingent reinforcement, other competing stimulation, and liquid rescheduling for the treatment of rumination. *Behavioral Treatments, 12,* 55–64.

Zangrillo, A. N., Fisher, W. W., Greer, B. D., Owen, T. M., & DeSouza, A. A. (2016). Treatment of escape-maintained challenging behavior using chained schedules: An evaluation of the effects of thinning positive plus negative reinforcement during functional communication training. *International Journal of Developmental Disabilities, 62,* 147–156.

Zarcone, J. R., Iwata, B. A., Vollmer, T. R., Jagtiani, S., Smith, R. G., & Mazaleski, J. L. (1993). Extinction of self-injurious escape behavior with and without instructional fading. *Journal of Applied Behavior Analysis, 26,* 353–360.

# CHAPTER 21

# Developing Function-Based Punishment Procedures for Problem Behavior

Dorothea C. Lerman and Lisa M. Toole

Numerous procedures based on the process of punishment are effective for treating problem behavior. When the contingent presentation of a stimulus decreases the future likelihood of a behavior, behavior analysts use the term *positive punishment*. Procedural variations of positive punishment examined in the applied literature include the contingent presentation of verbal reprimands, brief physical restraint, and demands. When the contingent removal of a stimulus decreases the future likelihood of a behavior, behavior analysts use the term *negative punishment*. We can divide negative punishment further into two procedures, *response cost* and *time out*. Response cost is the contingent removal of a specific amount of a positive reinforcer (e.g., loss of tokens), and time out is the contingent loss of access to reinforcement for a specific time (e.g., removal of reinforcement for 2 minutes).

Basic research findings on punishment conducted primarily with nonhumans have been instrumental for developing an effective technology of punishment. The voluminous applied literature on punishment, now spanning more than 45 years, has demonstrated the advantages and disadvantages of this treatment approach. The goal of this research has been to develop safe and effective punishers for the problem behavior of individuals with intellectual developmental disorder, particularly for the most severe forms of problem behavior—ones that place these individuals, their caregivers, or the environment at risk for significant harm.

However, numerous authors over the last several decades have noted that both basic and applied research on punishment is declining (e.g., Baron, 1991; Crosbie, 1998; Kahng, Iwata, & Lewin, 2002; Lydon, Healy, Moran, & Foody, 2015; Pelios, Morren, Tesch, & Axelrod, 1999). Although the use of punishment has been controversial for many years, authors have attributed the decrease in applied research to advances in the functional analysis of problem behavior and greater use of function-based treatment (Kahng et al., 2002; Pelios et al., 1999). Despite advances in treatment with extinction and reinforcement (see Vollmer, Athens, & Fernand, Chapter 19, and Fisher, Greer, & Bouxsein, Chapter 20, this volume), research findings suggest that punishment remains an important option for caregivers of individuals with severe forms of problem behavior as defined above. Punishment may be indicated clinically when a behavior analyst cannot identify or control the reinforcers maintaining problem behavior (e.g., Fisher et al., 1993; Hagopian, Rooker, & Zarcone, 2015; Lindberg, Iwata, & Kahng, 1999; Raulston, Hansen, Machalicek, McIntyre, & Carnett, 2019; Saini, Greer, & Fisher, 2015), or when function-based treatments do not produce acceptable outcomes (e.g., Fisher et al., 1993; Hagopian, Fisher, Thibault-Sullivan, Acquisto, & LeBlanc, 1998; Hanley, Piazza, Fisher, & Maglieri, 2005; Wacker et al., 1990). For example, results of several large-*N* studies on treatment with functional-communication training showed that punishment was sometimes necessary to maintain treatment effects under practical schedules of reinforcement for the communication response (Hagopian et al., 1998; Rooker, Jessel, Kurtz, & Hagopian, 2013). Punishment also may be the treatment of choice for life-threatening behavior that a behavior analyst must decrease rapidly to prevent physical harm (e.g., Foxx, 2003).

Advances in the functional analysis of problem behavior, however, should lead to improvements in the selection and use of punishers in clinical settings. The term *function-based punishment* may seem counterintuitive, because clinicians are more likely to use punishment when the function of behavior is unknown. However, as we discuss in more detail below, clinicians should only prescribe punishment with some knowledge of the consequences that may be relevant to and irrelevant to the maintenance of the problem behavior. For the purposes of this chapter, *function-based punishers* are those that are likely to be effective, given this information. The objectives of this chapter are to provide an overview of punishment procedures, approaches for selecting punishment procedures, factors that influence the effects of punishment, and strategies for using punishment effectively.

## TYPES OF PUNISHMENT PROCEDURES

Punishment may be indicated clinically if (1) initial interventions based on reinforcement, extinction, and establishing operations do not produce clinically acceptable decreases in problem behavior; or (2) the problem behavior warrants immediate intervention with procedures likely to produce rapid decreases in responding, which might include punishment. As described in the following sections, a myriad of safe and effective punishers is available for clinical use. Although we often classify these procedural variations of punishment by form (such as overcorrection), function (such as time out), or both, many commonly used procedures include multiple potential punishing stimuli. For example, clinicians frequently combine time out with some type of physical restraint (e.g., Fisher, Piazza, Bowman, Kurtz, et al., 1994). In ad-

dition, we classify a procedure as punishment by its effects on behavior. Thus, although researchers have found that the various procedures described below function as punishment for some individuals, they may have different functions for others. We discuss these alternative functions later in the chapter (see "Selecting Punishment Procedures").

Below, we have divided the procedures into two groups for organizational purposes. The positive-punishment group consists of procedures that include the presentation of an aversive stimulus contingent on behavior. The negative-punishment group consists of procedures that include the removal of preferred or reinforcing stimuli contingent on behavior. The purpose of this section is to provide a brief description and summary of research findings on these clinical variations of punishment.

## Positive-Punishment Procedures

Researchers have shown that a variety of stimuli decrease problem behavior when presented contingent on the behavior. These stimuli include verbal reprimands, demands, physical contact, water mist, certain tastes and smells, noise, and shock. Some of these stimuli have been evaluated in relatively few studies on punishment.

### Verbal Reprimands

Brief statements of disapproval or instruction may function as an effective punisher for many problem behaviors, including self-injurious behavior (SIB), aggression, pica, rumination, and stereotypy. In several studies, for example, caregivers delivered a stern "No," or "Don't do that, you'll hurt yourself," contingent on problem behavior to reduce the frequency of the behavior (e.g., Dominguez, Wilder, Cheung, & Rey, 2014; Maglieri, DeLeon, Rodriguez-Catter, & Sevin, 2000; Richman, Lindauer, Crosland, McKerchar, & Morse, 2001; Thompson, Iwata, Conners, & Roscoe, 1999; Van Houten, Nau, MacKenzie-Keating, Sameoto, & Colavecchia, 1982). Results of a few studies indicate that behavior analysts can establish a reprimand as an effective conditioned punisher (e.g., Dorsey, Iwata, Ong, & McSween, 1980). Several studies have evaluated factors that influence the reductive effects of reprimands. Verbal reprimands were more effective when paired with eye contact and physical contact (e.g., a firm grasp on the shoulder), when the person delivering the reprimand was physically near the target of the reprimand, and when reprimands were provided contingent on the problem behavior of other individuals (e.g., Richman et al., 2001; Van Houten et al., 1982).

### Response Blocking and Physical Restraint

Various punishment procedures involve physical contact between the caregiver and the behaver. These procedures differ in terms of the amount and duration of the contact. *Response blocking* is the use of brief physical contact to prevent a response from occurring and is the least intrusive of these procedures (e.g., Giles, St. Peter, Pence, & Gibson, 2012; Lalli, Livezey, & Kates, 1996; Lerman & Iwata, 1996; Reid, Parsons, Phillips, & Green, 1993). In Reid et al. (1993) and Lerman and Iwata (1996), for example, the therapist blocked hand mouthing by placing his or her hand approximately 2 centimeters from the participant's mouth. This behavior prevented the participant from inserting his or her hand into the mouth (i.e., the back of the therapist's hand contacted the individual's hand). However, the reductive effects of response blocking may be due to extinction rather than to punishment in some cases (Smith, Russo, & Le, 1999).

*Physical restraint* restricts or limits an individual's movement, unlike response blocking, which only prevents the response. Results of several studies have shown that numerous variations of physical restraint effectively reduce problem behavior. Restraint procedures have included *hands down*, in which the therapist holds the individual's hands to the side or in the lap for a specified time (Bitgood, Crowe, Suarez, & Peters, 1980; Hagopian et al., 1998; Lerman, Iwata, Shore, & DeLeon, 1997; Thompson et al., 1999); *baskethold*, in which the therapist stands behind the individual, crosses the individual's arms across the chest, and holds them above the wrists for a specified time (Fisher, Piazza, Bowman, Kurtz, et al., 1994), and *movement suppression time out*, in which the therapist uses the least amount of physical contact necessary to keep the individual motionless while standing in a corner (Rolider & Van Houten, 1985).

In most studies, the therapist used brief physical contact, such as 30–60 seconds, and implemented physical restraint in conjunction with other potential punishers (e.g., verbal reprimands, time out; Thompson et al., 1999). In fact, time out from positive reinforcement was a likely component of any physical-restraint procedure if access to reinforcing stimuli was unavailable while the therapist restrained the individual. Furthermore, therapists commonly used some form of physical contact or restraint with many of the punishers described in this section (e.g., overcorrection, aversive smells, time out; e.g., Cipani, Brendlinger, McDowell, & Usher, 1991). Researchers have not sufficiently explored the contribution of physical contact or restraint to the efficacy of other procedures.

### Overcorrection and Other Forms of Contingent Effort

Several procedural variations of punishment are similar, in that the behavior analyst requires the individual to engage in an effortful response following problem behavior. This type of punisher is *overcorrection* if the contingent response is topographically like the problem behavior or related to the problem behavior in some other manner (e.g., an appropriate replacement behavior). Foxx and Azrin (1972) developed overcorrection, and it consists of two procedural components that the behavior analyst implements alone or in combination, depending on the problem behavior. *Restitutional overcorrection* requires the individual to restore the physical environment to a better state than its original state if problem behavior produced disruption to the physical environment. For example, a behavior analyst would require an individual who turned over a garbage can in the dining room to pick up the garbage can and the trash, and then to sweep and mop the entire dining-room floor. *Positive-practice overcorrection* requires the individual to repeatedly practice an appropriate, related behavior. For example, a behavior analyst would require the individual who turned over a garbage can in the dining room to repeatedly place the garbage can gently on the floor. Researchers have implemented positive practice alone in numerous studies with behavior that does not disrupt the environment, such as stereotypic behavior (e.g., Anderson & Le, 2011; Cipani et al., 1991; Foxx & Azrin, 1973; Peters & Thompson, 2013). For example, in Peters and Thompson (2013), the therapist interrupted motor stereotypy and physically prompted the participants to engage appropriately with leisure materials for 30 seconds. The direct and indirect effects of overcorrection are like those associated with other contingent-effort procedures described below, despite some claims to the contrary (see MacKenzie-Keating & McDonald, 1990, for a discussion). For example, results of studies examining the effects of overcorrection on the practiced response have been inconsistent, showing increases, decreases, and no change (e.g., Peters & Thompson, 2013).

Similar procedures that behavior analysts do not typically classify as overcorrection include *contingent demands,* in which researchers required individuals to complete tasks that were unrelated to the problem behavior (Fischer & Nehs, 1978; Fisher et al., 1993; Watson, 1993); *negative practice,* in which the researchers required the individuals to exhibit the problem behavior repeatedly (Azrin, Nunn, & Frantz, 1980); and *contingent exercise,* in which the researchers required the individuals to perform motor movements that were unrelated to the problem behavior (Kahng, Abt, & Wilder, 2001; Luce, Delquadri, & Hall, 1980). *Response interruption and redirection* is a well-studied intervention for vocal stereotypy that resembles contingent-effort procedures (Ahearn, Clark, MacDonald, & Chung, 2007). In Ahearn et al. (2007), for example, the therapist delivered questions or instructions requiring vocal responses contingent on occurrences of vocal stereotypy; the questions or instructions continued until a participant exhibited three correct responses without engaging in vocal stereotypy. Results of research suggest that response interruption and redirection functions as punishment in some cases (e.g., Ahrens, Lerman, Kodak, Worsdell, & Keegan, 2011; Shawler & Miquel, 2015).

## Water Mist

Researchers have used contingent water mist to decrease problem behavior in individuals with developmental disabilities in a few studies (e.g., Arntzen & Werner, 1999; Dorsey et al., 1980; Friman, Cook, & Finney, 1984; Singh, Watson, & Winton, 1986). A therapist generally implemented the procedure by standing in front of an individual with a squeeze-type bottle containing room-temperature water, holding the water bottle at a slant to avoid spraying water directly into the individual's eyes, and delivering one mist of water for each instance of problem behavior.

## Aversive Tastes and Smells

Results of studies have shown that the contingent delivery of an *aversive taste,* such as vinegar or lemon juice, or *aversive smell,* such as aromatic ammonia, successfully treats problem behavior. In several studies, for example, a therapist squirted a small amount of unsweetened concentrated lemon juice or vinegar into the mouth contingent on self-stimulatory behavior (Cipani et al., 1991; Friman et al., 1984), chronic rumination (Sajwaj, Libet,

& Agras, 1974), public masturbation (Cook, Altman, Shaw, & Blaylock, 1978), and pica (Paisey & Whitney, 1989). The therapist applied aromatic ammonia (i.e., smelling salts) by breaking an ammonia capsule and holding it under the individual's nose for a specified time. Researchers have used this treatment for SIB (Altman, Haavik, & Cook, 1978; Singh, Dawson, & Gregory, 1980a; Tanner & Zeiler, 1975), aggression (Doke, Wolery, & Sumberc, 1983), and breath holding and hyperventilation (Singh, 1979; Singh, Dawson, & Gregory, 1980b). Researchers have not reported on the clinical use of other types of aromatics.

## Noise

Researchers have used the contingent presentation of noise as a punisher for finger and thumb sucking (Stricker, Miltenberger, Garlinghouse, Deaver, & Anderson, 2001; Stricker, Miltenberger, Garlinghouse, & Tulloch, 2003), hair pulling (Rapp, Miltenberger, & Long, 1998), and auditory hallucinations (Fonagy & Slade, 1982). In Stricker et al. (2001), for example, participants wore a device that automatically detected when a participant's hand moved toward the mouth and produced a 65-decibel tone when that occurred. The procedure reduced the thumb sucking of the two participants to near-zero levels. Although the researchers attributed the findings to an increase in the participants' awareness of thumb sucking, the tone may have functioned as a punishing stimulus. Results of a subsequent study with the same device were consistent with a punishment interpretation, because a 90-decibel tone was necessary to reduce the finger sucking (Stricker et al., 2003).

## Shock

Society considers *contingent electric shock* the most intrusive and controversial of the punishment procedures, but research has shown that it produces rapid and durable reductions in severe SIB (Duker & Seys, 1996; Linscheid, Iwata, Ricketts, Williams, & Griffin, 1990; Salvy, Mulick, Butter, Bartlett, & Linscheid, 2004) and aggression (Ball, Sibbach, Jones, Steele, & Frazier, 1975; Foxx, 2003). In previous studies, researchers delivered brief, moderate intensity electric shock (e.g., 84 volts) to the participant's extremity (e.g., leg) via electrodes that a movement detection device activated (e.g., the Self-Injurious Behavior Inhibiting System; Linscheid et al., 1990) or remotely by a caregiver or therapist. Research findings indicate that shock does not increase the risk of undesirable side effects and can be a safe alternative to other punishment procedures (e.g., Linscheid, Pejeau, Cohen, & Footo-Lenz, 1994).

## Negative-Punishment Procedures

### Time Out from Positive Reinforcement

*Time out,* one of the most common forms of punishment, is the contingent loss of access to positive reinforcers or withdrawal of the opportunity to earn positive reinforcers for a period. Researchers have removed reinforcement typically by moving an individual to a less reinforcing environment, such as a barren room, partitioned area, or corner (*exclusionary* or *seclusionary* time out), or by discontinuing reinforcement in the current environment (*nonexclusionary* time out). Toole, Bowman, Thomason, Hagopian, and Rush (2003), for example, used exclusionary time out to treat the severe aggression of a 15-year-old girl with intellectual developmental disorder. The participant had access to several highly preferred items and activities throughout the day. A therapist guided her to a padded treatment room, using the least amount of physical assistance necessary, following each instance of aggression. The therapist required the participant to stay in the room for 5 minutes. Research has examined a wide range of time-out durations (e.g., 15 seconds to 30 minutes); however, results of studies on the relation between this parameter and treatment efficacy have produced inconsistent outcomes (see Matson & DiLorenzo, 1984, for a review). Furthermore, research comparing the effectiveness of fixed-duration time-out lengths to those based on the absence of problem behavior during time out (i.e., contingent release) suggests that the latter does not confer any additional benefits (e.g., Donaldson & Vollmer, 2011; Mace, Page, Ivancic, & O'Brien, 1986).

Researchers have developed numerous procedural variations of nonexclusionary time out to restrict reinforcement access following problem behavior without removing the participant from the immediate environment. These variations include the *visual screen,* in which a researcher placed a hand, mask, or cloth over an individual's eyes (Mitteer, Romani, Greer, & Fisher, 2015; Singh et al., 1986; Rush, Crockett, & Hagopian, 2001); the *time-out ribbon,* in which a researcher removed a ribbon a participant wore, and reinforcement was unavailable when the participant did not have the ribbon (Foxx & Shapiro, 1978; Salend & Gordon,

1987); *contingent observation,* in which a researcher required a participant to remain near the reinforcing environment (Porterfield, Herbert-Jackson, & Risely, 1976); and *item removal,* in which a researcher terminated ongoing stimulation sources, such as music, leisure materials, and food (Dupuis, Lerman, Tsami, & Shireman, 2015; Falcomata, Roane, Hovanetz, Kettering, & Keeney, 2004; Keeney, Fisher, Adelinis, & Wilder, 2000; Ritschl, Mongrella, & Presbie, 1972). In Falcomata et al. (2004), for example, the therapist removed continuous access to a radio for 5 seconds contingent on inappropriate vocalizations. Researchers have called this latter form of time out *response cost* in some studies. However, we typically classify procedures that produce time-based reinforcement loss as time out. During response cost, by contrast, participants earn reinforcement for appropriate behavior rather than the passage of time, and clinicians do not return lost reinforcers.

Researchers have often combined physical restraint with exclusionary or nonexclusionary time out. For example, a researcher might use a baskethold to restrain a participant or physically guide the participant to remain in a prescribed stance while sitting or standing in the corner of a room (e.g., Fisher, Piazza, Bowman, Kurtz, et al., 1994; Matson & Keyes, 1990; Rolider & Van Houten, 1985). No studies have examined the contribution of potentially aversive aspects of physical contact to the efficacy of these procedures.

### Response Cost

The contingent removal of a specific amount of reinforcement, such as tokens, can function as an effective punisher. Typically, the participant obtains reinforcement via appropriate behavior, as in differential reinforcement of alternative behavior, or independently of behavior, as in noncontingent reinforcement, and loses these reinforcers contingent on problem behavior. Researchers have conducted much of the research on response cost in the context of token-economy systems (e.g., LeBlanc, Hagopian, & Maglieri, 2000; Truchlicka, McLaughlin, & Swain, 1998). However, participants have lost other reinforcers via response cost, including books and audiotapes (Kahng, Tarbox, & Wilke, 2001), money (Epstein & Masek, 1978; Long, Miltenberger, Ellingson, & Ott, 1999), and participation in tournaments (e.g., Allen, 1998). Kahng, Tarbox, and Wilke (2001), for example, gave a young boy who engaged in food refusal access to highly preferred items, such as books and audiotapes. The therapist removed the items if the boy refused to accept a bite of food or engaged in problem behavior, and returned the items contingent on bite acceptance. Surprisingly little research has evaluated methods for determining the most appropriate amount and type of reinforcers to remove in a response cost intervention.

## SELECTING PUNISHMENT PROCEDURES

Although researchers have evaluated numerous punishers for clinical use, efficient approaches for prescribing specific punishment procedures have received less attention in the literature. Ethical guidelines mandate that behavior analysts should give priority to the least restrictive procedure that is clinically effective (e.g., Behavior Analysis Certification Board, 2016; Van Houten et al., 1988; Vollmer et al., 2011). Inherent in this approach to intervention selection is the need to arrange punishment procedures hierarchically according to their degree of restrictiveness or intrusiveness (i.e., how much each procedure limits individual freedom or intrudes into an individual's life in some manner) or aversiveness (i.e., how much each procedure produces discomfort, pain, or distress). We typically consider nonexclusionary time out and response cost as the least restrictive of the procedures, followed by exclusionary time out, overcorrection, and other physical punishers. We sometimes refer to this hierarchical arrangement as a *levels system* and use it to guide intervention evaluation and selection. Readers can find case examples and guidelines in several sources for using this approach to identify effective punishment procedures (e.g., Alberto & Troutman, 2006; Barton, Brulle, & Repp, 1983; Cooper, Heron, & Heward, 1987; Couvillon, Kane, Peterson, Ryan, & Scheuermann, 2019; Foxx, 1982; Gaylord-Ross, Weeks, & Lepner, 1980; Gross, Wright, & Drabman, 1981; Lovaas & Favell, 1987; Repp & Deitz, 1978). Some states have adopted policies that explicitly categorize procedures by restrictiveness level (Spreat & Lipinski, 1986).

Nonetheless, attempts to apply the least restrictive treatment model may themselves raise ethical concerns. Clinicians using a hierarchical system typically evaluate punishment procedures on a trial basis, starting with the least restrictive procedure that may be effective and moving to more restrictive procedures until they identify an effective intervention. To illustrate, a clinician may initially evaluate a 5-minute time-out procedure to reduce a child's disruption, because the literature has demonstrated the efficacy of this intervention (e.g., Clark, Rowbury, Baer, & Baer, 1973). If this intervention does not reduce the child's behavior, the clinician may increase the time-out duration. The clinician may try a more restrictive procedure, such as overcorrection, if the lengthier time out is ineffective. The clinician may continue to evaluate increasingly restrictive procedures, such as restraint, until he or she identifies an effective procedure.

This process can be time-consuming, delay the onset of treatment, and produce prolonged exposure to multiple intrusive procedures. The assumption that a more restrictive procedure has a greater likelihood of success than a less restrictive procedure has no empirical support. The hierarchical approach emphasizes the topography of an intervention versus its function; it ignores the possibility that an intrusive procedure might function as a punisher for some people but as a reinforcer for others, such as water mist for some participants in Fisher, Piazza, Bowman, Kurtz, et al. (1994). In fact, intrusiveness level is subjective. Of concern is the chance that exposure to progressively intrusive interventions could promote habituation to putative punishers, decreasing the effectiveness of punishment. Finally, clinicians should consider a variety of additional factors when selecting a punishment procedure, including the immediacy of effects, relevance to behavioral function, severity of the behavior, and caregivers' willingness to use the procedure (Iwata, Vollmer, & Zarcone, 1990; Van Houten et al., 1988; Vollmer & Iwata, 1993).

Assessment procedures that reliably identify effective interventions would permit clinicians to select punishment procedures based on other concerns, such as restrictiveness level, behavior severity, and caregivers' willingness to implement the procedure. Such an assessment would avoid the trial-and-error approach clinicians commonly use to select interventions. As discussed in the following sections, researchers have evaluated several potential assessments. When combined with a functional analysis, these strategies may provide clinicians with a more reliable, efficient approach for determining the least restrictive procedure that is effective.

### Functional Analysis

Knowing the function of problem behavior is especially important once a clinician has decided to include punishment in treatment. Several punishment procedures are uniquely indicated or contra-indicated for particular behavioral functions. Punishment will also be more effective if the clinician combines it with extinction and differential reinforcement of alternative behavior (e.g., Azrin & Holz, 1966; Holz, Azrin, & Ayllon, 1963; Rawson & Leitenberg, 1973; Thompson et al., 1999). Thus clinicians should withhold identified functional reinforcers for problem behavior and deliver those reinforcers for appropriate behavior whenever possible.

Iwata, Dorsey, Slifer, Bauman, and Richman (1982/1994) described a comprehensive functional-analytic approach that is useful for identifying viable options when a clinician is considering punishment as a treatment component. As Saini, Fisher, Betz, and Piazza (Chapter 13, this volume) describe, the experimental functional analysis effectively identifies the function of problem behavior for most participants. Furthermore, although behavior analysts use the assessment to test putative reinforcers for problem behavior, results will reveal sensitivity or lack thereof to consequences that could function as punishers for the behavior. The experimental functional analysis tests the effects of two commonly used procedural variations of punishment (verbal reprimands and time out) in the *attention* and *demand* conditions, respectively. Thus examination of assessment outcomes may indicate whether a procedure is likely to be effective, unlikely to be effective, or specifically contraindicated for the problem behavior.[1]

For example, Figure 21.1 illustrates three possible outcomes for the attention condition of the functional analysis. Verbal reprimands and physical contact delivered during this condition may have no effect on problem behavior, which would exclude them as punishment (see upper panel). Alternatively, lower levels of problem behavior in the attention condition than in the control condition (see middle panel) provide some indication that this consequence may be an effective intervention. Finally, results may show that problem behavior is sensitive to attention as a reinforcer (see lower panel). In this case, punishment procedures that increase verbal or physical attention contingently, such as blocking, overcorrection, and physical restraint, may be contraindicated as

punishment for problem behavior. On the other hand, punishment procedures with a contingent decrease in attention, such as time out, may be indicated (Hagopian et al., 1998).

Figure 21.2 shows similar outcomes for the demand condition. This condition directly tests contingent removal of interaction and instructional materials. If levels of problem behavior are like those in the control condition (see upper panel), attention or material loss (i.e., time out) may not be effective. On the other hand, time out may be viable if levels of problem behavior are lower in

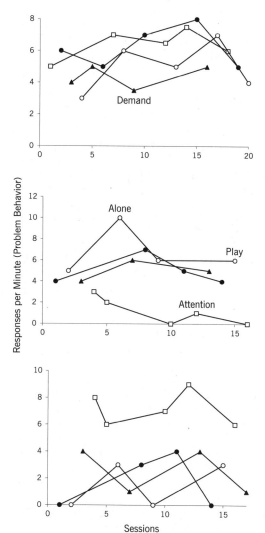

**FIGURE 21.1.** Three possible outcomes for the attention condition of the functional analysis that would provide important information about potential punishers (see text for further details).

[1] We can determine the punishing effects of these consequences only if the behavior occurs during the conditions under which we test them (so that the behavior contacts the contingencies), and if levels are lower than those in an appropriate control condition.

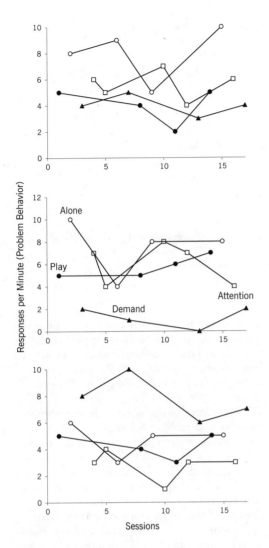

**FIGURE 21.2.** Three possible outcomes for the demand condition of the functional analysis that would provide important information about potential punishers (see text for further details).

the demand condition than in the control condition (see middle panel). Results showing that escape from demands functions as reinforcement for problem behavior would indicate that punishment procedures that remove or delay demands, such as time out, physical restraint, or protective equipment, may be contraindicated (Magee & Ellis, 2001). Procedures with a contingent increase in demands, such as additional work, exercise, and overcorrection, may be indicated for escape-maintained problem behavior (Hagopian et al., 1998).

We summarize the relation between the various punishment procedures described in the previous section and each behavioral function in Table 21.1. However, further research is needed to test these predictions. Results of a quantitative review of applied research on punishment found similar treatment outcomes, regardless of whether the researchers conducted a functional analysis before treatment (Lydon et al., 2015). Whether the researchers selected punishers based on functional-analytic results was not clear. Furthermore, automatic reinforcement maintained problem behavior in most cases, particularly in studies published since 2000. Automatic reinforcement is a function that has less relevance to selection of a punishment procedure.

Although results of the functional analysis may help narrow the list of viable intervention options, additional assessments will typically be warranted to identify the most appropriate, effective intervention. We describe approaches that applied research has examined in the following sections. However, further research is needed on the predictive validity and clinical utility of these assessments. In fact, Lydon et al. (2015) found that just 8.5% of studies on punishment reported how the researchers selected the punisher. Of those, a little more than half reported using a controlled assessment before intervention implementation.

## Stimulus Avoidance Assessment

Fisher and colleagues described an efficient approach for identifying potential punishers (Fisher, Piazza, Bowman, Hagopian, & Langdon, 1994; Fisher, Piazza, Bowman, Kurtz, et al., 1994). The researcher evaluated participants' responses to various punishment procedures by using a procedure like the one Pace, Ivancic, Edwards, Iwata, and Page (1985) developed for identifying potential reinforcers. Fisher, Piazza, Bowman, Kurtz, et al. (1994) included water mist and procedural variations of time out, restraint, and contingent effort in the evaluation. The researchers presented each potential punisher independently of responding for 15–180 seconds across 10 trials, with a buzzer preceding the onset of each trial to decrease the likelihood of superstitious conditioning. Observers measured avoidance responses (e.g., dropping to the floor), negative vocalizations (e.g., crying), and positive vocalizations (e.g., laughing) during these exposures. The researchers predicted that procedures associated with the highest rates of avoidance responses and negative vocalizations were most likely to function as punishers. They subsequently compared the clinical efficacy of

**TABLE 21.1.  Predicted Effectiveness of Punishment Procedures in Relation to Behavioral Function**

| Punisher | Maintaining reinforcer | | | |
| --- | --- | --- | --- | --- |
| | Attention | Tangibles | Escape | Automatic |
| Verbal reprimand | Contraindicated | — | — | — |
| Response blocking/ physical restraint | Contraindicated | Indicated | Contraindicated | Indicated |
| Overcorrection/ contingent effort | Contraindicated | — | Indicated | — |
| Water mist | — | — | — | — |
| Aversive taste/smell | — | — | — | — |
| Shock | — | — | — | — |
| Time out | Indicated | Indicated | Contraindicated | Contraindicated |
| Response cost | — | Indicated | — | — |

*Note.* Dashes indicate that the procedure is neither indicated nor contraindicated.

procedures with low, medium, and high levels of these responses in a multielement design for each participant. The assessment had good predictive validity. This procedure may be useful for assessing other types of procedures (e.g., withdrawal of preferred items) and certain parameters of punishment (e.g., magnitude).

An advantage of this approach is that it empirically evaluates multiple potential punishers in a short time. Behavior analysts can combine assessment results with other important considerations, such as restrictiveness and caregiver preference, to prescribe the most appropriate intervention. Fisher, Piazza, Bowman, Hagopian, and Langdon (1994), for example, asked caregivers to rate each of nine potential punishers as acceptable or unacceptable. The researchers excluded those rated as unacceptable from the stimulus avoidance assessment. Furthermore, the researchers evaluated ease of implementation for each procedure by measuring escape responses during the avoidance assessment (i.e., the number of times the participants successfully prevented implementation). These data may indicate whether (1) a high level of treatment integrity would be possible if caregivers implemented the punisher in the participant's natural environment, and (2) caregivers would find the procedure acceptable for clinical use. Both factors are important to consider in selecting interventions.

## Brief Punisher Assessment

Brief assessments of punishers, conducted in conjunction with or instead of avoidance assessments, have been useful for identifying effective interven-

tions. Researchers evaluate one or more potential punishers during brief sessions to predict the effectiveness of the procedure(s) when implemented over lengthier periods. For example, Fisher and colleagues (Fisher, Piazza, Bowman, Hagopian, & Langdon, 1994; Fisher, Piazza, Bowman, Kurtz, et al., 1994) compared the effects of three punishment procedures on problem behavior by implementing each procedure during three to six 10-minute sessions, alternated in a multielement design. Results showed that the assessment had good predictive validity when they evaluated the punisher associated with the lowest levels of problem behavior throughout the day in an intervention package.

Thompson et al. (1999) evaluated the effects of several procedures on SIB in a brief assessment with AB designs. They conducted an extended evaluation with the least restrictive procedure that correlated with a 75% or greater reduction in SIB with and without reinforcement. Punishment alone was effective in reducing SIB below baseline levels for three of four participants, providing some support for the predictive validity of the brief assessment. However, the researchers provided few procedural details, such as the number and length of sessions or the range of punishers evaluated, because the brief assessment was not the focus of the investigation. Similarly, Verriden and Roscoe (2018) found that a punisher assessment was necessary to decrease the occurrence of automatically reinforced problem behavior, following unsuccessful treatment attempts with reinforcement-based approaches.

Like stimulus avoidance assessments (Fisher, Piazza, Bowman, Hagopian, & Langdon, 1994;

Fisher, Piazza, Bowman, Kurtz, et al., 1994), brief punisher assessments provide information about the potential efficacy of multiple punishment procedures in an efficient manner. Clinicians can also obtain other measures relevant to intervention selection, such as the immediacy of effects, ease of implementation, and potential for side effects, while conducting the assessment.

## Activity Assessment

A few studies have described another potential strategy for identifying effective punishers, based on work by Terhune and Premack (1970, 1974) and Allison and Timberlake (1974). In this assessment approach, baseline observations determined the relative lengths of time for which participants engaged in various freely available activities. Results of some studies predicted that an activity associated with a low probability of engagement would function as a punisher. The contingency arrangement required the participant to engage in the low-probability activity following instances of the targeted (high-probability) behavior. Krivacek and Powell (1978), for example, required three students with intellectual developmental disorder to engage in low-probability activities, such as running, tracing letters, and playing with a ball, contingent on problem behavior. The researchers selected activities in which participants rarely engaged spontaneously. Although problem behavior decreased during intervention, the researchers did not remove engagement time for the low-probability activity from the total session time in the results. As such, the findings are difficult to interpret, because participants had less opportunity to engage in the target behavior during intervention than during baseline.

Other researchers have predicted that any activity may function as a punisher if the contingency requires a participant to engage in the activity at higher than desired levels (Dougher, 1983; Holburn & Dougher, 1986; Realon & Konarski, 1993). This *response satiation* approach to intervention selection suggests that even activities with similar or high levels of engagement relative to the target behavior can function as punishers. Realon and Konarski (1993), for example, required two participants with developmental disabilities to manipulate leisure materials for 5–15 seconds following each occurrence of SIB. The researchers selected the punishment duration by examining baseline levels of SIB and item manipulation. During a control condition, the researchers required 1 second of item manipulation for each occurrence

of SIB—a contingency that did not establish response satiation. Although only the contingency that produced response satiation was effective, the physical contact needed to ensure that participants manipulated the items for the required time may have functioned as punishment. Thus differences in the duration of physical contact confounded the analysis of response satiation. Results of other studies, however, suggest that response satiation may be a viable method for identifying and arranging punishment contingencies (e.g., Dougher, 1983; Holburn & Dougher, 1986).

Although further research is needed, activity assessments are appealing, because they broaden the range of potential punishers available for clinical use. This approach increases the likelihood of successful intervention with procedures based on contingent effort. Caregivers may find these procedures more acceptable than other punishers, especially if the contingent response is appropriate and functional.

## Choice Assessments

Behavior analysts can use additional assessments of caregiver or client preference to guide intervention selection when multiple effective punishers are available. Behavior analysts can assess caregiver preference by obtaining verbal report or ratings of acceptability (e.g., opinions about appropriateness and willingness to implement procedures), or by asking caregivers to choose among the available interventions. Surprisingly few studies have evaluated the acceptability of interventions after caregivers or staff members have implemented them in the natural environment (Armstrong, Ehrhardt, Cool, & Poling, 1997; see Mueller, Edwards, & Trahant, 2003, for a notable exception). Research findings suggest that many factors influence acceptability ratings, including knowledge of or experience with a procedure, intrusiveness of the procedure, procedural complexity or ease of use, number of previously unsuccessful attempts to treat the behavior, and client characteristics such as age and problem severity (for reviews, see Foxx, McHenry, & Bremer, 1996; Lennox & Miltenberger, 1990; O'Brien & Karsh, 1990). Thus having caregivers implement each procedure during brief punisher assessments before rating the acceptability of or choosing an intervention may be beneficial.

In selecting an intervention, behavior analysts can also consider the preferences of the individuals whose behavior they are targeting for reduction. Several studies have evaluated methods for assessing preferences of individuals with limited expressive-communication skills for interventions (Giles et al., 2012; Hanley, Piazza, Fisher, Contrucci, & Maglieri, 1997; Hanley et al., 2005). Individuals with developmental disabilities chose among two or three different interventions by activating one of three switches or touching one of two pictures paired with each procedure. In Hanley et al. (2005), for example, two children chose between differential reinforcement alone, differential reinforcement plus punishment, and punishment alone. Interestingly, both children showed a clear preference for differential reinforcement plus punishment by allocating most responding to the choice associated with this procedure.

## USING PUNISHMENT EFFECTIVELY

Research findings indicate that punishment can be highly effective for treating many behavior disorders and is more effective than treatment with reinforcement or extinction (e.g., Barton, Matson, Shapiro, & Ollendick, 1981; Grace, Kahng, & Fisher, 1994; Hagopian et al., 1998; Wacker et al., 1990). However, the relative efficacy of extinction, reinforcement, and punishment may be difficult to predict in application, because various factors related to the use of these procedures can influence clinical outcomes.

In fact, results of basic research suggest that the ways clinicians commonly implement punishment in applied settings can undermine these interventions' effectiveness. Punishment may not produce immediate, substantial, or sustained reductions in problem behavior if the consequence is delayed, intermittent, relatively mild, paired with reinforcement for problem behavior, or preceded by exposure to a less intense form or type of punisher, or if punishment reduces the amount of reinforcement received (see Lerman & Vorndran, 2003, for a review). Punishment may also be associated with many undesirable side effects. We provide a brief overview of factors related to the use of punishment below, together with a discussion of current applied findings on strategies for using punishment effectively.

### Contiguity of the Punisher

In most applied studies of punishment, a therapist delivered a consequence immediately after instances of problem behavior. Such contiguity was probably critical to the interventions' effectiveness, although few applied studies have compared the effects of immediate and delayed punishment directly. In a notable exception, Abramowitz and O'Leary (1990) found that verbal reprimands were more effective in decreasing off-task behavior in schoolchildren when a teacher delivered a reprimand immediately after the onset of the behavior, rather than after the behavior had occurred continuously for 2 minutes. Basic studies with humans and nonhumans indicate that punishment procedures can fail to suppress responding when the consequence is delayed by just 10–30 seconds (e.g., Banks & Vogel-Sprott, 1965; Goodall, 1984; Trenholme & Baron, 1975). When a punisher is delayed, other responses or multiple instances of the target behavior are likely to occur before the consequence is delivered, weakening the contingency between the response and its consequence.

Nonetheless, some applied studies have shown that delayed punishment is effective (e.g., Azrin & Powers, 1975; Maglieri et al., 2000; Van Houten & Rolider, 1988). Maglieri et al. (2000) used delayed verbal reprimands to reduce the consumption of prohibited food items by a girl with Prader–Willi syndrome. Consumption decreased to zero when the therapist delivered a verbal reprimand after a 10-minute session in which the girl consumed prohibited food. The researchers did not evaluate the procedural components responsible for the efficacy of the delayed punisher (e.g., therapist instructions, recent history with immediate punishment). Results of two studies (Rolider & Van Houten, 1985; Van Houten & Rolider, 1988) suggest that delayed punishment may be effective if a consequence is paired with stimuli associated with engaging in the behavior. Contingent on earlier instances of the target behavior, the researchers in these studies required participants to engage in the response (aggression, theft) or listen to audiotape recordings of their behavior (disruption). A therapist or caregiver then immediately delivered the punisher (verbal reprimands, physical restraint). Both procedures were highly effective in decreasing problem behavior. Although the researchers did not evaluate the effect of the delayed punisher alone for most participants, this approach may have prevented the adventitious punishment of any untargeted responses that occurred before the delivery of the consequence. Products of the behavior also may have acquired conditioned aversive properties due to this pairing procedure. Researchers should evaluate other stimuli that might bridge the interval between a response and its consequence, such as instructions and conditioned punishers, in further applied research (Trenholme & Baron, 1975).

## Schedule of Punishment

Results of basic and applied studies suggest that punishment is more likely to be effective if the punisher is delivered contingent on each occurrence of the target behavior, rather than intermittently (e.g., Azrin, Holz, & Hake, 1963; Calhoun & Matherne, 1975; Lerman et al., 1997; Thomas, 1968). Nonetheless, several applied studies have demonstrated successful treatment of problem behavior with intermittent punishment schedules (e.g., Barton et al., 1987; Cipani et al., 1991; Clark et al., 1973; Dominguez et al., 2014; Romanczyk, 1977). Researchers have used a variety of schedules, including variable-ratio (VR) and fixed-interval (FI) schedules, as well as the differential punishment of high response rates. For example, a VR 4 schedule of time out was as effective in decreasing disruption as a continuous schedule in Clark et al. (1973). The generality of applied findings on intermittent punishment is unclear, however, because punishment appeared to be confounded with extinction or other potential punishers (e.g., verbal reprimands) in most studies.

Punishing every instance of behavior may often be impractical, especially if the rate of responding is relatively high. However, gradually thinning the schedule of punishment may be possible after obtaining clinically significant reductions in problem behavior under a continuous schedule (e.g., Barton et al., 1987; Lerman et al., 1997). In Lerman et al. (1997), for example, the therapist successfully thinned the schedule of punishment with time out or restraint from fixed-ratio (FR) 1 to FI 300 seconds for two participants who engaged in SIB maintained by automatic reinforcement. Nevertheless, they could not increase the schedule beyond FR 1 for two other participants, limiting the generality of the findings. Further research is needed on strategies for improving the effectiveness of intermittent punishment.

## Magnitude of the Punisher

Basic research conducted primarily with electric shock indicates that a larger amount or intensity of punishment will produce larger reductions in behavior if the magnitude is not increased gradually over time (e.g., Cohen, 1968; Terris & Barnes, 1969). Some applied studies have shown that the intensity or duration of punishment influ-

ences treatment efficacy (e.g., Hobbs, Forehand, & Murray, 1978; Richman et al., 2001; Stricker et al., 2003; Williams, Kirkpatrick-Sanchez, & Iwata, 1993). Richman et al. (2001), for example, showed a positive relation between the loudness of verbal reprimands and reductions in breath holding exhibited by a teenager with intellectual developmental disorder. In Williams et al. (1993), a high-intensity shock (18.5 milliamperes) was more effective in decreasing SIB than a low-intensity shock (3.5 milliamperes). Nonetheless, results of applied research have been inconsistent relative to basic findings on magnitude. Lengthier durations of time out, overcorrection, and restraint have not produced larger and more reliable reductions in problem behavior than shorter durations (e.g., Cole, Montgomery, Wilson, & Milan, 2000; Singh, Dawson, & Manning, 1981).

Thus increasing the magnitude of an ineffective punisher may have limited clinical utility and may even promote resistance to punishment (e.g., Cohen, 1968; Terris & Barnes, 1969). Lengthier durations of punishment per se also may lead to habituation. For these reasons, clinicians should use punishers that are effective when presented briefly and at magnitudes that are in the range of those reported in applied studies.

## Availability of Alternative Sources of Reinforcement

Basic and applied research also indicates that punishment will be more effective if reinforcement is available readily for engaging in alternative responses (e.g., Holz et al., 1963; Rawson & Leitenberg, 1973; Thompson et al., 1999) or independently of responding (e.g., DeRosa, Roane, Bishop, & Silkowski, 2016). Thompson et al. (1999), for example, found that levels of SIB maintained by automatic reinforcement were much lower when they combined punishment with reinforcement of toy manipulation than when they used either punishment or reinforcement alone. Results of basic studies have shown that increased deprivation for the reinforcer maintaining the punished behavior reduces the effectiveness of punishment (e.g., Azrin et al., 1963). Basic findings further suggest that the total amount of reinforcement obtained from other sources should meet or exceed that obtained before punishment (i.e., when the individual could freely engage in the unpunished response; Fantino, 1973). As such, punishment may be most effective when the participant can obtain the maintaining reinforcer(s) for problem behavior or reinforcers that are highly substitutable for the functional reinforcer(s) through many sources (e.g., both contingent on and independently of responding).

## Reinforcement of the Punished Response

Many applied studies have shown that punishment can be effective in the absence of extinction (e.g., Fisher, Piazza, Bowman, Hagopian, & Langdon, 1994; Keeney et al., 2000; Lerman et al., 1997; Thompson et al., 1999). In fact, clinicians are more likely to use punishment when the reinforcer maintaining behavior is unknown or cannot be controlled. Nonetheless, basic research indicates that punishment will be more effective if a behavior analyst withholds or infrequently delivers reinforcement for the target behavior (Azrin & Holz, 1966). The punisher may even acquire discriminative or conditioned reinforcing properties if a behavior consistently produces both punishment and reinforcement under certain conditions (e.g., Holz & Azrin, 1961). Thus behavior analysts should combine punishment with extinction or other procedures to reduce the amount of reinforcement available for the punished response whenever possible (see Vollmer et al., Chapter 20, this volume).

## Antecedent Control of the Punished Response

Results of at least three applied studies have shown that establishing discriminative control over the punished response by pairing a stimulus with punishment for engaging in the behavior enhances an intervention's effectiveness (e.g., Maglieri et al., 2000; McKenzie, Smith, Simmons, & Soderlund, 2008; Piazza, Hanley, & Fisher, 1996). In these studies, the researcher delayed or omitted the punisher while the researchers evaluated the effects of the antecedent. In a study mentioned earlier, Maglieri et al. (2000) used discrimination training to treat the food stealing of a young girl with Prader–Willi syndrome. The researchers placed an orange sticker on one of two containers of prohibited food in a refrigerator. The researchers established the sticker as a discriminative stimulus by reprimanding the girl when she consumed food from the container with the sticker, and by providing no differential consequences when she consumed food from the container without the sticker. As expected, the girl consumed food from the container without the sticker, but not from the container with the sticker. Food stealing immediately decreased to zero when the researchers placed the sticker on both containers and on containers in a different refrigerator.

Piazza et al. (1996) exposed a man with developmental disabilities who engaged in cigarette pica to discrimination training with two different-colored cards. The researchers punished pica with response interruption in the presence of a purple card, but not in the presence of a yellow card. No pica occurred in the presence of the purple card when the researchers subsequently evaluated stimulus control in the absence of the punishment contingency. Finally, McKenzie et al. (2008) delivered reprimands for eye poking when a participant with intellectual developmental disorder wore wristbands, and withheld punishment when the participant did not wear the wristbands. Subsequently, the participant did not engage in eye poking when she wore the wristbands in other settings, even though the researchers provided no differential consequences for the behavior. Further research is needed to evaluate the long-term effectiveness of antecedent-control techniques.

## Use of Conditioned Punishers

Behavior analysts may enhance the effectiveness of intermittent, mild, or delayed punishers by establishing and using conditioned aversive stimuli in treatment. Results of basic and applied studies indicate that stimuli that are neutral or ineffective as punishers may function as punishers after they are associated with punishing stimuli (e.g., Dixon, Helsel, Rojahn, Cipolone, & Lubestsky, 1989; Dorsey et al., 1980; Hake & Azrin, 1965; Salvy et al., 2004; Vorndran & Lerman, 2006). For example, a verbal reprimand alone was effective in suppressing problem behavior after the researchers paired the word *no* with an effective punisher such as shock or water mist contingent on responding in several applied studies (e.g., Dorsey et al., 1980; Lovaas & Simmons, 1969). Establishing and using conditioned punishers may be especially beneficial when the caregiver withholds or delays the primary (unconditioned) punisher periodically. Furthermore, conditioning may permit caregivers to maintain intervention effects with less intrusive procedures if they occasionally pair the conditioned punisher with the original punisher (e.g., Vorndran & Lerman, 2006). However, we need further research on the long-term maintenance of conditioned punishment.

## Maintenance of Punishment Effects

Several applied studies have reported the long-term efficacy of punishment with electric shock, overcorrection, physical restraint, verbal reprimands, and water mist, among others (e.g., Altman et al., 1978; Arntzen & Werner, 1999; Iwata, Rolider, & Dozier, 2009; Kazdin, 1971; Richman et al., 2001; Rolider, Williams, Cummings, & Van Houten, 1991; Salvy et al., 2004; Zegiob, Jenkins, Becker, & Bristow, 1976). Researchers typically collected data from 6 to 12 months after the initial application of punishment, during which time they continued, faded, or withdrew the original treatment. Researchers have reported successful clinical outcomes across longer periods, from several years to 25 years after treatment (Duker & Seys, 1996; Foxx, Bittle, & Faw, 1989; Foxx & Livesay, 1984; McGlynn & Locke, 1997). However, the reliability and validity of longer-term outcomes are less clear, due to a reliance on anecdotal information, archival records, indirect measures of outcome, and/or circumscribed observations.

Despite numerous examples of long-term maintenance, problem behavior sometimes reemerges during and following treatment withdrawal (e.g., Arntzen & Werner, 1999; Duker & Seys, 1996; Iwata et al., 2009; Williams et al., 1993). For example, Ricketts, Goza, and Matese (1993) and Williams et al. (1993) reported relapses in treatment with contingent electric shock 6 months and 31 months, respectively, after the initiation of treatment. In fact, we cannot determine the likelihood that treatment with punishment will produce long-term effects by examining the literature, because researchers generally do not submit and journals generally do not publish treatment failures. More important, few studies have directly evaluated strategies that might promote successful maintenance.

Nonetheless, factors that have correlated with specific cases of successful and unsuccessful maintenance may suggest some potential approaches for ensuring that punishment effects maintain over the long run. Researchers have attributed relapses to habituation or tolerance to the punisher, problems with intervention consistency or integrity, restricted opportunities to receive reinforcement for appropriate behavior, and continued reinforcement of the punished behavior (e.g., Duker & Seys, 1996; Foxx & Livesay, 1984; Ricketts et al., 1993). Habituation to the punisher may be less likely to occur with limited or infrequent exposure to the punishing stimulus. Using brief punishers that are highly effective in reducing problem behavior, or randomly alternating among several effective punishers (e.g., Charlop, Burgio, Iwata, & Ivancic, 1988; Toole et al., 2004), would restrict an individual's contact with the punishing stimulus. Ensuring that caregivers continue to implement the intervention correctly and consistently, combining punishment with dense schedules of alternative reinforcement, and removing or reducing reinforcement for problem behavior should also increase the likelihood of successful maintenance (e.g., Foxx, 2003; Foxx & Livesay, 1984; Linscheid, Hartel, & Cooley, 1993).

A complex or labor-intensive intervention may be difficult for staff or caregivers to sustain over time, possibly leading to relapse. Nevertheless, fading or modifying components of the original procedure to simplify implementation may decrease the effectiveness of the intervention. Several studies by Foxx and colleagues have demonstrated a systematic approach for successfully fading punishment (see Foxx, 2003, for a review). Foxx et al. (1989), for example, successfully treated the severe aggression exhibited by a man with a dual diagnosis across 52 months. The initial intervention included punishment with contingent electric shock, escape extinction, and reinforcement of compliance. As part of the maintenance program, the researchers replaced contingent electric shock with a nonexclusionary time-out procedure by first combining the two punishers and then discontinuing the shock after 12 months. They only withdrew shock after the participant had been responding regularly to positive reinforcers in his home and work settings. Over the next 30 months, the researchers gradually decreased the time-out duration from 3 hours to 15 minutes, and aggression remained low. The researchers noted that the time-out procedure had been ineffective before treatment with contingent electric shock. These results suggest that a gradual, highly systematic plan for fading intervention is a key component of long-term maintenance.

## Stimulus Generalization of Punishment Effects

Unlike the research on maintenance, research on stimulus generalization of punishment effects has found that such effects rarely generalize beyond the intervention setting or context (e.g., Doke & Epstein, 1975; Lovaas & Simmons, 1969; Marholin & Townsend, 1978; Rollings, Baumeister, & Baumeister, 1977). Reductions in problem behavior typically failed to occur in contexts that were not associated with punishment, despite attempts to promote such transfer (e.g., Birnbrauer, 1968; Corte, Wolf, & Locke, 1971; Tate & Baroff, 1966). Basic studies with humans have also had difficulty demonstrating generalization (e.g., O'Donnell & Crosbie, 1998; O'Donnell, Crosbie, Williams, & Saunders, 2000).

However, researchers have conducted surprisingly few studies in this area. Further research is needed on strategies to promote generalization, because caregivers are often unable to closely monitor behavior or implement interventions across settings and situations. Problem behavior is likely to emerge wherever a caregiver withholds a punisher, especially if the behavior continues to produce reinforcement. Current knowledge about generalization suggests that punishment effects may be more likely to transfer to contexts that closely resemble the intervention setting or situation (e.g., Guttman & Kalish, 1956; Hoffman & Fleshler, 1965; Honig & Slivka, 1964). In fact, the presence of stimuli that have acquired tight control over responding may help ensure that problem behavior rarely occurs in the absence of the punishment contingency (see Rollings & Baumeister, 1981).

Results of three studies described previously suggest that researchers can establish discriminative control over the punished response by pairing a stimulus with punishment for engaging in the behavior (Maglieri et al., 2000; McKenzie et al., 2008; Piazza et al., 1996). In these studies, problem behavior did not occur when the researchers introduced the discriminative stimulus (a sticker, colored card, or wristbands) in settings that had never been associated with punishment. Although these findings are promising, we need further research on the durability of this strategy, because the researchers examined generalization in only a few sessions.

Finally, generalization may be more likely to occur if the intervention conditions are modified systematically to resemble those present in the generalization contexts. For example, a behavior analyst could fade the magnitude, schedule, immediacy, or type of punishment gradually (Foxx et al., 1989) and could incorporate stimuli from the generalization setting (i.e., people, activities, materials) into the intervention setting before testing for generalization.

## Indirect Effects of Punishment

The most commonly described disadvantages of punishment include the risk of elicited and operant aggression; other emotional responses, such as crying; decreases in appropriate behavior or generalized response suppression; escape from or avoidance of the punishing agent or situation; and

caregivers' misuse of punishment (e.g., Kazdin, 2001). Although basic and applied studies have reported these indirect effects, researchers have conducted few systematic analyses with clinical problems. Nonetheless, research findings indicate that punishment can produce short-lived increases or decreases in unpunished appropriate and inappropriate responses. For example, although several studies have reported increases in aggression or crying during treatment with punishment (e.g., Duker & Seys, 1996; Hagopian & Adelinis, 2001), other studies have shown collateral decreases in unpunished topographies of targeted problem behavior, such as stereotypy (Cook, Rapp, Gomes, Frazer, & Lindblad, 2014), as well as increases in positive affect or appropriate behavior, such as compliance and toy play (e.g., Koegel, Firestone, Kramme, & Dunlap, 1974; Rolider et al., 1991; Toole et al., 2003). Interestingly, researchers have reported that some of these response forms, such as aggression, crying, and toy play, decrease under punishment (Bitgood et al., 1980; Lerman, Kelley, Vorndran, & Van Camp, 2003; Linscheid et al., 1990; Thompson et al., 1999). Thus the likelihood of obtaining indirect effects and the forms that they may take may be difficult to predict in application.

Basic findings suggest that aggression and emotional responses may be more likely to occur when individuals are exposed to unavoidable, intense aversive stimulation (e.g., Azrin, Hutchinson, & Hake, 1966; Hunt & Brady, 1995). Collateral changes also may occur among unpunished responses that (1) are functionally equivalent to the punished behavior (e.g., Baker, Woods, Tait, & Gardiner, 1986; St. Peter, Byrd, Pence, & Foreman, 2016), (2) occur in the same context as the punished behavior (e.g., Bolles, Holtz, Dunn, & Hill, 1980), or (3) tend to immediately follow the punished behavior (e.g., Dunham, 1977, 1978). Both basic and applied studies suggest that minimizing exposure to the punishing stimulus with brief punishers that are highly effective, combining punishment with rich reinforcement schedules for alternative behavior, and withholding reinforcement for functionally equivalent problem behavior may decrease the likelihood of increases in aggression and other undesirable indirect effects.

## CONCLUSIONS

Numerous procedural variations of punishment produce durable reductions in problem behavior, even when the contingencies maintaining the behavior are unknown. Knowledge of behavioral function, however, should increase the likelihood of selecting an effective punisher, obtaining long-term reductions in behavior, and successfully fading treatment. Furthermore, basic and applied findings suggest that we can improve the effectiveness of punishment by (1) selecting punishers via pretreatment avoidance, choice, or activity assessments; (2) delivering the consequence immediately after each instance of the behavior; (3) ensuring that alternative reinforcement sources are available readily; (4) establishing discriminative control over the punished response; and (5) developing and using conditioned punishers. Nonetheless, we need further research on strategies to promote the long-term and generalized effects of punishment in applied settings.

# REFERENCES

Abramowitz, A. J., & O'Leary, S. G. (1990). Effectiveness of delayed punishment in an applied setting. *Behavior Therapy, 21,* 231–239.

Ahearn, W. H., Clark, K. M., MacDonald, R. P. F., & Chung, B. I. (2007). Assessing and treating vocal stereotypy in children with autism. *Journal of Applied Behavior Analysis, 40,* 263–275.

Ahrens, E. N., Lerman, D. C., Kodak, T., Worsdell, A. S., & Keegan, C. (2011). Further evaluation of response interruption and redirection as treatment for stereotypic behavior. *Journal of Applied Behavior Analysis, 44,* 95–108.

Alberto, P. A., & Troutman, A. C. (2006). *Applied behavior analysis for teachers* (7th ed.). Upper Saddle River, NJ: Pearson/Merrill Prentice Hall.

Allen, K. D. (1998). The use of an enhanced simplified habit reversal procedure to reduce disruptive outbursts during athletic performance. *Journal of Applied Behavior Analysis, 31,* 489–492.

Allison, J., & Timberlake, W. (1974). Instrumental and contingent saccharin licking in rats: Response deprivation and reinforcement. *Learning and Motivation, 5,* 231–247.

Altman, K., Haavik, S., & Cook, J. W. (1978). Punishment of self-injurious behavior in natural settings using contingent aromatic ammonia. *Behaviour Research and Therapy, 16,* 85–96.

Anderson, J., & Le, D. D. (2011). Abatement of intractable vocal stereotypy using an overcorrection procedure. *Behavior Interventions, 26,* 134–146.

Armstrong, K. J., Ehrhardt, K. E., Cool, R. T., & Poling, A. (1997). Social validity and treatment integrity data: Reporting in articles published in the *Journal of Developmental and Physical Disabilities, 1992–1995. Journal of Developmental and Physical Disabilities, 9,* 359–367.

Arntzen, E., & Werner, S. B. (1999). Water mist punishment for two classes of problem behaviour. *Scandinavian Journal of Behaviour Therapy, 28,* 88–93.

Azrin, N. H., & Holz, W. C. (1966). Punishment. In W. K. Honig (Ed.), *Operant behavior: Areas of research and application* (pp. 380–447). New York: Appleton.

Azrin, N. H., Holz, W. C., & Hake, D. F. (1963). Fixed-ratio punishment. *Journal of the Experimental Analysis of Behavior, 6,* 141–148.

Azrin, N. H., Hutchinson, R. R., & Hake, D. F. (1966). Extinction induced aggression. *Journal of the Experimental Analysis of Behavior, 9,* 191–204.

Azrin, N. H., Nunn, R. G., & Frantz, S. E. (1980). Habit reversal vs. negative practice treatment of nailbiting. *Behaviour Research and Therapy, 18,* 281–285.

Azrin, N. H., & Powers, M. A. (1975). Eliminating classroom disturbances of emotionally disturbed children by positive practice procedures. *Behavior Therapy, 6,* 525–534.

Baker, A. G., Woods, W., Tait, R., & Gardiner, K. (1986). Punishment suppression: Some effects on alternative behavior. *Quarterly Journal of Experimental Psychology: Comparative and Physiological Psychology, 38B,* 191–215.

Ball, T. S., Sibbach, L., Jones, R., Steele, B., & Frazier, L. (1975). An accelerometer-activated device to control assaultive and self-destructive behaviors in retardates. *Journal of Behavior Therapy and Experimental Psychiatry, 6,* 223–228.

Banks, R. K., & Vogel-Sprott, M. (1965). Effect of delayed punishment on an immediately rewarded response in humans. *Journal of Experimental Psychology, 70,* 357–359.

Baron, A. (1991). Avoidance and punishment. In I. H. Iverson & K. A. Lattal (Eds.), *Experimental analysis of behavior* (Pt. 1, pp. 173–217). Amsterdam: Elsevier Science.

Barton, L. E., Brulle, A. R., & Repp, A. C. (1987). Effects of differential schedule of time-out to reduce maladaptive responding. *Exceptional Children, 53,* 351–356.

Barton, R. P., Matson, J. L., Shapiro, E. S., & Ollendick, T. H. (1981). A comparison of punishment and DRO procedures for treating stereotypic behavior of mentally retarded children. *Applied Research in Mental Retardation, 2,* 247–256.

Behavior Analyst Certification Board. (2014). BACB professional and ethical compliance code for behavior analysts. Retrieved March 30, 2019, from *www.bacb.com/wp-content/uploads/BACB-Compliance-Code-english_190318.pdf*.

Birnbrauer, J. S. (1968). Generalization of punishment effects. A case study. *Journal of Applied Behavior Analysis, 1,* 201–211.

Bitgood, S. C., Crowe, M. J., Suarez, Y., & Peters, R. D. (1980). Immobilization: Effects and side effects on stereotyped behavior in children. *Behavior Modification, 4,* 187–208.

Bolles, R. C., Holtz, R., Dunn, T., & Hill, W. (1980).

Comparisons of stimulus learning and response learning in a punishment situation. *Learning and Motivation, 11,* 78–96.

Calhoun, K. S., & Matherne, P. (1975). The effects of varying schedules of time-out on aggressive behavior of a retarded girl. *Journal of Behavior Therapy and Experimental Psychiatry, 6,* 139–143.

Charlop, M. H., Burgio, L. D., Iwata, B. A., & Ivancic, M. T. (1988). Stimulus variation as a means of enhancing punishment effects. *Journal of Applied Behavior Analysis, 21,* 89–95.

Cipani, E., Brendlinger, J., McDowell, L., & Usher, S. (1991). Continuous vs. intermittent punishment: A case study. *Journal of Developmental and Physical Disabilities, 3,* 147–156.

Clark, H. B., Rowbury, T., Baer, A. M., & Baer, D. M. (1973). Timeout as a punishing stimulus in continuous and intermittent schedules. *Journal of Applied Behavior Analysis, 6,* 443–455.

Cohen, P. S. (1968). Punishment: The interactive effects of delay and intensity of shock. *Journal of the Experimental Analysis of Behavior, 11,* 789–799.

Cole, G. A., Montgomery, R. W., Wilson, K. M., & Milan, M. A. (2000). Parametric analysis of overcorrection duration effects: Is longer really better than shorter? *Behavior Modification, 24,* 359–378.

Cook, J. L., Rapp, J. T., Gomes, L. A., Frazer, T. J., & Lindblad, T. L. (2014). Effects of verbal reprimands on targeted and untargeted stereotypy. *Behavioral Interventions, 29,* 106–124.

Cook, J. W., Altman, K., Shaw, J., & Blaylock, M. (1978). Use of contingent lemon juice to eliminate public masturbation by a severely retarded boy. *Behaviour Research and Therapy, 16,* 131–134.

Cooper, J. O., Heron, T. E., & Heward, W. L. (1987). *Applied behavior analysis.* Columbus, OH: Merrill.

Corte, H. E., Wolf, M. M., & Locke, B. J. (1971). A comparison of procedures for eliminating self-injurious behavior of retarded adolescents. *Journal of Applied Behavior Analysis, 4,* 201–213.

Couvillon, M. A., Kane, E. J., Peterson, R. L., Ryan, J. B., & Scheuermann, B. (2019). Policy and program considerations for choosing crisis intervention programs. *Journal of Disability Policy Studies, 30,* 35–45.

Crosbie, J. (1998). Negative reinforcement and punishment. In K. A. Lattal & M. Perone (Eds.), *Handbook of research methods in human operant behavior* (pp. 163–189). New York: Plenum Press.

DeRosa, N. M., Roane, H. S., Bishop, J. R., & Silkowski, E. L. (2016). The combined effects of noncontingent reinforcement and punishment on the reduction of rumination. *Journal of Applied Behavior Analysis, 49,* 680–685.

Dixon, M. J., Helsel, W. J., Rojahn, J., Cipollone, R., & Lubetsky, M. J. (1989). Aversive conditioning of visual screening with aromatic ammonia for treating aggressive and disruptive behavior in a developmentally disabled child. *Behavior Modification, 13,* 91–107.

Doke, L. A., & Epstein, L. H. (1975). Oral overcorrection: Side effects and extended applications. *Journal of Experimental Child Psychology, 20,* 496–511.

Doke, L. A., Wolery, M., & Sumberc, C. (1983). Treating chronic aggression: Effects and side effects of response-contingent ammonia spirits. *Behavior Modification, 7,* 531–556.

Dominguez, A., Wilder, D. A., Cheung, K., & Rey, C. (2014). The use of a verbal reprimand to decrease rumination in a child with autism. *Behavioral Interventions, 29,* 339–345.

Donaldson, J. M., & Vollmer, T. R. (2011). An evaluation and comparison of time-out procedures with and without release contingencies. *Journal of Applied Behavior Analysis, 44,* 693–705.

Dorsey, M. F., Iwata, B. A., Ong, P., & McSween, T. E. (1980). Treatment of self-injurious behavior using a water mist: Initial response suppression and generalization. *Journal of Applied Behavior Analysis, 13,* 343–353.

Dougher, M. J. (1983). Clinical effects of response deprivation and response satiation procedures. *Behavior Therapy, 14,* 286–298.

9Duker, P. C., & Seys, D. M. (1996). Long-term use of electrical aversion treatment with self-injurious behavior. *Research in Developmental Disabilities, 17,* 293–301.

Dunham, P. J. (1977). The nature of reinforcing stimuli. In W. K. Honig & J. E. R. Staddon (Eds.), *Handbook of operant behavior* (pp. 98–124). Englewood Cliffs, NJ: Prentice-Hall.

Dunham, P. J. (1978). Changes in unpunished responding during response-contingent punishment. *Animal Learning and Behavior, 6,* 174–180.

Dupuis, D. L., Lerman, D. C., Tsami, L., & Shireman, M. L. (2015). Reduction of aggression evoked by sounds using noncontingent reinforcement and time-out. *Journal of Applied Behavior Analysis, 48,* 669–674.

Epstein, L. H., & Masek, B. J. (1978). Behavioral control of medicine compliance. *Journal of Applied Behavior Analysis, 11,* 1–9.

Falcomata, T. S., Roane, H. S., Hovanetz, A. N., Kettering, T. L., & Keeney, K. M. (2004). An evaluation of response cost in the treatment of inappropriate vocalizations maintained by automatic reinforcement. *Journal of Applied Behavior Analysis, 37,* 83–87.

Fantino, E. (1973). Aversive control. In J. A. Nevin & G. S. Reynolds (Eds.), *The study of behavior: Learning, motivation, emotion, and instinct* (pp. 239–279). Glenview, IL: Scott, Foresman.

Fischer, J., & Nehs, R. (1978). Use of a commonly available chore to reduce a boy's rate of swearing. *Journal of Behavior Therapy and Experimental Psychiatry, 9,* 81–83.

Fisher, W. W., Piazza, C. C., Bowman, L. G., Hagopian, L. P., & Langdon, N. A. (1994). Empirically derived consequences: A data-based method for prescribing treatments for destructive behavior. *Research in Developmental Disabilities, 15,* 133–149.

Fisher, W. W., Piazza, C. C., Bowman, L. G., Kurtz, P. F.,

Sherer, M. R., & Lachman, S. R. (1994). A preliminary evaluation of empirically derived consequences for the treatment of pica. *Journal of Applied Behavior Analysis, 27,* 447–457.

Fisher, W. W., Piazza, C. C., Cataldo, M. F., Harrell, R., Jefferson, G., & Conner, R. (1993). Functional communication training with and without extinction and punishment. *Journal of Applied Behavior Analysis, 26,* 23–36.

Fonagy, P., & Slade, P. (1982). Punishment vs. negative reinforcement in the aversive conditioning of auditory hallucinations. *Behaviour Research and Therapy, 20,* 483–492.

Foxx, R. M. (1982). *Decreasing behaviors of retarded and autistic persons.* Champaign, IL: Research Press.

Foxx, R. M. (2003). The treatment of dangerous behavior. *Behavioral Interventions, 18,* 1–21.

Foxx, R. M., & Azrin, N. H. (1972). Restitution: A method of eliminating aggressive–disruptive behavior of retarded and brain damaged patients. *Behaviour Research and Therapy, 10,* 15–27.

Foxx, R. M., & Azrin, N. H. (1973). The elimination of autistic self-stimulatory behavior by overcorrection. *Journal of Applied Behavior Analysis, 6,* 1–14.

Foxx, R. M., Bittle, R. G., & Faw, G. D. (1989). A maintenance strategy for discontinuing aversive procedures: A 32-month follow-up of the treatment of aggression. *American Journal on Mental Retardation, 94,* 27–36.

Foxx, R. M., & Livesay, J. (1984). Maintenance of response suppression following overcorrection: A 10-year retrospective examination of eight cases. *Analysis and Intervention in Developmental Disabilities, 4,* 65–79.

Foxx, R. M., McHenry, W. C., & Bremer, B. A. (1996). The effects of a video vignette on increasing treatment acceptability. *Behavioral Interventions, 11,* 131–140.

Foxx, R. M., & Shapiro, S. T. (1978). The timeout ribbon: A nonexclusionary timeout procedure. *Journal of Applied Behavior Analysis, 11,* 125–136.

Friman, P. C., Cook, J. W., & Finney, J. W. (1984). Effects of punishment procedures on the self-stimulatory behavior of an autistic child. *Analysis and Intervention in Developmental Disabilities, 4,* 39–46.

Gaylord-Ross, R. J., Weeks, M., & Lipner, C. (1980). An analysis of antecedent, response, and consequence events in the treatment of self-injurious behavior. *Education and Training of the Mentally Retarded, 15,* 35–42.

Giles, A. F., St. Peter, C. C., Pence, S. T., & Gibson, A. B. (2012). Preference for blocking or response redirection during stereotypy treatment. *Research in Developmental Disabilities, 33,* 1691–1700.

Goodall, G. (1984). Learning due to response-shock contingency in signaled punishment. *Quarterly Journal of Experimental Psychology, 36B,* 259–279.

Grace, N. C., Kahng, S. W., & Fisher, W. W. (1994). Balancing social acceptability with treatment effectiveness of an intrusive procedure: A case report. *Journal of Applied Behavior Analysis, 27,* 171–172.

Gross, A. M., Wright, B., & Drabman, R. S. (1980). The empirical selection of a punisher for a retarded child's self-injurious behavior: A case study. *Child Behavior Therapy, 2,* 59–65.

Guttman, N., & Kalish, H. I. (1956). Discriminability and stimulus generalization. *Journal of Experimental Psychology, 51,* 79–88.

Hagopian, L. P., & Adelinis, J. D. (2001). Response blocking with and without redirection for the treatment of pica. *Journal of Applied Behavior Analysis, 34,* 527–530.

Hagopian, L. P., Fisher, W. W., Thibault-Sullivan, M., Acquisto, J., & LeBlanc, L. A. (1998). Effectiveness of functional communication training with and without extinction and punishment: A summary of 21 inpatient cases. *Journal of Applied Behavior Analysis, 31,* 211–235.

Hagopian, L. P., Rooker, G. W., & Zarcone, J. R. (2015). Delineating subtypes of self-injurious behavior maintained by automatic reinforcement. *Journal of Applied Behavior Analysis, 48,* 523–543.

Hake, D. F., & Azrin, N. H. (1965). Conditioned punishment. *Journal of the Experimental Analysis of Behavior, 8,* 279–293.

Hanley, G. P., Piazza, C. C., Fisher, W. W., Contrucci, S. A., & Maglieri, K. A. (1997). Evaluation of client preference for function-based treatment packages. *Journal of Applied Behavior Analysis, 30,* 459–473.

Hanley, G. P., Piazza, C. C., Fisher, W. W., & Maglieri, K. A. (2005). On the effectiveness of and preference for punishment and extinction components of function-based interventions. *Journal of Applied Behavior Analysis, 38,* 51–65.

Hobbs, S. A., Forehand, R., & Murray, R. G. (1978). Effects of various durations of timeout on the noncompliant behavior of children. *Behavior Therapy, 9,* 652–656.

Hoffman, H. S., & Fleshler, M. (1965). Stimulus aspects of aversive controls: The effects of response contingent shock. *Journal of the Experimental Analysis of Behavior, 8,* 89–96.

Holburn, C. S., & Dougher, M. J. (1986). Effects of response satiation procedures in the treatment of aerophagia. *American Journal of Mental Deficiency, 91,* 72–77.

Holz, W. C., & Azrin, N. H. (1961). Discriminative properties of punishment. *Journal of the Experimental Analysis of Behavior, 4,* 225–232.

Holz, W. C., Azrin, N. H., & Ayllon, T. (1963). Elimination of behavior of mental patients by response-produced extinction. *Journal of the Experimental Analysis of Behavior, 6,* 407–412.

Honig, W. K., & Slivka, R. M. (1964). Stimulus generalization of the effects of punishment. *Journal of the Experimental Analysis of Behavior, 7,* 21–25.

Hunt, H. F., & Brady, J. V. (1995). Some effects of punishment and intercurrent "anxiety" on a single operant. *Journal of Comparative and Physiological Psychology, 48,* 305–310.

Iwata, B. A., Dorsey, M. F., Slifer, K. J., Bauman, K. E., & Richman, G. S. (1994). Toward a functional analysis of self-injury. *Journal of Applied Behavior Analysis, 27,* 197–209. (Reprinted from *Analysis and Intervention in Developmental Disabilities, 2,* 3–20, 1982)

Iwata, B. A., Rolider, N. U., & Dozier, C. L. (2009). Evaluation of timeout programs through phased withdrawal. *Journal of Applied Research in Intellectual Disabilities, 22*(2), 203–209.

Iwata, B. A., Vollmer, T. R., & Zarcone, J. R. (1990). The experimental (functional) analysis of behavior disorders: Methodology, applications, and limitations. In A. C. Repp & N. N. Singh (Eds.), *Perspectives on the use of nonaversive and aversive interventions for persons with developmental disabilities* (pp. 301–330). Sycamore, IL: Sycamore.

Kahng, S., Abt, K. A., & Wilder, D. (2001). Treatment of self-injury correlated with mechanical restraints. *Behavioral Interventions, 16,* 105–110.

Kahng, S., Iwata, B. A., & Lewin, A. B. (2002). Behavioral treatment of self-injury, 1964 to 2000. *American Journal on Mental Retardation, 107,* 212–221.

Kahng, S., Tarbox, J., & Wilke, A. E. (2001). Use of a multicomponent treatment for food refusal. *Journal of Applied Behavior Analysis, 34,* 93–96.

Kazdin, A. E. (1971). The effect of response cost in suppressing behavior in a pre-psychotic retardate. *Journal of Behavior Therapy and Experimental Psychiatry, 2,* 137–140.

Kazdin, A. E. (2001). *Behavior modification in applied settings* (6th ed.). Belmont, CA: Wadsworth/Thomson Learning.

Keeney, K. M., Fisher, W. W., Adelinis, J. D., & Wilder, D. A. (2000). The effects of response cost in the treatment of aberrant behavior maintained by negative reinforcement. *Journal of Applied Behavior Analysis, 33,* 255–258.

Koegel, R. L., Firestone, P. B., Kramme, K. W., & Dunlap, G. (1974). Increasing spontaneous play by suppressing self-stimulation in autistic children. *Journal of Applied Behavior Analysis, 7,* 521–528.

Krivacek, D., & Powell, J. (1978). Negative preference management: Behavioral suppression using Premack's punishment hypothesis. *Education and Treatment of Children, 1,* 5–13.

Lalli, J. S., Livezey, K., & Kates, K. (1996). Functional analysis and treatment of eye poking with response blocking. *Journal of Applied Behavior Analysis, 29,* 129–132.

LeBlanc, L. A., Hagopian, L. P., & Maglieri, K. A. (2000). Use of a token economy to eliminate excessive inappropriate social behavior in an adult with developmental disabilities. *Behavioral Interventions, 15,* 135–143.

Lennox, D. B., & Miltenberger, R. G. (1990). On the conceptualization of treatment acceptability. *Education and Training in Mental Retardation, 25,* 211–224.

Lerman, D. C., & Iwata, B. A. (1996). A methodology for distinguishing between extinction and punishment effects associated with response blocking. *Journal of Applied Behavior Analysis, 29,* 231–234.

Lerman, D. C., Iwata, B. A., Shore, B. A., & DeLeon, I. G. (1997). Effects of intermittent punishment on self-injurious behavior: An evaluation of schedule thinning. *Journal of Applied Behavior Analysis, 30,* 187–201.

Lerman, D. C., Kelley, M. E., Vorndran, C. M., & Van Camp, C. M. (2003). Collateral effects of response blocking during the treatment of stereotypic behavior. *Journal of Applied Behavior Analysis, 36,* 119–123.

Lerman, D. C., & Vorndran, C. M. (2002). On the status of knowledge for using punishment: Implications for treating behavior disorders. *Journal of Applied Behavior Analysis, 35,* 431–464.

Lindberg, J. S., Iwata, B. A., & Kahng, S. (1999). On the relation between object manipulation and stereotypic self-injurious behavior. *Journal of Applied Behavior Analysis, 32,* 51–62.

Linscheid, T. R., Hartel, F., & Cooley, N. (1993). Are aversive procedures durable?: A five year follow-up of three individuals treated with contingent electric shock. *Child and Adolescent Mental Health Care, 3,* 67–76.

Linscheid, T. R., Iwata, B. A., Ricketts, R. W., Williams, D. E., & Griffin, J. C. (1990). Clinical evaluation of the Self-Injurious Behavior Inhibiting System (SIBIS). *Journal of Applied Behavior Analysis, 23,* 53–78.

Linscheid, T. R., Pejeau, C., Cohen, S., & Footo-Lenz, M. (1994). Positive side effects in the treatment of SIB using the Self-Injurious Behavior Inhibiting System (SIBIS): Implications of operant and biochemical explanations of SIB. *Research in Developmental Disabilities, 15,* 81–90.

Long, E. S., Miltenberger, R. G., Ellingson, S. A., & Ott, S. M. (1999). Augmenting simplified habit reversal in the treatment of oral–digital habits exhibited by individuals with mental retardation. *Journal of Applied Behavior Analysis, 32,* 353–365.

Lovaas, O. I., & Favell, J. E. (1987). Protection of clients undergoing aversive/restrictive interventions. *Education and Treatment of Children, 10,* 311–325.

Lovaas, O. I., & Simmons, J. Q. (1969). Manipulation of self-destruction in three retarded children. *Journal of Applied Behavior Analysis, 2,* 143–157.

Luce, S. C., Delquadri, J., & Hall, R. V. (1980). Contingent exercise: A mild but powerful procedure for suppressing inappropriate verbal and aggressive behavior. *Journal of Applied Behavior Analysis, 13,* 583–594.

Lydon, S., Healy, O., Moran, L., & Foody, C. (2015). A quantitative examination of punishment research. *Research in Developmental Disabilities, 36,* 470–484.

Mace, F. C., Page, T. J., Ivancic, M. T., & O'Brien, S. (1986). Effectiveness of brief time-out with and without contingent delay: A comparative analysis. *Journal of Applied Behavior Analysis, 19*(1), 79–86.

MacKenzie-Keating, S. E., & McDonald, L. (1990). Overcorrection: Reviewed, revisited, and revised. *Behavior Analyst, 13*, 39–48.

Magee, S. K., & Ellis, J. (2001). The detrimental effects of physical restraint as a consequence for inappropriate classroom behavior. *Journal of Applied Behavior Analysis, 34*, 501–504.

Maglieri, K. A., DeLeon, I. G., Rodriguez-Catter, V., & Sevin, B. M. (2000). Treatment of covert food stealing in an individual with Prader–Willi syndrome. *Journal of Applied Behavior Analysis, 33*, 615–618.

Marholin, D., & Townsend, N. M. (1978). An experimental analysis of side effects and response maintenance of a modified overcorrection procedure. *Behavior Therapy, 9*, 383–390.

Matson, J. L., & DiLorenzo, T. M. (1984). *Punishment and its alternatives: New perspectives for behavior modification.* New York: Springer.

Matson, J. L., & Keyes, J. B. (1990). A comparison of DRO to movement suppression time-out and DRO with two self-injurious and aggressive mentally retarded adults. *Research in Developmental Disabilities, 11*, 111–120.

McGlynn, A. P., & Locke, B. J. (1997). A 25-year follow-up of a punishment program for severe self-injury. *Behavioral Interventions, 12*, 203–207.

McKenzie, S. D., Smith, R. G., Simmons, J. N., & Soderlund, M. J. (2008). Using a stimulus correlated with reprimands to suppress automatically maintained eye poking. *Journal of Applied Behavior Analysis, 41*, 255–259.

Mitteer, D. R., Romani, P. W., Greer, B. D., & Fisher, W. W. (2015). Assessment and treatment of pica and destruction of holiday decorations. *Journal of Applied Behavior Analysis, 48*, 912–917.

Mueller, M. M., Edwards, R. P., & Trahant, D. (2003). Translating multiple assessment techniques into an intervention selection model for classrooms. *Journal of Applied Behavior Analysis, 36*, 563–573.

O'Brien, S., & Karsh, K. G. (1990). Treatment acceptability: Consumer, therapist, and society. In A. C. Repp & N. N. Singh (Eds.), *Perspectives on the use of nonaversive and aversive interventions for persons with developmental disabilities* (pp. 503–516). Sycamore, IL: Sycamore.

O'Donnell, J., & Crosbie, J. (1998). Punishment generalization gradients with humans. *Psychological Record, 48*, 211–232.

O'Donnell, J., Crosbie, J., Williams, D. C., & Saunders, K. J. (2000). Stimulus control and generalization of point-loss punishment with humans. *Journal of the Experimental Analysis of Behavior, 73*, 261–274.

Pace, G. M., Ivancic, M. T., Edwards, G. L., Iwata, B. A., & Page, T. J. (1985). Assessment of stimulus preference and reinforcer value with profoundly retarded individuals. *Journal of Applied Behavior Analysis, 18*, 249–255.

Paisey, T. L., & Whitney, R. B. (1989). A long-term case study of analysis, response suppression, and treatment maintenance involving life-threatening pica. *Behavioral Residential Treatment, 4*, 191–211.

Pelios, L., Morren, J., Tesch, D., & Axelrod, S. (1999). The impact of functional analysis methodology on treatment choice for self-injurious and aggressive behavior. *Journal of Applied Behavior Analysis, 32*, 185–195.

Peters, L. C., & Thompson, R. H. (2013). Some indirect effects of positive practice overcorrection. *Journal of Applied Behavior Analysis, 46*, 613–625.

Piazza, C. C., Hanley, G. P., & Fisher, W. W. (1996). Functional analysis and treatment of cigarette pica. *Journal of Applied Behavior Analysis, 29*, 437–450.

Porterfield, J. K., Herbert-Jackson, E., & Risley, T. R. (1976). Contingent observation: An effective and acceptable procedure for reducing disruptive behavior of young children in a group setting. *Journal of Applied Behavior Analysis, 9*, 55–64.

Rapp, J. T., Miltenberger, R. G., & Long, E. S. (1998). Augmenting simplified habit reversal with an awareness enhancement device: Preliminary findings. *Journal of Applied Behavior Analysis, 31*, 665–668.

Raulston, T. J., Hansen, S. G., Machalicek, W., McIntyre, L. L., & Carnett, A. (2019). Interventions for repetitive behavior in young children with autism: A survey of behavioral practices. *Journal of Autism and Developmental Disorders, 49*, 3047–3059.

Rawson, R. A., & Leitenberg, H. (1973). Reinforced alternative behavior during punishment and extinction with rats. *Journal of Comparative and Physiological Psychology, 85*, 593–600.

Realon, R. E., & Konarski, E. A. (1993). Using decelerative contingencies to reduce the self-injurious behavior of people with multiple handicaps: The effects of response satiation? *Research in Developmental Disabilities, 14*, 341–357.

Reid, D. H., Parsons, M. B., Phillips, J. F., & Green, C. W. (1993). Reduction of self-injurious hand mouthing using response blocking. *Journal of Applied Behavior Analysis, 26*, 139–140.

Repp, A. C., & Deitz, D. E. D. (1978). On the selective use of punishment: Suggested guidelines for administrators. *Mental Retardation, 16*, 250–254.

Richman, D. M., Lindauer, S. E., Crosland, K. A., McKerchar, T. L., & Morse, P. S. (2001). Functional analysis and treatment of breath holding maintained by nonsocial reinforcement. *Journal of Applied Behavior Analysis, 34*, 531–534.

Ricketts, R. W., Goza, A. B., & Matese, M. (1993). A 4-year follow-up of treatment of self-injury. *Journal of Behavior Therapy and Experimental Psychiatry, 24*, 57–62.

Ritschl, C., Mongrella, J., & Presbie, R. J. (1972). Group time-out from rock and roll music and out-of-seat behavior of handicapped children while riding a school bus. *Psychological Reports, 31*, 967–973.

Rolider, A., & Van Houten, R. (1985). Suppressing tantrum behavior in public places through the use of delayed punishment mediated by audio recordings. *Behavior Therapy, 16*, 181–194.

Rolider, A., Williams, L., Cummings, A., & Van Houten, R. (1991). The use of a brief movement restriction procedure to eliminate severe inappropriate behavior. *Journal of Behavior Therapy and Experimental Psychiatry, 22,* 23–30.

Rollings, J. P., & Baumeister, A. A. (1981). Stimulus control of stereotypic responding: Effects on target and collateral behavior. *American Journal of Mental Deficiency, 86,* 67–77.

Rollings, J. P., Baumeister, A. A., & Baumeister, A. A. (1977). The use of overcorrection procedures to eliminate the stereotyped behaviors of retarded individuals: An analysis of collateral behaviors and generalization of suppressive effects. *Behavior Modification, 1,* 29–46.

Romanczyk, R. G. (1977). Intermittent punishment of self-stimulation: Effectiveness during application and extinction. *Journal of Consulting and Clinical Psychology, 45,* 53–60.

Rooker, G. W., Jessel, J., Kurtz, P. F., & Hagopian, L. P. (2013). Functional communication training with and without alternative reinforcement and punishment: An analysis of 58 applications. *Journal of Applied Behavior Analysis, 46,* 708–722.

Rush, K. S., Crockett, J. L., & Hagopian, L. P. (2001). An analysis of the selective effects of NCR with punishment targeting problem behavior associated with positive affect. *Behavioral Interventions, 16,* 127–135.

Saini, V., Greer, B. D., & Fisher, W. W. (2015). Clarifying inconclusive functional analysis results: Assessment and treatment of automatically reinforced aggression. *Journal of Applied Behavior Analysis, 48,* 315–330.

Sajwaj, T., Libet, J., & Agras, S. (1974). Lemon-juice therapy: The control of life-threatening rumination in a six-month-old infant. *Journal of Applied Behavior Analysis, 7,* 557–563.

Salend, S. J., & Gordon, B. D. (1987). A group-oriented timeout ribbon procedure. *Behavioral Disorders, 12,* 131–137.

Salvy, S., Mulick, J. A., Butter, E., Bartlett, R. K., & Linscheid, T. R. (2004). Contingent electric shock (SIBIS) and a conditioned punisher eliminate severe head banging in a preschool child. *Behavioral Interventions, 19,* 59–72.

Shawler, L. A., & Miquel, C. F. (2015). The effects of motor and vocal response interruption and redirection on vocal stereotypy and appropriate vocalizations. *Behavioral Interventions, 30,* 112–134.

Singh, N. N. (1979). Aversive control of breath-holding. *Journal of Behavior Therapy and Experimental Psychiatry, 10,* 147–149.

Singh, N. N., Dawson, M. J., & Gregory, P. R. (1980a). Self-injury in the profoundly retarded: Clinically significant versus therapeutic control. *Journal of Mental Deficiency Research, 24,* 87–97.

Singh, N. N., Dawson, M. J., & Gregory, P. R. (1980b). Suppression of chronic hyperventilation using response-contingent aromatic ammonia. *Behavior Therapy, 11,* 561–566.

Singh, N. N., Dawson, M. J., & Manning, P. J. (1981). The effects of physical restraint on self-injurious behavior. *Journal of Mental Deficiency Research, 25,* 207–216.

Singh, N. N., Watson, J. E., & Winton, A. S. W. (1986). Treating self-injury: Water mist spray versus facial screening or forced arm exercise. *Journal of Applied Behavior Analysis, 19,* 403–410.

Smith, R. G., Russo, L., & Le, D. D. (1999). Distinguishing between extinction and punishment effects of response blocking: A replication. *Journal of Applied Behavior Analysis, 32,* 367–370.

Spreat, S., & Lipinski, D. P. (1986). A survey of state policies regarding use of restrictive/aversive behavior modification procedures. *Behavioral Residential Treatment, 1,* 137–152.

St. Peter, C. C., Byrd, J. D., Pence, S. T., & Foreman, A. P. (2016). Effects of treatment-integrity failures on a response-cost procedure. *Journal of Applied Behavior Analysis, 49,* 308–328.

Stricker, J. M., Miltenberger, R. G., Garlinghouse, M. A., Deaver, C. M., & Anderson, C. A. (2001). Evaluation of an awareness enhancement device for the treatment of thumb sucking in children. *Journal of Applied Behavior Analysis, 34,* 77–80.

Stricker, J. M., Miltenberger, R. G., Garlinghouse, M., & Tulloch, H. E. (2003). Augmenting stimulus intensity with an awareness enhancement device in the treatment of finger sucking. *Education and Treatment of Children, 26,* 22–29.

Tanner, B. A., & Zeiler, M. (1975). Punishment of self-injurious behavior using aromatic ammonia as the aversive stimulus. *Journal of Applied Behavior Analysis, 8,* 53–57.

Tate, B. G., & Baroff, G. S. (1966). Aversive control of self-injurious behavior in a psychotic boy. *Behaviour Research and Therapy, 4,* 281–287.

Terhune, J. G., & Premack, D. (1970). On the proportionality between the probability of not-running and the punishment effect of being forced to run. *Learning and Motivation, 1,* 141–149.

Terhune, J. G., & Premack, D. (1974). Comparison of reinforcement and punishment functions produced by the same contingent event in the same subject. *Learning and Motivation, 5,* 221–230.

Terris, W., & Barnes, M. (1969). Learned resistance to punishment and subsequent responsiveness to the same and novel punishers. *Psychonomic Science, 15,* 49–50.

Thomas, J. R. (1968). Fixed-ratio punishment by timeout of concurrent variable-interval behavior. *Journal of the Experimental Analysis of Behavior, 11,* 609–616.

Thompson, R. H., Iwata, B. A., Conners, J., & Roscoe, E. M. (1999). Effects of reinforcement for alternative behavior during punishment of self-injury. *Journal of Applied Behavior Analysis, 32,* 317–328.

Toole, L. M., Bowman, L. G., Thomason, J. L., Hagopian, L. P., & Rush, K. S. (2003). Observed increases in positive affect during behavioral treatment. *Behavioral Interventions, 18,* 35–42.

Toole, L. M., DeLeon, I. G., Kahng, S., Ruffin, G. E., Pletcher, C. A., & Bowman, L. G. (2004). Re-evaluation of constant versus varied punishers using empirically derived consequences. *Research in Developmental Disabilities, 25,* 577–586.

Trenholme, I. A., & Baron, A. (1975). Immediate and delayed punishment of human behavior by loss of reinforcement. *Learning and Motivation, 6,* 62–79.

Truchlicka, M., McLaughlin, T. F., & Swain, J. C. (1998). Effects of token reinforcement and response cost on the accuracy of spelling performance with middle-school special education students with behavior disorders. *Behavioral Interventions, 13,* 1–10.

Van Houten, R., Axelrod, S., Bailey, J. S., Favell, J. E., Foxx, R. M., Iwata, B. A., et al. (1988). The right to effective behavioral treatment. *Journal of Applied Behavior Analysis, 21,* 381–384.

Van Houten, R., Nau, P. A., MacKenzie-Keating, S. E., Sameoto, D., & Colavecchia, B. (1982). An analysis of some variables influencing the effectiveness of reprimands. *Journal of Applied Behavior Analysis, 15,* 65–83.

Van Houten, R., & Rolider, A. (1988). Recreating the scene: An effective way to provide delayed punishment for inappropriate motor behavior. *Journal of Applied Behavior Analysis, 21,* 187–192.

Verriden, A. L., & Roscoe, E. M. (2018). An evaluation of a punisher assessment for decreasing automatically reinforced problem behavior. *Journal of Applied Behavior Analysis, 52,* 205–226.

Vollmer, T. R., Hagopian, L. P., Bailey, J. S., Dorsey, M. F., Hanley, G. P., Lennox, D., et al. (2011). The Association for Behavior Analysis International position statement on restraint and seclusion. *Behavior Analyst, 34,* 103–110.

Vollmer, T. R., & Iwata, B. A. (1993). Implications of a functional analysis technology for the use of restrictive behavioral interventions. *Child and Adolescent Mental Health Care, 3,* 95–113.

Vorndran, C. M., & Lerman, D. C. (2006). Establishing and maintaining treatment effects with less intrusive consequences via a pairing procedure. *Journal of Applied Behavior Analysis, 39,* 35–48.

Wacker, D. P., Steege, M. W., Northup, J., Sasso, G., Berg, W., Reimers, T., et al. (1990). A component analysis of functional communication training across three topographies of severe behavior problems. *Journal of Applied Behavior Analysis, 23,* 417–429.

Watson, T. S. (1993). Effectiveness of arousal and arousal plus overcorrection to reduce nocturnal bruxism. *Journal of Behavior Therapy and Experimental Psychiatry, 24,* 181–185.

Williams, D. E., Kirkpatrick-Sanchez, S., & Iwata, B. A. (1993). A comparison of shock intensity in the treatment of longstanding and severe self-injurious behavior. *Research in Developmental Disabilities, 14,* 207–219.

Zegiob, L. E., Jenkins, J., Becker, J., & Bristow, A. (1976). Facial screening: Effects on appropriate and inappropriate behaviors. *Journal of Behavior Therapy and Experimental Psychiatry, 7,* 355–357.

# CHAPTER 22

# Token Economies

David Reitman, Kyle Boerke, and Areti Vassilopoulos

Researchers developed the first token-economy programs in the early 1960s, and these represented some of the earliest applications of experimental and conceptual innovations in applied behavior analysis (Ferster & Skinner, 1957; Skinner, 1953). A general dissatisfaction with the quality of care provided to individuals in institutionalized settings, and a desire to construct environments that would be more conducive to the development and maintenance of adaptive behavior in these individuals (i.e., a "total motivating environment"; Ayllon & Azrin, 1968, p. 24), inspired the development of token economies. Ayllon and Azrin (1965) were among the first to report positive results with a token-based reward program. Allyon and Azrin initially implemented a token economy at Anna State Hospital in Illinois with individuals with severe impairments such as schizophrenia. They showed that the contingent delivery of token reinforcement increased work and self-care behavior, but that noncontingent delivery of tokens or program discontinuation resulted in drastic reductions in adaptive behavior. Ayllon and Azrin (1968) reported their extended findings in *The Token Economy: A Motivational System for Therapy and Rehabilitation*.

## DEFINING THE TOKEN ECONOMY

*Token economies* are formal descriptions of *contingency relations*, defined here as antecedents, behaviors, and consequences that modify or influence behavior through the delivery of conditioned reinforcement (Hackenberg, 2018). *Antecedents* (i.e., discriminative stimuli or cues) are events preceding a behavior that indicate that an individual should perform a behavior specified as part of a token economy. *Behaviors* are the actions specified in the contingency relations. *Consequences* in the form of backup reinforcers should follow the performance of the behavior reliably. Often the performance of the behavior signals the delivery of both immediate consequences and progress toward long-term, larger incentives.

A key feature of a token economy is the delivery of symbolic or token reinforcers (e.g., poker chips, points) after the performance of the specified behavior (Miltenberger, 2001). Most conditioned reinforcers lack inherent value and influence behavior by affording individuals opportunities to exchange them for backup reinforcers, such as special privileges, edibles, and activities (Fiske, Isenhower, Bamond, & Lauderdale-Littin, 2020; Leon, Borrero, & DeLeon, 2016; Russell, Ingvarsson, Haggar, & Jessel, 2018). Thus the purpose of tokens and conditioned reinforcers generally is to bridge the delay between delivery of backup reinforcers and performance of the behavior (Clark, Lachowicz, & Wolf, 1968; Dickerson, Tenhula, & Green-Paden, 2005; Jones, Downing, Latkowski, Ferre, & McMahon, 1992; Kazdin & Bootzin, 1972).

The following elements seem to be common features of well-formulated contingency management or token-economy programs (Ivy, Meindi, Overley, & Robson, 2017). First, a behavior analyst sets goals and specifies behaviors in observable terms. Second, the behavior analyst identifies potential reinforcers and punishers, if applicable. Third, the behavior analyst or his or her designee monitors target behaviors frequently and delivers consequences consistently. Fourth, the behavior analyst develops a program that is flexible and can change as the needs of the individual or program change. Finally, collaboration among all parties, a written agreement, and formal monitoring processes are other program elements considered necessary to maximize effectiveness (Miltenberger, 2001). The goal of a token-economy program is to strengthen adaptive or desirable behavior and decrease problem behavior simultaneously (Miltenberger, 2001). Stokes and Baer (1977) recommended that behavior analysts fade token-economy programs as rapidly as possible after the programs are successful. Interestingly, a meta-analysis of prize-based reinforcement programs for persons with substance abuse problems revealed that consistent monitoring and ongoing praise were needed to sustain gains after program fading. Although token-economy programs yielded abstinence in the immediate postintervention follow-up, the participants did not maintain abstinence at a 6-month follow-up (Benishek et al., 2014).

## Identify and Define Behavior

The first and arguably most important step in implementing a token-economy program is to identify and define the target behavior objectively. In fact, Ayllon and Azrin (1968) dedicated 28 pages of their groundbreaking text to the topic. Ambiguous or poorly described behavior promotes misunderstanding and confusion regarding program objectives and could fail to cue the consistent delivery of reinforcement for appropriate behavior. One study showed that classroom teachers provided inconsistent feedback on students' behaviors and infrequent reinforcement for positive classroom behaviors before they implemented a token economy. Both teacher behaviors improved immediately after token-economy implementation (Kowalewicz & Coffee, 2014).

Moore, Tingstrom, Doggett, and Carlyon (2001) further examined problems with the specification of the target behavior and feedback. The researchers first analyzed an ineffective token economy at the request of a unit psychiatrist. Their analysis revealed ambiguous target behaviors, such as *following directions*, *being nice*, and *being where you are supposed to be*. The researchers also noted that lengthy delays between the delivery and redemption of tokens reduced program effectiveness. The researchers recommended the development of operational definitions for each target behavior. For example, they defined *following directions* as "making eye contact with the speaker and initiating compliance within 5–7 seconds of the request." Staff delivered backup reinforcement based on points each patient earned the previous day in the original program. Instead, the researchers divided days into four blocks, and behavior during one block determined the privileges during the next block. These adjustments produced substantial reductions in time out and an increase in points earned for target behavior such as following directions, but did not reduce problem behavior directly.

## Identify Conditioned Reinforcers

Researchers have used tokens, imitation dollar bills, buttons, stickers, and poker chips as conditioned reinforcers (Reynolds & Kelley, 1997). The selection of conditioned reinforcers should be sensitive to the implementation context. Handing a poker chip to a student who is working on an academic task, such as writing an essay, could disrupt the behavior (Drabman & Tucker, 1974). Some researchers have delivered checkmarks, smiley faces, or stars on a chart to reduce the potential disruption of token delivery (Anhalt, McNeil, & Bahl, 1998; Higgins, Williams, & McLaughlin, 2001; McGinnis, Friman, & Carlyon, 1999; Sullivan & O'Leary, 1990). For example, Higgins et al. (2001) developed a token economy for a third-grade student with learning disabilities, in which a teacher recorded a checkmark contingent on appropriate behavior on a piece of paper taped to the top left-hand corner of the student's desk. Thus the student could receive performance feedback without significant interruption. Hupp, Reitman, Northup, O'Callaghan, and LeBlanc (2002) modified Pringles potato chip containers and attached them to clipboards. Researchers delivered tokens after the students demonstrated the ready position during kickball games. A key feature of token delivery was that students could hear the token as it reached the bottom of the cylinder, but did not need to divert attention from the game to receive or retain the token.

Inclusion of response cost also may influence choice of conditioned reinforcers (Jowett Hirst, Dozier, & Payne, 2016). This consideration is important, because many token programs include such a contingency (see Musser, Bray, Kehle, & Jenson, 2001). Token programs with response cost may include conditioned reinforcers that the caregiver can remove easily, because conflict may ensue when the caregiver removes tokens. Erasing a point from a blackboard, flipping a card, or taking a chip from a container may be easier than removing a token from a client's hand or pocket. For example, Salend and Allen (1985) used 2.5-centimeter × 7.6-centimeter strips of paper taped to the tops of second graders' desks in a study evaluating the difference between externally managed and self-managed response cost programs. The teacher removed the strips of paper contingent on the performance of problem behavior during the externally managed condition.

Most authors recommend pairing verbal praise with conditioned reinforcement, although the empirical merits of verbal praise and its role in fading conditioned reinforcement is unknown (Alberto & Troutman, 2006; Drabman & Lahey, 1974; Drabman & Tucker, 1974; Kirby & Shields, 1972; Paul & Lentz, 1977). Finally, behavior analysts may base the selection of conditioned reinforcement on safety or health issues, because individuals may swallow small tokens, and circulating tokens may facilitate the spread of illness.

### Identify Backup Reinforcers

*Backup reinforcers* are items, activities, or privileges that the individual can exchange for conditioned reinforcers (Kazdin, 2001). There are several considerations in their selection. First, backup reinforcers should have established reinforcing properties. One common method of identifying backup reinforcers is to ask the target individual about preferred consequences. However, some have questioned the validity of verbal assessment methods (Northup, 2000). Furthermore, verbal assessments are not always feasible for the target population. For instance, stimulus preference assessments that measure participant approaches to stimuli presented individually (Pace, Ivancic, Edwards, Iwata, & Page, 1985) or in pairs (Fisher et al., 1992) may be more informative than verbal methods for individuals with intellectual developmental disorder. Behavior analysts may also use behavioral observation to identify backup reinforcers (Ayllon & Azrin, 1968). Specifically, Premack (1959) noted

that "any stimulus to which the species responds can be used as a reinforcer, provided only that the rate of the response governed by the stimulus is greater than that of some other response" (p. 227). The Premack principle became the basis for Allyon and Azrin's (1968) rule about the probability of behavior, which suggests that we ought to "observe what the individual does when the opportunity exists. Those activities that are probable at a given time will serve as reinforcers" (Ayllon & Azrin, 1968, p. 60).

*Satiation*, a reduction in reinforcement efficacy after the repeated delivery of the reinforcer, can lead to the failure of any token-economy program. One method of preventing reinforcer satiation is to make conditioned reinforcers exchangeable for a variety of backup reinforcers (Ayllon & Azrin, 1968; Bowman, Piazza, Fisher, Hagopian, & Kogan, 1997; Egel, 1980, 1981; Reese, Sherman, & Sheldon, 1998). For example, Sran and Borrero (2010) assigned children to no-selection, single-selection, or varied-reinforcer-selection conditions in a token program. Results indicated that children preferred conditions in which researchers gave them the option to select from a variety of reinforcers. The best outcomes were associated with maximum variety.

Another method of preventing or delaying reinforcer satiation is to make the achievement of the backup reinforcers effortful. A study by DeLeon et al. (2011) revealed that stimuli associated with high or moderate effort were more preferred and retained their value longer than stimuli without an earning requirement. Nevertheless, reevaluation of backup reinforcers may be necessary as often as once a week in certain contexts (Drabman & Tucker, 1974).

### Establish a Schedule of Reinforcement and Exchange Rate

There are two methods of manipulating the delivery of backup reinforcers to maximize a token economy's effectiveness. The first involves manipulation of the reinforcement schedule to reduce the effects of reinforcer satiation. Specifically, a behavior analyst generally uses continuous reinforcement, such as a fixed-ratio 1 schedule, during the initiation of a token economy to establish a high rate of behavior. Next, the behavior analyst should introduce intermittent reinforcement based on either ratio or variable-time schedules after behavior stabilizes on the continuous-reinforcement schedule (see Kazdin, 2001). We could find little empirical support, however, for a body of research that clearly demonstrates the utility of fading reinforcement from continuous to intermittent schedules in token economies. Another approach is to manipulate the amount of the conditioned reinforcer needed to obtain the backup reinforcer (i.e., the exchange rate). A behavior analyst usually sets the rate of reinforcement in the token economy by measuring the natural rate of the appropriate behavior during baseline, which ensures that the individual will contact the reinforcement contingency (Ayllon & Azrin, 1968). Observing the baseline rate allows the behavior analyst to gauge the number of tokens a client will earn during a given period. For example, Salend and Allen (1985) reported that they gave participants "a set amount of tokens that represented the established number of problem behaviors that the subject could engage in before losing reinforcement" (p. 61). Thus they based the number of tokens available to each participant on baseline levels of performance. The behavior analyst then assigns the price of the backup reinforcers and creates a menu of rewards with a range of backup reinforcers—some inexpensive (easy to earn), others more costly (difficult to earn), and still others priced at the intermediate level.

Establishing the value of conditioned reinforcers may be challenging especially for younger clients or clients with developmental delays. Researchers have developed several procedures to address this problem. Having clients observe others during token exchange can sometimes establish tokens as conditioned reinforcers (Ayllon & Azrin, 1968). The noncontingent delivery of tokens followed immediately by an opportunity to exchange the tokens for backup reinforcers may be effective if difficulties arise (Kazdin, 2001).

Delays between cash-out or redemption periods, delivery of conditioned reinforcers, the performance of the behavior, or some combination of these variables may reduce the effectiveness of a putative reinforcer for some clients. In these cases, reducing the delay between task performance and token delivery may be sufficient to improve performance (Field, Nash, Handwerk, & Friman, 2004). Field et al. (2004) showed that reducing the number of tokens needed to earn privileges and doubling exchange times by half resulted in a decrease in intense behavioral episodes and an increase in points earned compared to baseline. By contrast, Reed and Martens (2011) found that extended delays between the disbursement of tokens and cashing out did not reduce the effectiveness of a token

economy. Indeed, the behavior of children with lower levels of impulsivity improved even when exchange delays were relatively long.

In an extension of earlier work, Hupp et al. (2002) examined the separate and combined effects of medication and a token economy on the symptoms of young children with attention-deficit/hyperactivity disorder (ADHD) during a kickball game. More importantly, the study also compared the effects of promised delayed reward to actual delayed reward aided by immediate token delivery. Researchers supplied tokens contingent on "sportsman-like" behavior. Results indicated that delay of promised rewards did not increase sportsman-like behavior during the kickball games, although delayed rewards delivered via tokens increased sportsman-like behavior for all five children observed. Interestingly, stimulant medication had little to no positive effect on sportsman-like behavior in this sample of young children.

More recently, Pelham et al. (2014) assessed the effects of medication (i.e., methylphenidate) and behavioral treatment in various doses and combinations. Researchers assigned children diagnosed with ADHD in a summer program to either high-intensity, moderate-intensity, or low-intensity behavioral treatment with a token economy, or no behavioral treatment and high-dose, moderate-dose, or low-dose medication or placebo. Results indicated that the token economy and medication produced substantial improvements in child compliance. More importantly, a combination of low doses of the two modalities had large beneficial effects on child behavior. In addition, the highest dose of medication produced only minimal added benefits when combined with high-intensity behavioral treatment.

## Keep Records

Creating a daily or weekly chart may have many benefits, including provision of a visual record of client improvement that may enhance compliance with therapy-related tasks (Reitman & Drabman, 1996). Indeed, research suggests that persons implementing token economies and other types of behavior management programs may not recognize the improvements of their clients without such aids. For example, Reitman, Murphy, Hupp, and O'Callaghan (2004) found that a classroom teacher's ratings of child behavior generally remained unchanged, although a token program significantly reduced classroom behavior problems. By contrast, the use of periodic reviews of graphs or similar behavioral data in the presence of the clients may serve to facilitate more robust changes in behavior, or perhaps more consistent changes in the perceptions of those who interact with persons in behavioral interventions. During the chart review, the professionals or paraprofessionals (in the case of parents, supervisors, or others) can provide the clients with praise and feedback concerning progress, compliance with recommendations, or both. Following such consultation, therapists and clients, including persons like classroom teachers and administrators, may decide jointly to alter the treatment plan based on performance feedback (Hawkins & Mathews, 1999).

## Decide If Response Cost Is Warranted

*Response cost* or *behavior penalty* (Clark, 1996) is a negative-punishment procedure in which the implementer removes conditioned token reinforcers in a response-contingent fashion (Azrin & Holz, 1966). Clinicians and researchers have long used response cost in token economies to reduce the frequency of problem behavior (Eluri, Andrade, Trevino, & Mahmoud, 2016; Kazdin, 1971, 1972; Miltenberger, 2001; Reynolds & Kelley, 1997; Witt & Elliot, 1982). Response cost does not restrict access to reinforcement directly, unlike many other reductive techniques (e.g., time out; Reynolds & Kelley, 1997). Indeed, participants in a token-economy program may continue to earn conditioned reinforcers for the performance of adaptive behaviors, despite losing tokens when they perform problem behaviors.

An important step in implementing a token-economy program is to determine whether the use of response cost is necessary to effect behavior change. In deciding whether to use response cost, a behavior analyst should ask whether a client's problem behavior is inhibiting the performance of adaptive behavior. If the answer is yes, response cost is likely to be beneficial in reducing the performance of the problem behavior. However, Miltenberger (2001) warns that token programs using a behavior penalty may fail if the behavior analyst does not establish the token program before the implementation of response cost. One further consideration is that the penalty must result in removal of tokens and access to backup reinforcers without resulting in the complete loss of tokens. Complete loss of earned tokens and the loss of opportunities to exchange tokens for backup reinforcers may cause the program to fail (Kazdin, 1972; Miltenberger, 2001).

Over the past 50 years, most studies have suggested equivalence between programs that do and do not use response cost. Kaufman and O'Leary (1972) examined the differential effects of reward and response cost on academic and social behavior. Researchers randomly assigned adolescents in a hospital to a reward condition in which the adolescents began each session with no tokens and could earn tokens throughout the period, or to a response cost condition in which the adolescents began the period with 10 tokens, which researchers removed after rule infractions. The adolescents could exchange tokens for backup reinforcers from the school store. Interestingly, the two conditions were equally effective in reducing problem behavior. A more recent study by Donaldson, DeLeon, Kahng, and Fisher (2014) evaluated the effectiveness of an *earn* condition (i.e., token economy), a *loss* condition (i.e., response cost), and a *choice* condition in which students could select one of the conditions. In the earn condition, students began with zero tokens and could earn tokens for remaining on task and for engaging in nondisruptive behavior. During the loss condition, students began with 10 tokens and lost a token for engaging in off-task or disruptive behavior. As in earlier research, both the earn and loss conditions reduced the students' disruptive behaviors to near-zero levels. Interestingly, students seemed to prefer the loss condition, and the authors noted significant advantages for the loss condition relative to the time required to maintain the token program.

## Engage Participants and Train Staff

Implementation of token programs typically begins with a formal explanation of the rules of the token economy to clients. A behavior analyst should consult clients during program development well in advance of implementation. A formal meeting ensures that clients understand how to earn tokens, when and where to redeem tokens, what tokens can be exchanged for, and how much backup reinforcers cost. Finally, the behavior analyst must inform clients about which behaviors result in token gain and loss.

Although behavior analysts regard consistent token delivery as a key component for behavior change, researchers have yet to establish the precise level of consistency needed to achieve effectiveness. On the other hand, research on treatment fidelity has revealed that some interventions implemented with less than 100% fidelity (Noell, Gresham, & Gansle, 2002; Northup, Fisher,

Kahng, & Harrell, 1997) can retain effectiveness. Whatever the exact level of consistency needed, improvements in integrity may require extensive staff training (e.g., hospital personnel, teachers, parents). Thus ongoing staff supervision and an additional level of contingency management may be necessary to maximize the likelihood of success. This may entail praise and other incentives for staff members who consistently deliver conditioned and backup reinforcers; constructive feedback for errors; and periodic staff retraining to eliminate drift (Miltenberger, 2001).

Staff training looms as a unique opportunity to improve the generality of treatment effects for behavioral interventions, including response cost. However, researchers have devoted only limited attention to this important topic. Suffice it to say that token programs are likely to vary greatly in the fidelity of implementation and effectiveness (see Noell et al., 2005).

## Phase Out the Program

Teachers periodically ask us how we could recommend to them that they "bribe" students to behave. They also ask us, "What message would that teach them when they enter the real world? How could we, as professionals, recommend that we teach students to work only when they know we will reward them?" Notwithstanding the observation that few if any adults work without compensation, we believe that we are unlikely to persuade persons strongly opposed to extrinsic reinforcement to accept it (see Reitman, 1988, for an extended discussion of this issue). Instead, we typically suggest that the best token programs are those that we phase out deliberately.

Paul and Lentz (1977) presented one of the best examples of such phasing out. In their now-classic study, the researchers worked with patients institutionalized for psychosis from four state hospitals in central Illinois. The researchers assigned patients to one of three treatment groups with 28 patients in each group: milieu therapy, social-learning therapy with a token program, and a control group. The researchers followed patients for over 10 years. They offered a unique option to patients in the social-learning group to reduce dependence on the token program. In a token program with a conventional levels system, individuals earn opportunities to participate in more reinforcing environments but remain participants in the token economy. In a unique twist, Paul and Lentz decreased the amount of required program

time as patients advanced through the levels of the program, and patients at the highest level, Level 4, could buy themselves out of the program. Specifically, patients on Level 1, the entrance level, engaged in 6 hours of scheduled classes and activities each day and earned tokens for adaptive behavior (e.g., self-care, bed making, and appropriate mealtime behavior). Patients who progressed to Level 2 attended 3 hours of classes and activities, and engaged in individual assignments for the other 3 hours. Patients at Levels 3 and 4 engaged in 4–6 hours of individual assignments and did not attend scheduled classes and activities. Patients had the opportunity to earn more tokens, and the criterion for earning tokens shifted upward at each level. Patients at Level 4 could purchase a "credit card" that gave them unlimited access to reinforcers if they continued to meet Level 4 requirements. The researchers also included a fading component to enhance the success of the program. The program included a delay-to-reinforcement "payday" in which patients received a lump sum of tokens as they graduated from Level 1 to Level 2. This component taught the patients to plan as they would outside the hospital setting. Furthermore, Paul and Lentz supplied staff and patients with rules about the implementation and use of the token program.

Several effective techniques exist for reducing reliance on extrinsic or arbitrary contingencies and promoting the generalization and maintenance of behavior change (O'Callaghan, Reitman, Northup, Hupp, & Murphy, 2003; Stokes & Baer, 1977). For example, a behavior analyst may employ *indiscriminable contingencies* to facilitate generalization of a token program's contingencies. The behavior analyst must "make unclear the limits of training contingencies; in particular, conceal, when possible, the point at which those contingencies stop operating, if possible by delayed reinforcement" (Stokes & Baer, 1977, p. 287). Intermittent reinforcement (e.g., variable-ratio or variable-time schedules) also appears to facilitate generalization (Ferster & Skinner, 1957). Increasing the cost of the backup reinforcers or delaying the opportunity to redeem tokens are other approaches to fading token programs. We encourage readers to consult Stokes and Baer (1977) for a complete list of techniques for promoting generalization.

Finally, Sullivan and O'Leary (1990) used a reversal design to study the efficacy of fading procedures for both token and response cost programs. Results suggested that the two types of programs were equally effective for increasing duration of on-task behavior. Only half the children in the token program showed high levels of maintenance, however.

## ADDITIONAL CONSIDERATIONS

### Treatment Acceptability

Theodore, Bray, and Kehle (2004) found that although teacher ratings did not reflect changes in behavior that were apparent through direct observation, teachers reported a favorable experience with the token program. Reitman et al. (2004) reported similar results. McGoey and DuPaul (2000) suggested that an all-positive-reinforcement token program and a response cost program were about equally effective in reducing disruptive classroom behavior. Interestingly, teacher acceptability ratings favored the response cost procedure. When questioned, some teachers commented that this procedure was far less time-consuming than "catching the children being good." We discuss the relative merits of response-cost-only programs at greater length toward the end of this chapter.

### Individual versus Group Contingencies

Drabman, Spitalnik, and Spitalnik (1974) conducted one of the earliest studies exploring the relative efficacy of group and individual contingencies. They included four experimental conditions: individual reinforcement; group reinforcement determined by the most disruptive child in the group; group reinforcement determined by the least disruptive child in the group; and group reinforcement determined by a randomly chosen child in the group. Although the conditions were equally effective at reducing disruptive behavior, the teacher preferred group reinforcement determined by a randomly selected child in the group, because it was the least time-consuming and easiest to use. Children, by contrast, ranked group reinforcement determined by the least disruptive child in the group as most preferred; however, the teacher disliked that procedure. Neither the teacher nor the students preferred the individual-reinforcement condition. Children and teachers preferred an interdependent group contingency with response cost over one with reward in a study by Lee, Penrod, and Price (2017).

Reitman et al. (2004) provided additional data on the effectiveness of individual versus group contingencies. Children earned opportunities to play the Rewards Target Game (see Anhalt et al., 1998), in which chances to throw a Velcro ball at a target permitted access to several reinforcing activities, and the researchers made tangibles contingent on the behavior of either randomly selected children; the group; or one of the three target or "star" children, the individual contingency. During baseline, the teacher received training and explained the token program to her class. The token program also contained a response cost in which the teacher could move a marker down (which was the negative consequence), contingent on disruptive behavior. Although initial rates of disruptive behavior were somewhat low (M = 15% of intervals for each of the three participants), the results indicated that the token economy reduced rates of classroom rule violations for both individual and group contingencies. A study by Kowalewicz and Coffee (2014) used a changing-criterion design to show that a group interdependent contingency based on a mystery motivator as part of a Tier 1 intervention in an elementary school improved behavior. Importantly, effects were maintained at follow-up. Seven of the eight classroom teachers indicated that they would be likely to use the group contingency intervention again, as it required minimal training, and the data collection and time requirements were practical.

### Follow-Up, Maintenance, and Generalization

LePage et al. (2003) used a token economy on an acute inpatient psychiatric unit to reduce assaults on staff and patients. Patients voluntarily enrolled in the program, and they earned stamps for performing behavior necessary for successful transition to the community. Examples of such behavior included taking medication, timely appointment keeping, and showering. Researchers implemented response cost for major violations of safety rules requiring a police presence on the unit, such as hitting another person or destroying property. Patients redeemed tokens for privileges such as off-ground passes, movies, stereo rental, or items from the token store (e.g., snacks, drinks, phone cards). The program was effective at a 2-year follow-up. Patient-to-patient and employee injuries decreased by 48% and 21%, respectively. Finally, a study by O'Callaghan et al. (2003) used training modifications based on the work of Stokes and Baer (1977) to facilitate generalization of social skills to games without token programs.

Drabman and Tucker's (1974) critique and recommendations concerning failures of token programs provide an unusually comprehensive account of shortcomings and potential fixes for frequently encountered implementation problems in school settings. They identified three major classes of failures: *program-based*, *teacher-based*, and *setting-based*. Program-based failures included poor definition or poor monitoring of target behavior, or both. Teacher- or personnel-based problems included failure to reward approximations of the behavior (shaping), altering programs without consulting the data, and ignoring disruptive behavior that produced social reinforcement from classmates. Setting-based failures included problems with discriminating changes in behavior for many children simultaneously. Most importantly, Drabman and Tucker offered recommendations for choosing and distributing tokens and managing day-to-day changes in a classroom-based token program.

Although many years have passed since the introduction of the token economy, questions remain about its efficacy. Specifically, Maggin, Chafouleas, Goddard, and Johnson (2011) conducted a critical review, using criteria developed through the What Works Clearinghouse, to evaluate the experimental rigor of existing research on token programs. Maggin et al. concluded that token economies in academic settings did not meet evidence-based standards, although they concluded that the data were supportive of its use. Specifically, they recommended the development of systematic procedures for evaluating implementation fidelity and guidelines for staff training.

## CHALLENGES: PROBLEMS OF APPLICATION

There are many limitations of token programs, and most are like those of behavior modification procedures more generally (see Reitman, Hupp, & O'Callaghan, 2005). One of the more durable but less devastating is the *no-cure criticism* (Kendall, 1989)—the notion that treatment effects typically do not persist after treatment withdrawal. Of course, we can apply this criticism with equal measure to psychotropic medications regarded as highly efficacious, such as stimulant medication. Another concern relates to the ethical issues raised by the imposition of contingencies on vulnerable groups, such as children and adults with intellectual developmental disorder. Fortunately, most behavior analysts seek to minimize this risk by fostering a collaborative process between a treater and client in which both parties contribute equally, or as equally as the client's disability or status may permit. Another factor to consider is the right to effective treatment, which may dictate the short-term use of behavior change strategies to facilitate the long-term goal of greater freedom and independence (Reitman, 1988).

The implementation of a token program may present considerable training and resource challenges. For example, persons charged with the administration of a token economy must comply with the terms of the agreement or contract. Teachers or staff providing direct care must guard against reacting to noncompliance or aggression in ways that are inconsistent with the rules of the token program. Response cost requires the dispassionate removal of points or tokens from a potentially volatile person. Emotional reactions from the program administrator may undermine the token program by supplying social or attention-based reinforcers for problem behavior. Thus administrators may become unable or unwilling to continue a token program, because they may require caregivers and staff to endure significant antisocial behavior and commit material resources to support the token program's contingencies. Behavior analysts should seek support from relatives, counselors, or other staff for a caregiver, staff person, or teacher who appears overwhelmed.

Although an additional challenge is somewhat beyond the scope of this chapter, some researchers have argued that a failure to account for *motivating operations* (events that influence the effectiveness of conditioned stimuli as reinforcers) may compromise the effectiveness of contingency management procedures (Laraway, Snycerski, Michael, & Poling, 2003). For example, receiving $20 for cutting a neighbor's lawn would reduce the likelihood of a child's completing chores at home if the child was participating in a home-based program based primarily on monetary reinforcers. Earlier researchers have noted that failure to consider deprivation, satiation, and competing sources of reinforcement has doomed many a token program (Allyon & Azrin, 1968; Drabman & Tucker, 1974).

Most token programs require well-developed repertoires of organizational, communication, and negotiation skills. Thus persons charged with administering token programs must either teach the prerequisite skills as needed or modify the token program to reduce demands on persons implementing the program. The data suggest, however, that token programs can be beneficial even in the most difficult circumstances (see Ayllon & Azrin, 1968; Drabman & Tucker, 1974; Field et al., 2004).

## RESPONSE-COST-ONLY PROGRAMS

Researchers have pursued less resource-intensive approaches to token-economy programs, such as programs involving response cost only (Donaldson et al., 2014), or group rather than individualized programs (Kowalewicz & Coffee, 2014; Mikami et al., 2013; Reed & Martens, 2011). For example, results of a study by Conyers et al. (2004) suggested that implementers may favor response-cost-only programs over more complex and resource-intensive positive programs. Conyers et al. supplied participants with tokens and subsequently removed tokens contingent on disruptive behaviors (e.g., crying or noncompliance). Disruptive behavior decreased from 67% during baseline to 5% after response cost was implemented. In the replication phase of the study, disruptive behavior increased to a mean of 52% and subsequently returned to 5% after reinstatement of the response cost.

One possible flaw in response-cost-only programs stems from the often-repeated maxim that punishment procedures do not teach appropriate responding (Reitman, 1998). In addition, Azrin and Holz (1966) noted in their extensive review that punishment often elicits an escape-related response from the target individual. Nevertheless, researchers should continue to explore ways to simplify the delivery and improve the real-world effectiveness of token-economy programs. Several aspects of response-cost-only programs are appealing from an effectiveness perspective. First, the use of punishment (negative punishment, in this case) is commonplace in society. For example, late-return charges for library books, speeding or parking tickets, overdraft charges at the bank, or extra charges for exceeding cellphone minutes are everyday examples of response cost (Kazdin, 2001; Miltenberger, 2001). So, although punishment-based procedures certainly have their detractors (see Sidman, 1989), familiarity may be an asset in promoting acceptability and adherence.

## SUMMARY AND DIRECTIONS FOR FUTURE RESEARCH

Researchers have used token programs successfully in homes, prisons, recreational settings, educational settings, hospitals, businesses, and industry (Drabman et al., 1974; Gendreau, Listwan, Kuhns, & Exum, 2014; Hupp et al., 2002; Kahng, Boscoe, & Byrne, 2003; Kazdin, 2001; McNamara, 1971). We can distinguish token programs in these settings by the selected consequences (reinforcers and punishers), the identity of the contractors (e.g., the helping professional, parent, teacher, peer, sibling), and the intervention setting (e.g., school, mental health clinic, hospital). Tokens programs have addressed a wide range of problems, such as schizophrenia, intellectual developmental disorder, ADHD, oppositional defiant disorder, and autism spectrum disorder.

Researchers also have used token programs with children and adolescents to influence behaviors that would not justify a psychiatric diagnosis, such as social interaction, school attendance, academic productivity, and time on task (Kowalewicz & Coffee, 2014; Miltenberger, 2001; Truchlicka, McLaughlin, & Swain, 1998). Researchers have used token programs with adults to reduce positive cocaine and marijuana tests (Budney, Higgins, Delany, Kent, & Bickel, 1991), decrease workplace injuries (Fox, Hopkins, & Anger, 1987), improve safe driving practices among pizza delivery drivers (Ludwig & Geller, 1991), and increase adherence to medical or rehabilitative regimens (Gottlieb, 2000).

Token economies have been represented well in academic settings. For example, Staats, Staats, Schutz, and Wolf (1962) increased reading proficiency with a program in which individuals could exchange tokens for small trinkets and edibles. This study established that both immediately delivered tangible reinforcers and token reinforcers could decrease escape-related behaviors in an academic context. O'Leary and Becker (1967) also evaluated the effectiveness of token-economy programs in classrooms. O'Leary, Becker, Evans, and Saudargas (1969) examined how classroom context influenced the effectiveness of token programs designed to reduce children's deviant behavior. They evaluated factors such as a program itself, rules, lesson structure, and social reinforcement. The token programs decreased disruptive behavior for nearly 86% of the participants, whereas the other experimental conditions produced no significant difference.

Finally, although the field has regarded the efficacy of token economies as about as well established as any in the behavioral literature (Kazdin, 2001), researchers conducted many of the original studies before the application of more recent, rigorous standards for empirical research. Thus claims about the efficacy of token programs require additional empirical support (Maggin et al., 2011). Either way, implementation and dissemination challenges still abound. Chief among the challenges are intervention integrity, training, and consultation—subjects of great relevance for bringing effective treatments to the public with greater regularity. Reitman and colleagues conducted a series of studies to evaluate whether they could use token programs to increase appropriate social behavior in athletic settings (see Reitman et al., 2005). For example, Hupp and Reitman (1999) implemented a token economy during a basketball camp for children diagnosed with ADHD. Tokens consisted of "B-Ball Bucks" that the researchers delivered contingent on sportsman-like behavior, such as cheering for peers, and children could exchange them for a variety of backup reinforcers. The token program improved sportsman-like behavior, whereas discussions about the value of good sportsmanship did not. Perhaps more importantly, reinforcing appropriate behavior appeared to decrease un-sportsman-like behavior, even though the researchers did not target un-sportsman-like behavior (e.g., verbal or physical aggression) directly. Clearly, further studies are necessary to establish whether social skills learned and mastered in the context of a sports setting can be generalized to and maintained in nonathletic settings. Consult Conner-Smith and Weisz (2003), Noell et al. (2005), or both for excellent introductions to these topics.

## BASIC RESEARCH AND CLINICAL FOLKLORE

Although this chapter has reviewed a substantial number of studies evaluating the efficacy of token and contingency management procedures and their application to a variety of human behaviors, a surprising amount of speculation and clinical folklore seems to guide much of the application of this popular procedure. For example, researchers often extrapolate from basic research that conditioned reinforcers may become powerful reinforcers in their own right (e.g., Jones et al., 1992). Yet few, if any, rigorous experimental studies support this assertion. Additionally, little research on exactly how token economies exert their influence exists, even though researchers hypothesize that token programs may heighten awareness of the target individual's appropriate behavior, possibly conferring conditioned reinforcing properties on the behavior manager (see Risley, 2005). The fact that many contingency management procedures also rely extensively on verbal stimuli complicates this issue (see Hayes, 1989).

Additional bridge studies are needed to inform issues such as identification of reinforcing stimuli and the point(s) at which satiation for those stimuli occurs. Many stimulus preference methods are available, but consensus about which methods are best suited to which populations is lacking. Similarly, some stimuli that function as reinforcement may be impractical (e.g., a hospital setting in which patients may earn iPods as backup reinforcers) or require considerable staff resources to deliver consistently (e.g., rewarding a child with 15 minutes of a staff person's time during each school day). Even relatively straightforward issues of reinforcer satiation (e.g., frequency of reinforcer variation, satiation monitoring in applied settings) appear under researched, thus leaving the behavior analyst with little practical research-informed guidance. Fortunately, recent work by applied behavior analysts has begun to take a fresh look at token programs, with an eye toward blending elements of basic and applied research. These studies could lead to greater clarity concerning how to maximize the clinical yield and practicality of token programs in applied settings (cf. DeLeon et al., 2011; Donaldson et al., 2014; Reed & Martens, 2011; Sran & Borrero, 2010).

On a final note, Paul and Lentz (1977) conducted a groundbreaking longitudinal study of the impact of a level-based token program. Over 40 years later, it remains one of the few studies to have reported long-term, socially meaningful impact from a token-based instructional program. Moreover, the researchers' emphasis on fading to promote maintenance and generalization of the program has remained surprisingly novel. A cursory examination of the many classrooms that employ token programs is likely to reveal little attention to efforts to fade such programs over the course of the school year, or to do so systematically across the school years. Thus, although this chapter has documented an extensive literature concerned with the token economy, its many variations, and the many settings in which researchers and clinicians use it suggest that there is an ongoing need for evaluation of this well-known intervention.

## REFERENCES

Alberto, P. A., & Troutman, A. C. (2006). *Applied behavior analysis for teachers* (7th ed.). Upper Saddle River, NJ: Pearson/Merrill Prentice Hall.

Anhalt, K., McNeil, C. B., & Bahl, A. B. (1998). The ADHD classroom kit: A whole-classroom approach for managing disruptive behavior. *Psychology in the Schools, 35,* 67–79.

Ayllon, T., & Azrin, N. H. (1965). The measurement

and reinforcement of behavior of psychotics. *Journal of the Experimental Analysis of Behavior, 8,* 357–383.

Ayllon, T., & Azrin, N. H. (1968). *The token economy: A motivational system for therapy and rehabilitation.* New York: Appleton-Century-Crofts.

Azrin, N. H., & Holz, W. C. (1966). Punishment. In W. K. Honig (Ed.), *Operant behavior: Areas of research and application* (pp. 790–826). New York: Appleton-Century-Crofts.

Benishek, L. A., Dugosh, K. L., Kirby, K. C., Matejkowski, J., Clements, N. T., Seymour, B. L., et al. (2014). Prize-based contingency management for the treatment of substance abusers: A meta-analysis. *Addiction, 109,* 1426–1436.

Bowman, L. G., Piazza, C. C., Fisher, W. W., Hagopian, L. P., & Kogan, J. S. (1997). Assessment of preference for varied versus constant reinforcers. *Journal of Applied Behavior Analysis, 30,* 451–458.

Budney, A. J., Higgins, S. T., Delany, D. D., Kent, L., & Bickel, W. K. (1991). Contingent reinforcement of abstinence with individuals abusing cocaine and marijuana. *Journal of Applied Behavior Analysis, 24,* 657–665.

Clark, L. (1996). *SOS!: Help for parents.* Bowling Green, KY: Parents Press.

Clark, M., Lachowicz, J., & Wolf, M. (1968). A pilot basic education program for school dropouts incorporating a token reinforcement system. *Behaviour Research and Therapy, 6,* 183–188.

Conner-Smith, J. K., & Weisz, J. R. (2003). Applying treatment outcome research in clinical practice: Techniques for adapting interventions to the real world. *Child and Adolescent Mental Health, 8,* 3–10.

Conyers, C., Miltenberger, R., Maki, A., Barenz, R., Jurgens, M., Sailer, A., et al. (2004). A comparison of response cost and differential reinforcement of other behavior to reduce disruptive behavior in a preschool classroom. *Journal of Applied Behavior Analysis, 37,* 411–415.

DeLeon, I. G., Gregory, M. K., Frank-Crawford, M. A., Allman, M. J., Wilke, A. E., Carreau-Webster, A. B., et al. (2011). Examination of the influence of contingency on changes in reinforcer value. *Journal of Applied Behavior Analysis, 44*(3), 543–558.

Dickerson, F. B., Tenhula, W. N., & Green-Paden, L. D. (2005). The token economy for schizophrenia: Review of the literature and recommendations for future research. *Schizophrenia Research, 75,* 405–416.

Donaldson, J. M., DeLeon, I. G., Kahng, S., & Fisher, A. B. (2014). Effects of and preference for conditions of token earn versus token loss. *Journal of Applied Behavior Analysis, 47*(3), 537–548.

Drabman, R. S., & Lahey, B. B. (1974). Feedback in the classroom behavior modification: Effects on the target and her classmates. *Journal of Applied Behavior Analysis, 7,* 591–598.

Drabman, R. S., Spitalnik, R., & Spitalnik, K. (1974). Sociometric and disruptive behavior as a function of four types of token reinforcement programs. *Journal of Applied Behavior Analysis, 7,* 93–101.

Drabman, R. S., & Tucker, R. D. (1974). Why classroom token economies fail. *Journal of School Psychology, 12,* 178–188.

Egel, A. L. (1980). The effects of constant vs. varied reinforcer presentation on responding by autistic children. *Journal of Experimental Child Psychology, 30,* 455–463.

Egel, A. L. (1981). Reinforcer variation: Implications for motivating developmentally disabled children. *Journal of Applied Behavior Analysis, 14,* 345–350.

Eluri, Z., Andrade, I., Trevino, N., & Mahmoud, E. (2016). Assessment and treatment of problem behavior maintained by mand compliance. *Journal of Applied Behavior Analysis, 49,* 383–387.

Ferster, C. B., & Skinner, B. F. (1957). *Schedules of reinforcement.* New York: Appleton-Century-Crofts.

Field, C. E., Nash, H. M., Handwerk, M. L., & Friman, P. C. (2004). A modification of the token economy for nonresponsive youth in family-style residential care. *Behavior Modification, 28,* 438–457.

Fisher, W., Piazza, C. C., Bowman, L. G., Hagopian, L. P., Owens, J. C., & Slevin, I. (1992). A comparison of two approaches for identifying reinforcers for persons with severe and profound disabilities. *Journal of Applied Behavior Analysis, 25,* 491–498.

Fiske, K. E., Isenhower, R. W., Bamon, M. J., & Lauderdale-Littin, S. (2020). An analysis of token reinforcement using a multiple-schedule assessment. *Journal of Applied Behavior Analysis, 53,* 563–571.

Fox, D. K., Hopkins, B. L., & Anger, W. K. (1987). The long-term effects of a token economy on safety performance in open-pit mining. *Journal of Applied Behavior Analysis, 20,* 215–224.

Gendreau, P., Listwan, S. J., Kuhns, J. B., & Exum, M. L. (2014). Making prisoners accountable: Are contingency management programs the answer? *Criminal Justice and Behavior, 41*(9), 1079–1102.

Gottlieb, H. (2000). Medication nonadherence: Finding solutions to a costly medical problem. *Drug Benefit Trends, 12,* 57–62.

Hackenberg, T. D. (2018). Token reinforcement: Translational research and application. *Journal of Applied Behavior Analysis, 51,* 393–435.

Hawkins, R. P., & Mathews, J. R. (1999). Frequent monitoring of clinical outcomes: Research and accountability in clinical practice. *Education and Treatment of Children, 22,* 117–135.

Hayes, S. C. (Ed.). (1989). *Cognition, contingencies and rule-governed behavior.* New York: Plenum Press.

Higgins, J. W., Williams, R. L., & McLaughlin, T. F. (2001). The effects of a token economy employing instructional consequences for a third-grade student with learning disabilities: A data-based case study. *Education and Treatment of Children, 24,* 99–106.

Hupp, S. D. A., & Reitman, D. (1999). Improving sports skills and sportsmanship in children diagnosed with attention deficit/hyperactivity disorder. *Child and Family Behavior Therapy, 21,* 35–51.

Hupp, S. D. A., Reitman, D., Northup, J., O'Callaghan, P., & LeBlanc, M. (2002). The effects of delayed rewards, tokens, and stimulant medication on sportsmanlike behavior with ADHD-diagnosed children. *Behavior Modification, 26,* 148–162.

Ivy, J. W., Meindl, J. N., Overley, E., & Robson, K. M. (2017). Token economy: A systematic review of procedural descriptions. *Behavior Modification, 41,* 708–737.

Jones, R. N., Downing, R. H., Latkowski, M. E., Ferre, R. C., & McMahon, W. M. (1992). Levels systems as shaping and fading procedures: Use in a child inpatient psychiatry setting. *Child and Family Behavior Therapy, 14,* 15–37.

Jowett Hirst, E. S., Dozier, C. L., & Payne, S. W. (2016). Efficacy and preference for reinforcement and response cost in token economies. *Journal of Applied Behavior Analysis, 49,* 329–345.

Kahng, S. W., Boscoe, J. H., & Byrne, S. (2003). The use of an escape contingency and a token economy to increase food acceptance. *Journal of Applied Behavior Analysis, 36,* 349–353.

Kaufman, K. F., & O'Leary, K. D. (1972). Reward, cost, and self-evaluation procedures for disruptive adolescents in a psychiatric hospital school. *Journal of Applied Behavior Analysis, 5,* 293–309.

Kazdin, A. E. (1971). The effect of response cost in suppressing behavior in a pre-psychotic retardate. *Journal of Behavior Therapy and Experimental Psychiatry, 2,* 137–140.

Kazdin, A. E. (1972). Response cost: The removal of conditioned reinforcers for therapeutic change. *Behavior Therapy, 3,* 533–546.

Kazdin, A. E. (2001). *Behavior modification in applied settings* (6th ed.). Pacific Grove, CA: Brooks/Cole.

Kazdin, A. E., & Bootzin, R. R. (1972). The token economy: An evaluative review. *Journal of Applied Behavior Analysis, 5,* 343–372.

Kendall, P. C. (1989). The generalization and maintenance of behavior change: Comments, considerations, and the "no-cure" criticism. *Behavior Therapy, 20,* 357–364.

Kirby, F. D., & Shields, F. (1972). Modification of arithmetic response rate and attending behavior in a seventh-grade student. *Journal of Applied Behavior Analysis, 5,* 79–84.

Kowalewicz, E. A., & Coffee, G. (2014). Mystery motivator: A Tier 1 classroom behavioral intervention. *School Psychology Quarterly, 29*(2), 138–156.

Laraway, S., Snycerski, S., Michael, J., & Poling, A. (2003). Motivating operations and terms to describe them: Some further refinements. *Journal of Applied Behavior Analysis, 36,* 407–414.

Lee, K., Penrod, B., & Price, J. N. (2017). A comparison of cost and reward procedures with interdependent group contingencies. *Behavior Modification, 41,* 21–44.

Leon, Y., Borrero, J. C., & DeLeon, I. G. (2016). Parametric analysis of delayed primary and conditioned reinforcers. *Journal of Applied Behavior Analysis, 49,* 639–655.

LePage, J. P., Delben, K., Pollard, S., McGhee, M., Van-

horn, L., Murphy, J., et al. (2003). Reducing assaults on an acute psychiatric unit using a token economy: A 2-year follow-up. *Behavioral Interventions, 18,* 179–190.

Ludwig, T. D., & Geller, E. S. (1991). Improving the driving practices of pizza deliverers: Response generalization and moderating effects of driving history. *Journal of Applied Behavior Analysis, 24,* 31–44.

Maggin, D. M., Chafouleas, S. M., Goddard, K. M., & Johnson, A. H. (2011). A systematic evaluation of token economies as a classroom management tool for students with challenging behavior. *Journal of School Psychology, 49*(5), 529–553.

McGinnis, J. C., Friman, P. C., & Carlyon, W. D. (1999). The effect of token rewards on "intrinsic" motivation for doing math. *Journal of Applied Behavior Analysis, 32,* 375–379.

McGoey, K. E., & DuPaul, G. J. (2000). Token reinforcement and response cost procedures: Reducing the disruptive behavior of preschool children with attention-deficit/hyperactivity disorder. *School Psychology Quarterly, 15,* 330–343.

McNamara, J. R. (1971). Teacher and students as sources for behavior modification in the classroom. *Behavior Therapy, 2,* 205–213.

Mikami, A. Y., Griggs, M. S., Lerner, M. D., Emeh, C. C., Reuland, M. M., Jack, A., et al. (2013). A randomized trial of a classroom intervention to increase peers' social inclusion of children with attention-deficit/hyperactivity disorder. *Journal of Consulting and Clinical Psychology, 81*(1), 100–112.

Miltenberger, R. G. (2001). *Behavior modification: Principles and procedures* (2nd ed.). Belmont, CA: Wadsworth/Thomson Learning.

Moore, J. W., Tingstrom, D. H., Doggett, R. A., & Carlyon, W. D. (2001). Restructuring an existing token economy in a psychiatric facility for children. *Child and Family Behavior Therapy, 23,* 53–59.

Musser, E. H., Bray, M. A., Kehle, T. J., & Jenson, W. R. (2001). Reducing disruptive behaviors in students with serious emotional disturbance. *School Psychology Review, 30,* 294–304.

Noell, G. H., Gresham, F. M., & Gansle, K. A. (2002). Does treatment integrity matter?: A preliminary investigation of instructional implementation and mathematics performance. *Journal of Behavioral Education, 11,* 51–67.

Noell, G. H., Witt, J. C., Slider, N. J., Connell, J. E., Gatti, S. L., Williams, K., et al. (2005). Treatment implementation following behavioral consultation in schools: Comparison of three follow-up strategies. *School Psychology Review, 34,* 87–106.

Northup, J. (2000). Further evaluation of the accuracy of reinforcer surveys: A systematic replication. *Journal of Applied Behavior Analysis, 33,* 335–338.

Northup, J., Fisher, W. W., Kahng, S. W., & Harrell, R. T. (1997). An assessment of the necessary strength of behavioral treatments for severe behavior problems. *Journal of Developmental and Physical Disabilities, 9,* 1–16.

O'Callaghan, P. M., Reitman, D., Northup, J., Hupp, S. D. A., & Murphy, M. A. (2003). Promoting social skills generalization with ADHD-diagnosed children in a sports setting. *Behavior Therapy, 34,* 313–330.

O'Leary, K. D., & Becker, W. C. (1967). Behavior modification of an adjustment class: A token reinforcement program. *Exceptional Children, 9,* 637–642.

O'Leary, K. D., Becker, W. C., Evans, M. B., & Saudargas, R. A. (1969). A token reinforcement program in a public school: A replication and systematic analysis. *Journal of Applied Behavior Analysis, 2,* 3–13.

Pace, G. M., Ivancic, M. T., Edwards, G. L., Iwata, B. A., & Page, T. J. (1989). The use of behavioral assessment to prescribe and evaluate treatments for severely handicapped children. *Journal of Applied Behavior Analysis, 18,* 173–178.

Paul, G. L., & Lentz, R. J. (1977). *Psychosocial treatment of chronic mental patients: Milieu versus social-learning programs.* Cambridge, MA: Harvard University Press.

Pelham, W. E., Burrows-MacLean, L., Gnagy, E. M., Fabiano, G. A., Coles, E. K., Wymbs, B. T., et al. (2014). A dose-ranging study of behavioral and pharmacological treatment for children with ADHD. *Journal of Abnormal Child Psychology, 42*(6), 1019–1031.

Premack, D. (1959). Toward empirical behavioral laws: 1. Positive reinforcement. *Psychological Review, 66,* 219–233.

Reed, D. D., & Martens, B. K. (2011). Temporal discounting predicts student responsiveness to exchange delays in a classroom token system. *Journal of Applied Behavior Analysis, 44*(1), 1–18.

Reese, M. R., Sherman, J. A., & Sheldon, J. B. (1998). Reducing disruptive behavior of a group home resident with autism and mental retardation. *Journal of Autism and Developmental Disorders, 28,* 159–165.

Reitman, D. (1998). Punished by misunderstanding: A critical evaluation of Kohn's *Punished by Rewards* and its implications for behavioral interventions with children. *Behavior Analyst, 21,* 143–157.

Reitman, D., & Drabman, R. S. (1996). Read my fingertips: A procedure for enhancing the effectiveness of time-out with argumentative children. *Child and Family Behavior Therapy, 18,* 35–40.

Reitman, D., Hupp, S. D. A., & O'Callaghan, P. M. (2005). Sport skill training. In A. M. Gross & R. S. Drabman (Eds.), *Encyclopedia of behavior modification and cognitive behavior therapy: Vol. 2. Clinical child applications* (pp. 1050–1054). Thousand Oaks, CA: SAGE.

Reitman, D., Murphy, M. A., Hupp, S. D. A., & O'Callaghan, P. M. (2004). Behavior change and perceptions of change: Evaluating the effectiveness of a token economy. *Child and Family Behavior Therapy, 26,* 17–36.

Reynolds, L. K., & Kelley, M. L. (1997). The efficacy of a response cost-based treatment package for managing aggressive behavior in preschoolers. *Behavior Modification, 21,* 216–230.

Risley, T. (2005). Montrose M. Wolf (1935–2004). *Journal of Applied Behavior Analysis, 38,* 279–287.

Russell, D., Ingvarsson, E. T., Haggar, J. L., & Jessel, J. (2018). Using progressive ratio schedules to evaluate tokens as generalized conditioned reinforcers. *Journal of Applied Behavior Analysis, 51,* 40–52.

Salend, S. J., & Allen, E. M. (1985). Comparative effects of externally managed and self-managed response-cost systems on inappropriate classroom behavior. *Journal of School Psychology, 23,* 59–67.

Sidman, M. (1989). *Coercion and its fallout.* Boston: Authors Cooperative.

Skinner, B. F. (1953). *Science and human behavior.* New York: Macmillan.

Sran, S. K., & Borrero, J. C. (2010). Assessing the value of choice in a token system. *Journal of Applied Behavior Analysis, 43*(3), 553–557.

Staats, A. W., Staats, C. K., Schutz, R. E., & Wolf, M. (1962). The conditioning of textual responses using "extrinsic" reinforcers. *Journal of the Experimental Analysis of Behavior, 5,* 33–40.

Stokes, T. F., & Baer, D. M. (1977). An implicit technology of generalization. *Journal of Applied Behavior Analysis, 10,* 349–367.

Sullivan, M. A., & O'Leary, S. G. (1990). Maintenance following reward and cost token programs. *Behavior Therapy, 21,* 139–149.

Theodore, L. A., Bray, M. A., & Kehle, T. J. (2004). A comparative study of group contingencies and randomized reinforcers to reduce disruptive classroom behavior. *School Psychology Quarterly, 19,* 253–271.

Truchlicka, M., McLaughlin, T. F., & Swain, J. C. (1998). Effects of token reinforcement and response cost on the accuracy of spelling performance of middle school special education students with behavior disorders. *Behavioral Interventions, 13,* 1–10.

Witt, J. C., & Elliot, S. N. (1982). The response cost lottery: A time efficient and effective classroom intervention. *Journal of School Psychology, 20,* 155–161.

# SUBSPECIALTIES IN APPLIED BEHAVIOR ANALYSIS

We have reorganized the order of chapters in Part VII in this edition of the *Handbook of Applied Behavior Analysis*. In addition, there are three new chapters on the subspecialties of pediatric feeding disorders, teacher consultation, and telehealth. Chapter 23 by Kodak, Grow, and Bergman opens Part VII with a review of behavioral treatments of autism spectrum disorder (ASD). Kodak et al. discuss the changes in the criteria for diagnosing ASD and behaviors that are associated with a diagnosis of ASD. The chapter also provides a summary of the most recent research on the effects of applied-behavior-analytic treatments, which readers are sure to find instructive. Chapter 24 by Friman provides the reader with an insightful summary of the contributions applied behavior analysts can make to the field of pediatric medicine. He discusses three routine behavior problems that pediatricians commonly confront—bedtime problems, enuresis, and encopresis—and describes relevant behavior-analytic interventions to illustrate his points. Chapter 25 by Piazza and Kirkwood presents a behavior-analytic conceptualization of pediatric feeding disorders. The authors also address many practical considerations associated with assessment and treatment of feeding disorders in children.

Martens, Daly, Begeny, and Sullivan have organized their Chapter 26 discussion of behavioral approaches to education around a model called the *learning/instructional hierarchy*. This model promotes the dynamic development of proficient skill performance. The authors have provided a historical context for behavioral approaches to education, in addition to describing more recent studies evaluating strategies for effective teaching. Chapter 27 by DiGennaro Reed, Hagermoser Sanetti, and Codding on teacher consultation is a new and welcome addition to the *Handbook of Applied Behavior Analysis*. The authors introduce their topic within the framework of federal legislation that has altered the landscape of public education. The authors define *behavioral consultation*, discuss different models of consultation, and provide guidance on procedures to maximize the effectiveness of consultation. Miltenberger, Gross, Valbuena, and Sanchez use the exemplar of firearms to introduce the reader to the behavioral literature on safety skills training in Chapter 28. These authors provide a comprehensive overview of the factors that contribute to firearms injuries and death, such as the prevalence of gun ownership, gun storage practices, and laws that regulate gun purchasing, to name a few. The authors then review the literature on firearm safety training and the empirical support for the various interventions.

In Chapter 29, Silverman, Holtyn, Jarvis, and Subramaniam provide an updated discussion of the behavior analysis and treatment of drug addiction. The authors describe early studies on interventions for drug addiction that form the framework for more recent work. They then explicitly outline what advances researchers have made on interventions for drug addiction since the publication of their chapter in the first edition of the handbook. Baker, LeBlanc, MacNeill, and Raetz address the topic of behavioral gerontology in Chapter 30. These authors believe that behavior analysts will conduct research that is more valuable to the aging community at large if they use the non-behavior-analytic literature to inform their research. The authors review recent advances in behavior-analytic assessment and assessment-informed interventions for older persons, and describe how these assessments and interventions can have a positive social impact. Wacker, Schieltz, Suess, and Lindgren describe the telehealth services they have delivered at the University of Iowa since the 1990s in Chapter 31. These pioneers in the area of telehealth service delivery describe the ways in which other disciplines have used telehealth and describe a service delivery model for applied behavior analysts.

The chapters in Part VII up to this point focus on interventions for individual recipients. Wilder and Gravina, by contrast, discuss the application of behavior-analytic principles to groups and organizations in Chapter 32. They define *organizational behavior management,* describe the differences between organizational behavior management and industrial–organizational psychology, provide the reader with a history of the field, and explain how behavior analysts can apply the principles of their field to groups and organizations.

In sum, Part VII of the handbook showcases the depth and breadth of behavior analysis and the significant contributions behavior analysts can make to many socially important issues.

# CHAPTER 23

# Behavioral Treatment of Autism Spectrum Disorder

Tiffany Kodak, Laura L. Grow, and Samantha C. J. Bergmann

Autism spectrum disorder (ASD) is a neurodevelopmental disorder that is evident in early childhood. Standard classification systems previously included ASD in a category of related diagnoses, including autistic disorder, Asperger's disorder, Rett's disorder, childhood disintegrative disorder, and pervasive developmental disorder not otherwise specified. Currently, clinicians base the diagnosis of ASD on diagnostic criteria established by the *Diagnostic and Statistical Manual of Mental Disorders*, fifth edition (DSM-5; American Psychiatric Association, 2013). DSM-5 no longer includes differential diagnoses such as Asperger's disorder or pervasive developmental disorder not otherwise specified. Clinicians diagnose individuals with ASD if they meet the revised diagnostic criteria described below.

Individuals diagnosed with ASD demonstrate two core areas of impairment (American Psychiatric Association, 2013). First, these individuals display persistent impairment in reciprocal social communication and social interaction that may cause difficulties in social and emotional reciprocity, reduced affect, and unresponsiveness to social interactions. Deficits in social communication include odd and repetitive speech patterns and markedly delayed speech and language skills, and may include a complete lack of spoken language.

Individuals with ASD may also have difficulties with eye contact, relationships with peers, and play skills. The second core area of impairment consists of marked abnormalities in behavior patterns, characterized by restricted, repetitive, or stereotyped interests or activities. Children with ASD may engage in repetitive behavior, such as repeatedly placing items in lines and stereotyped body movements, such as rocking and hand flapping. They may display restricted activities, such as consuming only certain foods (e.g., chicken nuggets, chips); engaging in problem behavior if activities do not occur in a particular order; or resisting changes in the environment, such as having a tantrum if a driver takes a different route to school. Individuals with ASD may also display hyper- or hyporeactivity to sensory stimulation (e.g., plugging ears in the presence of loud sounds, increased pain tolerance). Clinicians can specify ASD severity at three levels (Level 1, *Requiring support*; Level 2, *Requiring substantial support*; or Level 3, *Requiring very substantial support*), based on the degree of impairment in social communication and interaction and the severity of restricted, repetitive behaviors (American Psychiatric Association, 2013).

Over the past 30 years, the prevalence of ASD has increased. Recent prevalence estimates indicate that ASD occurs in 1 in 54 children (Centers for Disease Control and Prevention, 2020). This prevalence estimate is much higher than estimates obtained in the 1980s and early 2000s (Burd, Fisher, & Kerbeshian, 1987; Centers for Disease Control and Prevention, 2020). Several factors may influence the apparent increasing trends in ASD diagnoses, including heightened awareness of the disorder's characteristics, better assessment tools, early diagnosis, expansion of diagnostic criteria to include cases that were subthreshold according to DSM-IV-TR criteria (American Psychiatric Association, 2000, 2013), confusion regarding measures of prevalence versus incidence, and issues about the design of studies evaluating the prevalence of ASD (Hill, Zuckerman, & Fombonne, 2015; Volkmar, Lord, Bailey, Schultz, & Klin, 2004). Because of these problems, we do not know whether the apparent growth in ASD prevalence reflects an actual increase in the proportion of children affected by the disorder.

## ASSOCIATED FEATURES OF ASD

Several medical conditions and behavioral excesses or deficits correlate with a diagnosis of ASD (American Psychiatric Association, 2013). Although certain characteristics or conditions may be more common in individuals with ASD, the associated features are not part of ASD diagnostic criteria. The features we review below include sleeping and feeding disorders, delays in toilet training, severe behavior problems, and genetic and medical conditions (Zwaigenbaum et al., 2015).

### Sleep Problems

Individuals with ASD display a higher incidence of sleep problems, including increased daytime sleep (Piazza, Fisher, Kieswetter, Bowman, & Moser, 1990) and decreased total sleep, bedtime tantrums, and frequent night wakings (Kodak & Piazza, 2008). Sleep problems can cause decreased cognitive functioning, increased levels of self-injurious behavior and other severe problem behavior, and increased levels of parental stress (Kodak & Piazza, 2008; McStay, Dissanayake, Scheeren, Koot, & Begeer, 2014). As a result, many individuals with ASD would benefit from treatment for sleep problems, given the negative impact these problems can have on both the children and their caregivers. A description of behaviorally based treatments for sleep problems is outside the scope

of this chapter. Refer to Kodak and Piazza (2008) for a detailed description of treatments that researchers have used to treat the sleep problems of individuals with ASD and other developmental disabilities.

### Feeding Disorders

The prevalence of feeding disorders is substantially higher in individuals diagnosed with ASD than in typically developing children, and up to 90% of children with ASD display at least some inappropriate mealtime behavior (DeMeyer, 1979; Sharp et al., 2013). Food selectivity is one type of feeding problem that is common in individuals with ASD, perhaps due to the rigid and restricted interests characteristic of this population (Schreck, Williams, & Smith, 2004). Children who display food selectivity may consume enough food to meet their overall caloric needs, but they may not meet their daily nutritional needs because of limited consumption of foods high in macro- and micronutrients (Piazza, 2008). Treatments based on the principles of applied behavior analysis (ABA) have been highly effective in increasing the variety of foods consumed and in decreasing inappropriate mealtime behavior in individuals with food selectivity. For a description of effective behavioral interventions for children with feeding disorders, refer to Kodak and Piazza (2008), Volkert and Piazza (2012), and two recent randomized clinical trials by Piazza and colleagues (Peterson, Piazza, Ibanez, & Fisher, 2019; Peterson, Piazza, & Volkert, 2016).

### Delayed Toilet Training

Many individuals with developmental disabilities do not complete toilet training successfully before the age of 6. In fact, over half of parents of children with ASD report concerns regarding toilet training and incontinence (Williams, Oliver, Allard, & Sears, 2003). Azrin and Foxx (1971) developed an intensive behavioral treatment package for toilet training for adults with developmental disabilities; it includes reinforcement for voids on the toilet, fluid loading, scheduled toilet trips, and overcorrection. Numerous studies have evaluated variations of this treatment package with individuals with ASD and other developmental disabilities (e.g., LeBlanc, Carr, Crossett, Bennett, & Detweiler, 2005).

Despite the effectiveness of the procedures developed by Azrin and Foxx (1971) 50 years ago, researchers have raised concerns regarding the appropriateness of using punishment procedures in toileting treatments (Cicero & Pfadt, 2002). As a result, researchers have developed novel treatments that include antecedent manipulations and reinforcement-based procedures to increase the frequency of continent voids (e.g., Hagopian, Fisher, Piazza, & Wierzbicki, 1993) and stools (Piazza, Fisher, Chinn, & Bowman, 1991). Hagopian et al. (1993) used a water-prompting procedure to increase urinary continence in a young male with intellectual developmental disorder. Results indicated that the water-prompting procedure increased continent voids, while maintaining low levels of self-injurious behavior that had occurred during other toileting treatments.

Many toilet-training treatment packages include multiple components, such as scheduled sits and wearing underwear. Greer, Neidert, and Dozier (2015) conducted toilet training with 20 children ages 19–39 months, including one child diagnosed with ASD. The researchers implemented a toilet-training package that included a dense schedule of toilet sits, wearing underwear, and differential reinforcement for remaining dry with 6 of the 20 children, including the child with ASD. Two of these children, including the child with ASD, showed improved toileting with the package. The remaining 14 children participated in a component analysis and began toilet training with either the dense schedule of toilet sits, underwear, or differential reinforcement; researchers subsequently added components if accidents did not decrease. Wearing underwear improved urinating on the toilet for two of the four participants. Neither the dense schedule of toilet sits nor differential reinforcement for remaining dry improved urinating on the toilet for any participant. Overall, results indicated that replacing diapers or pull-ups with underwear improved toileting behavior, but we need additional research to identify components that might strengthen this effect.

Future research might focus on comparing the relative effectiveness of different approaches to toilet training and measuring potential side effects or issues that arise with each intervention. For example, overcorrection or frequent scheduled sits may evoke problem behavior, and a water prompt may be difficult to fade.

## Severe Problem Behavior

Individuals with ASD are more likely to engage in severe problem behavior, including self-injurious,

aggressive, and disruptive behavior; noncompliance; elopement; and pica (American Psychiatric Association, 2000). Researchers have used functional-analysis procedures to identify the environmental variables that maintain the problem behavior of individuals with developmental disabilities (e.g., Iwata, Dorsey, Slifer, Bauman, & Richman, 1982/1994). Researchers then use the results of these procedures to inform treatment. Although the assessment and treatment of severe problem behavior is critical to intervention programs for many individuals with ASD, other chapters in this book review functional analysis and treatment of problem behavior. Saini, Fisher, Betz, and Piazza (Chapter 13) describe experimental functional analysis; Vollmer, Athens, and Fernand (Chapter 19) describe function-based extinction treatments; Fisher, Greer, and Bouxsein (Chapter 20) describe function-based reinforcement treatments; and Lerman and Toole (Chapter 21) describe function-based punishment treatments.

## Associated Conditions and Genetic Disorders

Individuals with ASD may have some level of intellectual impairment, although the proportion of individuals with comorbid intellectual impairment varies across studies, with estimates ranging from 18% (Levy et al., 2010) to 70% (Matson & Shoemaker, 2009). In addition, several medical conditions and genetic syndromes are more common in individuals with ASD. Approximately 16% of individuals with ASD are diagnosed with epilepsy (Levy et al., 2010), with the onset of seizures occurring during childhood or adolescence (Rutter, 1970). Genetic disorders, including tuberous sclerosis and fragile X syndrome, are also associated with ASD. Refer to Volkmar et al. (2004) for more information on the relation between these genetic disorders and ASD.

## EARLY INTENSIVE BEHAVIORAL INTERVENTION

Early intensive behavioral intervention (EIBI) is a comprehensive treatment approach for children with ASD (Roane, Fisher, & Carr, 2016). It includes a comprehensive, hierarchically arranged curriculum implemented for several years, with the goal of improving a child's overall functioning (Smith, 1999). Behavior analysts develop procedures for EIBI programs based on principles of operant conditioning, such as reinforcement, stimulus control, and generalization, to increase adaptive behavior and reduce problem behavior. The EIBI therapist provides numerous learning opportunities to the child, using carefully programmed instructional and reinforcement procedures. The program targets multiple areas of functioning in a developmental sequence to improve several broad skill areas. Educational targets for EIBI programming often include preacademic and academic skills, verbal behavior, social skills, and independent-play skills. Typically, EIBI programs last 25–40 hours per week for 2–3 years and include individualized instruction in many settings, such as the home, community, and school (National Autism Center, 2009, 2015). Results of surveys of caregivers and service providers show that EIBI is one of the most common and requested treatments for children with ASD (Green et al., 2006; Stahmer, Collings, & Palinkas, 2005).

The University of California at Los Angeles (UCLA) Young Autism Project is a landmark outcome study that documented substantial improvements in approximately 47% of children with ASD receiving EIBI (Lovaas, 1987), and those gains in functioning were maintained through adolescence (McEachin, Smith, & Lovaas, 1993). The success of initial studies on EIBI led to additional research and widespread dissemination. EIBI is the most studied comprehensive treatment model for young children with ASD (Reichow, 2012). To date, research has compared (1) different intensities of EIBI (e.g., Smith, Eikeseth, Klevstrand, & Lovaas, 1997), (2) EIBI and other treatments (e.g., Eikeseth, Smith, Jahr, & Eldevik, 2002; Howard, Sparkman, Cohen, Green, & Stanislaw, 2005), and (3) clinic- versus caregiver-managed models (e.g., Sallows & Graupner, 2005; Smith, Groen, & Wynn, 2000).

Researchers have established criteria to review the empirical support for EIBI in experimental studies (e.g., Horner et al., 2005; Reichow, Volkmar, & Cicchetti, 2008; Reichow & Wolery, 2009). Although specific criteria differ somewhat, the criteria for experimental rigor, verification of diagnosis, and measures of procedural integrity have overlapped considerably. Meta-analyses conducted with various criteria have sought to identify variables that predict the outcome of behavioral interventions with young children with ASD. Overall, research on the relation between a child's IQ at the start of treatment and whether the child benefits from EIBI has produced mixed or negligible results (Reichow, 2012). Characteristics of EIBI programs that produce better outcomes, such as higher IQ scores, improved adaptive behavior, and increased

language skills, include greater treatment intensity (Makrygianni & Reed, 2010; Virues-Ortega, 2010), longer treatment duration (Makrygianni & Reed, 2010; Virues-Ortega, 2010), inclusion of caregiver training (Makrygianni & Reed, 2010), and supervisor training with the UCLA model (Reichow & Wolery, 2009).

Results of meta-analyses and systematic reviews have produced strong consensus that EIBI is an effective treatment for many behavioral deficits and excesses of ASD (Reichow & Wolery, 2009). The National Standards Project identified EIBI, which it called *comprehensive behavioral treatment for young children*, as an established intervention for children with ASD (National Autism Center, 2009, 2015). An established intervention has sufficient available evidence to permit investigators to determine *confidently* that the intervention produces positive outcomes for individuals with ASD (National Autism Center, 2015, p. 34). EIBI has the most empirical support of all comprehensive treatment models for children with ASD (Reichow, 2012).

## ABA-Based Models of Early Intervention

Researchers have developed several intervention models based on ABA principles to improve outcomes for children with ASD. The models described below have demonstrated effectiveness in studies published in peer-reviewed journals, and their authors have published commercially available treatment manuals. We review each model in detail and describe key differences between the models. Finally, we provide recommendations for integrating the models to maximize learning.

### Natural Environment Training

The essential features of *natural environment training* are the emphasis on child-directed interactions, techniques that increase motivation to respond, and generalization of skills. Behavior analysts typically conduct natural environment training—also called *natural language approaches* (LeBlanc, Esch, Sidener, & Firth, 2006) and *naturalistic-teaching strategies* (National Autism Center, 2015)—in natural settings such as the home, with an emphasis on training caregivers to promote learning opportunities during playtime. This model capitalizes on naturally occurring establishing operations to teach functional-language skills, although the literature on the model does not describe establishing operations as a component. Natural environment training incorporates choice-making opportunities, frequent preference assessments, and reinforcer variation across trials to increase the likelihood of occasioning vocalizations. Natural environment training intersperses mastered tasks to maintain a child's motivation to respond. The behavior analyst programs training in free-play-like settings, to decrease the similarity between the training setting and typical academic or work settings. Natural environment training typically targets requests for items in the initial portion of treatment to establish a functional relation between the vocal response (e.g., *dinosaur*) and associated reinforcers (e.g., brief access to a toy dinosaur).

Natural environment training uses recommendations from Stokes and Baer (1977) to train and promote generalization. Thus the approach emphasizes training multiple exemplars, training across settings and therapists, and use of intermittent contingencies to promote generalization of language (LeBlanc et al., 2006). After the child demonstrates an established verbal repertoire, the behavior analyst programs intermittent contingencies that more closely approximate the contingencies in natural settings (e.g., school). The child is more likely to use his or her newly acquired language in many settings, due to natural environment training's emphasis on generalization of language skills across settings and therapists. Natural environment training includes several teaching strategies, such as the natural language paradigm and pivotal-response training.

## Incidental Teaching

Hart and Risley (1968) developed *incidental-teaching* strategies from their experiences teaching language to preschool children in natural settings. The therapist conducts incidental-teaching strategies in unstructured settings such as free-play time in a classroom. Incidental teaching is child-directed, and a therapist uses a child's initiation as a learning opportunity. The goal is to teach the child to respond to multiple cues in the natural environment with spontaneous language.

Incidental-teaching programs incorporate discriminative stimuli that signal the availability of adult attention for language attempts (Hart & Risley, 1975). This discrimination is important, because the child's attempts to communicate are unlikely to produce reinforcement unless an adult is attending to the child's vocalizations. The therapist initiates a learning trial when the child shows interest in an item by pointing or gesturing to it. The therapist physically approaches the child, engages in eye contact, and exhibits a questioning look (Hart & Risley, 1975). If the child does not emit a spontaneous vocalization, the therapist provides a prompt. For example, if the child does not say, "Toy, please," after looking at a toy on the shelf, the therapist delivers the prompt "Say 'Toy, please.'" The therapist then fades prompts as the child responds accurately after less intrusive prompts. Hart and Risley (1975) recommend rotating among a few prompts that are context-specific, such as "What is this?" or "What do you want?" Limiting prompt variety ensures that the prompt functions as a discriminative stimulus for the correct vocal response. For example, the prompt "What is this?" requires the child to provide a label for the indicated stimulus, and the prompt "What do you want?" requires the child to provide a label for the stimulus that is of interest to the child (Hart & Risley, 1975). Limited prompt variation is one variable that distinguishes incidental teaching from other natural environment training procedures.

Previous research showed that incidental teaching with disadvantaged preschool children was effective in producing variability in verbal responses, generalization to novel therapists (Hart & Risley, 1975), and preference for play activities that incorporated incidental teaching (Hart & Risley, 1968). Research on incidental teaching with children with ASD indicated that training produced generalization of language (e.g., McGee, Krantz, Mason, & McClannahan, 1983).

McGee, Krantz, and McClannahan (1985) compared incidental-teaching and traditional-teaching procedures (e.g., teaching at a desk in a private room with minimal distractions). They employed both strategies to train children to use prepositions, and results indicated that acquisition of target prepositions did not vary across teaching procedures. Incidental-teaching sessions were longer than traditional-teaching sessions, but incidental teaching produced more correct preposition use during generalization sessions than traditional teaching. This study highlights the need for additional research comparing teaching strategies to identify procedures that produce (1) rapid acquisition, (2) higher levels of attending, (3) generalization of skills across settings and therapists, and (4) the least amount of instructional time necessary to produce mastery of target skills. Future research also should identify child preferences for language-training strategies, such as those conducted with other behavioral interventions (Hanley, Piazza, Fisher, Contrucci, & Maglieri, 1997; Hanley, Piazza, Fisher, & Maglieri, 2005; Schmidt, Hanley, & Layer, 2009).

Incidental teaching includes only one learning trial per teaching episode, which is a major limitation. Prolonged intertrial intervals may occur, depending on the latency to the child's initiation of the next trial. Charlop-Christy and Carpenter (2000) developed a revised teaching procedure called *multiple incidental-teaching sessions* to address this limitation. The procedure is like incidental teaching, but includes multiple learning or practice trials after the child initiates an interaction. The therapist presents two practice trials after the first child-initiated trial, to provide additional learning opportunities to the child. In this regard, multiple incidental-teaching sessions combine incidental-teaching and discrete-trial-training procedures. Research on multiple incidental-teaching sessions is limited; thus we need additional studies on its effectiveness and efficiency.

## Natural Language Paradigm

Koegel, O'Dell, and Koegel (1987) developed the *natural language paradigm* as a combination of language training and play, to make learning fun for a child and therapist. Training begins with the therapist providing the child with choices between high-preference stimuli. A learning opportunity begins when the child selects a preferred item (e.g., a toy lion). The therapist restricts access to the preferred item and models a short phrase (e.g., "Lion roars"), while concomitantly modeling an appropriate motor activity (e.g., opening the lion's mouth). The therapist uses shaping to reinforce closer approximations to the target vocalization across trials. Thus the therapist initially provides reinforcement for attempts to echo the therapist's model—for example, if the child makes the sound "Rrrr" after the therapist says, "Lion roars." The therapist provides brief access to the preferred item (e.g., 3–5 seconds) after a correct response, and pairs social reinforcement (e.g., praise) with play opportunities. The therapist typically repeats the target vocalization multiple times during the reinforcement interval. For example, the therapist says, "Lion roars," several times while the child plays with the lion. After the brief reinforcement interval, the therapist restricts access to the item and models a different phrase (e.g., "Yellow lion"). If the child does not emit a vocalization after two models of the target response, the therapist removes the item and provides the child with choic-

es between high-preference stimuli (Charlop-Christy & Kelso, 1997). The goal of reinforcement variation is to prevent satiation and to maintain the child's motivation to respond during learning trials.

Therapists often use a graduated prompt-delay procedure to promote spontaneous language (Walker, 2008). The therapist inserts a pause between discriminative-stimulus presentation (e.g., the toy lion) and the therapist's model (e.g., "Lion roars"). The therapist increases the length of the pause as the child's language skills improve. Spontaneous language should emerge as the child emits appropriate vocalizations before the therapist's delayed model. The graduated prompt-delay procedure aids the transfer of stimulus control from the therapist's model to the appropriate antecedent stimuli (Walker, 2008).

Natural language paradigm training involves repeated turn taking with toys between the therapist and child in a setting that approximates play conditions in the natural environment. Training also facilitates generalization by targeting multiple responses across different stimulus exemplars in novel play settings. For example, the therapist may model, "Lion roars," with the lion, but may say, "Bear roars," with a bear. Furthermore, the therapist provides many descriptors for each stimulus, so the child learns multiple vocal responses for one toy. Variations in modeled responses may decrease the likelihood that the child engages in repetitive vocalizations with items (e.g., always saying, "Yellow lion," when the child sees a toy lion).

Research on the natural language paradigm shows that children rapidly acquire targeted language skills and generalize language across settings (Gianoumis, Seiverling, & Sturmey, 2012; Koegel et al., 1987; Laski, Charlop, & Schreibman, 1988). However, several procedural variables warrant additional consideration. Shaping target responses may be difficult when multiple therapists implement the natural language paradigm at different times, because the paradigm does not delineate the criteria for identifying targets to reinforce and targets to extinguish. The natural language paradigm also does not have clear operational definitions for target behavior, and data collection may interrupt the flow of training. That is, the therapist may have difficulty collecting data on his or her modeled response and the child's response without substantially disrupting the flow of the play-like session.

Laski et al. (1988) and Gillett and LeBlanc (2007) trained caregivers to implement the natural language paradigm with their children, and results indicated that the participants' vocalizations increased. Gillett and LeBlanc also found that vocalizations that were prompted in the beginning of the study became spontaneous after intervention. Similarly, Spector and Charlop (2018) trained siblings of children with ASD to accurately implement the natural language paradigm, and two of the three children with ASD showed improved speech. Thus children may benefit from the natural language paradigm, despite its limitations. However, we need more research on the efficacy of this paradigm with children who require extensive shaping to acquire vocal verbal behavior or receive intervention to improve play skills.

### Pivotal-Response Training

Another natural environment training strategy is called *pivotal-response training* because it focuses on *pivotal areas,* which are skills that produce collateral improvement in other skill areas. Intervention typically occurs in natural settings such as the child's home. Most intervention opportunities capitalize on naturally occurring environmental stimuli and establishing operations. For example, if a child approaches a swing set, sits on the swing, and waits for an adult to push him or her, the adult models a vocalization (e.g., "Swing") and pushes the swing when the child imitates the modeled response. Thereafter, the adult may momentarily stop the swing by holding it in the air, give an expectant look, and provide an independent opportunity for the child to say, "Swing." If the child emits a relevant vocalization, the adult continues pushing the child on the swing.

Caregivers and teachers implement pivotal-response training across many settings. Research shows that caregivers, teachers, and other school personnel can implement pivotal-response training with high integrity after training via a video-training package, ongoing feedback, and a self-directed learning model (Nefdt, Koegel, Singer, & Gerber, 2010; Robinson, 2011; Schreibman & Koegel, 2005). Although studies show that researchers have trained caregivers and educators to implement pivotal-response training successfully, we need more research to identify efficacious and cost-effective training strategies.

### Applied-Verbal Behavior

The applied-verbal behavior approach to early intervention for ASD is based on Skinner's (1957) functional approach to verbal behavior. Skinner's functional approach defines a verbal operant on the basis of its topographical characteristics (e.g., a child saying, "Red"), antecedent events that occasion or evoke the response (e.g., a parent pointing to a picture of a red ball), and the consequent events that reinforce the response (e.g., a parent saying, "Good job, the ball is red.").

Skinner's (1957) taxonomy of verbal behavior includes seven elementary verbal operants, and early intervention programs typically focus on five of these: *mand, tact, echoic, intraverbal,* and *autoclitic.* Treatment typically begins with mand training, because this verbal operant has the most direct benefit to the speaker (Skinner, 1957). A *mand* is a verbal operant (e.g., "Drink, please") that a relevant establishing operation evokes (e.g., walking outside on a hot day) and delivery of the requested consequence reinforces (e.g., giving the child a drink). Behavior analysts should conduct mand training by using the appropriate antecedent and consequent events; that is, mand training tends to be most effective when the relevant establishing operations are present or presumed to be present, and the consequence related to the child's mand is available following an appropriate response.

Therapists using an applied-verbal behavior approach are also concerned with stimulus control. Mands should occur in the presence of the relevant establishing operations and discriminative stimuli (e.g., a listener who typically responds to the child's vocalization). However, these therapists often include antecedent prompts that are components of other verbal operants early in training. For example, an applied-verbal behavior therapist may include an intraverbal prompt (e.g., "What do you want?) or an echoic prompt (e.g., "Drink"), to increase the likelihood that the child will emit the target response (e.g., the child saying, "Drink") and that the target response will contact the relevant reinforcer (e.g., delivery of the drink). Over time, the therapist quickly fades these prompts to establish a *pure* verbal operant.

Once the child acquires multiple mands, the therapist combines antecedents that control trained verbal operants with other antecedents to teach additional functions of language (e.g., combined mand–tact training). The therapist programs these antecedents into learning opportunities to produce the target response, and uses fading to transfer control of the verbal response from one set of stimulus conditions to another. Numerous studies have shown that therapists can transfer stimulus control from one verbal operant (e.g., a tact) to another (e.g., an intraverbal) during training (e.g., Miguel, Petursdottir, & Carr,

2005). In addition, Skinner (1957) described most vocal verbal behavior as impure or under multiple sources of control. Thus studies that evaluate ways to promote the emergence of untrained operants following intervention, or that develop verbal behavior under multiple sources of control, should guide treatment practices in verbal behavior (e.g., Finn, Miguel, & Ahearn, 2012; Michael, Palmer, & Sundberg, 2011).

Skinner's (1957) account of verbal behavior has improved communication-training procedures by placing an emphasis on initial mand training and highlighting the need for intraverbal training (Sundberg & Michael, 2001). Prior approaches to communication training focused primarily on tact training and largely neglected intraverbal-behavior training. That is, researchers taught individuals with ASD to tact most items in their environment, but the children could not converse with others. This limited training procedure did not teach the skills necessary for individuals with ASD to function in typical settings or to establish peer relationships. As such, Skinner's conceptualization and the inclusion of mand and intraverbal training have advanced the quality of treatment provided to children in communication-training programs (Sundberg & Michael, 2001).

### Discrete-Trial Training

Lovaas and colleagues developed discrete-trial training in the early 1970s as a behavioral intervention for children with ASD (Lovaas, Koegel, Simmons, & Long, 1973). This model emphasizes a highly structured approach to teaching, in which the child and therapist sit at a table, and the therapist trains various skills during discrete-learning trials with brief intervals between trials. The therapist breaks the skills into components and teaches those components until the child masters them. The therapist subsequently teaches the child to combine components into larger behavior sequences. The therapist delivers highly preferred items (usually small edible items) and praise to the child following correct responses. Sessions, sometimes referred to as *drills*, consist of a specific number of trials that may involve presenting the same discriminative stimulus in a massed-trial format (e.g., repeatedly presenting trials of "Touch dog" throughout a session).

Early studies evaluating discrete-trial training for young children with ASD reported substantial increases in IQ scores, decreases in inappropriate behavior (e.g., self-stimulatory and problem behavior), and increases in spontaneous social interactions (Lovaas, 1987; Lovaas et al., 1973). Discrete-trial training often produces rapid skill acquisition, because it allows fast-paced instruction to maximize the number of learning opportunities in a brief period.

Discrete-trial training has several additional advantages relative to other early-intervention models. First, it involves well-defined and straightforward training procedures, which are easy to teach to inexperienced staff members. Second, discrete-trial training may be well suited for teaching certain verbal operants (e.g., tacts, echoics), because it is like the format of typical classroom instruction (e.g., sitting at a desk and answering questions) than other intervention models. Finally, data collection during learning trials may be easier with this approach than with other models (Sundberg & Partington, 1999).

### Unique Features of Early-Intervention Models

Many behaviorally based early-intervention models have different language-training approaches, teaching methods, and terminology. Natural environment training and applied-verbal behavior both emphasize naturalistic-training procedures that focus on teaching requests (natural environment training) or mands (applied-verbal behavior) under conditions in which a child is motivated to obtain the requested item. The procedures maximize the effects of the relevant establishing operations by conducting frequent preference assessments, restricting access to the items outside of teaching trials, or both. Skills taught in discrete-trial training vary from those of natural environment training and applied-verbal behavior, because discrete trials incorporate specific, verbal discriminative stimuli (e.g., "What is it?") instead of programming trials to bring responding under antecedent control (Skinner, 1957). Discrete-trial training may produce correct responding on each trial, but extensive training may be necessary to generalize these skills to other, less structured settings. Thus proponents of natural environment training and applied-verbal behavior have stated that discrete-trial training may not promote skill generalization as much as other early-intervention models do (Sundberg & Michael, 2001).

Each model uses different terminology. Natural environment training and discrete-trial training make a distinction between teaching receptive and expressive language. Teaching *receptive* language typically refers to training auditory–visual conditional discriminations (e.g., teaching a child point to a picture following the presentation of an auditory stimulus). Proponents of applied-verbal behavior refer to this type of training as *teaching listener behavior.* Teaching *expressive* language typically refers to teaching children to tact an item in the presence of a nonverbal stimulus (e.g., a picture) and a verbal stimulus (e.g., "What is it?"). The distinction between receptive and expressive language is consistent with a structural approach to language development (Leaf & McEachin, 1999; Maurice, Green, & Luce, 1996; see Petursdottir & Carr, 2011 for a review). Alternatively, applied-verbal behavior therapists approach communication training from a functional perspective and consider the antecedent and consequent events for verbal behavior during teaching (Lerman et al., 2005).

The intervention setting also varies substantially, particularly early in training. Natural environment training and applied-verbal behavior language training occurs in natural settings and focuses on establishing mand repertoires. This teaching occurs during free-play time, such as the loosely structured activities in preschool classrooms. In discrete-trial training, by contrast, a child is not trained in the natural environment until the child masters several prerequisite skills during one-on-one seatwork (e.g., attending, compliance). That is, discrete-trial training teaches verbal operants (typically tacts and echoics) during one-on-one activities at a desk for the first year or two of treatment, followed by practice in other, less structured settings later in treatment (e.g., the second year of early intervention).

Differences in the language-training setting substantially alter the way each approach addresses motivational issues. Natural environment training describes motivation as a child's willingness to respond for preferred items. A therapist provides frequent choices between highly preferred items to encourage the child to participate in treatment. The applied-verbal behavior approach involves establishing operations that momentarily increase the effectiveness of a reinforcing stimulus and increase the likelihood of behavior that has produced the stimulus in the past. Thus the therapist programs naturally occurring establishing operations into mand training, such as conducting training after the child has not had access to several highly preferred items for a period (Kelley, Shillingsburg, Castro, Addison, & LaRue, 2007). Finally, discrete-trial training provides highly preferred items (e.g., food) following correct responses during each trial. Discrete-trial training places less emphasis on motivational variables, and a therapist typically does not conduct frequent preference assessments during trials. Instead, the therapist alternates several highly preferred food items across trials to decrease the likelihood of satiation.

## Combining Early-Intervention Models

Each approach to early intervention has unique strengths that therapists can use in an eclectic approach that includes several empirically validated, ABA-based interventions. For example, a therapist can use natural environment training to teach social skills, such as turn taking and sharing toys. The therapist can train the functions of verbal operants using the applied-verbal behavior approach in the natural environment, while the child acquires other skills (such as attending behavior and instruction following) during discrete-trial training. The therapist can capitalize on naturally occurring establishing operations by only using certain highly preferred items during language training and restricting them at other times. The therapist can implement tact training during discrete-trial training to increase the child's mean length of utterance in the context of the function of the vocalization (applied-verbal behavior). For example, training might focus on teaching tacts and corresponding autoclitic frames while constructing toys during learning trials (e.g., "That's a tail"; Finn et al., 2012).

The therapist can incorporate Skinner's (1957) taxonomy of verbal behavior to teach skills with natural environment training or discrete-trial training. For example, a therapist may teach *yes* and *no* as a mand–intraverbal operant with an applied-verbal behavior approach. The therapist can ask the child whether he or she wants to watch highly preferred videos on some trials or nonpreferred videos on other trials. The therapist can use discrete-trial training and program the relevant antecedents and consequences in the training context. Combining discrete-trial training with other early-intervention models capitalizes on the strengths of several models by incorporating naturally occurring establishing operations, and the learning trials are more child-driven because the therapist offers the child preferred or nonpreferred videos before each trial.

## CLINICAL CONSIDERATIONS AND FUTURE RESEARCH

### Establishing a Reinforcing Environment

In many cases, the identification of reinforcing stimuli is a critical factor in the success of behavior acquisition programs. Behavior analysts commonly conduct systematic preference assessments to identify a hierarchy of potentially reinforcing items or activities. Much research has focused on developing effective and efficient methods for assessing preferences for stimuli among individuals with developmental disabilities (see Saini, Retzlaff, et al., Chapter 10, this volume).

A preference assessment can provide opportunities for individuals to select the reinforcers for upcoming teaching sessions in an early-intervention program. Although behavioral experts recommend frequent, systematic preference assessments to control for potential fluctuations in preference for reinforcers over time, early-intervention programs vary widely in how often they assess preferences. A study by Love, Carr, Almason, and Petursdottir (2009) found that most early-intervention programs (i.e., 65%) assessed preference multiple times per day, whereas a few programs (i.e., 19%) conducted preference assessments quarterly or annually. Research indicates that frequent, brief preference assessments are more effective than less frequent, comprehensive assessments for identifying potential reinforcers (DeLeon et al., 2001). Despite research supporting the use of frequent preference assessments, some early-intervention programs may conduct preference assessments less often because of time or resource constraints. Researchers have responded to this clinical issue by developing brief preference assessments that are more time-efficient to implement in natural settings (e.g., Carr, Nicolson, & Higbee, 2000). In addition, researchers have developed self-instruction packages to assist staff members who do not have access to expert trainers to conduct preference assessments with children accurately (Graff & Karsten, 2012).

In conjunction with frequent preference assessments, clinicians can intersperse choice-making opportunities throughout educational programming to increase the reinforcing properties of instruction in general (Laski et al., 1988; Toussaint, Kodak, & Vladescu, 2016). Moreover, research suggests that individuals may prefer instructional contexts that incorporate opportunities to make choices among reinforcers to environments that provide identical reinforcers selected by a therapist (Tiger, Hanley, & Hernandez, 2006). There are multiple opportunities to integrate choices into a typical teaching session during early intervention (e.g., task and reinforcer selection). Previous research has demonstrated that providing choices between tasks may produce increased task engagement (Dunlap et al., 1994) and decreased problem behavior (Romaniuk et al., 2002). Choice between reinforcers also can lead to more efficient skill acquisition (Toussaint et al., 2016). Several reinforcement parameters, such as reinforcement rate, quality, immediacy, and magnitude, may influence an individual's choice and alter the efficacy of the reinforcing stimuli included in early-intervention learning trials. Future research should determine the extent to which choice variables influence the acquisition of new skills.

## Assessing and Identifying Target Skills

A behavior analyst should assess an individual's current skill level in several domains to select appropriate targets for intervention. Information from a formal assessment of skills allows the clinician to (1) measure several important behavioral repertoires, (2) identify areas that would benefit from intervention, and (3) track educational progress over time. Several formal assessment programs are commercially available to clinicians and researchers.

### Assessment of Basic Learning and Language Skills— Revised

The Assessment of Basic Learning and Language Skills—Revised (ABLLS-R) is a tool for identifying areas that require intervention for children with autism and other developmental disabilities (Partington, 2006). The ABLLS-R includes educational skills grouped into 25 areas (e.g., social skills, motor skills). Skinner's (1957) account of verbal behavior forms the basis for the language components of the ABLLS-R. The ABLLS-R has guidelines clinicians can use to develop goals for individualized education plans. The author of the ABLLS-R also co-wrote a book, *Teaching Language to Children with Autism or Other Developmental Disabilities* (Sundberg & Partington, 1998), as a companion treatment manual for many skills the ABLLS-R assesses. The ABLLS-R collects information (1) during interviews of caregivers and other individuals who are familiar with the child (e.g., teachers), (2) during naturalistic observations, and (3) in tests of specific skills.

### Verbal Behavior Milestones Assessment and Placement Program

The Verbal Behavior Milestones Assessment and Placement Program (VB-MAPP) assesses the current level of several language and related behaviors to identify educational target skills in individuals with ASD and other developmental disabilities (Sundberg, 2008). The VB-MAPP includes three main sections: the Milestones Assessment, the Barriers Assessment, and the Transition Assessment. Like the ABLLS-R, the VB-MAPP includes information gathered by (1) interviewing caregivers and others who are familiar with the child, (2) collecting data during naturalistic observations, and (3) conducting tests of specific skills.

The Milestones Assessment evaluates the child's current behavioral repertoire along 16 dimensions of behavior (e.g., listener responding) arranged in a developmental sequence across three levels. The three levels measure skills that are typical for children between the ages of 0 and 18 months, 18 and 30 months, and 30 and 48 months, respectively. The Barriers Assessment assesses 24 language and learning barriers (e.g., prompt dependency) that may interfere with progress during educational programming. The behavior analyst should address barriers identified during this assessment before focusing on other objectives. The Transition Assessment gathers information on specific skills needed to make educational gains in less restrictive environments. The assessment has three main categories. Category 1 measures academic independence (e.g., group skills) and determines the level of support the child needs. Category 2 assesses learning patterns (e.g., rate of skill acquisition) and determines the child's readiness for acquiring skills outside of one-on-one instruction. Category 3 evaluates self-help skills (e.g., toileting skills), spontaneity (e.g., adaptability to change), and self-direction (e.g., independent play skills).

### Promoting the Emergence of Advanced Knowledge Relational Training System

The Promoting the Emergence of Advanced Knowledge (PEAK) Relational Training System is an assessment and curriculum tool that is based on the principles of ABA. It includes four modules, each of which contains 184 skills. The modules are divided by the author's conceptualization of distinct learning modalities, which include direct contingency learning in the Direct Training Module, generalization of skills to novel stimuli and learning contexts in the Generalization Module, the formation of stimulus equivalence classes in the Equivalence Module, and the transformation of relational frames to more complex derived re-

lational responses in the Transformation Module. The behavior analyst completes PEAK assessments for each module in either an indirect (survey) or direct (actual client interaction) modality. The behavior analyst assesses a skill directly if the caregiver does not know whether the child has mastered the skill. The equivalence and transformation modules also contain a preassessment of arbitrary-stimulus relations to evaluate whether a child can derive novel-stimulus relations after receiving information from the behavior analyst. The assessment duration can range from 1 to 4 hours, depending on the size and complexity of the child's verbal repertoire.

Following the assessment, the behavior analyst provides the therapists with goals and brief instructions on how to teach the deficit skills the assessment has identified. Most published research on PEAK has focused on the first module, the Direct Training Module. Researchers have reported correlations between the Direct Training Module and IQ, expressive and receptive language, and other behavioral assessments of language like the VB-MAPP (Dixon et al., 2014, 2015). A study of PEAK implementation showed that direct-care professionals with no history of ABA or discrete-trial training implemented PEAK with 60–80% accuracy after reviewing the manual. After one to four sessions of behavioral-skills training lasting 10–45 minutes, the same staff implemented PEAK with 100% accuracy (Belisle, Rowsey, & Dixon, 2016).

### Autism Curriculum Encyclopedia

Developed by professionals at the New England Center for Children, the Autism Curriculum Encyclopedia (ACE) is an educational software package of 2,000 skills (*www.acenecc.org*). The ACE includes three assessments: the Core Skills Assessment, the ACE Skills Assessment, and the Preference Assessment. The Core Skills Assessment measures 52 basic skills such as picture–object matching, requesting assistance, and following one-step directions. The ACE Skills Assessment identifies specific targets for individual learners, and it includes links to protocols that behavior analysts can use to teach targeted skills. Finally, the Preference Assessment includes 12 assessments, instructions and data sheets for each assessment, and a tool to assist practitioners in selecting an ideal assessment to conduct. The ACE includes procedures to track student progress and measure outcomes across years.

## Early-Intervention Curricular Manuals

Several early-intervention curricular manuals based on ABA principles are commercially available (e.g., Leaf & McEachin, 1999; Lovaas, 2003). Many of the recommendations and strategies in published curricula are rooted in the original treatment manual associated with the UCLA Young Autism Project, *Teaching Developmentally Disabled Children: The ME Book* (Lovaas, 1981), which used discrete-trial training as a primary instructional strategy (e.g., Leaf & McEachin, 1999). By contrast, the Sundberg and Partington (1998) manual references Skinner's (1957) analysis of verbal behavior as the conceptual framework for language training. Most early-intervention supervisors use more than one published manual when designing a curriculum for a given client, even though different manuals recommend different training methods (Love et al., 2009).

## Instructional Procedures

### Identifying Effective and Efficient Instructional Strategies

Developing the most effective, efficient teaching procedures for learners with ASD is an important and growing area of research. One way to improve a teaching program is to use assessments to identify strategies that produce the best outcomes for each learner. Whereas structured evaluations (e.g., the VB-MAPP and ABLLS-R) are available to assess a learner's current repertoire of skills and track progress over time, these assessments may not identify a specific intervention or the critical components of intervention to teach missing skills. Research suggests that learners respond idiosyncratically to different prompts, prompt-fading strategies, and error correction procedures (e.g., McGhan & Lerman, 2013; Seaver & Bourret, 2014). In such cases, the behavior analyst should base the selection of teaching strategies on the results of an assessment designed to match teaching procedures to the individual.

Researchers have evaluated several types of assessment-based instruction with individuals with ASD. Some assessments evaluate skills that may be components of more advanced skills (i.e., prerequisites; Kodak et al., 2015). Results of skills assessment could inform instructional programming to promote effective instruction. Other assessments identify particular instructional strategies to teach a specific skill. For example, McGhan and Lerman (2013) and Carroll, Joachim, St. Peter, and Rob-

inson (2015) designed and evaluated assessments to identify effective and efficient error correction procedures for learners with ASD and attention-deficit/hyperactivity disorder (ADHD). The results of both studies validated and demonstrated the clinical utility of these assessments to select error correction procedures. Similarly, Kodak, Clements, and LeBlanc (2013) evaluated a rapid assessment to identify which teaching strategies led to acquisition of auditory–visual conditional discriminations (e.g., receptive identification) with learners with ASD.

Initial studies examining assessment-based instruction have been positive; nevertheless, the generality of the assessment results across tasks or learner characteristics remain unclear. Although researchers have begun to address this topic (Bourret, Vollmer, & Rapp, 2004; Fisher, Kodak, & Moore, 2007; Kodak et al., 2015; Kodak, Fisher, Clements, Paden, & Dickes, 2011; Lerman, Vorndran, Addison, & Kuhn, 2004; Seaver & Bourret, 2014), we need more research on empirical methods for matching instructional strategies to learner characteristics. Future research should explore the utility of these assessment-based strategies as components of comprehensive EIBI programs.

### Identifying Effective Prompting Strategies

Behavior analysts frequently use response or stimulus prompts to increase the likelihood of a correct response. Evaluating and selecting effective prompts are best practices, and both require careful consideration of learner and task variables (Wolery & Gast, 1984). Before initiating an intervention, a behavior analyst should assess whether a learner has the relevant prerequisite skills for particular prompts to occasion correct responses. For example, model prompts are most appropriate for learners who display an imitation repertoire. In addition, prompts may be differentially effective, depending on the task (Lerman et al., 2004; McComas et al., 1996). For instance, a picture schedule may be more effective for activities such as making a snack, whereas a gestural prompt may better facilitate social initiations.

Research has sought to develop and evaluate assessments to identify effective prompting strategies, components of instruction, and consequences for individuals with ASD. For example, Seaver and Bourret (2014) developed an assessment that compared (1) prompts for individual learners, (2) prompt-fading strategies, and (3) the most and least effective prompts and fading strategies with a novel skill. These researchers found that effective prompts and prompt-fading strategies varied across individuals, but the assessment accurately identified ideal strategies for learners across tasks. Lerman et al. (2004) found differential efficacy of prompts across types of skills. For example, one participant required physical prompts to acquire auditory–visual conditional discriminations of numbers and completion of puzzles, but differential reinforcement without prompts was sufficient to produce acquisition of matching numbers. Future research should examine the generality of the results of assessment-based instruction across skills and types of prompts. In addition, future research might focus on identifying specific learner skills or deficits predictive of the relative efficacy of various stimulus and response prompts.

## Identifying Prompt-Fading Strategies

Behavior analysts typically incorporate response and stimulus prompts into instructional procedures during initial teaching sessions and fade the prompts as quickly as possible (i.e., prompt fading). The purpose of prompt fading is to transfer stimulus control from therapist-delivered prompts to stimuli in the natural environment that should evoke appropriate responses (Walker, 2008). Researchers have developed and evaluated multiple prompt-fading procedures (e.g., least-to-most prompting; Horner & Keilitz, 1975). Numerous studies have compared the relative effectiveness and efficiency of prompt-fading techniques (e.g., Seaver & Bourret, 2014). In general, research indicates that most prompt-fading procedures are effective for teaching many new skills (Ault, Wolery, Doyle, & Gast, 1989). However, the efficiency of the procedures varies; that is, the number of sessions required to teach new skills varies considerably across different prompting procedures. The specific skills of the learner or the task may affect the efficiency of the prompting procedures (Wolery & Gast, 1984). For example, within-stimulus fading may be ideal for learners who attend to irrelevant features of stimuli (i.e., faulty stimulus control), whereas an identity-matching prompt may be well suited for learners who have poor attending skills (Fisher et al., 2007). Another consideration is that of the training and effort required to implement various prompt-fading techniques. For example, within-stimulus fading requires extensive preparation and materials. Future research might evaluate how the learner's skill level, features of the task, and practical considerations (e.g., time and effort) influence the efficiency of various prompt-fading strategies.

## Maintenance and Generalization

A primary goal of early intervention is for a child to exhibit previously learned skills during direct instruction (i.e., maintenance of the skills over time) and engage in these skills in many settings and in novel situations (i.e., generalization of skills). Unfortunately, many early-intervention programs fail to program adequately for maintenance and generalization of skills (Smith, 1999). Furthermore, the educational gains achieved during intervention often do not generalize to other response topographies (e.g., learning to add the -*ing* ending to a novel word) or to response variations required in other settings (Charlop, Schreibman, & Thibodeau, 1985). As such, future research should evaluate variables that promote and interfere with maintenance and generalization of skills acquired through early intervention.

*Maintenance.* Maurice et al. (1996) recommend assessing maintenance once per week for 3–6 weeks to measure whether a child continues to exhibit the recently mastered skill. When data demonstrate that the child has maintained a target skill (e.g., correct responses during weekly maintenance probes), the child may continue to practice the skill at relevant times, but without additional data collection on the mastered skill.

Many early-intervention manuals recommend modifications to ongoing teaching procedures to increase the likelihood that children with ASD will show skill maintenance after training. For example, Lovaas (2003) recommended modifying both the schedule and the type of reinforcement provided for correct responses—procedures that can also promote generalization. In addition, when the behavior analyst uses arbitrary reinforcers (e.g., food) to train a new task, he or she should program naturally occurring reinforcers (e.g., praise, high fives) into treatment and maintenance, to ensure that behavior is not extinguished in the natural environment once the delivery arbitrary reinforcers ceases.

*Generalization.* Generalization occurs when a child displays skills acquired in one setting or with one person in other settings or with other people without direct training. Stokes and Baer (1977) described seven techniques to evaluate and promote generalization. The specific techniques most relevant to early intervention include training sufficient exemplars and using indiscriminable contingencies. Training sufficient exemplars involves (1) teaching multiple responses to the same stimulus, such as teaching multiple ways to deliver a compliment; and (2) teaching the child to engage in the correct response across many different, relevant stimuli, such as teaching the child to tact *dog* in the presence of different examples of dogs that share some features. Sometimes generalization can occur when the behavior analyst includes as few as two response exemplars, therapists, or settings during training (e.g., Stokes, Baer, & Jackson, 1974), but more exemplars are required at other times (e.g., Wunderlich, Vollmer, Donaldson, & Phillips, 2014). Future research should focus on determining the optimal conditions to achieve stimulus generalization.

Another behavioral technique that is highly relevant to training for generalization is the use of indiscriminable contingencies. When using indiscriminable contingencies, the behavior analyst typically provides reinforcement for appropriate behavior on an intermittent schedule (e.g., variable-interval 30 seconds). For example, Freeland and Noell (2002) evaluated whether completion of math problems was maintained when correct responding no longer produced reinforcement following a phase in which (1) each correct response produced reinforcement or (2) correct responding produced intermittent reinforcement. Results indicated that responding was maintained only following a phase of intermittent reinforcement. Although most behavior analysts typically thin the schedule of reinforcement after a child masters skills in early-intervention programs, few studies have evaluated the reinforcement schedule necessary to maintain skills in settings other than the training setting.

## Treatment Integrity

Many studies demonstrating the efficacy of early-intervention models involved rigorous experimental protocols in which highly trained clinicians served as therapists. However, most direct-service providers in practice have less education and experience than the therapists in the published research. Thus therapists in practice are unlikely to implement ABA interventions with the same integrity levels as those reported in the literature (e.g., Reed, Osborne, & Corness, 2007; Smith, Flanagan, Garon, & Bryson, 2015).

The impact of treatment integrity on the effectiveness of behavioral interventions has received increased attention in recent years (Fryling, Wallace, & Yassine, 2012). Carroll, Kodak, and Fisher (2013) conducted an initial study to identify the prevalence of treatment integrity failures when classroom teachers of children with ASD implemented discrete-trial training. The results showed that teachers and paraprofessionals made frequent errors during discrete-trial training: (1) only correcting approximately 40% of errors following incorrect responses; (2) not providing clear instructions during approximately 50% of teaching trials; and (3) not delivering reinforcement consistently (teachers delivered reinforcement for only about 20% of correct responses). Although the frequent occurrence of instructional errors during classroom-based discrete-trial training is a cause for concern, whether these errors negatively affected learning was unclear. Therefore, Carroll et al. (2013) conducted a second experiment to evaluate the impact of these common instructional errors on children's learning. The authors compared high-integrity instruction (in which the therapist made no errors) to low-integrity instruction (in which the therapist made errors during 67% of trials) and to a no-instruction control condition. The researchers based the low-integrity instruction percentage on the mean number of errors teachers and paraprofessionals made using discrete-trial training with children with ASD during classroom observations. The results showed that participants rapidly acquired skills in the high-integrity instruction condition, but did not acquire similar skills in the low-integrity instruction condition. In fact, most participants did not learn targeted skills during low-integrity instruction, despite three times the number of instructional sessions. Participants acquired the skills when the researchers used high-integrity instruction with those skills initially assigned to the low-integrity condition.

Similar studies evaluating decrements in treatment integrity found that errors occurring in 33–100% of trials affected learning (e.g., DiGennaro Reed, Reed, Baez, & Maguire, 2011; Jenkins, Hirst, & DiGennaro Reed, 2015; Noell, Gresham, & Gansle, 2002). However, whether these controlled studies that manipulated specific components of instruction represent the types and frequency of errors occurring during the implementation of ABA interventions in homes, schools, and clinics is unclear. Additional research should evaluate the minimum amount of treatment integrity necessary to produce positive treatment outcomes. Investigations like these can assist in developing guidelines for treatment integrity in practice.

## CONCLUSION

Early intervention based on the principles of ABA is a critical component of any comprehensive treatment for children diagnosed with ASD. Although several behavioral early-intervention strategies have produced impressive results with small groups of children with ASD, most outcome studies evaluating the large-scale implementation of early-intervention procedures have focused on the UCLA-based model (i.e., discrete-trial training; e.g., Smith et al., 2000). Thus researchers should conduct randomized controlled trials of other behavioral early-intervention models, such as natural environment training and applied-verbal behavior, to identify additional effective strategies. In addition, many practitioners combine various behaviorally based early-intervention models. Future research might examine the utility of combining the behavioral early-intervention approaches to take advantage of unique features of each model.

Despite an increase in early-intervention research in the past 40 years, we need considerably more research to delineate optimal teaching strategies for children with ASD. For example, we need research to evaluate the impact of learner and task variables on the effectiveness of particular intervention strategies. Future research might focus on developing systematic evaluations of potential variables that interact with the effectiveness of acquisition procedures. Information from an assessment of this type might lead to better identification of procedures that result in rapid skill acquisition. Improving our existing teaching technologies and developing new ones are likely to improve the outcomes for children with ASD treated with early intervention.

## REFERENCES

American Psychiatric Association. (2000). *Diagnostic and statistical manual of mental disorders* (4th ed., text rev.). Washington, DC: Author.

American Psychiatric Association. (2013). *Diagnostic and statistical manual of mental disorders* (5th ed.). Arlington, VA: Author.

Ault, M. J., Wolery, M., Doyle, P. M., & Gast, D. L. (1989). Review of comparative studies in the instruction of students with moderate and severe handicaps. *Exceptional Children, 55,* 346–356.

Azrin, N. H., & Foxx, R. M. (1971). A rapid method of toilet training the institutionalized retarded. *Journal of Applied Behavior Analysis, 4,* 89–99.

Belisle, J., Rowsey, K. E., & Dixon, M. R. (2016). The

use of *in situ* behavioral skills training to improve staff implementation of the peak relational training system. *Journal of Organizational Behavior Management, 36,* 71–79.

Bourret, J., Vollmer, T. R., & Rapp, J. T. (2004). Evaluation of a vocal mand assessment and vocal mand training procedures. *Journal of Applied Behavior Analysis, 37,* 129–144.

Burd, L., Fisher, W., & Kerbeshian, J. (1987). A prevalence study of pervasive developmental disorders in North Dakota. *Journal of the American Academy of Child and Adolescent Psychiatry, 26,* 700–703.

Carr, J. E., Nicolson, A. C., & Higbee, T. S. (2000). Evaluation of a brief multiple-stimulus preference assessment in a naturalistic context. *Journal of Applied Behavior Analysis, 33,* 352–357.

Carroll, R. A., Joachim, B. T., St. Peter, C. C., & Robinson, N. (2015). A comparison of error-correction procedures on skill acquisition during discrete-trial instruction. *Journal of Applied Behavior Analysis, 48*(2), 257–273.

Carroll, R. A., Kodak, T., & Fisher, W. W. (2013). An evaluation of programmed treatment-integrity errors during discrete-trial instruction. *Journal of Applied Behavior Analysis, 46,* 379–394.

Centers for Disease Control and Prevention. (2020, March 25). Data and statistics on autism spectrum disorder. Retrieved from *www.cdc.gov/ncbddd/autism/data.html*.

Charlop, M. H., Schreibman, L., & Thibodeau, M. G. (1985). Increasing spontaneous verbal responding in autistic children using a time delay procedure. *Journal of Applied Behavior Analysis, 18,* 155–166.

Charlop-Christy, M. H., & Carpenter, M. H. (2000). Modified incidental teaching sessions: A procedure for parents to increase spontaneous speech in their children with autism. *Journal of Positive Behavior Interventions, 2,* 98–112.

Charlop-Christy, M. H., & Kelso, S. E. (1997). *How to treat the child with autism: A guide to treatment at the Claremont Autism Center.* Claremont, CA: Claremont McKenna College.

Cicero, F. R., & Pfadt, A. (2002). Investigation of a reinforcement-based toilet training procedure for children with autism. *Research in Developmental Disabilities, 23,* 319–331.

DeLeon, I. G., Fisher, W. W., Rodriguez-Catter, V., Maglieri, K., Herman, K., & Marhefka, J. (2001). Examination of relative reinforcement of stimuli identified through pretreatment and daily brief preference assessments. *Journal of Applied Behavior Analysis, 34,* 463–473.

DeMeyer, M. K. (1979). *Parents and children in autism.* New York: Wiley.

DiGennaro Reed, F. D., Reed, D. D., Baez, C. N., & Maguire, H. (2011). A parametric analysis of errors of commission during discrete-trial training. *Journal of Applied Behavior Analysis, 44,* 611–615.

Dixon, M. R., Belisle, J., Stanley, C. R., Rowsey, K. E.,

Daar, J. H., & Szelkey, S. (2015). Toward a behavior analysis of complex language: Evaluating the relationship between PEAK and the VB-MAPP. *Journal of Developmental and Physical Disabilities, 27,* 223–233.

Dixon, M. R., Carman, J., Tyler, P. A., Whiting, S. W., Enoch, M., & Daar, J. H. (2014). Peak relational training system for children with autism and developmental disabilities: Correlation with Peabody Picture Vocabulary Test and assessment reliability. *Journal of Developmental and Physical Disabilities, 26,* 603–614.

Dunlap, G., dePerczel, M., Clarke, S., Wilson, D., White, R., & Gomez, A. (1994). Choice making to promote adaptive behavior for students with emotional and behavioral challenges. *Journal of Applied Behavior Analysis, 27,* 505–518.

Eikeseth, S., Smith, T., Jahr, E., & Eldevik, S. (2002). Intensive behavioral treatment at school for 4- to 7-year-old children with autism: A 1-year comparison controlled study. *Behavior Modification, 26,* 49–68.

Finn, H. E., Miguel, C. F., & Ahearn, W. H. (2012). The emergence of untrained mands and tacts in children with autism. *Journal of Applied Behavior Analysis, 45,* 265–280.

Fisher, W. W., Kodak, T., & Moore, J. W. (2007). Embedding an identity-matching task within a prompting hierarchy to facilitate acquisition of conditional discriminations in children with autism. *Journal of Applied Behavior Analysis, 40,* 489–499.

Freeland, J. T., & Noell, G. H. (2002). Programming for maintenance: An investigation of delayed intermittent reinforcement and common stimuli to create indiscriminable contingencies. *Journal of Behavioral Education, 11,* 5–18.

Fryling, M. J., Wallace, M. D., & Yassine, J. N. (2012). Impact of treatment integrity on intervention effectiveness. *Journal of Applied Behavior Analysis, 45,* 449–453.

Gianoumis, S., Seiverling, L., & Sturmey, P. (2012). The effects of behavior skills training on correct teacher implementation of natural language paradigm teaching skills and child behavior. *Behavioral Interventions, 27,* 57–74.

Gillett, J. N., & LeBlanc, L. A. (2007). Parent-implemented natural language paradigm to increase language and play in children with autism. *Research in Autism Spectrum Disorders, 1*(3), 247–255.

Graff, R. B., & Karsten, A. M. (2012). Evaluation of a self-instruction package for conducting stimulus preference assessments. *Journal of Applied Behavior Analysis, 45,* 69–82.

Green, V. A., Pituch, K. A., Itchon, J., Choi, A., O'Reilly, M., & Sigafoos, J. (2006). Internet survey of treatments used by parents of children with autism. *Research in Developmental Disabilities, 27,* 70–84.

Greer, B. D., Neidert, P. L., & Dozier, C. L. (2016). A component analysis of toilet-training procedures recommended for young children. *Journal of Applied Behavior Analysis, 49,* 69–84.

Hagopian, L. P., Fisher, W., Piazza, C. C., & Wierzbicki, J. J. (1993). A water-prompting procedure for the treatment of urinary incontinence. *Journal of Applied Behavior Analysis, 26,* 473–474.

Hanley, G. P., Piazza, C. C., Fisher, W. W., Contrucci, S. A., & Maglieri, K. A. (1997). Evaluation of client preference for function-based treatment packages. *Journal of Applied Behavior Analysis, 30,* 459–473.

Hanley, G. P., Piazza, C. C., Fisher, W. W., & Maglieri, K. A. (2005). On the effectiveness of and preference for punishment and extinction components of function-based interventions. *Journal of Applied Behavior Analysis, 38,* 51–65.

Hart, B. M., & Risley, T. R. (1968). Establishing use of descriptive adjectives in the spontaneous speech of disadvantaged preschool children. *Journal of Applied Behavior Analysis, 1,* 109–120.

Hart, B., & Risley, T. R. (1975). Incidental teaching of language in the preschool. *Journal of Applied Behavior Analysis, 8,* 411–420.

Hill, A. P., Zuckerman, K., & Fombonne, E. (2015). Epidemiology of autism spectrum disorders. In M. D. Robinson-Agramonte (Ed.), *Translational approaches to autism spectrum disorder* (pp. 13–38). Cham, Switzerland: Springer International.

Horner, R. D., & Keilitz, I. (1975). Training mentally retarded adolescents to brush their teeth. *Journal of Applied Behavior Analysis, 25,* 491–498.

Horner, R. H., Carr, E. G., Halle, J., McGee, G., Odom, S., & Wolery, M. (2005). The use of single-subject research to identify evidence-based practice in special education. *Exceptional Children, 71,* 165–179.

Howard, J. S., Sparkman, C. R., Cohen, H. G., Green, G., & Stanislaw, H. (2005). A comparison of intensive behavior analytic and eclectic treatments for young children with autism. *Research in Developmental Disabilities, 26,* 359–383.

Iwata, B. A., Dorsey, M. F., Slifer, K. J., Bauman, K. E., & Richman, G. S. (1994). Toward a functional analysis of self-injury. *Journal of Applied Behavior Analysis, 27,* 197–209. (Reprinted from *Analysis and Intervention in Developmental Disabilities, 2,* 3–20, 1982)

Jenkins, S. R., Hirst, J. M., & DiGennaro Reed, F. D. (2015). The effects of discrete-trial training commission errors on learner outcomes: An extension. *Journal of Behavioral Education, 24,* 196–209.

Kelley, M. E., Shillingsburg, M. A., Castro, M. J., Addison, L. R., & LaRue, R. H., Jr. (2007). Further evaluation of emerging speech in children with developmental disabilities: Training verbal behavior. *Journal of Applied Behavior Analysis, 40,* 431–445.

Kodak, T., Clements, A., & LeBlanc, B. (2013). A rapid assessment of instructional strategies to teach auditory-visual conditional discriminations to children with autism. *Research in Autism Spectrum Disorders, 7,* 801–807.

Kodak, T., Clements, A., Paden, A. R., LeBlanc, B., Mintz, J., & Toussaint, K. A. (2015). Examination of the relation between an assessment of skills and performance on auditory–visual conditional discriminations for children with autism spectrum disorder. *Journal of Applied Behavior Analysis, 48,* 52–70.

Kodak, T., Fisher, W. W., Clements, A., Paden, A. R., & Dickes, N. (2011). Functional assessment of instructional variables: Linking assessment and treatment. *Research in Autism Spectrum Disorders, 5,* 1059–1077.

Kodak, T., & Piazza, C. C. (2008). Assessment and behavioral treatment of feeding and sleeping disorders in children with autism spectrum disorders. *Child and Adolescent Psychiatric Clinics of North America, 17,* 887–905.

Koegel, R. L., O'Dell, M. C., & Koegel, L. K. (1987). A natural language paradigm for teaching non-verbal autistic children. *Journal of Autism and Developmental Disorders, 17,* 187–199.

Laski, K. E., Charlop, M. H., & Schreibman, L. (1988). Training parents to use the natural language paradigm to increase their autistic children's speech. *Journal of Applied Behavior Analysis, 21,* 391–400.

Leaf, R., & McEachin, J. (1999). *A work in progress: Behavior management strategies and a curriculum for intensive behavior treatment of autism.* New York: DRL Books.

LeBlanc, L. A., Carr, J. E., Crossett, S. E., Bennett, C. M., & Detweiler, D. D. (2005). Intensive outpatient behavioral treatment of primary urinary incontinence of children with autism. *Focus on Autism and Other Developmental Disabilities, 20,* 98–105.

LeBlanc, L. A., Esch, J., Sidener, T. M., & Firth, A. M. (2006). Behavioral language interventions for children with autism: Comparing applied verbal behavior and naturalistic teaching approaches. *Analysis of Verbal Behavior, 22,* 49–60.

Lerman, D. C., Parten, M., Addison, L. R., Vorndran, C. M., Volkert, V. M., & Kodak, T. (2005). A methodology for assessing the functions of emerging speech in children with autism. *Journal of Applied Behavior Analysis, 38,* 303–316.

Lerman, D. C., Vorndran, C., Addison, L., & Kuhn, S. A. (2004). A rapid assessment of skills in young children with autism. *Journal of Applied Behavior Analysis, 37,* 11–26.

Levy, S., Giarrelli, E., Li-Ching, L., Schieve, L., Kirby, R., Cunniff, C., et al. (2010). Autism spectrum disorder and co-occurring developmental, psychiatric, and medical conditions among children in multiple populations of the United States. *Journal of Developmental and Behavioral Pediatrics, 31,* 267–275.

Lovaas, O. I. (1981). *Teaching developmentally disabled children: The ME book.* Baltimore: University Park Press.

Lovaas, O. I. (1987). Behavioral treatment and normal educational and intellectual functioning in young autistic children. *Journal of Consulting and Clinical Psychology, 55,* 3–9.

Lovaas, O. I. (2003). *Teaching individuals with developmental delays: Basic intervention techniques.* Austin, TX: PRO-ED.

Lovaas, O. I., Koegel, R., Simmons, J. Q., & Long, J. (1973). Some generalization and follow-up measures on autistic children in behavior therapy. *Journal of Applied Behavior Analysis, 6,* 131–166.

Love, J. R., Carr, J. E., Almason, S. M., & Petursdottir, A. I. (2009). Early and intensive behavioral intervention for autism: A survey of clinical practices. *Research in Autism Spectrum Disorders, 3,* 421–428.

Makrygianni, M. K., & Reed, P. (2010). A meta-analytic review of the effectiveness of behavioural early intervention programs for children with autism spectrum disorders. *Research in Autism Spectrum Disorders, 4,* 577–593.

Matson, J. L., & Shoemaker, M. (2009). Intellectual disability and its relationship to autism spectrum disorders. *Research in Developmental Disabilities, 30,* 1107–1114.

Maurice, C., Green, G., & Luce, S. C. (1996). *Behavioral intervention for young children with autism: A manual for parents and professionals.* Austin, TX: PRO-ED.

McComas, J. J., Wacker, D. P., Cooper, L. J., Asmus, J. M., Richman, D., & Stoner, B. (1996). Brief experimental analysis of stimulus prompts for accurate responding on academic tasks in an out-patient clinic. *Journal of Applied Behavior Analysis, 29,* 397–401.

McEachin, J. J., Smith, T., & Lovaas, O. I. (1993). Long-term outcome for children with autism who received early intensive behavioral treatment. *American Journal on Mental Retardation, 97,* 359–372.

McGee, G. G., Krantz, P. J., Mason, D., & McClannahan, L. E. (1983). A modified incidental-teaching procedure for autistic youth: Acquisition and generalization of receptive object labels. *Journal of Applied Behavior Analysis, 16,* 329–338.

McGee, G. G., Krantz, P. J., & McClannahan, L. E. (1985). The facilitative effects of incidental teaching on preposition use by autistic children. *Journal of Applied Behavior Analysis, 18,* 17–31.

McGhan, A. C., & Lerman, D. C. (2013). An assessment of error-correction procedures for learners with autism. *Journal of Applied Behavior Analysis, 46,* 626–639.

McStay, R. L., Dissanayake, C., Scheeren, A., Koot, H. M., & Begeer, S. (2014). Parenting stress and autism: The role of age, autism severity, quality of life and problem behaviour of children and adolescents with autism. *Autism, 18,* 502–510.

Michael, J., Palmer, D. C., & Sundberg, M. L. (2011). The multiple control of verbal behavior. *Analysis of Verbal Behavior, 27,* 3–22.

Miguel, C. F., Petursdottir, A. I., & Carr, J. E. (2005). The effects of multiple-tact and receptive-discrimination training on the acquisition of intraverbal behavior. *Analysis of Verbal Behavior, 21,* 27–41.

National Autism Center. (2009). *National Standards Project.* Randolph, MA: Author.

National Autism Center. (2015). *Findings and conclusions: National Standards Project, Phase 2.* Randolph, MA: Author.

Nefdt, N., Koegel, R., Singer, G., & Gerber, M. (2010).

The use of a self-directed learning program to provide introductory training in pivotal response treatment to parents of children with autism. *Journal of
Positive Behavioral Interventions, 12,* 23–32.

Noell, G. H., Gresham, F. M., & Gansle, K. A. (2002).
Does treatment integrity matter?: A preliminary
investigation of instructional implementation and
mathematics performance. *Journal of Behavioral Education, 11,* 51–67.

Partington, J. W. (2006). *Assessment of Basic Language
and Learning Skills—Revised.* Pleasant Hill, CA: Behavior Analysts.

Peterson, K. M., Piazza, C. C., Ibañez, V. F., & Fisher, W.
W. (2019). Randomized controlled trial of an applied
behavior analysis intervention for food selectivity in
children with autism spectrum disorder. *Journal of
Applied Behavior Analysis, 52,* 895–917.

Peterson, K. M., Piazza, C. C., & Volkert, V. M. (2016).
A comparison of a modified sequential oral sensory
approach to an applied behavior-analytic approach
in the treatment of food selectivity in children with
autism spectrum disorder. *Journal of Applied Behavior
Analysis, 49,* 485–511.

Petursdottir, A. I., & Carr, J. E. (2011). A review of recommendations for sequencing receptive and expressive language instruction. *Journal of Applied Behavior
Analysis, 44,* 859–876.

Piazza, C. C. (2008). Feeding disorders and behavior:
What have we learned? *Developmental Disabilities
Research Reviews, 14,* 174–181.

Piazza, C. C., Fisher, W., Chinn, S., & Bowman, L.
(1991). Reinforcement of incontinent stools in the
treatment of encopresis. *Clinical Pediatrics, 30,* 28–32.

Piazza, C. C., Fisher, W., Kiesewetter, K., Bowman, L.,
& Moser, H. (1990). Aberrant sleep patterns in children with Rett syndrome. *Brain and Development, 12,*
488–493.

Reed, P., Osborne, L. A., & Corness, M. (2007). The
real-world effectiveness of early teaching interventions for children with autism spectrum disorder. *Exceptional Children, 73,* 417–433.

Reichow, B. (2012). Overview of meta-analyses on early
intensive behavioral intervention for young children
with autism spectrum disorders. *Journal of Autism and
Developmental Disorders, 42,* 512–530.

Reichow, B., Volkmar, F. R., & Cicchetti, D. V. (2008).
Development of the evaluative method for evaluating
and determining evidence-based practices in autism.
*Journal of Autism and Developmental Disorders, 38,*
1311–1319.

Reichow, B., & Wolery, M. (2009). Comprehensive
synthesis of early intensive behavioral interventions
for young children with autism based on the UCLA
Young Autism Project. *Journal of Autism and Developmental Disorders, 39,* 23–41.

Roane, H. S., Fisher, W. W., & Carr, J. E. (2016). Applied behavior analysis as treatment for autism spectrum disorder. *Journal of Pediatrics, 175,* 27–32.

Robinson, S. E. (2011). Teaching paraprofessionals of
students with autism to implement pivotal response
treatment in inclusive school settings, using a brief
video feedback treatment package. *Focus on Autism
and Other Developmental Disabilities, 26,* 105–118.

Romaniuk, C., Miltenberger, R., Conyers, C., Jenner,
N., Jurgens, M., & Ringenberg, C. (2002). The influence of activity choice on problem behaviors maintained by escape versus attention. *Journal of Applied
Behavior Analysis, 35,* 349–362.

Rutter, M. (1970). Psychological development: Predictions from infancy. *Journal of Child Psychology and
Psychiatry, 11,* 49–62.

Sallows, G. O., & Graupner, T. D. (2005). Intensive
behavioral treatment for children with autism: Four-
year outcome and predictors. *American Journal on
Mental Retardation, 110,* 417–438.

Schmidt, A. C., Hanley, G. P., & Layer, S. A. (2009).
A further analysis of the value of choice: Controlling for illusory discriminative stimuli and evaluating
the effects of less preferred items. *Journal of Applied
Behavior Analysis, 42,* 711–716.

Schreck, K. A., Williams, K., & Smith, A. F. (2004).
A comparison of eating behaviors between children
with and without autism. *Journal of Autism and Developmental Disorders, 34,* 433–438.

Schreibman, L., & Koegel, R. L. (2005). Training for
parents of children with autism: Pivotal responses,
generalization, and individualization of intervention.
In E. D. Hibbs & P. S. Jensen (Eds.), *Psychosocial
treatments for child and adolescent disorders: Empirically based strategies for clinical practice* (pp. 605–631).
Washington, DC: American Psychological Association.

Seaver, J. L., & Bourret, J. C. (2014). An evaluation of
response prompts for teaching behavior chains. *Journal of Applied Behavior Analysis, 47,* 777–792.

Sharp, W. G., Berry, R. C., McCracken, C., Nuhu, N.
N., Marvel, E., et al. (2013). Feeding problems and
nutrient intake in children with autism spectrum disorders: A meta-analysis and comprehensive review of
the literature. *Journal of Autism and Developmental
Disorders, 43,* 2159–2173.

Skinner, B. F. (1957). *Verbal behavior.* New York: Appleton-Century-Crofts.

Smith, I. M., Flanagan, H. E., Garon, N., & Bryson, S.
E. (2015). Effectiveness of community-based early
intervention based on pivotal response treatment.
*Journal of Autism and Developmental Disorders, 45,*
1858–1872.

Smith, T. (1999). Outcome of early intervention for
children with autism. *Clinical Psychology: Science and
Practice, 6,* 33–49.

Smith, T., Eikeseth, S., Klevstrand, M., & Lovaas, O. I.
(1997). Intensive behavioral treatment for preschoolers with severe mental retardation and pervasive
developmental disorder. *American Journal on Mental
Retardation, 102,* 238–249.

Smith, T., Groen, A., & Wynn, J. (2000). Randomized
trial of intensive early intervention for children with

pervasive developmental disorder. *American Journal on Mental Retardation, 105,* 269–285.

Spector, V., & Charlop, M. H. (2018). A sibling-mediated intervention for children with autism spectrum disorder: Using the natural language paradigm (NLP). *Journal of Autism and Developmental Disorders, 48*(5), 1508–1522.

Stahmer, A. C., Collings, N. M., & Palinkas, L. A. (2005). Early intervention practices for children with autism: Descriptions from community providers. *Focus on Autism and Other Developmental Disabilities, 20,* 66–79.

Stokes, T. F., & Baer, D. M. (1977). An implicit technology of generalization. *Journal of Applied Behavior Analysis, 10,* 349–367.

Stokes, T. F., Baer, D. M., & Jackson, R. L. (1974). Programming the generalization of a greeting response in four retarded children. *Journal of Applied Behavior Analysis, 7,* 599–610.

Sundberg, M. L. (2008). *Verbal Behavior Milestones Assessment and Placement Program.* Concord, CA: AVB Press.

Sundberg, M. L., & Michael, J. (2001). The benefits of Skinner's analysis of verbal behavior for children with autism. *Behavior Modification, 25,* 698–724.

Sundberg, M. L., & Partington, J. W. (1998). *Teaching language to children with autism or other developmental disabilities.* Pleasant Hill, CA: Behavior Analysts.

Sundberg, M. L., & Partington, J. W. (1999). The need for both discrete trial and natural environment language training for children with autism. In P. M. Ghezzi, W. L. Williams, & J. E. Carr (Eds.), *Autism: Behavior analytic perspectives* (pp. 139–156). Reno, NV: Context Press.

Tiger, J. H., Hanley, G. P., & Hernandez, E. (2006). An evaluation of the value of choice with preschool children. *Journal of Applied Behavior Analysis, 39,* 1–16.

Toussaint, K. A., Kodak, T., & Vladescu, J. C. (2016). An evaluation of choice on instructional efficacy and individual preferences among children with autism. *Journal of Applied Behavior Analysis, 49*(1), 170–175.

Virues-Ortega, J. (2010). Applied behavior analytic intervention for autism in early childhood: Meta-analysis, meta-regression and dose-response meta-analysis of multiple outcomes. *Clinical Psychology Review, 30,* 387–399.

Volkert, V. M., & Piazza, C. C. (2012). Pediatric feeding disorders. In P. Sturmey & M. Hersen (Eds.), *Handbook of evidence-based practice in clinical psychology* (pp. 323–338). Hoboken, NJ: Wiley.

Volkmar, F. R., Lord, C., Bailey, A., Schultz, R. T., & Klin, A. (2004). Autism and pervasive developmental disorders. *Journal of Child Psychology and Psychiatry, 45,* 135–170.

Walker, G. (2008). Constant and progressive time delay procedures for teaching children with autism: A literature review. *Journal of Autism and Developmental Disorders, 38,* 261–275.

Williams, G., Oliver, J. M., Allard, A. M., & Sears, L. (2003). Autism and associated medical and familial factors: A case control study. *Journal of Developmental and Physical Disabilities, 15,* 335–349.

Wolery, M., & Gast, D. L. (1984). Effective and efficient procedures for the transfer of stimulus control. *Topics in Early Childhood Special Education, 4,* 52–77.

Wunderlich, K. L., Vollmer, T. R., Donaldson, J. M., & Phillips, C. L. (2014). Effects of serial and concurrent training on acquisition and generalization. *Journal of Applied Behavior Analysis, 47,* 1–15.

Zwaigenbaum, L., Bauman, M. L., Choueiri, R., Kasari, C., Carter, A., Granpeesheh, D., et al. (2015). Early intervention for children with autism spectrum disorder under 3 years of age: Recommendations for practice and research. *Pediatrics, 136*(Suppl. 1), S60–S81.

# CHAPTER 24

# Behavioral Pediatrics
## Integrating Applied Behavior Analysis with Pediatric Medicine

Patrick C. Friman

Few children in the United States have a mental health care provider, but all have a medical health care provider. The medical care provided falls under the general rubric of pediatric primary care, and a pediatric primary care provider is the first professional a caregiver concerned about his or her child's behavior problems contacts. About one-fourth of the children seen in primary care have symptoms that meet criteria for a behavioral or emotional disorder (Costello, Edelbrock, et al., 1988; Horwitz, Leaf, Leventhal, Forsyth, & Speechley, 1992), and another 40% or more may exhibit subclinical behaviors or emotions that cause their caregivers concern (Costello & Shugart, 1992). These proportions are found in urban (e.g., Costello, Edelbrock, et al., 1988) and rural (Polaha, Dalton, & Allen, 2011) settings. As a result, researchers have referred to pediatricians as "gatekeepers" for child mental health services (Dulcan et al., 1990; Costello, Burns, et al., 1988), and to the locus of their practices as "de facto mental health settings" (Green et al., 2017; Jenssen, Buttenheim, & Fiks, 2019; Regier, Goldberg, & Taube, 1978; cf. Polaha et al., 2011). *Applied behavior analysis* (ABA) is a powerful science that specializes in behavior, its analysis, and the development of methods for influencing it in socially adaptive ways. *Behavioral pediatrics* is the branch of pediatrics that focuses on the relation between behavior and pediatric health care (Blum & Friman, 2000; Christophersen, 1982; Friman, 2005a, 2008; Friman & Blum, 2003). The central message of this chapter is that integrating ABA and behavioral pediatrics extends the scope of ABA, expands effective practice, and improves pediatric health care for children.

Behavioral pediatrics is a broad field that includes four primary domains of research and practice: (1) the evaluation and treatment of high-frequency, low-intensity (routine) child behavior problems presenting in primary health care settings; (2) the influence of physiological variables on child behavior problems; (3) the influence of behavioral variables on child medical problems; and (4) contextual variables that are central to the first three domains. The high prevalence of behavioral problems presenting in pediatric settings, and the increasing recognition of the reciprocal relationship between medical concerns and child behavior problems, have led to dramatic growth in behavioral pediatrics over the past 40 years. ABA has made significant contributions over that time, and these, coupled with the continuing growth of behavioral pediatrics, provide multiple opportunities for applied behavior analysts to work in child health care settings.

## RELATIONSHIP BETWEEN PEDIATRICS AND ABA

As indicated above, primary care providers (several subspecialties provide primary care for children but the most common by far is pediatrics; hereafter, I use the term *pediatrician* to refer to the providers and *pediatrics* to the settings) are the professionals who are most likely to provide initial interventions for children's behavioral or emotional problems (Christophersen, 1982; Costello, Burns, et al., 1988; Costello, Edelbrock, 1988; Dulcan et al., 1990). They are most likely to use supportive counseling, prescriptive behavioral treatment, or referral (Blum & Friman, 2000; Friman & Blum, 2003; Friman, 2005a, 2008). ABA has contributed substantially to the development, implementation, and evaluation of pediatric interventions, especially prescriptive behavioral treatment, for many of the behavior problems children present initially in primary care (Christophersen, 1982; Friman, 2005a, 2008; Friman & Blum, 2003). The cardinal principle informing these interventions—that behavior is influenced by its current and historical circumstances—is familiar to and accepted by most pediatricians. Thus primary care pediatricians have incorporated many of these interventions into practice, including interventions for child discipline, incontinence, sleep disorders, habit disorders, and symptoms of attention-deficit/hyperactivity disorder (e.g., Blum & Friman, 2000; Blum, Williams, Friman, & Christophersen, 1995; Christophersen & Friman, 2010; Christophersen & Mortweet, 2013; Friman, 2002; Friman & Schmitt, 1989).

In this chapter, I discuss four problems that behavior analysts treat, study, or treat and study, one representing each of the four primary domains of behavioral pediatrics: (1) bedtime struggles, representing routine behavior problems; (2) constipation and retentive encopresis, representing physiological influences on behavior; (3) nocturnal enuresis, representing behavioral influences on medical problems, and (4) adherence to medical regimens, representing contextual variables central to problems in the first three domains.

## ROUTINE BEHAVIOR PROBLEMS

The pediatrician is one of the most trusted professionals in the United States. Almost all families have pediatric care providers for their children—and, contrary to the stigma that results from contacting a mental health care provider about a child's problem, stigma results from *not* contacting a pediatric care provider about a child's problem. Therefore, the pediatrician is almost always the first professional to learn of child behavior problems. Most of these are low-intensity, high-frequency problems that are not necessarily representative of true pathology. But by caregivers' reports, they are often disruptive to families and difficult to solve (Christophersen, 1982; Earls, 1980; Friman, 2005a, 2008). Additionally, a significant percentage of them will deteriorate into more serious conditions if left unsolved. A classic example involves bedtime problems.

### Bedtime Problems

Teaching children to go to bed, go to sleep, and stay asleep throughout the night is difficult for many families in mainstream North American culture, in that at least 30% of families contend with sleep problems three or more nights a week (Friman & Schnoes, 2020; Lozoff, Wolf, & Davis, 1985). The difficulties caregivers report include bedtime struggles like resistance to going to bed; fussing and crying while in bed; and night waking with fussing, crying, and unauthorized departures from the bedroom. Pediatricians often address these problems by prescribing soporific drugs, but these medications produce side effects, and treatment gains are often lost when the medication is withdrawn (Christophersen & Mortweet, 2013; Edwards & Christophersen, 1994).

### Behavioral Treatment for Bedtime Problems

The primary component of the most effective behavioral interventions for bedtime problems involves one of the first documented and most frequently used ABA-informed procedures: extinction. As children develop sleep habits, they often learn to associate specific environmental factors with self-quieting and the induction of sleep. Misinformed caregiver efforts to help children sleep (e.g., soothe, cuddle, or lie down with the child until sleep onset occurs) often result in problematic sleep associations that mitigate the process of falling asleep. Unfortunately, when such a caregiver is absent at bedtime, the child is left without the stimulus that is most powerfully associated with sleep. The child's response to the caregiver's absence typically involves prolonged and intensive crying that resembles an extinction burst (Blampied & Bootzin, 2013; Edwards & Christophersen, 1994; Ferber, 2006; Friman, 2005b; Friman &

Schnoes, 2020). This response usually motivates the caregiver to intervene either by further soothing or by disciplining the child—both of which, unfortunately, usually worsen the problem. Soothing responses to crying can reinforce it, disciplinary responses to crying often provoke more crying, and both caregiver responses interfere with the child's learning to self-quiet (Blampied & Bootzin, 2013; Friman, 2005b; Friman & Schnoes, 2020; Lozoff et al., 1985; Schnoes & Reimers, 2009). Not surprisingly, after failed attempts to solve the problem themselves, caregivers whose children exhibit bedtime problems often ask their pediatricians for advice. I have described the four procedures professionals are most likely to prescribe below, which were all ABA-derived.

*Extinction.* The extinction approach to bedtime problems involves no visits by the caregiver to the child's bedroom after the child has gone to bed. In effect, the child is left to cry it out. Generally, extinction works more rapidly than other approaches, but it presents problems that mitigate its overall effectiveness: (1) Crying can be highly aversive to caregivers, especially during the first nights of treatment; (2) crying and screaming can draw attention from the neighbors, with predictably problematic consequences; and (3) extended crying and screaming differentially affects caregivers, which can cause marital/couple discord (Adams & Rickert, 1989; Edwards & Christophersen, 1994; Rickert & Johnson, 1988). Thus extinction is a straightforward behavioral approach to child bedtime problems that has limited social validity. To improve social validity, sleep researchers have developed other multicomponent methods that employ extinction but include other procedures to decrease its intensity and aversiveness for caregivers.

*Graduated Extinction.* Graduated extinction involves advising caregivers to ignore bedtime problem behavior for specific time intervals that gradually increase, usually beginning with a 5-minute interval at the first episode, 10 minutes at the second, and 15 minutes for subsequent episodes on Night 1 (e.g., Adams & Rickert, 1989). These intervals increase over the course of a week, ending with 35 minutes for the first episode on Night 7, 40 minutes for the second, and 45 minutes for all subsequent episodes and nights. Although children can have tantrums for longer than 45 minutes at night, research (Adams & Rickert, 1989; see also Edwards & Christophersen, 1994)

and a large amount of clinical experience that Ferber (2006) has described suggest that very few do. Although the mechanism responsible for the effectiveness of graduated extinction is unknown, one possible explanation is that increasing the response requirement to 45 minutes of crying may lean the schedule so much that the reinforcing effects of sleep supersede the reinforcing effects of caregiver visitation.

*Positive Routines.* The positive-routines procedure involves a hybrid of extinction and a reinforcing bedtime ritual. In this procedure, a caregiver decides on a preferred bedtime for the child and establishes the time at which the child typically falls asleep. Beginning shortly before the time the child typically falls asleep, the caregiver engages the child in several quiet activities lasting no longer than 20 minutes total. During the activities, the caregiver issues easily followed instructions and richly supplies reinforcement for compliance. These are followed by the terminal instruction "Now get in bed and go to sleep," or something equivalent—a procedure consistent with the high-probability instructional sequence in research on behavioral momentum (Mace et al., 1988). If the child leaves the bed at any time after the completion of the routines and the terminal instruction, the caregiver places him or her back in bed, telling the child that the routine is over and it is time for bed. The caregiver ignores crying or verbalizations. At specified intervals (e.g., 1 week), the caregiver moves the positive routine back in time 5–10 minutes. This backward movement continues until the caregiver arrives at the preferred bedtime for the child, which can take 6–8 weeks or more. Experimental comparison of the positive-routines procedure with scheduled extinction showed that both improved bedtime behavior for children, but the caregivers using positive routines reported significantly improved marital relations, suggesting a more socially valid procedure (Adams & Rickert, 1989).

*The Bedtime Pass.* The bedtime pass program involves (1) requiring the child to get into bed; (3) providing the child with a small object (e.g., a laminated note card) exchangeable for one "free" trip out of the bedroom or one visit by the caregiver after being put to bed to satisfy an acceptable request (e.g., for a drink, hug, or visit to the bathroom); (3) having the child surrender the pass after using it; and (4) using extinction thereafter (Schnoes, 2011). In the initial study, the program eliminated the high rates of crying out, calling out, and coming out of the bedroom after bedtime that two children (ages 3 and 10 years) exhibited. Additionally, caregivers achieved these successful results without an accompanying "extinction burst" during initial intervention periods, and a large group of sample caregivers rated the intervention as more acceptable than extinction alone (Friman et al., 1999). Investigators replicated results of the bedtime pass program in a single-subject analysis of four 3-year-old children (Freeman, 2006) and a randomized trial involving 19 children ages 3–6 years (Moore, Fruzetti, & Friman, 2007). The bedtime pass may achieve its effectiveness through differential reinforcement of alternative behavior (Vollmer & Iwata, 1992), in which the request and surrender of the pass allow the child to access potent bedtime reinforcers, and the caregiver places bedtime problems on extinction.

This brief discussion of child bedtime problems and their treatment is by no means complete. It merely involves four ABA-derived interventions that professionals use most frequently and have the most empirical support (for other interventions, see Burke, Kuhn, & Peterson, 2004; Friman, 2005b; Friman & Schnoes, 2020; Honaker & Meltzer, 2014).

## INFLUENCE OF PHYSIOLOGICAL VARIABLES ON CHILD BEHAVIOR PROBLEMS

The fundamental assumption of ABA is that behavior occurs as a function of environmental circumstances, but this position does not exclude the influence of physiological variables. Rather, many physiological variables may be causal but are the results of environmental contingencies that occurred in a phylogenetic context (Skinner, 1966). Physiological variables often play an initiating role in behavior problems that present in pediatrics. For example, child stomach pain caused by physiological variables (e.g., a flu virus) can lead to missing school. While home from school, reinforcers such as avoidance of schoolwork and contact with sympathetic responses from caregivers influence the child's behavior. These influences can in turn result in complaints of stomach pain that do not involve physiological variables, a condition sometimes referred to as *recurrent abdominal pain* (Finney, Lemanek, Cataldo, Katz, & Fuqua, 1989). There are many other examples, but the one I want to discuss here is constipation—a physio-

logical variable that can cause toileting problems, ranging from resistance to a bona fide diagnostic category known as *retentive encopresis*.

### Retentive Encopresis

#### Definition

Functional encopresis, a common presenting complaint in pediatrics (representing 3–5% of referrals), is a disorder in which children either voluntarily or involuntarily pass feces into or onto an inappropriate location, usually their clothing (Christophersen & Friman, 2010; Friman, 2017, 2019). Encopresis is not diagnosed if the problem is exclusively due to an anatomical or neurological abnormality that prevents continence. The current criteria from the *Diagnostic and Statistical Manual of Mental Disorders*, fifth edition (DSM-5; American Psychiatric Association, 2013) are as follows: (1) inappropriate passage of feces at least once a month for at least 3 months; (2) chronological or developmentally equivalent age of at least 4 years; and (3) not due exclusively to the direct physiological effects of a substance (e.g., a laxative) or a general medical condition, except through a mechanism involving constipation. DSM-5 distinguishes two subtypes of encopresis: one with constipation and overflow incontinence, and one without these symptoms. I focus on encopresis with constipation and overflow, because this subtype has a physiological cause (i.e., constipation). The etiology of encopresis without constipation remains unknown (Beaudry-Bellefeuille, Booth, & Lane, 2017).

#### Relevant Physiology

The large intestine or colon is the distal end of the alimentary tract, which is composed sequentially of the esophagus, stomach, small intestine, and colon. I provide a rudimentary description of the system here, because behavior analysts should understand the physiology that supplies the logic of effective treatment (for more thorough reviews, see Weinstock & Clouse, 1987; Whitehead & Schuster, 1985). The colon is a tube-shaped organ with a muscular wall. It connects the small intestine to the rectum and anus. It has three primary functions: fluid absorption, storage, and evacuation. Extended storage and planned evacuation are the defining features of fecal continence. Muscular contractions of the colon walls, called *peristalsis*, produce a wave-like motion that moves waste through the colon; various external events (e.g., a meal, moving about) stimulate these movements. The colon absorbs moisture from the waste that moves through it, creating semisolid feces.

The rectum, a hollow receptacle at the distal end of the colon, usually contains little or no feces until muscular contractions in the colonic wall propel feces into it, which produces distension. Distension stimulates sensory receptors in the rectal mucosa and in the muscles of the pelvic floor, resulting in relaxation of the internal sphincter, which facilitates defecation. This process is involuntary, but a child can constrict the anal canal and inhibit defecation by contracting the external anal sphincter and the functionally related puborectalis muscle. When the child suppresses the urge to defecate, the rectum accommodates the retained stool through the adaptive pliance of its structure and terminates the reflex relaxation of the internal sphincter. The urge gradually decays, and some of the fecal matter in the rectum returns to the descending colon by retroperistalsis.

## Etiology

Physicians can trace between 80 and 95% of encopresis cases to a primary causal variable, constipation (Hatch, 1988; Levine, 1982). Although definitions for constipation vary, children who frequently go 2 or more days without a bowel movement are probably prone to constipation. Caregivers of children with encopresis commonly complain that the children deliberately soil their clothing, but this attribution is usually false (Levine, 1982). The primary cause of soiling is fecal retention (constipation), which is generally not caused by characterological or psychopathological problems (Friman, 2002; Friman, Mathews, Finney, & Christophersen, 1988; Gabel, Hegedus, Wald, Chandra, & Chaponis, 1986). Retention is usually the result of a constellation of factors, many of which are beyond a child's immediate control (Levine, 1982). These factors include a constitutional predisposition (i.e., slow gastrointestinal transit time); diet; insufficient leverage for passage of hard stools; and occasional or frequent painful passage of hard stools, resulting in negative reinforcement for holding stools. In rare cases, retention may be related to sexual abuse. Some children—especially those with extreme constipation, treatment failure, or both—have an increased threshold of awareness of rectal distension, a possibly weak internal sphincter, a tendency to contract the external sphincter during the act of defeca-

tion, or a combination of these factors (Meunier, Marechal, & De Beaujeu, 1979; Wald, Chandra, Chiponis, & Gabel, 1986). The combined effects of these factors are a lowered probability of voluntary stool passage and a heightened probability of fecal retention.

Chronic fecal retention causes fecal impaction, which enlarges the colon, produces decreased motility of the bowel system, and occasionally results in involuntary passage of large stools and soiling due to seepage of soft fecal matter. Physicians often refer to the seepage as *paradoxical diarrhea*, because the children retain large masses of stool and are functionally constipated, but their colon allows passage of soft stool around the mass, which results in diarrhea (Levine, 1982). The relation of fecal impaction to encopresis is well established, and 80% of patients show fecal impaction accompanying fecal incontinence at the first clinic visit via clinical exam and 90% on X-ray of the lower abdomen (Davidson, 1958; Levine, 1982).

## Evaluation

Either before or directly after the initial visit, the behavior analyst should refer a child with encopresis to the pediatrician for a medical examination; this usually includes a routine check of history, abdominal palpation, rectal examination, and sometimes an X-ray of the abdomen to determine the extent of fecal impaction. A barium enema is rarely necessary unless features of the exam suggest Hirschsprung's disease. Rare anatomical and neurological problems can cause fecal retention and soiling; neurological problems include Hirschsprung's disease, and anatomical defects include a variety of malformations and locations of the anus that a physical exam can detect and that require medical management (Hatch, 1988).

In addition to routine behavior assessments, the behavioral interview for encopresis should include questions related to constipation. These include asking whether (1) there is ever a long period between bowel movements; (2) bowel movements are atypically large (e.g., stop up the toilet); (3) fecal matter ever has an unusually foul odor; (4) fecal matter is ever hard, difficult, or painful to pass; (5) the child ever complains of not being able to feel the movement or make it to the toilet on time; and (6) the child ever hides soiled underwear. An affirmative answer to one or more of these questions is highly suggestive of retentive encopresis, and hiding underwear suggests a history that includes some form of punishment.

Encopresis is not well understood outside the medical community, and characterological and psychopathological interpretations prevalent in Western culture are likely to influence a caregiver's interpretation of the condition, which may influence how the child views the problem. The behavior analyst can begin encopresis treatment during the evaluation by providing accurate information that "demystifies" the problem. Lastly, the evaluation should include questions about diet and timing of meals. Low-fiber diets and irregular meals can contribute to encopresis (Koppen et al., 2016).

## Treatment

During the past 40 years, several descriptive and controlled experimental studies have supported a multicomponent approach to treatment of chronic retentive encopresis, partly derived from the pioneering work of Davidson (1958), Christophersen and Rainey (1976), Levine (1982), and Wright (1975). The behavior analyst can address the first component during the evaluation by demystifying the entire elimination process and its disordered manifestations. Generally, this means providing information about bowel dynamics and the relation of the problem to constipation. Second, the caregiver should remove fecal impaction with enemas, laxatives, or both under the direction of the pediatrician. Third, the child should sit on the toilet for about 5 minutes once or twice a day. Fourth, the caregivers should promote proper toileting with encouragement and not with coercion. Additionally, they should not reserve their praise and affection for proper elimination; caregivers should provide praise for just sitting on the toilet. Fifth, caregivers should give the child a stool softener like mineral oil or MiraLAX™ under the pediatrician's direction, to ease the passage of hard stools. Sixth, the caregiver should increase the child's dietary fiber. Seventh, the caregiver should arrange for and encourage the child to increase his or her activity level and fluid intake, to increase and maintain colon motility. Eighth, the child's feet should be on a flat surface during toileting episodes. Foot placement is crucial to the Valsalva maneuver, which is the grunting push necessary to produce a bowel movement. Ninth, the caregiver should reward the child for bowel movements in the toilet. See Christophersen and Friman (2010) and Friman (2019) for reviews discussing these recommendations in greater depth.

The literature on this approach or variations thereof has progressed sufficiently to lead to group trials (e.g., Stark et al., 1997). For example, in a study of 58 children with encopresis, 60% were completely continent after 5 months, and those who did not achieve full continence averaged a 90% decrease in accidents (Lowery, Srour, Whitehead, & Schuster, 1985). However, not all children succeed with the conventional approach, and researchers have developed augmentative methods for these children. In a manner typical of ABA, developing these augmentative methods began with the study of behaviors associated with treatment failure (Stark, Spirito, Lewis, & Hart, 1990). Incorporating behavior management methods relevant to the behaviors, teaching caregivers to use them, and delivering treatment in a group format produced an 83% decrease in accidents in 18 treatment-resistant children with encopresis, and the children maintained decreased accidents or even improved at a 6-month follow-up (Stark, Owens-Stively, Spirito, Lewis, & Guevremont, 1990).

The general premise of this section—that physiological variables can influence or cause behavior problems—is not controversial even within ABA, a science dedicated to environmental variables. Constipation is one such variable, and there are many others (e.g., anorexia due to gastroesophageal reflux, restricted activities due to pain). Because of the physiological component of these problems, serious health consequences of unsuccessful treatment often compound the behavioral components that contribute to the problem. For example, extreme fecal retention can be life-threatening, and even routine cases can seriously decrease social standing and increase social isolation in affected children. Because of the behavioral components of these problems, a solely medical intervention is insufficient for effective treatment. A method that delivers or aids the delivery of the medical components of treatment while addressing the behavioral components is needed, and thus behavioral pediatrics is an ideal context. Additionally, although many types of behavior problems stem from physiological influences, the most frequently occurring problem is some form of noncompliance with a treatment regimen for the physiological dimensions. As an example, cooperation with prescribed treatment for encopresis is so necessary for success that instructional control training is frequently a component of treatment (Christophersen & Friman, 2010; Friman, 2017, 2019). Furthermore, although researchers have made progress in improving pediatric compliance, it remains one of the most chronic problems in pediatric medicine (see the discussion of adherence below). Therefore, this domain of behavioral pediatrics provides many opportunities for applied behavior analysts interested in working in pediatric health care settings.

## INFLUENCE OF BEHAVIORAL VARIABLES ON CHILD MEDICAL PROBLEMS

In this section, I discuss the influence of behavior on physiological variables, with emphasis on the behavioral treatment of physiologically based behavior problems that pediatricians frequently see. For decades, health-based sciences have demonstrated relations between child behavior and health. As examples, eating nutritious food and engaging in modest exercise can improve children's cardiovascular health; obtaining sufficient sleep can improve children's emotional resiliency and adaptability; and maintaining adequate personal hygiene can decrease children's susceptibility to infectious disease. Historically, ABA has demonstrated a variety of healthful outcomes from behavior changes (e.g., Friman & Christophersen, 1986; Finney et al., 1993; Irwin, Cataldo, Matheny, & Peterson, 1992; Stark et al., 1993). An updated review of this literature is beyond the scope of this chapter. Here I merely focus on biofeedback, a treatment involving the manipulation of behavioral variables to improve health, and use treatment of nocturnal enuresis as the primary example.

*Biofeedback* involves the use of electrical or electromechanical equipment to measure and increase the salience of stimuli associated with pertinent physiological processes and training patients to discriminate and control them to improve their own health. The penultimate goal of biofeedback is to train patients to alter the physiological processes in healthful directions, and the ultimate goal is to train them to do so without biofeedback (Culbert, Kajander, & Reaney, 1996). Most biofeedback treatments (e.g., anorectal manometry combined with electromyography for treatment of fecal incontinence) require sophisticated instrumentation and specialized training to use them; thus pediatricians may not incorporate them into primary care practices readily. However, nocturnal enuresis, a physiologically based behavior problem that is one of the most frequent presenting behavioral complaints in primary care pediatrics, is highly responsive to urine alarm treatment—a minimally technical, uncomplicated form of biofeedback that is used readily in primary care settings (Christophersen & Friman, 2010; Friman, 2017, 2019). Below I briefly review nocturnal enuresis, its relevant physiology, and its alarm-based treatment.

## Nocturnal Enuresis

### Definition

The current criteria for nocturnal and diurnal enuresis from DSM-5 (American Psychiatric Association, 2013) are as follows: (1) repeated urination into bed or clothing; (2) at least two occurrences per week for at least 3 months, or a sufficient number of occurrences to cause clinically significant impairment or distress; (3) chronological age of 5 years, or for children with developmental delays, a mental age of at least 5; and (4) not due exclusively to the direct effects of a substance (e.g., diuretics) or a general medical condition (e.g., diabetes). There are three subtypes of enuresis—nocturnal only, diurnal only, and mixed nocturnal and diurnal. There are two courses: The primary course includes children who have never established continence, and the secondary course involves children who resume having accidents after establishing continence. Here I primarily discuss nocturnal enuresis, which researchers estimate occurs in as many as 20% of first-grade children (Christophersen & Friman, 2010; Friman, 2017, 2019).

### Relevant Physiology

The bladder is an elastic, hollow organ with a wall consisting of detrusor muscle. Its shape resembles an upside-down balloon with a long narrow neck; it has two primarily mechanical functions, storage and release of urine (Vincent, 1974). Extended storage and volitional release are the defining properties of urinary continence. In infancy, distension of the bladder leads to contraction of the bladder and automatic (nonvolitional) urine evacuation. As children mature, the capacity of the central nervous system to inhibit bladder contraction increases, which typically coincides with the development of continence in early childhood (Berk & Friman, 1990; Koff, 1995).

The components of the urogenital system that are under volitional control to establish continence are the muscles of the pelvic floor. Except during imminent or actual urination, these muscles remain in a state of tonus or involuntary partial contraction, which maintains the bladder neck in an elevated and closed position (Vincent, 1974). Even after initiation of urination has begun, contraction of the pelvic-floor muscles can raise the bladder neck abruptly and terminate urination. These urinary inhibitory responses are either not present or sporadic for children with nocturnal enuresis (Christophersen & Friman, 2010; Friman, 2017, 2019; also see Houts, 1991).

## Etiology

Although nocturnal enuresis has a strong genetic basis, its exact cause is unknown. For decades, researchers attempted to link it to causal psychopathology, but contemporary research (Friman, Handwerk, Swearer, McGinnis, & Warzak, 1998) and several reviews of older research (Christophersen & Friman, 2010; Friman, 2017, 2019) suggest that most children with enuresis do not exhibit clinically significant psychopathology, and psychopathology is more likely to be an outcome than a cause of nocturnal enuresis when they do. Physiologically oriented studies of nocturnal enuresis suggest that some affected children may have difficulty concentrating their urine during the night and produce more urine nocturnally than their nonenuretic peers (Lackgren, Neveus, & Stenberg, 1997; Rittig, Knudsen, Norgaard, Pedersen, & Djurhuus, 1989). The overall importance of this factor, however, is controversial, because the proportion of children with enuresis who have urine concentration problems may be small (Eggert & Kuhn, 1995). Nocturnal enuresis is usually most productively viewed as a deficit in the skills necessary to prevent urination while asleep (Christophersen & Friman, 2010; Friman, 2017, 2019; Houts, 1991).

## Evaluation

As for a child with encopresis, the behavior analyst should refer a child with nocturnal enuresis to a pediatrician for a medical evaluation before initiation of treatment. Although pathophysiological causes of nocturnal enuresis are very rare, they are real and should be ruled out. There are several other elements necessary for a complete evaluation of nocturnal enuresis, but these are well documented in other sources. I refer the reader to them because the intention of this section is merely to describe alarm-based treatment (e.g., Christophersen & Friman, 2010; Friman, 2017, 2019).

## Treatment

The most common treatments for nocturnal enuresis are the urine alarm and the two medications, desmopressin acetate (DDAVP) and imipramine. These medications can provide symptomatic relief (approximately 25–40% of children will be dry most nights when taking them); however, the enuresis usually returns when the medications are stopped (Moffatt, 1997). More importantly, both medications have been associated with adverse side effects. For imipramine, just the common side effects give one pause, as they range across systems from extrapyramidal symptoms in the central nervous system to urticaria and pruritus of the skin (Skidmore-Roth, 2010). For DDAVP, the most serious side effects are hyponatremia, seizures, and death; the occurrence of these has led the U.S. Food and Drug Administration to rule against use of the most widely used DDAVP formula (nasal spray) for treatment of enuresis (Hatti, 2007).

The urine alarm is a moisture-sensitive switching system that sounds when the child urinates. Researchers have reported that repeated pairing of awakening by the alarm with episodes of wetting is the single most effective treatment for enuresis (Christophersen & Friman, 2010; Friman, 2017, 2019). Its success rate is higher (approximately 75%) and its relapse rate lower (approximately 41%) than those for any other drug or skill-based treatment (Shepard, Poler, & Grabman, 2017).

The urine alarm is a simple form of biofeedback treatment, because its primary function is to provide feedback for a physiological event (urination) that occurs beneath awareness. The feedback, the alarm ringing, increases the salience of urination and aids the child to ultimately establish urinary self-control. The mechanism by which the alarm improves enuresis, however, is still unknown. Changes in secretion of hormones that affect the ability to concentrate urine or alterations in the brain's inhibition of bladder contraction are at least theoretically possible, but have not been investigated. The current prevailing account involves a combination of classical conditioning of pelvic-floor muscles and operant conditioning of volitional behaviors related to continence via avoidance of the alarm (Christophersen & Friman, 2010; Friman, 2017, 2019; Houts, 1991). In this account, children are not necessarily trained to awaken to the alarm, merely to engage their urination-inhibiting system even if they are asleep—

a skill that would be difficult to teach without the sensory feedback the alarm provides.

The enuresis alarm produces cures slowly, and during the first few weeks of alarm use, waking occurs only after a complete voiding if it occurs at all. One study using the size of the urine stain on the soiled sheets as the dependent measure showed that before accident-free nights, the stain grew increasingly smaller on successive nights, suggesting a gradual process of continence attainment (Ruckstuhl & Friman, 2003). In other words, the feedback properties of the alarm gradually but inexorably strengthened the skills necessary to avoid it. The core skill involves contraction of the pelvic-floor muscles, causing sustained elevation of the bladder neck, which stops or prevents urination. Increased sensory awareness of urinary need and waking to urinate are possible outcomes, but are less likely and actually inferior to sustained, accident-free sleep throughout the night.

Increasing sensory awareness of urinary need before daytime accidents, however, is a key component in the most empirically supported treatment for diurnal enuresis. Only two studies are available, as researchers have studied diurnal enuresis minimally, and the first used a much simpler conceptualization (Halliday, Meadow, & Berg, 1987). Specifically, this early study merely suggested that the alarm served as a reminder for urination. A colleague and I (Friman & Vollmer, 1995) conducted a subsequent study using the biofeedback conceptualization with a young girl who was initially unresponsive to urinary urge and onset, but who rapidly became responsive with use of the alarm. The decreasing latency between alarm onset and appropriate response was characteristic of learning curves during alarm-based treatment for nocturnal enuresis and biofeedback treatments in general.

Most biofeedback treatments are much more technically complex than the urine alarm, and clinicians use them for a broad range of physiologically based behavioral concerns that often initially present in pediatric settings. Among the physiological processes that we can monitor are muscle tension, skin temperature, respiratory rate, blood pressure, and skin moisture (perspiration) (Friman, 2009). Researchers and clinicians have used biofeedback devices sensitive to these processes in treating a variety of disorders, including headaches, other varieties of chronic pain, asthma, bruxism, anxiety disorders, sleep disorders, and dysfunction of the autonomic nervous system

(Culbert et al., 1996). Additionally, evidence that biofeedback can generate operant responses that lead to control over physiological processes long thought to be outside volition, like skin temperature and blood pressure, is mounting. For example, researchers have used verbally based awareness enhancement methods to alter the level of mediators of the immune system in saliva (Olness, Culbert, & Uden, 1989) and to decrease the recurrence of chronic mouth ulcers (Andrews & Hall, 1990). Collectively, the large body of research documenting the effectiveness of the urine alarm, and the even larger literature on the effectiveness of biofeedback treatment for a broad range of medical conditions, underscore the research and clinical potential represented by the influence of behavioral variables on physiology. This potential, in turn, represents an excellent opportunity for applied behavior analysts interested in working in pediatric settings.

## CONTEXTUAL VARIABLES

A broad range of contextual variables influence the effectiveness of health care and its delivery. These variables are not specific to any particular problem that presents in a health care delivery system, but they have the capacity to influence all of them. For example, doctor communication is central, but not specific, to care for problems treated in health care settings, although its role can vary depending on the problem at hand. For example, effective communication may be less critical for treatments like "the tincture of time" (e.g., "Let's just watch this for a while and see if the child grows out of it") than it would be for a complex medical intervention. A directly related contextual variable is patient communication. For example, if patients incompletely report symptoms or do not ask critical questions, the care they receive may be inadequate (e.g., Finney et al., 1990). I have chosen treatment adherence for this chapter as the exemplar of a contextual variable that affects care.

### Treatment Adherence

#### Definition

Treatment adherence is so central to pediatric medicine that this chapter probably should have begun with it. True, routine behavior problems are very frequently concerns in pediatric medicine, but treatment adherence is always a concern because it begins with adhering to the pediatric appointment itself. Treatment effectiveness is a moot issue if families do not keep appointments or do not follow prescribed treatments. Estimated rates of nonadherence hover around 50% for both psychological (Kazdin, 1996) and medical (Rapoff, 2010) services. Although treatment adherence is problematic across clinical populations, it is particularly challenging with children and adolescents, because there are usually at least two sources of nonadherence: the children/adolescents and their caregivers (Watson, Foster, & Friman, 2006). Thus establishing acceptable levels of adherence requires examining child and caregiver variables that either facilitate or impede it.

The relevant literature highlights three salient terms: *adherence, compliance,* and *integrity. Compliance* and *adherence* are basically synonymous, but *adherence* has gained favor in recent years (see Rapoff, 2010), and I use it here. *Adherence* and *integrity,* however, are not synonymous, because treatment integrity refers to the fidelity with which a clinician delivers treatment. Adherence refers to the extent to which patients keep appointments and accurately and consistently follow the steps of prescribed treatments. For example, a routine prescription for functional retentive encopresis includes increases in fluid, fiber, scheduled toilet sits, stool softeners, and incentives, as well as decreases in dairy products, processed foods, coercion, punishment, and irregular or extended toilet sits. Assessing treatment adherence involves determining the number of prescribed steps actually followed (accuracy) and the regularity of applications (consistency).

Although patient nonadherence has always been the primary focus in treatment adherence research, clinicians and researchers alike now realize that treatment integrity among clinicians should also be a target. Clinician communication about treatment has a significant effect on the probability of adherence, and accuracy and consistency are dimensions of the communication. Additional variables include clinician training and experience, interpersonal skill, capacity to manifest authority without instigating resistance, and sense of timing. Other not so self-evident and possibly more manipulable variables include the specificity of treatment recommendations; the standardization of treatment protocols; and the provision of supportive instructional aids like handouts, audio and video recordings, and e-mail or web-based communications. For example, as described above, incontinence is a problem that frequently presents in pediatrics, and there are empirically supported treatment protocols for its most commonly presenting forms (enuresis and encopresis). These treatments include information on relevant physiology, diet, toileting schedules, behavioral contingencies, activity levels, and caregiver involvement. To maximize integrity, a clinician would verbally deliver information covering these details and supplement the delivery with supportive instructional aids. Other examples include regimens for chronic diseases and empirically supported treatment protocols for behavior disorders.

### Assessment of Adherence

Adherence is an observable and measurable behavior, and thus well suited to behavioral assessment. The primordial adherence behavior is appointment keeping, and its assessment is straightforward: Did the patient keep the appointment? The other adherence behaviors to be assessed are determined by the nature of the problem to be treated. For acute problems like otitis media or strep throat, the behaviors of primary concern are relatively simple; they typically involve rest and taking prescribed medication for an abbreviated time. For chronic diseases, the behaviors of concern are usually more complex. They typically involve multiple timelines and classes of behavior. The vast literature on behavioral assessment offers some guidance on selection of target behaviors that can readily inform how and what to assess when adherence to a complex regimen for a chronic condition is the focus (e.g., Friman, 2009).

A complete review of assessment is far beyond the scope of this chapter. I merely provide a cursory description. There are at least four options for selecting target regimen behaviors. The first is the most straightforward, but probably the most difficult, and this is to measure all behaviors that are relevant to regimen adherence. The second involves targeting only those behaviors that are most problematic or aversive to others. For example, children with enuresis are often less bothered by soiled bedding than their caregivers are. The third involves targeting behaviors that are the most immediately crucial to a patient's health and well-being. For example, compliance with daily insulin injections is more immediately critical to health maintenance in diabetes than foot care is. The fourth involves targeting those behaviors that are easiest to change; the rationale here is to build up momentum for larger changes (cf. Mace et al., 1988).

The next issue involves who does the assessing and who is assessed—questions particularly important in pediatrics, because although children are the targets of treatment, their caregivers are usually the recipients of the regimen and are always partly and often fully responsible for carrying it out. Thus both a child and a caregiver can often be the focus of assessment. Additionally, as is typical in most branches of medicine, there are multiple sources of information, including physicians, nurses, therapists, and support staff. For example, in our early appointment-keeping research, the staff at the outpatient check-in desk supplied critical assessment data (Friman, Finney, Rapoff, & Christophersen, 1985).

The final issue involves how to assess adherence, and the literature describes multiple strategies. Here, I briefly discuss only the most common. However, this dimension of adherence assessment would seem to be limited only by the resources, ingenuity, and creativity of investigators. In short, how best to assess adherence presents a growth potential for behavior analysts. The types I list here include drug assays, direct observation, electronic monitoring, pill counts, provider estimates, and patient and caregiver reports (Rapoff, 2010). There are advantages and disadvantages to each. I then discuss functional assessment of adherence and some general concerns about procedures.

*Drug Assays.* Drug assays range in sophistication from observing a bioavailable marker that is either part of or added to a drug to various kinds of testing, ranging from determining simple blood sugar levels (something the patient or patient's caregivers do) to testing for various metabolites (something that only a lab technician can do). However, proper interpretation of a drug assay virtually always involves some basic knowledge of clinical pharmacology, especially as it pertains to absorption, distribution, and elimination of medications in (or not in) the body. The advantages of assays include objective quantification, clinical utility, and information on dose–response relations. Their disadvantages include abbreviated time horizons, expense, invasiveness, need for expert readings, and variability of readings due to various causes (e.g., enteric coatings, contents of the stomach, presence of other drugs, age, gender, habits).

*Observation.* Although direct observation is considered a sine qua non for behavior-analytic research, it is actually limited in research on ad-

herence. Most measures are indirect, like assays (see above) or pill counts (see below). But the limited use of direct observation is not so much an obstacle as it is an opportunity. The indirect measures are likely to dominate the field, but direct observation can supplement them when this is feasible. However, expanding assessment to include direct observation will usually require observers other than those on the research team, because although treatments are prescribed in clinical settings, they are usually carried out elsewhere (e.g., home, school). The most likely candidates are family members or school personnel, but there are other possibilities. For example, a study on dietary compliance used camp counselors as observers (Lorenz, Christensen, & Pitchert, 1985). Validity is the primary advantage of direct observations. They are direct measures of adherence, and they accrue all the scientific advantages that behavior analysts have touted for decades (e.g., Johnston & Pennypacker, 2009; Rapoff, 2010). Their disadvantages primarily involve access. As indicated above, little of the typical treatment regimen is carried out in the clinic setting. Regimen requirements are distributed temporally across the patients' days and nights, and situationally across the settings of their lives. The cost of resources necessary to carry out representative direct observations of adherence behaviors necessary for most regimens is prohibitive. Nonetheless, when accessibility is not a significant concern, behavior analysts should include direct observation in adherence assessment.

*Electronic Monitors.* The revolution in electronic technology that has occurred over the past few decades has significantly expanded assessment options for adherence researchers. For example, researchers can now monitor whether a patient retrieves pills or liquids from medication bottles or an inhalant from an inhaler, and researchers can store the obtained data electronically and retrieve it later for analysis. The research on electronic monitoring is so extensive that a pediatric psychology task force has identified it as a *well-established* measure (Quittner, Modi, Lemanek, Levers-Landis, & Rapoff, 2008). The primary advantage of electronic monitoring is that it can provide objective measures of a broad spectrum of adherence behaviors continuously (if necessary) in real time. No other method has this advantage. The primary disadvantage is that data from electronic monitoring provide only an indirect measure of adherence behavior. A patient may not take pills retrieved from a bottle, may not swallow liquid from a dispenser, and may dispense mist from an inhaler into the air rather than inhale it into the lungs. Thus, independent of other measures indicating that the patient ingested the medicine, the behavior analyst is likely to consider electronic monitoring only as a supplementary measure.

*Pill Counts.* The long-standing tradition of using pill counts as a measure of adherence began to fade with the advent of electronic monitoring. Their use is simple: The researcher merely counts the pills remaining in the medication container and compares it against the prescribed regimen. Obviously, this is a primitive method, compared to the real-time data available from electronic monitoring. Thus, although pill counts are a measure of adherence behavior and any measure is better than no measure, they share none of the advantages of electronic monitoring and all their disadvantages.

*Provider Estimates.* Obtaining provider estimates typically involves asking medical providers to complete scales that assess adherence. The most common involve Likert-type scales whose items pertain to judgments about the likelihood adherence has occurred and its extent. In a more primitive form, providers merely answer *yes* or *no* when asked whether they believe a patient has or will follow a regimen. The primary advantage of provider estimates is feasibility. They require little effort or expense. A small amount of evidence suggests that they are more accurate than global ratings from patients and their caregivers. The disadvantages will be obvious to behavior analysts. Provider estimates merely involve asking for providers' opinions, and opinions, even from well-established experts, are subject to bias and other well-known threats to validity (Rapoff, 2010). Moreover, outside of some forms of social validity, opinions are wholly unsatisfactory as a primary measure for behavior analysts.

*Patient and Caregiver Reports.* Patient and caregiver reports are merely variations on self-reports—a method fundamental to research in mainstream psychology, psychiatry, some related social sciences, and clinical medical research. Yet, outside of social validity, behavior analysts virtually never use them as a primary source of assessment data. The reasons are immediately evident to behavior analysts: Behavior is the subject under consideration, and reports of behavior are only considered as behavior, not as measures of behavior. Although

some well-respected behavior analysts have acknowledged the potential utility of self-reports and have suggested methods for increasing their rigor (e.g., reducing bias, heightening validity; Critchfield, Tucker, & Vuchinich, 1998), behavior-analytic researchers remain skeptical of their use as a source of data. Non-behavior-analytic researchers studying adherence are much less skeptical, and they have developed multiple self-report methods, including global rating scales, structured interviews, and daily diaries. As just one example, sleep diaries are a staple of clinical and scientific approaches to pediatric sleep problems (e.g., Ferber & Kryger, 1995). The behavior analyst contemplating research that involves assessment of adherence should consider coupling self-report measures with the more objective measures favored in behavior analysis. Doing so could expand the scope of the research and the possibility of having behavior-analytically oriented adherence research accepted in mainstream medical journals. Although the research (or at least a portion of it) could strain the credulity of behavior analysts, the advantage of exporting the behavior-analytic dimension of the research into mainstream medicine could—and would, in my opinion—be worth the cost.

*Functional Assessment.* There is little mention of function in the adherence literature. Once again, behavior analysts should see this as an opportunity rather than as a reason to avoid this important area of investigation. Although what follows is elementary to behavior analysts, it bears mentioning nonetheless: Determining the function of a behavior, whether it involves self-injury or nonadherence, is a well-established method for designing treatments that are informed by the identified functions.

*General Concerns about Procedures.* There are multiple issues to address in the pursuit of adherence research that I only briefly mention here, but the brevity of my remarks is inversely related to their importance. Beyond limited space, the reason for brief mention of these concerns is that they are central to all methods deployed to measure human behavior. The first is reactivity. All measurement systems are reactive, and the portion of data resulting from the reactivity is not reflective of the behavior being measured. Second, the measures employed must be representative of that behavior (in this instance, adherence). For example, pills missing from a pill container are not necessarily an accurate representation of medication consumed. Direct measures, when possible and feasible, are always preferred over indirect measures, because they more completely and accurately capture the essence of adherence. For example, directly observing a patient walking into a clinic is superior to asking a caregiver whether his or her child kept his or her appointment. Standards of measurement, especially reliability and validity, are essential considerations in all measurement systems, and assessment of adherence is no exception. Interpretation is important, because the data do not speak for themselves. Learning that a patient took a pill means little without information about the importance, meaning, and relevance (to the regimen) of that pill. Adherence to a medical regimen is a clinical activity, and its assessment data should have demonstrable clinical utility. As a counterexample, much of the information solicited in the packets that patients receive in medical settings has little or no bearing on their medical condition or its treatment.

### Improving Adherence

*Health Education.* There are two forms of intervention in behavioral pediatrics, and health education is one of them (prescriptive treatment is the other). Some amount of health education accompanies all treatment prescribed in pediatrics (e.g., see the discussions of bedtime problems, encopresis, and enuresis above), and a major portion of it pertains to the importance of following the treatment regimen. As one example, health education messages about the importance of completing the regimen are now a standard part of prescribed antibiotic regimens. This was not always the case. Patients often discontinued the regimen as soon as their symptoms receded. Premature discontinuation, however, can lead to symptom recurrence and treatment resistance. In pediatric studies evaluating the use of health education to increase adherence, among the most typical targets are antibiotic regimens for otitis media; the results are mixed, with only about half of available studies showing a significant benefit (Rapoff, 2010). However, this 50% failure rate may be more a reflection of educational methods than of health education itself. For example, a test of three educational methods to promote adherence to a regimen for reducing dangerous infant behavior showed that an educational video with modeling was as effective as an in-home demonstration, and more effective than educational materials supplied by the American Academy of Pediatrics (Linnerooth et al., 2002).

The point for behavior analysts is that health education is a primordial component of pediatric medicine, and that one of its central purposes is to promote adherence. The extent to which it does so in its currently employed forms, the extent to which those forms could be improved, and the development of new behaviorally informed methods are all rich opportunities for behavior-analytic research.

*Monitoring.* Monitoring, whether its target is subatomic dynamics (Heisenberg, 1958/1999) or human behavior (Friman, 2009), affects the behavior of the object monitored. The direction of the change in human behavior is determined by its social valence: Socially acceptable behaviors tend to increase in frequency, and socially unacceptable behaviors tend to decrease in frequency (Nelson, 1977). As a thought experiment, imagine the amount and direction of behavior change that would result from pointing a video camera at a group. In pediatric medicine, the primary monitor is almost always a caregiver. Researchers have used monitoring to enhance adherence across a broad range of programs, from functional encopresis (O'Brien, Ross, & Christophersen, 1986) to diet and exercise (Rapoff, 2010).

*Prompts and Reminders.* Although prompts and reminders can play a role across virtually all medical regimens, professionals use them more for appointment keeping than for any other dimension of pediatric medicine. Reminder phone calls are now a basic part of virtually all medical subspecialties that involve prescriptive treatment, although this was not always the case. For example, Outpatient Pediatrics at the University of Kansas School of Medicine routinely reported high no-show rates for pediatric visits. The department had not used prompts or reminders. Our research group implemented an intervention involving mailed and telephoned reminders, and it resulted in approximately a 20% increase in appointments kept and a 20% decrease in appointments not kept (cancellations were not included in the database). These improvements in appointment keeping were accompanied by substantial cost savings (Friman et al., 1985). We replicated these results in a training clinic staffed by pediatric residents (Friman, Glasscock, Finney, & Christophersen, 1987). Studies like these have led to the virtually universal use of reminder systems in modern medicine and stand as evidence that behaviorally based research on prompting can exert a significant influence on how professionals address nonadherence in medical settings. That influence extends far beyond appointment keeping. Some form of prompting could potentially improve adherence to any medical regimen to be followed outside a clinic setting. As just one example of potential research in this area, research on smartphone-based prompting applications to improve adherence is limited. But the ubiquity of smartphones coupled with their almost limitless capacity for applications presents an opportunity for enterprising behavior analysts to assess their potential for increasing adherence to appointments and medical regimens.

*Incentives.* Presumably the most powerful incentive for adhering to a medical regimen involves negative reinforcement in the form of rapid relief from symptoms. However, not all appointments result in treatment, and not all treatment results in rapid relief. As just one example of the latter, the regimen for juvenile diabetes requires multiple behaviors that are effortful (e.g., dietary restrictions, foot care), painful (e.g., insulin shots, blood sugar tests), or both, but that do not provide immediate symptom relief. Thus the addition of positive reinforcement in the form of tangible incentives can be helpful. One example involves token systems to promote adherence to regimens in juvenile rheumatoid arthritis. The basic form involves four primary components: (1) task-analyzing the regimen into readily executable steps, (2) supplying tokens contingent upon completion of steps, (3) withdrawing tokens contingent upon failure to complete steps, and (4) arranging for regular exchange of tokens for agreed-upon rewards. One of the most difficult regimens to follow involves abstaining from addictive substances, and incentive programs have been more effective than virtually any other method for accomplishing this outcome (e.g., Higgins, Heil, & Sigmon, 2013). Despite this extraordinary range of documented effective applications, ranging from performing simple steps in a juvenile rheumatoid arthritis regimen to complying with prescribed abstinence from the most addictive substances known to humankind, incentive programs for improving adherence to medical regimens has received only modest attention from researchers in general and even less from behavior analysts in particular.

*Miscellaneous Approaches.* There are various other approaches to promoting adherence in pediatric populations, although research directly evaluating them is scant. Disciplinary interven-

tion is one example. The literature showing that behaviorally based disciplinary interventions (e.g., time out, time in) can improve compliance is so well established that it need not be cited here. Nonadherence to a medical regimen is a form of noncompliance, and child resistance is frequently a factor. The extent to which disciplinary strategies can improve adherence is a subject worthy of behavior-analytic investigation.

Rule governance is another aspect of behavior that almost certainly plays a significant role in adherence. Skinner (1969) described rules as contingency-specifying stimuli, and Hayes (1989) has characterized rule-governed behavior as behavior under the control of verbal stimuli. When cognitively oriented investigators refer to *self-management* for promoting adherence (cf. Rapoff, 2010), they are really referring to rule-governed behavior. However, the cognitive account places emphasis on the self as agent and deemphasizes the role of the environment (i.e., verbal community). This may explain why there is so little research showing that self-management can improve adherence. Why there is no behavior-analytic research examining the role rule governance plays in adherence awaits an explanation.

A final option involves various forms of psychotherapy. From a cognitive perspective, mental illness involves some combination of cognitive distortion and neurotransmitter levels. Despite being highly theoretical at this stage of its development, this perspective appears to operate at the level of dogma in mainstream psychology and psychiatry. From a behavioral perspective, mental illness involves maladaptive verbal behavior and environmental contingencies. Regardless of perspective, the so-called illness can interfere with adherence when present. Conventional approaches (e.g., cognitive) employ some combination of medication and direct psychotherapy to resolve the illness and increase compliance. Behavioral approaches employ health education to correct the problematic rule governance (e.g., vaccines do not cause autism spectrum disorder) and contingency management to improve behaviors related to adherence. Testing these approaches to improving adherence against each other could be interesting.

This section on adherence is cursory. Nonadherence to medical regimens is the single greatest threat to the health and well-being of children in the United States. This problem is so well recognized that it typically receives book-length treatment (e.g., O'Donohue & Levensky, 2006; Rapoff,

2010; Stuart, 1982). Although the section ends this chapter on behavioral pediatrics, it should probably have been the introductory section (as noted earlier), because the treatments discussed in the first three dimensions of behavioral pediatrics are moot if patients do not keep appointments or follow regimens. One of the major concerns of behavior analysts in the 21st century is how to bring our field more into the mainstream of everyday life. Almost all U.S. children have a primary care physician. Thus any research or intervention that targets pediatrics in general, as adherence does, is by definition, mainstream. Enterprising behavior analysts might consider taking that route.

## CONCLUSIONS

Behavioral pediatrics is a diverse field that includes research and treatment of common child behavior problems, research on the interactions between physiology and behavior that affect child health, and treatments derived from the findings of that research. ABA is a science that conducts research on interactions between environmental and behavioral variables and evaluates interventions for socially significant problems that have been derived from that research. The integration of behavioral pediatrics and ABA not only benefits both fields, but actually extends the effectiveness of pediatricians—the primary guardians of child health in this country—and thereby contributes to the health of children. I have confined my discussion to four problem areas, each representing one domain of behavioral pediatrics. This represents a much-abbreviated review of behavioral pediatrics and the potential role of ABA, and there are many aspects of behavioral pediatrics that I have not addressed (e.g., infant colic, oppositional behaviors, habit disorders, anxiety and depressive disorders, chronic illnesses, and pain). For a broader sample, please refer to various source documents (e.g., Allen, Barone, & Kuhn, 1993; Blum & Friman, 2000; Christophersen, 1982; Friman, 2005a, 2008; Friman & Blum, 2003).

Despite its many contributions to behavioral pediatrics, ABA is still not widely available and accepted in the pediatric medical community. Remedying the problem of limited availability is a primary purpose of this chapter; I hope to increase the number of applied behavior analysts interested in behavioral pediatrics. Remedying the problem of limited acceptance is an important concern,

but a subsidiary one in this chapter. Nonetheless, I suggest a few tactics that could help. For example, applied behavior analysts interested in collaborating with pediatricians at a local level should attend and present at pediatric conferences and lectures. They should also attend case management discussions in pediatric settings and offer to help physicians implement behavioral assessments and treatments. If these contacts result in a referral, promptly sending data-based feedback on the effects of the ABA interventions to the referring pediatrician for inclusion in the patient's medical chart not only mirrors standard practice between physicians in all domains of medicine; it is also likely to lead to more referrals. Additionally, the increasing demands by third-party payers for documentation of treatment and its effects can make data-based feedback necessary for continued reimbursement for costs accruing from needed ongoing treatment. This fact, coupled with the value ABA places on ongoing data collection, makes applied behavior analysts increasingly attractive as collaborators in pediatric medicine. Applied behavior analysts could also become more involved in medical professional organizations and thereby provide a community resource for questions pertaining to behavior. More systemically, incorporating the clinical phenomena referred to by hypothetical constructs like depression, anxiety, or temperament into behavior-analytic theories, and making those phenomena the focus of ABA assessments and interventions, could advance the field and increase its acceptance (e.g., Friman, Hayes, & Wilson, 1998; see also Friman, 2010). Lastly, and consistent with the primary purpose of this chapter, designing and testing treatments for problems that frequently present in pediatric settings contributes to the recognition of ABA as a resource and acceptance of it by pediatricians as a valuable science (Riley & Freeman, 2019). Perhaps more than any other subspecialty in medicine, pediatrics is a pragmatic specialty, and effective and efficient treatments readily trump ideological differences.

In conclusion, the large and mounting body of evidence documenting the many ways ABA has been found to influence behavior, coupled with the mutually determinative role played by behavior and physiology, suggests that a partnership between applied behavior analysts and pediatricians would benefit the health of children in the United States. I have argued in this chapter that behavioral pediatrics is the ideal locus for this partnership.

# REFERENCES

Adams, L. A., & Rickert, V. I. (1989). Reducing bedtime tantrums: Comparison between positive routines and graduated extinction. *Pediatrics, 84,* 756–761.

Allen, K. D., Barone, V. J., & Kuhn, B. R. (1993). A behavioral prescription for promoting applied behavior analysis within pediatrics. *Journal of Applied Behavior Analysis, 26,* 493–502.

American Psychiatric Association. (2013). *Diagnostic and statistical manual of mental disorders* (5th ed.). Arlington, VA: Author.

Andrews, V. H., & Hall, H. R. (1990). The effect of relaxation/imagery training on recurrent apthous stomatitis. *Psychosomatic Medicine, 52,* 526–535.

Beaudry-Bellefeuille, I., Booth, D., & Lane, S. J. (2017). Defecation-specific behavior in children with functional defecation issues: A systematic review. *Permanente Journal, 21,* 17–47.

Berk, L. B., & Friman, P. C. (1990). Epidemiologic aspects of toilet training. *Clinical Pediatrics, 29,* 278–282.

Blampied, N. M., & Bootzin, R. R. (2013). Sleep: A behavioral account. In G. Madden (Ed.), *Handbook of behavior analysis* (pp. 425–454). Washington, DC: American Psychological Association.

Blum, N., & Friman, P. C. (2000). Behavioral pediatrics: The confluence of applied behavior analysis and pediatric medicine. In J. Carr & J. Austin (Eds.), *Handbook of applied behavior analysis* (pp. 161–186). Reno, NV: Context Press.

Blum, N., Williams, G., Friman, P. C., & Christophersen, E. R. (1995). Disciplining young children: The role of verbal instructions and reason. *Pediatrics, 96,* 336–341.

Burke, R. V., Kuhn, B. R., & Peterson, J. L. (2004). A "storybook" ending to children's bedtime problems: The use of a rewarding social story to reduce bedtime resistance and frequent night waking. *Journal of Pediatric Psychology, 29,* 389–396.

Christophersen, E. R. (1982). Incorporating behavioral pediatrics into primary care. *Pediatric Clinics of North America, 29,* 261–295.

Christophersen, E. R., & Friman, P. C. (2010). *Elimination disorders.* Cambridge, MA: Hogrefe.

Christophersen, E. R., & Mortweet, S. M. (2013). *Treatments that work with children* (2nd ed.). Washington, DC: American Psychological Association.

Christophersen, E. R., & Rainey, S. K. (1976). Management of encopresis through a pediatric outpatient clinic. *Journal of Pediatric Psychology, 4,* 38–41.

Costello, E. J., Burns, B. J., Costello, A. J., Edelbrock, C., Dulcan, M., & Brent, D. (1988). Service utilization and psychiatric diagnosis in pediatric primary care: The role of the gatekeeper. *Pediatrics, 82,* 435–441.

Costello, E. J., Edelbrock, C., Costello, A. J., Dulcan, M., Burns, B. J., & Brent, D. (1988). Psychopathology in pediatric primary care: The new hidden morbidity. *Pediatrics, 82,* 415–424.

Costello, E. J., & Shugart, M. A. (1992). Above and below the threshold: Severity of psychiatric symptoms and functional impairment in a pediatric sample. *Pediatrics, 90,* 359–368.

Critchfield, T. S., Tucker, J. A., & Vuchinich, R. E. (1998). Self-report. In A. Lattal & M. Perone (Eds.), *Handbook of research methods in human operant behavior* (pp. 435–470). New York: Plenum Press.

Culbert, T. P., Kajander, R. L., & Reaney, J. B. (1996). Biofeedback with children and adolescents: Clinical observations and patient perspectives. *Journal of Developmental and Behavioral Pediatrics, 17,* 342–350.

Davidson, M. (1958). Constipation and fecal incontinence. *Pediatric Clinics of North America, 5,* 749–757.

Dulcan, M. K., Costello, E. J., Costello, A. J., Edelbrock, C., Brent, D., & Janiszewski, S. (1990). The pediatrician as gatekeeper to mental healthcare for children: Do caregivers' concerns open the gate? *Journal of the American Academy of Child and Adolescent Psychiatry, 29,* 453–458.

Earls, F. (1980). Prevalence of behavior problems in 3-year-old children: A cross national replication. *Archives of General Psychiatry, 37,* 1153–1157.

Edwards, K. J., & Christophersen, E. R. (1994). Treating common bedtime problems of young children. *Journal of Developmental and Behavioral Pediatrics, 15,* 207–213.

Eggert, P., & Kuhn, B. (1995). Antidiuretic hormone regulation in patients with primary nocturnal enuresis. *Archives of Diseases in Childhood, 73,* 508–511.

Ferber, R. (2006). *Solve your child's bedtime problems: New and expanded edition.* New York: Fireside.

Ferber, R., & Kryger, M. (1995). *Principles and practice of sleep medicine in the child.* Philadelphia: Saunders.

Finney, J. W., Brophy, C. J., Friman, P. C., Golden, A. S., Richman, G. S., & Ross, A. F. (1990). Promoting parent–provider interaction during child health supervision visits. *Journal of Applied Behavior Analysis, 23,* 207–214.

Finney, J. W., Lemanek, K. L., Cataldo, M. F., Katz, H. P., & Fuqua, R. W. (1989). Pediatric psychology in primary health care: Brief targeted therapy for recurrent abdominal pain. *Behavior Therapy, 20,* 283–291.

Finney, J. W., Miller, K. M., & Adler, S. P. (1993). Changing protective and risky behaviors to prevent child-to-parent transmission of cytomegalovirus. *Journal of Applied Behavior Analysis, 26,* 471–472.

Freeman, K. A. (2006). Treating bedtime resistance with the bedtime pass: A systematic replication and component analysis with 3-year-olds. *Journal of Applied Behavior Analysis, 39,* 423–428.

Friman, P. C. (2002). *The psychopathological interpretation of common child behavior problems: A critique and related opportunity for behavior analysis.* Invited address at the 28th annual convention of the Association for Behavior Analysis, Toronto, ON, Canada.

Friman, P. C. (2005a). Behavioral pediatrics. In M. Hersen (Ed.), *Encyclopedia of behavior modification and therapy* (Vol. 2, pp. 731–739). Thousand Oaks, CA: SAGE.

Friman, P. C. (2005b). *Good night, we love you, we will miss you, now go to bed and go to sleep: Managing bedtime problems in young children.* Boys Town, NE: Girls and Boys Town Press.

Friman, P. C. (2008). Primary care behavioral pediatrics. In M. Hersen & A. Gross (Eds.), *Handbook of clinical psychology* (Vol. 2, pp. 728–758). Hoboken, NJ: Wiley.

Friman, P. C. (2009). Behavioral assessment. In M. Hersen, D. Barlow, & M. Nock (Eds.), *Single case experimental designs* (3rd ed., pp. 91–143). Boston: Allyn & Bacon.

Friman, P. C. (2010). Come on in, the water is fine: Achieving mainstream relevance through integration with primary medical care. *Behavior Analyst, 33,* 19–36.

Friman, P. C. (2017). Incontinence. In A. Wetzel (Ed.), *The SAGE encyclopedia of abnormal and clinical psychology* (pp. 1296–1298). Thousand Oaks, CA: SAGE.

Friman, P. C. (2019). Incontinence in the child: A biobehavioral perspective. In T. H. Ollendick, S. W. White, & B. A. White (Eds.), *The Oxford handbook of clinical child and adolescent psychology* (pp. 367–381). New York: Oxford University Press.

Friman, P. C., & Blum, N. J. (2003). Primary care behavioral pediatrics. In M. Hersen & W. Sledge (Eds.), *Encyclopedia of psychotherapy* (pp. 379–399). New York: Academic Press.

Friman, P. C., & Christophersen, E. R. (1986). Biobehavioral prevention in primary care. In N. Krasnegor, J. D. Arasteh, & M. F. Cataldo (Eds.), *Child health behavior: A behavioral pediatrics perspective* (pp. 254–280). New York: Wiley.

Friman, P. C., Finney, J. W., Rapoff, M. A., & Christophersen, E. R. (1985). Improving pediatric appointment keeping: Cost effectiveness and social validation of reminders and reduced response requirement. *Journal of Applied Behavior Analysis, 18,* 315–323.

Friman, P. C., Glasscock, S. G., Finney, J. W., & Christophersen, E. R. (1987). Reducing effort with reminders and a parking pass to improve appointment keeping for patients of pediatric residents. *Medical Care, 25,* 83–86.

Friman, P. C., Handwerk, M. L., Swearer, S. M., McGinnis, C., & Warzak, W. J. (1998). Do children with primary nocturnal enuresis have clinically significant behavior problems? *Archives of Pediatrics and Adolescent Medicine, 152,* 537–539.

Friman, P. C., Hayes, S. C., & Wilson, K. (1998). Why behavior analysts should study emotion: The example of anxiety. *Journal of Applied Behavior Analysis, 31,* 137–156.

Friman, P. C., Hoff, K. E., Schnoes, C., Freeman, K. A., Woods, D. W., & Blum, N. (1999). The bedtime pass: An approach to bedtime crying and leaving the room. *Archives of Pediatric and Adolescent Medicine, 153,* 1027–1029.

Friman, P. C., Mathews, J. R., Finney, J. W., & Christophersen, E. R. (1988). Do children with encopresis have clinically significant behavior problems? *Pediatrics, 82,* 407–409.

Friman, P. C., & Schmitt, B. D. (1989). Thumb sucking: Guidelines for pediatricians. *Clinical Pediatrics, 28,* 438–440.

Friman, P. C., & Schnoes, C. (2020). Pediatric prevention: Sleep dysfunction. *Pediatric Clinics of North America, 67,* 559–571.

Friman, P. C., & Vollmer, D. (1995). Successful use of the nocturnal urine alarm for diurnal enuresis. *Journal of Applied Behavior Analysis, 28,* 89–90.

Gabel, S., Hegedus, A. M., Wald, A., Chandra, R., & Chaponis, D. (1986). Prevalence of behavior problems and mental health utilization among encopretic children. *Journal of Developmental and Behavioral Pediatrics, 7,* 293–297.

Green, C., Storfer-Isser, A., Stein, R. E. K., Garner, A. S., Kerker, B. D., Szilagyi, M., et al. (2017). Which pediatricians comanage mental health conditions? *Academic Pediatrics, 17,* 479–486.

Halliday, S., Meadow, S. R., & Berg, I. (1987). Successful management of daytime enuresis using alarm procedures: A randomly controlled trial. *Archives of Diseases in Children, 62,* 132–137.

Hatch, T. F. (1988). Encopresis and constipation in children. *Pediatric Clinics of North America, 35,* 257–281.

Hatti, M. (2007). 2 deaths spur bed-wetting drug warning: FDA warns that some patients taking desmpopressin may be at risk of seizure and death. Retrieved July 11, 2016, from *www.webmd.com/children/news/20071204/2-deaths-spur-bedwetting-drug-warning.*

Hayes, S. C. (1989). *Rule-governed behavior: Cognition, contingencies, and instructional control.* New York: Plenum Press.

Heisenberg, W. (1999). *Physics and philosophy.* Amherst, NY: Prometheus. (Original work published 1958)

Higgins, S. T., Heil, S. H., & Sigmon, S. C. (2013). Voucher based contingency management in the treatment of substance abuse disorders. In G. Madden (Ed.), *APA handbook of behavior analysis* (pp. 481–500). Washington, DC: American Psychiatric Association.

Honaker, S. M., & Meltzer, L. J. (2014). Bedtime problems and night wakings in young children: An update of the evidence. *Pediatric Respiratory Reviews, 15,* 333–339.

Horwitz, S. M., Leaf, P. J., Leventhal, J. M., Forsyth, B., & Speechley, K. N. (1992). Identification and management of psychosocial and developmental problems in community-based, primary care pediatric practices. *Pediatrics, 89,* 480–485.

Houts, A. C. (1991). Nocturnal enuresis as a biobehavioral problem. *Behavior Therapy, 22,* 133–151.

Irwin, C. E., Cataldo, M. F., Matheny, A. P., & Peterson, L. (1992). Health consequences of behaviors: Injury as a model. *Pediatrics, 90,* 798–807.

Jenssen, B. P., Buttenheim, A. M., & Fiks, A. G. (2019). Using behavioral economics to encourage parent behavior change: Opportunities to improve clinical effectiveness. *Academic Pediatrics, 19,* 4–10.

Johnston, J. M., & Pennypacker, H. S. (2009). *Strategies and tactics of behavioral research* (3rd ed.). New York: Routledge.

Kazdin, A. E. (1996). Dropping out of child therapy: Issues for research and implications for clinical practice. *Clinical Child Psychology and Psychiatry, 1,* 133–156.

Koff, S. A. (1995). Why is desmopressin sometimes ineffective at curing bed wetting. *Scandinavian Journal of Urology and Nephrology, Supplementum, 173,* 103–108.

Koppen, I. J., von Gontard, A., Chase, J., Cooper, C. S., Rittig, C. S., Bauer, S. B., et al. (2016). Management of functional nonretentive fecal incontinence in children: Recommendations from the International Children's Continence Society. *Journal of Pediatrics, 12,* 56–64.

Lackgren, G., Neveus, T., & Stenberg, A. (1997). Diurnal plasma vasopressin and urinary output in adolescents with monosymptomatic nocturnal enuresis. *Acta Paediatrica, 86,* 385–390.

Levine, M. D. (1982). Encopresis: Its potentiation, evaluation, and alleviation. *Pediatric Clinics of North America, 29,* 315–330.

Linnerooth, P. J. N., Walsh, M., Spear, S., Niccols, R., Maestretti, J., Pulido, L., et al. (2002). *Reducing infant potentially dangerous behavior: A randomized controlled trial of three interventions for preventing unintentional child injury.* Paper presented at the 36th annual convention of the Association for Advancement of Behavior Therapy, Reno, NV.

Lorenz, R. A., Christensen, N. K., & Pitchert, J. W. (1985). Diet related knowledge, skill, and adherence among children with insulin dependent diabetes mellitus. *Pediatrics, 75,* 872–876.

Lowery, S., Srour, J., Whitehead, W. E., & Schuster, M. M. (1985). Habit training as treatment of encopresis secondary to chronic constipation. *Journal of Pediatric Gastroenterology and Nutrition, 4,* 397–401.

Lozoff, B., Wolf, A. W., & Davis, N. S. (1985). Bedtime problems seen in pediatric practice. *Pediatrics, 75,* 477–483.

Mace, F., Hock, M. L., Lalli, J. S., West, B. J., Belfiore, P., Pinter, E., et al. (1988). Behavioral momentum in the treatment of noncompliance. *Journal of Applied Behavioral Analysis, 21,* 123–142.

Meunier, P., Marechal, J. M., & De Beaujeu, M. J. (1979). Rectoanal pressures and rectal sensitivity in chronic childhood constipation. *Gastroenterology, 77,* 330–336.

Moffatt, M. E. (1997). Nocturnal enuresis: A review of the efficacy of treatments and practical advice for clinicians. *Journal of Developmental and Behavioral Pediatrics, 18,* 49–56.

Moore, B. A., Fruzetti, A. E., & Friman, P. C. (2007).

Evaluating the Bedtime Pass Program for child resistance to bedtime: A randomized controlled trial. *Journal of Pediatric Psychology, 32,* 283–287.

Nelson, R. (1977). Assessment and therapeutic functions of self-monitoring. In M. Hersen, R. M. Eisler & P. M. Miller (Eds.), *Progress in behavior modification* (Vol. 5, pp. 263–308). New York: Academic Press.

O'Brien, S., Ross, L. V., & Christophersen, E. R. (1986). Primary encopresis: Evaluation and treatment. *Journal of Applied Behavior Analysis, 19,* 137–145.

O'Donohue, W. T., & Levensky, E. R. (2006). *Promoting treatment adherence.* London: SAGE.

Olness, K., Culbert, T., & Uden, D. (1989). Self-regulation of salivary immunoglobulin A by children. *Pediatrics, 83,* 66–71.

Polaha, J., Dalton, W. T., & Allen, S. (2011). The prevalence of emotional and behavior problems in pediatric primary care serving rural children. *Journal of Pediatric Psychology, 36,* 652–660.

Quittner, A. L., Modi, A. C., Lemanek, K. L., Levers-Landis, C. E., & Rapoff, M. A. (2008). Evidence-based assessment of adherence to medical treatments in pediatric psychology. *Journal of Pediatric Psychology, 33,* 916–936.

Rapoff, M. A. (2010). *Adherence to pediatric medical regimens* (2nd ed.). New York: Springer.

Regier, D. A., Goldberg, I. D., & Taube, C. A. (1978). The de facto US mental health system. *Archives of General Psychiatry, 35,* 685–693.

Rickert, V. I., & Johnson, M. (1988). Reducing nocturnal awaking and crying episodes in infants and young children: A comparison between scheduled awakenings and systematic ignoring. *Pediatrics, 81,* 203–212.

Riley, A. R., & Freeman, K. A. (2019). Impacting pediatric primary care: Opportunities and challenges for behavioral research in a shifting healthcare landscape. *Behavior Analysis, 19,* 23–38.

Rittig, S., Knudsen, U. B., Norgaard, J. P., Pedersen, E. B., & Djurhuus, J. C. (1989). Abnormal diurnal rhythm of plasma vasopressin and urinary output in patients with enuresis. *American Journal of Physiology, 256,* F644–F671.

Ruckstuhl, L. E., & Friman, P. C. (2003). *Evaluating the effectiveness of the vibrating urine alarm: A study of effectiveness and social validity.* Paper presented at the 29th annual convention of the Association for Behavior Analysis, San Francisco, CA.

Schnoes, C. J. (2011). The bedtime pass. In M. Perlis, M. Aloia, & B. Kuhn (Eds.), *Behavioral treatments for sleep disorders: A comprehensive primer of behavioral sleep medicine interventions* (pp. 293–298). Boston: Elsevier.

Schnoes, C. J., & Reimers, T. M. (2009). Assessment and treatment of child and adolescent sleep disorders. In D. McKay & E. A. Storch (Eds.), *Cognitive-behavior therapy for children: Treating complex and refractory cases* (pp. 293–324). New York: Springer.

Shepard, J. A., Poler, J. E., & Grabman, J. H. (2017).

Evidence-based psychosocial treatments for pediatric elimination disorders. *Journal of Clinical Child and Adolescent Psychology, 46*, 767–797.

Skidmore-Roth, L. (2010). *Mosby's nursing drug reference* (23rd ed.). St. Louis, MO: Elsevier.

Skinner, B. F. (1966). The phylogeny and ontogeny of behavior. *Science, 153*, 1205–1213.

Skinner, B. F. (1969). *Contingencies of reinforcement.* New York: Appleton-Century-Crofts.

Stark, L. J., Knapp, L. G., Bowen, A. M., Powers, S. W., Jelalian, E., Evans, S., et al. (1993). Increasing caloric consumption in children with cystic fibrosis: Replication with 2-year follow-up. *Journal of Applied Behavior Analysis, 26*, 435–450.

Stark, L. J., Opipari, L. C., Donaldson, D. L., Danovsky, D. A., Rasile, D. A., & DelSanto, A. F. (1997). Evaluation of a standard protocol for retentive encopresis: A replication. *Journal of Pediatric Psychology, 22*, 619–633.

Stark, L. J., Owens-Stively, J. A., Spirito, A., Lewis, A. V., & Guevremont, D. (1990). Group behavioral treatment of retentive encopresis. *Journal of Pediatric Psychology, 15*, 659–671.

Stark, L. J., Spirito, A., Lewis, A. V., & Hart, K. J. (1990). Encopresis: Behavioral parameters associated with children who fail medical management. *Child Psychiatry and Human Development, 20*, 169–179.

Stuart, R. B. (1982). *Adherence, compliance, and generalization in medicine.* New York: Brunner/Mazel.

Vincent, S. A. (1974). Mechanical, electrical and other aspects of enuresis. In J. H. Johnston & W. Goodwin (Eds.), *Reviews in pediatric urology* (pp. 280–313). New York: Elsevier.

Vollmer, T. R., & Iwata, B. A. (1992). Differential reinforcement as treatment for behavior disorders: Procedural and functional variations. *Research in Developmental Disabilities, 13*, 393–417.

Wald, A., Chandra, R., Chiponis, D., & Gabel, S. (1986). Anorectal function and continence mechanisms in childhood encopresis. *Journal of Pediatric Gastroenterology and Nutrition, 5*, 346–351.

Watson, T. S., Foster, N., & Friman, P. C. (2006). Treatment adherence in children and adolescents. In W. T. Odonohue & E. R. Levensky (Eds.), *Promoting treatment adherence* (pp. 343–351). London: SAGE.

Weinstock, L. B., & Clouse, R. E. (1987). A focused overview of gastrointestinal physiology. *Annals of Behavioral Medicine, 9*, 3–6.

Whitehead, W. E., & Schuster, M. M. (1985). *Gastrointestinal disorders: Behavioral and physiological basis for treatment.* New York: Academic Press.

Wright, L. (1975). Outcome of a standardized program for treating psychogenic encopresis. *Professional Psychology, 6*, 453–456.

# CHAPTER 25

# A Behavior-Analytic Approach to Pediatric Feeding Disorders

Cathleen C. Piazza and Caitlin A. Kirkwood

Feeding is unique relative to other behaviors discussed in this book, because food[1] functions as an appetitive stimulus, and feeding is ubiquitous across species. Organisms require relatively constant caloric intake, and metabolic output cannot exceed caloric intake for long. Many organisms have adapted unique mechanisms for the habitat in which they feed that promote consistent acquisition of calories and nutrients. For example, the hyacinth macaw, a native parrot of South America, has a beak that can exert hundreds of pounds of pressure per square inch; this beak is ideal for cracking the hard shells of the palm nuts that are a major component of the bird's diet (Borsari & Ottoni, 2005). Some organisms have adaptations that allow them to reduce metabolic needs, store nutrients, or both to respond to predictable changes in their habitat that affect food availability. For example, black bears suppress their basal metabolic rate by 25% during the 5–7 months per year that they hibernate (Toien et al., 2011). Despite an organism's adaptations to feed in a specific habitat or during predictable environmental changes, unpredictable changes in environmental conditions, such as drought, may threaten the organism's ability to access calories and nutrients consistently.

Not surprisingly, nature has even provided some organisms with the ability to adapt to unpredictable changes in food availability. For example, some bird species that typically exhibit a narrow range of foraging behavior develop strategies to identify alternative food sources when the food in their typical habitat becomes scarce (Diquelou, Griffin, & Sol, 2016).

Even when changes occur that disrupt food availability, motivation to feed is typically not disrupted (Diquelou et al., 2016). In fact, professionals in the United States are often so confident about the reinforcing properties of food that their response to a caregiver of a poorly growing child is "The child will eat when he [or she] gets hungry." But are there exceptions to this time-worn adage? And if so, why does this happen and what are the stimulus conditions under which it occurs?

## DEFINITION

We use the term *feeding disorder* for children who do not consume sufficient calories, hydration, or nutrition to gain weight and grow, to maintain hydration, or to meet their nutritional needs for macro- and micronutrients. Feeding disorders are heterogeneous and may include refusal to eat; refusal to eat certain types or textures of food;

---

[1] We use the term *food* here to mean an organism's source of energy (kilocalories) and nutrients.

dependence on a limited or developmentally in-appropriate source of nutrition, such as bottle de-pendence in a 3-year-old child; and skill deficits, such as inability to self-feed or transition to age- or developmental-stage-appropriate textures. The *Diagnostic and Statistical Manual of Mental Disorders,* fifth edition (DSM-5; American Psychiatric Association, 2013) uses the term *avoidant/restrictive food intake disorder* to refer to the following: (1) A child exhibits a feeding or eating disturbance characterized by persistent failure to meet appropriate nutritional needs, energy needs, or both, with significant weight loss, significant nutritional deficiency, need for enteral feeding or oral nutritional supplements, or obvious interference with psychosocial functioning; (2) the disturbance is not better explained by a lack of available food or by an associated culturally permissible practice; (3) the eating disturbance does not occur only during the course of anorexia nervosa or bulimia nervosa, and there is no evidence of a disturbance in the child's experience of body weight or shape; and (4) the eating disturbance is not attributed to a con-current medical condition or better explained by another mental disorder, and if the eating distur-bance occurs in the context of another condition or disorder, its severity exceeds what is routinely associated with that condition or disorder and warrants additional clinical attention.

A diagnostic nosology such as DSM-5 is help-ful in describing the characteristics of a feeding disorder, but it tells us little about why feeding disorders occur or how to develop effective inter-ventions. Although multiple children may have the same topographical expression of a feeding disorder, such as poor weight gain, the etiology of the feeding disorder may be different across chil-dren. For example, one poorly growing child may have delayed gastric emptying, complain of being full, and refuse to eat after consuming a small amount of food (Stein, Everhart, & Lacy, 2015). Another child, by contrast, may have oral–motor skill deficits. Although the child eats frequently and appears motivated to eat (e.g., asks for food), meals are lengthy, and the child cannot consume sufficient calories to gain weight and grow. A third child may vomit frequently, and poor weight gain is an indirect result of gastroesophageal reflux dis-ease. Within those broad topographical presenta-tions of feeding disorders, individual children may exhibit different behaviors that contribute to their feeding disorders, such as excessive saliva produc-tion, inability to chew, inability to lateralize the tongue, an open-mouth posture, persistent tongue thrust, pocketing food, poor lip closure, refusal, spitting out food, and vomiting (Arvedson & Brodsky, 2002).

## DEPENDENT VARIABLES

Feeding consists of a complex chain of behav-iors that includes placing bites or drinks into the mouth; lateralizing the food to the molars and chewing, if necessary; forming a bolus (a mass of food or drink) on the tongue; elevating the tongue; and propelling the bolus to the pharynx (Derkay & Schechter, 1998). A child with a feeding disor-der may have difficulties with one or more of the behaviors in the chain. Thus intervention may target one or more problematic feeding behaviors, and intervention for one behavior may affect the occurrence of other behaviors. We provide the reader with operational definitions and a discus-sion of dependent variables that researchers have used; we realize that the list is not exhaustive and that the field does not have standard operational definitions for these behaviors.

*Acceptance,* the occurrence of the bite or drink entering the mouth, is often the first in the chain of feeding behaviors that researchers target for in-tervention. In LaRue et al. (2011), observers scored the occurrence of acceptance if a child leaned to-ward the spoon or cup and opened his or her mouth in the absence of negative vocalizations and inap-propriate behavior, so that the feeder could deposit the entire bolus of food (except for an amount smaller than the size of a pea) or any amount of liq-uid in the mouth within 5 seconds of presentation. Notice that LaRue et al.'s definition included qual-ifiers such as "leaned toward the spoon or cup in the absence of negative vocalizations" and "within 5 seconds of presentation." LaRue et al. included these qualifiers to ensure that observers were measuring children's rather than feeders' behav-ior. Observers scored acceptance if a child leaned forward soon after the bite or drink presentation and opened his or her mouth so that the feeder could put the bite or drink in the child's mouth. By contrast, observers did not score acceptance if the child's mouth was open because he or she was crying, which gave the feeder the opportunity to put the bite or drink in the mouth. Ideally, in-tervention increases feeding compliance, and dis-tinguishing between child compliance and feeder behavior is important for determining progress. Observers in LaRue et al. scored the occurrence of acceptance for each bite or drink presentation and converted occurrences to a percentage after dividing the occurrences of acceptance by the number of presented bites or drinks.

Children in Peterson, Piazza, and Volkert (2016) self-fed, and "observers scored the occurrence of acceptance when the child used the utensil or his fingers to put the entire bite of food in his mouth within 8 s of presentation, not including placement of the bite in the mouth during re-presentation" (p. 5). Peterson et al. converted occurrences of acceptance to a percentage after dividing the number of accepted bites by the number of presented bites. Peterson et al. described the bite presentation as one piece of food measuring 0.6 × 0.6 × 0.6 centimeters, and the feeder restricted the operant by presenting only one bite at a time. Observers scored acceptance only if the child put the entire bite in his mouth within 8 seconds of the feeder placing the bite in front of the child. Acceptance, in this case, conveyed information about how much food entered the child's mouth, and it accounted for the number of bites available to the child to accept from session to session.

*Inappropriate mealtime behavior* may refer to numerous behaviors that disrupt feeding and that differ along many dimensions. Some researchers have addressed this dilemma by conceptualizing inappropriate mealtime behavior as behavior a child emits with his or her external body parts, such as the head, hands, arms, and legs, that prevents solids, liquids, or both from entering or remaining in the mouth. These researchers have separated inappropriate mealtime behavior from behaviors the child emits with his or her mouth, such as expulsion and packing, and behaviors that have a putative physiological basis, such as coughing, gagging, and vomiting. For example, observers in Ibañez, Piazza, and Peterson (2019) scored inappropriate mealtime behavior "when the utensil was in arm's reach of the child and the child turned his head 45° or greater away from the utensil during a bite or drink presentation; used his hand to contact the utensil, food or drink, or the feeder's hand or arm anywhere from the elbow down while the feeder was presenting the bite or drink; threw food, liquids, or utensils; or blocked his mouth with his hand, bib, or toys" (p. 1009). Notice that Ibañez et al.'s operational definition qualifies that the utensil must be in arm's reach of the child, because the defined behavior can occur only when a utensil is present. Observers scored the frequency of inappropriate mealtime behavior and converted it to a rate by dividing the number of inappropriate mealtime behaviors by the duration the utensil was in arm's reach of the child. Controlling for the presence of the utensil may be important in cases where the duration of utensil presence may differ markedly from phase to phase or from condition to condition.

*Expulsion* is food or liquid exiting the mouth. For example, Wilkins, Piazza, Groff, and Vaz (2011) defined expulsion for liquids as each time any amount of liquid (pea size or larger) that the child had not swallowed was visible outside the lips after any amount of liquid had passed the plane of the lips; and expulsion for solids as each time any amount of food (pea size or larger) that the child had not swallowed was visible outside the lips after the entire bolus of food had passed the plane of the lips. Observers in Wilkins et al. scored the frequency of expulsion and presented the data as expulsions per bite. As with many feeding behaviors, the opportunity to engage in expulsion will affect rates of expulsion, and the clinician should consider which method of data presentation is most appropriate to address the clinical problem or research question. For example, the clinician might calculate expulsions per bite if opportunity to expel is fixed (e.g., based on number of presented bites), but expulsions per opportunity if opportunity to expel varies, such as during re-presentation.

*Mouth clean* is a product measure of swallowing that we often use, because swallowing is difficult to measure reliably in our clinical experience. For example, observers in Kadey, Piazza, Rivas, and Zeleny (2013) scored "mouth clean if no food larger than a pea was in [the child's] mouth, unless the absence of food was the result of expulsion" (p. 540). The feeder in Kadey et al. checked the child's mouth 30 seconds after the bite entered the mouth by saying, "Show me." The mouth check gave observers the opportunity to score mouth clean or *pack*, which is the converse of mouth clean. For example, observers in Wilkins et al. (2014) scored "pack if the entire bite (with the exception of food smaller than a pea) entered the child's mouth, and food larger than a pea was in the child's mouth at the 30-s check" (p. 4). Kadey et al. and Wilkins et al. converted mouth clean or pack, respectively, to a percentage after dividing the number of occurrences of mouth clean or pack, respectively, by the number of bites that entered the child's mouth. Note that the denominator in Kadey et al. and Wilkins et al. was number of bites that entered the mouth, meaning that no opportunities for mouth clean or pack occurred if no bites entered the child's mouth; this is important for readers to remember when interpreting data from studies that use this measure. Note also that Kadey et al. and Wilkins et al. included a caveat that the child could have a mouth clean if a small amount of food remained in the mouth, because even typical feeders may have residue in the mouth after swallowing. The researchers based the size of the residue (pea size in these studies) on the amount of presented food. In both studies, bolus sizes were a level small maroon spoon for six children, a half-level small maroon spoon for four children, and a level baby spoon for two children in Wilkins et al., and a level small maroon spoon for the child in Kadey et al. The size of the acceptable residue might change if the presented bolus was larger or smaller. For example, the acceptable residue in Volkert, Peterson, Zeleny, and Piazza (2014) was the size of a grain of rice, because the presented bolus was a piece of food measuring 0.6 × 0.6 × 0.6 centimeters.

Although chewing is an important feeding skill, there is a relative dearth of applied-behavior-analytic research on teaching children with feeding disorders to chew. In a notable exception, Volkert et al. (2014) scored a *chew* "each time the child's teeth and/or jaw completed one up-and-down motion with the teeth parted at least 1.3 cm following a verbal or model prompt while food was visible anywhere in the mouth except the center of the tongue or between the front teeth" (p. 708). One limitation of this definition is that it did not differentiate rotary chews from an immature chewing pattern such as munching (Volkert, Piazza, Vaz, & Frese, 2013). One unique and important feature of Volkert et al. (2014), however, was that the researchers included a measure of mastication. They defined *mastication* as food with pieces no larger than 0.2 × 0.2 centimeters in a liquid medium at the mastication check. The mastication check was like the mouth check described by Kadey et al. (2013), but observers determined whether the child had masticated rather than swallowed the bite. One important future direction for research on pediatric feeding disorders is to develop more sophisticated measures of chewing, perhaps using automated methods (Hadley, Krival, Ridgel, Hahn, & Tyler, 2015), which will allow investigators to determine whether a child's chewing skills are appropriate for the child's age, developmental level, or a combination.

## ETIOLOGY

Research has suggested that the etiology of feeding disorders is complex and multifactorial (Rommel, Meyer, Feenstra, & Veereman-Wauters, 2003). For example, Rommel et al. (2003) characterized the feeding disorders of 700 children referred for assessment and treatment of severe feeding difficulties as medical (86%), oral–motor (61%), and/or behavioral (18%). Combined causes, such as medical, behavioral, and/or oral–motor, for the feeding disorder occurred in over 60% of children. Other researchers have found that feeding disorders have neurological (62%), structural (53%), behavioral (43%), cardiorespiratory (34%), and metabolic (12%) causes, with most children having causes in two or more categories simultaneously (Burklow, McGrath, Valerius, & Rudolph, 2002; Davis, Bruce, Cojin, Mousa, & Hyman, 2010). Feeding disorders are also prevalent among specific diagnostic groups, such as children with autism spectrum disorder, cerebral palsy, and Down syndrome (Bandini et al., 2010).

The high prevalence of medical conditions and oral–motor dysfunction in children with feeding disorders suggests that biological factors play an important role in the etiology and maintenance of feeding disorders. Children with chronic medical problems that affect the digestive system directly, such as congenital defects of the gastrointestinal tract, delayed gastric emptying, food allergies, gastroesophageal reflux disease, malabsorption, or metabolic disorders, may associate eating with fatigue, nausea, pain, or a combination. For example, children with gastroesophageal reflux disease may associate eating with the pain that occurs when excess acid erupts into the esophagus. Nausea plays an important role in the development of food aversions (Schafe & Bernstein, 1996), and when nausea is paired with eating, aversions to tastes may develop after only one or a few trials, may generalize to different foods, and may be highly treatment-resistant.

Researchers estimate that feeding disorders occur in 40–70% of children with chronic medical conditions (Davis et al., 2010; Douglas & Byron, 1996; Lukens & Silverman, 2014; Thommessen, Heiberg, Kase, Larsen, & Riis, 1991), suggesting that the presence of other chronic medical problems, such as bronchopulmonary dysplasia, may contribute to the etiology of feeding disorders. Infants with complex medical histories are subject to numerous invasive diagnostic tests and procedures that involve manipulation of the face and mouth, such as laryngoscopy. Such a child may come to associate the presentation of items to the mouth with discomfort, pain, or both. From the child's perspective, a spoon may be indistinguishable from a laryngoscope or other devices that professionals use during invasive medical procedures and tests.

Caregivers of chronically hospitalized and medically fragile children often report oral aversions that affect feeding and other activities associated with the face and mouth, such as face washing and tooth brushing.

Oral–motor dysfunction may include difficulties sucking, difficulties with bolus propulsion, inability to lateralize food from one side to another, difficulties swallowing, and tongue thrust, and these problems may affect a child's ability and motivation to eat (Darrow & Harley, 1998). The child's refusal to eat may cause or exacerbate preexisting oral–motor dysfunction and further contribute to the child's failure to develop appropriate oral–motor skills. That is, a child who refuses to eat does not have the opportunity to practice the skill of eating and does not develop the oral–motor skills to become a competent eater.

When eating is paired with an aversive experience, the child may develop refusal behavior such as batting at the spoon, head turning, or covering the mouth to avoid eating. These behaviors may increase in frequency as a function of caregiver responses to child behavior during meals. Borrero, Woods, Borrero, Masler, and Lesser (2010) conducted observations of 25 children with feeding disorders and their caregivers to describe and quantify the caregivers' responses to the children's inappropriate mealtime behavior. Researchers compared conditional probabilities of a caregiver providing attention, escape, or a tangible item following refusal or acceptance to the unconditioned probabilities of each event. Observations indicated that caregivers coaxed, removed the spoon, threatened to take away preferred items, presented preferred foods, or engaged in a combination of these events following refusal behavior. Escape in the form of spoon removal or meal termination and attention in the form of coaxing, reprimands, and statements of concern most frequently followed refusal behavior. Similarly, Piazza, Fisher, et al. (2003) observed caregivers and children with feeding disorders during meals. Caregivers responded to inappropriate mealtime behavior with one or more of the following consequences: (1) providing escape from bites of food or the meal, (2) coaxing or reprimanding (e.g., "Eat your peas, they are good for you"), or (3) providing a toy or preferred food.

## EVALUATION

A behavior analyst should consider referring a child with a feeding disorder for evaluation by an interdisciplinary team, given the evidence that the cause of feeding disorders is multifactorial (Rommel et al., 2003). The goal of evaluation should be to determine whether anatomical, medical, or oral–motor skill deficits contribute to the child's feeding disorder and whether the child is a safe oral feeder. Members of such a team might include a behavior analyst, a dietitian, a gastroenterologist or the child's primary physician, and an occupational or speech therapist. A behavior analyst should not underestimate the negative consequences of feeding a child before appropriate evaluation. At a minimum, the behavior analyst should consult the child's primary physician, describe the proposed course of assessment and treatment, and obtain medical clearance to start therapy. Failure to identify a medical condition or oral–motor skill deficits before beginning therapy could result in worsening of the feeding disorder or even death. For example, introducing food variety to promote proper nutrient intake is a reasonable goal for a child with a feeding disorder, but a reaction to an unidentified food allergy could cause anaphylaxis, which is a severe, potentially life-threatening event (Sicherer & Sampson, 2010). In addition, some children with oral–motor dysfunction do not manage specific consistencies of solids, liquids, or both, and other children are not safe oral feeders with solids or liquids of any consistency. Oral–motor dysfunction may be associated with aspiration due to solids or liquids entering the airway, which can cause medical problems such as pneumonia. An evaluation by a swallow specialist, usually an occupational or speech therapist, can determine whether oral–motor dysfunction may be causing or contributing to a child's feeding disorder and determine whether the child is a safe oral feeder (Schwarz, Corredor, Fisher-Medina, Cohen, & Rabinowitz, 2001). A dietitian calculates the child's caloric, hydrational, and nutritional needs and determines whether the child requires diet modifications. For example, a child with a glycogen storage disorder requires careful monitoring of blood sugar levels and a diet that restricts simple sugars. Drops in blood sugar levels may cause seizures, coma, and even death (Goto, Arah, Goto, Terauchi, & Noda, 2013).

Results of the interdisciplinary evaluation may indicate that the child needs medical treatment, consistency or texture manipulations, a special diet, or a combination, and these interventions may resolve the child's feeding disorder. Some children, however, may not start feeding or may not feed well even after interdisciplinary intervention, particularly if they engage in refusal behavior. In these cases, a qualified behavior analyst can manipulate mealtime antecedents and consequences to determine whether they affect the child's refusal behavior.

Piazza, Fisher, et al. (2003) used analogue functional analyses to assess the effects of caregiver consequences on child behavior. Inappropriate mealtime behavior, such as batting at the spoon and head turning, produced attention, such as coaxing and brief verbal reprimands, during the *attention* condition; a break from the bite or drink presentation during the *escape* condition; access to a tangible item, such as a preferred food, during the *tangible* condition; and no differential consequence during the *control* condition. Escape from bite or drink presentations functioned as negative reinforcement for the inappropriate mealtime behavior of 9 of the 10 children who showed differential responding during the functional analyses. Access to adult attention or tangible items functioned as positive reinforcement for the inappropriate mealtime behavior of 8 of the 10 children who showed differential responding during the functional analyses. Girolami and Scotti (2001) found that escape from food presentation and mealtime demands for two children, and contingent access to toys and attention for one child, functioned as reinforcement for mealtime behavior problems such as aggression and spitting out food. Najdowski et al. (2008) trained caregivers to conduct functional analyses in which a caregiver placed a plate of nonpreferred food on the table in front of a child in the attention, escape, and tangible conditions and preferred food in the control condition. The caregiver washed dishes in the attention and control conditions and provided attention following inappropriate mealtime behavior in the attention condition. The caregiver sat next to the child; provided continuous prompts to "Take a bite"; followed the child with the plate if the child left the chair; used three-step prompting; and removed the bite if the child engaged in inappropriate mealtime behavior in the demand condition. Unlike in the Piazza, Fisher, et al. (2003) and Girolami and Scotti (2001) studies, escape was the only reinforcer identified for inappropriate mealtime behavior. Najdowski et al. noted that the experimental preparation they used might have accounted for the difference in findings.

Bachmeyer, Kirkwood, Criscito, Mauzy, and Berth (2019) conducted two functional analyses with three children with feeding disorders: one with the procedure Piazza, Fisher, et al. (2003) described and one with the procedure Najdowski et al. (2008) described. Bachmeyer et al. then com-pared variations of extinction matched to the results of each functional analysis. Both analyses identified escape and attention as reinforcement for inappropriate mealtime behavior, and escape and attention extinction were necessary to achieve a clinically acceptable outcome for one participant. For the other two participants, the Piazza, Fisher, et al. procedure identified multiple reinforcers for inappropriate mealtime behavior, but the Najdowski et al. procedure identified only escape as the reinforcer for inappropriate mealtime behavior. For those two participants, the intervention matched to the reinforcers identified by the Piazza, Fisher, et al. procedure produced a clinically acceptable outcome, but the intervention matched to the reinforcer identified by the Najdowski et al. procedure did not.

The differential responding demonstrated by participants across test and control conditions in Bachmeyer et al. (2019), Girolami and Scotti (2001), Najdowski et al. (2008), and Piazza, Fisher, et al. (2003) suggest that even if the etiology of a pediatric feeding disorder is multiple and complex, environmental events may reinforce inappropriate mealtime behavior. This finding is important, because (1) we may not be able to identify the cause of the child's feeding disorder; (2) even if we identify the cause, that cause may be immutable, such as a history of prematurity; and (3) the underlying cause may not be related to the condition(s) that maintains the behavior (Iwata et al., 1982/1994). We can, however, change how we respond to the child's inappropriate mealtime behavior, and such changes may be effective as treatment.

## TREATMENT

Evaluations of treatments based on theories of operant conditioning have formed the bulk of the intervention research on pediatric feeding disorders. Kerwin (1999) surveyed peer-reviewed medical and psychological journals to identify studies that reported on psychosocial or behavioral interventions for pediatric feeding disorders. She used the modified criteria of the Task Force on Promotion and Dissemination of Psychological Procedures (1995) to identify methodologically rigorous studies that met the criteria and to classify interventions for pediatric feeding disorders that were well established, probably efficacious, or promising. Analysis of the 29 studies that met the criteria indicated that the only well-established interventions were behavioral interventions that included

(1) positive reinforcement of appropriate feeding behavior and ignoring inappropriate mealtime behavior, and (2) positive reinforcement of appropriate feeding behavior and physical guidance of the appropriate feeding behavior (e.g., Ahearn, Kerwin, Eicher, Shantz, & Swearingin, 1996; Kerwin, Ahearn, Eicher, & Burd, 1995; Linscheid, Oliver, Blyler, & Palmer, 1978; Piazza, Anderson, & Fisher, 1993; Riordan, Iwata, Finney, Wohl, & Stanley, 1984; Riordan, Iwata, Wohl, & Finney, 1980; Stark, Powers, Jelalian, Rape, & Miller, 1994).

Volkert and Piazza (2012) extended Kerwin (1999), using the same criteria to identify studies of interventions for pediatric feeding disorders and to categorize the level of empirical support for those interventions. Volkert and Piazza identified 74 studies that met the inclusion criteria. Analysis of those studies showed that differential reinforcement of alternative behavior, escape extinction and putative escape extinction, and physical guidance for self-feeding were well-established interventions; non-nutritive sucking (Field et al., 1982; Sehgal, Prakash, Gupta, Mohan, & Anand, 1990) and oral stimulation (Fucile, Gisel, & Lau, 2002; Rocha, Moreira, Pimenta, Ramos, & Lucena, 2007) were probably efficacious interventions; and oral support (Boiron, Nobrega, Roux, Henrot, & Saliba, 2007; Einarsson-Backes, Deitz, Price, Glass, & Hays, 1994), stimulus fading (e.g., Shore, Babbit, Williams, Coe, & Snyder, 1998), and simultaneous presentation without escape extinction (e.g., Ahearn, 2003; Buckley & Newchok, 2005; Piazza et al., 2002) were promising interventions. Like Kerwin, Volkert and Piazza found that most empirically supported interventions were behavior-analytic. Unlike Kerwin, however, they found that three interventions (non-nutritive sucking, oral stimulation, and oral support) did not incorporate behavior-analytic principles or procedures. These studies appeared in journals from the fields of developmental medicine, occupational therapy, otorhinolaryngology, and pediatrics, and focused on increasing oral intake in premature infants. For the purposes of this chapter, we review interventions aimed at increasing acceptance, decreasing inappropriate mealtime behavior, decreasing expulsion, increasing mouth clean and decreasing packing, and teaching chewing skills.

## Acceptance

Results of the analysis by Volkert and Piazza (2012) showed that *differential reinforcement of alternative behavior* was a well-established intervention for pediatric feeding disorders. Researchers have used differential reinforcement in several ways that include, but are not limited to, immediate (Patel, Piazza, Martinez, Volkert, & Santana, 2002) or delayed (Kern & Marder, 1996; Riordan et al., 1984) reinforcement with stimuli that researchers selected arbitrarily (Kern & Marder, 1996; Casey, Cooper-Brown, Wacker, & Rankin, 2006) or with systematic preference assessments (Buckley, Strunck, & Newchok, 2005), or with tokens the child could exchange for meal discontinuation (Kahng, Boscoe, & Byrne, 2003). For example, Peterson, Volkert, and Zeleny (2015) used differential reinforcement for two children with a feeding disorder to increase self-drinking from a cup. Researchers conducted a multiple-stimulus-without-replacement assessment before each session and used the three most preferred stimuli as reinforcement for self-drinking. The researchers increased the amount of liquid in the cup after the child's self-drinking with the smaller amount increased with differential reinforcement.

Stark et al. (1996) randomly assigned nine children with cystic fibrosis to a behavioral intervention or a wait-list control group and used calories consumed and weight gain as the dependent variables. The multicomponent behavioral intervention included caregiver praise, a star chart, and access to privileges for appropriate feeding behavior. Caloric intake increased to 1,032 calories per day and mean weight gain was 1.7 kilograms for the group receiving the behavioral intervention, compared to 244 calories and 0 kilograms, respectively, for the control group. Participants maintained higher levels of caloric intake relative to baseline at 3- and 6-month follow-ups. Other researchers have used differential reinforcement alone and in combination with other procedures, such as response cost (Kahng, Tarbox, & Wilke, 2001), to increase acceptance of solids (Werle, Murphy, & Budd, 1993), liquids (Kelley, Piazza, & Fisher, 2003), or both (Roth, Williams, & Paul, 2010). One study demonstrated increased acceptance and decreased self-injurious behavior during noncontingent reinforcement (Wilder, Normand, & Atwell, 2005).

Manipulating antecedents is another method that researchers have used to increase the food or liquid acceptance of children with feeding disorders. For example, Meier, Fryling, and Wallace (2012) and Patel et al. (2007) used *high-probability instructions*, such as "Put an empty spoon in your mouth," that were like those of the target behavior (e.g., "Take a bite") to increase acceptance. *Simul-*

*taneous presentation* is an antecedent procedure in which the feeder presents preferred food and non-preferred food together, like a nonpreferred pea on a preferred chip. For example, Ahearn (2003) added condiments to increase vegetable consumption, and Tiger and Hanley (2006) added chocolate to milk to increase milk consumption. Piazza et al. (2002) compared *simultaneous* and *sequential* presentation in an extension of Kern and Marder (1996). The feeder presented a bite of nonpreferred food on a bite of preferred food in the simultaneous condition or presented the bite of preferred food if the child ate the bite of nonpreferred food in the sequential condition. Acceptance increased for two of three participants in the simultaneous but not the sequential condition. Acceptance for the third participant increased when the feeder implemented simultaneous presentation and physical guidance, but not when the feeder implemented sequential presentation and physical guidance.

### Acceptance and Inappropriate Mealtime Behavior

Before researchers began conducting functional analyses of inappropriate mealtime behavior, they developed procedures for putative escape extinction, based on the assumption that escape from bites or drinks functioned as negative reinforcement for inappropriate mealtime behavior. The procedures researchers have studied most often are *nonremoval of the spoon* (Hoch, Babbitt, Coe, Krell, & Hackbert, 1994) and *physical guidance* (Ahearn et al., 1996), and both involve discontinuing the hypothesized response–reinforcer relation. Ahearn et al. (1996) showed that nonremoval of the spoon and physical guidance increased acceptance. During nonremoval of the spoon, the feeder held the bite near the child's lips until the feeder could deposit the bite into the mouth. During physical guidance, the feeder applied gentle pressure to the mandibular junction of the jaw to open the mouth and deposited the bite if the child did not accept it. Ahearn et al. assessed caregiver acceptability for the interventions by asking each caregiver which treatment he or she preferred. All caregivers chose physical guidance, which was associated with fewer corollary behaviors (such as disruptions) for all children and with shorter meal durations for two of the three children.

Studies by Hoch et al. (1994) and Ahearn et al. (1996) are representative of other studies on putative escape extinction, in that researchers included differential or noncontingent reinforcement (Cooper et al., 1995) in an intervention package. Piazza, Patel, Gulotta, Sevin, and Layer (2003) attempted to clarify the relative contributions of positive reinforcement and putative escape extinction. Differential positive reinforcement of mouth clean, in which the feeder provided attention and tangible items for mouth clean and inappropriate mealtime behavior produced escape, was not effective for increasing acceptance or decreasing inappropriate mealtime behavior. Acceptance increased and inappropriate mealtime behavior decreased only when the feeder implemented putative escape extinction. Inappropriate mealtime behavior and negative vocalizations were lower for some children during differential reinforcement and putative escape extinction relative to putative escape extinction alone, but the differences were often small or not replicated in subsequent phases. Piazza, Patel, et al. concluded that putative escape extinction was necessary to increase acceptance and decrease inappropriate mealtime behavior, but that differential positive reinforcement for mouth clean may have contributed to lower levels of inappropriate mealtime behavior, negative vocalizations, or both for some children when combined with putative escape extinction. A study by Reed et al. (2004) produced similar results for noncontingent reinforcement and putative escape extinction, except that the effects of noncontingent reinforcement on inappropriate mealtime behavior and negative vocalizations were less robust than those for differential positive reinforcement in Piazza, Patel, et al. (2003).

Peterson, Piazza, Ibañez, and Fisher (2019) conducted a randomized controlled trial to evaluate the effects of a behavior-analytic intervention (noncontingent reinforcement and nonremoval of the spoon) relative to a wait-list control to determine whether the food selectivity of young children with autism spectrum disorder would resolve over time without intervention. The researchers randomly assigned three children to the behavior-analytic intervention and three children to the wait-list control group. Consumption increased for the three children in the behavior-analytic group, but not for the children in the wait-list control group.

Researchers based the behavior-analytic interventions described above on the assumption that escape from bites or drinks would function as reinforcement for inappropriate mealtime behavior in the absence of a formal functional analysis (Ahearn et al., 1996; Cooper et al., 1995; Hoch et al., 1994). By contrast, Bachmeyer et al. (2009) used a functional analysis to determine that escape from bites or drinks and adult attention reinforced the inappropriate mealtime behavior of four children with feeding disorders. Bachmeyer et al. then evaluated the effects of variations of extinction that matched one or both functional reinforcers: (1) escape extinction and attention following inappropriate mealtime behavior, (2) attention extinction and escape following inappropriate mealtime behavior, and (3) escape extinction and attention extinction. Results showed that variations of extinction that discontinued delivery of the reinforcers for inappropriate mealtime behavior identified by the functional analysis (escape and attention), were necessary to reduce inappropriate mealtime behavior to clinically acceptable rates and to increase acceptance to high, stable levels. LaRue et al. (2011) tested the effects of a negative-reinforcement-based intervention (differential negative reinforcement and nonremoval of the spoon with re-presentation) with 11 children whose inappropriate mealtime behavior was maintained by escape. Mouth clean produced a 30-second break from bite or drink presentations during differential negative reinforcement. Acceptance increased and inappropriate mealtime behavior decreased when the feeder implemented nonremoval of the spoon and re-presentation; differential negative reinforcement for mouth clean had no effect on behavior, either alone or in combination with nonremoval of the spoon and re-presentation.

The studies on escape extinction reviewed above included consequence manipulations such as differential reinforcement for acceptance and nonremoval of the spoon (e.g., Piazza, Patel, et al., 2003; Reed et al., 2004). Researchers also have tested antecedent manipulations with escape extinction or putative escape extinction to increase acceptance. Patel et al. (2006) combined high-probability instructions that were like those for the low-probability instruction with nonremoval of the spoon to increase acceptance. Dawson et al. (2003), by contrast, showed that high-probability instructions did not differentially affect levels of acceptance when combined with nonremoval of the spoon.

Mueller, Piazza, Patel, Kelley, and Pruett (2004) used *blending*, a variation of simultaneous presentation, with differential or noncontingent positive reinforcement and nonremoval of the spoon to increase consumption for two children with a feeding disorder. Blending or mixing preferred and nonpreferred foods, such as preferred yogurt mixed with nonpreferred green-bean puree, produced an increase in acceptance and mouth clean and decreased inappropriate mealtime behavior. The researchers gradually increased the ratio of nonpreferred to preferred food until the children were consuming the nonpreferred food alone.

Mueller et al. (2004) used a *fading* component to achieve the targeted outcome; other researchers have used various fading procedures with nonremoval of the spoon or physical guidance. Groff, Piazza, Volkert, and Jostad (2014) used a syringe to deposit solids and liquids into the mouth of a child who clenched his teeth during presentation, gradually increased the volume of solids and liquids in the syringe, and then faded from syringe to spoon for solids and syringe to cup for liquids. During fading, the researchers taped the syringe to a spoon or a cup, so the tip of the syringe protruded from the tip of the spoon or lip of the cup by 5 centimeters, and moved the tip of the syringe and the tip of the spoon or lip of the cup closer together. The child began eating from a spoon and drinking from the cup without the syringe during probe sessions the feeder conducted between fading steps. Other dimensions on which researchers have conducted fading include bite number (Najdowski, Wallace, Doney, & Ghezzi, 2003), bottle to spoon (Johnson & Babbitt, 1993), high- to low-probability demands (Penrod, Gardella, & Fernand, 2012), liquid to baby food (Bachmeyer, Gulotta, & Piazza, 2013), preferred to nonpreferred liquid type (Luiselli, Ricciardi, & Gilligan, 2005), liquid volume (Hagopian, Farrell, & Amari, 1996), portion size (Freeman & Piazza, 1998), spoon distance (Rivas, Piazza, Patel, & Bachmeyer, 2010), food variety (Valdimarsdottir, Halldorsdottir, & Sigurådóttir, 2010), spoon to cup (Babbitt, Shore, Smith, Williams, & Coe, 2001), and texture (Luiselli & Gleason, 1987; Shore et al., 1998).

## Alternative Interventions

Recent research has compared the effects of behavior-analytic interventions for pediatric feeding disorders to ones that are popular among non-behavior-analytic professionals. For example, Addison et al. (2012) compared the effects of a behavior-analytic intervention to a *sensory-integration intervention*. A speech therapist and two occupational therapists developed individualized sensory-integration interventions for the two participants. Acceptance and amount consumed increased and inappropriate mealtime behavior decreased during the behavior-analytic but not the sensory-integration intervention. Peterson et al. (2016) conducted a randomized controlled trial of a behavior-analytic versus a modified *sequential-oral-sensory approach* to treat the food selectivity of six young children with autism spectrum disorder. Peterson et al. randomly assigned three children to the behavior-analytic intervention and three children to the modified sequential-oral-sensory intervention, compared the effects across novel, healthy target foods, and tested for generalization of intervention effects. Consumption of novel, healthy target foods increased for the children in the behavior-analytic intervention group, but not for the children in the modified sequential-oral-sensory group. Peterson et al. then implemented the behavior-analytic intervention with the children previously assigned to the modified sequential-oral-sensory intervention group. Consumption of novel, healthy target foods increased during the behavior-analytic intervention, and Peterson et al. observed a potential generalization effect for foods that had been exposed to the modified sequential-oral-sensory intervention.

## Expulsion

Results of functional analysis studies show that escape from bites or drinks functions as negative reinforcement for inappropriate mealtime behavior, but inappropriate mealtime behavior is probably not the only behavior that produces escape. For example, Coe et al. (1997) used nonremoval of the spoon to increase the acceptance of two children with a feeding disorder and observed simultaneous increases in expulsion. Coe et al. hypothesized that negative reinforcement in the form of escape from swallowing food reinforced expulsion. *Re-presentation*, or scooping up expelled food and placing it back into the mouth or getting a new bite of the same food, resulted in near-zero levels of expulsion.

Although Coe et al. (1997) and Sevin, Gulotta, Sierp, Rosica, and Miller (2002) demonstrated the effectiveness of re-presentation, others have found that re-presentation was not effective consistently. For example, Wilkins et al. (2011) added a *chin prompt* when nonremoval of the spoon plus re-presentation did not decrease expulsion. During the chin prompt, the feeder placed gentle upward pressure on the child's chin as the feeder deposited the bite or drink during re-presentation, which reduced expulsion. Shalev, Milnes, Piazza, and Kozisek (2018) compared a *modified chin prompt*, in which the feeder waited for the child's jaw to relax and then placed gentle upward pressure on the chin while depositing the drink, with *reclined*

*seating*, in which the feeder reclined the highchair from its upright position. Expulsion decreased and was equivalent for the two interventions. Patel, Piazza, Santana, and Volkert (2002) evaluated the effects of *type and texture of food* (Munk & Repp, 1994) on expulsion. Rates of expulsion were higher when the feeder presented meat relative to other foods, and expulsion decreased when the researchers lowered the texture of meat.

*Utensil manipulation* is another strategy researchers have used to decrease expulsion (Dempsey, Piazza, Groff, & Kozisek, 2011; Gulotta, Piazza, Patel, & Layer, 2005; Hoch, Babbitt, Coe, Duncan, & Trusty, 1995; Volkert, Vaz, Piazza, Frese, & Barnett, 2011). For example, Girolami, Boscoe, and Roscoe (2007) showed that presenting and re-presenting bites on a Nuk, which is a bristled utensil caregivers use to initiate toothbrushing with infants, reduced expels relative to presentation and re-presentation of bites on a spoon or on a spoon and a Nuk, respectively. Wilkins et al. (2014) compared presentation of bites on a spoon or a Nuk with 12 children during initial intervention. Acceptance increased and inappropriate mealtime behavior decreased for 8 of 12 children. Five of the 8 had lower levels of expulsion, and 4 of the 8 had higher levels of mouth clean, when the feeder presented bites on the Nuk.

## Mouth Clean and Pack

Hoch et al. (1994) proposed that the feeder should provide reinforcement for a behavior that occurs early in the chain of feeding behaviors, such as acceptance, and then shift reinforcement to a behavior that occurs later in the chain, such as swallowing. To that end, Patel, Piazza, Martinez, et al. (2002) compared the effects of differential positive reinforcement for acceptance versus mouth clean. When differential reinforcement did not increase acceptance or mouth clean, the feeder added putative escape extinction. Acceptance and mouth clean increased and inappropriate mealtime behavior decreased. Patel et al. concluded that the point in the chain in which the feeder provided differential reinforcement was not as important as putative escape extinction for increasing acceptance and mouth clean and decreasing inappropriate mealtime behavior.

Two consequence-based interventions researchers have used to increase mouth clean and decrease packing are *redistribution* (Girolami et al., 2007; Gulotta et al., 2005; Levin, Volkert, & Piazza, 2014; Sevin et al., 2002; Stubbs, Volkert, Rubio, & Ottinger, 2017) and a *chaser* (Vaz, Piazza, Stewart, Volkert, & Groff, 2012). For example, Sevin et al. (2002) used a Nuk brush during redistribution to remove packed food from the participant's mouth and place the food on the tongue. Redistribution increased mouth clean and decreased packing. Volkert et al. (2011) obtained similar results by using a *flipped spoon* during redistribution. The feeder removed packed food with a spoon, inserted the spoon with the bite into the participant's mouth, turned the spoon 180°, and dragged the bowl of the spoon along the tongue toward the lips to deposit the previously packed bite. The feeder in Vaz et al. (2012) gave the child a chaser (a liquid or solid the child consistently accepted and swallowed) to reduce packing. The feeder presented the chaser either immediately after he or she deposited the target bite into the child's mouth for two children, or 15 seconds after he or she deposited the target bite for a third child.

Researchers in the studies described above used a Nuk or a flipped spoon to redistribute packed food. Researchers have also evaluated the effects of utensil manipulation as an antecedent intervention (Dempsey et al., 2011; Sharp, Odom, & Jaquess, 2012; Stubbs et al., 2017). For example, Sharp, Harker, and Jaquess (2010) compared the effects of presentation on an upright spoon, a flipped spoon, or a Nuk. Levels of mouth clean increased for the flipped spoon and Nuk but were not clinically acceptable. Other studies have shown clinically acceptable increases in mouth clean and decreases in packing with flipped-spoon presentation (Rivas, Piazza, Kadey, Volkert, & Stewart, 2011; Sharp et al., 2012; Stubbs et al., 2017), Nuk presentation (Gulotta et al., 2005; Sevin et al., 2002), or a combination of flipped spoon and chin prompt (Dempsey et al., 2011).

Texture or food consistency is another antecedent variable that affects levels of mouth clean and pack (Bachmeyer et al., 2013; Kadey et al., 2013; Patel, Piazza, Layer, Coleman, & Swartzwelder, 2005; Sharp & Jaquess, 2009). For example, Kadey et al. (2013) assessed food texture and food type to identify potential causes of one young girl's packing. First, the researchers compared levels of mouth clean with chopped food (table food cut into small pieces), wet ground food (small chunks of food in a wet medium), and pureed food (table food blended until smooth). The results showed that levels of mouth clean were highest with pureed food, but even those levels were not acceptable clinically. When the researchers presented foods individually, they determined that the child

had mouth clean with some pureed foods but not others. The researchers pureed food in a smoothie blender during a second texture assessment, and levels of mouth clean were higher than with the other textures.

Finally, researchers have used fading to increase mouth clean and decrease pack. For example, the goal for the child in Patel, Piazza, Kelly, Ochsner, and Santana (2001) was to increase his intake of a calorically dense beverage, Carnation Instant Breakfast with whole milk. The child refused the breakfast drink, but he did drink water. Therefore, the researchers added and gradually increased the amount of the drink powder in water and subsequently replaced the water with milk. Other dimensions along which researchers have faded to increase mouth clean and decrease pack are liquid to baby food (Bachmeyer et al., 2013), spoon to cup (Groff, Piazza, Zeleny, & Dempsey, 2011), syringe to spoon, and syringe to cup (Groff et al., 2014).

## Chewing

Chewing is a skill that emerges in typically eating children as the caregiver increases the texture of presented food, which is usually around 12 months of age. In our experience, many children with feeding disorders do not begin chewing at or after 12 months of age when the caregiver increases food texture. Nevertheless, caregivers often base the texture of presented food on a child's age rather than the child's chewing skills. A mismatch between the texture of presented food and the child's chewing skills increases the risk of aspiration, particularly if the child swallows the food without masticating it sufficiently (Patel et al., 2005). Children who lack appropriate chewing skills may develop inappropriate compensatory behavior, such as using the tongue to push food against the roof of the mouth. We often see this behavior emerge when the caregiver presents meltable solids, such as cookies, crackers, and chips. The child learns that he or she can use the tongue to moisten and break apart the meltable solid, and this behavior does not change when the caregiver presents foods that do not melt or break apart with saliva, such as meats. These children reach an impasse in which they consume meltable solids and small amounts of more difficult foods, such as pizza, but they cannot advance any further. They often have excessive meal lengths and do not consume sufficient calories for weight gain and growth, because their chewing skills are not efficient and effective. We have found that teaching a child to chew is the strategy that is most effective for advancing texture.

For example, our group evaluated a multicomponent intervention to increase chews per bite, assess mastication, and eliminate early swallowing, which observers scored at the mastication check if no food was visible in the mouth and the food was not absent because of expulsion (Volkert et al., 2014). Caregivers served as feeders and used graduated verbal, model, and physical prompting to teach the children in sequential steps to chew (1) on an empty 7.6-centimeter piece of airline tubing that was 0.6 centimeters in diameter, (2) on a bite of food measuring $0.6 \times 0.6 \times 0.6$ centimeters in the tube, (3) on a strip of food measuring $0.6 \times 0.6 \times 5.1$ centimeters on half of a tube, and (4) on a strip of food measuring $0.6 \times 0.6 \times 5.1$ centimeters. Final steps included presenting a bite of food measuring $0.6 \times 0.6 \times 0.6$ centimeters and increasing bite size for one child.

Volkert et al. (2013) noted that one limitation of the chewing literature is that studies have not measured mastication. Ensuring that a child has masticated accepted food is important for minimizing aspiration risk. Volkert et al. used a vocal prompt, "Chew X times," for one child and provided praise if the child met the chew criterion. The feeder checked 30 seconds after the bite entered the child's mouth to determine if the child masticated the bite, which Volkert et al. defined as food with pieces no larger than $0.2 \times 0.2$ centimeters in a liquid medium after chewing. Chews per bite and mastication increased during the intervention.

### Caregiver Training

Caregiver training is one of the most, if not the most, important aspect of intervention for pediatric feeding disorders, as caregivers typically serve as feeders or are present at mealtime. Werle et al. (1993) used several training techniques, such as discussion, handouts, role plays, behavioral rehearsal, verbal feedback, and occasional videotape review, to train three caregivers to use specific and general prompts and positive reinforcement. Results indicated increased offerings of target foods and specific prompts for two caregivers, with an additional increase in positive attention for a third caregiver. Werle et al. observed a simultaneous increase in acceptance of target foods across children and decreases in food refusal as training continued.

Anderson and McMillan (2001) trained two caregivers of a child with a feeding disorder to implement a feeding intervention with above 90% integrity; the researchers used verbal and written instructions, modeling, video review, and performance feedback during and after in-home feeding services. Mueller et al. (2003) evaluated four different multicomponent training packages to increase intervention integrity for caregivers implementing pediatric feeding interventions. In Study 1, written protocols, verbal instructions, therapist modeling, and rehearsal training increased caregivers' intervention integrity to high levels. Mueller et al. then examined the effects of the training package's components in Study 2. Mueller et al. assigned six caregivers to one of three training conditions with two caregivers per condition: written protocols and verbal instructions; written protocols, verbal instructions, and modeling; and written instructions, verbal instructions, and rehearsal. Each training package produced high levels of intervention integrity and maintenance over a 3-month period. Other researchers have taught caregivers to use general and specific prompts (Pangborn, Borrero, & Borrero, 2013; Werle et al., 1993), functional-analysis procedures (Najdowski et al., 2003, 2008), intervention (e.g., demand fading, differential reinforcement, escape extinction; Anderson & McMillan, 2001; Najdowski et al., 2003, 2010; Pangborn et al., 2013; Seiverling, Williams, Sturmey, & Hart, 2012), and data collection (Najdowski et al., 2003).

### CONCLUSION

The negative health consequences of a feeding disorder can be serious and substantial and may include dehydration, growth limitation, severe malnourishment, and substantial weight loss (Babbitt et al., 2001; Palmer & Horn, 1978; Piazza & Carroll-Hernandez, 2004). Deficits in calories, nutrition, or both can cause long-term behavior, health, and learning problems (Freedman, Dietz, Srinivasan, & Berenson, 1999). Young children may be at greatest risk for the negative impact of a feeding disorder, as the most damaging effects of inadequate caloric intake, poor nutrition, or both occur before age 5, which is a period of critical brain development (Winick, 1969). Feeding disorders may also affect a child's social development, as children with feeding disorders often miss important social opportunities, such as birthday parties, because of their inability or unwillingness to eat. Feeding disorders often have a negative impact on families as well, as they may cause caregiver stress and depression (Franklin & Rodger, 2003; Singer, Sing, Hill, & Jaffe, 1990) and are financially costly to the families and to society (Nebraska Legislature, 2009; Williams, Riegel, Gibbons, & Field, 2007).

The etiology of feeding disorders is multiply controlled and complex (Rommel et al., 2003), and the behaviors that constitute a feeding disorder are heterogeneous. Current diagnostic nosologies describe the characteristics of a feeding disorder but are not prescriptive. Historically, researchers have hypothesized that escape from feeding functions as negative reinforcement for inappropriate mealtime behavior, based on the results of studies in which putative escape extinction was effective for increasing acceptance and decreasing inappropriate mealtime behavior (Cooper et al., 1995; Hoch et al., 1994; Kerwin et al., 1995; Patel, Piazza, Martinez, et al., 2002; Piazza, Patel, et al., 2003; Reed et al., 2004). Functional analysis studies have confirmed that escape functioned as negative reinforcement for the inappropriate mealtime behavior of most children in those studies (Allison et al., 2012; Bachmeyer et al., 2009; Girolami & Scotti, 2001; Kirkwood, Piazza, & Peterson, in press; LaRue et al., 2011; Najdowski et al., 2008; Piazza, Fisher, et al., 2003), but some studies have found that adult attention and tangible items functioned as reinforcement too (Bachmeyer et al., 2009; Girolami & Scotti, 2001; Piazza, Fisher, et al., 2003). There are only a few studies of function-based interventions (Allison et al., 2012; Bachmeyer et al., 2009; Bachmeyer et al., 2019; Kirkwood et al., in press; LaRue et al., 2011; Najdowski et al., 2003). Results of these studies suggest that we can use the results of a functional analysis of inappropriate mealtime behavior to prescribe effective interventions to increase acceptance and decrease inappropriate mealtime behavior.

The complexity of feeding disorders, however, necessitates that we refine our functional-analysis procedures to identify the characteristics of the feeding environment that establish escape or other stimuli as reinforcement. Results of studies on fading suggest that we can alter the properties of stimuli associated with high levels of acceptance and low levels of inappropriate mealtime behavior to produce appropriate feeding. Can we identify those antecedent variables a priori? Most children emit some form of appropriate behavior. How can we identify that behavior and use it to prescribe an effective feeding intervention?

Similarly, although behavior analysts have evaluated procedures to reduce expulsion and packing,

we know little about what causes these behaviors. Are they part of a chain of escape and avoidance behaviors, and as we extinguish one behavior, does another behavior emerge to take its place? Are they the result of an oral–motor skill deficit, in which the child lacks the skills to manage solids or liquids effectively? Are they the result of a combined etiology? The systematic, data-based approach that behavior analysts use is ideal for answering these questions, but we have yet to apply them to pediatric feeding disorders.

Finally, intervention for a feeding disorder requires knowledge that extends far beyond applied behavior analysis. A behavior analyst should recognize when to consult with another professional, such as an allergist, pediatric gastroenterologist, or speech and language pathologist. Inadequate training can lead to mistakes in therapy that can have serious consequences, such as anaphylaxis due to cross-contamination, aspiration when a child is not a safe oral feeder for the presented food or liquid, or choking because the presented texture is inappropriate for the child's chewing skills. "Knowing what you don't know" is an essential skill for behavior analysts working with children with feeding disorders.

## REFERENCES

Addison, L. R., Piazza, C. C., Patel, M. E., Bachmeyer, M. H., Rivas, K. M., Milnes, S. M., et al. (2012). A comparison of sensory integrative and behavioral therapies as treatment for pediatric feeding disorders. *Journal of Applied Behavior Analysis, 45,* 455–471.

Ahearn, W. H. (2003). Using simultaneous presentation to increase vegetable consumption in a mildly selective child with autism. *Journal of Applied Behavior Analysis, 36,* 361–365.

Ahearn, W. H., Kerwin, M. E., Eicher, P. S., Shantz, J., & Swearingin, W. (1996). An alternating treatments comparison of two intensive interventions for food refusal. *Journal of Applied Behavior Analysis, 29,* 321–332.

Allison, J., Wilder, D. A., Chong, I., Lugo, A., Pike, J., & Rudy, N. (2012). A comparison of differential reinforcement and noncontingent reinforcement to treat food selectivity in a child with autism. *Journal of Applied Behavior Analysis, 45,* 613–617.

American Psychiatric Association. (2013). *Diagnostic and statistical manual of mental disorders* (5th ed.). Arlington, VA: Author.

Anderson, C. M., & McMillan, K. (2001). Parental use of escape extinction and differential reinforcement to treat food selectivity. *Journal of Applied Behavior Analysis, 34,* 511–515.

Arvedson, J. C., & Brodsky, L. (2002). *Pediatric swallowing and feeding: Assessment and management* (2nd ed.). Albany, NY: Singular.

Babbitt, R. L., Shore, B. A., Smith, M., Williams, K. E., & Coe, D. A. (2001). Stimulus fading in the treatment of adipsia. *Behavioral Interventions, 16,* 197–207.

Bachmeyer, M. H., Gulotta, C. S., & Piazza, C. C. (2013). Liquid to baby food fading in the treatment of food refusal. *Behavioral Interventions, 28,* 281–298.

Bachmeyer, M. H., Kirkwood, C. A., Criscito, A. B., Mauzy, C. R., & Berth, D. P. (2019). A comparison of functional analysis methods of inappropriate mealtime behavior. *Journal of Applied Behavior Analysis, 52,* 603–621.

Bachmeyer, M. H., Piazza, C. C., Frederick, L. D., Reed, G. K., Rivas, K. D., & Kadey, H. J. (2009). Functional analysis and treatment of multiply controlled inappropriate mealtime behavior. *Journal of Applied Behavior Analysis, 42,* 641–658.

Bandini, L. G., Anderson, S. E., Curtin, C., Cermak, S., Evans, E. W., Scampini, R., et al. (2010). Food selectivity in children with autism spectrum disorders and typically developing children. *Journal of Pediatrics, 157,* 259–264.

Boiron, M., Nobrega, L. D., Roux, S., Henrot, A., & Saliba, E. (2007). Effects of oral stimulation and oral support on non-nutritive sucking and feeding performance in preterm infants. *Developmental Medicine and Child Neurology, 49,* 439–444.

Borrero, C. S. W., Woods, J. N., Borrero, J. C., Masler, E. A., & Lesser, A. D. (2010). Descriptive analysis of pediatric food refusal and acceptance. *Journal of Applied Behavior Analysis, 43,* 71–88.

Borsari, A., & Ottoni, E. B. (2005). Preliminary observations of tool use in captive hyacinth macaws (*Anodorhynchus hyacinthinus*). *Animal Cognition, 8,* 48–53.

Buckley, S. D., & Newchok, D. K. (2005). An evaluation of simultaneous presentation and differential reinforcement with response cost to reduce packing. *Journal of Applied Behavior Analysis, 38,* 405–409.

Buckley, S. D., Strunck, P. G., & Newchok, D. K. (2005). A comparison of two multicomponent procedures to increase food consumption. *Behavioral Interventions, 20,* 139–146.

Burklow, K. A., McGrath, A. M., Valerius, K. S., & Rudolph, C. (2002). Relationships between feeding difficulties, medical complexity, and gestational age. *Nutrition in Clinical Practice, 17,* 373–378.

Casey, S. D., Cooper-Brown, L. J., Wacker, D. P., & Rankin, B. E. (2006). The use of descriptive analysis to identify and manipulate schedules of reinforcement in the treatment of food refusal. *Journal of Behavioral Education, 15,* 41–52.

Coe, D. A., Babbitt, R. A., Williams, K. E., Hajimihalis, C., Snyder, A. M., Ballard, C., et al. (1997). Use of extinction and reinforcement to increase food consumption and reduce expulsion. *Journal of Applied Behavior Analysis, 30,* 581–583.

Cooper, L. J., Wacker, D. P., McComas, J. J., Brown, K.,

Peck, S. M., Richman, D., et al. (1995). Use of component analyses to identify active variables in treatment packages for children with feeding disorders. *Journal of Applied Behavior Analysis, 28,* 139–153.

Darrow, D. H., & Harley, C. M. (1998). Evaluation of swallowing disorders in children. *Otolaryngologic Clinics of North America, 31,* 405–418.

Davis, A. M., Bruce, A., Cocjin, J., Mousa, H., & Hyman, P. (2010). Empirically supported treatments for feeding difficulties in young children. *Current Gastroenterology Reports, 12,* 189–194.

Dawson, J. E., Piazza, C. C., Sevin, B. M., Gulotta, C. S., Lerman, D., & Kelley, M. L. (2003). Use of the high-probability instructional sequence and escape extinction in a child with food refusal. *Journal of Applied Behavior Analysis, 36,* 105–108.

Dempsey, J., Piazza, C. C., Groff, R. A., & Kozisek, J. M. (2011). A flipped spoon and chin prompt to increase mouth clean. *Journal of Applied Behavior Analysis, 44,* 961–965.

Derkay, C. S., & Schechter, G. L. (1998). Anatomy and physiology of pediatric swallowing disorders. *Otolaryngologic Clinics of North America, 31,* 397–404.

Diquelou, M. C., Griffin, A. S., & Sol, G. D. (2016). The role of motor diversity in foraging innovations: A cross-species comparison in urban birds. *Behavioral Ecology, 27,* 584–591.

Douglas, J. E., & Byron, M. (1996). Interview data on severe behavioural eating difficulties in young children. *Archives of Disease in Childhood, 75,* 304–308.

Einarsson-Backes, L. M., Dietz, J., Price, R., Glass, R., & Hays, R. (1994). The effect of oral support on sucking efficiency in preterm infants. *American Journal of Occupational Therapy, 48,* 490–498.

Field, T., Ignatoff, E., Stinger, S., Brennan, J., Greenberg, R., Widmayer, S., et al. (1982). Nonnutritive sucking during tube feedings: Effects on preterm neonates in an intensive care unit. *Pediatrics, 70,* 381–384.

Franklin, L., & Rodger, S. (2003). Parents' perspectives on feeding medically compromised children: Implications for occupational therapy. *Australian Occupational Therapy Journal, 50,* 137–147.

Freedman, D. S., Dietz, W. H., Srinivasan, S. R., & Berenson, G. S. (1999). The relation of overweight to cardiovascular risk factors among children and adolescents: The Bogalusa Heart Study. *Pediatrics, 103,* 1175–1182.

Freeman, K. A., & Piazza, C. C. (1998). Combining stimulus fading, reinforcement, and extinction to treat food refusal. *Journal of Applied Behavior Analysis, 31,* 691–694.

Fucile, S., Gisel, E., & Lau, C. (2002). Oral stimulation accelerates the transition from tube to oral feeding in preterm infants. *Journal of Pediatrics, 141,* 230–236.

Girolami, P. A., Boscoe, J. H., & Roscoe, N. (2007). Decreasing expulsions by a child with a feeding disorder: Using a brush to present and re-present food. *Journal of Applied Behavior Analysis, 40,* 749–753.

Girolami, P. A., & Scotti, J. R. (2001). Use of analog functional analysis in assessing the function of mealtime problem behavior. *Education and Training in Mental Retardation and Developmental Disabilities, 36,* 207–223.

Goto, A., Arah, O. A., Goto, M., Terauchi, Y., & Noda, M. (2013). Severe hypoglycemia and cardiovascular disease: Systematic review and meta-analysis with bias analysis. *British Journal of Medicine, 347,* 1–11.

Groff, R. A., Piazza, C. C., Volkert, V. M., & Jostad, C. M. (2014). Syringe fading as treatment for feeding refusal. *Journal of Applied Behavior Analysis, 47,* 834–839.

Groff, R. A., Piazza, C. C., Zeleny, J. R., & Dempsey, J. R. (2011). Spoon-to-cup fading as treatment for cup drinking in a child with intestinal failure. *Journal of Applied Behavior Analysis, 44,* 949–954.

Gulotta, C. S., Piazza, C. C., Patel, M. R., & Layer, S. A. (2005). Using food redistribution to reduce packing in children with severe food refusal. *Journal of Applied Behavior Analysis, 38,* 39–50.

Hadley, A. J., Krival, K. R., Ridgel, A. L., Hahn, E. C., & Tyler, D. J. (2015). Neural network pattern recognition of lingual–palatal pressure for automated detection of swallow. *Dysphagia, 30,* 176–187.

Hagopian, L. P., Farrell, D. A., & Amari, A. (1996). Treating total liquid refusal with backward chaining and fading. *Journal of Applied Behavioral Analysis, 29,* 573–575.

Hoch, T. A., Babbitt, R. L., Coe, D. A., Duncan, A., & Trusty, E. M. (1995). A swallow induction avoidance procedure to establish eating. *Journal of Behavior Therapy and Experimental Psychiatry, 26,* 41–50.

Hoch, T. A., Babbitt, R. L., Coe, D. A., Krell, D. M., & Hackbert, L. (1994). Contingency contacting: Combining positive reinforcement and escape extinction procedures to treat persistent food refusal. *Behavior Modification, 18,* 106–128.

Ibañez, V. F., Piazza, C. C., & Peterson, K. M. (2019). A translational evaluation of renewal of inappropriate mealtime behavior. *Journal of Applied Behavior Analysis, 52,* 1005–1020.

Iwata, B. A., Dorsey, M. F., Slifer, K. J., Bauman, K. E., & Richman, G. S. (1994). Toward a functional analysis of self-injury. *Journal of Applied Behavior Analysis, 27,* 197–209. (Reprinted from *Analysis and Intervention in Developmental Disabilities, 2,* 3–20, 1982)

Johnson, C. R., & Babbitt, R. L. (1993). Antecedent manipulation in the treatment of primary solid food refusal. *Behavior Modification, 17,* 510–521.

Kadey, H., Piazza, C. C., Rivas, K. M., & Zeleny, J. (2013). An evaluation of texture manipulations to increase swallowing. *Journal of Applied Behavior Analysis, 46,* 539–543.

Kahng, S., Boscoe, J. H., & Byrne, S. (2003). The use of an escape contingency and a token economy to increase food acceptance. *Journal of Applied Behavior Analysis, 36,* 349–353.

Kahng, S., Tarbox, J., & Wilke, A. E. (2001). Use of a multicomponent treatment for food refusal. *Journal of Applied Behavior Analysis, 34,* 93–96.

Kelley, M. E., Piazza, C. C., & Fisher, W. W. (2003). Acquisition of cup drinking using previously refused foods as positive and negative reinforcement. *Journal of Applied Behavior Analysis, 36,* 89–93.

Kern, L., & Marder, T. J. (1996). A comparison of simultaneous and delayed reinforcement as treatments for food selectivity. *Journal of Applied Behavior Analysis, 2,* 243–246.

Kerwin, M. E. (1999). Empirically supported treatments in pediatric psychology: Severe feeding problems. *Journal of Pediatric Psychology, 24,* 193–214.

Kerwin, M. E., Ahearn, W. H., Eicher, P. S., & Burd, D. M. (1995). The costs of eating: A behavioral economic analysis of food refusal. *Journal of Applied Behavior Analysis, 28,* 245–260.

Kirkwood, C. A., Piazza, C. C., & Peterson, K. M. (in press). A comparison of function- and nonfunction-based extinction for inappropriate mealtime behavior. *Journal of Applied Behavior Analysis.*

LaRue, R. H., Stewart, V., Piazza, C. C., Volkert, V. M., Patel, M. R., & Zeleny, J. (2011). Escape as reinforcement and escape extinction in the treatment of feeding problems. *Journal of Applied Behavior Analysis, 44,* 719–735.

Levin, D. S., Volkert, V. M., & Piazza, C. C. (2014). A multi-component treatment to reduce packing in children with feeding and autism spectrum disorders. *Behavior Modification, 38,* 940–963.

Linscheid, T. R., Oliver, J., Blyler, E., & Palmer, S. (1978). Brief hospitalization for the behavioral treatment of feeding problems in the developmentally disabled. *Journal of Pediatric Psychology, 12,* 451–459.

Luiselli, J. K., & Gleason, D. L. (1987). Combining sensory reinforcement and texture fading procedures to overcome chronic food refusal. *Journal of Behavior Therapy and Experimental Psychiatry, 18,* 149–155.

Luiselli, J. K., Ricciardi, J. N., & Gilligan, K. (2005). Liquid fading to establish milk consumption by a child with autism. *Behavioral Interventions, 20,* 155–163.

Lukens, C. T., & Silverman, A. H. (2014). Systematic review of psychological interventions for pediatric feeding problems. *Journal of Pediatric Psychology, 39,* 903–917.

Meier, A. E., Fryling, M. J., & Wallace, M. D. (2012). Using high-probability foods to increase the acceptance of low-probability foods. *Journal of Applied Behavior Analysis, 45,* 149–153.

Mueller, M. M., Piazza, C. C., Moore, J. W., Kelley, M. E., Bethke, S. A., Pruett, A., et al. (2003). Training parents to implement pediatric feeding protocols. *Journal of Applied Behavior Analysis, 36,* 545–562.

Mueller, M. M., Piazza, C. C., Patel, M. R., Kelley, M. E., & Pruett, A. (2004). Increasing variety of foods consumed by blending nonpreferred foods into preferred foods. *Journal of Applied Behavior Analysis, 37,* 159–170.

Munk, D. D., & Repp, A. C. (1994). Behavioral assessment of feeding problems of individuals with severe disabilities. *Journal of Applied Behavior Analysis, 27,* 241–250.

Najdowski, A. C., Wallace, M. D., Doney, J. K., & Ghezzi, P. M. (2003). Parental assessment and treatment of food selectivity in natural settings. *Journal of Applied Behavior Analysis, 36,* 383–386.

Najdowski, A. C., Wallace, M. D., Penrod, B., Tarbox, J., Reagon, K., & Higbee, T. S. (2008). Caregiver-conducted experimental functional analyses of inappropriate mealtime behavior. *Journal of Applied Behavior Analysis, 41,* 459–465.

Najdowski, A. C., Wallace, M. D., Reagon, K., Penrod, B., Higbee, T. S., & Tarbox, J. (2010). Utilizing a home-based parent training approach in the treatment of food selectivity. *Behavioral Interventions, 25,* 89–107.

Nebraska Legislature. (2009). *Fiscal note: Legislative fiscal analyst estimate.* LB 243, Revision 01.

Palmer, S., & Horn, S. (1978). Feeding problems in children. In S. Palmer & S. Ekvall (Eds.), *Pediatric nutrition in developmental disorders* (pp. 107–129). Springfield, IL: Charles C Thomas.

Pangborn, M. M., Borrero, C. S. W., & Borrero, J. C. (2013). Sequential application of caregiver training to implement pediatric feeding protocols. *Behavioral Interventions, 28,* 107–130.

Patel, M. R., Piazza, C. C., Kelley, M. L., Ochsner, C. A., & Santana, C. M. (2001). Using a fading procedure to increase fluid consumption in a child with feeding problems. *Journal of Applied Behavior Analysis, 34,* 357–360.

Patel, M. R., Piazza, C. C., Layer, S. A., Coleman, R., & Swartzwelder, D. M. (2005). A systematic evaluation of food textures to decrease packing and increase oral intake in children with pediatric feeding disorders. *Journal of Applied Behavior Analysis, 38,* 89–100.

Patel, M. R., Piazza, C. C., Martinez, C. J., Volkert, V. M., & Santana, C. M. (2002). An evaluation of two differential reinforcement procedures with escape extinction to treat food refusal. *Journal of Applied Behavior Analysis, 35,* 363–374.

Patel, M. R., Piazza, C. C., Santana, C. M., & Volkert, V. M. (2002). An evaluation of food type and texture in the treatment of a feeding problem. *Journal of Applied Behavior Analysis, 35,* 183–186.

Patel, M. R., Reed, G. K., Piazza, C. C., Bachmeyer, M. H., Layer, S. A., & Pabico, R. S. (2006). An evaluation of a high-probability instructional sequence to increase acceptance of food and decrease inappropriate behavior in children with pediatric feeding disorders. *Research in Developmental Disabilities, 27,* 430–442.

Patel, M. R., Reed, G. K., Piazza, C. C., Mueller, M., Bachmeyer, M. H., & Layer, S. A. (2007). Use of a high-probability instructional sequence to increase compliance to feeding demands in the absence of escape extinction. *Behavioral Interventions, 22,* 305–310.

Penrod, B., Gardella, L., & Fernand, J. (2012). An evaluation of a progressive high-probability instructional sequence combined with low-probability demand fading in the treatment of food selectivity. *Journal of Applied Behavior Analysis, 45,* 527–537.

Peterson, K. M., Piazza, C. C., Ibañez, V. F., & Fisher, W. W. (2019). Randomized controlled trial of an applied behavior analysis intervention for food selectivity in children with autism spectrum disorder. *Journal of Applied Behavior Analysis, 52,* 895–917.

Peterson, K. M., Piazza, C. C., & Volkert, V. M. (2016). Comparison of a modified sequential oral sensory approach to an applied behavior analytic approach in the treatment of food selectivity in children with autism spectrum disorders. *Journal of Applied Behavior Analysis, 49,* 485–511.

Peterson, K. M., Volkert, V. M., & Zeleny, J. R. (2015). Increasing self-drinking for children with feeding disorders. *Journal of Applied Behavior Analysis, 48,* 436–441.

Piazza, C. C., Anderson, C., & Fisher, W. W. (1993). Teaching self-feeding skills to patients with Rett syndrome. *Developmental Medicine and Child Neurology, 35,* 991–996.

Piazza, C. C., & Carroll-Hernandez, T. A. (2004) Assessment and treatment of pediatric feeding disorders. In R. E. Tremblay, R. G. Barr, & R. Peters (Eds.), *Encyclopedia on early childhood development* [Online]. Montreal: Centre of Excellence for Early Childhood Development. Retrieved July 29, 2013, from *www.excellence-earlychildhood.ca/documents/Piazza-Carroll-HernandezANGxp.pdf.*

Piazza, C. C., Fisher, W. W., Brown, K. A., Shore, B. A., Patel, M. R., Katz, R. M., et al. (2003). Functional analysis of inappropriate mealtime behaviors. *Journal of Applied Behavior Analysis, 36,* 187–204.

Piazza, C. C., Patel, M. R., Gulotta, C. S., Sevin, B. M., & Layer, S. A. (2003). On the relative contribution of positive reinforcement and escape extinction in the treatment of food refusal. *Journal of Applied Behavior Analysis, 36,* 309–324.

Piazza, C. C., Patel, M. R., Santana, C. M., Goh, H., Delia, M. D., & Lancaster, B. M. (2002). An evaluation of simultaneous and sequential presentation of preferred and nonpreferred food to treat food selectivity. *Journal of Applied Behavior Analysis, 35,* 259–270.

Reed, G. K., Piazza, C. C., Patel, M. R., Layer, S. A., Bachmeyer, M. H., Bethke, S. D., et al. (2004). On the relative contributions of noncontingent reinforcement and escape extinction in the treatment of food refusal. *Journal of Applied Behavior Analysis, 37,* 27–41.

Riordan, M. M., Iwata, B. A., Finney, J. W., Wohl, M. K., & Stanley, A. E. (1984). Behavioral assessment and treatment of chronic food refusal in handicapped children. *Journal of Applied Behavior Analysis, 17,* 327–341.

Riordan, M. M., Iwata, B. A., Wohl, M. K., & Finney, J.

W. (1980). Behavioral treatment of food refusal and selectivity in developmentally disabled children. *Applied Research in Mental Retardation, 1,* 95–112.

Rivas, K. D., Piazza, C. C., Kadey, H. J., Volkert, V. M., & Stewart, V. (2011). Sequential treatment of a feeding problem using a pacifier and flipped spoon. *Journal of Applied Behavior Analysis, 44,* 387–391.

Rivas, K. D., Piazza, C. C., Patel, M. R., & Bachmeyer, M. H. (2010). Spoon distance fading with and without escape extinction as treatment for food refusal. *Journal of Applied Behavior Analysis, 43,* 673–683.

Rocha, A. D., Moreira, M. E. L., Pimenta, H. P., Ramos, J. R. M., & Lucena, S. L. (2007). A randomized study of the efficacy of sensory–motor–oral stimulation and non-nutritive sucking in very low birthweight infant. *Early Human Development, 83,* 385–388.

Rommel, N., DeMeyer, A. M., Feenstra, L., & Veereman-Wauters, G. (2003). The complexity of feeding problems in 700 infants and young children presenting to a tertiary care institution. *Journal of Pediatric Gastroenterology and Nutrition, 37,* 75–84.

Roth, M. P., Williams, K. E., & Paul, C. M. (2010). Treating food and liquid refusal in an adolescent with Asperger's disorder. *Clinical Case Studies, 9,* 260–272.

Schafe, G. E., & Bernstein, I. L. (1996). Taste aversion learning. In E. D. Capaldi (Ed.), *Why we eat what we eat: The psychology of eating* (pp. 31–51). Washington, DC: American Psychological Association.

Schwarz, S. M., Corredor, J., Fisher-Medina, J., Cohen, J., & Rabinowitz, S. (2001). Diagnosis and treatment of feeding disorders in children with developmental disabilities. *Pediatrics, 108,* 671–676.

Sehgal, S. K., Prakash, O., Gupta, A., Mohan, M., & Anand, N. K. (1990). Evaluation of beneficial effects of nonnutritive sucking in preterm infants. *Indian Pediatrics, 27,* 263–266.

Seiverling, L., Williams, K., Sturmey, P., & Hart, S. (2012). Effects of behavioral skills training on parental treatment of children's food selectivity. *Journal of Applied Behavior Analysis, 45,* 197–203.

Sevin, B. M., Gulotta, C. S., Sierp, B. J., Rosica, L. A., & Miller, L. J. (2002). Analysis of response covariation among multiple topographies of food refusal. *Journal of Applied Behavior Analysis, 35,* 65–68.

Shalev, R. A., Milnes, S. M., Piazza, C. C., & Kozisek, J. M. (2018). Treating liquid expulsion in children with feeding disorders. *Journal of Applied Behavior Analysis, 51,* 70–79.

Sharp, W. G., Harker, S., & Jaquess, D. L. (2010). Comparison of bite-presentation methods in the treatment of food refusal. *Journal of Applied Behavior Analysis, 43,* 739–743.

Sharp, W. G., & Jaquess, D. L. (2009). Bite size and texture assessments to prescribe treatment for severe food selectivity in autism. *Behavioral Interventions, 24,* 157–170.

Sharp, W. G., Odom, A., & Jaquess, D. L. (2012). Comparison of upright and flipped spoon presentations to guide treatment of food refusal. *Journal of Applied Behavior Analysis, 45,* 83–96.

Shore, B. A., Babbitt, R. L., Williams, K. E., Coe, D. A., & Snyder, A. (1998). Use of texture fading in the treatment of food selectivity. *Journal of Applied Behavior Analysis, 31,* 621–633.

Sicherer, S. H., & Sampson, H. A. (2010). Food allergy. *Journal of Allergy and Clinical Immunology, 125,* S116–S125.

Singer, L. T., Sing, L. Y., Hill, B. P., & Jaffe, A. C. (1990). Stress and depression in mothers of failure to thrive children. *Journal of Pediatric Psychology, 15,* 711–720.

Stark, L. J., Mulvihill, M. M., Powers, S. W., Jelaliàn, E., Keating, K., Creveling, S., et al. (1996). Behavioral intervention to improve calorie intake of children with cystic fibrosis: Treatment versus wait list control. *Journal of Pediatric Gastroenterology and Nutrition, 22,* 240–253.

Stark, L. J., Powers, S. W., Jelalian, E., Rape, R. N., & Miller, D. L. (1994). Modifying mealtime interactions of children with cystic fibrosis and their parents via behavioral parent training. *Journal of Pediatric Psychology, 19,* 751–768.

Stein, B., Everhart, K. K., & Lacy, B. E. (2015). Gastroparesis: A review of current diagnosis and treatment options. *Journal of Clinical Gastroenterology, 49,* 550–558.

Stubbs, K. H., Volkert, V. M., Rubio, E. K., & Ottinger, E. (2017). A comparison of flipped-spoon presentation and redistribution to decrease packing in children with feeding disorders. *Learning and Motivation, 62,* 103–111.

Task Force on Promotion and Dissemination of Psychological Procedures. (1995). Training in and dissemination of empirically validated treatments: Report and recommendations. *Clinical Psychologist, 48,* 3–23.

Thommessen, M., Heiberg, A., Kase, B. F., Larsen, S., & Riis, G. (1991). Feeding problems, height and weight in different groups of disabled children. *Acta Paediatrica, 5,* 527–533.

Tiger, J. H., & Hanley, G. P. (2006). Using reinforcer pairing and fading to increase the milk consumption of a preschool child. *Journal of Applied Behavior Analysis, 39,* 399–403.

Toien, O., Blake, J., Edgar, D. M., Grahn, D. A., Heller, H. G., & Barnes, B. M. (2001). Hibernation in black bears: Independence of metabolic suppression from body temperature. *Science, 331,* 906–909.

Valdimarsdottir, H., Halldorsdottir, L. Y., & Sigurådóttir, Z. G. (2010). Increasing the variety of foods consumed by a picky eater: Generalization of effects across caregivers and settings. *Journal of Applied Behavior Analysis, 43,* 101–105.

Vaz, P. C. M., Piazza, C. C., Stewart, V., Volkert, V. M., & Groff, R. A. (2012). Using a chaser to decrease packing in children with feeding disorders. *Journal of Applied Behavior Analysis, 45,* 97–105.

Volkert, V. M., Peterson, K. M., Zeleny, J. R., & Piazza,

C. C. (2014). A clinical protocol to increase chewing and assess mastication in children with feeding disorders. *Behavior Modification, 38,* 705–729.

Volkert, V. M., & Piazza, C. C. (2012). Pediatric feeding disorders. In P. Sturmey & M. Hersen (Eds.), *Handbook of evidence-based practice in clinical psychology: Vol. 1. Child and adolescent disorders* (pp. 323–337). Hoboken, NJ: Wiley.

Volkert, V. M., Piazza, C. C., Vaz, P. C. M., & Frese, J. (2013). A pilot study to increase chewing in children with feeding disorders. *Behavior Modification, 37,* 391–408.

Volkert, V. M., Vaz, P. C. M., Piazza, C. C., Frese, J., & Barnett, L. (2011). Using a flipped spoon to decrease packing in children with feeding disorders. *Journal of Applied Behavior Analysis, 44,* 617–621.

Werle, M. A., Murphy, T. B., & Budd, K. S. (1993). Treating chronic food refusal in young children: Home-based parent training. *Journal of Applied Behavior Analysis, 26,* 421–433.

Wilder, D. A., Normand, M., & Atwell, J. (2005). Noncontingent reinforcement as treatment for food refusal and associated self-injury. *Journal of Applied Behavior Analysis, 38,* 549–553.

Wilkins, J. W., Piazza, C. C., Groff, R. A., & Vaz, P. C. M. (2011). Chin prompt plus re-presentation as treatment for expulsion in children with feeding disorders. *Journal of Applied Behavior Analysis, 44,* 513–522.

Wilkins, J. W., Piazza, C. C., Groff, R. A., Volkert, J. M., Kozisek, J. M., & Milnes, S. M. (2014). Utensil manipulation during initial treatment of pediatric feeding problems. *Journal of Applied Behavior Analysis, 47,* 1–16.

Williams, K. E., Riegel, K., Gibbons, B., & Field, D. G. (2007). Intensive behavioral treatment for severe feeding problems: A cost-effective alternative to tube feeding? *Journal of Developmental and Physical Disabilities, 19,* 227–235.

Winick, M. (1969). Malnutrition and brain development. *Journal of Pediatrics, 74,* 667–679.

# CHAPTER 26

# Behavioral Approaches to Education

Brian K. Martens, Edward J. Daly III, John C. Begeny, and William E. Sullivan

The power and precision with which early behavior analysts used operant-conditioning principles to change behavior resulted in almost immediate applications to education. For example, Skinner's (1954) model of programmed instruction used teaching machines to provide students with immediate feedback and reinforcement for correct responding across many tightly sequenced tasks (e.g., arithmetic facts). Frequent reinforcement, self-paced practice, and prompting and fading—what Skinner originally called *vanishing*—produced learning that was enjoyable, occurred quickly, and involved few errors (Skinner, 1984). Keller (1968) showed how to apply these same principles to create a personalized system of instruction for college students. Curriculum materials for Keller's personalized system of instruction courses consisted of 30 or more small content units, each associated with its own set of study questions and exercises. Students were free to study and attend lectures whenever they wanted, but the system prescribed brief examinations on the material in each "unit." Instructors graphed performance on these unit tests and required mastery before moving forward in the curriculum.

The examples above suggest that behavioral approaches to education are characterized by an emphasis on *doing* rather than *knowing*. The first and most important feature of behavioral skill training is repeated measurement of student responding.

Measuring responding accuracy and then fluency (responding accurately, quickly, and in different contexts) allows the teacher to evaluate learning outcomes in relation to instructional goals and provides the basis for varying instruction (Christ, Zopluoglu, Monaghen, & Van Norman, 2013; Fuchs & Fuchs, 1986; Reschly, 2004). With a focus on responding as the basic unit of analysis, the student's task becomes one of emitting gradually more refined, coordinated, and effective response repertoires under increasingly demanding and naturalistic stimulus conditions (Martens, Daly, & Ardoin, 2015). The teacher acts more as a trainer or coach than as a lecturer or educator, to promote high rates of correct independent responding by the student (Keller, 1968). That is, the teacher facilitates learning by arranging repeated opportunities to respond in the presence of diverse curricular materials; sometimes with modeling, prompting, and error correction; and always with differential reinforcement for correct or desired responding (Martens et al., 2015). From the perspective of both teacher and student, behavioral approaches to skill training make learning active, fast-paced, relatively error-free, and more reinforcing than punishing (Miltenberger, 2016).

The fundamentals of behavioral skill training have remained unchanged since their inception: (1) well-sequenced stimulus materials that are linked horizontally across related skills and vertically by difficulty; (2) brief, repeated opportunities to respond in the presence of these stimuli; (3) modeling, prompting, and feedback by the teacher to increase the likelihood of correct responding; (4) differential reinforcement to establish and strengthen stimulus control over correct responding; and (5) frequent performance monitoring to inform instructional planning and evaluate learning outcomes (Fuchs, Fuchs, & Speece, 2002; Martens & Witt, 2004).

Professionals consider behavioral approaches to skill training standard practice when teaching daily living, communication, and other adaptive behaviors to individuals with developmental disabilities (e.g., Carroll, Joachim, St. Peter, & Robinson, 2015; Lerman, Hawkins, Hillman, Shireman, & Nissen, 2015; Marion, Martin, Yu, Buhler, & Kerr, 2012), and when remediating deficits in children's basic academic skills (Daly, Martens, Barnett, Witt, & Olson, 2007; Daly, Neugebauer, Chafouleas, & Skinner, 2015). Researchers have applied behavioral instruction approaches to athletic performance (e.g., Brobst & Ward, 2002; Kladopoulos & McComas, 2001; Tai & Miltenberger, 2017), in secondary and higher education (Cavanaugh, Heward, & Donelson, 1996; Saville, Zinn, Neef, Van Norman, & Ferreri, 2006; Stocco, Thompson, Hart, & Soriano, 2017), during in-service teacher training (DiGennaro, Martens, & McIntyre, 2005; Hogan, Knez, & Kahng, 2015; Luck, Lerman, Wu, Dupuis, & Hussein, 2018), and in teaching children important safety skills (Dickson & Vargo, 2017; Houvouras & Harvey, 2014). Although the effectiveness of these techniques has led to the development of comprehensive behavioral instruction- and performance-monitoring programs (e.g., Direct Instruction, Precision Teaching), public schools do not use the programs or their component techniques (Begeny & Martens, 2006; Lindsley, 1992; Saville et al., 2006).

We have organized the material in the present chapter loosely around a model for the dynamic development of proficient skill performance known as the *learning/instructional hierarchy* (Daly, Lentz, & Boyer, 1996; Haring, Lovitt, Eaton, & Hansen, 1978; Martens & Witt, 2004). Consistent with this model, we begin with a discussion of stimulus control as the basis of proficient performance, instructional strategies for initial skill acquisition, and the components of discrete-trial training. We then discuss (1) ways to strengthen both responding and stimulus control through fluency building, (2) ways to present curricular materials in a free-operant format and arrange reinforcement for productive practice, and (3) the benefits of fluent responding for maintaining performance under more demanding conditions. The next section discusses challenges that behavioral educators face when attempting to program for skill generalization, and ways of further refining instruction and performance assessment to produce generative-response repertoires. From a somewhat narrow perspective on behavioral skill instruction, we then broaden the focus of the chapter to discuss three examples of behaviorally oriented instruction programs/systems: the Helping Early Literacy with Practice Strategies program, Direct Instruction, and the Morningside Model of Generative Instruction, including research supporting their effectiveness. We also address whether teachers use or receive training in these and other empirically supported techniques in this section. The last section of the chapter describes how behavioral skill training and progress monitoring form the basis of a tiered service delivery model known as *response to intervention*, which teachers use widely in schools before they determine that children are eligible for special education (e.g., Balu et al., 2015).

## STRATEGIES OF EFFECTIVE TEACHING

### The Learning/Instructional Hierarchy as a Dynamic Teaching Model

Haring et al. (1978) proposed the learning/instructional hierarchy to describe how children's performance of skills improves over time with training and how teachers should modify instructional procedures as performance improves. Although often referred to as a stage model, the learning/instructional hierarchy is perhaps better characterized as a dynamic approach to teaching that involves closely monitoring the proficiency with which a student performs a skill and then tailoring instruction and reinforcement to strengthen student responding. The teacher defines the target skill and its controlling stimuli. For example, a goal might be oral reading of 150-word passages at the third-grade level. The teacher tightly controls training stimuli initially and measures how the student performs the skills (Martens et al., 2015; Martens & Eckert, 2007). The goal is to increase responding gradually along a continuum as accurate, rapid, sustained, and generalized reading comes under stimulus control—that is, as reading becomes accurate and fluent. During later stages of training, when the teacher uses more diverse and naturalistic stimuli to occasion responding, he or she measures proficiency by *when* the student performs a skill or by the range of conditions under which the student continues to exhibit proficient performance.

Once the teacher identifies a student's strength of responding, the teacher uses the learning/instructional hierarchy to select training and reinforcement procedures that previous research has shown best promote learning. For example, one student may read tentatively with low accuracy, and another student may read with high accuracy and fluency during brief performance runs. The learning/instructional hierarchy provides the framework for Direct Instruction (Gersten, Carnine, & White, 1984), discussed later in the chapter, and researchers have used it to design, implement, and evaluate interventions for many academic performance problems (e.g., Szadokierski, Burns, & McComas, 2017; Daly & Martens, 1994).

## Stimulus Control

Fundamental to proficient performance of any skill is the development of *stimulus control*, or bringing the student's response under control of key stimuli in the environment. Failing to write the correct answer in response to a math problem or dictated spelling word signifies a lack of stimulus control. Failing to write the correct answer when working in a noisy classroom suggests that stimulus control may not be strong enough for performance to remain stable in the face of distraction. The first goal of skill training, then, is to establish stimulus control by providing the student with opportunities to respond with modeling, prompting, and feedback, plus differential reinforcement for correct responding. As practice trials accumulate, the student's need for assistance decreases, stimulus control increases, performance of the behavior becomes more efficient, and the student better discriminates the conditions under which behavior produces reinforcement.

For example, Chafouleas, Martens, Dobson, Weinstein, and Gardner (2004) evaluated the effects of three interventions involving practice, feedback, and reinforcement with children who exhibited different baseline levels of oral reading fluency. The two students whose oral reading was under stimulus control of the printed words benefited most from practice alone via repeated readings. These were the students with the highest fluency and lowest error rates at baseline. The students with the highest baseline error rates benefited more from practice combined with either performance feedback or feedback plus reinforcement. These students had the weakest strength of responding, and the intervention likely was effective because the additional intervention components helped bring rapid and accurate reading under stimulus control of the text.

## Acquisition

Acquisition-level training focuses on providing students with enough assistance to perform a skill correctly that was not in their repertoire previously, and then differentially reinforcing accurate performance of the skill in the presence of its evoking stimuli. Accuracy is the first and most basic performance criterion a student must meet when learning any skill. Promoting stimulus control with reinforcement for correct responding may be as simple as praising a child for saying, "Red!" after the teacher shows the child an apple and asks him or her to say its color, or as complex as giving a student a grade of A on a composition about the Civil War in response to a homework assignment in history. Three-term acquisition trials (i.e., antecedent–behavior–consequence) may occur in the natural environment when opportunities to model and reinforce a target skill present themselves, such as in incidental teaching, or in isolation under control of a trainer, such as in discrete-trial training (Wolery, Bailey, & Sugai, 1988).

Research has shown that discrete-trial training is effective for teaching many skills and involves presentation of (1) a command and a discriminative stimulus in the presence of which we expect the student to emit the response, (2) a prompt to increase the likelihood of a correct response, (3) an opportunity to emit the response, (4) corrective feedback for incorrect responses, and (5) differential reinforcement for correct responding. Many children with developmental disabilities such as autism spectrum disorder do not imitate adults, exhibit repetitive or stereotypic behavior, pay little attention to social cues, have limited communication, and may not mand for (i.e., request) information (Marion et al., 2012; Smith, 2001). As a result, these children may not acquire skills through exploring, playing, imitating, and talking in the same manner as their typically developing peers. Behavior analysts often use discrete-trial training to teach these children important social, communication, and self-help skills (e.g., Valentino, LeBlanc, Veazey, Weaver, & Raetz, 2019). Discrete-trial training includes teaching skills in isolation; prompting, guiding, and reinforcing the correct response; and conducting many learning trials per session.

Once a student can perform a skill accurately with assistance, the teacher withdraws or gradually fades assistance to transfer control to the discriminative stimulus. Procedures for systematically fading prompts may involve intermittently withdrawing or gradually reducing their intensity, increasing the latency to their presentation, or using progressively less intrusive prompts (Cengher, Budd, Farrell, & Fienup, 2018; Wolery et al., 1988). One strategic concern during acquisition is how to fade or withdraw prompts in a way that maintains correct responding (Cividini-Motta & Ahearn, 2013). Teachers typically address this concern by measuring correct responses and errors at each prompt level and by altering the prompt's intrusiveness based on the resulting performance data. For example, if accuracy is high when the teacher provides assistance, then fading assistance may be necessary to promote independent responding. If accuracy is low with no improvement over time, the student may need more assistance, or the teacher should teach the skill using easier materials (Wolery et al., 1988). If only errors occur, then the teacher may need to teach prerequisite or component skills before continuing. Conversely, if accuracy is high and stable in the absence of assistance, then the teacher may need to restructure the training situation to build fluency.

## Fluency

Once the student has met the desired criterion for accuracy of responding with discrete-trial training (e.g., 90% correct trials over three consecutive sessions), training shifts to fluency building. Binder (1996) defined *fluency* as "the fluid combination of accuracy plus speed that characterizes competent performance" (p. 164). By virtue of its emphasis on response rate, fluency building requires free-operant rather than discrete-trial training arrangements (Johnson & Layng, 1996). In a free-operant arrangement, the teacher gives students enough stimulus materials, such as a worksheet of 30 addition problems, for them to practice timed performance runs during which they are free to emit as many or as few responses as they wish. During free-operant performance runs, accurate rate of responding, such as words read correctly per minute, replaces percentage of correct trials as a measure of student performance. A key feature of fluency building is the differential reinforcement of in-creasingly efficient and fluent performance, which strengthens stimulus control. Research has suggested that productive skill practice should include (1) tasks, materials, or both to which the student can respond with high accuracy and minimal assistance (i.e., instructionally matched materials); (2) brief, repeated practice opportunities with feedback and reinforcement; (3) monitoring and charting performance; and (4) performance criteria for increasing the difficulty of material (Daly et al., 2007).

A strategic concern with fluency building, which involves exposure to material that increases in difficulty, is exactly where in a vertically linked curriculum sequence to begin practice. Depending on the skill, the teacher may determine the starting point when the student reaches a fluency criterion on less difficult material, such as passage reading (Daly, Martens, Kilmer, & Massie, 1996), or material that differs in the ratio of known to unknown items, such as word-list training (MacQuarrie, Tucker, Burns, & Hartman, 2002). As an example, Martens et al. (2007) evaluated the effects of a fluency-based after-school reading program with 15 low-achieving second- and third-grade students. The curriculum included four passages at each of six grade levels, sequenced by difficulty both within and across grades. The researchers required students to meet a retention criterion of reading 100 words correctly per minute in the absence of practice 2 days after training to advance to a more difficult passage in the curriculum. Training occurred 3 times a week and consisted of phrase drill–error correction for words missed at pretest, listening to a passage preview, and three repeated readings of the passage. Additional components of the program included goal setting, charting, and token reinforcement for meeting the fluency criterion. Results showed that after the equivalent of 5½ weeks of training, children advanced between two and three grade levels on average in the difficulty of passages they could read above the retention criterion. The researchers also observed significant pre- to postintervention gains for children at each grade level on untrained, generalization passages.

## Maintenance and Generalization

Once the student reaches a desired level of fluency during relatively brief performance runs, such as 2 minutes of math computation or 1 minute of oral reading, the teacher can strengthen performance further by modifying the training conditions to more closely approximate the natural environment. The progression from fluency building to maintenance to generalization involves strengthening stimulus control and programming stimulus diversity. The teacher strengthens stimulus control through differential reinforcement of correct and then rapid responding to discriminative stimuli (such as two-digit numbers and the sign for multiplication), over time and under many stimulus conditions (such as alone with the trainer, in class during a group exercise, or at home for homework). The teacher also programs stimulus diversity by systematically varying features of the discriminative stimuli (such as presenting math computation problems vertically in worksheets or horizontally in story problems).

A basic assumption of response-to-intervention models is that students will show individual differences in benefiting from instructional trials. Research has shown that for some students, strength of responding following intervention will increase enough to produce generalized oral reading fluency (Daly, Martens, et al., 1996), whereas for others it may not (e.g., Daly, Martens, Hamler, Dool, & Eckert, 1999). Generalization is an important outcome of intervention and often requires explicit programming (Stokes & Baer, 1977). Researchers have examined several strategies for promoting generalized oral reading fluency, which include training loosely with multiple low-word-overlap passages; training with common stimuli, such as high-word-overlap passages or color-coded rimes; training with passages containing multiple exemplars of key or frequent words; training to functional fluency aims, such as 100 words read correctly per minute; and training broadly applicable skills such as phoneme blending (Ardoin, McCall, & Klubnik, 2007; Bonfiglio, Daly, Martens, Lan-Hsiang, & Corsaut, 2004; Daly, Chafouleas, Persampieri, Bonfiglio, & LaFleur, 2004; Daly, Martens, et al., 1996; Martens et al., 2007; Martens, Werder, Hier, & Koenig, 2013; Martens et al., 2019; Mesmer et al., 2010).

Three questions arise with respect to fluency building: (1) What rate of performance should we require to promote maintenance and generalization of a skill; (2) how should we design fluency-building activities for more complex or composite skills; and (3) how should we arrange reinforcement to support practice over time? Advocates of precision teaching adopted and subsequently abandoned three *norm-referenced* approaches to answering the first question. These approaches included comparisons to typical peers, competent peers, and competent adults (Johnson & Layng, 1996). The norm-referenced fluency aims were problematic because they did not always predict generalization—fluent performance over time in different circumstances, with different materials, or on more complex tasks (Binder, 1996). As a result, researchers developed *functional* fluency aims, indicating performance levels above which students would be likely to maintain fluency under more demanding practice conditions. Summarized by the acronym RESAA, researchers have used these aims to predict *retention* in the absence of practice; *endurance* over longer performance runs; *stability* in the face of distraction; *application* to more complex tasks; and *adduction*, which is spontaneous emergence of new skill forms (Johnson & Layng, 1996). For example, McDowell and Keenan (2001) trained a 9-year-old boy with attention-deficit/hyperactivity disorder (ADHD) to say phonemes displayed on flash cards at increasing levels of fluency. Before performance reached a fluency aim of 60–80 sounds correct per minute, probes for endurance showed decreases in fluency and on-task behavior. The boy maintained on-task behavior and fluency at high levels after he achieved the fluency aim.

With respect to the second question, one implication of the learning/instructional hierarchy is that students should practice prerequisite or component skills to high levels of fluency before teachers require students to combine them into more complex or composite skills (Binder, 1996). This may be relatively easy to accomplish when a teacher is training simple or basic skills the first time they appear in a curriculum sequence, if the teacher can build sufficient time for practice into the instructional day. For building fluency in more complex skills, however, the situation becomes more challenging. Consider oral reading fluency, for example. Even after the teacher has identified a starting point for fluency building in the curriculum, deficits in one or more component skills may mitigate the effects of practice and reinforcement with connected text. For example, the teacher may identify a starting point as end-of-first-grade passages for a third grader with significant reading difficulties, but the student's problems with reading sight word vocabulary and decoding may prevent her from achieving fluency. In such a case, the teacher may need to provide fluency- or even acquisition-level training in isolation on the deficient component skills, along with opportunities to practice the composite skill. Research has shown that cumulative dysfluency is "perhaps the single most important factor in long-term student failure" (Binder, 1996, p. 184), and cumulative fluency accelerates the learning process and even leads to the spontaneous emergence of new skills, as we discuss in the next section.

Previous research has shown that teachers can maintain high rates of academic performance by using intermittent fixed-ratio schedules to support practice (McGinnis, Friman, & Carlyon, 1999), multiple-ratio schedules where the magnitude of reinforcement progressively increases as completion rate increases (Lovitt & Esveldt, 1970), and even lottery schedules where chances of reinforcement are as low as 50% (Martens et al., 2002). Preliminary evidence also suggests that students may prefer different reinforcement contingencies as their skill proficiency increases. For example, Lannie and Martens (2004) gave students the opportunity to complete two sets of math problems, either both easy or both difficult. The completion of problems from each set produced a different reinforcement contingency. Students could earn rewards for on-task behavior at specified intervals while working one set of problems, or for the number of problems completed correctly from the other set. Students in the study chose reinforcement for time on task when working difficult problems, but switched to reinforcement for the number of problems completed correctly when working easy problems, as this contingency maximized the amount of reinforcement per session.

## THE ROLE AND ANALYSIS OF GENERATIVE-RESPONSE REPERTOIRES

As suggested in the previous section, student responding in a classroom should be highly predictable to anyone familiar with the curriculum. In a well-sequenced curriculum, response demands will be repetitive for many of the behavioral repertoires taught early in the curriculum, such as reading text or basic math calculations, as teachers incorporate them into increasingly complex behavioral repertoires that they presume will prepare students for life beyond the classroom (e.g., preparing reports). Although response demands may be predictable, the academic stimuli that occasion them are continually changing as time, exemplars, and settings change. Some of these stimulus changes occur naturally, but a teacher should program them.

One limitation that teachers face, however, is that they cannot teach all possible stimulus–response relations as they prepare students for future

academic behavior. Alessi's (1987) conceptualization of the teacher's task is most insightful for understanding how to promote and analyze generalization of academic responding. An economical and efficient approach to teaching is to train *generative-response repertoires*, which allow students to respond and even combine trained responses in novel ways to differing configurations of stimuli and task demands. These response repertoires are generative in the sense that a student is now capable of applying previously learned responses in ways that a teacher has not instructed. These response repertoires also may be *recombinative* in that the student may combine responses in novel ways, thereby generating a new response repertoire. The results are new and more sophisticated behavioral repertoires for responding adaptively to varying stimulus conditions. The teacher, therefore, should strive to teach a generative set of responses as a subset of all possible responses (the universal set of all possible stimulus–response combinations for the response class). Trained responses are generative and functional if they contribute to the student's ability to respond appropriately in the presence of untaught stimuli. After the teacher brings the student's responding under stimulus control for the generative set, stimulus generalization proceeds until the student reaches a threshold of responding with the generative set that correlates with increases in correct responding for items from the universal set. The teacher conducts measurement with the generative-response set to assess mastery and with samples from the universal set to assess generalization (Alessi, 1987).

### Generative Repertoires in Oral Reading Fluency

This conceptualization of generalization is perhaps most appropriate for the basic academic skills that serve as the foundation for all other skills in a curriculum. Oral reading fluency and phoneme blending are examples of basic academic skills that have gained prominence in the wider educational community. Authoritative documents such as reports from the National Reading Panel (2000) and the National Research Council (Snow, Burns, & Griffin, 1998) have established their critical role in reading development. In the case of oral reading fluency, a student's word reading should come under the stimulus control of the text, which consists of varying configurations of letters separated by spaces and punctuation marks. Those letters, of course, are organized into words that the student must read or decode rapidly to understand or to provide a verbal report of the content of the text. Words appear in different orders in texts, with grammatical conventions constraining the order somewhat, and the student must be able to read words fluently across texts for functional word reading. The curriculum defines the generative set of response repertoires, and the teacher applies different strategies to bring student responding under the control of texts, which become progressively difficult throughout the curriculum. If the teacher simply measures student performance on the instructional texts, he or she does not know whether responding for instructed words will occur in other texts that contain the same words. If the student fails to generalize word reading to other texts, reading will not become a functional skill for other tasks the student will need to perform (e.g., reading to prepare for a history exam).

Researchers have analyzed generalization of word reading by manipulating word overlap in two passages and measuring student responding (Daly, Martens, et al., 1996; Martens et al., 2019). Two passages have *high word overlap* if many of the same words appear in the two passages, but the stories are different and have different word orders (Daly, Martens, et al., 1996). Manipulating word overlap between texts can facilitate the measurement of generalized oral reading fluency. For example, Daly, Martens, et al. (1996) found greater generalization for instruction to high-word-overlap passages than to low-word-overlap passages of equal difficulty. Word overlap interacted with difficulty level, so that greater gains were observed for easier materials than for harder materials.

Researchers have analyzed generalized reading fluency based on word overlap to identify potentially effective reading interventions through brief experimental analyses (Daly, Bonfiglio, Mattson, Persampieri, & Foreman-Yates, 2005; Daly et al., 1999). For example, Daly, Persampieri, McCurdy, and Gortmaker (2005) conducted brief experimental analyses using a single-case experimental design to evaluate whether the reading deficits of two students were skill-based, performance-based, or both. They used the results of the brief experimental analyses to identify individualized interventions. One intervention was an instructional strategy that included repeated readings, listening-passage preview, phrase drill–error correction, and syllable segmentation–error correction. The other intervention was a reward contingency. Initially, they combined the instructional strategy and reward conditions in an intervention package and alternated the intervention package with a control

condition. Next, they compared the effects of the individual interventions alone by alternating the instructional strategy and the reward condition. Finally, they compared the intervention package with the individual intervention that produced the highest level of responding when they evaluated the effects of the instructional strategy and reward conditions alone. In this type of brief experimental analysis, a behavior analyst compares performance in high-word-overlap passages to equal-difficulty-level, low-word-overlap passages and evaluates the differences across interventions. Low-word-overlap passages serve as controls for difficulty level and extraneous variables that might affect responding over time. Assessment of oral reading fluency is sufficiently sensitive that it can detect differences during rapidly alternating conditions. The resulting interventions are more robust and more likely to produce generalized improvements over time, because the analysis is a direct measure of generalized responding (Daly, Persampieri, et al., 2005).

Daly, Persampieri, et al. (2005) used the results of the brief experimental analysis to identify the most efficient intervention that produced the highest level of responding. The reward contingency was most effective for one student. The intervention that combined instructional strategies with the reward contingency was most effective for the second student. The researchers taught the students to self-manage the reading intervention, and they measured correctly read words per minute during continuous monitoring of student performance. Both students demonstrated substantial improvements in oral reading fluency in an independent reading series.

The prior conceptual analysis of generative responding suggests that word reading should generalize not only to untaught configurations of instructed words, such as the same words in novel texts, but also to untaught words. The universal word set should include all words that might appear in texts of the appropriate difficulty for a given level in the curriculum (e.g., first grade vs. second grade). Many of these words may not share stimulus properties with the generative set. Nonetheless, students should be able to read them. Teachers can sample this set by using equal-difficulty-level but low-word-overlap passages. For example, Daly, Persampieri, et al. (2005) used one reading series for measurement over time and an independent series for instruction. They used the universal set to evaluate the effectiveness of the empirically derived instructional interventions, which permitted subsequent conclusions regarding generalization of word-reading fluency to untaught reading materials.

Gortmaker, Daly, McCurdy, Persampieri, and Hergenrader (2007) used a brief experimental analysis to identify potential parent-tutoring interventions for three students with learning disabilities. Researchers presented high- and low-word-overlap passages relative to the intervention passages in a multiple-probe design and in a multiple-baseline-across-participants design, respectively, during the brief experimental analysis. Results of the brief experimental analysis identified reading interventions that parents would use. Improvements as a function of parent tutoring in high- and low-word-overlap passages validated the effectiveness of the tutoring intervention. The intervention improved students' generalized reading fluency to instructed words in novel order (as measured by performance in the high-word-overlap passages) and to uninstructed words in novel texts (as measured in low-word-overlap passages).

### Generative Repertoires in Phonological Awareness

The ability to manipulate sounds in words is an even more basic skill than word reading. Blending phonemes, the basic units of speech, to form words is critical to a student's success in becoming a reader (National Reading Panel, 2000). Experiential deficits in phoneme blending put students at significant risk for classification as having a learning disability (Vellutino, Scanlon, & Tanzman, 1998). As a prerequisite skill to reading words, a student's ability to blend sounds to form words in response to textual stimuli is a highly generalizable skill when the student attains proficiency. Combining responses allows the student to read a word he or she has been unable to read previously. Phoneme blending is an excellent example of a recombinative, generative-response repertoire, because students are required to combine sounds based on textual stimuli as a basis for becoming good readers. We can think of phonemic responding as a *minimal-response repertoire* (Alessi, 1987; Skinner, 1957), because (1) there is a point-to-point correspondence between the textual stimulus and the response, and (2) the verbal response is the smallest response under the stimulus control of the textual display.

Daly et al. (2004) demonstrated the superiority of bringing phonemes versus whole words under stimulus control for improving generalized word reading. In this study, they compared two conditions that they equated for response opportunities,

differential reinforcement, and degree of overlap in phonemes between trained words and generalization words. They made assessment and reinforcement opportunities indiscriminable across conditions, so that students could not associate words with a condition. The critical difference between the two conditions was the size of the response that the researchers brought under stimulus control. They trained phonemes in the phoneme-blending condition and sight words in the sight-word-reading condition. They rearranged the letters corresponding to phonemes in unknown words to measure generalization across both conditions. Thus the researchers trained the students to read a nonsense variant of each unknown word that contained the same phonemes. Students mastered many more words in the phoneme-blending condition than in the sight-word-reading condition. This method of measuring generalization for phoneme blending represents a solid point of departure for working out future experimental analyses of how these minimal-response repertoires may ultimately enable the student to read and understand connected text.

## ACADEMIC INSTRUCTIONAL PROGRAMS BASED ON THE PRINCIPLES OF BEHAVIOR ANALYSIS

The applications of behavior analysis in effective academic instructional programs and intervention are far-reaching, and a discussion of each program or intervention that integrates elements of behavioral instruction is beyond the scope of this chapter. In fact, many program designers and educators in general may not view a program or intervention as behavior-analytically derived, even if it integrates behavioral principles. Instead, most educators and education researchers commonly discuss effective instructional practices as evidence-based, scientifically based, or research-based practices (e.g., Brownell, Smith, Crockett, & Griffin, 2012; National Reading Panel, 2000; Wood & Blanton, 2009), rather than attributing those practices to a particular educational or psychological paradigm. Clearly, however, many practices educators describe as evidence-based incorporate several key elements from a behavior-analytic paradigm; thus we could consider them as falling within a general framework of behavioral instruction.

To illustrate, research evidence for at least the past 20 years has called for systematic and explicit instruction in phonics at the early grade levels, particularly for children at risk for developing later reading difficulties (Archer & Hughes, 2011; National Reading Panel, 2000). Reading programs such as Open Court Reading (Adams et al., 2005) and Sound Partners (Vadasy et al., 2000) are two examples that provide such instruction. Although researchers did not develop these programs solely from behavior-analytic principles, many key elements of these programs, such as explicit instruction, systematic prompts, and frequent opportunities to respond, undoubtedly map onto the characteristics of behavioral skill instruction. We describe three examples that combine behavioral techniques with comprehensive instructional programs, curricula, models, or systems designed to improve students' academic skills. We discuss the effectiveness of each program and provide estimates regarding educators' training and use of them.

## Helping Early Literacy with Practice Strategies

Helping Early Literacy with Practice Strategies (HELPS) offers two structured reading programs specifically designed to improve students' reading fluency. Teachers can implement the programs either in a one-on-one (Begeny, 2009) or a small-group (Begeny, Ross, Greene, Mitchell, & Whitehouse, 2012) context, and materials are currently available in English and Spanish. The HELPS programs integrate each of the five characteristics listed at the beginning of the chapter that are most central to behavioral approaches to instruction, and they integrate specific tools for monitoring and promoting strong implementation fidelity. Researchers based the instructional components of HELPS on existing research on reading fluency instruction and intervention (e.g., Chard, Vaughn, & Tyler, 2002; National Reading Panel, 2000; Morgan & Sideridis, 2006; Therrien, 2004), and the development process used iterative methods and other principles of design-based research (e.g., Anderson & Shattuck, 2012; Shernoff et al., 2011). The HELPS programs include repeated reading of instructionally appropriate text, modeling, phrase drill–error correction, verbal cueing procedures for students to read with fluency and for comprehension, goal setting, performance feedback with graphing, and a motivational reward system.

Implementation of HELPS sessions requires 8–12 minutes apiece. The program includes a teacher's manual and an online training video, together with three primary protocols to assist educators with implementation fidelity: (1) a flowchart that visually displays each instructional component and the proper sequence; (2) brief, scripted instructions the educator provides to the student(s); and (3) a tips and reminders sheet. The flowchart and scripted instructions promote strong implementation fidelity of the core procedures, and the tips and reminders sheet assists the educator with implementation quality (e.g., high-quality implementation of each core procedure, and use of behaviors that are most likely to engage and motivate each student). The HELPS programs also include a series of 100 systematically sequenced reading passages, a placement assessment to match curriculum passages with the student's skill level, and other materials to assist educators with achieving high implementation fidelity.

Research shows that the HELPS program can improve oral reading fluency and comprehension for many populations, including average readers, students with reading difficulties or disabilities, and English-language-learner students when a teacher, a teacher assistant, a school volunteer, or a parent implements it approximately three times per week (e.g., Begeny, Braun, et al., 2012; Begeny et al., 2010; Begeny, Mitchell, Whitehouse, Samuels, & Stage, 2011; Begeny, Ross, et al., 2012; Mitchell & Begeny, 2014). Research also supports the implementation fidelity (Begeny, Easton, Upright, Tunstall, & Ehrenbock, 2014; Begeny, Upright, Easton, Ehrenbock, & Tunstall, 2013) and progress-monitoring (Begeny et al., 2015) materials that supplement or are built directly into the HELPS implementation procedures.

## Direct Instruction

As was the case for the Open Court Reading and Sound Partners programs mentioned previously, the researchers who developed Direct Instruction did not base it specifically on principles of behavior analysis, though this approach to instruction clearly falls within a behavioral framework (Becker, 1992; Fredrick, Deitz, Bryceland, & Hummel, 2000). According to Becker (1992), Direct Instruction is "a systematic approach to the design and delivery of a range of procedures for building and maintaining basic cognitive skills" (p. 71). Specifically, Direct Instruction is a skill-based instructional curriculum in which teachers promote the sequential development of student competencies by following scripted instructional routines (Becker, 1992; Gersten et al., 1984). Teachers generally use small-group instruction and instructional strategies, such as modeling, and positive reinforcement, such as praise, for accurate responding. Furthermore, Direct Instruction lessons ensure that teachers allow students to obtain sufficient practice with targeted material and receive frequent opportunities to respond with corrective feedback.

In Project Follow Through, one of the largest educational experiments ever conducted, Direct Instruction was one of several instructional programs independently used with thousands of students representing various socioeconomic levels and ethnicities throughout the United States. This large-scale project aimed to assess each program by comparing pre- and posttest scores on various measures to a similar control group (see Watkins, 1997, for a detailed review of the study). Although Project Follow Through had important limitations, such as an inconsistent use of experimental-design elements, data analyses suggested that students receiving Direct Instruction performed better than those receiving any other instructional program on basic skill measures, comprehension measures, and affective measures such as self-esteem (Becker, 1992; Watkins, 1997). Adams and Engelmann (1996) subsequently conducted a meta-analytic review of 37 studies that examined the effectiveness of Direct Instruction after Project Follow Through concluded. The authors reported that "Direct Instruction interventions have been shown to produce superior performance with preschool, elementary, and secondary regular and special education students and adults. Direct Instruction has also produced superior results with various minority populations, including non-English speakers" (p. 3).

A more recent review of Direct Instruction by the U.S. Institute of Education's What Works Clearinghouse (WWC) found only two studies that met their *evidence standards* (i.e., their research methodology standards) for review. The WWC reported that one Direct Instruction study had "no discernible effects on the oral language, print knowledge, cognition, and math skills of special education students" (WWC, 2007), and that the other study, a review of the Direct Instruction curriculum Reading Mastery, had "potentially positive effects on the reading achievement of English-language[-learner] students" (WWC, 2006). We describe educators' use of and training in Direct Instruction later.

## Morningside Model of Generative Instruction

The Morningside Model of Generative Instruction (Johnson & Street, 2004, 2012, 2013) is an instructional model developed from the work of Johnson and colleagues at Morningside Academy in Seattle, WA. Founded by Kent Johnson in 1980, Morningside Academy offers schooling for elementary and middle school students who have been academically unsuccessful at their previous schools. Core instructional components at Morningside Academy include (1) student groupings according to their entering repertoires and levels of instructional achievement; (2) a carefully sequenced curriculum of component and composite foundational academic skills (reading, writing, mathematics, reasoning, and problem solving); (3) explicit, direct instruction in components; and (4) daily measurement of performance, with a focus on building fluency in each of the skills outlined in the instructional sequence (Johnson & Street, 2013). The Morningside Model of Generative Instruction "hinges on the belief that complex behavioral repertoires emerge without explicit instruction when well selected component repertoires are appropriately sequenced, carefully instructed, and well-rehearsed" (Johnson & Street, 2004, p. 26). In other words, the Morningside Model of Generative Instruction explicitly seeks to build generative-response repertoires through appropriate instructional sequencing, effective instructional practices, and student mastery of skills.

Although conducting tightly controlled research on its educational programs is not a major goal of Morningside Academy, educators routinely gather pre- and postoutcome data on the instructional package, including implementation of the Morningside Model of Generative Instruction in 128 partner schools and school districts across the United States and Canada. Data collection ranges from daily criterion-referenced measures to yearly norm-referenced tests. Data collected over 35 years at Morningside Academy and its partner schools demonstrate that its educational model is effective, especially compared to typical educational programs. For instance, in one rural public school in British Columbia that implemented the Morningside model of generative instruction, the percentage of students performing at grade level in writing rose from 39 to 80% in 9 months. In a separate school in British Columbia, the number of students reading in the below-average range decreased by 24% in one school year, and the number of students reading in the above-average range increased by 35%. Johnson and Street (2004, 2012) described similar results across each of the major academic areas and across a range of grade levels and school types (e.g., rural, urban).

## Teachers' Training in and Use of Behavioral Instruction Practices and Programs

A few publications offer insight into educators' levels of training and usage of behavioral instruction practices. In the 1990s several authors observed that most teachers were not using such practices, particularly educators in regular education classrooms (e.g., Axelrod, 1996; Binder, 1991; Fredrick et al., 2000; Hall, 1991). The data presented earlier about HELPS, Direct Instruction, and the Morningside Model of Generative Instruction suggest that at least some behaviorally oriented programs are widely used, are included in professional development, or a combination. In addition, two more recent studies have addressed the topic through surveys.

Begeny and Martens (2006) asked master's-level elementary, secondary, and special education teachers in training to estimate how much coursework and applied training they received in various behavioral instruction and measurement practices during their undergraduate and graduate training. Results indicated that students in each type of degree program received little to no coursework or applied training in most of the instructional practices the survey listed (e.g., prompting, shaping, fading). Moreover, teachers' training in behavioral assessment practices (such as using graphs to make instructional decisions) and instructional programs (such as Direct Instruction) was particularly low, even for special educators.

Burns and Ysseldyke (2009) surveyed special education teachers (*N* = 174) and school psychologists (*N* = 333) a few years later about their use of eight different evidence-based practices with small, medium, and large effects in meta-analytic research. Special educators used a 5-point Likert scale to rate how frequently they used each practice. The researchers surveyed school psychologists because they work closely with special educators and could offer observations about teachers' use of the eight evidence-based practices in the survey. As such, the survey asked school psychologists to rank-order the practices by how often they observed the practices in classrooms for students with special needs. Findings showed that most special education teachers reported using applied behavior analysis almost every day (55% of the respondents) or at least once per week (16%). Also, 83% reported using direct instruction (the general approach, rather than the specific Direct Instruction program) almost every day. School psychologists indicated that they observed direct instruc-

tion most often of the eight practices in the survey, and they ranked applied behavior analysis fifth.

These findings suggest at least some evidence exists to indicate that behavioral instruction practices are prevalent in many U.S. classrooms. Because U.S. and state policies have emphasized the use of evidence-based practices, of which many integrate core characteristics that are consistent with the science of applied behavior analysis, continued or even more widespread use of and training in behavioral instruction practices in the near future seem plausible.

## SCHOOL-BASED RESPONSE-TO-INTERVENTION MODELS

Response-to-intervention models are becoming more prevalent in today's schools. Response to intervention is a multi-tiered prevention model in which the teacher matches evidence-based practices to students' instructional and behavioral needs (Ardoin, Wagner, & Bangs, 2016). These models are based on the notion that educators can order the severity of student problems along a continuum and deliver services in graduated tiers (Tilly, 2008). A comprehensive description of response to intervention is beyond the scope of this chapter; therefore, we discuss it solely from a behavior-analytic perspective. In so doing, we describe (1) legislative influences on response to intervention, (2) fundamental characteristics of response-to-intervention models, and (3) the role that behavior-analytic principles and procedures play in response-to-intervention implementation.

### Legislative Influences

The No Child Left Behind Act of 2001 and the Individuals with Disabilities Education Improvement Act of 2004 have led to important reforms in education practice by emphasizing the measurement of student performance for high-stakes decision making (Reschly & Bergstrom, 2009). Several provisions in the No Child Left Behind Act have aided in the development and implementation of response to intervention (Burns & Gibbons, 2008). Included among these are (1) frequent collection and review of data on student performance, (2) use of evidence-based instructional and intervention procedures, and (3) an emphasis on prevention and early identification of academic problems. These provisions have prompted schools to focus on student-learning outcomes by collecting data that teachers then use to make educational decisions (Tilly, 2008). Most notably, the No Child Left Behind Act has made schools accountable for student learning by creating contingencies, such as rewards and sanctions, for educational professionals for student outcomes.

The Individuals with Disabilities Education Improvement Act of 2004 introduced response to intervention as an alternative method for identifying students with specific learning disabilities. Historically, a discrepancy between a student's score on an individually administered measure of cognitive ability and academic achievement identified the student as having a learning disability. Educators have characterized this approach as a *wait-to-fail* model, because the child does not receive services until his or her achievement level falls significantly below that of same-grade or same-age peers. Gresham (2009) suggested that delaying services decreases their effectiveness. In addition to linking response to intervention with disability classification, the Individuals with Disabilities Education Improvement Act promoted the use of positive behavioral interventions and supports in the schools. Positive behavioral interventions and supports aligns with response to intervention to prevent behavior problems by teaching and reinforcing appropriate behaviors with evidence-based interventions that teachers apply systematically to students, based on the students' demonstrated levels of need (Sugai & Horner, 2009).

## Characteristics of Response to Intervention

Response to intervention is the practice of implementing evidence-based instruction and interventions, systematically evaluating student progress, and altering instruction and intervention to align with student needs (Buffman, Mattos, & Webber, 2009; Burns & Gibbons, 2008; Sugai & Horner, 2009). Although the recommended structure of response to intervention has varied somewhat in the literature, a consensus has emerged around a three-tiered model (Burns, Deno, & Jimerson, 2007) with six critical features (Fuchs & Fuchs, 1998; Fuchs et al., 2002; Sugai & Horner, 2009):

1. Interventions and instruction are evidence-based.
2. Educators match interventions to student needs along a graduated continuum that increases in intensity, frequency, duration, and individualization.
3. Educators use a standardized problem-solving protocol for assessment and educational decision making.
4. Educators use data-based decision rules for assessing student progress and altering current instruction, intervention, or both.
5. Educators deliver evidence-based instruction and interventions with high fidelity.
6. A system exists to screen and to identify students who are not making adequate progress.

Educators provide students with universal instruction and behavior management strategies that they implement with high fidelity at the prevention level, which is Tier 1. Approximately 10–20% of students will not respond adequately and will need more intensive intervention, given the continuum of student problems. Schools typically conduct *universal screening* (1) to evaluate the effectiveness of the instruction and interventions at Tier 1, (2) to identify struggling students so that the school can provide additional services immediately, and (3) to establish school-based norms to aid in evaluating student performance. Universal screening involves the assessment of students' basic academic skills at least three times per year, using standard curriculum-like probes (Buffman et al., 2009; Burns & Gibbons, 2008; Erchul & Martens, 2010; Tilly, 2008). Schools identify and monitor *at-risk* students who score below a criterion or percentile on a universal-screening measure, to determine whether these students are making adequate progress in Tier 1.

Typically, schools use a *dual-discrepancy* approach to determine whether a student is making adequate progress. A dual-discrepancy approach compares the student's *performance level* and *rate of progress* to those of peers. As an example, a school will identify a student as at risk if he or she scores below the 25th percentile in oral reading fluency during universal screening. The school then must repeatedly measure this student's reading skills over time. The school will label the student's progress inadequate if he or she continues to score below a criterion and to display a rate of progress significantly below that of typical peers (e.g., Burns & Senesac, 2005).

Students making inadequate progress at Tier 1 receive Tier 2 interventions. About 5–15% of the student population will need Tier 2 interventions to supplement Tier 1 supports. Note that Tier 2 services supplement rather than replace Tier 1 supports. Educators typically match Tier 2 interventions to specific student problems and implement them in a small-group format with high fidelity.

Ideally, these small groups consist of students with similar problems or instructional needs. Educators monitor students in Tier 2 at least monthly, and they again use the dual-discrepancy approach to evaluate intervention effectiveness and to determine whether a student needs more individualized intervention, more intensive intervention, or both. Educators remove Tier 2 interventions when a student's rates of skill acquisition and progress become equal to or exceed those of their peers (Buffman et al., 2009; Burns & Gibbons, 2008; Erchul & Martens, 2010; Tilly, 2008).

Finally, educators reserve Tier 3 interventions for students who show inadequate progress at Tier 2. Approximately 5% of the student population will receive Tier 3 interventions. An educator usually delivers these in a one-on-one format, with high fidelity and with greater intensity, duration, and frequency than Tier 2 interventions. Again, Tier 3 interventions supplement rather than replace Tier 1 support. Educators monitor students' progress weekly at Tier 3 and use the dual-discrepancy approach. Educators return students who make adequate progress in Tier 3 to Tier 1 or 2, and provide more intensive interventions or make a referral for a special education evaluation for any student who continues to show inadequate progress in Tier 3.

## Applied Behavior Analysis and Response-to-Intervention Implementation

Response to intervention and applied behavior analysis are related closely, as both emphasize student behavior, modification of instructional antecedents and consequences, and measurement of behavior change when educators manipulate these variables systematically (Ardoin et al., 2016). Essentially, applied behavior analysis provides a framework within which educators can identify target behaviors, develop and match interventions to those behaviors, and evaluate those interventions by measuring changes in behavior (Martens & Ardoin, 2010). In this section, we describe how educators apply principles of applied behavior analysis in the context of a response-to-intervention model in schools.

Ardoin et al. (2016) outlined several considerations for student support team members to consider when selecting target behaviors for a particular student. First, the team must consider the social significance of the target behaviors to the student, the school, and the family. Second, the team must select an appropriate replacement

behavior if the goal is to decrease problem behavior. The target behavior must not be more effortful than problem behavior and must produce the same consequences with similar quality, rate, and delay. Selecting target academic behaviors is somewhat more difficult. The goal of academic instruction is often for students to complete composite tasks that require several prerequisite skills. Therefore, team members must collect data on the composite task and on key prerequisite skills (Daly et al., 2007; Martens & Ardoin, 2010).

After selection of a target behavior, team members must consider an appropriate evidence-based intervention to improve student performance at Tier 2 or 3. They can make informed decisions about possible environmental modifications through direct assessment of student skills and behavior in the educational environment (Barnett, Daly, Jones, & Lentz, 2004; Gresham, Watson, & Skinner, 2001). Daly, Martens, Witt, and Dool (1997) suggested that students' deficits in academic performance may be related functionally to instructional variables in several ways: (1) lack of motivation, (2) insufficient opportunities to practice the skill, (3) inadequate assistance in how to perform the skill, (4) failure to vary curriculum materials to promote generalization, and (5) use of material that is too difficult for a student's skill level.

Researchers have implemented brief experimental analyses to test academic interventions matched to these hypothesized functions (Daly et al., 1997; Daly, Murdoch, Lillenstein, Webber, & Lentz, 2002; Martens, Eckert, Bradley, & Ardoin, 1999). Single-case experimental designs may be uniquely suited to evaluating functional relations between instructional variables and student academic performance when used as part of a larger, data-based problem-solving model (Barnett et al., 2004). For example, Jones et al. (2009) described a systematic problem-solving approach for improving the oral reading fluency of six third- and fourth-grade students. *Problem identification* used the schoolwide Dynamic Indicators of Basic Early Literacy Skills passages as universal-screening measures to identify children at risk for reading failure. *Problem analysis* applied each of four evidence-based instructional components (rate-contingent reinforcement, repeated readings, listening-passage preview plus phrase drill–error correction, and training on easier material) to a different passage of equivalent difficulty in a brief experimental analysis with a reversal. Researchers conducted a 3- to 10-trial extended analysis after they had identified one or more effective instructional components. The extended analysis evaluated the effects of these strategies in combination. Researchers then implemented the most effective instructional package twice per week for the remainder of the school year as the final phase, *problem evaluation*. Students showed large increases in oral reading fluency during the extended analysis of intervention packages, and three of the six students showed gains consistently above an aim line of a one-word increase per week during problem evaluation.

Finally, repeated measurement of intervention effectiveness across tiers as part of a student's cumulative intervention history is vital to the health of any response-to-intervention model (Daly et al., 2007). Teams should measure student behavior continuously over time; otherwise, they may run the risk of continuing ineffective interventions (Ardoin et al., 2016). Teams should measure both inappropriate and appropriate behavior in the actual learning environment during behavioral interventions. Martens et al. (2015) suggests that teams measure direct effects of intervention on trained material and generalized effects on global outcome measures for academic performance. Examining both sets of data can help determine whether students are not responding to intervention or are responding to intervention but failing to generalize what they learn.

## CONCLUSION

Large numbers of U.S. children continue to have significant difficulties with basic academic skills. The National Center for Education Statistics (2015) reported that 31% of fourth graders read below the basic level, and the number of children classified as having learning disabilities increased by 351% from 1976 and 1977 to 1998 and 1999 (U.S. Department of Education, 2000). Many have cited the failure to adopt evidence-based practices for the relative ineffectiveness of the American public education system with low-achieving students (e.g., Lindsley, 1992; Snow et al., 1998). As noted by Carnine (1992), dogma rather than science has often dictated educational reform over the years, enabling fads to cycle through the schools with no demonstrable improvements in instruction. We have shown in this chapter that effective teaching methods based on the principles of behavior analysis are available to educators and have been for some time. The No Child Left Behind Act of 2001

and the Individuals with Disabilities Education Improvement Act of 2004 have created opportunities for behavior analysts to become more active in promoting adoption of these evidence-based practices, and we hope the material in this chapter will continue to prompt efforts in this direction.

## REFERENCES

Adams, G. L., & Engelmann, S. (1996). *Research on Direct Instruction: 25 years beyond DISTAR*. Seattle, WA: Educational Achievement Systems.

Adams, M., Adcock, I., Bereiter, C., Brown, A., Campione, J., Carruthers, I., et al. (2005). *Open Court Reading*. DeSoto, TX: SRA/McGraw-Hill.

Alessi, G. (1987). Generative strategies and teaching for generalization. *Analysis of Verbal Behavior, 5*, 15–27.

Anderson, T., & Shattuck, J. (2012). Design-based research: A decade of progress in education research? *Educational Researcher, 41*, 16–25.

Archer, A. L., & Hughes, C. A. (2011). *Explicit instruction: Effective and efficient teaching*. New York: Guilford Press.

Ardoin, S. P., McCall, M., & Klubnik, C. (2007). Promoting generalization of oral reading fluency: Providing drill versus practice opportunities. *Journal of Behavioral Education, 16*, 54–69.

Ardoin, S. P., Wagner, L., & Bangs, K. E. (2016). Applied behavior analysis: A foundation for response to intervention. In S. R. Jimerson, M. K. Burns, & A. M. VanDerHeyden (Eds.), *Handbook of response to intervention: The science and practice of multi-tiered systems of support* (2nd ed., pp. 29–42). New York: Springer.

Axelrod, S. (1996). What's wrong with behavior analysis? *Journal of Behavioral Education, 6*, 247–256.

Balu, R., Pei, Z., Doolittle, F., Schiller, E., Jenkins, J., & Gersten, R. (2015). *Evaluation of response to intervention practices for elementary school reading* (NCEE 2016-4000). Washington, DC: National Center for Education Evaluation and Regional Assistance, Institute of Education Sciences, U.S. Department of Education.

Barnett, D. W., Daly, E. J., Jones, K. M., & Lentz, F. E. (2004). Response to intervention empirically based special service decisions from single-case designs of increasing and decreasing intensity. *Journal of Special Education, 38*(2), 66–79.

Becker, W. C. (1992). Direct Instruction: A twenty year review. In R. P. West & L. A. Hamerlynck (Eds.), *Designs for excellence in education: The legacy of B. F. Skinner* (pp. 71–112). Longmont, CO: Sopris West.

Begeny, J. C. (2009). *Helping Early Literacy with Practice Strategies (HELPS): A one-on-one program designed to improve students' reading fluency*. Raleigh, NC: Helps Education Fund. Retrieved from *www.helpsprogram. org*.

Begeny, J. C., Braun, L. M., Lynch, H. L., Ramsay, A. C., & Wendt, J. M. (2012). Initial evidence for using the HELPS reading fluency program with small instructional groups. *School Psychology Forum: Research in Practice, 6*, 50–63.

Begeny, J. C., Easton, J. E., Upright, J. J., Tunstall, K. R., & Ehrenbock, C. A. (2014). The reliability and user-feasibility of materials and procedures for monitoring the implementation integrity of a reading intervention. *Psychology in the Schools, 51*, 517–533.

Begeny, J. C., Laugle, K. M., Krouse, H. E., Lynn, A. E., Tayrose, M. P., & Stage, S. A. (2010). A control-group comparison of two reading fluency programs: The Helping Early Literacy with Practice Strategies (HELPS) program and the Great Leaps K–2 reading program. *School Psychology Review, 39*, 137–155.

Begeny, J. C., & Martens, B. K. (2006). Assessing preservice teachers' training in empirically-validated behavioral instruction practices. *School Psychology Quarterly, 21*, 262–285.

Begeny, J. C., Mitchell, R. C., Whitehouse, M. H., Samuels, F. H.., & Stage, S. A. (2011). Effects of the HELPS reading fluency program when implemented by classroom teachers with low-performing second-grade students. *Learning Disabilities Research and Practice, 26*, 122–133.

Begeny, J. C., Ross, S. G., Greene, D. J., Mitchell, R. C., & Whitehouse, M. H. (2012). Effects of the Helping Early Literacy with Practice Strategies (HELPS) Reading Fluency program with Latino English language learners: A preliminary evaluation. *Journal of Behavioral Education, 21*, 134–149.

Begeny, J. C., Upright, J. J., Easton, J. E., Ehrenbock, C. A., & Tunstall, K. R. (2013). Validity estimates and functionality of materials and procedures used to monitor the implementation integrity of a reading intervention. *Journal of Applied School Psychology, 29*, 284–304.

Begeny, J. C., Whitehouse, M. H., Methe, S. A., Codding, R. S., Stage, S. A., & Neupert, S. (2015). Do intervention-embedded assessment procedures successfully measure student growth in reading? *Psychology in the Schools, 52*, 578–593.

Binder, C. V. (1991). Marketing measurably effective instructional methods. *Journal of Behavioral Education, 1*, 317–328.

Binder, C. (1996). Behavioral fluency: Evolution of a new paradigm. *Behavior Analyst, 19*, 163–197.

Bonfiglio, C. M., Daly, E. J., Martens, B. K., Lan-Hsiang, R. L., & Corsaut, S. (2004). An experimental analysis of reading interventions: Generalization across instructional strategies, time, and passages. *Journal of Applied Behavior Analysis, 37*, 111–114.

Brobst, B., & Ward, P. (2002). Effects of posting, goal setting, and oral feedback on the skills of female soccer players. *Journal of Applied Behavior Analysis, 35*, 247–257.

Brownell, M. T., Smith, S. J., Crockett, J. B., & Griffin, C. C. (2012). *Inclusive instruction: Evidence-based practices for teaching students with disabilities.* New York: Guilford Press.

Buffman, A., Mattos, M., & Webber, C. (2009). *Pyramid response to intervention: RTI, professional learning communities, and how to respond when kids don't learn.* Bloomington, IN: Solution Tree.

Burns, M. K., Deno, S. L., & Jimerson, S. R. (2007). Toward a unified response-to-intervention model. In S. R. Jimerson, M. K. Burns, & A. M. VanDer-Heyden (Eds.), *Handbook of response to intervention: The science and practice of assessment and intervention* (pp. 428–440). New York: Springer.

Burns, M. K., & Gibbons, K. A. (2008). *Implementing response-to-intervention in elementary and secondary schools: Procedures to assure scientific-based practices.* New York: Routledge.

Burns, M. K., & Senesac, B. V. (2005). Comparison of dual discrepancy criteria to assess response to intervention. *Journal of School Psychology, 43*, 393–406.

Burns, M. K., & Ysseldyke, J. E. (2009). Reported prevalence of evidence-based instructional practices in special education. *Journal of Special Education, 43*, 3–11.

Carnine, D. (1992). Expanding the notion of teachers' rights: Access to tools that work. *Journal of Applied Behavior Analysis, 25*, 13–19.

Carroll, R. A., Joachim, B. T., St. Peter, C., & Robinson, N. (2015). A comparison of error-correction procedures on skill acquisition during discrete-trial instruction. *Journal of Applied Behavior Analysis, 48*, 257–273.

Cavanaugh, R. A., Heward, W. L., & Donelson, F. (1996). Effects of response cards during lesson closure on the academic performance of secondary students in an earth science course. *Journal of Applied Behavior Analysis, 29*, 403–406.

Cengher, M., Budd, A., Farrell, N., & Fienup, D. M. (2018). A review of prompt-fading procedures: Implications for effective and efficient skill acquisition. *Journal of Developmental and Physical Disabilities, 30*, 155–173.

Chafouleas, S. M., Martens, B. K., Dobson, R. J., Weinstein, K. S., & Gardner, K. B. (2004). Fluent reading as the improvement of stimulus control: Additive effects of performance-based interventions to repeated reading on students' reading and error rates. *Journal of Behavioral Education, 13*, 67–81.

Chard, D. J., Vaughn, S., & Tyler, B. J. (2002). A synthesis of research on effective interventions for building reading fluency with elementary students with learning disabilities. *Journal of Learning Disabilities, 35*, 386–406.

Christ, T. J., Zopluoglu, C., Monaghen, B. D., & Van Norman, E. R. (2013). Curriculum-based measurement of oral reading: Multi-study evaluation of schedule, duration, and dataset quality on progress monitoring outcomes. *Journal of School Psychology, 51*, 19–57.

Cividini-Motta, C., & Ahearn, W. H. (2013). Effects

of two variations of differential reinforcement on prompt dependency. *Journal of Applied Behavior Analysis, 46*, 640–650.

Daly, E. J., III, Bonfiglio, C. M., Mattson, T., Persampieri, M., & Foreman-Yates, K. (2005). Refining the experimental analysis of academic skill deficits: Part I. An investigation of variables affecting generalized oral reading performance. *Journal of Applied Behavior Analysis, 38*, 485–498.

Daly, E. J., III, Chafouleas, S. M., Persampieri, M., Bonfiglio, C. M., & LaFleur, K. (2004). Teaching phoneme segmenting and blending as critical early literacy skills: An experimental analysis of minimal textual repertoires. *Journal of Behavioral Education, 13*, 165–178.

Daly, E. J., III, Lentz, F. E., & Boyer, J. (1996). The instructional hierarchy: A conceptual model for understanding the effective components of reading interventions. *School Psychology Quarterly, 11*, 369–386.

Daly, E. J., III, & Martens, B. K. (1994). A comparison of three interventions for increasing oral reading performance: Application of the instructional hierarchy. *Journal of Applied Behavior Analysis, 27*, 459–469.

Daly, E. J., III, Martens, B. K., Barnett, D., Witt, J. D., & Olson, S. C. (2007). Varying intervention delivery in response to intervention: Confronting and resolving challenges with measurement, instruction, and intensity. *School Psychology Review, 36*, 562–581.

Daly, E. J., III, Martens, B. K., Hamler, K. R., Dool, E. J., & Eckert, T. L. (1999). A brief experimental analysis for identifying instructional components needed to improve oral reading fluency. *Journal of Applied Behavior Analysis, 32*, 83–94.

Daly, E. J., III, Martens, B. K., Kilmer, A., & Massie, D. (1996). The effects of instructional match and content overlap on generalized reading performance. *Journal of Applied Behavior Analysis, 29*, 507–518.

Daly, E. J., III, Martens, B. K., Witt, J. C., & Dool, E. J. (1997). A model for conducting a functional analysis of academic performance problems. *School Psychology Review, 26*, 554–574.

Daly, E. J., III, Murdoch, A., Lillenstein, L., Webber, L., & Lentz, F. E. (2002). An examination of methods for testing treatments: Conducting brief experimental analyses of the effects of instructional components on oral reading fluency. *Education and Treatment of Children, 25*, 288–316.

Daly, E. J., III, Neugebauer, S. R., Chafouleas, S. M., & Skinner, C. H. (2015). *Interventions for reading problems: Designing and evaluating effective strategies* (2nd ed.). New York: Guilford Press.

Daly, E. J., III, Persampieri, M., McCurdy, M., & Gortmaker, V. (2005). Generating reading interventions through experimental analysis of academic skills: Demonstration and empirical evaluation. *School Psychology Review, 34*, 395–414.

Dickson, M. J., & Vargo, K. K. (2017). Training kindergarten students lockdown drill procedures using behavioral skills training. *Journal of Applied Behavior Analysis, 50*, 407–412.

DiGennaro, F. D., Martens, B. K., & McIntyre, L. L. (2005). Increasing treatment integrity through negative reinforcement: Effects on teacher and student behavior. *School Psychology Review, 34*, 220–231.

Erchul, W. P., & Martens, B. K. (2010). *School consultation: Conceptual and empirical bases of practice.* New York: Springer.

Fredrick, L. D., Deitz, S. M., Bryceland, J. A., & Hummel, J. H. (2000). *Behavior analysis, education, and effective schooling.* Reno, NV: Context Press.

Fuchs, L. S., & Fuchs, D. (1986). Effects of systematic formative evaluation: A meta-analysis. *Exceptional Children, 53*, 199–208.

Fuchs, L. S., & Fuchs, D. (1998). Treatment validity: A unifying construct for reconceptualizing the identification of learning disabilities. *Learning Disability Quarterly, 13*, 204–219.

Fuchs, L. S., Fuchs, D., & Speece, D. L. (2002). Treatment validity as a unifying construct for identifying learning disabilities. *Learning Disability Quarterly, 25*, 33–45.

Gersten, R., Carnine, D., & White, W. A. T. (1984). The pursuit of clarity: Direct instruction and applied behavior analysis. In W. L. Heward, T. E. Heron, D. S. Hill, & J. Trap-Porter (Eds.), *Focus on behavior analysis in education* (pp. 38–57). Columbus, OH: Merrill.

Gortmaker, V. J., Daly, E. J., III, McCurdy, M., Persampieri, M. J., & Hergenrader, M. (2007). Improving reading outcomes for children with learning disabilities: Using brief experimental analysis to develop parent-tutoring interventions. *Journal of Applied Behavior Analysis, 40*, 203–221.

Gresham, F. M. (2009). Using response to intervention for identification of specific learning disabilities. In A. Akin-Little, S. G. Little, M. A. Bray, & T. J. Kehle (Eds.), *Behavioral interventions in schools: Evidence-based positive strategies* (pp. 205–220). Washington, DC: American Psychological Association.

Gresham, F. M., Watson, T. S., & Skinner, C. H. (2001). Functional behavioral assessment: Principles, procedures, and future directions. *School Psychology Review, 30*(2), 156–172.

Hall, R. V. (1991). Behavior analysis and education: An unfulfilled dream. *Journal of Behavioral Education, 1*, 305–316.

Haring, N. G., Lovitt, T. C., Eaton, M. D., & Hansen, C. L. (1978). *The fourth R: Research in the classroom.* Columbus, OH: Merrill.

Hogan, A., Knez, N., & Kahng, S. (2015). Evaluating the use of behavioral skills training to improve school staffs' implementation of behavior intervention plans. *Journal of Behavioral Education, 24*, 242–254.

Houvouras, A. J., IV, & Harvey, M. T. (2014). Establishing fire safety skills using behavioral skills training. *Journal of Applied Behavior Analysis, 47*, 420–424.

Individuals with Disabilities Education Improvement Act of 2004, Pub. L. No. 108-446, 20 U.S.C. 1400 et seq. (2004).

Johnson, K. R., & Layng, T. V. J. (1996). On terms and procedures: Fluency. *Behavior Analyst, 19,* 281–288.

Johnson, K., & Street, E. M. (2004). *The Morningside Model of Generative Instruction: What it means to leave no child behind.* Concord, MA: Cambridge Center for Behavioral Studies.

Johnson, K., & Street, E. M. (2012). From the laboratory to the field and back again: Morningside Academy's 32 years of improving students' academic performance. *Behavior Analyst Today, 13,* 20–40.

Johnson, K., & Street, E. M. (2013). *Response to intervention and precision teaching: Creating synergy in the classroom.* New York: Guilford Press.

Jones, K. M., Wickstrom, K. F., Noltemeyer, A. L., Brown, S. M., Schuka, J. R., & Therrien, W. J. (2009). An experimental analysis of reading fluency. *Journal of Behavioral Education, 18,* 35–55.

Keller, F. S. (1968). "Good-bye teacher . . ." *Journal of Applied Behavior Analysis, 1,* 79–89.

Kladopoulos, C. N., & McComas, J. J. (2001). The effects of form training on foul-shooting performance in members of a women's college basketball team. *Journal of Applied Behavior Analysis, 34,* 329–332.

Lannie, A. L., & Martens, B. K. (2004). Effects of task difficulty and type of contingency on students' allocation of responding to math worksheets. *Journal of Applied Behavior Analysis, 37,* 53–65.

Lerman, D. C., Hawkins, L., Hillman, C., Shireman, M., & Nissen, M. A. (2015). Adults with autism spectrum disorder as behavior technicians for young children with autism: Outcomes of a behavioral skills training program. *Journal of Applied Behavior Analysis, 48,* 233–256.

Lindsley, O. R. (1992). Why aren't effective teaching tools widely adopted? *Journal of Applied Behavior Analysis, 25,* 21–26.

Lovitt, T. C., & Esveldt, K. A. (1970). The relative effects on math performance of single- versus multiple-ratio schedules: A case study. *Journal of Applied Behavior Analysis, 3,* 261–270.

Luck, K. M., Lerman, D. C., Wu, W. L., Dupuis, D. L., & Hussein, L. A. (2018). A comparison of written, vocal, and video feedback when training teachers. *Journal of Behavioral Education, 27,* 124–144.

MacQuarrie, L. L., Tucker, J. A., Burns, M. K., & Hartman, B. (2002). Comparison of retention rates using traditional, drill sandwich, and incremental rehearsal flash card methods. *School Psychology Review, 31,* 584–595.

Marion, C., Martin, G. L., Yu, C. T., Buhler, C., & Kerr, D. (2012). Teaching children with autism spectrum disorder to mand "Where?" *Journal of Behavioral Education, 21,* 273–294.

Martens, B. K., & Ardoin, S. P. (2010). Assessing disruptive behavior within a problem-solving model. In G. G. Peacock, R. A. Ervin, E. J. Daly, III, & K. W. Merrell (Eds.), *Practical handbook of school psychology: Effective practices for the 21st century* (pp. 157–174). New York: Guilford Press.

Martens, B. K., Ardoin, S. P., Hilt, A., Lannie, A. L., Panahon, C. J., & Wolfe, L. (2002). Sensitivity of children's behavior to probabilistic reward: Effects of a decreasing-ratio lottery system on math performance. *Journal of Applied Behavior Analysis, 35,* 403–406.

Martens, B. K., Daly, E. J., & Ardoin, S. P. (2015). Applications of applied behavior analysis to school-based instructional intervention. In H. S. Roane, J. L. Ringdahl, & T. S. Falcomata (Eds.), *Clinical and organizational applications of applied behavior analysis* (pp. 125–150). New York: Elsevier.

Martens, B. K., & Eckert, T. L. (2007). The instructional hierarchy as a model of stimulus control over student *and* teacher behavior: We're close but are we close enough? *Journal of Behavioral Education, 16,* 83–91.

Martens, B. K., Eckert, T. L., Begeny, J. C., Lewandowski, L. J., DiGennaro, F., Montarello, S., et al. (2007). Effects of a fluency-building program on the reading performance of low-achieving second and third grade students. *Journal of Behavioral Education, 16,* 39–54.

Martens, B. K., Eckert, T. L., Bradley, T. A., & Ardoin, S. P. (1999). Identifying effective treatments from a brief experimental analysis: Using single-case design elements to aid decision making. *School Psychology Quarterly, 14*(2), 163–181.

Martens, B. K., Werder, C. S., Hier, B. O., & Koenig, E. A. (2013). Fluency training in phoneme blending: A preliminary study of generalized effects. *Journal of Behavioral Education, 22,* 16–36.

Martens, B. K., & Witt, J. C. (2004). Competence, persistence, and success: The positive psychology of behavioral skill instruction. *Psychology in the Schools, 41,* 19–30.

Martens, B. K., Young, N. D., Mullane, M. P., Baxter, E. B., Sallade, S. J., Kellen, D., et al. (2019). Effects of word overlap on generalized gains from a repeated readings intervention. *Journal of School Psychology, 74,* 1–9.

McDowell, C., & Keenan, M. (2001). Developing fluency and endurance in a child diagnosed with attention deficit hyperactivity disorder. *Journal of Applied Behavior Analysis, 34,* 345–348.

McGinnis, J. C., Friman, P. C., & Carlyon, W. D. (1999). The effect of token rewards on "intrinsic" motivation for doing math. *Journal of Applied Behavior Analysis, 32,* 375–379.

Mesmer, E. M., Duhon, G. J., Hogan, K., Newry, B., Hommema, S., Fletcher, C., et al. (2010). Generalization of sight word accuracy using a common stimulus procedure: A preliminary investigation. *Journal of Behavior Education, 19,* 47–61.

Miltenberger, R. G. (2016). *Behavior modification: Principles and procedures* (6th ed.). Boston: Cengage Learning.

Mitchell, C., & Begeny, J. C. (2014). Improving student

reading through parents' implementation of a structured reading program. *School Psychology Review, 43,* 41–58.

Morgan, P. L., & Sideridis, G. D. (2006). Contrasting the effectiveness of fluency interventions for students with or at risk for learning disabilities: A multilevel random coefficient modeling meta-analysis. *Learning Disabilities: Research and Practice, 21,* 191–210.

National Center for Education Statistics. (2015). The nation's report card: Mathematics and reading assessments. Retrieved February 9, 2015, from *www. nationsreportcard.gov/reading_math_2015/#?grade=4.*

National Reading Panel. (2000). *Report of the National Reading Panel. Teaching children to read: An evidence-based assessment of the scientific research literature on reading and its implications for reading instruction* (NIH Publication No. 00-4769). Washington, DC: National Institute of Child Health and Human Development.

No Child Left Behind Act of 2001, Pub. L. No. 107-110, 20 U.S.C. 6301 (2002).

Reschly, D. J. (2004). Paradigm shift, outcomes, criteria, and behavioral interventions: Foundations for the future of school psychology. *School Psychology Review, 33,* 408–416.

Reschly, D. J., & Bergstrom, M. K. (2009). Response to intervention. In T. B. Gutkin & C. R. Reynolds (Eds.), *The handbook of school psychology* (4th ed., pp. 434–460). Hoboken, NJ: Wiley.

Saville, B. K., Zinn, T. E., Neef, N. A., Van Norman, R., & Ferreri, S. J. (2006). A comparison of interteaching and lecture in the college classroom. *Journal of Applied Behavior Analysis, 39,* 49–61.

Shernoff, E. S., Mariñez-Lora, A. M., Frazier, S. L., Jakobsons, L. J., Atkins, M. S., & Bonner, D. (2011). Teachers supporting teachers in urban schools: What iterative research designs can teach us. *School Psychology Review, 40,* 465–485.

Skinner, B. F. (1954). The science of learning and the art of teaching. *Harvard Educational Review, 24,* 86–97.

Skinner, B. F. (1957). *Verbal behavior.* Acton, MA: Copley.

Skinner, B. F. (1984). *A matter of consequences.* New York: New York University Press.

Smith, T. (2001). Discrete trial training in the treatment of autism. *Focus on Autism and Other Developmental Disabilities, 16,* 86–92.

Snow, C. E., Burns, M. S., & Griffin, P. (1998). *Preventing reading difficulties in young children.* Washington, DC: National Academy Press.

Stocco, C. S., Thompson, R. H., Hart, J. M., & Soriano, H. L. (2017). Improving the interview skills of college students using behavioral skills training. *Journal of Applied Behavior Analysis, 50,* 495–510.

Stokes, T. F., & Baer, D. M. (1977). An implicit technology of generalization. *Journal of Applied Behavior Analysis, 10,* 349–367.

Sugai, G., & Horner, R. H. (2009). Responsiveness-to-intervention and school-wide positive behavior supports: Integration of multi-tiered system approaches. *Exceptionality, 17*(4), 223–237.

Szadokierski, I., Burns, M. K., & McComas, J. J. (2017). Predicting intervention effectiveness from reading accuracy and rate measures through the instructional hierarchy: Evidence for a skill-by-treatment interaction. *School Psychology Review, 46,* 190–200.

Tai, S. S., & Miltenberger, R. G. (2017). Evaluating behavioral skills training to teach safe tackling skills to youth football players. *Journal of Applied Behavior Analysis, 50,* 849–855.

Therrien, W. J. (2004). Fluency and comprehension gains as a result of repeated reading: A meta-analysis. *Remedial and Special Education, 25,* 252–261.

Tilly, W. D. (2008). The evolution of school psychology to science-based practice: Problem solving and the three-tiered model. In A. Thomas & J. Grimes (Eds.), *Best practices in school psychology V* (pp. 17–35). Bethesda, MD: National Association of School Psychologists.

U.S. Department of Education. (2000). *Twenty-second annual report to Congress on the implementation of the Individual with Disabilities Education Act.* Washington, DC: U.S. Government Printing Office.

Vadasy, P. F., Wayne, S., O'Conner, R., Jenkins, J., Firebaugh, M., & Peyton, J. (2000). *Sound Partners* [Curriculum program]. Longmont, CO: Cambium Learning Group/Sopris West.

Valentino, A. L., LeBlanc, L. A., Veazey, S. E., Weaver, L. A., & Raetz, P. B. (2019). Using a prerequisite skills assessment to identify optimal modalities for mand training. *Behavior Analysis in Practice, 12,* 22–32.

Vellutino, F. R., Scanlon, D. M., & Tanzman, V. S. (1998). The case for early intervention in diagnosing specific reading disability. *Journal of School Psychology, 36,* 367–397.

Watkins, C. L. (1997). *Project Follow Through: A case study of contingencies influencing instructional practices of the educational establishment.* Concord, MA: Cambridge Center for Behavioral Studies.

What Works Clearinghouse (WWC). (2006). WWC intervention report: Reading Mastery/SRA/McGraw Hill. Retrieved February 2016, from *http://ies.ed.gov/ncee/wwc/pdf/intervention_reports/WWC_Reading_Mastery_092806.pdf.*

What Works Clearinghouse (WWC). (2007). WWC intervention report: Direct Instruction, DISTAR, and Language for Learning. Retrieved February 2016, from *http://ies.ed.gov/ncee/wwc/pdf/intervention_reports/WWC_Direct_Instruction_052107.pdf.*

Wolery, M., Bailey, D. B., & Sugai, G. M. (1988). *Effective teaching: Principles and procedures of applied behavior analysis with exceptional students.* Boston: Allyn & Bacon.

Wood, K. D., & Blanton, W. E. (2009). *Literacy instruction for adolescents: Research-based practice.* New York: Guilford Press.

# CHAPTER 27

# Teacher Consultation in Behavioral Assessment and Intervention

Florence D. DiGennaro Reed, Lisa M. Hagermoser Sanetti, and Robin S. Codding

The Individuals with Disabilities Education Improvement Act (IDEA) of 2004 requires states and local education agencies to offer students with disabilities a free appropriate public education in the least restrictive environment, and it emphasizes the right to a *high-quality* education. These and other educational reforms, such as the No Child Left Behind Act of 2001, mandate accommodations and modified instruction to ensure that students with disabilities participate in the general education curriculum to the maximum extent appropriate with fellow students without disabilities. Such mandates oblige teachers to support the educational needs of an increasingly diverse group of students with individualized needs (Putnam, Handler, Rey, & McCarty, 2005). Teachers already have many responsibilities for student learning, such as providing core curricular instruction; identifying individual learning needs; differentiating instruction; and creating a positive, safe, and engaging classroom environment for students. Teachers also assume an important role in promoting and supporting the use of evidence-based prevention and intervention strategies.

We cannot expect teachers to master the skills necessary to address the unique needs of every student they will educate during their career given the many responsibilities and pressures they

already face. In fact, 4.2% of children 17 years or younger in the United States were diagnosed with a disability in 2013 (Houtenville, Brucker, & Lauer, 2014); this percentage represents more than 3 million public school students who may require specialized services. Teachers often are primarily responsible for implementing preventative practices, such as effective classroom management, and academic and behavior intervention plans (Forman, Olin, Hoagwood, Crowe, & Saka, 2009; Fahmie & Luczynski, 2018; Forman et al., 2013; Long et al., 2016). Nevertheless, they would benefit from the expertise of a professional who has the training and experience to assess and treat academic and behavioral challenges in the classroom. Subsequently, the growing demands on educators and increased accountability for high-quality education have facilitated the development of school consultation as a service one or more professionals offer to educators (Luiselli & Diament, 2002).

*Behavioral consultation*—a model that relies on the principles of behavior analysis—has decades of empirical support and scientific evidence demonstrating its effectiveness and popularity (e.g., Sheridan et al., 2012; Sheridan, Welch, & Orme, 1996). Behavioral consultation is the most widely evaluated type of consultation (Sheridan et al.,

1996), with studies focused primarily on client outcomes (Kratochwill, Altschaefl, & Bice-Urbach, 2014). Researchers have documented improvements across many client outcomes (e.g., activities of daily living, academics, behavior, social-emotional challenges, mental health diagnoses) and settings (e.g., home, school, community; Sheridan et al., 1996). These results hold across many evaluation designs, including single-case designs (e.g., Beaulieu, Hanley, & Roberson, 2012), longitudinal evaluations (e.g., Kratochwill, Elliott, & Busse, 1995), and randomized controlled trials (e.g., Sheridan et al., 2012). Across time, new branches of research are emerging in behavioral consultation, such as teleconsultation (Machalicek et al., 2009) and peer consultation (Gormley & DuPaul, 2015), which will inform the next iteration of the various consultation models.

## WHAT IS BEHAVIORAL CONSULTATION?

Applied behavior analysis, behavior therapy, and assessment and intervention approaches from the behavioral theoretical school served as the initial basis for behavioral consultation (e.g., Kratochwill & Bergan, 1990). Three foundational features of behavioral consultation differentiate it from traditional service delivery. First, service delivery is indirect: The consultant (e.g., a behavior analyst) typically does not have direct contact with the client (e.g., student), but rather works with the consultee (e.g., a parent, teacher), who provides intervention services to the client. Second, the consultant uses problem-solving strategies to address the needs of the consultee and client. Finally, the consultant uses his or her knowledge of behavioral theory and consultation to make relevant information available to the consultee. The primary goal of behavioral consultation is to use a triadic, indirect model of service delivery to maximize the interdependent contributions of the consultant (expert in behavioral theory and consultation) and consultee (expert in the client and relevant environments) to produce change in client behavior (Kratochwill et al., 2014).

### Roles and Responsibilities of the Consultant, Consultee, and Client

Everyone in the consultation process—consultant, consultee, and client—has a role that includes specific responsibilities. We now describe these roles and the corresponding responsibilities.

### Consultant

Behavioral consultants have three primary responsibilities. First, they must be knowledgeable of and fluent in the consultation process. A consultant is responsible for skillfully guiding the consultee through and meeting the objectives for the model's stages (see below). Second, the consultant is responsible for providing needed information to the consultee. For example, the consultant may provide information about (1) the theory underlying the consultant's hypothesis that the intervention components are appropriate for a client, (2) assessment and intervention techniques, (3) expected latency to client outcomes, and/or (4) appropriate modifications to intervention components. Furthermore, the consultant is responsible for providing the consultee with resources to implement the assessment and intervention plan effectively and consistently (e.g., data sheets, intervention materials). The consultant may need to work with the consultee to obtain resources that are necessary but not in the consultee's immediate control, such as release time for the consultee to prepare for the intervention and the physical space to implement it. Finally, the consultant has an ethical and professional responsibility to ensure the consultee provides the intervention to the client as planned to maximize its potential benefit. In other words, consultation does not end after the consultant designs an intervention plan for a consultee; the consultant must continue to support the consultee in his or her implementation, ensuring the client is accessing the intervention as planned.

### Consultee

Consultees have up to four responsibilities during consultation. First, the consultee is responsible for specifying and describing the problem behavior(s). Given the behavioral focus of this consultation model, the consultant will expect the consultee to assist with operationally defining the problem behavior(s) and identifying antecedents, sequential conditions, and consequences. Second, the consultee is responsible for evaluating the intervention procedure (Is he or she sufficiently able to implement the intervention? Is the intervention acceptable?) and outcomes (Is the client showing progress? Has the client met the goals of consultation?). Third, the consultee is responsible for working with the client to implement the intervention, which is a critical responsibility. The client is not likely to benefit from the intervention if the consultee does not implement it. Finally, some consultees will be responsible for supervision of other individuals who assist with intervention implementation. For example, a teacher may supervise a paraprofessional who implements the intervention that a consultant and the teacher have developed for a student.

## Client

Clients typically have one responsibility in the consultation process, which is to respond to the intervention, thereby informing the goals of consultation. For example, if a client is improving, the goal of consultation may be to continue the intervention for a specified period and then develop a data-based, systematic plan for fading intervention or consultation supports. Alternatively, if a client is not progressing, or if his or her rate of progress is not acceptable, these data will inform the consultant and consultee that they need to reengage in the problem-solving process. Consultants and consultees may decide to engage clients who are able in the process of setting and evaluating their goals, which is an effective intervention technique (e.g., O'Leary & Dubey, 1979).

## Consultation Models

Researchers have developed and evaluated numerous models of behavioral consultation over the past 40-plus years. In addition, behavior analysts have published numerous texts outlining consultation strategies; perhaps the most popular of these is Bailey and Burch (2010). We have not reviewed these texts here, as they do not describe *empirically evaluated* consultation models, even though they may be informative. Rather, we note overlap between strategies and consultation models when applicable. We briefly describe three empirically supported consultation models that researchers have implemented most commonly.

## Problem-Solving Consultation

Historically, problem-solving consultation followed a four-stage process (Bergan & Kratochwill, 1990); however, researchers have identified a fifth stage as a best practice (Kratochwill et al., 2014). Although we present the stages in a linear order here, they are fluid in practice; stages often overlap, and consultants and consultees may return to a previous stage to meet the consultation goals (Gilles, Kratochwill, Felt, Schienebeck, & Vac-

carello, 2011). The first stage, *establishing relationships*, focuses on the importance of developing a productive relationship between the consultant and consultee. Research consistently demonstrates that trust, openness, flexibility, genuineness, and positive communication are essential to facilitating collaboration during the consultation process (Dinnebeil, Hale, & Rule, 1996; Gilles et al., 2011; Kratochwill et al., 2014). Although competence in problem identification and analysis are necessary to successful consultation, they may not be sufficient. The integration of technical expertise in consultation and behavioral theory with positive interpersonal skills is essential to maximizing consultation outcomes (Kratochwill et al., 2014). The second stage, *problem identification*, focuses on operationally defining the problem behavior, the expected behavior, and the discrepancy between these. Researchers consider this the most critical step, as accurate problem identification is predictive of effective planning and implementation (Bergan & Tombari, 1975, 1976). The third stage, *problem analysis*, includes analyzing the environmental conditions occasioning the problem behavior, developing hypotheses regarding the function(s) of that behavior, and designing an intervention plan. The consultant may recommend additional data collection, typically using behavioral assessment techniques (e.g., antecedent–behavior–consequence [A-B-C] recording, time sampling, direct observation, functional analysis). The fourth stage, *plan implementation*, focuses on the consultee's implementation of the intervention. The consultant (1) ensures the availability of materials, (2) ensures the consultee has the skills to implement the intervention, (3) monitors consultee implementation and client progress, (4) conducts regular check-ins or interacts with the consultee, (5) regularly analyzes data, and (6) makes data-based decisions about the need to revise the intervention. The fifth stage, *plan evaluation*, focuses on data-based evaluation of plan effectiveness and goal attainment. Plan evaluation is not necessarily the end of the consultation process, because the consultant may develop new goals for maintenance, generalization, other behaviors, or a combination of these.

## Integrated Model of School Consultation

The following sources inform the integrated model of school consultation: (1) Bergan and Kratochwill's (1990) model of behavioral consultation, (2) Caplan's (1963) model of mental health consultation, (3) research on relational communication (Erchul & Chewning, 1990), and (4) social-psychology research on social power and influence (Erchul & Martens, 2010). This model includes three stages: precursors to consultation, the consultation process, and consultation outcomes. During the precursors stage, a consultant must have or develop a general understanding of the operations of the consultation setting (i.e., schools and classrooms) and must fully and systematically enter the consultation setting. The consultant must understand the intervention and referral processes in the consultation setting, the consultee's expectations of the consultative relationship, previously implemented problem-solving efforts and interventions, and the consultee's perception of the factors that are responsible for the problem behavior (Erchul & Martens, 2010).

The consultation process begins after the consultant has gained entry to the consultation setting. In this model, the process centers on three interrelated tasks: problem solving, social influence, and support and development. The problem-solving process is based on Bergan and Kratochwill's model previously described. This model of consultation emphasizes the consultant's use of social influence during the problem-solving process because consultants often need to alter consultees' attitudes and beliefs to benefit clients. As outlined in the French and Raven (1959) model, there are six bases of social power: (1) *coercive power,* in which the consultee perceives that the consultant can punish the consultee if he or she doesn't comply; (2) *reward power,* in which the consultee perceives that the consultant can reward the consultee for compliance; (3) *legitimate power,* in which the consultee believes that the consultant has a legitimate right to influence the consultant's beliefs or attitudes based on his or her position; (4) *expert power,* in which the consultee perceives that the consultant has expertise in the area of interest to the consultee; (5) *referent power,* in which the consultant is able to influence the consultee via the consultee's real or perceived identification with the consultant; and (6) *informational power,* in which the consultant is able to influence the consultee by providing logical information to the consultee about the need for change. Researchers have used these bases of social power to develop numerous strategies for social influence, and consultants may use these strategies in the problem-solving process. A full review of social power and social influence is beyond the scope of this chapter; interested readers should see Erchul and Martens (2010).

Throughout the consultation process, the integrated model of school consultation emphasizes the importance of supporting consultees' efforts as teachers and intervention agents, while simultaneously empowering them to become capable and independent problem solvers (Witt & Martens, 1988). Doing so may include connecting consultees with resources, providing emotional supports, and developing their professional skills (e.g., assessment and intervention training).

### Conjoint Behavioral Consultation

Youth who demonstrate challenging behaviors often do so across multiple environments and contexts (e.g., home, school, community; Sheridan et al., 2012). Conjoint behavioral consultation is grounded in ecological-systems theory (Bronfenbrenner, 1979), in which the consultant actively involves caregivers as co-consultees with teachers, thereby addressing the unique perspectives and contributions of the primary environments in which youth develop. Conjoint behavioral consultation fosters positive caregiver–teacher relationships, incorporates data-based problem solving and collaboration, and implements evidence-based interventions across home and school settings (Sheridan et al., 2012).

Conjoint behavioral consultation includes four stages implemented in a collaborative manner among the consultant and caregiver and teacher consultees (Sheridan & Kratochwill, 2008). In the first stage, *conjoint needs identification,* the consultant and consultees work together to (1) identify the client's most pressing needs in home and school settings, (2) select and operationally define target behaviors, (3) choose the specific settings for and goals of consultation, and (4) collect baseline data across settings. The consultant's goals in this stage of conjoint behavioral consultation include developing the relationship between the caregiver(s) and teachers, and identifying the strengths and capacities of the client, family, and school to promote goal attainment. In the second stage, *conjoint needs analysis,* the consultant reviews data to identify environmental variables across settings that may influence target behavior, with a specific focus on setting events, ecological conditions, and cross-system variables. The consultant develops hypotheses about the function of the target behavior, and the consultant and consultees engage in a collaborative, strengths-based approach to developing an intervention plan across home and school settings. In the third stage, *cross-system plan implementation,* caregiver(s) and teachers implement the intervention plan in the home and school, with ongoing support from the consultant. Simultaneous implementation across settings increases the likelihood of generalization and maintenance as an outcome of conjoint behavioral consultation (Sheridan, Clarke, & Burt, 2008). In the fourth stage, *conjoint plan evaluation,* the behavioral data form the basis of a discussion among the consultant, caregiver(s), and teacher regarding next steps (e.g., identifying new goals, continuing intervention).

## TEACHER INVOLVEMENT WITH BEHAVIORAL ASSESSMENT AND INTERVENTION

Despite a mutually compatible interest in helping children become independent and effective learners, teachers encounter many barriers that consultants should consider. Increasing accountability standards and adoption of the Common Core State Standards Initiative have led to growing demands on teachers' time and have intensified and added teaching responsibilities (Maras, Splett, Reinke, Stormont, & Herman, 2014). These changes are occurring during a climate of persistent decreases in school budgets, leading to an ever-present notion of having to do more with less. Simultaneously, time allocated in the school day for planning and collaboration with other professionals is often minimal, even though teachers report desiring more opportunities for collaboration (Long et al., 2016; Maras et al., 2014). Bosworth Gingiss, Potthoff, and Roberts-Gray (1999) have identified these diminishing resources (i.e., materials, staff, funding, facilities, and time) as some of the most important predictors of effective implementation of school-based interventions.

Researchers have conducted surveys to assess teachers' training in behaviorally oriented practices (Begeny & Martens, 2006; Stormont, Reinke, & Herman, 2011a, 2011b). General education teachers in training at both primary and secondary levels report low levels of coursework and applied training in most instructional concepts, strategies, programs, and assessment practices that are behaviorally oriented. As many as 43% of teacher trainees indicated no training on the items assessed in one study (Begeny & Martens, 2006). For example, 40% or more of teachers reported receiving no coursework or applied training opportunities with direct instruction, personalized systems of instruction, curriculum-based measurement, graphing student performance, single-case design, use of timed trials for repeated practice of academic skills, strategies for promoting generalization of skills, or use of guided notes.

Most general education teachers reported a lack of familiarity with evidence-based behavioral interventions and programs, such as the Good Behavior Game (Barrish, Saunders, & Wolf, 1969) or the Olweus Bullying Prevention Program (Olweus, 1991). Only 57% knew whether professionals in their schools conducted functional behavioral assessments and implemented behavioral interventions (Stormont et al., 2011a). Many teachers also reported a need for more training in classroom management and behavioral interventions (Reinke, Stormont, Herman, Puri, & Goel, 2011). Across surveys, teachers and teachers in training in special education (1) reported significantly more coursework and applied training in academic assessment, (2) agreed at significantly higher rates that using evidence-based practices in behavioral intervention is important, and (3) rated non-evidence-based practices (e.g., having a discussion with a child following misbehavior) as less acceptable than teachers and teachers in training in general education rated them (Begeny & Martens, 2006; Stormont et al., 2011b).

Despite low levels of training on behavioral practices and limited familiarity with specific evidence-based programs, overwhelmingly teachers agree on the importance of using evidence-based behavioral intervention practices such as (1) identifying triggers and reinforcers for problem behavior; (2) teaching skills using examples, practice, and feedback; (3) reinforcing and practicing behavioral expectations; (4) adapting instructional strategies to increase engagement and opportunities for success; and (5) observing and recording behavior (Stormont et al., 2011b). Moreover, teachers largely agree that they should not use non-evidence-based practices, such as grade retention and suspension. Therefore, determining teachers' baseline knowledge of behavioral principles, concepts, and skills is important when the consultant is establishing his or her own and the teachers' responsibilities for intervention planning, development, and implementation. For example, given the limited opportunities teachers have had to graph data, this responsibility might be better suited for a consultant. Considering the barriers in the school, such as limited time and resources, working with teachers to mitigate those barriers through consultative support is important.

## Behavioral Assessment

The model of indirect service delivery that comprises behavioral consultation necessitates that teachers assume an active role in behavioral assessment. Decades of research has documented that consultants can train teachers to conduct behavioral assessment effectively (e.g., Watson, Ray, Sterling-Turner, & Logan, 1999), including stimulus preference assessments (e.g., Lerman, Tetreault, Hovanetz, Strobel, & Garro, 2008) and various techniques of functional behavioral assessment (e.g., Watson et al., 1999).

### Stimulus Preference Assessment

Identifying stimuli that serve as reinforcers increases the probability that reinforcement-based procedures will have desired effects. As a result, training teachers to conduct preference assessments, rather than relying on intuition or parental report, is a worthwhile endeavor. Lerman et al. (2008) successfully trained teachers with varied backgrounds and experience to conduct single-stimulus, paired-choice, and multiple-stimulus-without-replacement preference-assessment procedures. The researchers conducted training for 6 hours a day for 5 days; addressed many topics; and included lecture, discussion, modeling, role play, and additional practice with feedback. Teachers not only met mastery criteria during training, but also maintained skills for up to 6 months following training with only brief feedback. Research also has documented that teachers can train others to conduct preference assessments effectively using a pyramidal or train-the-trainer training model, consisting of instruction, modeling, practice, and feedback (Pence, St. Peter, & Tetreault, 2012).

### Functional Behavioral Assessment

Numerous studies have shown that consultants can train teachers and other school personnel to implement functional behavioral assessment procedures, including indirect and direct assessments (e.g., Loman & Horner, 2014; Maag & Larson, 2004) and functional analyses (e.g., Kunnavatana, Bloom, Samaha, & Dayton, 2013; Moore et al., 2002; Wallace, Doney, Mintz-Resudek, & Tarbox, 2004) in general and special education classrooms. Training formats included one-on-one instruction, workshops, and group formats (Wallace et al., 2004), as well as innovative technology uses such as video conferencing (Suess, Wacker, Schwartz, Lustig, & Detrick, 2016), even across continents (Alnemary, Wallace, Symon, & Barry, 2015). Training procedures have generally involved behavioral skills training, which we describe in detail in the next section. Research has demonstrated that experienced teachers can train their colleagues effectively to implement functional analyses (Pence, St. Peter, & Giles, 2014). These findings are especially important, considering federal mandates requiring schools to conduct functional behavioral assessments (IDEA, 2004) and research indicating greater reductions in student problem behavior when teachers use function-based interventions (Rispoli et al., 2015).

## Teachers as Effective Intervention Agents

A growing body of literature has documented that teachers can serve as highly effective change agents to improve student outcomes when provided with evidence-based training, effective consultation, and follow-up support. Researchers have used appropriate consultative supports to train general and special education teachers to implement multicomponent individualized behavior plans (e.g., Codding, Feinburg, Dunn, & Pace, 2005; DiGennaro, Martens, & McIntyre, 2005; DiGennaro Reed, Codding, Catania, & Maguire, 2010; Kaufman, Codding, Markus, Tryon, & Kyse, 2013; Mouzakitis, Codding, & Tryon, 2015; Sanetti, Collier-Meek, Long, Byron, & Kratochwill, 2015), increase behavior-specific praise statements (e.g., Jenkins, Floress, & Reinke, 2015), deliver discrete-trial instruction (e.g., Catania, Almeida, Liu-Constant, & DiGennaro Reed, 2009), use academic interventions (e.g., Gilbertson, Witt, Singletary, & VanDerHeyden, 2007; Noell et al., 2005), improve classroom management (e.g., Codding, Livanis, Pace, & Vaca, 2008; Codding & Smyth, 2008; Oliver, Wehby, & Nelson, 2015; Slider, Noell, & Williams, 2006), and enhance the problem-solving processes of teams of teachers (e.g., Burns, Peters, & Noell, 2008; Duhon, Mesmer, Gregerson, & Witt, 2009; Newton, Horner, Algozzine, Todd, & Algozzine, 2012).

### Training

In their meta-analysis, Joyce and Showers (2002) indicated that traditional in-service workshops that disseminate knowledge and raise awareness about educational practices do not translate into skills that teachers retain or use in classrooms. Rather, (1) didactic instruction on the intervention; (2) modeling of the intervention; (3) role plays and practice implementing the intervention, with immediate feedback and error correction; and (4) ongoing follow-up support facilitate successful intervention implementation.

Behavioral skills training is one approach to this training model (Parsons, Rollyson, & Reid, 2012; Sarokoff & Sturmey, 2004). During such training, the instructor (1) describes the target intervention, (2) provides a written protocol or brief description of the intervention, (3) demonstrates the intervention, (4) requires the teacher (or consultee) to practice the intervention, (5) provides feedback during practice, and (6) repeats Steps 4 and 5 until the teacher has achieved mastery. We recommend that a consultant tell a teacher the rationale for implementing an intervention. The consultant should tell the teacher how the intervention will help students achieve the expected goals and how the intervention is consistent with the school context and mission. The written protocol should include only the essential steps that a teacher needs to follow. Extraneous information or extensive explanations and examples may reduce the likelihood that teachers will use these written protocols. A posttraining test may be useful to assess the teacher's comprehension of the intervention (DiGennaro Reed et al., 2010).

The consultant should model implementation of the intervention for the teacher after introducing the verbal explanation and written protocol. The consultant can model the intervention conventionally or *in vivo*, using role plays during which the consultant serves as the implementer and the teacher serves as the confederate. The consultant can also use self-created or web-accessed videos (DiGennaro Reed et al., 2010; Slider et al., 2006). A postmodeling test may be useful to assess the teacher's comprehension of the intervention. The test might describe role-play scenarios and ask the teacher to identify errors of omission and commission (Slider et al., 2006).

The consultant should schedule time for the teacher to practice implementing the intervention during role plays, taking turns in the roles of implementer and student. The consultant can conduct these practice opportunities simultaneously with pairs or groups of teachers, or can have one pair or group model the intervention for the larger group participating in the training (Parsons et al., 2012). During this time, the consultant should circulate around the room to each pair or group and provide immediate error correction and feedback on intervention implementation. Given the importance of

this step, having more than one consultant to assist with providing feedback may be useful. Teachers benefit from receiving behavior-specific praise for correct intervention implementation, and corrective feedback with instruction and additional modeling for incorrect implementation.

The final aspect of behavioral skills training is to ensure that teachers meet a criterion level established by the consultant, trainer, or both. For example, having each teacher implement the behavioral intervention with 100% accuracy would be useful (Parsons et al., 2012). The consultant can arrange tests during training to assess performance in which each teacher practices implementing the intervention with the trainer or consultant, after two opportunities to practice the intervention with a partner. An alternative strategy is to video-record teachers practicing the intervention with one another and score their performance after the training (Sarokoff & Sturmey, 2004). The consultant can conduct additional training and proficiency tests with teachers who do not meet the mastery criterion.

Although these training procedures have improved intervention integrity, data from two meta-analyses suggest that training alone does not produce sustained implementation (Noell et al., 2014; Slider et al., 2006; Solomon, Klein, & Politylo, 2012). Noell et al. (2014) found that mean consultee intervention implementation was 36%, regardless of whether the consultant used behavioral skills training or other standard training procedures. These data are consistent with recommendations by Joyce and Showers (2002) indicating that teachers need ongoing follow-up support. Two novel antecedent strategies, intervention choice and implementation planning, have demonstrated promise for sustaining intervention adherence after training (Dart, Cook, Collins, Gresham, & Chenier, 2012; Sanetti, Kratochwill, & Long, 2013). We describe these two approaches below.

*"Test-Driving" Intervention Options and Choosing One.* Dart et al. (2012) conducted a study whereby teachers used one of three interventions (e.g., self-monitoring, check-in/check-out, and response cost). Teachers used each intervention once during a 30-minute interval that the teacher and consultant identified during a meeting. Teachers sampled each intervention over the course of 2 days with a target student in their classroom. Teachers then rank-ordered each intervention from least to most acceptable. Each teacher ultimately implemented the intervention he or she chose as most

acceptable. The opportunity to try different interventions and select the most acceptable produced sustained accurate intervention implementation.

*Implementation Planning for Logistics and Barriers.* Sanetti et al. (2013) have developed a model of training that emphasizes preimplementation planning. First, the teacher and consultant develop an action and a coping plan. During the action-planning process, the teacher and consultant (1) define the intervention steps; (2) adapt these steps to match the teacher's classroom context; (3) establish the logistical details of intervention delivery (i.e., when, how often, for how long, where, by whom); and (4) identify resources needed to facilitate implementation (Sanetti et al., 2013). Action planning crystallizes the roles of the consultant and teacher in a way that also ensures greater implementation feasibility. Coping planning requires the teacher and consultant to identify up to four barriers and develop strategies to address or mitigate each barrier. A consultant can conduct action and coping planning during one 20-minute meeting (Sanetti et al., 2015). Empirical findings suggest that implementation planning, when provided after standard consultation and training, results in higher intervention adherence and quality (Sanetti et al., 2015; Sanetti, Collier-Meek, Long, Kim, & Kratochwill, 2014; Sanetti et al., 2013).

## Ongoing Follow-Up Supports

The standard model of behavioral consultation assumes that consultants meet with teachers weekly and conduct interviews to evaluate how the plan is going (Bergan & Kratochwill, 1990). During this interview, a consultant asks a teacher whether he or she is implementing the plan and if the target student or students are improving. The consultant schedules time for teacher questions. The consultant does not review intervention protocols or data. This form of follow-up meeting is not effective for enhancing intervention implementation (Noell et al., 2005, 2014). Yet a robust finding in the literature is the benefit of ongoing consultative support after formal training. Three specific strategies that improve teachers' intervention implementation include performance feedback, self-monitoring, and coaching. We describe these strategies below.

*Performance Feedback.* Performance feedback has a rich literature base with evidence support-

ing its effectiveness at facilitating adherence to academic and behavioral intervention plans (Noell et al., 2014). In fact, researchers have established performance feedback as an evidence-based practice (Fallon, Collier-Meek, Maggin, Sanetti, & Johnson, 2015). Implementation outcomes with performance feedback *alone* are superior (Noell et al., 2014) to those of self-monitoring or variations of performance feedback (e.g., meeting cancelation, directed rehearsal). Consultants can deliver performance feedback on any schedule (e.g., daily, weekly) after direct observation of teachers' intervention integrity. Researchers have used performance feedback only when intervention integrity reaches a threshold (e.g., <75%). The interval between direct observations of intervention integrity and feedback to teachers can be as short as a few hours or up to 1 week without affecting intervention integrity outcomes (Solomon et al., 2012).

Consultants most often deliver performance feedback verbally during individual meetings with a teacher, but a consultant also can deliver performance feedback during team-based meetings or via email or written notes (DiGennaro, Martens, & Kleinmann, 2007; Fallon et al., 2015). Performance feedback includes (1) review of intervention adherence data with teachers, provided graphically, verbally, or both; (2) praise for intervention steps implemented accurately and with high quality; (3) corrective feedback for errors of omission and commission; (4) review of the intervention plan; and (5) an opportunity for teachers to ask questions and problem-solve barriers to implementation. The materials required for performance feedback include the intervention plan or protocol and observational data on intervention integrity. Consultants often review graphic displays of teacher implementation data, student data, or both. Performance feedback meetings can also include directed rehearsal, in which a teacher practices intervention components that he or she omitted or implemented incorrectly, and cancellation of performance feedback meetings contingent on accurate implementation that meets a criterion (e.g., DiGennaro et al., 2007; DiGennaro et al., 2005). Researchers have also embedded goal setting with performance feedback meetings (Codding & Smyth, 2008; Duchaine, Jolivette, & Fredrick, 2011; Hall & Macvean, 1997; Hawkins & Heflin, 2011; Myers, Simonsen, & Sugai, 2011).

*Self-Monitoring.* Self-monitoring is a promising alternative for enhancing teachers' implementation of discrete-trial instruction (Belfiore, Fritts, & Herman, 2008), token economies (Pelletier, Mc-Namara, Braga-Kenyon, & Ahearn, 2010; Petscher & Bailey, 2006; Plavnick, Ferreri, & Maupin, 2010) and behavior support plans (Mouzakitis et al., 2015). Self-monitoring requires teachers to record their own behavior; however, researchers have provided considerable support and training to ensure that teachers record implementation accuracy correctly. In these studies, teacher self-monitoring occurred (1) immediately after a pager signaled that a teacher implemented an intervention step, (2) after the teacher viewed a video of him- or herself implementing an intervention, (3) via completion of a checklist on the same day the teacher implemented the intervention, or (4) with a combination of these strategies. Researchers observed higher levels of implementation and greater consistency when they included additional supports, such as using a pager, prompting teachers to perform steps in the intervention plan, viewing a video of themselves, or following written performance feedback illustrating comparisons between the consultant's and the teacher's integrity data.

*Coaching.* The two common models of coaching are supervisory and side-by-side (i.e., *in vivo*; Blakely, 2001; Joyce & Showers, 1995). Supervisory coaching involves an observation of a teacher implementing a strategy or intervention followed by descriptive feedback to the teacher regarding strengths and challenges. During side-by-side coaching, the coach (1) models the intervention in the classroom; (2) provides immediate *in vivo* praise and corrective feedback after the teacher implements the intervention; (3) prompts the intervention steps when needed; and (4) provides additional modeling when needed. The consultant can implement coaching in any frequency or duration (e.g., one session, weekly). Systematic reviews suggest that coaching improves teachers' intervention implementation. Less evidence exists on whether these improvements translate into improved student outcomes, and only a small percentage of existing studies have analyzed fidelity of the coaching process (Kretlow & Bartholomew, 2010; Stormont, Reinke, Newcomer, Marchese, & Lewis, 2015).

### Fading Consultation Support by using a Data-Based Process

Teachers can maintain high levels of implementation integrity, particularly with performance feedback, after the consultant removes follow-up supports (Noell et al., 2014). Consultants can promote maintenance by fading intervention support or intensity. *Dynamic fading* is a common strategy that researchers have used (e.g., DiGennaro et al., 2007; DiGennaro et al., 2005; Kaufman et al., 2013); it is a thinning schedule of follow-up support contingent on teachers' intervention implementation. For example, let's assume that a consultant initially provides follow-up support twice weekly after each observation of a teacher. After the teacher demonstrates 100% accurate intervention implementation for three consecutive sessions, the consultant might provide follow-up support once weekly. The consultant could thin the schedule to once every other week when the teacher meets the criterion for a second time. Follow-up support returns to a richer schedule if the teacher cannot maintain high levels of accurate implementation. Gross, Duhon, and Doerksen-Klopp (2014) used a changing-criterion design to evaluate a variation of dynamic fading that the authors called *fading with indiscriminable contingencies*. The consultant initially provided follow-up support daily. The consultant decreased follow-up support to every other day and then to weekly each time the teacher's implementation integrity was 100% for 2 consecutive days.

Another option may be to *fade the intensity of follow-up support*. Mouzakitis et al. (2015) removed consultant-provided performance feedback after pairing performance feedback with self-monitoring. Two of three teachers maintained acceptable levels of intervention adherence when the consultant used self-monitoring only. The third teacher required both components of support to be successful.

## CONCLUSION

In this chapter, we have summarized empirically supported models of behavioral consultation and have outlined the roles and responsibilities of individuals in the consultation process. We have described the various barriers teachers encounter in the consultative relationship and advocate that consultants work alongside teachers to mitigate those barriers through consultative support. We have concluded the chapter with research documenting the effective use of teachers in behavioral assessment and intervention, which requires an evidence-based approach to training and ongoing follow-up support.

## REFERENCES

Alnemary, F. M., Wallace, M., Symon, J. B. G., & Barry, L. M. (2015). Using international videoconferencing to provide staff training on functional behavioral assessment. *Behavioral Interventions, 30,* 73–86.

Bailey, J., & Burch, M. (2010). *25 essential skills and strategies for the professional behavior analyst: Expert tips for maximizing consulting effectiveness.* New York: Routledge.

Barrish, H. H., Saunders, M., & Wolf, M. M. (1969). Good Behavior Game: Effects of individual contingencies for group consequences on disruptive behavior in a classroom. *Journal of Applied Behavior Analysis, 2,* 119–124.

Beaulieu, L., Hanley, G. P., & Roberson, A. A. (2012). Effects of responding to a name and group call on preschoolers' compliance. *Journal of Applied Behavior Analysis, 45*(4), 685–707.

Begeny, J. C., & Martens, B. K. (2006). Assessing preservice teachers' training in empirically validated behavioral instruction practices. *School Psychology Quarterly, 21,* 262–285.

Belfiore, P. J., Fritts, K. M., & Herman, B. C. (2008). The role of procedural integrity: Using self-monitoring to enhance discrete trial instruction (DTI). *Focus on Autism and Other Developmental Disabilities, 23*(2), 95–102.

Bergan, J. R., & Kratochwill, T. R. (1990). *Behavioral consultation and therapy.* New York: Plenum Press.

Bergan, J. R., & Tombari, M. L. (1975). The analysis of verbal interactions occurring during consultation. *Journal of School Psychology, 13,* 209–226.

Bergan, J. R., & Tombari, M. L. (1976). Consultant skill and efficiency and the implementation and outcomes of consultation. *Journal of School Psychology, 14,* 3–14.

Blakely, M. R. (2001). A survey of levels of supervisory support and maintenance of effects reported by educators involved in direct instruction implementation. *Journal of Direct Instruction, 1,* 73–83.

Bosworth, K., Gingiss, P. M., Potthoff, S., & Roberts-Gray, C. (1999). A Bayesian model to predict the success of the implementation of health and education innovations in school-centered programs. *Evaluation and Program Planning, 22,* 1–11.

Bronfenbrenner, U. (1979). *The ecology of human development: Experimental by nature and design.* Cambridge, MA: Harvard University Press.

Burns, M. K., Peters, R., & Noell, G. H. (2008). Using performance feedback to enhance implementation fidelity of the problem-solving team process. *Journal of School Psychology, 46,* 537–550.

Caplan, G. (1963). Types of mental health consultation. *American Journal of Orthopsychiatry, 3,* 470–481.

Catania, C. N., Almeida, D., Liu-Constant, B., & Di-Gennaro Reed, F. D. (2009). Video modeling to train staff to implement discrete trial instruction. *Journal of Applied Behavior Analysis, 42,* 387–392.

Codding, R. S., Livanis, A., Pace, G. M., & Vaca, L. (2008). Using performance feedback to improve intervention integrity of classwide behavior plans: An investigation of observer reactivity. *Journal of Applied Behavior Analysis, 41,* 417–422.

Codding, R. S., & Smyth, C. A. (2008). Using performance feedback to decrease classroom transition time and examine collateral effects on academic engagement. *Journal of Educational and Psychological Consultation, 18,* 325–345.

Codding, R. S., Feinburg, A. B., Dunn, E. K., & Pace, G. M. (2005). Effects of immediate performance feedback on implementation of behavior support plans. *Journal of Applied Behavior Analysis, 38,* 205–219.

Dart, E. H., Cook, C. R., Collins, T. A., Gresham, F. M., & Chenier, J. S. (2012). Test driving interventions to increase intervention integrity and student outcomes. *School Psychology Review, 41,* 467–481.

DiGennaro, F. D., Martens, B. K., & Kleinmann, A. E. (2007). A comparison of performance feedback procedures on teachers' intervention implementation integrity and students' inappropriate behavior in special education classrooms. *Journal of Applied Behavior Analysis, 40,* 447–461.

DiGennaro, F. D., Martens, B. K., & McIntyre, L. L. (2005). Increasing intervention integrity through negative reinforcement: Effects on teacher and student behavior. *School Psychology Review, 34,* 220–231.

DiGennaro Reed, F. D., Codding, R., Catania, C., & Maguire, H. (2010). Effects of video modeling on intervention integrity of behavior support plans. *Journal of Applied Behavior Analysis, 43,* 291–295.

Dinnebeil, L. A., Hale, L. M., & Rule, S. (1996). A qualitative analysis of parents' and service coordinators' descriptions of variables that influence collaborative relationships. *Topics in Special Education, 16,* 322–347.

Duchaine, E. L., Jolivette, K., & Fredrick, L. D. (2011). The effect of teacher coaching with performance feedback on behavior-specific praise in inclusion classrooms. *Education and Treatment of Children, 34,* 209–227.

Duhon, G. J., Mesmer, E. M., Gregerson, L., & Witt, J. C. (2009). Effects of public feedback during RTI team meetings on teacher implementation integrity and student academic performance. *Journal of School Psychology, 47,* 19–37.

Erchul, W. P., & Chewning, T. G. (1990). Behavioral consultation from a request-centered relational communication perspective. *School Psychology Quarterly, 5,* 1–20.

Erchul, W. P., & Martens, B. K. (2010). *School consultation: Conceptual and empirical bases of practice.* New York: Springer.

Fahmie, T. A., & Luczynski, K. C. (2018). Preschool life skills: Recent advancements and future directions. *Journal of Applied Behavior Analysis, 51,* 183–188.

Fallon, L. M., Collier-Meek, M. A., Maggin, D. M., Sanetti, L. M. H., & Johnson, A. J. (2015). Is performance feedback an evidence-based practice?: A systematic review and evaluation. *Exceptional Children, 81,* 227–246.

Forman, S. G., Olin, S. S., Hoagwood, K. E., Crowe, M., & Saka, N. (2009). Evidence-based intervention in schools: Developers' views of implementation barriers and facilitators. *School Mental Health, 1,* 26–36.

Forman, S. G., Shapiro, E. S., Codding, R. S., Gonzales, J. E., Reddy, L. A., Rosenfield, S. A., et al. (2013). Implementation science and school psychology. *School Psychology Quarterly, 28*(2), 77–100.

French, J. R. P., & Raven, B. H. (1959). The bases of social power. In D. Carwright (Ed.), *Studies in social power* (pp. 159–167). Ann Arbor, MI: Institute for Social Research.

Gilbertson, D., Witt, J. C., Singletary, L. L., & VanDer-Heyden, A. (2007). Supporting teacher use of intervention: Effects of response dependent performance feedback on teacher implementation of a math intervention. *Journal of Behavioral Education, 16,* 311–326.

Gilles, C. N. R., Kratochwill, T. R., Felt, J. N., Schienebeck, C. J., & Vaccarello, C. A. (2011). Problem solving consultation: Applications in evidence-based prevention and intervention. In M. A. Bray & T. J. Kehle (Eds.), *The Oxford handbook of school psychology* (pp. 666–667). New York: Oxford University Press.

Gormley, M. J., & DuPaul, G. J. (2015). Teacher-to-teacher consultation: Facilitating consistent and effective intervention across grade levels for students with ADHD. *Psychology in the Schools, 52*(2), 124–138.

Gross, T., Duhon, G. J., & Doerksen-Klopp, B. (2014). Enhancing intervention integrity maintenance through fading with indiscriminable contingencies. *Journal of Behavioral Education, 23,* 108–131.

Hall, L. J., & Macvean, M. L. (1997). Increases in the communicative behaviours of students with cerebral palsy as a result of feedback to, and the selection of goals by, paraprofessionals. *Behaviour Change, 14,* 174–184.

Hawkins, S. M., & Heflin, L. J. (2011). Increasing secondary teachers' behavior-specific praise using a video self-modeling and visual performance feedback intervention. *Journal of Positive Behavior Interventions, 1,* 97–108.

Houtenville, A. J., Brucker, D. L., & Lauer, E. A. (2014). *Annual compendium of disability statistics: 2014.* Durham: University of New Hampshire, Institute on Disability.

Individuals with Disabilities Education Improvement Act (IDEA) of 2004, Pub. L. No. 108-446, 20 U.S.C. 1400 et seq. (2004).

Jenkins, L. N., Floress, M. T., & Reinke, W. (2015). Rates and types of teacher praise: A review and future directions. *Psychology in the Schools, 52,* 463–476.

Joyce, B., & Showers, B. (1995). The evolution of peer coaching. *Improving Professional Practice, 53*(6), 12–16.

Joyce, B., & Showers, B. (2002). *Student achievement through staff development.* Alexandria, VA: Association for Supervision and Curriculum Development.

Kaufman, D., Codding, R. S., Markus, K. A., Tryon, G. S., & Kyse, E. N. (2013). Effects of verbal and written performance feedback on intervention adherence: Practical application of two delivery formats. *Journal of Educational and Psychological Consultation, 23,* 264–299.

Kratochwill, T. R., Altschaefl, M. R., & Bice-Urbach, B. (2014). Best practices in problem-solving consultation: Applications in prevention and intervention systems. In P. L. Harrison & A. Thomas (Eds.), *Best practices in school psychology: Data-based and collaborative decision making* (pp. 461–482). Bethesda, MD: National Association of School Psychologists.

Kratochwill, T. R., & Bergan, J. R. (1990). *Behavioral consultation in applied settings: An individual guide.* Boston: Kluwer Academic.

Kratochwill, T. R., Elliott, S. N., & Busse, R. T. (1995). Behavior consultation: A five-year evaluation of consultant and client outcomes. *School Psychology Quarterly, 10*(2), 87–117.

Kretlow, A. G., & Bartholomew, C. C. (2010). Using coaching to improve the fidelity of evidence-based practices: A review of studies. *Teacher Education and Special Education, 33,* 279–299.

Kunnavatana, S. S., Bloom, S. E., Samaha, A. L., & Dayton, E. (2013). Training teachers to conduct trial-based functional analyses. *Behavior Modification, 37,* 707–722.

Lerman, D. C., Tetreault, A., Hovanetz, A., Strobel, M., & Garro, J. (2008). Further evaluation of a brief, intensive teacher-training model. *Journal of Applied Behavior Analysis, 41,* 243–248.

Loman, S. L., & Horner, R. H. (2014). Examining the efficacy of a basic functional behavioral assessment training package for school personnel. *Journal of Positive Behavior Interventions, 16,* 18–30.

Long, A. C. J., Hagermoser Sanetti, L. M., Collier-Meek, M. A., Gallucci, J., Altschaefl, M., & Kratochwill, T. R. (2016). An exploratory investigation of teachers' intervention planning and perceived implementation barriers. *Journal of School Psychology, 55,* 1–26.

Luiselli, J. K., & Diament, C. (Eds.). (2002). *Behavior psychology in the schools: Innovations in evaluation, support, and consultation.* West Hazleton, PA: Haworth Press.

Maag, J. W., & Larson, P. J. (2004). Training a general education teacher to apply functional assessment. *Education and Treatment of Children, 27,* 26–36.

Machalicek, W., O'Reilly, M., Chan, J. M., Rispoli, M., Lang, R., Davis, T., et al. (2009). Using videoconferencing to support teachers to conduct preference assessments with students with autism and developmental disabilities. *Research in Autism Spectrum Disorders, 3,* 32–41.

Maras, M. A., Splett, J. W., Reinke, W. M., Stormont, M., & Herman, K. C. (2014). School practitioners' perspectives on planning, implementing, and evaluating evidence-based practices. *Children and Youth Services Review, 47*, 314–322.

Moore, J. W., Edwards, R. P., Sterling-Turner, H. E., Riley, J., DuBard, M., & McGeorge, A. (2002). Teacher acquisition of functional analysis methodology. *Journal of Applied Behavior Analysis, 35*, 73–77.

Mouzakitis, A., Codding, R. S., & Tryon, G. (2015). The effects of self-monitoring and performance feedback on the intervention integrity of behavior support plan implementation. *Journal of Positive Behavior Interventions, 17*, 223–234.

Myers, D. M., Simonsen, B., & Sugai, G. (2011). Increasing teachers' use of praise with a response-to-intervention approach. *Education and Treatment of Children, 34*, 35–59.

Newton, S. J., Horner, R. H., Algozzine, B., Todd, A. W., & Algozzine, K. (2012). A randomized wait-list controlled analysis of the implementation integrity of team-initiated problem solving processes. *Journal of School Psychology, 50*, 421–441.

No Child Left Behind Act of 2001, Pub. L. No. 107-110, 20 U.S.C. 6301 (2002).

Noell, G. H., Gansle, K. A., Mevers, J. L., Knox, R. M., Mintz, J. C., & Dahir, A. (2014). Improving intervention plan implementation in schools: A meta-analysis of single subject design studies. *Journal of Behavioral Education, 23*, 168–191.

Noell, G. H., Witt, J. C., Slider, N. J., Connell, J. E., Gatti, S. L., Williams, K. L., et al. (2005). Treatment implementation following behavioral consultation in schools: A comparison of three follow-up studies. *School Psychology Review, 34*, 87–107.

O'Leary, S. G., & Dubey, D. R. (1979). Applications of self-control procedures by children: A review. *Journal of Applied Behavior Analysis, 12*(3), 449–465.

Oliver, R. M., Wehby, J. H., & Nelson, J. R. (2015). Helping teachers maintain classroom management practices using a self-monitoring checklist. *Teaching and Teacher Education, 51*, 113–120.

Olweus, D. (1991). Bully/victim problems among schoolchildren: Basic facts and effects of a school-based intervention program. In D. J. Pepler & K. H. Rubin (Eds.), *The development and intervention of childhood aggression* (pp. 411–448). Hillsdale, NJ: Erlbaum.

Parsons, M. B., Rollyson, J. H., & Reid, D. H. (2012). Evidence-based staff training: A guide for practitioners. *Behavior Analysis in Practice, 5*(2), 2–11.

Pelletier, K., McNamara, B., Braga-Kenyon, P., & Ahearn, W. H. (2010). Effect of video self-monitoring on procedural integrity. *Behavioral Interventions, 25*, 261–274.

Pence, S. T., St. Peter, C. C., & Giles, A. F. (2014). Teacher acquisition of functional analysis methods using pyramidal training. *Journal of Behavioral Education, 23*, 132–149.

Pence, S. T., St. Peter, C. C., & Tetreault, A. S. (2012). Increasing accurate preference assessment implementation through pyramidal training. *Journal of Applied Behavior Analysis, 45*, 345–359.

Petscher, E. S., & Bailey, J. S. (2006). Effects of training, prompting, and self-monitoring on staff behavior in a classroom for students with disabilities. *Journal of Applied Behavior Analysis, 39*, 215–226.

Plavnick, J. B., Ferreri, S. J., & Maupin, A. N. (2010). The effects of self-monitoring on the procedural integrity of a behavioral intervention for young children with developmental disabilities. *Journal of Applied Behavior Analysis, 43*, 315–320.

Putnam, R. F., Handler, M. W., Rey, J., & McCarty, J. (2005). The development of behaviorally based public school consultation services. *Behavior Modification, 29*, 521–537.

Reinke, W. M., Stormont, M., Herman, K. C., Puri, R., & Goel, N. (2011). Supporting children's mental health in schools: Teacher perceptions of needs, roles, and barriers. *School Psychology Quarterly, 26*, 1–12.

Rispoli, M., Ninci, J., Burke, M. D., Zaini, S., Hatton, H., & Sanchez, L. (2015). Evaluating the accuracy of results for teacher implemented trial-based functional analyses. *Behavior Modification, 39*, 627–653.

Sanetti, L. M. H., Collier-Meek, M. A., Long, A. C. J., Byron, J., & Kratochwill, T. R. (2015). Increasing teacher intervention integrity of behavior support plans through consultation and implementation planning. *Journal of School Psychology, 53*, 209–229.

Sanetti, L. M. H., Collier-Meek, M. A., Long, A. C. J., Kim, J., & Kratochwill, T. R. (2014). Using implementation planning to increase teachers' adherence and quality to behavior support plans. *Psychology in the Schools, 51*, 879–895.

Sanetti, L. M. H., Kratochwill, T. R., & Long, A. C. J. (2013). Applying adult behavior change theory to support mediator-based intervention implementation. *School Psychology Quarterly, 28*, 47–62.

Sarokoff, R. A., & Sturmey, P. (2004). The effects of behavioral skills training on staff implementation of discrete-trial teaching. *Journal of Applied Behavior Analysis, 37*, 535–538.

Sheridan, S. M., Bovaird, J. A., Glover, T. A., Garbacz, A., Witte, A., & Kwon, K. (2012). A randomized trial examining the effects of conjoint behavioral consultation and the mediating role of the parent–teacher relationship. *School Psychology Review, 41*, 23–46.

Sheridan, S. M., Clarke, B. L., & Burt, J. D. (2008). Conjoint behavioral consultation: What do we know and what do we need to know? In W. P. Erchul & S. M Sheridan (Eds.), *Handbook of research in school consultation* (pp. 171–202). Mahwah, NJ: Erlbaum.

Sheridan, S. M., & Kratochwill, T. R. (2008). *Conjoint behavioral consultation: Promoting family–school connections and interventions* (2nd ed.). New York: Springer.

Sheridan, S. M., Welch, M., & Orme, S. F. (1996). Is consultation effective?: A review of outcome research. *Remedial and Special Education, 17*, 341–354.

Slider, N. J., Noell, G. H., & Williams, K. L. (2006). Providing practicing teachers classroom management professional development in a brief study format. *Journal of Behavioral Education, 15,* 215–228.

Solomon, B. G., Klein, S. K., & Polityo, B. C. (2012). The effect of performance feedback on teachers' intervention integrity: A meta-analysis of single-case literature. *School Psychology Review, 41,* 160–175.

Stormont, M., Reinke, W., & Herman, K. (2011a). Teachers' characteristics and ratings for evidence-based behavioral interventions. *Behavioral Disorders, 37,* 19–29.

Stormont, M., Reinke, W., & Herman, K. (2011b). Teachers' knowledge of evidence-based interventions and available school resources for children with emotional and behavioral problems. *Journal of Behavioral Education, 20,* 138–147.

Stormont, M., Reinke, W. M., Newcomer, L., Marchese, D., & Lewis, C. (2015). Coaching teachers' use of social behavior interventions to improve children's outcomes: A review of the literature. *Journal of Positive Behavior Interventions, 17,* 69–82.

Suess, A. N., Wacker, D. P., Schwartz, J. E., Lustig, N., & Detrick, J. (2016). Preliminary evidence on the use of telehealth in an outpatient behavior clinic. *Journal of Applied Behavior Analysis, 49,* 686–692.

Wallace, M. D., Doney, J. K., Mintz-Resudek, C. M., & Tarbox, R. S. F. (2004). Training educators to implement functional analyses. *Journal of Applied Behavior Analysis, 37,* 89–92.

Watson, T. S., Ray, K. P., Sterling-Turner, H., & Logan, P. (1999). Teacher-implemented functional analysis and intervention: A method for linking assessment to intervention. *School Psychology Review, 28,* 292–302.

Witt, J. C., & Martens, B. K. (1988). Problems with problem-solving consultation: A re-analysis of assumptions, methods, and goals. *School Psychology Review, 17,* 211–226.

# CHAPTER 28

# Teaching Safety Skills to Children

Raymond G. Miltenberger, Amy C. Gross, Diego Valbuena, and Sindy Sanchez

Children may encounter numerous threats to personal safety in their lives. Safety experts divide these threats into two categories: (1) frequently occurring situations in which a child has repeated opportunities to engage in safe behavior, and (2) low-incidence but life-threatening situations in which the child may have only one opportunity to engage in safe behavior successfully (Miltenberger, 2008). Examples of frequently occurring situations that require safe behavior include riding in an automobile, riding a bike, and crossing the street. Examples of safe behavior in these situations include using a seatbelt, wearing a helmet, and looking both ways before crossing, respectively. Examples of low-incidence but life-threatening situations include attempted abduction, home fires (e.g., Garcia, Dukes, Brady, Scott, & Wilson, 2016), and finding an unattended firearm. Examples of safe behavior in these situations include saying, "No," leaving the area, and telling an adult; immediately evacuating the house; and not touching the firearm, leaving the area, and telling an adult, respectively. A child's use of safe behavior in such situations could save his or her life. Many safety threats require a child to emit multiple responses to maintain his or her safety, and we refer to those responses as *safety skills*.

Although use of safety skills during frequently occurring safety threats is important for preventing accidental injury or death, we focus in this chapter on safety skills for low-incidence but life-threatening safety threats. In particular, we focus on teaching appropriate safety skills in the presence of an unattended firearm (Maxfield, Miltenberger, & Novotny, 2019). We review the problem of firearm injuries and deaths, and discuss two approaches to prevention of these: modifying parent behavior to promote safe storage of firearms (Violano et al., 2018), and teaching children appropriate safety skills in the presence of an unattended firearm, with an emphasis on behavioral skills training.

## FIREARM INJURIES AND DEATHS

### Prevalence of Firearm Injuries and Deaths

Firearms injure or kill hundreds of children in the United States (Parikh, Silver, Patel, Iqbal, & Goyal, 2017). Between 2009 and 2013, an average of 3,061 children ages 0–19 years survived unintentional firearm injuries, and 951 children ages 0–19 years died from suicide or unintentional shootings (Brady Campaign to Prevent Gun Violence, n.d.-a). Childhood firearm injuries and deaths are often not deliberate. The American Academy of Pediatrics (AAP, 2000) reported that the percentages of unintentional deaths caused by firearms for children under age 5, ages 5–9, ages 10–14, and ages 15–19 were 24%, 26%, 21%, and 5%, respectively. A firearm accidentally killed over

1,500 children between 1996 and 2001 (Common Sense about Kids and Guns, n.d.). Only vehicular accidents caused more unintentional deaths than firearms did (Kellerman, 1993; Zavoski, Lapidus, Lerer, & Banco, 1995).

Handguns, which are firearms designed to be held and fired with one hand, cause more unintentional firearm injuries and deaths than do shotguns and rifles, which are firearms designed to be held and fired with both hands (AAP, 2000; Grossman, Reay, & Baker, 1999; Knight-Bohnhoff & Harris, 1998; Zavoski et al., 1995). Easy access to firearms increases the risk of accidental firearm injuries and fatalities (Hemenway & Solnick, 2015; Miller, Azrael, & Hemenway, 2001; Miller, Azrael, Hemenway, & Vriniotis, 2005; Ordog et al., 1988). In fact, most incidents occur in the homes of the victims or of friends or family members of the victims (Common Sense about Kids and Guns, n.d.; DiScala & Sege, 2004; Eber, Annest, Mercy, & Ryan, 2004; Grossman et al., 1999; Kellerman & Reay, 1986; Wintemute, Teret, Kraus, Wright, & Bradfield, 1987).

## Prevalence of Gun Ownership

Reported rates of firearm ownership vary, with 20–40% of households owning at least one firearm (Common Sense about Kids and Guns, n.d.; Haught, Grossman, & Connell, 1995; National Opinion Research Center, 2014; Schuster, Franke, Bastian, Sor, & Halfon, 2000; Senturia, Christoffel, & Donovan, 1994). Owning one firearm increases the likelihood of owning another firearm fivefold (Senturia et al., 1994), and households containing a male member are more likely to have a firearm than those without a male (Knight-Bohnhoff & Harris, 1998; Schuster et al., 2000). More than half of firearm-owning households own a handgun. Parents are more likely to have a rifle, a shotgun, and a handgun, respectively (Schuster et al., 2000). Handgun owners cite protection most often as the reason for keeping the firearm in the home (AAP, 2000; Dresang, 2001; Haught et al., 1995; Wiley & Casey, 1993). However, a firearm in the home is far more likely to kill a family member or friend than to protect the family from a stranger (AAP, 2000; Dresang, 2001; Kellerman, 1993; Kellerman & Reay, 1986).

## Risk Factors for Firearm Injuries and Deaths

Two important risk factors associated with unintentional firearm injuries to and deaths of children are unsafe storage practices (i.e., the owner stores the firearm unlocked, loaded, near ammunition) and children's tendencies to play with firearms they find (Himle & Miltenberger, 2004). Several investigators have documented that many firearm owners fail to store their firearms safely (e.g., Azreal, Cohen, Salhi, & Miller, 2018; Azrael, Miller, & Hemenway, 2000; Crifasi, Doucette, McGinty, Webster, & Barry, 2018), and that children often play with firearms when they find them (Hardy, 2002; Hardy, Armstrong, Martin, & Strawn, 1996; Jackman, Farah, Kellerman, & Simon, 2001).

## Parental Behavior and Beliefs about Firearms

### Firearm Storage Behavior

Many parents do not store their firearms safely, even though access to firearms is so closely associated with childhood firearm injuries and deaths. Fewer than half of parents reported storing their firearms in the safest manner—that is, locked, unloaded, and separate from ammunition (Farah & Simon, 1999; Stennies, Ikeda, Leadbetter, Houston, & Sacks, 1999; Wiley & Casey, 1993). More importantly, 13–30% of parents reported storing their firearms both unlocked and loaded, which is the most unsafe storage practice (Common Sense about Kids and Guns, n.d.; Farah & Simon, 1999; Hemenway, Solnick, & Azrael, 1995; Miller et al., 2005; Schuster et al., 2000; Senturia et al., 1994; Stennies et al., 1999). Many firearm owners reported storing their firearms in a manner between these two extremes (Stennies et al., 1999). Nearly half of firearm owners reported storing ammunition separately from firearms (Haught et al., 1995; Hendricks & Reichert, 1996).

Investigators have shown that childproof safety devices for firearms prevent firearm injuries and deaths. The General Accounting Office (1991) reviewed medical examiners' and coroners' reports and concluded that childproof safety devices and loading indicators could have prevented about 8% and 23% of unintentional injuries and deaths, respectively. Vernick et al. (2003) determined that one or more of three safety devices—personalized firearms (Crifasi, O'Dwyer, McGinty, Webster, & Barry, 2019), loaded chamber indicators, and magazine safeties—could have prevented 45% of unintentional deaths. Unfortunately, fewer than half of firearm-owning parents use such safety devices (Common Sense about Kids and Guns, n.d.; Haught et al., 1995; Schuster et al., 2000).

## Firearm Safety Beliefs

Results of surveys have shown that firearm-owning and non-firearm-owning parents differ in their firearm safety beliefs. Knight-Bohnhoff and Harris (1998) interviewed firearm-owning and non-firearm-owning parents about their knowledge and beliefs regarding unintentional firearm injuries and deaths. Firearm-owning parents reported that education-based safety training was a sufficient strategy for avoiding unintentional firearm injuries and deaths (Knight-Bohnhoff & Harris, 1998), whereas non-firearm-owning parents were more likely to believe that keeping firearms out of the house was the best way to avoid such injuries and deaths (Farah & Simon, 1999). Firearm-owning parents preferred to obtain safety information from a firearm organization, whereas non-firearm-owning parents preferred to obtain safety information from the police. Firearm-owning parents stated that they (1) would be willing to talk to their pediatrician about firearms, and (2) believed statistics regarding the greater risks than benefits of owning firearms. Nevertheless, these parents did not remove firearms from their household, although most reported that they would follow advice to keep firearms locked and unloaded (Webster, Wilson, Duggan, & Pakula, 1992). Non-firearm-owning parents stated that information from their pediatrician would make them less likely to buy a firearm in the future.

Webster et al. (1992) surveyed parents in a pediatrician's office and found that firearm owners were more willing than nonowners to trust children with firearms at a much younger age. Fourteen percent of firearm owners were willing to trust a child under 12 years of age with a firearm, and 39% were willing to trust a child between 12 and 15 years of age with a firearm. Twenty-six percent of firearm owners said that they would never trust a child with a firearm. By contrast, only 3% of nonowners were willing to trust a child under 12 years of age with a firearm, and 9% were willing to trust a child between 12 and 15 years of age with a firearm. Forty-two percent of nonowners said that they would never trust a child with a firearm (Webster et al., 1992). Firearm-owning and non-firearm-owning parents combined said that they would trust their own children with a firearm at an average age of 9, but that they would not trust other children until age 21 (Farah & Simon, 1999). Firearm-owning parents were more likely than non-firearm-owning parents to believe that children could discriminate between real and toy firearms at an earlier age, and

were also more likely to think that their own children could make this judgment reliably (Farah & Simon, 1999; Webster et al., 1992).

Many parents, regardless of firearm ownership status, were confident that their children would not touch or play with a firearm if the opportunity arose (Common Sense about Kids and Guns, n.d.; Farah & Simon, 1999). Parents reported talking to their children about firearm safety (Farah & Simon, 1999; Knight-Bohnhoff & Harris, 1998), but most reported not discussing firearm ownership with parents of their children's friends (Brady Campaign to Prevent Gun Violence, n.d.-b). Of those who had not discussed the issue with the friends' parents, most said that they had not thought about it; some assumed that there were no firearms in the households of the friends' parents, or that the friends' parents stored their firearms safely (Brady Campaign to Prevent Gun Violence, n.d.-b).

## Child Behavior

Although parents tend to believe that their children will not touch or play with a firearm, this is often not the case. Hardy et al. (1996) found that 19% of children whose parents owned a firearm reported playing with it without their parents' knowledge. In addition, 24% more children than parents verified that the children were aware that their parents kept a firearm in the house, and 67% of children stated that they knew where the firearm was located and had access to it (Hardy et al., 1996). Hardy (2002) asked parents and children similar questions about firearm safety. When investigators asked parents if their children would play with a firearm, 41% said yes, 32% said no, and 27% were unsure. Interestingly, 40% of children whose parents answered no had played with a firearm, as did 59% of children of the unsure parents. Furthermore, when investigators placed children in a room with various toys, toy firearms, and real but disabled firearms, the children often touched and played with the real firearms (Hardy, 2002; Jackman et al., 2001).

Jackman et al. (2001) sent pairs or trios of 8- to 12-year-old boys into a room in which the investigators had placed a firearm in a drawer. Jackman et al. found that at least one child handled the firearm in 76% of the groups, and at least one child pulled the trigger in 48% of the groups. Only once (5%) did a child leave the room and report finding the firearm to an adult. Nearly all children who touched the firearm (93%) and pulled the trigger

(94%) had received firearm safety information at some point. Hardy (2002) obtained similar results: 53% of children played with the firearm in the room, and only 1 child out of 70 reported finding the firearm to an adult. Furthermore, children were not able to discriminate between real and toy firearms as well as parents believed. In fact, about half the children who found the firearm were not sure whether it was real or a toy (Hardy, 2002; Jackman et al., 2001). Children were more likely to identify a firearm as a toy when it was real than to identify it as real when it was a toy (Hardy, 2002).

## PREVENTION OF CHILDHOOD FIREARM INJURIES AND DEATHS

The two major risk factors for childhood firearm injuries and deaths are accessible firearms and children's tendencies to play with firearms they find. Therefore, two approaches to preventing firearm injuries are (1) to promote safe storage of firearms by parents and (2) to assess and teach child safety skills.

### Promoting Safe Storage Practices

Investigators and community members have used various strategies to promote safe storage of firearms. These strategies have included legislation making storing a firearm where it is accessible to children a felony, as well as efforts by pediatricians, physicians, the mass media, and others to educate parents about the dangers of firearms and the need for safe storage (e.g., Himle & Miltenberger, 2004; Jostad & Miltenberger, 2004).

### Gun Legislation

Florida was the first state to implement a law that punished those who stored or left a loaded firearm where a child could access it. The Child Access Prevention Law had positive results in Florida during its first year of implementation, with a 50% drop in firearm deaths. As of 1997, 19 other states had adopted similar laws (Cummings, Grossman, Rivara, & Koepsell, 1997). Cummings et al. (1997) evaluated whether these laws were effective in decreasing the death rate of children under 15 years of age. Overall, the death rate was 23% lower than expected in states that adopted safe storage laws. The study also found that the decrease in deaths was greater for children under 10 years of age than for those between 10 and 14 years of age.

Webster and Starnes (2000) also evaluated the effectiveness of the Child Access Prevention Law in decreasing firearm deaths. They found no change in firearm death rates in states where the penalty was a misdemeanor, but a decrease in such deaths in states where the penalty was a felony. However, when they excluded Florida's data from the analysis, the decrease in firearm death rates after the implementation of the Child Access Prevention Law was not statistically significant. Florida may have been so successful because it was the first state to implement the law; therefore, the law received much publicity. Florida also had the most severe penalty, and the death rate before implementation was quite high, so there was more room for change. Researchers continue to hypothesize about reasons for the success in Florida but not in other states (Webster & Starnes, 2000).

### Parent Education

Grossman, Mang, and Rivara (1995) evaluated family physicians' and pediatricians' beliefs and practices regarding firearm safety and safe storage practices. They found that many family physicians and pediatricians agreed that they should be responsible for counseling families about firearms, yet it was low on their list of priorities. About one-third stated that they did not know what to tell parents, and one-half admitted that they had never counseled a family on firearm safety. Family physicians were more likely to promote teaching children safe firearm use when the children were "old enough," and pediatricians were more likely to agree that individuals should not keep firearms in homes with children. Pediatricians were more willing to suggest removal of firearms to parents, yet both groups doubted that families would follow this advice. Both family physicians and pediatricians said that they would tell parents to store ammunition and firearms separately, and thought parents would be receptive to this suggestion (Grossman et al., 1995).

Grossman et al. (2000) evaluated the effectiveness of physician education, written materials about safe storage, and a discount coupon for purchasing safe storage devices on parents' firearm ownership and storage behavior. The program did not produce any significant changes in ownership or storage behavior compared to that of controls. Sidman et al. (2005) evaluated the effects of a media campaign and discount coupons for lock boxes on the storage practices of firearm owners in King County, Washington. The authors conducted telephone surveys to assess storage practices in the intervention county and nine control counties in different states, and found that the intervention did not produce statistically significant changes in safe storage practices.

Coyne-Beasley, Schoenbach, and Johnson (2001) evaluated the effectiveness of the Love Our Kids, Lock Your Guns program on participants' safe storage practices. The investigators gave a survey, individualized counseling, safety information, and a firearm lock with instructions at no expense to individuals in the parking lot of a mall. Coyne-Beasley et al. evaluated the effectiveness of the program after 6 months. Almost all participants thought the program was helpful. At follow-up, 77% of participants said that they locked their firearms, compared to 48% at baseline; 72% said that they used the firearm lock, compared to none at baseline; and only 7% stored their firearms loaded and unlocked, compared to 18% at baseline. After the program, participants who had children were more likely than those without children to lock their firearms.

Although the research by Coyne-Beasley et al. (2001) illustrates a program that was successful in promoting safe storage of firearms, the investigators made personal contact with individual firearm owners and gave away firearm locks; this is a time- and resource-intensive practice that communities are not likely to apply on a wide scale. In general, research on changing firearm storage practices has produced mixed results, with many programs producing no changes. Furthermore, this research used self-reports of storage practices, so we need to interpret the results cautiously. McGee, Coyne-Beasley, and Johnson (2003) concluded that what interventions or intervention components increase the likelihood of safe firearm storage is not clear. Clearly, the field needs more research to evaluate strategies for promoting safe storage practices by firearm owners. Safe firearm storage would decrease the threat to child safety and the need to teach children firearm safety skills.

## Assessing and Teaching Child Safety Skills

### Assessing Child Safety Skills

Given that methods for promoting safe firearm storage have not been successful, an alternative approach is to teach firearm safety skills to children. Investigators have used three methods to evaluate whether teaching approaches are effective: self-report, role play, and *in situ* assessments. The tar-

get behaviors are the same across assessment and teaching procedures: "Stop what you are doing, do not touch the firearm, leave the area, and tell an adult." Most investigators have used a 0–3 rating scale (0 = *touched the firearm, regardless of completing further steps*; 1 = *did not touch the firearm*; 2 = *did not touch the firearm and immediately left the room*; and 3 = *did not touch the firearm, immediately left the room, and told an adult that he or she found the firearm*). Across assessment methods, a teacher (or other evaluator) does not provide feedback to a child about his or her responses during the assessment, as the purpose is to observe and measure what the child does either before or after teaching.

*Self-Report.* Self-report is a method in which a child states what he or she would do when encountering an unattended firearm. The teacher describes a situation in which the child encounters an unattended firearm (e.g., "Imagine that you are at your friend's house playing in the basement, while your friend's parents are upstairs. You are playing hide and seek, and when you open a closet to hide in, you see a firearm in the closet. What would you do?"). The child then responds by telling the teacher what he or she would do (e.g., "I would stop playing and not touch the firearm; then I would go upstairs and tell my friend's parents right away").

Although self-report assessments are time-efficient relative to assessments in which a child performs the behavior, their limitations outweigh their benefits. That is, a child may describe the safety skill vocally, but may not demonstrate the skills when he or she encounters a firearm (e.g., Gatheridge et al., 2004; Himle, Miltenberger, Gatheridge, & Flessner, 2004). Given the potential of self-reports to produce false positives in which the child states that he or she would perform the correct skills but does not perform them in the actual situation, we do not recommend self-report to evaluate firearm safety skills.

*Role Play.* During role-play assessments, the teacher presents the child with a scenario and asks him or her to demonstrate what he or she would in that situation. For example, the teacher might place a disabled firearm or a toy firearm on top of a desk and say to the child, "Pretend that you walked into your parents' office and found a firearm on top of their desk. Now pretend that I'm your dad, and show me what you would do." The teacher then would walk to another room and wait for the child to demonstrate what he or she would do.

Researchers consider role-play assessments superior to self-reports, as the child must demonstrate what he or she would do in the presence of a firearm. However, research shows that the behavior the child demonstrates during role play may not match what he or she does when he or she encounters a firearm (e.g., Gatheridge et al., 2004; Himle, Miltenberger, Gatheridge, et al., 2004). We do not recommend role-play assessments, given the danger of a child's finding an unattended firearm, and the false positives associated with role-play assessments.

*In Situ Assessments.* In situ assessments represent the most valid method for evaluating safety skills (Miltenberger, Sanchez, & Valbuena, 2015). Three essential features must be present during an *in situ* assessment of firearm safety skills. First, the child must encounter an unattended firearm in the natural environment. Second, the child must not know that someone is observing him or her. Third, the child must not be in the presence of an adult when he or she finds the firearm. Importantly, investigators and clinicians should use a disabled firearm or realistic replica to ensure the child's safety. *In situ* assessments simulate a real-life situation and capture whether child behavior is under the stimulus control of the firearm rather than the observer. We recommend that investigators and clinicians use *in situ* assessments of firearm safety skills, because of the shortcomings of self-report and role-play assessments as described above (e.g., Himle, Miltenberger, Gatheridge, et al., 2004; Gatheridge et al., 2004).

## Teaching Safety Skills to Children

Investigators have used two approaches to teach firearm safety skills to children. One is informational, and the other is active learning. In an informational approach, the teacher talks about the dangers of firearms and describes the safety skills associated with firearms, often with the child vocally rehearsing the safety skills. Live or video modeling is often part of the informational approach. The safety skills associated with a firearm are not to touch it, to get away from it, and to report its presence to an adult (e.g., Gatheridge et al., 2004; Himle, Miltenberger, Gatheridge, et al., 2004; Kelso, Miltenberger, Waters, Egemo-Helm, & Bagne, 2007). In an active-learning approach, the teacher provides instructions and modeling, and the child practices the safety skills in simulated situations. The teacher praises correct performance and gives corrective feedback for incorrect performance (Gatheridge et al., 2004; Himle, Miltenberger, Flessner, & Gatheridge, 2004; Miltenberger et al., 2004).

*Informational Training.* Hardy et al. (1996) evaluated an informational-training approach to teach firearm safety skills by surreptitiously videotaping children as they found a firearm in a playroom before and after receiving firearm safety information. The pre- and postteaching assessments consisted of two children playing in a room that contained a disabled firearm, a toy firearm, and other toys. The intervention was a 30-minute session in which a police officer told children and parents that a child should never touch a firearm without permission from parents; a child should tell an adult if he or she finds a firearm or if another child is playing with a firearm; and all firearms are dangerous unless an adult says otherwise. Hardy et al. found that children in the training group were just as likely to touch and play with the real firearm after training as children in the control group were. Hardy (2002) reported similar results.

The Eddie Eagle GunSafe Program is a commonly used training program for children, distributed by the National Rifle Association (Himle, Miltenberger, Gatheridge, et al., 2004). This program uses various materials and activities (such as posters, coloring books, videos, cutting materials, sequencing cards with the safety motto, and certificates and stickers to use as rewards) to provide information about firearm safety skills. During training, children receive information, recite the safety motto, and verbally respond with the safety motto to "what if" scenarios during five 15-minute training sessions. We consider this an informational approach because the child does not actually perform the target behaviors (stop, do not touch, leave the area, and tell an adult) in a situation in which he or she finds an unattended firearm. The Eddie Eagle GunSafe Program has trained well over 15 million children, yet there are few studies evaluating its effectiveness.

Himle, Miltenberger, Gatheridge, et al. (2004) found that 4- and 5-year-old children trained with the Eddie Eagle GunSafe Program could tell the investigator what they were supposed to do when they found a firearm during a self-report assessment. However, they did not perform better than untrained children when the investigator asked them to role-play what they would do if they found an unattended firearm. Furthermore, the trained children did not perform the correct safety skills during *in situ* assessments. Gatheridge et al. (2004) also evaluated the Eddie Eagle GunSafe Program's effectiveness with 6- and 7-year-old children. These children performed well on the self-report assessment and did slightly better on role-play assessments than children in the control group. However, trained children did not perform the safety skills during *in situ* assessments.

Research has shown that the informational approaches reviewed above may not be effective for teaching children firearm safety skills. This finding is consistent with research showing that informational approaches are not effective for teaching safety skills for other safety threats, such as abduction and sexual abuse (e.g., Beck & Miltenberger, 2009; Miltenberger et al., 2013; Miltenberger & Hanratty, 2013; Poche, Yoder, & Miltenberger, 1988).

*Behavioral Skills and* In Situ *Training.* The ineffectiveness of informational approaches for teaching safety skills should not be surprising, because they do not require children to perform the safety skill correctly during training (Gatheridge et al., 2004; Hardy, 2000; Hardy et al., 1996; Himle, Miltenberger, Gatheridge, et al., 2004). On the other hand, behavioral skills training is an approach that requires active child rehearsal until the child masters the skills across a range of simulated situations. Research has shown that behavioral skills training is effective for training abduction prevention skills (Carroll-Rowan & Miltenberger, 1994; Johnson et al., 2005, 2006; Marchand-Martella & Huber, 1996; Olsen-Woods, Miltenberger, & Forman, 1998; Poche, Brouwer, & Swearingen, 1981; Poche et al., 1988), sexual abuse prevention skills (Lumley, Miltenberger, Long, Rapp, & Roberts, 1998; Miltenberger et al., 1999; Miltenberger & Thiesse-Duffy, 1988; Miltenberger, Thiesse-Duffy, Suda, Kozak, & Bruellman, 1990), pedestrian safety skills (Yeaton & Bailey, 1978), and fire safety skills (Jones, Kazdin, & Haney, 1981; Jones, Ollendick, McLaughlin, & Williams, 1989).

Behavioral skills training involves instructions, modeling, rehearsal, and feedback. The teacher gives instructions describing the safety threat and the safety skills to use in response to the threat. Next, the teacher models the safety skills in simulated situations of the safety threat. Then the child rehearses the safety skills during a role play. The teacher provides praise for correct performance and corrective feedback for incorrect performance. Rehearsal and feedback continue until the child performs the safety skills correctly and immediately when the teacher presents the

child with a range of simulated safety threats (e.g., Himle & Miltenberger, 2004; Miltenberger, 2008). As a result, the child should engage in the safety skills when faced with a real-life situation involving a similar safety threat.

Research evaluating behavioral skills training for teaching safety skills to children and adults with intellectual disabilities has produced many findings. First, behavioral skills training is effective in producing skill acquisition, although the skills are not always generalized to other settings or maintained over time (Marchand-Martella & Huber, 1996; Miltenberger et al., 2004; Poche et al., 1981). Second, behavioral skills training appears to be more effective with individuals rather than groups of children (Carroll-Rowan & Miltenberger, 1994; Johnson et al., 2005; Miltenberger & Olsen, 1996). Third, behavioral skills training is not effective in some instances until investigators add *in situ* training; that is, children learn the skills with behavioral skills training, but do not use them until training occurs in the natural setting (Johnson et al., 2005; Miltenberger et al., 1999). Fourth, behavioral skills training is more effective than informational approaches that do not involve performing the behavior in the context in which it may occur (Gatheridge et al., 2004; Himle, Miltenberger, Gatheridge, et al., 2004). Finally, behavioral skills training can be time-intensive, because some children require numerous sessions before acquiring and generalizing the skills (Johnson et al., 2005; Miltenberger et al., 1999).

Researchers have used *in situ* training with behavioral skills training in situations where behavioral skills training alone has not been effective at teaching firearm safety skills. *In situ* training has the same components as behavioral skills training (i.e., instructions, modeling, rehearsal, and feedback), but the investigator or clinician conducts the training immediately after a failed *in situ* assessment. The moment the child fails to perform the safety skill, the investigator enters the area, terminates the assessment, and begins the *in situ* training. The investigator discusses the safety threat, reviews the correct and incorrect aspects of the performance, and asks the child to rehearse the skills while providing additional feedback (e.g., Miltenberger et al., 2004, 2005, 2009, 2013).

Miltenberger and colleagues have evaluated behavioral skills training for teaching firearm safety skills to children, extending the existing literature on behavioral skills training in threat situations such as abduction and sexual abuse (Gatheridge et al., 2004; Himle, Miltenberger, Flessner, et al., 2004; Himle, Miltenberger, Gatheridge, et al., 2004; Miltenberger et al., 2004, 2005, 2009). Himle, Miltenberger, Gatheridge, et al. (2004) compared the firearm safety skills of 4- and 5-year-olds assigned to behavioral skills training, the Eddie Eagle GunSafe Program, or a control group. The investigators kept training time consistent across the two types of training by conducting training during five brief sessions. Investigators conducted the Eddie Eagle program with small groups, consistent with the instructions in the Eddie Eagle training materials. Similarly, investigators provided instructions and modeling to small groups of children assigned to the behavioral skills training group. Children in the behavioral skills training group rehearsed the skills and received individual feedback in scenarios in which they found a real but disabled firearm in the home to promote generalization. After training, the investigators conducted self-report, role-play, and *in situ* assessments and found that children in both training groups scored significantly higher than children in the control group on the self-report measure. That is, children in both training groups could say what to do when they found a firearm. Children in the behavioral skills training group scored significantly higher than children in the Eddie Eagle and control groups on the role-play assessment. In fact, all children in the behavioral skills training group did not touch the firearm, left the room, and reported finding the firearm to an adult. Finally, the skills did not generalize to *in situ* assessments for children in any group; the *in situ* assessment scores were similar for all three groups.

This study highlights the importance of multiple assessment procedures to examine the breadth of skill acquisition and generalization (Himle, Miltenberger, Gatheridge, et al., 2004). The results also suggest that the failure of children in the training groups to perform the skills either in the role-play assessments (the Eddie Eagle group) or the *in situ* assessments (both training groups) may have reflected a performance rather than a skill deficit. That is, children in both training groups could self-report the correct safety skills, and children in the behavioral skills training group could role-play the correct safety skills. By contrast, children in the Eddie Eagle group did not perform the safety skills during either role-play or *in situ* assessments, and children in the behavioral skills training group did not perform the skills during the *in situ* assessment. Other studies of safety skills training have reported similar findings (Lumley et al., 1998; Miltenberger et al., 1999).

Himle, Miltenberger, Flessner, et al. (2004) evaluated procedures to promote generalization of firearm safety skills from training sessions to *in situ* assessments with 4- and 5-year-olds. The investigators trained eight children individually in two 30-minute behavioral skills training sessions. In each session, the trainer gave the child instructions and modeled the safety skills. The child rehearsed the skills in various scenarios in which he or she found a firearm. The trainer provided praise and corrective feedback until the child performed the skills correctly five consecutive times. Investigators then assessed safety skills during an *in situ* assessment. Investigators conducted up to three booster training sessions if a child did not perform the skills correctly during the *in situ* assessment. The booster sessions were like the initial training sessions. Investigators implemented *in situ* training if a child still did not engage in the correct safety skills after the third booster session. Immediately after the child did not engage in the correct firearm safety skills during an *in situ* assessment, the investigator entered the assessment situation, vocally repeated and modeled the safety skills, and prompted the child to rehearse the safety skill until he or she performed it correctly five consecutive times. No children performed the correct safety skills during baseline. Three children performed the correct skills after behavioral skills training and booster sessions. The other five children performed the correct skills only after the addition of *in situ* training. Follow-up assessments occurred in each child's home between 2 weeks and 2 months after training. All children performed the correct skills during follow-up, except for one child who did not report the firearm to an adult. This child exhibited the correct skills during a subsequent assessment (Himle, Miltenberger, Flessner, et al., 2004).

In a similar study, Miltenberger et al. (2004) evaluated individual behavioral skills training with *in situ* training as needed for teaching safety skills to six children ages 6 and 7 years. Three of the children performed the correct skills during *in situ* assessments after two to four behavioral skills training sessions, but the other three children required *in situ* training before exhibiting the skills consistently during *in situ* assessments. All children generalized the skills to their homes and maintained them 5 months after training. The results of Himle, Miltenberger, Flessner, et al. (2004) and Miltenberger et al. (2004) demonstrated the importance of *in situ* training for teaching safety skills to children: *In situ* training produced correct performance for all children when behavioral skills training alone was not effective.

Gatheridge et al. (2004) compared the effectiveness of the Eddie Eagle GunSafe Program and behavioral skills training implemented in small groups of 6- and 7-year-olds. In addition, they evaluated *in situ* training with children who did not exhibit the skills after the Eddie Eagle GunSafe Program or behavioral skills training. The results showed that children in the Eddie Eagle and behavioral skills training groups had higher safety skills scores than children in the control group on a self-report assessment; that is, children in both training groups could tell the investigator what to do upon finding a firearm. Children in both training groups also performed significantly better than those in the control group during role-play assessments, in which the investigator described a scenario where a child finds an unattended firearm and told the child to act out what he or she would do in that scenario. Children in the behavioral skills training group performed significantly better than children in the Eddie Eagle group during role-play assessments, because all children in the behavioral skills training group engaged in the correct safety skills. These findings were consistent with those of Himle, Miltenberger, Gatheridge, et al. (2004) for 4- and 5-year-olds in the Eddie Eagle group relative to the behavioral skills training groups. Children in the behavioral skills training group in the Gatheridge et al. study also performed significantly better than children in the Eddie Eagle and control groups during *in situ* assessments. Most children in the behavioral skills training group in Gatheridge et al. performed the correct safety skills during *in situ* assessments. By contrast, the 4- and 5-year-olds in Himle, Miltenberger, Gatheridge et al. did not perform the correct safety skills during *in situ* assessments. Almost all children in the Eddie Eagle group in Gatheridge et al. did not demonstrate correct safety skills until they participated in *in situ* training, whereas most children in the behavioral skills training group demonstrated correct safety skills without *in situ* training.

Research results suggest that children often do not demonstrate correct safety skills during *in situ* assessment after behavioral skills training, but do demonstrate generalization of safety skills after the addition of *in situ* training (Himle, Miltenberger, Flessner, et al., 2004; Miltenberger et al., 2004). Consequently, Miltenberger et al. (2005) implemented two behavioral skills training sessions, followed by an *in situ* assessment within 30 minutes of the second training session, with 10 children ages 4 and 5 years. If a child did not perform the safety skills during the *in situ* assessment, a novel trainer entered the assessment situation and conducted *in situ* training. The results showed that all 10 children performed the skills after receiving two behavioral skills training sessions followed by an *in situ* assessment, and the skills were generalized and maintained over a 3-month follow-up period. Furthermore, 5 of the children participated in a dyad *in situ* assessment in which they found the firearm while accompanied by a peer, and all five engaged in the correct safety skills. These results suggest that the inclusion of *in situ* training earlier in training may improve the effectiveness and efficiency of behavioral skills training (Miltenberger et al., 2005). An alternative explanation is that *in situ* training alone would have been effective.

Although no study has evaluated *in situ* training alone to teach firearm safety skills, Miltenberger et al.'s (2009) results may provide an indication of the effects of *in situ* training alone. In this research, one group received behavioral skills training; one group received simulated *in situ* training with the same components as behavioral skills training, plus discussion of real-life scenarios during instruction, video clips of children encountering firearms alone and with a peer challenge, and rehearsal with a peer challenge; and one group received no training. In the first posttraining assessment, investigators found no differences in the scores among the three groups, suggesting that neither training procedure was effective. The investigators then conducted one *in situ* training session for those children in the three groups who did not engage in the correct skills. The children in all three groups demonstrated the safety skills, with no significant differences between groups after *in situ* training. These results suggest that *in situ* training alone may be sufficient for teaching safety skills, as the children in the control group acquired the skills after *in situ* training alone. Miltenberger et al. (2013) obtained similar results, in that *in situ* training alone was effective for teaching abduction prevention skills to children who were part of a no-treatment control group. Although these results are promising, the field needs more research to evaluate *in situ* training as a stand-alone intervention.

## CONCLUSIONS

We can draw several conclusions from the results of the studies evaluating behavioral skills training for teaching firearm safety skills to children. First, behavioral skills training, an approach in which a child practices the target safety skills and receives feedback, is superior to the Eddie Eagle GunSafe Program, an informational approach without practice or feedback components. This finding is consistent with other research demonstrating that practice of skills with feedback is necessary for training programs to be effective (e.g., Beck & Miltenberger, 2009; Poche et al., 1988). Table 28.1 shows the sequence of steps in behavioral skills training for teaching firearm safety skills to children.

Second, the number of behavioral skills training sessions required for children to perform the safety skills varies. In some cases, children performed the skills after two training sessions; in other cases, children did not perform the skills after five training sessions. This finding was consistent across 4- to 7-year-old children and suggests that investigators must repeat safety skills assessments to determine how many training sessions children require to demonstrate generalized use of skills.

Third, some children do not perform safety skills until they participate in *in situ* training. All children who participated in *in situ* training performed safety skills after one to three training sessions (most after just one session), regardless of how many behavioral skills training sessions preceded the *in situ* training. The behavioral mechanism that underlies the effectiveness of *in situ* training is not clear. One possibility is that it simply involves reinforcing instances of generalization—a known strategy for promoting generalization (Stokes & Baer, 1977). Another possibility is that being observed exhibiting the incorrect behavior and having to rehearse the safety skills repeatedly functions as punishment for incorrect behavior, and avoidance of observation and rehearsal functions as negative reinforcement of safety skills.

Fourth, children's responses to different assessments were not consistent, showing that different repertoires are involved in a child's (1) vocally describing the appropriate safety skills, (2) demonstrating the skills in the presence of the investigator, and (3) using the skills during *in situ* assessments. Results of research show that children may demonstrate safety skills in role plays, yet fail to perform safety skills during *in situ* assessments. As such, we view the failure to perform the skills during *in situ* assessments as a performance deficit, not a skills deficit. We hypothesize that *in situ* training functions as contingency management rather than as skills training. Therefore, behavioral skills training may be most appropriate for teaching skills, whereas *in situ* training may be most appropriate for reinforcing use of skills, but investigators should evaluate this hypothesis in future studies.

### TABLE 28.1. Steps in Teaching Firearm Safety Skills to Children

1. Provide instructions.
   a. Describe the dangers of playing with firearms and the safety skills to use when finding an unattended firearm ("Don't touch it, get away, and tell an adult").
   b. Give examples to illustrate the safety skills in different situations.

2. Model the safety skills.
   a. Simulate a situation in which you find a firearm (using a disabled firearm or a replica of a real firearm), and demonstrate the safety skills: "Don't touch it, run away from the firearm, and tell an adult about the firearm."
   b. Describe the importance of the skills after modeling them.

3. Provide the opportunity for rehearsal.
   a. Set up a scenario in which the child could find a firearm (e.g., on a shelf in the parents' bedroom), and place a firearm (a disabled firearm or a replica of a real firearm) in the simulated situation.
   b. Ask the child to show you the safety skills.
   c. During the rehearsal, set up the situation so that the child has to run out of the room and tell an adult in another room about finding the firearm.

4. Provide praise and feedback.
   a. Provide descriptive praise for correct rehearsal of the safety skills or for any aspect of the skills that the child executed correctly.
   b. Provide further instruction for improvement (feedback) if the child executed any aspect of the safety skills incorrectly.

5. Repeat with a variety of scenarios.
   a. Have the child rehearse the safety skills with praise and feedback in a variety of different scenarios.
   b. Create each scenario to represent a situation in which the child could find a firearm in his or her home or the home of a friend.

6. Conduct *in situ* assessment.
   a. Conduct *in situ* assessment by placing a disabled firearm or replica in a location where the child will find it, and recording the child's behavior.
   b. *In situ* assessment must occur without the child's knowledge.

7. Conduct *in situ* training as needed.
   a. If the child fails to use the skills during the *in situ* assessment, enter the room and conduct training.
   b. Review the safety skills.
   c. Have the child rehearse three to five times correctly in the situation.

## FUTURE DIRECTIONS

There are several areas for future research to improve methods for teaching safety skills to children. One direction for such research is to evaluate factors that influence the effectiveness of behavioral skills training. Research results to date suggest that behavioral skills training is superior to informational approaches, and that an individual format for behavioral skills training is superior to a group format. However, future research should investigate (1) whether there are age-related differences in the effectiveness of behavioral skills training; (2) whether modifications of behavioral skills training would enhance its effectiveness for children of different ages; (3) what the most efficient method of safety skills training is; and (4) what the single and interactive effects of behavioral skills training and *in situ* training are.

Future investigators might evaluate whether skill deficits, performance deficits, or both underlie why children do not use safety skills during *in situ* assessments. Identification of the factors that contribute to demonstrating safety skills in training sessions but not during *in situ* assessment may inform training procedures. For example, reinforcement contingencies for firearm play (e.g., automatic positive reinforcement from firearm play, automatic negative reinforcement in the form of avoidance of peer ridicule for demonstrating safety skills) may override reinforcement contingencies for performing correct safety skills. Rule-governed behavior (e.g., a child believes that a negative consequence would occur for reporting the firearm) also might function to suppress demonstration of safety skills. These explanations are speculative, but could be directions for future research.

Another area for future research is to incorporate dyad assessments and peer challenges into training and assessment. Except for two studies (Miltenberger et al., 2005, 2009), research to date has focused on skills assessment when the child finds the firearm while alone. Nevertheless, children may find a firearm while with other children. Future studies could evaluate scenarios in which a target child in a dyad or group of children who are research confederates finds a firearm. Investigators could program the confederates to respond in various ways (e.g., a confederate child challenges the target child to play with the firearm; Miltenberger et al., 2009).

One other topic for future research might be to evaluate strategies to improve the efficiency of behavioral skills training and increase its accessibility. In research studies, trained investigators (e.g., graduate students in behavior analysis) conduct behavioral skills training with individual children or small groups, typically in a handful of sessions. This method requires the presence of trained individuals who have the time to conduct the required training. Communities are not likely to implement this training widely unless it becomes more efficient. Peer training is one potential strategy to improve the efficiency of safety skills training. Jostad, Miltenberger, Kelso, and Knudson (2008) used behavioral skills training to teach four 6- and 7-year-old children to use behavioral skills training to teach safety skills to six 4- and 5-year-old children. The 6- and 7-year-olds conducted two to five behavioral skills training sessions and *in situ* training, if needed, with the 4- and 5-year-olds. Both groups of children correctly engaged in the safety skills during assessment. These results and those of a similar study by Tarasenko, Miltenberger, Brower-Breitwieser, and Bosch (2010) suggest that peer training may be an effective method of teaching safety skills; however, the field needs more research.

Training parents or teachers to be trainers might be another alternative to improve the efficiency of safety skills training. More children could receive training if teachers and parents could teach safety skills to their students and children, respectively. For example, the Eddie Eagle GunSafe Program is designed to teach parents or teachers to conduct training. Unfortunately, research conducted to date has not shown that it is effective (Gatheridge et al., 2004; Himle, Miltenberger, Gatheridge, et al., 2004; Kelso et al., 2007). Promising results from Gross, Miltenberger, Knudson, Bosch, and Brower-Breitwieser (2007) provide preliminary support for the effectiveness of an instructional program to teach parents to use behavioral skills training to teach safety skills to their children. Gross et al. demonstrated that three of four parents who read an instructional manual and watched a modeling video used behavioral skills and *in situ* training correctly to teach safety skills to their 4- to 7-year-old children. Vanselow and Hanley (2014) evaluated a computerized behavioral skills training program to teach an array of safety skills. Although the results showed that the computerized training was effective for only a few children, this represents an interesting use of technology to increase the accessibility of safety skills training programs. Hanratty, Miltenberger, and Florentino (2016) evaluated a training manual for teaching a preschool teacher to conduct behavioral skills training to teach safety skills to her 3- and 4-year-old students. This training was not effective. Investigators then implemented *in situ* training and incentives, including access to leisure activities, and the children demonstrated the skills. Additional research is needed to develop and evaluate the effectiveness of such programs, with the ultimate goal of promoting wide-scale dissemination.

# REFERENCES

American Academy of Pediatrics (AAP), Committee on Injury and Poison Prevention. (2000). Firearm-related injuries affecting the pediatric population. *Pediatrics, 105,* 888–895.

Azrael, D., Cohen, J., Salhi, C., & Miller, M. (2018). Firearm storage in gun-owning households with children: Results of a 2015 national survey. *Journal of Urban Health, 95,* 295–304.

Azrael, D., Miller, M., & Hemenway, D. (2000). Are household firearms stored safely?: It depends whom you ask. *Pediatrics, 106,* e31–e36.

Beck, K., & Miltenberger, R. (2009). Evaluation of a commercially available abduction prevention program. *Journal of Applied Behavior Analysis, 42,* 761–772.

Brady Campaign to Prevent Gun Violence. (n.d.-a). Sensible gun laws save lives. Retrieved July 28, 2015, from *www.bradycampaign.org.*

Brady Campaign to Prevent Gun Violence. (n.d.-b). Firearm facts. Retrieved June 1, 2015, from *www.bradycampaign.org.*

Carroll-Rowan, L., & Miltenberger, R. (1994). A comparison of procedures for teaching abduction prevention to preschoolers. *Education and Treatment of Children, 17,* 113–128.

Common Sense about Kids and Guns. (n.d.). Fact file. Retrieved July 28, 2015, from *www.kidsandguns.org.*

Coyne-Beasley, T., Schoenbach, V. J., & Johnson, R. M. (2001). "Love Our Kids, Lock Your Guns": A community-based firearm safety counseling and gun lock distribution program. *Archives of Pediatrics and Adolescent Medicine, 155,* 659–664.

Crifasi, C. K., Doucette, M. L., McGinty, E. E., Webster, D. W., & Barry, C. L. (2018). Storage practice of US gun owners in 2016. *American Journal of Public Health, 108,* 532–537.

Crifasi, C. K., O'Dwyer, J. K., McGinty, E. E., Webster, D. W., & Barry, C. L. (2019). Desirability of personalized guns among current gun owners. *American Journal of Preventive Medicine, 57,* 191–196.

Cummings, P., Grossman, D. C., Rivara, F. P., & Koepsell, T. D. (1997). State gun safe storage laws and child mortality due to firearms. *Journal of the American Medical Association, 278,* 1084–1086.

DiScala, C., & Sege, R. (2004). Outcomes in children and young adults who are hospitalized for firearms-related injuries. *Pediatrics, 113,* 1306–1312.

Dresang, L. T. (2001). Gun deaths in rural and urban settings: Recommendations for prevention. *Journal of the American Board of Family Practice, 14,* 107–115.

Eber, G. B., Annest, J. L., Mercy, J. A., & Ryan, G. W. (2004). Nonfatal and fatal firearm-related injuries among children aged 14 years and younger: United States, 1993–2000. *Pediatrics, 113,* 1686–1692.

Farah, M. M., & Simon, H. K. (1999). Firearms in the home: Parental perceptions. *Pediatrics, 104,* 1059–1063.

Garcia, D., Dukes, C., Brady, M. P., Scott, J., & Wilson, C. L. (2016). Using modeling and rehearsal to teach fire safety to children with autism. *Journal of Applied Behavior Analysis, 49,* 699–704.

Gatheridge, B. J., Miltenberger, R. G., Huneke, D. F., Satterlund, M. J., Mattern, A. R., Johnson, B. M., et al. (2004). Comparison of two programs to teach firearm injury prevention skills to 6- and 7-year-old children. *Pediatrics, 114,* 294–299.

General Accounting Office. (1991). Accidental shootings: Many deaths and injuries caused by firearms could be prevented. Retrieved August 6, 2020, from *www.gao.gov/assets/160/150353.pdf.*

Gross, A., Miltenberger, R., Knudson, P., Bosch, A., & Brower-Breitwieser, C. (2007). Preliminary evaluation of a parent training program to prevent gun play. *Journal of Applied Behavior Analysis, 40,* 691–695.

Grossman, D. C., Cummings, P., Koepsell, T. D., Marshall, J., D'Ambrosio, L., Thompson, R. S., et al. (2000). Firearm safety counseling in primary care pediatrics: A randomized, controlled trial. *Pediatrics, 106,* 22–26.

Grossman, D. C., Mang, K., & Rivara, F. P. (1995). Firearm injury prevention counseling by pediatricians and family physicians. *Archives of Pediatrics and Adolescent Medicine, 149,* 973–977.

Grossman, D. C., Reay, D. T., & Baker, S. A. (1999). Self-inflicted and unintentional firearm injuries among children and adolescents: The source of the firearm. *Archives of Pediatrics and Adolescent Medicine, 1538,* 875–882.

Hanratty, L., Miltenberger, R., & Florentino, S. (2016). Evaluating the effectiveness of a teaching package utilizing behavioral skills training and *in situ* training to teach gun safety skills in a preschool classroom. *Journal of Behavioral Education, 25,* 310–323.

Hardy, M. S. (2002). Teaching firearm safety to children: Failure of a program. *Developmental and Behavioral Pediatrics, 23,* 71–76.

Hardy, M. S., Armstrong, F. D., Martin, B. L., & Strawn, K. N. (1996). A firearm safety program for children: They just can't say no. *Journal of Developmental and Behavioral Pediatrics, 17,* 216–221.

Haught, K., Grossman, D., & Connell, F. (1995). Parents' attitudes toward firearm injury prevention counseling in urban pediatric clinics. *Pediatrics, 96,* 649–653.

Hemenway, D., & Solnick, S. J. (2015). Children and unintentional firearm death. *Injury Epidemiology, 2,* 26.

Hemenway, D., Solnick, S. J., & Azrael, D. R. (1995). Firearm training and storage. *Journal of the American Medical Association, 273,* 46–50.

Hendricks, C. M., & Reichert, A. (1996). Parents' self-reported behaviors related to health and safety of very young children. *Journal of School Health, 66,* 247–251.

Himle, M., & Miltenberger, R. (2004). Preventing unintentional firearm injury in children: The need for behavioral skills training. *Education and Treatment of Children, 27,* 161–177.

Himle, M. B., Miltenberger, R. G., Flessner, C., & Gatheridge, B. (2004). Teaching safety skills to children to prevent gun play. *Journal of Applied Behavior Analysis, 37,* 1–9.

Himle, M. B., Miltenberger, R. G., Gatheridge, B., & Flessner, C. (2004). An evaluation of two procedures for training skills to prevent gun play in children. *Pediatrics, 113,* 70–77.

Jackman, G. A., Farah, M. M., Kellerman, A. L., & Simon, H. K. (2001). Seeing is believing: What do boys do when they find a real gun? *Pediatrics, 107,* 1247–1250.

Johnson, B. M., Miltenberger, R. G., Egemo-Helm, K., Jostad, C. J., Flessner, C., & Gatheridge, B. (2005). Evaluation of behavioral skills training for teaching abduction-prevention skills to young children. *Journal of Applied Behavior Analysis, 38,* 67–78.

Johnson, B. M., Miltenberger, R. G., Knudson, P., Egemo-Helm, K., Kelso, P., Jostad, C., et al. (2006). A preliminary evaluation of two behavioral skills training procedures for teaching abduction prevention skills to school-age children. *Journal of Applied Behavior Analysis, 39,* 25–34.

Jones, R. T., Kazdin, A. E., & Haney, J. I. (1981). Social validation and training of emergency fire safety skills for potential injury prevention and life saving. *Journal of Applied Behavior Analysis, 14,* 249–260.

Jones, R. T., Ollendick, T. H., McLaughlin, K. J., & Williams, C. E. (1989). Elaborative and behavioral rehearsal in the acquisition of fire emergency skills and the reduction of fear of fire. *Behavior Therapy, 20,* 93–101.

Jostad, C. M., & Miltenberger, R. G. (2004). Firearm injury prevention skills: Increasing the efficiency of training with peer tutoring. *Child and Family Behavior Therapy, 26,* 21–35.

Jostad, C. M., Miltenberger, R. G., Kelso, P., & Knudson, P. (2008). Peer tutoring to prevent gun play: Acquisition, generalization, and maintenance of safety skills. *Journal of Applied Behavior Analysis, 41,* 117–123.

Kellerman, A. L. (1993). Preventing firearm injuries: A review of epidemiologic research. *American Journal of Preventive Medicine, 9*(Suppl. 1), 12–15.

Kellerman, A. L., & Reay, D. T. (1986). Protection or peril?: An analysis of firearm-related deaths in the home. *New England Journal of Medicine, 314,* 1557–1560.

Kelso, P., Miltenberger, R., Waters, M., Egemo-Helm, K., & Bagne, A. (2007). Teaching skills to second and third grade children to prevent gun play: A comparison of procedures. *Education and Treatment of Children, 30,* 29–48.

Knight-Bohnhoff, K., & Harris, M. B. (1998). Parent's behaviors, knowledge, and beliefs related to unintentional firearm injuries among children and youth in the Southwest. *Journal of Pediatric Health Care, 12,* 139–146.

Lumley, V. A., Miltenberger, R. G., Long, E. S., Rapp, J. T., & Roberts, J. A. (1998). Evaluation of a sexual abuse prevention program for adults with mental retardation. *Journal of Applied Behavior Analysis, 31,* 91–101.

Marchand-Martella, N., & Huber, G. (1996). Assessing the long-term maintenance of abduction prevention skills by disadvantaged preschoolers. *Education and Treatment of Children, 19,* 55–58.

Maxfield, T. C., Miltenberger, R. G., & Novotny, M. A. (2019). Evaluating small-scale simulation for training firearm safety skills. *Journal of Applied Behavior Analysis, 52,* 491–498.

McGee, K. S., Coyne-Beasley, T., & Johnson, R. M. (2003). Review of evaluations of educational approaches to promote safe storage of firearms. *Injury Prevention, 9,* 108–111.

Miller, M., Azrael, D., & Hemenway, D. (2001). Firearm availability and unintentional firearm deaths. *Accident Analysis and Prevention, 33,* 477–484.

Miller, M., Azrael, D., Hemenway, D., & Vriniotis, M. (2005). Firearm storage practices and rates of unintentional firearm deaths in the United States. *Accident Analysis and Prevention, 37,* 661–667.

Miltenberger, R. (2008). Teaching safety skills to children: Prevention of firearm injury as an exemplar of best practice in assessment, training, and generalization of safety skills. *Behavior Analysis in Practice, 1,* 30–36.

Miltenberger, R. G., Flessner, C., Gatheridge, B., Johnson, B., Satterlund, M., & Egemo, K. (2004). Evaluation of behavioral skills training procedures to prevent gun play in children. *Journal of Applied Behavior Analysis, 37,* 513–516.

Miltenberger, R., Fogel, V., Beck, K., Koehler, S., Graves, R., Noah, J., et al. (2013). Examining the efficacy of the Stranger Safety abduction prevention program and parent conducted *in situ* training. *Journal of Applied Behavior Analysis, 46,* 817–820.

Miltenberger, R. G., Gatheridge, B. J., Satterlund, M., Egemo-Helm, K. R., Johnson, B. M., Jostad, C., et al. (2005). Teaching safety skills to prevent gun play: An evaluation of *in situ* training. *Journal of Applied Behavior Analysis, 38,* 395–398.

Miltenberger, R., Gross, A., Knudson, P., Jostad, C., Bosch, A., & Brower Breitwieser, C. (2009). Evaluating behavioral skills training with and without simulated *in situ* training for teaching safety skills to children. *Education and Treatment of Children, 32,* 63–75.

Miltenberger, R., & Hanratty, L. (2013). Teaching sexual abuse prevention skills to children. In D. S. Bromberg & W. T. O'Donohue (Eds.), *Handbook of child and adolescent sexuality: Developmental and forensic psychology* (pp. 419–447). London: Elsevier.

Miltenberger, R. G., & Olsen, L. A. (1996). Abduction prevention training: A review of findings and issues for future research. *Education and Treatment of Children, 19*(1), 69–82.

Miltenberger, R. G., Roberts, J. A., Ellingson, S., Galensky, T., Rapp, J. T., Long, E. S., et al. (1999). Training and generalization of sexual abuse prevention skills for women with mental retardation. *Journal of Applied Behavior Analysis, 32*, 385–388.

Miltenberger, R., Sanchez, S., & Valbuena, D. (2015). Teaching safety skills to children. In H. S. Roane, J. E. Ringdahl, & T. S. Falcomata (Eds.), *Clinical and organizational applications of applied behavior analysis* (pp. 477–499). London: Elsevier.

Miltenberger, R., & Thiesse-Duffy, E. (1988). Evaluation of home-based programs for teaching personal safety skills to children. *Journal of Applied Behavior Analysis, 21*, 81–88.

Miltenberger, R. G., Thiesse-Duffy, E., Suda, K. T., Kozak, C., & Bruellman, J. (1990). Teaching prevention skills to children: The use of multiple measures to evaluate parent versus expert instruction. *Child and Family Behavior Therapy, 12*, 65–87.

National Opinion Research Center. (2014). General Social Survey final report: Trends in gun ownership in the United States, 1972–2014. Retrieved August 1, 2014, from *www.norc.org/PDFs/GSS%20 Reports/GSS_Trends%20in%20Gun%20Ownership_ US_1972-2014.pdf*.

Olsen-Woods, L. A., Miltenberger, R. G., & Forman, G. (1998). Effects of correspondence training in an abduction prevention training program. *Child and Family Behavior Therapy, 20*, 15–34.

Ordog, G. J., Wasserberger, J., Schatz, I., Owens-Collins, D., English, K., Balasubramanian, S., et al. (1988). Gunshot wounds in children under 10 years of age: A new epidemic. *American Journal of Diseases of Children, 142*, 618–622.

Parikh, K., Silver, A., Patel, S. J., Iqbal, S. F., & Goyal, M. (2017). Pediatric firearm-related injuries in the United States. *Hospital Pediatrics, 7*, 303–312.

Poche, C., Brouwer, R., & Swearingen, M. (1981). Teaching self-protection to young children. *Journal of Applied Behavior Analysis, 14*, 169–176.

Poche, C., Yoder, P., & Miltenberger, R. (1988). Teaching self-protection to children using television techniques. *Journal of Applied Behavior Analysis, 21*, 253–261.

Schuster, M. A., Franke, T. M., Bastian, A. M., Sor, S., & Halfon, N. (2000). Firearm storage patterns in US homes with children. *American Journal of Public Health, 90*, 588–594.

Senturia, Y. D., Christoffel, K. K., & Donovan, M. (1994). Children's household exposure to guns: A pediatric practice-based survey. *Pediatrics, 93*, 469–475.

Sidman, E. A., Grossman, D. C., Koepsell, T. D., D'Ambrosio, L., Britt, J., Simpson, E. S., et al. (2005). Evaluation of a community-based handgun safe-storage campaign. *Pediatrics, 115*, e654–e661.

Stennies, G., Ikeda, R., Leadbetter, S., Houston, B., & Sacks, J. (1999). Firearm storage practices and children in the home, United States, 1994. *Archives of Pediatrics and Adolescent Medicine, 153*, 586–590.

Stokes, T. F., & Baer, D. M. (1977). An implicit technology of generalization. *Journal of Applied Behavior Analysis, 10*, 349–367.

Tarasenko, M. A., Miltenberger, R. G., Brower-Breitwieser, C., & Bosch, A. (2010). Evaluation of peer training for teaching abduction prevention skills. *Child and Family Behavior Therapy, 32*, 219–230.

Vanselow, N. R., & Hanley, G. P. (2014). An evaluation of computerized behavior skills training to teach safety skills to young children. *Journal of Applied Behavior Analysis, 47*, 51–69.

Vernick, J. S., O'Brien, M., Hepburn, L. M., Johnson, S. B., Webster, C. W., & Hargarten, S. W. (2003). Unintentional and undetermined firearm related deaths: A preventable death analysis for three safety devices. *Injury Prevention: Journal of the International Society for Child and Adolescent Injury, 9*, 307–311.

Violano, P., Bonne, S., Duncan, T., Pappas, P., Christmas, A. B., Goldberg, S., et al. (2018). Prevention of firearm injuries with gun safety devices and storage: An Eastern Association for the Surgery of Trauma systemic review. *Journal of Trauma and Acute Care Surgery, 84*, 1003–1011.

Webster, D. W., & Starnes, M. (2000). Reexamining the association between child access prevention gun laws and unintentional shooting deaths of children. *Pediatrics, 106*, 1466–1469.

Webster, D. W., Wilson, M. E. H., Duggan, A. K., & Pakula, L. C. (1992). Parents' beliefs about preventing gun injuries to children. *Pediatrics, 89*, 908–914.

Wiley, C. C., & Casey, R. (1993). Family experiences, attitudes, and household safety practices regarding firearms. *Clinical Pediatrics, 32*, 71–76.

Wintemute, G. J., Teret, S. P., Kraus, J. F., Wright, M. A., & Bradfield, G. (1987). When children shoot children: 88 unintended deaths in California. *Journal of the American Medical Association, 257*, 3107–3109.

Yeaton, W. H., & Bailey, J. S. (1978). Teaching pedestrian safety skills to young children: An analysis and one-year follow-up. *Journal of Applied Behavior Analysis, 11*, 315–329.

Zavoski, R. W., Lapidus, G. D., Lerer, T. J., & Banco, L. I. (1995). A population-based study of severe firearm injury among children and youth. *Pediatrics, 96*, 278–282.

# CHAPTER 29

# Behavior Analysis and Treatment of Drug Addiction

## Recent Advances in Research on Abstinence Reinforcement

Kenneth Silverman, August F. Holtyn, Brantley P. Jarvis, and Shrinidhi Subramaniam

Extensive evidence in animals and in humans, in basic laboratory research and randomized clinical trials, suggests that drug addiction is an operant behavior that is maintained and modifiable by its consequences (Silverman, DeFulio, & Everly, 2011). This body of research serves as a rich foundation for applying the principles of operant conditioning to the treatment of drug addiction. Researchers have applied operant principles to drug addiction treatment in a variety of ways, but they have applied it most directly and arguably with the greatest effectiveness in the direct reinforcement of drug abstinence. Under abstinence reinforcement procedures, patients receive a desirable consequence contingent on providing objective evidence of drug abstinence. A chapter in the first edition of this handbook provided the context and overview of about 40 years of research on the development and evaluation of abstinence reinforcement interventions for drug addiction (Silverman, Kaminski, Higgins, & Brady, 2011). In the present chapter, we provide a brief overview of the earlier chapter, and then provide a qualitative and selective summary and discussion of the research that investigators have published since we wrote the original chapter.

## AN OVERVIEW OF RESEARCH ON ABSTINENCE REINFORCEMENT TO 2011

For over 40 years, researchers have applied abstinence reinforcement interventions to treat drug addiction in diverse populations of adults and adolescents who have used many different commonly abused drugs (Silverman, Kaminski, et al., 2011).

### Early Studies

Early studies applied abstinence reinforcement interventions to treat so-called "Skid Row alcoholics"; adults enrolled in methadone treatment who continued to use opiates, benzodiazepines, and alcohol during methadone treatment; health care professionals who abused various drugs; and cigarette smokers (Silverman, Kaminski, et al., 2011). Although these early studies differed considerably in the settings and procedures used to apply abstinence reinforcement contingencies, they "established a firm scientific foundation for the development of abstinence reinforcement interventions, and illustrated a range of creative and useful applications of an abstinence reinforcement technology" (Silverman, Kaminski, et al., 2011, p. 453).

## Voucher-Based Reinforcement

Higgins et al. (1991) developed and tested an abstinence reinforcement intervention to treat adults addicted to cocaine. The intervention offered participants monetary vouchers exchangeable for goods and services for providing routine urine samples that were negative for cocaine. Importantly, the voucher intervention used a schedule of escalating pay for sustained abstinence, in which the value of the vouchers increased as the number of consecutive cocaine-negative urine samples increased. This voucher-based abstinence reinforcement intervention proved effective and versatile. Over the next 20 years, researchers applied and evaluated the effectiveness of the voucher intervention in promoting cocaine abstinence in adults with primary cocaine dependence; adults and patients receiving methadone treatment who continued to use cocaine during this treatment; opiate abstinence in patients who continued to use opiates during methadone treatment; smoking cessation in diverse populations of cigarette smokers; and abstinence from marijuana use (Silverman, Kaminski, et al., 2011).

Petry, Martin, Cooney, and Kranzler (2000) developed a variation of the voucher-based abstinence reinforcement intervention, in which participants earned the opportunity to draw prizes from a fishbowl contingent on alcohol-negative breath or drug-negative urine samples. The possible prizes had small, large, jumbo, or no monetary values, and a participant had a chance of drawing one prize value on any given occasion. To reinforce sustained abstinence, the researchers used a schedule of escalating reinforcement for sustained abstinence in which the number of draws increased as the number of consecutive alcohol- or drug-negative samples increased. The prize-based abstinence reinforcement procedure was effective, and the National Institute on Drug Abuse's Clinical Trials Network evaluated the procedure in two multisite randomized controlled clinical trials (Peirce et al., 2006; Petry, Alessi, Marx, Austin, & Tardif, 2005).

Dallery and Glenn (2005) developed a novel Internet-based approach to reinforce smoking cessation that proved both effective and convenient. Under that system, participants provided breath carbon monoxide (CO) samples in front of a video camera connected to the Internet. The video, which included the reading on the CO meter, was time-stamped, transmitted across the Internet, and evaluated by staff. Participants received a monetary voucher if the CO level displayed on the CO meter met the criterion for reinforcement.

## Reviews and Meta-Analyses

Reviews and meta-analyses have shown that abstinence reinforcement interventions are among the most effective psychosocial interventions for the treatment of drug addiction (e.g., Dutra et al., 2008; Lussier, Heil, Mongeon, Badger, & Higgins, 2006; Pilling, Strang, Gerada, & National Institute for Clinical Excellence [NICE], 2007). One meta-analysis, for example, examined 34 controlled studies that evaluated the effectiveness of abstinence reinforcement interventions (called *contingency management* in that paper); relapse prevention; general cognitive-behavioral therapy; and treatments combining cognitive-behavioral therapy and contingency management. In that meta-analysis, the strongest effect was for contingency management interventions (Dutra et al., 2008).

## Improving Outcomes

Abstinence reinforcement interventions are clearly effective in promoting abstinence from most commonly abused drugs and in diverse populations. However, the interventions have two main limitations: (1) They are not effective for all patients, and (2) many patients resume drug use when the abstinence reinforcement intervention ends (Silverman, Kaminski, et al., 2011). As described in the original chapter, the effectiveness of abstinence reinforcement interventions can vary as a function of familiar parameters of operant conditioning that affect any operant-reinforcement contingency.

### Increasing Effectiveness

Conclusions from reviews and meta-analyses suggest that parameters such as immediacy and frequency of reinforcement and response requirements (i.e., abstinence from single vs. multiple drugs) alter the effectiveness of abstinence reinforcement interventions. However, individual studies show most clearly that the magnitude of reinforcement determines the effectiveness of these interventions (Silverman, Kaminski, et al., 2011). One study, for example, demonstrated that some patients who used cocaine during methadone treatment did not initiate cocaine abstinence when offered a standard voucher intervention in which they could earn up to about $1,150 in vouchers for providing cocaine-negative urine samples three times per week for 12 weeks. In a subsequent within-patient cross-over period, many of those treatment-refractory patients did initiate sustained cocaine abstinence when offered a high-magnitude voucher intervention in which they could earn up to $3,400 in vouchers for providing cocaine-negative urine samples three times per week for 9 weeks. Importantly, they achieved significantly higher rates of cocaine abstinence than during low- and zero-magnitude reinforcement conditions (Silverman, Chutuape, Bigelow, & Stitzer, 1999). One study also showed that an abstinence reinforcement intervention could become ineffective if reinforcement magnitude decreased too much (Petry et al., 2004).

### Preventing Relapse

Relapse to drug use is common after drug abuse treatment, independent of the type of treatment (McLellan, Lewis, O'Brien, & Kleber, 2000). Relatively few studies have evaluated interventions that could prevent relapse to drug use after an abstinence reinforcement intervention ends, even though researchers have observed relapse reliably since the earliest studies of such interventions (Silverman, Kaminski, et al., 2011). Several studies examined whether abstinence reinforcement would produce lasting effects if researchers combined it with cognitive-behavioral relapse prevention therapy, a counseling intervention designed to prevent relapse. Results of those studies showed that voucher-based abstinence reinforcement produced higher rates of abstinence during treatment than the cognitive-behavioral therapy when researchers presented each alone, and the combined treatment did not increase rates of abstinence compared to the voucher intervention alone either during or after treatment (Silverman, Kaminski, et al., 2011).

Results of a few studies have suggested that researchers could use abstinence reinforcement as a maintenance intervention to sustain abstinence and prevent relapse, at least while the abstinence reinforcement intervention continued (e.g., Preston, Umbricht, & Epstein, 2002; Silverman, Robles, Mudric, Bigelow, & Stitzer, 2004). One study, for example, showed that methadone-maintained patients could maintain cocaine abstinence for up to a year if the abstinence reinforcement contingency was in place for that period (Silverman et al., 2004).

## Dissemination

At the time we wrote our earlier chapter, professionals in the community had not used abstinence reinforcement interventions widely (Silverman, Kaminski, et al., 2011). Most efforts to apply such interventions sought to integrate those contingencies into substance abuse treatment clinics.

Resources available to substance abuse treatment clinics constrained applications of abstinence reinforcement interventions in those clinics. Researchers had attempted to "use reinforcers that [were] available in clinics, to devise ways to pay for reinforcers, and to use low-cost reinforcers" (Silverman, Kaminski, et al., 2011, p. 464). Take-home methadone doses for patients receiving methadone treatment proved to be one reinforcer that clinics could provide at relatively little additional cost. Researchers had used deposit contracts, in which patients deposited money at the start of treatment that they could earn back by achieving and maintaining drug abstinence during treatment, since the earliest days of research on abstinence reinforcement interventions (Elliott & Tighe, 1968).

Researchers tried to reduce the magnitude of reinforcement to make the interventions more practical; however, reducing reinforcement magnitude had the undesirable effect of reducing and possibly eliminating the effectiveness of the interventions (e.g., Glasgow, Hollis, Ary, & Boles, 1993; Petry et al., 2004). The National Institute on Drug Abuse Clinical Trials Network conducted large-scale multisite investigations in which the researchers effectively used higher-magnitude abstinence reinforcement that were effective in previous controlled studies (e.g., Peirce et al., 2006). These studies illustrated both the effectiveness of abstinence reinforcement interventions and the willingness of community treatment programs to apply these interventions, at least when external sources funded the reinforcers. The United Kingdom provided the greatest evidence that communities could adopt abstinence reinforcement interventions. Based on a rigorous review of psychosocial treatments for drug addiction, the NICE recommended routine use of voucher-based-reinforcement interventions for the treatment of drug addiction (substance misuse) in the United Kingdom's National Health Service (Pilling et al., 2007). This resulted in the National Health Service's offering voucher-based reinforcement as one of its interventions for drug addiction treatment.

Several researchers sought to use reinforcers available outside of the standard clinic setting for drug addiction treatment (Silverman, Kaminski, et al., 2011). Three research programs on this method stand out. Milby et al. (1996) investigated the use of abstinence-contingent housing and work therapy to promote abstinence in homeless cocaine-dependent adults. Ries et al. (2004) used U.S. Social Security Disability benefits in a contingent fashion to promote drug abstinence in adults with severe mental illness. Finally, Silverman (2004) used abstinence-contingent access to employment in a series of studies to initiate and maintain drug abstinence in unemployed adults with long histories of drug addiction.

## RECENT ADVANCES IN RESEARCH ON ABSTINENCE REINFORCEMENT

At the time the earlier chapter was written, conclusions about research on abstinence reinforcement interventions were relatively simple (Silverman, Kaminski, et al., 2011): (1) These interventions promoted abstinence from most commonly abused drugs and in diverse populations and settings; (2) a need existed to develop procedures to increase the proportion of patients who achieved abstinence when exposed to these interventions; (3) a need existed to develop procedures that promoted long-term abstinence and prevented relapse; and (4) a need existed to develop practical applications of abstinence reinforcement interventions that ensured the widespread application of these procedures in society. In the remainder of this chapter, we review studies conducted since we completed the earlier chapter, with special attention to whether recent research has confirmed and extended our earlier conclusions.

### General Utility of Abstinence Reinforcement Interventions

Reviews and meta-analyses published in the last several years have confirmed that abstinence reinforcement interventions are highly effective in promoting abstinence from most commonly abused drugs and in diverse populations (Benishek et al., 2014; Cahill, Hartmann-Boyce, & Perera, 2015; Castells et al., 2009; Davis et al., 2016). These reviews and meta-analyses also confirmed that such interventions are not always effective and rarely produce effects that are evident after the interventions end.

Two analyses of these interventions highlight key and consistent findings about their effectiveness (Benishek et al., 2014; Davis et al., 2016). First, the duration of abstinence reinforcement interventions is relatively short, with a mean of 12 weeks in both Davis et al. (2016) and Benishek et al. (2014), and a median of 8 and 12 weeks in Davis et al. and Benishek et al., respectively. Davis et al. reviewed voucher- and money-based contingency management interventions for substance use disorders from 2009 through 2014; they reported that 43 of 51 studies (84%) showed significant effects of the abstinence reinforcement interventions, and the rest (16%) did not produce significant effects. Of the 22 studies that produced significant effects while the abstinence reinforcement interventions were in effect and assessed posttreatment abstinence, only 7 (32%) showed a statistically significant effect at follow-up. Benishek et al. conducted a meta-analysis of prize-based abstinence reinforcement interventions from 2000 through 2013. Results were like those Davis et al. reported. Eighteen of the 19 studies (95%) reported a significant effect while the prize-based interventions were in effect. The effects of these interventions decreased in the 6 months after discontinuation of the interventions. Six of the nine studies (66%) with a 3-month follow-up assessment showed a significant effect of the prize-based abstinence reinforcement interventions. Two of the six studies (33%) with a 6-month follow-up assessment showed a significant intervention effect. An analysis that combined data from the 6-month follow-up showed that the overall effects of the prize-based interventions were not detectable at that time.

The more recent reviews and meta-analyses document the effectiveness of operant-conditioning principles in the treatment of drug addiction. Abstinence reinforcement interventions significantly increase drug abstinence while the interventions are in effect and occasionally after they end (Benishek et al., 2014; Cahill et al., 2015; Castells et al., 2009; Davis et al., 2016). However, these reviews and meta-analyses summarize the literature by statistical significance and effect sizes, but they do not fully highlight the clinical importance and limitations of abstinence reinforcement interventions: What proportion of patients fail to respond to such interventions? Do these interventions serve a clinically useful role if they do not maintain abstinence over time? Has recent research identified methods of promoting abstinence in treatment-resistant patients and promoting long-term abstinence? In this section, we summarize the results of selected studies to shed some light on these questions.

## Cigarette Smoking

One of the greatest challenges of applying abstinence reinforcement interventions to smoking cessation is the practical problem of collecting frequent breath CO samples from participants. The short half-life of breath CO is the reason for this problem. As described in our earlier chapter, Dallery and colleagues (e.g., Dallery & Glenn, 2005) developed a novel intervention including an Internet-based video technology to solve this practical problem. Participants use that system to provide breath CO samples in front of a video camera connected to the Internet. The software transmits the video of the participant providing the breath sample and the CO level displayed on the CO meter to the investigator. The participant receives a monetary voucher if the CO level displayed on the meter meets the criterion for abstinence reinforcement. At the time of the previous chapter, limited evidence had demonstrated the effectiveness of this approach, but two more recent randomized controlled clinical trials have provided rigorous and real-world evidence (Dallery, Raiff, & Grabinski, 2013; Dallery et al., 2017). In one study (Dallery et al., 2013), researchers randomly assigned cigarette smokers who were interested in quitting smoking to a contingent-CO or noncontingent-CO group. Participants in the contingent-CO group could earn up to $530 in vouchers for providing two breath CO samples per day that confirmed recent abstinence from smoking over a 7-week period. Noncontingent-CO (control) participants earned vouchers regardless of the CO levels of their breath samples. Contingent-CO participants provided significantly more CO-negative breath samples than participants in the noncontingent-CO group. As in previous abstinence reinforcement studies, the smoking cessation intervention was not effective for all participants, and participants did not maintain the effects at 3- and 6-month follow-ups.

As reported in the earlier chapter, voucher-based abstinence reinforcement can have profound effects in pregnant women who smoke cigarettes during pregnancy. Pregnant women in the abstinence reinforcement intervention initially earned vouchers for providing CO-negative breath samples and then for providing urine samples that were negative for cotinine. That intervention was effective in promoting smoking cessation in pregnant women and produced significant increases in fetal growth (Heil et al., 2008). A more recent analysis that combined data collected in three studies confirmed that the voucher-based abstinence reinforcement intervention was effective in promoting smoking cessation in a larger sample of pregnant women; it also extended the findings of the earlier research by showing that the voucher-based intervention produced significantly increased birth weight for babies and reduced the percentage of low-birth-weight babies (Higgins et al., 2010). Again as in previous abstinence reinforcement studies, the voucher-based intervention was not effective for all participants. For example, 34% of women were abstinent at the end of treatment. The combined analysis showed that the effects of the voucher-based abstinence reinforcement intervention were still evident and statistically significant after the intervention ended, although the rates of abstinence decreased progressively over the 12- and 24-week period after delivery. By 24 weeks postpartum, only 14% of women exposed to the voucher-based intervention were abstinent from smoking.

Researchers also have used abstinence reinforcement to promote smoking cessation in patients in a residential substance abuse treatment program (Alessi & Petry, 2014), in opioid-maintained patients (Dunn, Saulsgiver, & Sigmon, 2011), in smokers in Spain (Secades-Villa, Garcia-Rodriguez, Lopez-Nunez, Alonso-Perez, & Fernandez-Hermida, 2014), and in pregnant Indigenous women in New Zealand (Glover, Kira, Walker, & Bauld, 2015). Two related studies assessed the effects of financial incentives in promoting smoking cessation in socioeconomically disadvantaged adults (Kendzor et al., 2015) and homeless adults (Businelle et al., 2014). These studies generally confirmed prior findings that the abstinence reinforcement interventions (1) were effective in promoting smoking cessation, (2) were not effective for all participants, and (3) did not prevent postintervention relapse reliably. Some studies showed that the abstinence reinforcement interventions could produce effects that were still evident and statistically significant in the weeks after termination (e.g., Kendzor et al., 2015; Secades-Villa et al., 2014). Rates of abstinence after the abstinence reinforcement ended, however, were consistently lower than such rates while the abstinence reinforcement was in effect. Thus, even in the studies with significant postintervention effects on smoking cessation, smoking relapse after discontinuation of an abstinence reinforcement intervention remains a problem.

## Opioids

Three studies evaluated the effects of prize-based reinforcement on opiate abstinence and retention in methadone treatment for patients in China. One randomized study showed clear effects of the prize-based reinforcement on retention of patients in methadone treatment in one of two clinics, but the prize-based system did not affect opiate abstinence rates either in the clinic or overall (Hser et al., 2011). A second study randomly assigned methadone-treated patients to standard methadone maintenance with or without prize-based reinforcement of opiate abstinence and retention (Jiang et al., 2012). This study showed that the prize-based reinforcement intervention had no effect on treatment retention or opiate abstinence. A final study randomly assigned clinics to prize-based reinforcement for opiate abstinence and retention in methadone treatment or to standard methadone maintenance, and found a small but significant effect of prize-based reinforcement on both treatment retention and opiate abstinence (Chen et al., 2013). Thus these studies on the prize-based reinforcement intervention on opiate abstinence in China produced mixed effects on opiate abstinence. Only one of the studies showed that prize-based reinforcement increased opiate abstinence. As with other studies, prize-based reinforcement of opiate abstinence was not effective for all participants, and the only study that showed an increase in opiate abstinence during the intervention did not assess postintervention effects.

## Stimulants (Cocaine, Amphetamine, or Methamphetamine)

One study evaluated the effects of prize-based reinforcement on cocaine abstinence in a relatively small sample ($N = 19$) of cocaine-dependent adults receiving treatment in an outpatient mental health clinic (Petry, Alessi, & Rash, 2013). The participants were randomly assigned to receive prize-based reinforcement of cocaine abstinence or not over an 8-week period. The study showed mixed effects on cocaine abstinence. Results were significant only for most consecutive weeks of cocaine abstinence and proportion of expected samples that were cocaine-negative. Results were not significant for proportion of submitted samples that were cocaine-negative. The study did not assess postintervention effects.

In another study, 60 patients in an outpatient unit of a psychiatric hospital in Switzerland were randomly assigned to receive cognitive-behavioral therapy with or without prize-based reinforcement of cocaine abstinence over a 24-week period (Petitjean et al., 2014). The study did not show effects of the prize-based reinforcement intervention on several measures of cocaine abstinence, but it did show effects on the percentage of cocaine-negative urine samples at selected weeks during the study. There were no significant differences between groups at the 6-month follow-up assessment.

In one study, 127 men who routinely had sex with men and who used methamphetamine were randomly assigned to a 12-week voucher-based abstinence reinforcement intervention or to a control condition (Menza et al., 2010). Participants in the voucher-based intervention could earn up to about $450 in vouchers over the 12-week intervention for providing methamphetamine-free urine samples two or three times per week. The study failed to show a significant effect of the voucher intervention on methamphetamine use during or after treatment.

One study randomly assigned 176 outpatients with serious mental illness and stimulant dependence to a 12-week intervention in which they received either prize-based reinforcement for stimulant-negative urine samples or noncontingent prizes (McDonell et al., 2013). During treatment, participants assigned to receive the prize-based intervention provided significantly more stimulant-negative urine samples (over 80% negative) than the participants assigned to the noncontingent (control) condition (equal to or less than 70% negative). Participants assigned to the contingent prizes appeared to provide significantly more stimulant-negative urine samples (46%) than participants assigned to noncontingent prizes (35%) 16, 20, and 24 weeks after the intervention ended. Results of this study were limited, however, because of the high levels of missing data during the follow-up period, and the significant differences between groups were not maintained across all methods of handling missing urine samples.

Another study evaluated the effects of flexible methadone dosing and a voucher intervention that reinforced cocaine abstinence in patients in a methadone treatment program (Kennedy et al., 2013). After a 6-week baseline, participants who continued to use opiates and cocaine were randomly assigned to one of four conditions: voucher-based reinforcement of cocaine abstinence, flexible methadone dosing, flexible methadone dosing and voucher-based reinforcement of cocaine abstinence, or a no-treatment control group. Participants in the voucher intervention could earn up to $1,418 in vouchers for providing cocaine-free urine samples every Monday, Wednesday, and Friday over 16 weeks. Although the study examined the effects of flexible methadone dosing and voucher-based reinforcement of cocaine abstinence on opiate and cocaine use, we review only the effects of the voucher-based intervention here. The group exposed to the voucher-based intervention had significantly higher rates of cocaine-negative urine samples during treatment than the group that received neither intervention. Surprisingly, the group exposed to both flexible dosing and voucher-based cocaine abstinence reinforcement did not provide significantly more cocaine-negative urine samples than the group that received neither intervention. As in other studies, although the voucher-based intervention increased cocaine abstinence, not all participants responded to the intervention. Only about half the urine samples of participants in the group exposed to the voucher-based intervention alone were cocaine-negative. This study did not assess posttreatment results.

### Marijuana

Litt, Kadden, and Petry (2013) assigned 215 marijuana-dependent adults to one of three 9-week outpatient treatments: a case management (control) condition; a condition combining motivational-enhancement therapy, cognitive-behavioral therapy, and prize-based reinforcement for homework completion; and a condition combining motivational-enhancement therapy, cognitive-behavioral therapy, and prize-based reinforcement for abstinence from marijuana. The study evaluated the effects of those interventions on self-reported marijuana use in the months after the intervention ended. Neither of the experimental interventions that included prize-based reinforcement increased self-reported marijuana abstinence relative to the control condition; however, the intervention that included prize-based reinforcement for marijuana abstinence produced transient increases in marijuana abstinence in Months 5–8, compared to prize-based reinforcement of homework completion. There were no significant differences between groups at the latest follow-up time at Months 11–14.

Three controlled studies evaluated the effects of abstinence reinforcement interventions on marijuana use in adolescents. In the first of these studies, 31 adolescents with primary marijuana use

disorder who were enrolled in an outpatient treatment program were randomly assigned to receive usual care or usual care plus prize-based abstinence reinforcement (Killeen, McRae-Clark, Waldrop, Upadhyaya, & Brady, 2012). After a 2-week washout period, participants in the prize-based abstinence reinforcement group could earn the opportunity to draw prizes for providing alcohol-free breath samples and urine samples that were negative for marijuana, cocaine, opiates, methamphetamine, and amphetamine; control participants earned two prize draws for providing samples, independent of the breath or urinalysis results. The prize intervention was in effect for 10 weeks. The study showed no difference in urinalysis results between the two groups on any measure of drug use. Although this study included other drug use in the abstinence reinforcement intervention and in the outcome measures, marijuana was the predominant drug participants used in this study, and there were very low levels of drug use other than marijuana in both groups.

In a second study, 59 adolescents between the ages of 14 and 18 who met *Diagnostic and Statistical Manual of Mental Disorders,* fourth edition (DSM-IV) criteria for cannabis abuse or dependence and showed recent evidence of marijuana use, but no use of substances other than alcohol and tobacco, were randomly assigned to one of two conditions: cognitive-behavioral therapy and voucher-based abstinence reinforcement, or cognitive-behavioral therapy and noncontingent vouchers. The voucher condition started in Week 3 and continued until Week 10, and participants could earn up to $242 in vouchers for providing drug-free urine samples. Researchers tested urine samples for cannabis, cocaine, opioids, benzodiazepines, amphetamines, and methamphetamine. Participants exchanged voucher earnings for gift cards. There were no significant differences between groups on measures of marijuana use either during or after treatment.

In a final study, 153 adolescents between the ages of 12 and 18 who met DSM-IV criteria for cannabis abuse or dependence and showed recent evidence of marijuana use, but were not dependent on another substance, were randomly assigned to one of three groups (Stanger, Ryan, Scherer, Norton, & Budney, 2015). All groups received motivational-enhancement therapy and cognitive-behavioral therapy for 14 weeks. Two groups received an additional contingency management intervention, one with a parent-training component and one without parent training. After a 2-week washout period, participants in the contingency management groups began the contingency management intervention (Weeks 3–14). During this intervention, participants could earn voucher-based reinforcement for urine samples collected twice per week that were negative for all drugs assessed (cannabis, cocaine, opioids, benzodiazepines, amphetamine, and methamphetamine). Participants in the voucher condition could earn up to $590 in vouchers that were exchangeable for gift cards for providing drug-free urine samples. In addition, participants received a prize-based abstinence reinforcement intervention in which they could earn up to about $135 in prizes for providing drug-free urine samples during Weeks 1–4. Finally, parents could earn prize draws for developing and using a substance-abuse-monitoring contract. The contingency management intervention produced significant increases in abstinence from marijuana during treatment and at the end of treatment. Forty-eight percent of participants in the two groups exposed to the contingency management intervention achieved 4 or more weeks of continuous abstinence during treatment, whereas only 30% of participants in the group not exposed to the contingency management intervention did so. Abstinence rates decreased between the end of treatment and the 3-month follow-up, and the three groups had similar rates of abstinence at the 3-month follow-up.

## Alcohol

Researchers have conducted limited research on abstinence reinforcement interventions for alcohol use, at least in part because measures have not been available to detect alcohol use reliably beyond a relatively brief window of several hours since the last drink. Researchers can use breath alcohol tests, but participants can test alcohol-negative on these by remaining abstinent from alcohol for several hours before providing a breath sample.

Since our earlier chapter appeared, three studies have evaluated the effectiveness of using a transdermal alcohol sensor bracelet as a part of an abstinence reinforcement intervention for alcohol use. A participant wears this bracelet, called the Secure Continuous Remote Alcohol Monitor (SCRAM), locked on the ankle. The participant can wear the bracelet continuously, including in the shower. The bracelet includes features that detect removal and tampering. One of the studies used the bracelet in a contingency management intervention, but did not include an adequate experimental design to evaluate its effectiveness (Barnett, Tidey, Murphy, Swift, & Colby, 2011).

The second study used a within-participant cross-over design to evaluate the effectiveness of a contingency management intervention, including use of the SCRAM bracelet, in promoting alcohol abstinence (Dougherty et al., 2014). In that study, participants ($N = 26$) were exposed to $0 and $25 contingency management conditions in counterbalanced order, followed by a $50 contingency management condition. Each condition was in effect for 4 weeks. In the $0 condition, researchers did not give participants any instructions about alcohol consumption. During the $25 and $50 conditions, participants could earn $25 and $50 per week, respectively, if their transdermal alcohol concentration never exceeded 0.03 grams per decaliter (g/dl; this concentration corresponded to light to moderate drinking) on any day during the week. The $25 incentive condition significantly reduced drinking episodes and heavy drinking, relative to the $0 condition. In addition, participants exposed to the $25 condition followed by the $0 condition had less frequent drinking and less heavy drinking in the $0 condition than participants exposed to the $0 condition followed by the $25 condition. This result demonstrated that the $25 condition produced some lasting carryover effects on drinking that persisted after the $25 condition ended. There were few differences on drinking outcomes between the $25 and $50 conditions, except that the $50 condition was more effective in reducing heavy weekend drinking than the $25 condition.

A third study using the SCRAM technology enrolled 80 alcohol-dependent adults in a three-phase study that included an observation phase, a contingency management phase, and a follow-up phase (Dougherty, Karns, et al., 2015). At each weekly clinic visit during the observation and contingency management phases and monthly during the follow-up phase, participants completed Timeline Follow-Back interviews about drinking. During the initial observation phase, each participant wore a SCRAM bracelet with no explicit consequences for drinking. During the contingency management phase, a participant earned $50 each week if the SCRAM bracelet showed that the participant's transdermal alcohol concentration stayed below 0.03 g/dl every day of the week. During the follow-up phase, participants returned to the clinic every month for 3 months and completed Timeline Follow-Back interviews about drinking in the past 28 days. Transdermal alcohol concentration data showed that heavy drinking was significantly lower during the contingency phase than during the observation phase (Dougherty, Karns, et al., 2015). Self-reported days of drinking and heavy drinking were significantly lower during the contingency phase and follow-up phases than during the observation phase (Dougherty, Lake, et al., 2015). Although the study appeared to show that the effects of the contingency management intervention on participants' drinking were maintained in the follow-up period, the study did not include a rigorous experimental design that would have allowed clear demonstration of its effectiveness.

A small study evaluated the use of ethyl glucuronide, a metabolite of alcohol, in a voucher-based abstinence reinforcement intervention (McDonell et al., 2012). Laboratories can measure ethyl glucuronide in urine samples. This measure may be useful in abstinence reinforcement interventions, because it provides a longer window of detection than breath alcohol samples do. This study used a within-participant reversal design to evaluate the effectiveness of the voucher-based intervention in promoting abstinence from alcohol in 10 adults who met DSM-IV criteria for alcohol dependence. Four of the 10 participants did not complete the return-to-baseline condition, which limits the value of the research design. Given that limitation, the study provided some preliminary evidence of the effectiveness of reinforcing ethyl-glucuronide-negative urine samples in promoting abstinence from alcohol in study participants.

Another study evaluated the effectiveness of using cellphone technology to observe, record, and reinforce negative breath alcohol tests on a breathalyzer (Alessi & Petry, 2013). In this study, 30 participants who regularly used alcohol were randomly assigned to monitoring only or to monitoring plus contingency management. Researchers gave cellphones and breathalyzers to participants in both groups, and instructed each participant to use the cellphone to video-record him- or herself providing a breath sample in the breathalyzer within an hour of receiving a text message to provide a sample. Researchers told participants they would receive a text three times per day, and paid participants for providing valid (i.e., with the breathalyzer reading recorded on the video) breath samples within an hour of receiving a text. In addition, participants in the monitoring-plus-contingency-management group received vouchers for providing valid on-time samples indicating recent abstinence from alcohol (i.e., negative breath alcohol, <0.02 g/dl) under an escalating schedule for sustained alcohol abstinence. The voucher intervention was in effect for 4 weeks, and participants could earn up to $340 in vouchers for providing alcohol-negative breath tests. Both groups provided comparable rates of breath samples, but participants in the monitoring-plus-contingency-management group provided significantly more alcohol-negative breath samples (87%) than participants in the monitoring-only group (67%). Researchers did not assess rates of alcohol use after voucher-based abstinence reinforcement ended.

### Polydrug Use

Petry, Weinstock, and Alessi (2011) evaluated the effects of a group contingency management intervention on use of multiple substances. In that study, 239 outpatients enrolled in two community-based substance abuse treatment clinics were randomly assigned to standard care or to contingency management. Both groups provided two urine and breath samples per week for 12 weeks. Participants in the contingency management group received a prize-based reinforcement intervention in which they could earn draws for prizes for attending the clinic and for providing urine and breath samples that were negative for cocaine, methamphetamine, opioids, and alcohol. The researchers drew slips of paper with the participants' names from a hat to identify participants who could draw for prizes. The number of each participant's slips increased as the duration the participant attended clinic and provided drug-negative samples increased. The first five participants whose names were selected drew for one prize each; the sixth person whose name was selected drew for five prizes. This contingency management intervention significantly increased the number of days attended, continuous weeks of attendance, and longest duration of abstinence from all drugs and from each of the drugs tested. There was no effect on the percentage of drug-negative samples during or after treatment.

In another study, 170 adults living with HIV who met DSM-IV criteria for cocaine or opioid abuse or dependence, and who were members of an HIV drop-in center, were randomly assigned to a Twelve-Step facilitation group or to a contingency management group (Petry, Weinstock, Alessi, Lewis, & Dieckhaus, 2010). Both groups provided weekly breath samples tested for alcohol, and urine samples tested for opioids and cocaine, for 24 weeks. Participants in the contingency management condition received a prize-based reinforcement intervention in which they could draw for prizes contingent on completion of health activities and for submitting drug-free breath and urine samples. Participants in the contingency management condition achieved significantly longer durations of sustained abstinence from all drugs and from cocaine in particular during treatment. There was no effect on the percentage of drug-negative samples during or after treatment.

One study randomly assigned 305 adolescents with alcohol and other substance use disorders in a residential treatment program to one of four conditions: a usual-care control condition, a contingency management condition, an assertive continuing-care condition, or a condition that combined contingency management and assertive continuing care (Godley et al., 2014). Adolescents in the contingency management condition earned prize-based reinforcement for completing prosocial activities and for providing urine and breath samples negative for alcohol, amphetamine/methamphetamine, marijuana, cocaine, and opiates over 12 weeks. Participants assigned to the contingency management group achieved significantly higher percentages of self-reported days abstinent from drugs and alcohol during the 12 months after discharge from the residential treatment program (65%) than participants assigned to the usual-care control condition (53%). Oddly, the group exposed to both the contingency management and assertive continuing-care interventions did not differ from the usual-care control condition.

Holtyn et al. (2014a, 2014b) evaluated the effects of an employment-based abstinence reinforcement intervention in promoting abstinence from heroin and cocaine in out-of-treatment adults who injected drugs. Researchers invited unemployed out-of-treatment adults who injected drugs to attend a therapeutic workplace and referred them to methadone treatment. After a 4-week induction period, researchers invited participants to attend the workplace for 26 weeks and randomly assigned them to a work reinforcement group; a methadone and work reinforcement group; or an abstinence, methadone, and work reinforcement group. Work reinforcement participants could work in the therapeutic workplace independently of whether they enrolled in methadone treatment or provided drug-free urine samples. Methadone and work reinforcement participants had to enroll in methadone treatment to gain access to the workplace and to maintain maximum pay. Abstinence, methadone, and work reinforcement participants

had to enroll in methadone treatment to gain access to the workplace, and they also had to provide urine samples negative for opiates and cocaine to maintain maximum pay in the workplace. An intent-to-treat analysis showed that not all participants responded to the abstinence reinforcement contingencies, but that abstinence, methadone, and work reinforcement participants provided significantly more urine samples negative for opiates and for cocaine than work reinforcement participants did during treatment. Participants did not maintain those effects at the 6-month follow-up (Holtyn et al., 2014a). A within-group analysis of abstinence, methadone, and work reinforcement participants confirmed that abstinence from opiates and cocaine increased when abstinence reinforcement contingencies for those two drugs were applied sequentially (Holtyn et al., 2014b).

## Improving Outcomes

At the time we wrote the earlier chapter, researchers clearly needed to develop procedures to increase the proportion of patients who achieve abstinence when exposed to abstinence reinforcement interventions and procedures that promote long-term abstinence and prevent relapse. The studies published since that earlier review and described above confirm the need to increase the proportion of such patients. This section reviews selected studies that researchers have conducted since our earlier chapter to address these issues.

### Increasing Effectiveness

*Changing Reinforcement Parameters.* Festinger, Dugosh, Kirby, and Seymour (2014) evaluated the potential benefits of offering cash as opposed to vouchers for cocaine abstinence reinforcement. They randomly assigned 222 consecutive admissions to a Philadelphia methadone treatment program who met DSM-IV criteria for cocaine dependence to a usual-care control, a cash-based abstinence reinforcement intervention, or a voucher-based abstinence reinforcement intervention. They asked participants to provide urine samples three times per week for 12 weeks. Participants in the cash-based and voucher-based abstinence reinforcement groups could earn up to about $1,000 for providing cocaine-free urine samples over the 12-week period in cash or vouchers, respectively. Participants in both abstinence reinforcement groups achieved significantly longer durations of cocaine abstinence (6 weeks for each group) than participants in the usual-care control group did (4 weeks), but the two abstinence reinforcement groups did not differ significantly from each other. This study showed that cash-based and voucher-based reinforcement were both effective in promoting cocaine abstinence, but cash did not provide any benefit over vouchers.

Two studies examined the potential benefit of increasing the magnitude of reinforcement at the beginning of an abstinence reinforcement intervention, to increase the overall percentage of participants that achieve sustained abstinence. Higgins et al. (2014) evaluated the benefit of increasing the magnitude of reinforcement at the beginning of an intervention promoting smoking cessation in pregnant cigarette-smoking women. They randomly assigned 130 women to receive the revised voucher-based abstinence reinforcement intervention, the usual abstinence reinforcement intervention, or noncontingent vouchers. Participants in both abstinence reinforcement groups received vouchers under the same schedule of escalating reinforcement for sustained abstinence that previous studies have used. Participants in the revised voucher-based intervention received large bonus vouchers for smoking cessation during the first 6 weeks of the intervention. To keep the total earnings comparable between the two abstinence reinforcement groups, participants in the revised voucher-based condition received less frequent assessments and vouchers late in treatment. Both voucher-based abstinence reinforcement interventions increased point-prevalence smoking cessation early in pregnancy, the percentage of negative samples, and the mean number of consecutive negative samples, compared to the control condition; however, the two interventions did not differ from each other on those measures. Overall, the revised voucher-based intervention did not appear to improve outcomes over the usual voucher-based intervention. Neither abstinence reinforcement intervention significantly increased smoking cessation at the 24-week postpartum assessment after the interventions ended.

Similarly, Ledgerwood, Arfken, Petry, and Alessi (2014) attempted to improve the effectiveness of prize-based reinforcement for smoking cessation by increasing the probability of reinforcement early in the treatment period. They randomly assigned cigarette-smoking participants ($N = 81$) to receive standard care, traditional prize-based reinforcement for smoking cessation, or an enhanced prize-based reinforcement intervention for smoking cessation in which the probability of

reinforcement increased early in treatment. Both abstinence reinforcement interventions increased smoking cessation during treatment, compared to the standard-care condition; however, the two reinforcement groups did not differ from each other in smoking cessation during or after treatment. Neither abstinence reinforcement intervention produced significant effects on smoking cessation, compared to standard care, that were evident at 2-month or 6-month follow-up after the interventions had ended.

In another study, 100 adults who injected drugs and smoked cigarettes were randomly assigned to a usual-care control group, to a contingency management group, to a lung age group, or to a group that received both a contingency management and lung age intervention (Drummond et al., 2014). Participants in the contingency management intervention received monetary incentives for CO samples that indicated recent abstinence from smoking; however, this intervention used a very low overall incentive magnitude and infrequent CO testing. Researchers told participants in the lung age intervention the age equivalence of their lungs, based on spirometric assessments. No intervention affected the 6-month biologically verified rates of smoking cessation.

In a study of individuals who were interested in quitting smoking, Lamb, Kirby, Morral, Glabicka, and Iguchi (2010) compared a fixed-reinforcement schedule in which the criterion for reinforcement was a constant CO value (CO < 4 parts per million [ppm]) to a percentile schedule in which the researchers adjusted the criterion for reinforcement gradually and individually to require progressively lower CO values for reinforcement. Overall, the two schedules did not produce differences in the overall rate of participants who were abstinent at the end of treatment or in the overall number of CO-negative breath samples. There was some evidence that the percentile schedule was more effective for a subset of hard-to-treat smokers.

Romanowich and Lamb conducted a series of studies to evaluate parametrically different abstinence reinforcement interventions to promote smoking cessation in adults who did (Romanowich & Lamb, 2014, 2015) and did not (Romanowich & Lamb, 2010, 2013) plan to stop smoking. One of the studies compared a fixed-reinforcement schedule in which the criterion for reinforcement was a constant CO value (CO < 3 ppm) to a percentile schedule in which the researchers adjusted the criterion for reinforcement gradually and individually to require progressively lower CO values for reinforcement (Romanowich & Lamb, 2014). Contrary to expectation, the study did not show an overall benefit of the percentile schedule. Another study compared the framing of incentives as either losses or gains (Romanowich & Lamb, 2013). Framing incentives as losses may have improved abstinence more than framing incentives as gains did, but framing incentives as losses did not produce statistically significant increases in overall abstinence rates compared to framing incentives as gains. Another study compared escalating versus descending schedules of reinforcement, in which the value of the monetary incentives for smoking cessation (CO < 3 ppm) either increased or decreased, respectively, with consecutive visits (Romanowich & Lamb, 2010). Missed samples or samples that did not meet the abstinence criterion did not affect the magnitude of the incentive, as they do in typical abstinence reinforcement schedules. The schedule of reinforcement (escalating vs. descending) did not affect the overall rates of smoking cessation. Finally, one study compared fixed magnitude of reinforcement for abstinence (CO < 3 ppm), escalating magnitude of reinforcement for sustained abstinence, and a control condition (Romanowich & Lamb, 2015). The two abstinence reinforcement conditions produced significantly more overall rates of smoking abstinence than the control group, but did not differ from each other on overall smoking abstinence. The escalating-reinforcement schedule, however, did produce longer periods of sustained abstinence than the fixed schedule.

Petry, Alessi, Barry, and Carroll (2015) compared the effectiveness of different magnitudes of prize and voucher reinforcement in promoting cocaine abstinence in methadone-treated patients. That study randomly assigned 240 methadone-maintained patients who used cocaine to a usual-care control group or to one of three abstinence reinforcement interventions: a $300 prize contingency management intervention, a $900 prize contingency management intervention, or a $900 voucher reinforcement intervention. All three abstinence reinforcement interventions increased cocaine abstinence (percentage of drug-negative urine samples and longest duration of abstinence), compared to the usual-care control group; however, the three interventions did not differ from each other. As in other studies, no abstinence reinforcement intervention promoted abstinence in all participants. The usual-care control intervention, the $300 prize contingency management intervention, the $900 prize contingency management intervention, the $900 prize contingency management

intervention, and the $900 voucher intervention produced 36%, 56%, 55%, and 59% drug-negative urine samples, respectively. As in most other studies, none of the groups differed from each other at the 12-month follow-up assessment.

*Combining Abstinence Reinforcement with Pharmacotherapy.* Researchers have designed several randomized controlled studies to determine whether pharmacotherapy can enhance the effects of an abstinence reinforcement intervention. Two studies evaluated the potential benefit of combining bupropion with abstinence reinforcement to promote smoking cessation. Tidey, Rohsenow, Kaplan, Swift, and Reid (2011) evaluated the effects of bupropion and abstinence reinforcement alone and in combination over 4 weeks in promoting smoking cessation in 57 adults with schizophrenia who were not seeking treatment for smoking cessation. Participants in the abstinence reinforcement intervention earned cash under an escalating schedule for sustained abstinence for providing urine samples three times per week showing a 25% reduction in cotinine levels from the previous sample or a value below 80 nanograms per milliliter (ng/ml; i.e., cotinine-negative). The value of the incentive started at $25 for the first cotinine-reduced or -negative urine sample and increased by $5 for each consecutive reduced or negative sample. The study showed that the abstinence reinforcement intervention increased smoking cessation compared to a noncontingent condition, but that bupropion did not increase smoking cessation compared to placebo and did not increase the effects of the abstinence reinforcement intervention.

Gray et al. (2011) evaluated the effects of bupropion and abstinence reinforcement alone and in combination over 6 weeks in promoting smoking cessation in 134 adolescents between the ages of 12 and 21 who were seeking treatment for smoking cessation. Participants in the abstinence reinforcement intervention could earn cash payments for providing objective evidence of smoking cessation at the end of the first week and then two times per week for the remaining 5 weeks. At the end of the first week, CO-negative breath samples (CO ≤ 7 ppm) confirmed smoking cessation. Thereafter, abstinence was based on self-reported smoking cessation and urine cotinine (≤100 ng/ml). The value of the cash payments started at $10 and increased by $3 for each consecutive sample that met the abstinence criteria. Participants could earn $275 in total. Control participants (those not assigned to the abstinence reinforcement intervention) earned $10 for attending each visit. All participants also were randomly assigned to receive either bupropion SR or a placebo. The study failed to show any effect of abstinence reinforcement alone compared to the control condition (when combined with placebo) or of bupropion alone compared to placebo (when combined with control). Bupropion combined with abstinence reinforcement produced higher rates of smoking cessation than did placebo combined with abstinence reinforcement during Weeks 3 and 4, but not during Weeks 5 and 6. As with other studies, results did not show any effects of the abstinence reinforcement intervention at the 12-week follow-up assessment.

Three studies assessed the potential benefit of combining medication with abstinence reinforcement to promote cocaine abstinence. Schmitz, Lindsay, Stotts, Green, and Moeller (2010) compared levodopa–carbidopa to placebo under three different voucher-based reinforcement conditions: reinforcement for attendance, reinforcement for medication adherence, and reinforcement for abstinence. The participants were adults who met DSM-IV criteria for cocaine dependence and enrolled in outpatient treatment. Participants in all three conditions could earn vouchers every Monday, Wednesday, and Friday for the assigned target behavior in their condition (attendance, medication adherence, or cocaine abstinence, respectively). Participants could earn vouchers worth $2.50 initially. The value of the vouchers increased by $1.25 for every consecutive occurrence of the target behavior. Participants also could earn a $10 bonus for three consecutive occurrences of the target behavior. The voucher intervention was in effect for 12 weeks, and participants could earn up to $997.50. Levodopa–carbidopa did not affect cocaine-negative urine samples in participants who earned vouchers for attendance or medication adherence; however, the medication appeared to increase cocaine abstinence relative to placebo in participants who earned vouchers for cocaine-negative urine samples. Although these results suggest that levodopa–carbidopa may enhance the effectiveness of voucher reinforcement in promoting cocaine abstinence, there were high rates of attrition in this study (only 35% of participants were still in treatment by the end of the 12 weeks), which limit the conclusions we can draw from the study.

Winstanley, Bigelow, Silverman, Johnson, and Strain (2011) evaluated the effectiveness of combining fluoxetine with voucher-based reinforcement of cocaine abstinence in cocaine-dependent adults enrolled in methadone treatment. Participants in the voucher intervention condition could earn up to $1,155 in vouchers for providing cocaine-negative urine samples every Monday, Wednesday, and Friday for 12 weeks. Participants were randomly assigned to receive voucher-based reinforcement of cocaine abstinence, fluoxetine, both voucher-based reinforcement of cocaine abstinence and fluoxetine, or neither. Voucher-based reinforcement alone appeared to increase cocaine abstinence, but the addition of fluoxetine did not increase cocaine abstinence and may have decreased abstinence. The group receiving placebo plus voucher-based reinforcement of cocaine abstinence achieved the highest percentage of cocaine-negative urine samples; this group provided 69% cocaine-negative urine samples, compared to 35% cocaine-negative urine samples in the placebo group.

Umbricht et al. (2014) evaluated the effectiveness of topiramate and voucher-based abstinence reinforcement in promoting cocaine abstinence in cocaine-dependent methadone-maintained patients. Participants in the voucher intervention could earn up to $1,155 in vouchers for providing cocaine-negative urine samples every Monday, Wednesday, and Friday for 12 weeks. Participants were randomly assigned to receive voucher-based reinforcement of cocaine abstinence, topiramate, both voucher-based reinforcement of cocaine abstinence and topiramate, or neither. Although study retention was high, neither topiramate nor the voucher intervention affected cocaine use in this study.

*Group Contingencies.* Dallery and colleagues conducted a series of studies to evaluate the potential benefit of arranging contingencies for smoking cessation in which each participant's earnings were contingent on the behavior of the group (Dallery, Meredith, Jarvis, & Nuzzo, 2015; Meredith & Dallery, 2013; Meredith, Grabinski, & Dallery, 2011). They used this contingency to recruit social reinforcement and to test whether the combination of financial and social reinforcement would increase abstinence rates. The researchers gave participants access to online forums and encouraged them to offer support to their group members to foster communication and social reinforcement.

In one study, participants assigned to a no-voucher control condition provided significantly fewer CO-negative breath samples (35%) than when they were exposed to a condition in which they could earn vouchers for CO-negative breath samples, independent of whether the voucher reinforcement was independent (56%) or dependent (53%) on the CO results of other participants in their group (Meredith & Dallery, 2013). The addition of social contingencies by arranging financial reinforcement for CO-negative samples based on the group results did not increase the percentage of participants who stopped smoking, nor did having access to the online forum. Another study randomly assigned participants to receive all vouchers contingent on smoking cessation (CO-negative samples) of all members of the group (full group), or to receive some vouchers contingent on each participant's smoking cessation and some vouchers contingent on the group's smoking cessation (mixed group). Arranging all reinforcement contingent on the group's smoking cessation did not affect the smoking cessation outcomes either during the intervention (full group, 18% CO-negative; mixed group, 29% CO-negative) or after it ended (full group, 9% CO-negative; mixed group, 14% CO-negative). Another study (Halpern et al., 2015), described in detail below, also failed to show any benefit of a group-based incentive intervention.

## Preventing Relapse

*Combining Abstinence Reinforcement with Counseling Interventions.* Some researchers have hypothesized that combining abstinence reinforcement interventions with cognitive-behavioral relapse prevention therapy might prevent or reduce relapse after the abstinence reinforcement interventions end. Although early studies failed to demonstrate such effects (Silverman, Kaminski, et al., 2011), several studies published since our earlier chapter appeared have investigated this possibility. Carroll et al. (2012) randomly assigned 127 adults who met DSM-IV criteria for current cannabis dependence to four groups: cognitive-behavioral therapy alone, prize-based abstinence reinforcement alone, cognitive-behavioral therapy with reinforcement for treatment adherence (attending counseling sessions and completing homework), or cognitive-behavioral therapy plus prize-based abstinence reinforcement. In all prize-based reinforcement interventions, participants could earn up to about $250 in prizes over 12 weeks. In the abstinence reinforcement interventions, participants could earn prize draws for providing urine samples that tested negative for cannabis at 12

weekly assessments. The abstinence reinforcement intervention alone did not produce better outcomes than cognitive-behavioral therapy alone did. Also, cognitive-behavioral therapy did not improve outcomes when added to the abstinence reinforcement intervention, either during treatment or during the year-long follow-up period. In fact, the addition of cognitive-behavioral therapy may have had a deleterious effect on cannabis use outcomes.

Krishnan-Sarin et al. (2013) conducted a 4-week randomized controlled trial that compared cognitive-behavioral therapy alone, abstinence reinforcement alone, and cognitive-behavioral therapy plus abstinence reinforcement in 72 high school students who smoked cigarettes. Researchers determined abstinence with CO-negative breath samples and cotinine-negative urine samples, daily during Weeks 1 and 2 and every other day in Weeks 3 and 4. The CO cutoff was <7 ppm. The cutoff for cotinine initially required a decrease from the last reading or <100 ng/ml and then switched to the fixed requirement of <100 ng/ml. During treatment, the groups receiving abstinence reinforcement alone and cognitive-behavioral therapy plus abstinence reinforcement achieved higher rates of smoking cessation than the group receiving cognitive-behavioral therapy alone, but did not differ from each other. The combination of cognitive-behavioral therapy with the abstinence reinforcement intervention did not increase abstinence during the follow-up period. In fact, participants exposed to the abstinence reinforcement intervention alone had the highest rates of posttreatment abstinence of all three groups.

Ling, Hillhouse, Ang, Jenkins, and Fahey (2013) randomly assigned 202 opioid-dependent adults enrolled in treatment with sublingual buprenorphine to four different 16-week treatment conditions: cognitive-behavioral therapy, prize-based reinforcement of opioid abstinence, both cognitive-behavioral therapy and prize-based reinforcement of opioid abstinence, or neither (medical management). The study failed to show any difference in the rates of opioid abstinence among any of the conditions, either during treatment or at the follow-up assessments after the 16-week conditions ended.

McKay et al. (2010) randomly assigned 100 adults who met DSM-IV criteria for current cocaine dependence and who maintained 2 weeks of regular attendance in intensive outpatient treatment to four treatment conditions: treatment as usual, voucher-based reinforcement of cocaine abstinence, cognitive-behavioral relapse prevention counseling, or voucher-based reinforcement of cocaine abstinence plus cognitive-behavioral relapse prevention counseling. The main analyses showed that voucher-based reinforcement of cocaine abstinence produced significant increases in abstinence, but that cognitive-behavioral relapse prevention counseling had no effect on abstinence. The addition of cognitive-behavioral relapse prevention counseling to voucher-based reinforcement of cocaine abstinence thus did not produce significant increases in abstinence compared to voucher-based reinforcement of cocaine abstinence alone, either during or after treatment.

Two studies by Tevyaw et al. (2009) evaluated the benefit of combining motivational-enhancement therapy with abstinence reinforcement. In one study, researchers randomly assigned 110 college students who smoked but were not seeking treatment to receive a 3-week abstinenc reinforcement intervention for smoking cessation, motivational-enhancement therapy, noncontingent reinforcement, or both abstinence reinforcement intervention and motivational-enhancement therapy. During treatment, the abstinence reinforcement intervention increased smoking cessation, but motivational-enhancement therapy produced no beneficial effects, either alone or when combined with the abstinence reinforcement intervention. None of the groups differed at postintervention follow-up.

In a second study, 184 adults in 28-day residential treatment who met DSM-IV criteria for substance use disorder and smoked at least 10 cigarettes per day were randomly assigned to receive voucher-based reinforcement for smoking cessation, motivational-enhancement therapy, noncontingent reinforcement, or both voucher-based reinforcement and motivational-enhancement therapy (Rohsenow et al., 2015). During treatment, voucher-based reinforcement increased smoking cessation rates, but motivational-enhancement therapy had no effect on smoking cessation, either alone or when combined with voucher-based reinforcement. During the follow-up period after the interventions ended, there was no main effect of either the voucher-based reinforcement or motivational-enhancement intervention, and very few participants (≤7.5%) in any group were abstinent at follow-up.

Two studies evaluated benefits of combining community reinforcement therapy with abstinence reinforcement. One study randomly assigned 170 opioid-dependent adults in buprenorphine treatment to receive voucher-based reinforcement of opioid and cocaine abstinence for 12 weeks, or voucher-based reinforcement of opioid and cocaine abstinence plus counseling with the community reinforcement approach (Christensen et al., 2014). The combination of voucher-based abstinence reinforcement with counseling increased treatment retention and the total number of drug-free urine samples, compared to voucher-based abstinence reinforcement only. Whether the differential rates of treatment retention across the two groups confounded the measure of abstinence was unclear. The two groups did not differ in the longest period of continuous abstinence.

Schottenfeld, Moore, and Pantalon (2011) randomly assigned 145 cocaine-dependent women who were either pregnant or had custody of young children to receive voucher-based reinforcement of cocaine abstinence plus counseling with the community reinforcement approach, noncontingent vouchers plus counseling with the community reinforcement approach, Twelve-Step facilitation plus noncontingent vouchers, or Twelve-Step facilitation plus voucher-based abstinence reinforcement. Voucher-based reinforcement of cocaine abstinence increased abstinence compared to noncontingent vouchers, both during and after treatment. Counseling with the community reinforcement approach did not affect cocaine abstinence compared to Twelve-Step facilitation. There was no interaction between the type of counseling and voucher-based abstinence reinforcement.

*Abstinence Reinforcement as a Maintenance Intervention.* Several studies assessed whether arranging extended exposure to abstinence reinforcement could promote long-term abstinence and prevent relapse (Aklin et al., 2014; DeFulio & Silverman, 2011; Kirby et al., 2013; Roll, Chudzynski, Cameron, Howell, & McPherson, 2013). These studies extended research on the idea that abstinence reinforcement could be used as a maintenance intervention (DeFulio, Donlin, Wong, & Silverman, 2009; Silverman, 2004; Silverman, Kaminski, et al., 2011; Silverman, Robles, Mudric, Bigelow, & Stitzer, 2004). DeFulio et al. (2009) evaluated employment-based reinforcement as a maintenance intervention in the treatment of drug addiction. In that study, researchers invited adults who had used cocaine while enrolled in community methadone treatment to attend an initial 6-month phase of a therapeutic-workplace intervention to initiate drug abstinence and establish needed job skills. During this phase, researchers required participants to provide cocaine-free and opiate-free urine samples to gain and maintain access to the workplace. Participants who initiated cocaine and opiate abstinence and acquired needed skills during this initial 6-month phase were hired in a model data-entry business for 1 year and randomly assigned to an employment-only group or an abstinence-contingent employment group. As employees, participants could work 30 hours per week and were paid biweekly. Participants assigned to the employment-only condition could work regardless of their urinalysis results, as in typical employment. By contrast, researchers required participants assigned to abstinence-contingent employment to provide drug-free urine samples in order to work and to maintain maximum pay. Analyses of monthly urine samples collected from participants in both groups throughout the year of employment in the data-entry business showed that abstinence-contingent-employment participants provided significantly more cocaine-negative samples than employment-only participants.

In a more recent report, DeFulio and Silverman (2011) reported the abstinence outcomes for the year during and the year after employment in the model data-entry business, based on urine samples collected at 6-month intervals. During the year of employment, abstinence-contingent-employment participants provided significantly more cocaine-negative urine samples than employment-only controls (83% vs. 54%). However, during the follow-up year when the employment-based abstinence reinforcement contingency ended, the two groups provided similar rates of cocaine-negative urine samples (44% vs. 50%). This study showed that researchers could use abstinence reinforcement to maintain cocaine abstinence for as long as a year, but that the effects of the abstinence reinforcement intervention did not persist after it ended.

Three other studies confirmed that researchers could extend the effects of an abstinence reinforcement intervention by extending the duration of the abstinence reinforcement contingencies (Aklin et al., 2014; Kirby et al., 2013; Roll et al., 2013). The study by Kirby et al. (2013) is particularly important, because it experimentally evaluated the effect of duration of voucher-based abstinence reinforcement on abstinence outcomes. That study randomly assigned 130 cocaine-dependent, methadone-maintained patients to standard 12-week cocaine abstinence reinforcement or to extended 36-week cocaine abstinence reinforcement. There was no significant difference between the two

groups in cocaine abstinence during the initial 12 weeks, when both groups received voucher-based reinforcement. The participants exposed to the extended intervention achieved significantly more cocaine abstinence during the following 24 weeks than those in the 12-week program who were no longer receiving vouchers. Importantly, the two groups did not differ in cocaine abstinence during a 12-week follow-up period when neither group received voucher-based reinforcement.

## Dissemination

Dissemination of abstinence reinforcement interventions has remained relatively limited since the publication of our earlier chapter. However, two large-scale applications deserve mention. First, the U.S. Department of Veterans Affairs (VA) disseminated prize-based abstinence reinforcement as an evidence-based practice for substance use disorders and implemented it throughout the VA treatment system (Petry, DePhilippis, Rash, Drapkin, & McKay, 2014). The VA implemented prize-based contingency management interventions in over 70 substance abuse treatment clinics in the United States. This program illustrates the adoption and dissemination of abstinence reinforcement into real-world clinical settings.

Two studies by Halpern et al. (2015, 2018) represent important large-scale applications of incentives in real-world settings. The study by Halpern et al. (2015) evaluated the effectiveness of financial incentives in promoting smoking cessation in 2,538 CVS Caremark employees or their relatives and friends across the United States. Participants were randomly assigned to a usual-care control group or to one of four abstinence reinforcement interventions to promote smoking cessation: an individual-rewards group, a collaborative-rewards group, an individual-deposit group, or a competitive-deposit group. Participants in the collaborative-rewards and the competitive-deposit groups were placed in groups of six each and could communicate with other group members through a web-based chat room. Participants in the individual-deposit and competitive-deposit groups had to submit a $150 deposit to participate in their respective conditions. Participants in the two individual-incentives groups could earn $200 for providing biochemically confirmed evidence of smoking cessation at 14 days, 30 days, and 6 months, plus a bonus of $200 for evidence of smoking cessation at 6 months. Participants in the collaborative-rewards group who provided the biochemically confirmed measure of smoking cessation at the 14-day, 30-day, and 6-month assessments earned $100 for each of six members in the group who met the cessation criterion at that time (i.e., up to $600 per time). In addition, participants in this condition earned a bonus of $200 for providing evidence of smoking cessation at 6 months. Participants in the competitive-deposit group could earn up to $1,200 at each time for providing the biochemically confirmed measure of smoking cessation, but the amount earned was divided by the number of participants who provided the biochemically confirmed measure of smoking cessation.

The study by Halpern et al. (2015) illustrates several key points. First, the individual-rewards and collaborative-rewards interventions promoted significantly more smoking cessation than the usual-care control group, including the 12-month follow-up assessment that researchers conducted 6 months after the incentive interventions ended. These results confirm the general finding that abstinence reinforcement interventions can be effective. Second, although the individual-rewards and collaborative-rewards interventions were effective in promoting smoking cessation, they were effective in only about one-quarter of the participants at most, and the percentage of participants who sustained smoking cessation decreased over time. This result confirms the general finding that although abstinence reinforcement can be effective, many people do not respond to such interventions. Third, although the rates of smoking cessation for participants in the individual-rewards and collaborative-rewards groups were still significantly higher than those for participants in the usual-care control group at the 12-month follow-up, the percentage of participants who were still abstinent in the two rewards groups had decreased substantially by that follow-up, and fewer than 9% of participants in those groups were still abstinent at that time. This result confirms the finding that even when abstinence reinforcement interventions produce long-term effects after the interventions end, many people continue to relapse into drug use in the subsequent weeks and months. Finally, although researchers have viewed deposits as a potentially viable way to fund incentive interventions, fewer than 20% of participants agreed to pay deposits, and the overall rates of smoking cessation were low and generally not significantly different from those for the usual-care control group. A secondary analysis showed that those who paid a deposit were likely to become abstinent, which

suggests that deposit contracts may be useful for a subset of the population. Nevertheless, based on an intent-to-treat analysis, deposit contracts were not a particularly useful way to fund abstinence reinforcement interventions.

## CONCLUSIONS

Reviews, meta-analyses, and detailed summaries of individual studies published in the last several years have confirmed that abstinence reinforcement interventions are highly effective in promoting abstinence from most commonly abused drugs and in diverse populations. Yet we still must improve these interventions. As detailed in this chapter, studies have not shown consistently that abstinence reinforcement interventions are effective. Studies that showing that these interventions are effective also show that they are not effective for every participant, and the proportion of treatment failures is frequently large. Moreover, many studies show that the effects of abstinence reinforcement interventions do not persist after the interventions end. Even in studies finding that these interventions have detectable posttreatment effects, the proportion of patients remaining abstinent in the posttreatment period decreases reliably over time.

Efforts to increase the effectiveness of abstinence reinforcement interventions or to produce more lasting effects after the interventions end—by manipulating parameters of the interventions, combining the interventions with pharmacotherapies, or combining the interventions with psychosocial treatments—have met with very little success. As detailed in our earlier chapter (Silverman, Kaminski, et al., 2011) and in the current one, increasing the magnitude of reinforcement can substantially increase the effectiveness of abstinence reinforcement interventions, and arranging extended exposure to such interventions can prevent relapse and promote long-term abstinence, at least while the intervention continues.

The limitations of abstinence reinforcement interventions identified in this chapter raise questions about their clinical utility: What proportion of patients fail to respond to these interventions? Do such interventions serve a clinically useful role if they do not maintain abstinence over time? Not much has changed in our understanding of the benefits and limitations of abstinence reinforcement interventions in recent years. Overall, they can be effective in promoting abstinence in some patients, but they fail to address the needs of a substantial proportion of patients, and they almost always fail to promote abstinence that does not reverse when the intervention ends.

Given that the costs of abstinence reinforcement interventions can be minimal in patients who do not initiate abstinence, the failure to initiate abstinence in some patients is not a great cost to treatment providers and does not diminish the value of these interventions to patients who do respond. Finding ways to increase the proportion of patients who respond to these interventions is an important focus for the scientific community, but in the absence of those improvements, existing abstinence reinforcement interventions can still have value.

In some applications, abstinence reinforcement interventions that promote short-term abstinence can have profound effects on health (e.g., Higgins et al., 2010). Except in those instances in which short-term exposure to an intervention has clear health benefits, it is not clear that abstinence reinforcement interventions are clinically useful if they provide only a short-term break in drug use. Many view drug addiction as a chronic problem (McLellan et al., 2000). Relapse to drug use is common after most treatments end (McLellan et al., 2000), and abstinence reinforcement is obviously no exception to this pattern. Recognizing the chronic relapsing nature of drug addiction, Du-Pont, Compton, and McLellan (2015) have recommended a *5-year recovery* as a standard for assessing treatments for drug addiction for researchers and clinicians. A 5-year evaluation period would obviously place sizable financial and practical demands on researchers and funding agencies to arrange and support such long-term studies. Typical studies apply interventions that last 12 weeks and conduct 6- and 12-month follow-up assessments to examine the long-term effects of the intervention. Thus a 5-year evaluation period represents a significant challenge to the scientific community.

At this point, arranging abstinence reinforcement as a maintenance intervention appears to be the most likely means of maintaining long-term abstinence (DeFulio et al., 2009; Kirby et al., 2013; Silverman, DeFulio, & Sigurdsson, 2012; Silverman et al., 2004). Researchers have not identified practical methods of arranging long-term exposure to abstinence reinforcement interventions, however. Silverman and colleagues have attempted to use employment as a vehicle for maintaining long-term employment-based abstinence reinforcement (Silverman, 2004; Silverman et al., 2012;

Silverman, Holtyn, & Morrison, 2016), but other researchers have not adopted this method. Physician health programs require impaired physicians to undergo random drug testing for 5 years and stay abstinent throughout that time to continue practicing medicine. This model shows some real promise in addressing the chronic nature of drug addiction (DuPont, McLellan, White, Merlo, & Gold, 2009). Abstinence reinforcement interventions have great potential and could prove most useful in addressing the chronic, persistent problem of drug addiction if researchers can develop effective and practical methods that ensure long-term and lifelong abstinence ultimately.

## ACKNOWLEDGMENTS

Joseph V. Brady contributed to the version of this chapter in the first edition of the *Handbook of Applied Behavior Analysis.*

The National Institute on Drug Abuse and the National Institute of Allergy and Infectious Diseases of the National Institutes of Health, under Award Nos. R01DA037314, R01DA019497, R01AI117065, and T32DA07209, supported preparation of this chapter. The content is solely our responsibility and does not necessarily represent the official views of the National Institutes of Health.

## REFERENCES

Aklin, W. M., Wong, C. J., Hampton, J., Svikis, D. S., Stitzer, M. L., Bigelow, G. E., et al. 2014). A therapeutic workplace for the long-term treatment of drug addiction and unemployment: Eight-year outcomes of a social business intervention. *Journal of Substance Abuse Treatment, 47,* 329–338.

Alessi, S. M., & Petry, N. M. (2013). A randomized study of cellphone technology to reinforce alcohol abstinence in the natural environment. *Addiction, 108,* 900–909.

Alessi, S. M., & Petry, N. M. (2014). Smoking reductions and increased self-efficacy in a randomized controlled trial of smoking abstinence-contingent incentives in residential substance abuse treatment patients. *Nicotine and Tobacco Research, 16,* 1436–1445.

Barnett, N. P., Tidey, J., Murphy, J. G., Swift, R., & Colby, S. M. (2011). Contingency management for alcohol use reduction: A pilot study using a transdermal alcohol sensor. *Drug and Alcohol Dependence, 118,* 391–399.

Benishek, L. A., Dugosh, K. L., Kirby, K. C., Matejkowski, J., Clements, N. T., Seymour, B. L., et al. (2014). Prize-based contingency management for the treatment of substance abusers: A meta-analysis. *Addiction, 109*, 1426–1436.

Businelle, M. S., Kendzor, D. E., Kesh, A., Cuate, E. L., Poonawalla, I. B., Reitzel, L. R., et al. (2014). Small financial incentives increase smoking cessation in homeless smokers: A pilot study. *Addictive Behaviors, 39*, 717–720.

Cahill, K., Hartmann-Boyce, J., & Perera, R. (2015). Incentives for smoking cessation. *Cochrane Database of Systematic Reviews, 5*, CD004307.

Carroll, K. M., Nich, C., Lapaglia, D. M., Peters, E. N., Easton, C. J., & Petry, N. M. (2012). Combining cognitive behavioral therapy and contingency management to enhance their effects in treating cannabis dependence: Less can be more, more or less. *Addiction, 107*, 1650–1659.

Castells, X., Kosten, T. R., Capella, D., Vidal, X., Colom, J., & Casas, M. (2009). Efficacy of opiate maintenance therapy and adjunctive interventions for opioid dependence with comorbid cocaine use disorders: A systematic review and meta-analysis of controlled clinical trials. *American Journal of Drug and Alcohol Abuse, 35*, 339–349.

Chen, W., Hong, Y., Zou, X., McLaughlin, M. M., Xia, Y., & Ling, L. (2013). Effectiveness of prize-based contingency management in a methadone maintenance program in China. *Drug and Alcohol Dependence, 133*, 270–274.

Christensen, D. R., Landes, R. D., Jackson, L., Marsch, L. A., Mancino, M. J., Chopra, M. P., et al. (2014). Adding an Internet-delivered treatment to an efficacious treatment package for opioid dependence. *Journal of Consulting and Clinical Psychology, 82*, 964–972.

Dallery, J., & Glenn, I. M. (2005). Effects of an Internet-based voucher reinforcement program for smoking abstinence: A feasibility study. *Journal of Applied Behavior Analysis, 38*, 349–357.

Dallery, J., Meredith, S., Jarvis, B. P., & Nuzzo, P. A. (2015). Internet-based group contingency management to promote smoking abstinence. *Experimental and Clinical Psychopharmacology, 23*, 176–183.

Dallery, J., Raiff, B. R., & Grabinski, M. J. (2013). Internet-based contingency management to promote smoking cessation: A randomized controlled study. *Journal of Applied Behavior Analysis, 46*, 750–764.

Dallery, J., Raiff, B. R., Kim, S. J., Marsch, L. A., Stitzer, M., & Grabinski, M. J. (2017). Nationwide access to an Internet-based contingency management intervention to promote smoking cessation: A randomized controlled trial. *Addiction, 112*, 875–883.

Davis, D. R., Kurti, A. N., Skelly, J. M., Redner, R., White, T. J., & Higgins, S. T. (2016). A review of the literature on contingency management in the treatment of substance use disorders, 2009–2014. *Preventive Medicine, 92*, 36–46.

DeFulio, A., Donlin, W. D., Wong, C. J., & Silverman, K. (2009). Employment-based abstinence reinforce-

ment as a maintenance intervention for the treatment of cocaine dependence: A randomized controlled trial. *Addiction, 104*, 1530–1538.

DeFulio, A., & Silverman, K. (2011). Employment-based abstinence reinforcement as a maintenance intervention for the treatment of cocaine dependence: Post-intervention outcomes. *Addiction, 106*, 960–967.

Dougherty, D. M., Hill-Kapturczak, N., Liang, Y., Karns, T. E., Cates, S. E., Lake, S. L., et al. (2014). Use of continuous transdermal alcohol monitoring during a contingency management procedure to reduce excessive alcohol use. *Drug and Alcohol Dependence, 142*, 301–306.

Dougherty, D. M., Karns, T. E., Mullen, J., Liang, Y., Lake, S. L., Roache, J. D., et al. (2015). Transdermal alcohol concentration data collected during a contingency management program to reduce at-risk drinking. *Drug and Alcohol Dependence, 148*, 77–84.

Dougherty, D. M., Lake, S. L., Hill-Kapturczak, N., Liang, Y., Karns, T. E., Mullen, J., et al. (2015). Using contingency management procedures to reduce at-risk drinking in heavy drinkers. *Alcoholism: Clinical and Experimental Research, 39*, 743–751.

Drummond, M. B., Astemborski, J., Lambert, A. A., Goldberg, S., Stitzer, M. L., Merlo, C. A., et al. (2014). A randomized study of contingency management and spirometric lung age for motivating smoking cessation among injection drug users. *BMC Public Health, 14*, 761.

Dunn, K. E., Saulsgiver, K. A., & Sigmon, S. C. (2011). Contingency management for behavior change: Applications to promote brief smoking cessation among opioid-maintained patients. *Experimental and Clinical Psychopharmacology, 19*, 20–30.

DuPont, R. L., Compton, W. M., & McLellan A. T. (2015). Five-year recovery: A new standard for assessing effectiveness of substance use disorder treatment. *Journal of Substance Abuse Treatment, 58*, 1–5.

DuPont, R. L., McLellan, A. T., White, W. L., Merlo, L. J., & Gold, M. S. (2009). Setting the standard for recovery: Physicians' health programs. *Journal of Substance Abuse Treatment, 36*, 159–171.

Dutra, L., Stathopoulou, G., Basden, S. L., Leyro, T. M., Powers, M. B., & Otto, M. W. (2008). A meta-analytic review of psychosocial interventions for substance use disorders. *American Journal of Psychiatry, 165*, 179–187.

Elliott, R., & Tighe, T. (1968). Breaking the cigarette habit: Effects of a technique involving threatened loss of money. *Psychological Record, 18*, 503–513.

Festinger, D. S., Dugosh, K. L., Kirby, K. C., & Seymour, B. L. (2014). Contingency management for cocaine treatment: Cash vs. vouchers. *Journal of Substance Abuse Treatment, 47*, 168–174.

Glasgow, R. E., Hollis, J. F., Ary, D. V., & Boles, S. M. (1993). Results of a year-long incentives-based worksite smoking-cessation program. *Addictive Behaviors, 18*, 455–464.

Glover, M., Kira, A., Walker, N., & Bauld, L. (2015). Using incentives to encourage smoking abstinence among pregnant Indigenous women?: A feasibility study. *Maternal and Child Health Journal, 19,* 1393–1399.

Godley, M. D., Godley, S. H., Dennis, M. L., Funk, R. R., Passetti, L. L., & Petry, N. M. (2014). A randomized trial of assertive continuing care and contingency management for adolescents with substance use disorders. *Journal of Consulting and Clinical Psychology, 82,* 40–51.

Gray, K. M., Carpenter, M. J., Baker, N. L., Hartwell, K. J., Lewis, A. L., Hiott, D. W., et al. (2011). Bupropion SR and contingency management for adolescent smoking cessation. *Journal of Substance Abuse Treatment, 40,* 77–86.

Halpern, S. D., French, B., Small, D. S., Saulsgiver, K., Harhay, M. O., Audrain-McGovern, J., et al. (2015). Randomized trial of four financial-incentive programs for smoking cessation. *New England Journal of Medicine, 372,* 2108–2117.

Halpern, S. D., Harhay, M. O., Saulsgiver, K., Brophy, C., Troxel, A. B., & Volpp, K. G. (2018). A pragmatic trial of e-cigarettes, incentives, and drugs for smoking cessation. *New England Journal of Medicine, 378,* 2302–2310.

Heil, S. H., Higgins, S. T., Bernstein, I. M., Solomon, L. J., Rogers, R. E., Thomas, C. S., et al. (2008). Effects of voucher-based incentives on abstinence from cigarette smoking and fetal growth among pregnant women. *Addiction, 103,* 1009–1018.

Higgins, S. T., Bernstein, I. M., Washio, Y., Heil, S. H., Badger, G. J., Skelly, J. M., et al. (2010). Effects of smoking cessation with voucher-based contingency management on birth outcomes. *Addiction, 105,* 2023–2030.

Higgins, S. T., Delaney, D. D., Budney, A. J., Bickel, W. K., Hughes, J. R., Foerg, F., et al. (1991). A behavioral approach to achieving initial cocaine abstinence. *American Journal of Psychiatry, 148,* 1218–1224.

Higgins, S. T., Washio, Y., Lopez, A. A., Heil, S. H., Solomon, L. J., Lynch, M. E., et al. (2014). Examining two different schedules of financial incentives for smoking cessation among pregnant women. *Preventive Medicine, 68,* 51–57.

Holtyn, A. F., Koffarnus, M. N., DeFulio, A., Sigurdsson, S. O., Strain, E. C., Schwartz, R. P., et al. (2014a). The therapeutic workplace to promote treatment engagement and drug abstinence in out-of-treatment injection drug users: A randomized controlled trial. *Preventive Medicine, 68,* 62–70.

Holtyn, A. F., Koffarnus, M. N., DeFulio, A., Sigurdsson, S. O., Strain, E. C., Schwartz, R. P., et al. (2014b). Employment-based abstinence reinforcement promotes opiate and cocaine abstinence in out-of-treatment injection drug users. *Journal of Applied Behavior Analysis, 47,* 681–693.

Hser, Y. I., Li, J., Jiang, H., Zhang, R., Du, J., Zhang, C., et al. (2011). Effects of a randomized contingency management intervention on opiate abstinence and retention in methadone maintenance treatment in China. *Addiction, 106,* 1801–1809.

Jiang, H., Du, J., Wu, F., Wang, Z., Fan, S., Li, Z., et al. (2012). Efficacy of contingency management in improving retention and compliance to methadone maintenance treatment: A random controlled study. *Shanghai Archives of Psychiatry, 24,* 11–19.

Kendzor, D. E., Businelle, M. S., Poonawalla, I. B., Cuate, E. L., Kesh, A., Rios, D. M., et al. (2015). Financial incentives for abstinence among socioeconomically disadvantaged individuals in smoking cessation treatment. *American Journal of Public Health, 105,* 1198–1205.

Kennedy, A. P., Phillips, K. A., Epstein, D. H., Reamer, D. A., Schmittner, J., & Preston, K. L. (2013). A randomized investigation of methadone doses at or over 100 mg/day, combined with contingency management. *Drug and Alcohol Dependence, 130,* 77–84.

Killeen, T. K., McRae-Clark, A. L., Waldrop, A. E., Upadhyaya, H., & Brady, K. T. (2012). Contingency management in community programs treating adolescent substance abuse: A feasibility study. *Journal of Child and Adolescent Psychiatric Nursing, 25,* 33–41.

Kirby, K. C., Carpenedo, C. M., Dugosh, K. L., Rosenwasser, B. J., Benishek, L. A., Janik, A., et al. (2013). Randomized clinical trial examining duration of voucher-based reinforcement therapy for cocaine abstinence. *Drug and Alcohol Dependence, 132,* 639–645.

Krishnan-Sarin, S., Cavallo, D. A., Cooney, J. L., Schepis, T. S., Kong, G., Liss, T. B., et al. (2013). An exploratory randomized controlled trial of a novel high-school-based smoking cessation intervention for adolescent smokers using abstinence-contingent incentives and cognitive behavioral therapy. *Drug and Alcohol Dependence, 132,* 346–351.

Lamb, R. J., Kirby, K. C., Morral, A. R., Galbicka, G., & Iguchi, M. Y. (2010). Shaping smoking cessation in hard-to-treat smokers. *Journal of Consulting and Clinical Psychology, 78,* 62–71.

Ledgerwood, D. M., Arfken, C. L., Petry, N. M., & Alessi, S. M. (2014). Prize contingency management for smoking cessation: A randomized trial. *Drug and Alcohol Dependence, 140,* 208–212.

Ling, W., Hillhouse, M., Ang, A., Jenkins, J., & Fahey, J. (2013). Comparison of behavioral treatment conditions in buprenorphine maintenance. *Addiction, 108,* 1788–1798.

Litt, M. D., Kadden, R. M., & Petry, N. M. (2013). Behavioral treatment for marijuana dependence: Randomized trial of contingency management and self-efficacy enhancement. *Addictive Behaviors, 38,* 1764–1775.

Lussier, J. P., Heil, S. H., Mongeon, J. A., Badger, G. J., & Higgins, S. T. (2006). A meta-analysis of voucher-based reinforcement therapy for substance use disorders. *Addiction, 101,* 192–203.

McDonell, M. G., Howell, D. N., McPherson, S., Cameron, J. M., Srebnik, D., Roll, J. M., et al. (2012). Voucher-based reinforcement for alcohol abstinence using the ethyl-glucuronide alcohol biomarker. *Journal of Applied Behavior Analysis, 45*, 161–165.

McDonell, M. G., Srebnik, D., Angelo, F., McPherson, S., Lowe, J. M., Sugar, A., et al. (2013). Randomized controlled trial of contingency management for stimulant use in community mental health patients with serious mental illness. *American Journal of Psychiatry, 170*, 94–101.

McKay, J. R., Lynch, K. G., Coviello, D., Morrison, R., Cary, M. S., Skalina, L., et al. (2010). Randomized trial of continuing care enhancements for cocaine-dependent patients following initial engagement. *Journal of Consulting and Clinical Psychology, 78*, 111–120.

McLellan, A. T., Lewis, D. C., O'Brien, C. P., & Kleber, H. D. (2000). Drug dependence, a chronic medical illness: Implications for treatment, insurance, and outcomes evaluation. *Journal of the American Medical Association, 284*, 1689–1695.

Menza, T. W., Jameson, D. R., Hughes, J. P., Colfax, G. N., Shoptaw, S., & Golden, M. R. (2010). Contingency management to reduce methamphetamine use and sexual risk among men who have sex with men: A randomized controlled trial. *BMC Public Health, 10*, 774.

Meredith, S. E., & Dallery, J. (2013). Investigating group contingencies to promote brief abstinence from cigarette smoking. *Experimental and Clinical Psychopharmacology, 21*, 144–154.

Meredith, S. E., Grabinski, M. J., & Dallery, J. (2011). Internet-based group contingency management to promote abstinence from cigarette smoking: A feasibility study. *Drug and Alcohol Dependence, 118*, 23–30.

Milby, J. B., Schumacher, J. E., Raczynski, J. M., Caldwell, E., Engle, M., Michael, M., et al. (1996). Sufficient conditions for effective treatment of substance abusing homeless persons. *Drug and Alcohol Dependence, 43*, 39–47.

Peirce, J. M., Petry, N. M., Stitzer, M. L., Blaine, J., Kellogg, S., Satterfield, F., et al. (2006). Effects of lower-cost incentives on stimulant abstinence in methadone maintenance treatment: A national drug abuse treatment clinical trials network study. *Archives of General Psychiatry, 63*, 201–208.

Petitjean, S. A., Dursteler-MacFarland, K. M., Krokar, M. C., Strasser, J., Mueller, S. E., Degen, B., et al. (2014). A randomized, controlled trial of combined cognitive-behavioral therapy plus prize-based contingency management for cocaine dependence. *Drug and Alcohol Dependence, 145*, 94–100.

Petry, N. M., Alessi, S. M., Barry, D., & Carroll, K. M. (2015). Standard magnitude prize reinforcers can be as efficacious as larger magnitude reinforcers in cocaine-dependent methadone patients. *Journal of Consulting and Clinical Psychology, 83*, 464–472.

Petry, N. M., Alessi, S. M., Marx, J., Austin, M., & Tardif, M. (2005). Vouchers versus prizes: Contingency management treatment of substance abusers in community settings. *Journal of Consulting and Clinical Psychology, 73*, 1005–1014.

Petry, N. M., Alessi, S. M., & Rash, C. J. (2013). A randomized study of contingency management in cocaine-dependent patients with severe and persistent mental health disorders. *Drug and Alcohol Dependence, 130*, 234–237.

Petry, N. M., DePhilippis, D., Rash, C. J., Drapkin, M., & McKay, J. R. (2014). Nationwide dissemination of contingency management: The Veterans Administration initiative. *American Journal on Addictions, 23*, 205–210.

Petry, N. M., Martin, B., Cooney, J. L., & Kranzler, H. R. (2000). Give them prizes, and they will come: Contingency management for treatment of alcohol dependence. *Journal of Consulting and Clinical Psychology, 68*, 250–257.

Petry, N. M., Tedford, J., Austin, M., Nich, C., Carroll, K. M., & Rounsaville, B. J. (2004). Prize reinforcement contingency management for treating cocaine users: How low can we go, and with whom? *Addiction, 99*, 349–360.

Petry, N. M., Weinstock, J., & Alessi, S. M. (2011). A randomized trial of contingency management delivered in the context of group counseling. *Journal of Consulting and Clinical Psychology, 79*, 686–696.

Petry, N. M., Weinstock, J., Alessi, S. M., Lewis, M. W., & Dieckhaus, K. (2010). Group-based randomized trial of contingencies for health and abstinence in HIV patients. *Journal of Consulting and Clinical Psychology, 78*, 89–97.

Pilling, S., Strang, J., Gerada, C., & National Institute for Clinical Excellence (NICE). (2007). Psychosocial interventions and opioid detoxification for drug misuse: Summary of NICE guidance. *British Medical Journal, 335*, 203–205.

Preston, K. L., Umbricht, A., & Epstein, D. H. (2002). Abstinence reinforcement maintenance contingency and one-year follow-up. *Drug and Alcohol Dependence, 67*, 125–137.

Ries, R. K., Dyck, D. G., Short, R., Srebnik, D., Fisher, A., & Comtois, K. A. (2004). Outcomes of managing disability benefits among patients with substance dependence and severe mental illness. *Psychiatric Services, 55*, 445–447.

Rohsenow, D. J., Tidey, J. W., Martin, R. A., Colby, S. M., Sirota, A. D., Swift, R. M., et al. (2015). Contingent vouchers and motivational interviewing for cigarette smokers in residential substance abuse treatment. *Journal of Substance Abuse Treatment, 55*, 29–38.

Roll, J. M., Chudzynski, J., Cameron, J. M., Howell, D. N., & McPherson, S. (2013). Duration effects in contingency management treatment of methamphetamine disorders. *Addictive Behaviors, 38*, 2455–2462.

Romanowich, P., & Lamb, R. J. (2010). Effects of escalating and descending schedules of incentives on cigarette smoking in smokers without plans to quit. *Journal of Applied Behavior Analysis, 43,* 357–367.

Romanowich, P., & Lamb, R. J. (2013). The effect of framing incentives as either losses or gains with contingency management for smoking cessation. *Addictive Behaviors, 38,* 2084–2088.

Romanowich, P., & Lamb, R. J. (2014). The effects of percentile versus fixed criterion schedules on smoking with equal incentive magnitude for initial abstinence. *Experimental and Clinical Psychopharmacology, 22,* 348–355.

Romanowich, P., & Lamb, R. J. (2015). The effects of fixed versus escalating reinforcement schedules on smoking abstinence. *Journal of Applied Behavior Analysis, 48,* 25–37.

Schmitz, J. M., Lindsay, J. A., Stotts, A. L., Green, C. E., & Moeller, F. G. (2010). Contingency management and levodopa–carbidopa for cocaine treatment: A comparison of three behavioral targets. *Experimental and Clinical Psychopharmacology, 18,* 238–244.

Schottenfeld, R. S., Moore, B., & Pantalon, M. V. (2011). Contingency management with community reinforcement approach or Twelve-Step facilitation drug counseling for cocaine dependent pregnant women or women with young children. *Drug and Alcohol Dependence, 118,* 48–55.

Secades-Villa, R., Garcia-Rodriguez, O., Lopez-Nunez, C., Alonso-Perez, F., & Fernandez-Hermida, J. R. (2014). Contingency management for smoking cessation among treatment-seeking patients in a community setting. *Drug and Alcohol Dependence, 140,* 63–68.

Silverman, K. (2004). Exploring the limits and utility of operant conditioning in the treatment of drug addiction. *Behavior Analyst, 27,* 209–230.

Silverman, K., Chutuape, M. A., Bigelow, G. E., & Stitzer, M. L. (1999). Voucher-based reinforcement of cocaine abstinence in treatment-resistant methadone patients: Effects of reinforcement magnitude. *Psychopharmacology, 146,* 128–138.

Silverman, K., DeFulio, A., & Everly, J. J. (2011). Behavioral aspects. In P. Ruiz & E. C. Strain (Eds.), *Lowinson and Ruiz's substance abuse: A comprehensive textbook* (5th ed, pp. 88–106). Philadelphia: Lippincott Williams & Wilkins.

Silverman, K., DeFulio, A., & Sigurdsson, S. O. (2012). Maintenance of reinforcement to address the chronic nature of drug addiction. *Preventive Medicine, 55,* 46–53.

Silverman, K., Holtyn, A. F., & Morrison, R. (2016). The therapeutic utility of employment in treating drug addiction: Science to application. *Translational Issues in Psychological Science, 2,* 203–212.

Silverman, K., Kaminski, B. J., Higgins, S. T., & Brady, J. V. (2011). Behavior analysis and treatment of drug addiction. In W. W. Fisher, C. C. Piazza, & H. S. Roane (Eds.), *Handbook of applied behavior analysis* (pp. 451–471). New York: Guilford Press.

Silverman, K., Robles, E., Mudric, T., Bigelow, G. E., & Stitzer, M. L. (2004). A randomized trial of long-term reinforcement of cocaine abstinence in methadone-maintained patients who inject drugs. *Journal of Consulting and Clinical Psychology, 72,* 839–854.

Stanger, C., Ryan, S. R., Scherer, E. A., Norton, G. E., & Budney, A. J. (2015). Clinic- and home-based contingency management plus parent training for adolescent cannabis use disorders. *Journal of the American Academy of Child and Adolescent Psychiatry, 54,* 445–453.

Tevyaw, T. O., Colby, S. M., Tidey, J. W., Kahler, C. W., Rohsenow, D. J., Barnett, N. P., et al. (2009). Contingency management and motivational enhancement: A randomized clinical trial for college student smokers. *Nicotine and Tobacco Research, 11,* 739–749.

Tidey, J. W., Rohsenow, D. J., Kaplan, G. B., Swift, R. M., & Reid, N. (2011). Effects of contingency management and bupropion on cigarette smoking in smokers with schizophrenia. *Psychopharmacology, 217,* 279–287.

Umbricht, A., DeFulio, A., Winstanley, E. L., Tompkins, D. A., Peirce, J., Mintzer, M. Z., et al. (2014). Topiramate for cocaine dependence during methadone maintenance treatment: A randomized controlled trial. *Drug and Alcohol Dependence, 140,* 92–100.

Winstanley, E. L., Bigelow, G. E., Silverman, K., Johnson, R. E., & Strain, E. C. (2011). A randomized controlled trial of fluoxetine in the treatment of cocaine dependence among methadone-maintained patients. *Journal of Substance Abuse Treatment, 40,* 255–264.

# CHAPTER 30

# Behavioral Gerontology

Jonathan C. Baker, Linda A. LeBlanc, Brian MacNeill,
and Paige B. Raetz

Global and national demographics have shifted steadily toward an older population, with adults 65 years or older projected to account for 20% of the total U.S. population by the year 2030 and 24% by 2060 (Colby & Ortman, 2014). The group ages 85 and older is growing faster than any other group, with a disproportionate increase for women and minority groups (Colby & Ortman, 2014). These adults will need a range of medical and psychological services, because they are likely to experience declining health, sensory deficits (e.g., hearing loss), and cognitive impairments that will be costly, debilitating, and potentially socially isolating (Belsky, 1999). However, the infrastructure for providing these services is projected to be woefully inadequate as these individuals age and demand alternatives to traditional nursing homes (Molinari et al., 2003).

Due to the growing discrepancy between needs and infrastructure, enormous research and practice opportunities exist for behavior analysts interested in working with older adults. Behavior analysts have long advocated the use of environmental modifications to enhance the lives of older adults (Lindsley, 1964). Prominent behavior analysts have suggested that (1) natural contingencies for older adults support ineffective behavior (Skinner, 1983), (2) basic operant principles account for aging-related phenomena, and (3) many of the

declines in skills observed in older adults are reversible (Baltes & Barton, 1977). We use the term *behavioral gerontology* to refer to the application of behavior analysis to older adults in areas such as basic behavioral research, clinical applications, and organizational issues in service delivery agencies (Adkins & Mathews, 1999; Burgio & Burgio, 1986).

Since the mid-1980s, a small, stable number of publications on aging have appeared in behavioral journals (e.g., Baker & LeBlanc, 2011; Buchanan, Husfeldt, Berg, & Houlihan, 2011; Oleson & Baker, 2014; Pachis & Zonneveld, 2018; Raetz, LeBlanc, Baker, & Hilton, 2013; Trahan, Donaldson, McNabney, & Kahng, 2014; Virues-Ortega, Iwata, Nogales-González, & Frades, 2012), and a growing number of behavior-analytic studies have appeared in multidisciplinary aging journals (e.g., Altus, Engelman, & Mathews, 2002a, 2002b; Burgio et al., 2002; Feliciano, LeBlanc, & Feeney, 2010; Hussian & Brown, 1987; Ilem, Feliciano, & LeBlanc, 2015; Noguchi, Kawano, & Yamanaka, 2013). Despite the enormous potential for positive social impact, however, the field of behavioral gerontology has not grown at a rate commensurate with its potential (Burgio & Burgio, 1986).

Behavior analysts who publish in multidisciplinary aging journals have attempted to illustrate the advantages of a behavior-analytic approach to aging to nonbehavioral audiences (e.g., Noguchi et al., 2013). These benefits include a focus on environmental factors that promote or suppress behavior, and belief in the potential reversibility of decline and cost-effectiveness in a behavior-analytic intervention approach (Dupree & Schonfeld, 1998). Behavior-analytic researchers publishing in non-behavior-analytic journals also have benefited from contact with well-designed research that can inform behavioral gerontology, even though that research is not behavior-analytic per se.

Baker, Fairchild, and Seefeldt (2015) argue that non-behavior-analytic aging research provides a foundation for research and clinical considerations in behavioral gerontology. Behavior analysts who are aware of the current research topics on aging and pressing societal concerns for older adults are more likely to conduct research that the broader research community studying aging will value. For example, poor fluid intake is a common and life-threatening problem in older adults (Keller, Beck, & Namasivayam, 2015). Feliciano et al. (2010) provided an example of the application of behavior analysis to the problem of insufficient fluid intake in older adults. They developed the Hydration Interview, a functional assessment interview that identified risks for dehydration and barriers to hydration (e.g., questions regarding antecedent events, such as "When are you most likely to drink beverages?", and questions regarding consequences, such as "Would you drink more liquids if they tasted better?"). The interview guided the generation of potential hypotheses regarding environmental factors related to fluid intake. Feliciano et al. used the results of the assessment to develop interventions for two older adults. For example, if an individual indicated that he or she would drink more liquids if they tasted better, Felciano et al. conducted a preference assessment of liquids to identify preferred drinks. The function-based intervention package minimized variability in fluid intake for both participants. This study illustrates how behavior analysts can develop useful assessments for common aging-related health concerns that can inform intervention development and have a significant positive social impact on the lives of older adults.

This chapter provides a review of the literature on behavioral gerontology for behavior analysts who may not be familiar with the area. We have divided the chapter into two content areas, basic research and clinical application, with an emphasis on studies published in the past 10 years.

## BASIC BEHAVIOR-ANALYTIC RESEARCH ON AGING

The study of memory and cognition from an information-processing perspective has dominated basic research on aging (Birren & Schaie, 2001; Cherry & Smith, 1998); as a result, there is very little published literature from a behavior-analytic perspective (Derenne & Baron, 2002). The behavior-analytic experimental literature on aging focuses primarily on age-related changes in classically conditioned responses, responses to schedules of reinforcement, signal detection, and formation of stimulus equivalence classes. We summarize a few of the most consistent findings regarding age-related differences in learning and performance below, because applied work in gerontology that is not informed by these findings could lead to misinformed and ineffective intervention for clinical problems.

### Respondent Conditioning

A series of studies have documented clear age- and neurocognitive-disorder-related changes in classically conditioned (i.e., respondent) responses in both human and nonhuman species. We include both types of studies in this review, because both human and nonhuman animal research can inform our understanding of basic behavioral processes in classical conditioning.

A few studies have examined age-related differences in acquisition of classically conditioned responses, using *trace* and *delay* conditioning. Trace conditioning involves trials in which a brief interval separates the end of the conditioned stimulus and the beginning of the unconditioned stimulus. Delay conditioning involves onset of the conditioned stimulus before onset of the unconditioned stimulus, but both stimuli end simultaneously. Graves and Solomon (1985) noted the importance of using these two procedures. First, they summarized research suggesting that the two procedures result in the acquisition of conditioned responses (e.g., conditioned responses occurring during 80% of opportunities), but through two different neural systems. Although behavior analysts may not always focus on biological processes, researchers have shown that damage to the hippocampus has a negative impact on trace conditioning but not on delay conditioning. Age-related changes include deterioration of the hippocampus, which suggests that studies evaluating respondent conditioning in young and old organisms might show age-related differences with trace conditioning but not with delay conditioning. Second, Graves and Solomon noted that increases in the complexity of procedures are related inversely to the acquisition of conditioned responses for older organisms. Research on trace- and delay-conditioning procedures have shown that the trace procedure, where there is a gap between the end of the presentation of the conditioned stimulus and the beginning of the unconditioned stimulus, is a more complex procedure than the delay procedure, where the two stimuli overlap temporally and can affect the acquisition of conditioned responses.

Graves and Solomon (1985) examined the differences in trace and delay conditioning on the acquisition of conditioned responses in 6-month-old (young) and 36- to 60-month-old (old) albino rabbits. They defined acquisition of the conditioned response as those responses occurring during 4 trials of a 5-trial block or conditioned responses occurring during 8 trials of a 10-trial block. The older rabbits acquired the conditioned response between a mean of 700 and 800 trials, and the younger rabbits acquired the conditioned response between a mean of 430 and 470 trials in trace conditioning, but the investigators observed no differences during delay conditioning. Although this study did not differentiate between age-related differences associated with hippocampus damage versus complexity, it showed that a simple gap between the presentation of the conditioned stimulus and the presentation of the unconditioned stimulus resulted in older rabbits' requiring twice as many trials to acquire the response as when the two stimuli overlapped temporally. Other researchers have demonstrated similar differences in trace but not delay conditioning in older humans (e.g., Finkbiner & Woodruff-Pak, 1991), once again highlighting how a simple procedural difference can affect older but not younger organisms' acquisition of conditioned responses.

Younger humans have acquired conditioned responses when researchers combine delay and trace conditioning, which has led researchers to evaluate whether the same would be true for older humans. The question is whether interspersing delay conditioning with trace conditioning can improve the acquisition of conditioned responses for older organisms, so that it is more like that of younger organisms (Cheng, Faulkner, Disterhoft, & Desmond, 2010). Researchers using a combination of trace and delay conditioning to evaluate the acquisition of conditioned responses of younger (i.e., 20–25 years) and older (i.e., 60–68 years)

human participants showed not only that the performance of older participants was not like that of younger participants, but also that the combination resulted in almost no conditioned responses (Cheng et al., 2010). These results highlight that specific preparations can have an impact on responding in older adults. Respondent conditioning involves stimulus–stimulus pairing. The results of these studies indicate that researchers examining any procedures using stimulus–stimulus pairing with older adults need to be careful about drawing conclusions without a complete understanding of how those preparations can affect responding. These results also suggest that simple procedural variations could interact with age-related changes in performance and could affect findings from clinical approaches that seek to use stimulus–stimulus pairing, such as establishing conditioned reinforcement.

Researchers have evaluated differences among younger adults, older adults, and older adults with neurocognitive disorders (such as neurocognitive disorder due to Alzheimer's disease). As noted above, changes in classically conditioned response acquisition appear in later middle age (typically early 40s to early 60s) and progress into old age (over age 65) (Finkbiner & Woodruff-Pak, 1991; Woodruff-Pak & Jaeger, 1998; Woodruff-Pak & Thompson, 1988), with even greater changes observed for individuals with neurocognitive disorders. Acquisition of conditioned eyeblink responses and overall percentage of conditioned responses across trial blocks reliably differentiate typically aging individuals from those with vascular neurocognitive disorder and those with probable neurocognitive disorder due to Alzheimer's (Woodruff-Pak, 2001; Woodruff-Pak, Papka, Romano, & Li, 1996).

Taken together, the research described above supports that older adults acquire fewer conditioned responses or engage in fewer conditioned responses across trial blocks than younger adults do, and that older adults with neurocognitive disorder acquire, engage in, or acquire and engage in even fewer conditioned responses than healthy older adults. Researchers have posited that the differences in respondent conditioning between younger and older adults are related to changes in brain structure (Cheng et al., 2010; Woodruff-Pak, 2001), particularly cerebellar cortical atrophy, rather than to the mere passage of time. Furthermore, researchers have hypothesized that disease-related changes in the same cerebellar structure may be responsible for differences between healthy older adults and older adults with neurocognitive disorders (Cheng et al., 2010; Woodruff-Pak, 2001). Researchers have found that repeated exposure to conditioning procedures improves the performance of older adults. For example, Graves and Solomon (1985) showed that older adults could acquire conditioned responses in trace conditioning procedures eventually, and that procedural variations could also minimize age-related differences in procedures using delay versus trace conditioning.

Behavior analysts working in clinical settings with aging adults might not use respondent-conditioning procedures in their clinical practice, but much applied research in behavioral gerontology includes procedures to enhance stimulus control. These studies might inform clinical interventions that aim (1) to establish stimuli as reinforcement, such as pairing stimuli using a temporal overlap rather than attempting to present paired stimuli with temporal gaps; and (2) to ensure that discriminative stimuli are present throughout conditioning, rather than simply at the beginning of conditioning blocks. Using a trace-conditioning procedure directly, or expecting a stimulus to acquire reinforcing or evocative properties after a few pairings, may set up clinical procedures for failure. Until further research can evaluate whether the age-related effects found in respondent conditioning do not apply to operant conditioning, we advise behavior analysts to consider whether the literature on respondent conditioning might enhance their procedures.

## Operant Conditioning

Perhaps the two most studied areas in age-related basic research on operant conditioning are sensitivity to reinforcement and stimulus equivalence. Several studies have examined age-related sensitivity to reinforcement, because previous researchers have suggested that older adults' behavior was less sensitive to environmental changes than that of younger adults (Tripp & Alsop, 1999). Research in this area has produced interesting and sometimes conflicting results. Fisher and Noll (1996) found that when schedules of reinforcement varied, older adults' behavior was slower to change (i.e., to match the new schedule of reinforcement). However, their behavior matched relative reinforcement rates with increased exposure to reinforcement contingencies. Tripp and Alsop (1999) later compared responding of children, young adults, and older adults on different reinforcement sched-

ules, and found that older adults' behavior did not respond to schedules of reinforcement, regardless of exposure. Plaud, Plaud, and von Duvillard (1999) manipulated reinforcement magnitude on a computer-based task and found that older adults altered their responding accordingly, indicating that they were sensitive to changes in reinforcement schedules. That is, unlike Tripp and Alsop or Fisher and Noll, Plaud et al. found that older adults' behavior did change with schedule changes. Plaud et al. exposed older adults to extinction and found that they demonstrated persistent response bias (i.e., resistance to extinction), even when the researchers changed the contingencies.

Taken together, this line of research demonstrates that older adults' behavior is sensitive to changes in reinforcement. However, researchers classified the older adults' behavior as less sensitive to reinforcement than that of younger adults in almost every study. This research has several clinical implications, though clearly more research is needed before we can make definitive recommendations. Behavior analysts should take basic operant research findings into consideration when designing and implementing interventions for socially significant issues with aging adults. For example, basic research suggests that older adults may require increased exposure to intervention contingencies for socially appropriate behaviors to develop and be maintained when social stimuli maintain challenging behaviors, and when appropriate responses have produced limited or no reinforcement. Behavior analysts might provide higher-quality or higher-magnitude reinforcement for socially appropriate behaviors. Finally, based on the results of Plaud et al. (1999), behavior analysts should anticipate resurgence during periods of extinction when staff members implement interventions with poor integrity.

Several studies have examined age-related differences in responding in stimulus equivalence preparations and found generally weaker formation of equivalence classes for older adults. Stimulus equivalence preparations typically involve researchers' arbitrarily assigning stimuli to classes (e.g., Class A, Class B, Class C) and to groups within those classes (e.g., A1, A2, A3). Researchers then use match-to-sample preparations to teach relations (e.g., when a participant is presented with stimulus A1, the correct response out of an array of C2, A3, and B1 is B1). Wilson and Milan (1995) compared groups of older and younger adults, and found slower response times and poorer performance on posttests of equivalence relations for older adults. As a result, researchers have attempted to evaluate whether such a difference is due to the procedures or is age-related. Perez-Gonzalez and Moreno-Sierra (1999) found that older adults' performance on equivalence preparations was slightly better than that of Wilson and Milan's participants, but still found impaired formation of equivalence classes in older adults. Other studies have evaluated several methods for training equivalence class formation in older adults, to determine whether modifications in preparations could improve this formation. Saunders, Chaney, and Marquis (2005) found no difference in equivalence class formation when they used different numbers of samples (e.g., two-, three-, and four-choice match-to-sample configurations) and different training structures (e.g., linear series, many-to-one, and one-to-many training structures). Interestingly, their data suggested equivalence class formation in 75% of participants, compared to 45% of participants in Wilson and Milan. Researchers continue to evaluate the variables that are responsible for varying performance across age groups in match-to-sample preparations. For example, Steingrimsdottir and Arntzen (2014) showed that healthy older adults (ages 70–86) had shorter trials to criterion when (1) identity matching (i.e., classes were based on physical properties of stimuli) preceded arbitrary matching (i.e., classes were arbitrary), and (2) the procedure incorporated a 0-second delay (i.e., the sample stimulus disappeared as the response options appeared). Saunders et al. also found that a 0-second delay improved performance. The 0-second delay is contrasted with preparations in which the sample stimulus is present at the same time as the response options. The effectiveness of inserting a break between the sample stimulus and the response options seems to contradict the findings for effective manipulations in the literature on basic respondent conditioning. As noted earlier, researchers on respondent conditioning have shown that the trace preparation, where the conditioned stimulus ended before the unconditioned stimulus began, produced poorer acquisition of conditioned responses than the delay condition, where the conditioned and unconditioned stimulus overlapped.

Although further research is needed in both basic respondent and operant conditioning, researchers have identified age-related differences in behavior and procedural variations that can mitigate those differences. Basic research has uncovered age-related changes in basic behavioral pro-

cesses, such as the establishment of conditioned responses, sensitivity to changes in schedules of reinforcement, and formation of equivalence classes. As in classical-conditioning research, seemingly minor procedural variations can have an impact on responding in operant conditioning (e.g., changes in the stimulus delay in match-to-sample preparations). Behavior analysts who conduct research with or provide clinical services for older adults should evaluate whether procedural aspects of their interventions might have an impact on responsiveness.

## CLINICAL BEHAVIOR-ANALYTIC RESEARCH ON AGING

Clinical research in behavioral gerontology has focused primarily on mental health problems (e.g., depression, anxiety), health maintenance, and problems associated with neurocognitive disorders. The medical rather than the psychosocial model has been dominant, perhaps because 85% of older individuals have health concerns warranting regular medical visits (Butler, Finkel, Lewis, Sherman, & Sunderland, 1992). By contrast, few older adults have regular contact with mental health professionals (Belsky, 1999). However, evidence exists in each of these areas that change in the environment can produce change in behavior even when medical interventions cannot alter physical or cognitive status. For example, when researchers hold psychotropic medication constant, behavioral interventions can produce changes in behavior (Baker, Hanley, & Mathews, 2006). In this section, we review the effectiveness of behavioral interventions for mental and physical health issues, as well as recent advances in assessment, function-based intervention for behavioral excesses, non-function-based intervention for behavioral excesses, and intervention for behavioral deficits.

### Mental and Physical Health Issues

#### Mental Health

Depression and anxiety are common mental health problems for older adults (Sorocco, Kinoshita, & Gallagher-Thompson, 2005) and have been the subjects of investigation in extensive behavioral and cognitive-behavioral therapy research. Symptoms of depression include sadness, feelings of worthlessness and guilt, lethargy, sleep and appetite disturbances, and loss of interest in activities. Major depression occurs in 1–6% of older adults living in the community (Mojtabai & Olfson, 2004), 5–10% of medically ill or frail individuals (Dick & Gallagher-Thompson, 1996), 20–30% of individuals with neurocognitive disorders (Steinberg et al., 2003; Zarit & Zarit, 1998), and more than 50% of those living in nursing homes (Pellegrin, Peters, Lyketsos, & Marano, 2013). An additional 9–30% of older adults living in the community report symptoms of a duration or severity that do not meet the diagnostic criteria for major depression, but that still decrease quality of life significantly (Blazer, 1993; Thompson, Futterman, & Gallagher, 1988). Generalized anxiety disorder, the most common anxiety disorder, occurs in approximately 3–17% of older adults and is characterized by worry (Ladouceur, Leger, Dugas, & Freeston, 2004; Stein, 2004; Wild et al., 2010); an additional 15–43% of healthy older adults report anxiety symptoms that do not meet the diagnostic criteria for an anxiety disorder (Mehta et al., 2003).

Cognitive-behavioral therapy is an empirically supported intervention for depression and anxiety for older adults (Arean, 2004; Stanley, Diefenbach, & Hopko, 2004) when administered individually (Arean, 2004; Gallagher-Thompson & Thompson, 1996) or in groups (DeVries & Coon, 2002). Cognitive-behavioral therapy generally involves education about depression and anxiety; self-monitoring of negative or anxious thoughts and emotion states; replacement of dysfunctional beliefs and self-statements with functional ones; scheduling pleasant events; and training in such skills as problem solving, coping, and relaxation (Dick & Gallagher-Thompson, 1996; Dick, Gallagher-Thompson, & Thompson, 1996; Gatz et al., 1998).

Researchers have provided guidelines for how to use cognitive-behavioral therapy to address anxiety among older adults with neurocognitive disorders (Charlesworth, Sadek, Schepers, & Spector, 2015). Charlesworth et al. (2015) provided a description of an individually tailored approach to cognitive-behavioral therapy adapted for older adults with mild to moderate neurocognitive disorders. They described a 10-session approach including education, development of pretherapy skills (i.e., behaviors that research has shown must be present for the approach to work, such as awareness of emotions and ability to label emotions), self-monitoring, collaboration and goal setting, progressive muscle relaxation, and perspective taking. As an example of these modifications, Charlesworth et al. suggested

that evaluating and establishing pretherapy skills early in intervention are critical to the therapy process. Charlesworth et al. suggested that older adults with comorbid anxiety and neurocognitive disorders often lack pretherapy skills and may not be able to describe their emotional difficulties. Charlesworth et al. suggested modifying short-term cognitive-behavioral therapy to "focus more on developing the missing pre-therapy skills than to attempt to 'rush through' to goal-focused change material" (p. 392). Although Charlesworth et al. did not provide data on the effects of the approach, Tonga et al. (2015) presented three case examples to illustrate the challenges of using and modifying manual-based cognitive-behavioral therapy with older adults with neurocognitive disorders. The researchers tailored therapy to each client's presenting skills (e.g., use of technology-based memory aids, modified homework, slowed pace of progress through the manual); therefore, Tonga et al. also recommended that behavior analysts use individualized approaches.

### Physical Health Issues

Common physical health issues for older adults include diet, hydration, and continence. Other issues, such as compliance with health or medication recommendations, can affect health and create additional health issues. Compliance with health or medication recommendations is referred to as *intervention regimen adherence*, and the degree of compliance is typically a primary determinant of overall health status (Meichenbaum & Turk, 1987). Nonadherence to medical recommendations can have a direct impact on diet, hydration, and continence, which can then contribute to risk for cancer, diabetes, heart disease, delirium, urinary tract infections, and medication toxicity (Ho, Lee, & Meyskens, 1991; Kannel, 1986; Sanservo, 1997; Warren et al., 1994). Nonadherence (i.e., noncompliance) estimates for medication regimens by older adults range from 43 to 62%, despite evidence that the adults are aware of the benefits of the medication and the potentially dire consequences for nonadherence (Meichenbaum & Turk, 1987). Indeed, research suggests that education alone consistently produces little to no change in compliance (Sands & Holman, 1985). Interventions involving prompts and behavioral contingencies for adherence to diet and hydration recommendations have proven effective.

Stock and Milan (1993) compared the effects of two sets of behavioral interventions on dietary practices of older adults in a retirement community. Baseline involved prompts (i.e., researchers helped identify healthy foods), and the first intervention involved additional prompts (e.g., media, buttons, verbal reminders) with feedback (i.e., graphed percentage of healthy items) and praise when an individual reported selecting a healthy food. The second intervention incorporated a token-based lottery system with immediate and delayed reinforcement when the individual selected a healthy food. The additional prompts increased healthy selections from a baseline mean of 24% to an intervention mean of 65%, and the addition of the lottery system produced a marginal increase to 68% healthy selections.

Prompt systems have proven effective in increasing fluid consumption for older adults in nursing homes, but no studies have targeted community-dwelling elders. Nursing aides in Spangler, Risley, and Bilyew (1984) presented a cup and offered nursing home residents a choice of beverages every 1.5 hour. This intervention produced clinically and statistically significant improvements in hydration measured through urine. Simmons, Alessi, and Schnelle (2001) manipulated the frequency of prompts and beverage choices and found that 80% of nursing home residents increased their mean daily fluid intake with systematic prompts alone. The addition of choice of beverage produced an additional 21% increase in fluid intake and a decrease in the number of beverage refusals.

As described earlier, Feliciano et al. (2010) showed how behavior analysts could develop an assessment that informs intervention, and demonstrated the efficacy of that intervention. Feliciano et al. developed a functional assessment interview, the Hydration Interview, in which hydration was the target behavior. The interview evaluated risks of dehydration and then directed researchers to hypothesis-based interventions. Feliciano et al. showed that interventions produced increases in hydration measured through urine and increases in healthy fluid intake, with concomitant decreases in unhealthy fluid intake.

Urinary incontinence becomes more common with age, due to muscle weakness, decreased mobility, memory loss, and communication difficulties (Burgio & Locher, 1996). Older adults may restrict fluid intake to avoid accidents (Simmons et al., 2001), leading to dehydration, potential social stigma, and increased care requirements in nursing homes. Several interventions have proven effective in targeting incontinence, including psychoeducation and behavioral training, prompted voiding schedules, and the use of discriminative stimuli. Behavioral continence training consists of education about mechanisms of bladder control and specific recommendations, in-session practice of contracting and identifying relevant muscles, and assigned practice in contraction exercises (Burton, Pearce, Burgio, Engle, & Whitehead, 1988). This intervention produced an 82% reduction in incontinence, compared to a 79% reduction for community-dwelling participants who received behavioral training plus bladder sphincter biofeedback for practicing muscle contractions—an intrusive intervention in which a medical professional inserts a bladder into the body and fills it to simulate the feeling of an actual full bladder. Burgio et al. (2002) showed that reductions in incontinence for a group that received behavioral training exceeded reductions for a group that received behavioral training plus bladder sphincter biofeedback and for a group that received only written instructions (69%, 63%, and 58%, respectively).

Prompted-voiding schedules involve education, scheduled toilet visits with assistance, positive reinforcement for dry intervals and continent voids, and encouragement to resist urinary urges between scheduled visits (Fantol, Wyman, Harkins, & Hadley, 1990; Jeffcoate, 1961). Perhaps one of the most prolific researchers in the area, Schnelle and his colleagues have published many demonstrations of the efficacy of the intervention. For example, Schnelle et al. (2010) demonstrated that an intervention package with prompted voiding could decrease urinary incontinence and could increase physical activity and fluid intake for more than 100 participants in a randomized controlled trial.

In summary, researchers have demonstrated that behavioral assessments and interventions can effectively address mainstream gerontology issues. In addition to mental and physical health, a large body of behavioral gerontology research has focused on behavioral disturbances related to what are now called neurocognitive disorders (and were formerly known as dementia).

## Advances in Assessment and Assessment-Informed Interventions

Behavior analysts should be well informed about aging populations and proper preintervention assessments, which is similar to the expectations for behavior analysts working in other clinical specialties. Effective clinical approaches to behavioral gerontology must also incorporate population-specific behavioral assessments, such as those evaluating cognitive functioning, health, and diet.

## Stimulus Preference Assessment

The primary goals in care settings for older adults, such as day programming, assisted living, and neurocognitive care, are usually increased participation in and enjoyment of activities. Thus applied research on aging has focused on identifying strategies and stimuli for increasing engagement in leisure activities (LeBlanc, Raetz, & Feliciano, 2011; Williamson & Ascione, 1983). Increasing activity engagement helps to improve quality of life, maintain functioning, and prevent depression (Engelman, Altus, & Mathews, 1999; Engstrom, Mudford, & Brand, 2015; Garcia, Feliciano, & Ilem, 2018; LeBlanc et al., 2011; Teri, 1991). For older adults with neurocognitive disorders, increased engagement in leisure activities also reduces agitation and aggression (Feliciano, Steers, Elite-Marcandonatou, McLane, & Arean, 2009).

Historically, gerontologists have used surveys to identify preferred activities or have not attempted to identify preferences. The Pleasant Events Schedule—Alzheimer's Disease (Logsdon & Teri, 1997; Teri & Logsdon, 1991) is a survey assessment that prompts caregivers to identify examples of potentially preferred activities for older adults. Clinicians and researchers also have used the shortened version of this schedule (Logsdon & Teri, 1997) to assess preferences by asking the older adults with neurocognitive disorders a series of *yes–no* questions (e.g., "Do you enjoy reading magazines?"). One problem with the schedule is that the adults may respond, "Yes, I would like to do that," but may not engage in the activities they have endorsed when opportunities arise (LeBlanc, Raetz, Baker, Strobel, & Feeney, 2008).

Because of the limitations of surveys, researchers have begun to use direct observations to assess preferences. Both paired-stimulus (Fisher et al., 1992) and multiple stimulus without replacement (DeLeon & Iwata, 1996) preference assessments produce preference hierarchies that can predict the effects of stimuli as reinforcers for the behavior of older adults (e.g., LeBlanc, Cherup, Feliciano, & Sidener, 2006; Raetz et al., 2013). Most research with individuals with intellectual disabilities employs a fixed-ratio (FR) 1 schedule to examine the effects of contingent access to an activity on a target behavior (Hagopian, Long, & Rush, 2004). This research investigates whether presenting more preferred stimuli increases target behaviors more than presenting less preferred stimuli. Because therapeutic aging-care centers usually do not provide prompts or reinforcement for activity engagement, several studies on preference assessments with older adults with neurocognitive disorders have used engagement analyses rather than reinforcement analyses to evaluate the utility of preference assessments. Some studies have used selection-based reinforcement assessments. For the purposes of this review, an *engagement-based reinforcement assessment* measures duration of unprompted activity engagement, and a *selection-based reinforcement assessment* measures a participant's selection of one activity over another in a concurrent-operants arrangement to identify the relative reinforcing efficacy of stimuli.

LeBlanc et al. (2006) compared different methods of paired-stimulus presentation, such as tangible presentations, pictorial representations, printed text names, and vocally presented names, to evaluate the preferences of older adults with neurocognitive disorders or aphasia. Tangible presentations for one participant and vocal presentations for the other three participants produced higher subsequent independent engagement. LeBlanc et al. then used that optimal format for each participant to present choices between two activities, and the participant could engage in the chosen activity for up to 15 minutes (i.e., an engagement-based reinforcement assessment). Allowing the participants to select from activities identified in their prior preference assessment produced more engagement than when the researchers presented a standard list of leisure items.

Raetz et al. (2013) used an engagement-based reinforcement assessment to examine whether hierarchies of item preferences identified via a brief multiple stimulus without replacement assessment (i.e., three presentations of multiple-item arrays) would predict the subsequent engagement of older adults with neurocognitive disorders. Results of the multiple stimulus without replacement assessment generally predicted the level of subsequent engagement, although some participants engaged with items that were lower in the preference hierarchy. In addition, a single-array presentation from the multiple stimulus without replacement procedure (i.e., one presentation of the multiple-item array) correlated reasonably well with the results of the mean of the three arrays (i.e., standard brief multiple stimulus without replacement). The preferences identified for more than half the participants remained stable over a 3- to 5-month period.

Beattie, Wagner, and Baker (2019) compared a multiple stimulus without replacement assessment, which is a selection-based preference assessment (i.e., preference hierarchies based on order of selection), to a free-operant assessment (Roane, Vollmer, Ringdahl, & Marcus, 1998), which is an engagement-based preference assessment (i.e., preference hierarchies based on relative duration of engagement), with older adults with neurocognitive disorders. Beattie et al. also conducted two forms of reinforcement assessment. One was an engagement-based reinforcement assessment in which two items were available concurrently. The second was a selection-based reinforcement assessment in which four items were available, but a participant had to move to the area of the item. That is, after the participant selected an item, he or she had to leave the chosen item and move to engage with other items. The preference hierarchies of the multiple stimulus without replacement and the free-operant assessments positively correlated with the level of subsequent engagement during the engagement-based reinforcement assessment. In some cases, the results of the free-operant preference assessment better predicted subsequent engagement during the engagement-based reinforcement assessment. In other cases, the results of the multiple stimulus without replacement assessment better predicted subsequent selections during the selection-based reinforcement assessment. These results indicate that behavior analysts should attend to the types of preference assessments they are using, as different preference assessments produced different accuracy levels. Beattie et al. suggested that the differential results may have been due to the fact that the free-operant preference assessment is an engagement-based preference assessment, whereas the multiple stimulus without replacement assessment is a selection-based assessment.

Oleson and Baker (2014) used a free-operant preference assessment before using a concurrent-operants (i.e., selection-based) reinforcement assessment. During the concurrent-operants assessment, the researchers presented three items concurrently, provided each individual with the selected item, and removed the other items. They found that the free-operant assessment produced false negatives for one participant: One item the participant did not engage with showed reinforcing effects similar to those for an item the participant did engage with during the free-operant assessment in subsequent selection-based reinforcement assessments. The free-operant assessment also produced a false positive for the other participant: The item the participant engaged with most did not show a reinforcing effect.

Quick, Baker, and Ringdahl (2018) directly compared the multiple stimulus without replacement and free-operant assessments with older adults with neurocognitive disorders, to replicate and extend the Beattie et al. (2019) results. Quick et al.'s results suggested that although both assessments identified preferred items, only the multiple stimulus without replacement assessment produced a hierarchy of preferred items that was useful for reestablishing functional skills. Furthermore, they found that both selection-based and engagement-based assessments confirmed the results of the free-operant (for two of the three) and the multiple stimulus without replacement (for all three) assessments, though engagement-based reinforcement assessments yielded quicker results across participants.

Researchers also have used the paired-stimulus and multiple stimulus without replacement assessment procedures to identify items to reestablish functional skills, using a traditional contingent-access arrangement (an FR 1 schedule to examine the effects of contingent access to an activity on a target behavior; Hagopian et al., 2004). Virues-Ortega et al. (2012) showed that paired-stimulus assessments could identify leisure activities and edible items for use as reinforcement for arbitrary responses, such as pressing a lever, and significant responses, such as stacking blocks during physical therapy, for older adults with neurocognitive disorders. Although some research has shown that individuals with intellectual and developmental disabilities and autism spectrum disorder will select edible items over preferred leisure items when both are available, Virues-Ortega et al. found that older adults selected leisure items over edible items when both were available. Ritchie, Reuter-Yuill, Perez, and Baker (2019) obtained similar results, in that older adults selected leisure items over edibles when both were available. Although this difference in preference of leisure versus edible items might appear to be an age-related difference, a more parsimonious explanation might be related to the environment of and health-related changes in older adults. Food tends to be available readily in most aging-care settings, providing more than the necessary calories, given the lower levels of activity and reduced metabolism of older adults. As adults age, changes in olfactory senses and metabolism combine to decrease sensations of hunger and decrease enjoyable aspects of food. That is, their inability to taste and smell food decreases the value of the food. However, leisure activities are typically much less available (e.g., McClannahan & Risley, 1975). As such, the difference in the preference literature between older adults and individuals with intellectual and developmental disabilities and autism spectrum disorder may be due to physiological changes that abolish the value of food reinforcement, or may be due to the discriminability (Virues-Ortega et al., 2012) and availability (J. E. Ringdahl, personal communication, 2014) of different items in the older adults' environments.

Finally, researchers have evaluated preference assessments as an antecedent intervention to address behavioral excesses (Feliciano et al., 2009; Fisher & Buchanan, 2018). Feliciano et al. (2009) showed that providing items identified via a paired-stimulus choice assessment decreased depression and agitation in older adults with neurocognitive disorders. In some cases, the researchers identified when the target behavior, such as wandering, was likely to occur. They then developed a schedule that prompted staff members to provide preferred items before a target behavior occurred, to reduce the likelihood of occurrence. In other cases, the staff provided the preferred items during an activity choice-based redirection following the target behavior. In both cases, staff provided the preferred items as part of a multicomponent intervention plan that reduced target behaviors.

## Functional Assessment

Researchers have reported that function-based interventions reduce problematic or unsafe behaviors more effectively than non-function-based interventions do (Iwata, Pace, Cowdery, & Miltenberger, 1994). More recently, researchers have used functional assessments and function-based interventions (i.e., interventions that involve the manipulation of the response–reinforcement relation that maintains the target behavior) to address problematic or unsafe behaviors in older adults with neurocognitive disorders.

Several studies used functional assessments, such as interviewing staff members, direct observation, or experimental functional analysis, to guide the development of function-based interventions for older adults with neurocognitive disorders (e.g., Baker et al., 2006; Baker, LeBlanc, Raetz, & Hilton, 2011; Buchanan & Fisher, 2002; Burgio, Scilley, Hardin, Hsu, & Yancey, 1996; Dwyer-Moore & Dixon, 2007; Heard & Watson, 1999;

Moniz-Cook, Stokes, & Agar, 2003; Moniz-Cook, Woods, & Richards, 2001). Functional assessments have identified the most common socially mediated categories of reinforcement for the problematic behaviors of older adults with neurocognitive disorders, such as attention (e.g., Buchanan & Fisher, 2002; Dwyer-Moore & Dixon, 2007), access to tangibles (e.g., Heard & Watson, 1999), or escape from staff proximity (e.g., Baker et al., 2006). Researchers also have developed hypothesis-based interventions to address problematic behaviors maintained by nonsocially mediated consequences, such as providing items that produce sensory experiences like those produced by engaging in the problem behavior (Baker et al., 2011; Burgio et al., 1996).

Researchers have shown that function-based interventions are effective for older adults with neurocognitive disorders. One intervention is the noncontingent delivery of reinforcement at set intervals (e.g., Baker et al., 2006, Buchanan & Fisher, 2002). Other interventions with older adults with neurocognitive disorders have included teaching socially appropriate responses to produce reinforcement (i.e., differential reinforcement of alternative behaviors), while withholding reinforcement following problematic behaviors (e.g., Dwyer-Moore & Dixon, 2007). Function-based interventions have reduced many problematic behaviors effectively, including wandering (e.g., Dwyer-Moore & Dixon, 2007; Heard & Watson, 1999), aggression (Baker et al., 2006), disruptive vocalizations (Buchanan & Fisher, 2002), hoarding (Baker et al., 2011), and noncompliance (Moniz-Cook et al., 2003).

In addition to demonstrating the applicability of functional assessment in aging-care settings, researchers have conducted component analyses to identify the crucial components and experimental manipulations to include in functional-analytic conditions. Larrabee, Baker, and O'Neill (2018) evaluated the impact of researcher-programmed discriminative stimuli (which were stimuli that the researcher added to signal the condition, such as colored clothing and poster boards) in functional analyses for disruptive vocalizations among older adults with neurocognitive disorders. Larrabee et al. conducted multielement functional analyses with two versions of each condition, one with and one without programmed discriminative stimuli. They found that conditions without programmed discriminative stimuli produced levels of undifferentiated responding during test and control conditions similar to those reported in previous published studies (cf. Beaton, Peeler, & Harvey, 2006, who did not report any programmed stimuli associated with conditions and were unable to obtain differentiated results in their functional analyses). Larrabee et al. found that conditions with programmed discriminative stimuli produced differentiated responding during test and control conditions, which led to function-based interventions. Thus including programmed discriminative stimuli is important in functional analyses with older adults with cognitive impairments, to enhance these adults' ability to discriminate the experimental conditions; this should improve the efficacy and efficiency of the functional analysis.

### Assessment and Interventions for Verbal Behavior

Language disruptions among older adults are typically the results of stroke or neurocognitive degeneration (Baker, LeBlanc, & Raetz, 2008). Although the broader field of gerontology has studied changes in verbal behavior among older adults, Sundberg (1991) was among the first to point out the potential to understand, assess, and address changes in verbal behavior among older adults from a behavior-analytic perspective. Sundberg argued:

> It is a known fact that the verbal repertoires of elderly individuals tend to weaken. However, it is unclear what the crucial variables are. It is often assumed that biological deterioration is responsible for verbal problems, when quite possibly, it is environment deterioration that is the key variable. (p. 84)

Several studies in behavioral gerontology have provided evidence that supports Sundberg's claim. For example, Blackman, Howe, and Pinkston (1976), Carroll (1978), Quattrochi-Tubin and Jason (1980), Carstensen and Erickson (1986), and Bourgeois (1993) provided evidence that simple antecedent environmental manipulations (e.g., providing refreshments, rearranging rooms, providing memory books) resulted in increased interaction and verbal statements among older adults. However, Carstensen and Erickson argued that simply increasing the rate of interaction was not enough.

Henry and Horne (2000) were the first to apply Skinner's analysis to address language changes among older adults with neurocognitive disorders. The authors attempted to reestablish echoic (repeating what someone said), tact (labeling items), and mand compliance (complying with requests

from another individual) repertoires among five older adults with varying levels of cognitive impairment. Although the overall effects of the intervention were limited, Henry and Horne argued that replications were needed. Even though the participants had very few and weak remaining repertoires (e.g., one participant engaged only in echoic behavior), interventions produced increases in responding.

Baker et al. (2008) provided a behavioral conceptualization of aphasia to explain unusual patterns of skill loss common in older adults. Although not experimental in nature, this paper provided a behavioral framework for assessing language deficits and abilities (cf. Henry & Horne, 2000) that behavior analysts could use to program interventions. Gross, Fuqua, and Merritt (2013) expanded upon Baker et al. by developing and using an assessment to show evidence of verbal-operant deficits among older adults with neurocognitive disorders. They also demonstrated the functional independence of those deficits. For example, an older adult could not say, "Unicorn," in the presence of a picture of a horse with a spiraled horn on its head (a tact), but could say the word when asked to read the letters U-N-I-C-O-R-N (a textual). Such results are important, as functionally independent deficits mean that researchers can use responses that are still occurring (e.g., the textual response in the unicorn example) to prompt a response when it normally does not occur (e.g., the tact in the unicorn example) and then transfer stimulus control from one response to another. Oleson and Baker (2014) used a combination of the Baker et al. and Gross et al. assessments to evaluate mand repertoires. The assessments that Baker et al. and Gross et al. proposed constitute an important advancement in the science of behavioral gerontology. The behavior-analytic assessments incorporate ways to evaluate age-related changes that the larger field of gerontology and basic behavior-analytic research has identified, such as changes in stimulus control, and can inform intervention directly.

Several investigators have evaluated strategies to remediate language deficits, such as those observed in adults with aphasia and neurocognitive disorders. Most research has focused on establishing either echoic repertoires (e.g., Dixon, Baker, & Sadowski, 2011; Henry & Horne, 2000) or mand repertoires (i.e., requesting an item; e.g., Løkke, Granmo, Leirvick, & Lund, 2013; Oleson & Baker, 2014; Trahan et al., 2014). Baker et al. (2008) suggested that procedures for transfer of stimulus control might prove an effective way to reteach verbal behavior among older adults with language deficits. Oleson and Baker (2014) demonstrated that such an approach could be effective. Most recently, Ritchie et al. (2019) evaluated different transfer-of-stimulus-control procedures that might prove most useful. They compared time delays where they presented the prompt initially and subsequently delayed its presentation to a prompt–prompt–probe method.

Verbal behavior remains an important area for future research. Changes in verbal behavior are of great interest in the broader field of gerontology. However, most research has focused on assessing deficits that gerontologists believe have a biological etiology. Behavior analysis is poised well to provide a technology for intervening on and remediating verbal deficits among older adults where no other options exist.

## SUMMARY AND CONCLUSIONS

The broader field of gerontology highly values applications targeted toward the many socially important aging-related issues that researchers need to address. Current topics in mainstream gerontology research include health and diet, poor fluid intake, hospital readmission for acute health issues, ambulation, activities of daily living, disengagement in aging-care facilities, minimizing the use of physical and chemical restraints, and increasing the amount of meaningful activities that nursing homes offer residents (Drossel & Trahan, 2015; Fisher, Drossel, Yury, & Cherup, 2007; Kales, Gitlin, & Lyketsos, 2015; Tolson et al., 2011). However, most mainstream research is descriptive (Montgomery, 1996) or focused only on assessment, with little research on efficacious interventions for these issues. Behavior analysts interested in aging have almost unlimited potential for research and clinical opportunity, due to the growing demand by older adults for a range of services.

Although behavioral gerontology has enormous potential for positive social impact, several prominent behavior analysts have suggested that behavioral gerontology has not flourished as a subfield (Burgio & Burgio, 1986; Carstensen, 1988) and has not fully explored all potential applications of behavior analysis to aging (Derenne & Baron, 2002). Interested behavior analysts may have difficulty expanding into services for aging adults, due to the scope of their training and experience. Many applied behavior analysts receive training

primarily with children and young adults with autism spectrum disorder, with intellectual and developmental disabilities, or with both, rather than with older adults. Though the concepts and principles of behavior analysis are the same, numerous important clinical considerations involved in working with older adults necessitate specific training and supervision before marketing services to a new client base. LeBlanc, Heinicke, and Baker (2012) describe two tasks behavior analysts might focus on when considering expanding into aging services: (1) increasing professional competence with older adults, and (2) identifying and managing employment opportunities. LeBlanc et al. broke each task into component activities, such as reading the literature, pursuing supervision, and obtaining professional credentials, and provided guidance for engaging in the activities. The societal need is great, and we hope that at least some behavior analysts will become interested in pursuing a new area and will expand the impact of behavior analysis into aging services, making effective interventions available to more older adults.

Behavior analysts must continue to publish studies in aging journals and journals specific to other disciplines, such as nursing and occupational therapy, to introduce these groups to the benefits of the behavioral approach. However, behavior analysts also must continue to publish enough studies on behavioral gerontology in flagship behavior-analytic outlets to ensure that new behavior analysts become interested in the field. The field needs additional basic operant studies with humans for virtually every aspect of responding that age-related changes might impact. The applied area needs more studies that incorporate functional assessment and address health and mental health issues in community-dwelling older adults. There have been relatively few functional-analytic studies of older adults with neurocognitive disorders, compared to the thriving literature on functional analysis with individuals with developmental disabilities (Hanley, Iwata, & McCord, 2003), even though the adults with neurocognitive disorders are just as likely to have behaviors that staff members identify as challenging or difficult to manage. Though research suggests that function-based interventions are promising, little research has evaluated whether effective function-based interventions for problem behavior can reduce the need for medications, which is a concern in aging research now (Kales et al., 2015). Behavior analysts would do well to become familiar with the effects prescription medications can have on behavioral processes. Laraway, Snycerski, Michael, and Poling (2003) highlighted the varying effects that pharmaceutical interventions can have on motivating operations, particularly on establishing and abolishing operations for reinforcers and punishers. Additionally, Valdovinos and Kennedy (2004) noted that pharmacological studies primarily focus on unintended or unwanted side effects such as sweating, diarrhea, or tremors, but seldom discuss their effects on behavioral processes. Side effects of psychotropic medications could influence motivating variables, disrupt stimulus control, or establish new discriminative stimuli (Valdovinos & Kennedy, 2004).

## REFERENCES

Adkins, V. K., & Mathews, R. M. (1999). Behavioral gerontology: State of the science. *Journal of Clinical Geropsychology, 5*, 39–49.

Altus, D. E., Engelman, K. K., & Mathews, R. M. (2002a). Increasing mealtime participation and communication of persons with dementia. *Journal of Gerontological Nursing, 28*, 47–53.

Altus, D. E., Engelman, K. K., & Mathews, R. M. (2002b). Finding a practical method to increase engagement of residents of a dementia care unit. *American Journal of Alzheimer's Disease and Related Disorders, 17*, 245–248.

Arean, P. A. (2004). Psychosocial treatments for depression in the elderly. *Primary Psychiatry, 11*, 48–53.

Baker, J. C., Fairchild, K., & Seefeldt, D. (2015). Behavioral gerontology: Research and clinical considerations. In H. S. Roane, J. E. Ringdahl, & T. S. Falcomata (Eds.), *Clinical and organizational applications of applied behavior analysis* (pp. 425–450). San Diego, CA: Academic Press/Elsevier.

Baker, J., Hanley, G. P., & Mathews, R. M. (2006). Staff administered functional analysis and treatment of aggression by an elder with dementia. *Journal of Applied Behavior Analysis, 39*, 469–474.

Baker, J. C., & LeBlanc, L. A. (2011). Acceptability of interventions for aggressive behavior in long-term care settings: Comparing ratings and hierarchical selection. *Behavior Therapy, 42*, 30–41.

Baker, J. C., LeBlanc, L. A., & Raetz, P. B. (2008). A behavioral conceptualization of aphasia. *Analysis of Verbal Behavior, 24*, 147–158.

Baker, J. C., LeBlanc, L. A., Raetz, P. B., & Hilton, L. C. (2011). Assessment and treatment of hoarding in an individual with dementia. *Behavior Therapy, 42*, 135–142.

Baltes, M., & Barton, E. (1977). Behavioral analysis of aging: A review of the operant model and research. *Educational Gerontology: An International Quarterly, 2*, 383–405.

Beaton, S., Peeler, C. M., & Harvey, T. (2006). A functional analysis and treatment of the irrational and rational statements of an elderly woman with Alzheimer's disease. *Behavioral Interventions, 21*(1), 1–12.

Beattie, S., Wagner, S., & Baker, J. C. (2019). *Evaluation of preference and subsequent stimulus engagement among older adults with neurocognitive disorder.* Manuscript in preparation.

Belsky, J. (1999). *The psychology of aging: Theory, research, and interventions.* Belmont, CA: Brooks/Cole.

Birren, J. E., & Schaie, K. W. (Eds.). (2001). *Handbook of the psychology of aging* (5th ed.). San Diego, CA: Academic Press.

Blackman, D. K., Howe, M., & Pinkston, E. M. (1976). Increasing participation in social interaction of the institutionalized elderly. *Gerontologist, 16*, 69–76.

Blazer, D. (1993). *Depression in late life* (2nd ed.). St. Louis, MO: Mosby.

Bourgeois, M. (1993). Effects of memory aids on the dyadic conversations of individuals with dementia. *Journal of Applied Behavior Analysis, 26*, 77–87.

Buchanan, J. A., & Fisher, J. E. (2002). Functional assessment and noncontingent reinforcement in the treatment of disruptive vocalization in elderly dementia patients. *Journal of Applied Behavior Analysis, 35*, 99–103.

Buchanan, J., Husfeldt, J., Berg, T., & Houlihan, D. (2011). Publication trends in behavioral gerontology in the past 25 years: Are the elderly still an understudied population in behavioral research? *Behavioral Interventions, 23*, 65–74.

Burgio, K., & Locher, J. (1996). Urinary incontinence. In L. Carstensen, B. Edelstein, & L. Dornbrand (Eds.), *The practical handbook of clinical gerontology* (pp. 349–373). Thousand Oaks, CA: Sage.

Burgio, L. D., & Burgio, K. L. (1986). Behavioral gerontology: Application of behavioral methods to the problems of older adults. *Journal of Applied Behavior Analysis, 19*, 321–328.

Burgio, L., Scilley, K., Hardin, J. M., Hsu, C., & Yancey, J. (1996). Environmental "white noise": An intervention for verbally agitated nursing home residents. *Journal of Gerontology, 51B*, 364–373.

Burgio, L., Stevens, A., Burgio, K., Roth, D., Paul, P., & Gerstle, J. (2002). Teaching and maintaining behavior management in the nursing home. *Gerontologist, 42*, 487–496.

Burton, J. R., Pearce, K. L., Burgio, K. L., Engel, B. T., & Whitehead, W. E. (1988). Behavioral training for urinary incontinence in the elderly ambulatory patient. *Journal of the American Geriatrics Society, 36*, 693–698.

Butler, R. N., Finkel, S. I., Lewis, M. I., Sherman, F. T., & Sunderland, T. (1992). Aging and mental health: Primary care of the healthy older adult. A roundtable discussion: Part I. *Geriatrics, 47*, 54, 56, 61–65.

Carroll, P. S. (1978). The social hour for geropsychiatric patients. *Journal of American Geriatrics Society, 11*, 32–35.

Carstensen, L. L. (1988). The emerging field of behavioral gerontology. *Behavior Therapy, 19,* 259–281.

Carstensen, L. L., & Erickson, R. J. (1986). Enhancing the social environments of elderly nursing home residents: Are high rates of interaction enough? *Journal of Applied Behavior Analysis, 19,* 349–355.

Charlesworth, G., Sadek, S., Schepers, A., & Spector, A. (2015). Cognitive behavior therapy for anxiety in people with dementia: A clinician guideline for a person-centered approach. *Behavior Modification, 39,* 390–412.

Cheng, D. T., Faulkner, M. L., Disterhoft, J. F., & Desmond, J. E. (2010). The effects of aging in delay and trace human eyeblink conditioning. *Psychology and Aging, 25,* 684–690.

Cherry, K. E., & Smith, A. D. (1998). Normal memory aging. In M. Hersen & V. B. Van Hasselt (Eds.), *Handbook of clinical geropsychology* (pp. 87–110). New York: Plenum Press.

Colby, S. L., & Ortman, J. M. (2014). *Projections of the size and composition of the U.S. population: 2014 to 2060* (Current Population Reports, No. P25-1143). Washington, DC: U.S. Census Bureau. Retrieved from *www.census.gov/content/dam/Census/library/publications/2015/demo/p25-1143.pdf.*

DeLeon, I. G., & Iwata, J. C. (1996). Evaluation of a multiple-stimulus presentation format for assessing reinforcer preferences. *Journal of Applied Behavior Analysis, 29,* 519–533.

Derenne, A., & Baron, A. (2002). Behavior analysis and the study of human aging. *Behavior Analyst, 25,* 151–160.

DeVries, H. M., & Coon, D. W. (2002). Cognitive/behavioral group therapy with older adults. In F. W. Kaslow & T. Patterson (Eds.), *Comprehensive handbook of psychotherapy: Cognitive-behavioral approaches* (Vol. 2, pp. 547–576). New York: Wiley.

Dick, L. P., & Gallagher-Thompson, D. (1996). Late-life depression. In M. Hersen & V. B. Van Hasselt (Eds.), *Psychological treatment of older adults: An introductory text* (pp. 181–208). New York: Plenum Press.

Dick, L. P., Gallagher-Thompson, D., & Thompson, L. W. (1996). Cognitive-behavioral therapy. In R. T. Woods (Ed.), *Handbook of the clinical psychology of aging* (pp. 509–544). Chichester, UK: Wiley.

Dixon, M., Baker, J. C., & Sadowski, K. A. (2011). Applying Skinner's analysis of verbal behavior to persons with dementia. *Behavior Therapy, 42,* 120–126.

Drossel, C., & Trahan, M. A. (2015). Behavioral interventions are the first-line treatments for managing changes associated with cognitive decline. *Behavior Therapist, 38*(5), 126–131.

Dupree, L., & Schonfeld, L. (1998). The value of behavioral perspectives in treating older adults. In M. Hersen & V. B. Van Hasselt (Eds.), *Handbook of clinical geropsychology* (pp. 51–70). New York: Plenum Press.

Dwyer-Moore, K. J., & Dixon, M. R. (2007). Functional analysis and treatment of problem behavior of elderly adults in long-term care settings. *Journal of Applied Behavior Analysis, 40,* 679–684.

Engelman, K. K., Altus, D. E., & Mathews, R. M. (1999). Increasing engagement in daily activities by older adults with dementia. *Journal of Applied Behavior Analysis, 32,* 107–110.

Engstrom, E., Mudford, O. C., & Brand, D. (2015). Replication and extension of a check-in procedure to increase activity engagement among people with severe dementia. *Journal of Applied Behavior Analysis, 48,* 460–465.

Fantol, J. A., Wyman, J. F., Harkins, S. W., & Hadley, E. C. (1990). Bladder training in the management of lower urinary tract dysfunction in women: A review. *Journal of the American Geriatrics Society, 38,* 329–332.

Feliciano, L., LeBlanc, L. A., & Feeney, B. J. (2010). Assessment and management of barriers to fluid intake in community dwelling older adults. *Journal of Behavioral Health and Medicine, 1,* 3–14.

Feliciano, L., Steers, M. E., Elite-Marcandontou, A., McLane, M., & Areán, P. A. (2009). Applications of preference assessment procedures in depression and agitation management in elders with dementia. *Clinical Gerontologist, 32,* 239–259.

Finkbiner, R., & Woodruff-Pak, D. (1991). Classical eye-blink conditioning in adulthood: Effects of age and interstimulus interval on acquisition in the trace paradigm. *Psychology and Aging, 6,* 109–117.

Fisher, J. E., & Buchanan, J. A. (2018). Presentation of preferred stimuli as an intervention for aggression in a person with dementia. *Behavior Analysis: Research and Practice, 18,* 33–40.

Fisher, J. E., Drossel, C., Yury, C., & Cherup, S. (2007). A contextual model of restraint-free care for persons with dementia. In P. Sturmey (Ed.), *Functional analysis in clinical treatment* (pp. 211–237). Burlington, MA: Academic Press/Elsevier.

Fisher, J. E., & Noll, J. (1996). Age-associated differences in sensitivity to reinforcement frequency. *Journal of Clinical Geropsychology, 2,* 297–306.

Fisher, W., Piazza, C. C., Bowman, L. G., Hagopian, L. P., Owens, J. C., & Slevin, I. (1992). A comparison of two approaches for identifying reinforcers for persons with severe and profound disabilities. *Journal of Applied Behavior Analysis, 25,* 491–498.

Gallagher-Thompson, D., & Thompson, L. W. (1996). Applying cognitive-behavioral therapy to the psychological problems of later life. In S. H. Zarit & B. G. Knight (Eds.), *A guide to psychotherapy and aging: Effective clinical interventions in a life-stage context* (pp. 61–82). Washington, DC: American Psychological Association.

Garcia, S., Feliciano, L., & Ilem, A. A. (2018). Preference assessments in older adults with dementia. *Behavior Analysis: Research and Practice, 18,* 78–91.

Gatz, M., Fiske, A., Fox, L. S., Kaskie, B., Kasl-Godsley, J. E., McCallum, T. J., et al. (1998). Empirically validated psychological treatments for older adults. *Journal of Mental Health and Ageing, 4,* 9–46.

Graves, C. A., & Solomon, P. R. (1985). Age-related disruption of trace but not delay classical conditioning of the rabbit's nictitating membrane response. *Behavioral Neuroscience, 99,* 88–96.

Gross, A. C., Fuqua, R. W., & Merritt, T. A. (2013). Evaluation of verbal behavior in older adults. *Analysis of Verbal Behavior, 29,* 85–99.

Hagopian, L. P., Long, E. S., & Rush, K. S. (2004). Preference assessment procedures for individuals with developmental disabilities. *Behavior Modification, 28,* 668–677.

Hanley, G. P., Iwata, B. A., & McCord, B. E. (2003). Functional analysis of problem behavior: A review. *Journal of Applied Behavior Analysis, 36,* 147–185.

Heard, K., & Watson, T. S. (1999). Reducing wandering by persons with dementia using differential reinforcement. *Journal of Applied Behavior Analysis, 32,* 381–384.

Henry, L. M., & Horne, P. J. (2000). Partial remediation of speaker and listener behaviors in people with severe dementia. *Journal of Applied Behavior Analysis, 33,* 631–634.

Ho, E. E., Lee, F. C., & Meyskens, F. L. (1991). An exploratory study of attitudes, beliefs and practices related to the interim dietary guidelines for reducing cancer in the elderly. *Journal of Nutrition for the Elderly, 10,* 31–49.

Hussian, R. A., & Brown, D. (1987). Use of two-dimensional grid patterns to limit hazardous ambulation in demented patients. *Journal of Gerontology, 42,* 558–560.

Ilem, A., Feliciano, L., & LeBlanc L. A. (2015). Recognition of self-referent stimuli in people with dementia: Names and pictures as prosthetic memory aids. *Clinical Gerontologist, 38*(2), 157–169.

Iwata, B. A., Pace, G. M., Cowdery, G. E., & Miltenberger, R. G. (1994). What makes extinction work: An analysis of procedural form and function. *Journal of Applied Behavior Analysis, 27,* 131–144.

Jeffcoate, T. N. (1961). Functional disturbances of the female bladder and urethra. *Journal of the Royal College of Surgeons of Edinburgh, 7,* 28–47.

Kales, H. C., Gitlin, L. N., & Lyketsos, C. G. (2015). Assessment and management of behavioral and psychological symptoms of dementia. *British Medical Journal, 350,* h369.

Kannel, W. B. (1986). Nutritional contributors to cardiovascular disease in the elderly. *Journal of the American Geriatrics Society, 34,* 27–36.

Keller, H., Beck, A. M., & Namasivayam, A. (2015). Improving food and fluid intake for older adults living in long-term care: A research agenda. *Journal of the American Medical Directors Association, 16,* 93–100.

Ladouceur, R., Leger, E., Dugas, M., & Freeston, M. H. (2004). Cognitive-behavioral treatment of generalized anxiety disorder (GAD) for older adults. *International Psychogeriatrics, 16,* 195–207.

Laraway, S., Syncerski, S., Michael, J., & Poling, A. (2003). Motivating operations and terms to describe them: Some further refinements. *Journal of Applied Behavior Analysis, 36,* 407–414.

Larrabee, D., Baker, J. C., & O'Neill, D. (2018). Effects of programmed discriminative stimuli in a functional analysis on language disruptions in older adults with neurocognitive disorders. *Behavior Analysis: Research and Practice, 18*(1), 16–32.

LeBlanc, L. A., Cherup, S. M., Feliciano, L., & Sidener, T. M. (2006). Using choice-making opportunities to increase activity engagement in individuals with dementia. *American Journal of Alzheimer's Disease and Other Dementias, 21,* 318–325.

LeBlanc, L. A., Heineke, M., & Baker, J. C. (2012). Expanding your consumer base for behavior analytic services. *Behavior Analysis in Practice, 5,* 4–14.

LeBlanc, L. A., Raetz, P. B., Baker, J. C., Strobel, M. J., & Feeney, B. J. (2008). Assessing preference in elders with dementia using multimedia and verbal Pleasant Events Schedules. *Behavioral Interventions, 23,* 213–225.

LeBlanc, L. A., Raetz, P. B., & Feliciano, L. (2011). Behavioral gerontology. In W. W. Fisher, C. C. Piazza, & H. S. Roane (Eds.), *Handbook of applied behavior analysis* (pp. 472–488). New York: Guilford Press.

Lindsley, O. R. (1964). Geriatric behavioral prosthetics. In R. Kastenbaum (Ed.), *New thoughts in old age* (pp. 41–61). New York: Springer.

Logsdon, R. G., & Teri, L. (1997). The Pleasant Events Schedule—AD: Psychometric properties and relationship to depression and cognition in Alzheimer's disease patients. *Gerontologist, 37,* 40–45.

Løkke, J. A., Granmo, S., Leirvick, S. E. S., & Lund, P. A. (2013). Prompting and influence on manding in participants with Alzheimer's disease. *Norsk Tidsskrift for Atferdsanalyse, 40,* 189–195.

McClannahan, L. E., & Risley, T. R. (1975). Design of living environments for nursing-home residents: Increasing participation in recreation activities. *Journal of Applied Behavior Analysis, 8,* 261–268.

Mehta, K. M., Simonsick, E. M., Penninx, B., Schulz, R., Rubin, S., Scatterfield, S., et al. (2003). Prevalence and correlates of anxiety symptoms in well-functioning older adults: Findings from the Health Aging and Body Composition Study. *Journal of the American Geriatrics Society, 51,* 499–504.

Meichenbaum, D., & Turk, D. (1987). *Facilitating treatment adherence: A practitioner's guidebook.* New York: Plenum Press.

Mojtabai, R., & Olfson, M. (2004). Cognitive deficits and the course of major depression in a cohort of middle-aged and older community-dwelling adults. *Journal of the American Geriatrics Society, 52,* 1060–1069.

Molinari, V., Karel, M., Jones, S., Zeiss, A., Cooley, S. G., Wray, L., et al. (2003). Recommendations about the knowledge and skills required of psychologists working with older adults. *Professional Psychology: Research and Practice, 34,* 435–443.

Moniz-Cook, E., Stokes, G., & Agar, S. (2003). Difficult

behaviour and dementia in nursing homes: Five cases of psychosocial intervention. *Clinical Psychology and Psychotherapy, 10,* 197–208.

Moniz-Cook, E., Woods, R. T., & Richards, K. (2001). Functional analysis of challenging behaviour in dementia: The role of superstition. *International Journal of Geriatric Psychiatry, 16,* 45–56.

Montgomery, R. J. V. (1996). Advancing caregiver research: Weighing efficacy and feasibility of interventions. *Journal of Gerontology: Social Sciences, 51*(3), S109–S110.

Noguchi, D., Kawano, Y., & Yamanaka, K. (2013). Care staff training in residential homes for managing behavioral and psychological symptoms of dementia based on different reinforcement procedures of applied behavior analysis: A process research. *Psychogeriatrics, 13,* 108–117.

Oleson, C. R., & Baker, J. C. (2014). Teaching mands to older adults with dementia. *Analysis of Verbal Behavior, 30,* 113–127.

Pachis, J. A., & Zonneveld, K. L. M. (2019). Comparison of prompting procedures to teach Internet skills to older adults. *Journal of Applied Behavior Analysis, 52,* 173–187.

Pellegrin, L. D., Peters, M. E., Lyketsos, C. G., & Marano, C. M. (2013). Depression in cognitive impairment. *Current Psychiatry Reports, 15,* 383–391.

Perez-Gonzalez, L. A., & Moreno-Sierra, V. (1999). Equivalence class formations in elderly persons. *Psicothema, 11,* 325–336.

Plaud, J. J., Plaud, D. M., & von Duvillard, S. (1999). Human behavioral momentum in a sample of older adults. *Journal of General Psychology, 126,* 165–175.

Quattrochi-Tubin, S., & Jason, L. A. (1980). Enhancing social interactions and activity among the elderly through stimulus control. *Journal of Applied Behavior Analysis, 13,* 159–169.

Quick, M. J., Baker, J. C., & Ringdahl, J. E. (2018). Assessing the validity of engagement-based and selection-based preference assessments in elderly individuals with dementia. *Behavior Analysis: Research and Practice, 18*(1), 92–102.

Raetz, P. B., LeBlanc, L. A., Baker, J. C., & Hilton, L. (2013). Utility of the multiple stimulus without replacement procedure and stability of preferences of older adults with dementia. *Journal of Applied Behavior Analysis. 46,* 765–780.

Ritchie, H., Reuter-Yuill, L., Perez, A., & Baker, J. C. (2019). *Assessment and treatment of verbal behavior deficits with an older adult diagnosed with aphasia and a comparison of transfer of stimulus control procedures.* Manuscript accepted for publication.

Roane, H. S., Vollmer, T. R., Ringdahl, J. E., & Marcus, B. A. (1998). Evaluation of a brief stimulus preference assessment. *Journal of Applied Behavior Analysis, 31,* 605–620.

Sands, D., & Holman, E. (1985). Does knowledge enhance patient compliance? *Journal of Gerontological Nursing, 11,* 23–29.

Sanservo, A. C. (1997). Dehydration in the elderly: Strategies for prevention and management. *Nurse Practitioner, 22,* 41–70.

Saunders, R. R., Chaney, L., & Marquis, J. G. (2005). Equivalence class establishment with two-, three-, and four-choice matching to sample by senior citizens. *Psychological Record, 55,* 539–559.

Schnelle, J. F., Leung, F. W., Rao, S. S. C., Beusher, L., Keeler, M., Clift, J. W., et al. (2010). A controlled trial of an intervention to improve urinary/fecal incontinence and constipation. *Journal of the American Geriatrics Society, 58,* 1504–1511.

Simmons, S. F., Alessi, C., & Schnelle, J. F. (2001). An intervention to increase fluid intake in nursing home residents: Prompting and preference compliance. *Journal of the American Geriatrics Society, 49,* 926–933.

Skinner, B. F. (1983). Intellectual self-management in old age. *American Psychologist, 38,* 239–244.

Sorocco, K., Kinoshita, L., & Gallagher-Thompson, D. (2005). Mental health and aging: Current trends and future directions. In J. E. Maddux & B. A. Winstead (Eds.), *Psychopathology: Foundations for a contemporary understanding* (pp. 393–419). Mahwah, NJ: Erlbaum.

Spangler, P. F., Risley, T. R., & Bilyew, D. D. (1984). The management of dehydration and incontinence in nonambulatory geriatric patients. *Journal of Applied Behavior Analysis, 17,* 397–401.

Stanley, M. A., Diefenbach, G. J., & Hopko, D. R. (2004). Cognitive behavioral treatment for older adults with generalized anxiety disorders: A therapist manual for primary care settings. *Behavior Modification, 28,* 73–117.

Stein, M. B. (2004). Public health perspectives on generalized anxiety disorder. *Journal of Clinical Psychiatry, 65,* 3–7.

Steinberg, M., Sheppard, J., Tschanz, J. T., Norton, M. C., Steffens, D. C., Breitner, J. C. S., et al. (2003). The incidence of mental and behavioral disturbances in dementia: The Cache County study. *Journal of Neuropsychiatry and Clinical Neurosciences, 15,* 340–345.

Steingrimsdottir, H. S., & Arntzen, E. (2014). Performance by older adults on identity and arbitrary matching-to-sample tasks. *Psychological Record, 64,* 827–839.

Stock, L. Z., & Milan, M. A. (1993). Improving dietary practices of elderly individuals: The power of prompting, feedback, and social reinforcement. *Journal of Applied Behavior Analysis, 26,* 379–387.

Sundberg, M. L. (1991). 301 research topics from Skinner's book *Verbal Behavior. Analysis of Verbal Behavior, 9,* 81–96.

Teri, L. (1991). Behavioral assessment and treatment of depression in older adults. In P. Wisocki (Ed.), *Handbook of clinical behavior therapy with the elderly client* (pp. 225–240). New York: Plenum Press.

Teri, L., & Logsdon, R. G. (1991). Identifying pleasant activities for Alzheimer's disease patients: The

Pleasant Events Schedule—AD. *Gerontologist, 31,* 124–127.

Thompson, L. W., Futterman, A., & Gallagher, D. (1988). Assessment of late-life depression. *Psychopharmacology Bulletin, 24,* 577–586.

Tolson, D., Rolland, Y., Andrieu, S., Aquino, J. P., Beard, J., Benetos, A., et al. (2011). International association of gerontology and geriatrics: A global agenda for clinical research and quality of life in nursing homes. *Journal of the American Medical Directors Association, 12,* 184–189.

Tonga, J. B., Karlsoeen, B. B., Arnevik, E. A., Werheid, K., Korsnes, M. S., & Ulstein, I. D. (2015). Challenges with manual-based multimodal psychotherapy for people with Alzheimer's disease: A case study. *American Journal of Alzheimer's Disease and Other Dementias, 31*(4), 311–317.

Trahan, M. A., Donaldson, J. M., McNabney, M. K., & Kahng, S. (2014). Training and maintenance of a picture-based communication response in older adults with dementia. *Journal of Applied Behavior Analysis, 47,* 404–409.

Tripp, G., & Alsop, B. (1999). Age-related changes in sensitivity to relative reward frequency. *New Zealand Journal of Psychology, 28,* 30–36.

Valdovinos, M. G., & Kennedy, C. H. (2004). A behavior-analytic conceptualization of the side effects of psychotropic medication. *Behavior Analyst, 27,* 231–238.

Virues-Ortega, J., Iwata, B. A., Nogales-González, C., & Frades, B. (2012). Assessment of preference for edible and leisure items in individuals with dementia. *Journal of Applied Behavior Analysis, 45,* 839–844.

Warren, J. L., Bacon, W. E., Harris, T., McBean, A. M.,

Foley, D. J., & Phillips, C. (1994). The burden and outcomes associated with dehydration among U.S. elderly, 1991. *American Journal of Public Health, 84,* 1265–1269.

Wild, B., Eckl, A., Herzog, W., Niehoff, D., Lechner, S., Maatouk, I., et al. (2010). Assessing generalized anxiety disorder in elderly people using the GAD-7 and GAD-2 scales: Results of a validation study. *American Journal of Geriatric Psychiatry, 22,* 1029–1039.

Williamson, P. N., & Ascione, F. R. (1983). Behavioral treatment of the elderly: Implications for theory and therapy. *Behavior Modification, 7,* 583–610.

Wilson, K. M., & Milan, M. A. (1995). Age differences in the formation of equivalence classes. *Journal of Gerontology: Series B: Psychological Sciences and Social Sciences, 50B,* 212–218.

Woodruff-Pak, D. (2001). Eyeblink classical conditioning differentiates normal aging from Alzheimer's disease. *Integrative Physiological and Behavioral Science, 36,* 87–108.

Woodruff-Pak, D., & Jaeger, M. (1998). Predictors of eyeblink classical conditioning over the life span. *Psychology and Aging, 13,* 193–205.

Woodruff-Pak, D., Papka, M., Romano, S., & Li, Y. (1996). Eyeblink classical conditioning in Alzheimer's disease and cerebrovascular dementia. *Neurobiology of Aging, 17,* 505–512.

Woodruff-Pak, D., & Thompson, R. (1988). Classical conditioning of the eyeblink response in the delay paradigm in adults aged 18–23. *Psychology and Aging, 3,* 219–229.

Zarit, S., & Zarit, J. (1998). *Mental disorders in older adults: Fundamentals of assessment and treatment.* New York: Guilford Press.

# CHAPTER 31

# Telehealth and Applied Behavior Analysis

David P. Wacker, Kelly M. Schieltz, Alyssa N. Suess, and Scott D. Lindgren

Applied behavior analysts at the Center for Disabilities and Development and the Department of Pediatrics at The University of Iowa have used telehealth to assess and treat problem behavior since the late 1990s (see Barretto, Wacker, Harding, Lee, & Berg, 2006). The Center for Disabilities and Development has had a telehealth center for over 10 years. Federal grants and the Department of Pediatrics have supported our involvement in telehealth, which is part of a national movement to use telehealth services across all subdisciplines in medicine. Our hospital recently developed an e-health department, whose specific function is to advance telehealth services throughout Iowa while addressing issues ranging from reimbursement to technology. In this chapter, we first define telehealth and briefly describe how pediatric subspecialties and applied behavior analysts have used telehealth services nationally. We specifically describe the development of telehealth services at Iowa and current applications, and we discuss questions and concerns regarding further expansion of telehealth services. We conclude the chapter by suggesting some future directions that applied behavior analysts might consider.

## DEFINITION OF TELEHEALTH

*Telehealth* is an umbrella term that encompasses many health-related services using technology to exchange information from one site to another via electronic communications to improve health outcomes, lower costs, and provide better care (American Telemedicine Association, 2016; Center for Connected Health Policy, 2016; Committee on Pediatric Workforce, 2015). Throughout this chapter, we use the term *telehealth* interchangeably with the traditional term, *telemedicine*. Much of the telehealth literature demonstrates its application to healthcare in four broad categories: consultation, diagnosis, training, and intervention (see Figure 31.1). According to the Center for Connected Health Policy (2016), the electronic communications most commonly used in telehealth include *synchronous interactions*, *asynchronous interactions*, *remote patient monitoring*, and *mobile health*. Synchronous interactions (aka: live video or real time) are live, two-way interactions between a client (i.e., a patient, care provider, or professional) and a provider, whereas asynchronous interactions (aka: store and forward) are transmissions of prerecorded health information to a provider who evaluates the information later. Providers use remote patient monitoring and mobile health to track and monitor patient health outcomes and to provide health education and practice to promote healthy behavior, respectively.

Telehealth is not considered a replacement for in-person health care delivery, but rather a tool or supplement to deliver the same or an enhanced level of care typically provided at a distance. The

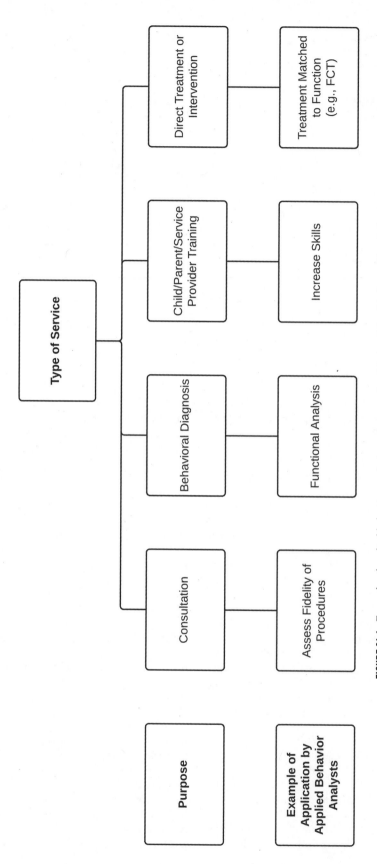

**FIGURE 31.1.** Example of applied behavior analysis services conducted via telehealth for problem behavior.

most common use of telehealth is the delivery of subspecialty consultation (Burke, Hall, & the Section on Telehealth Care, 2015; Committee on Pediatric Workforce, 2015). Variations occur in definition, reimbursement, and restrictions of telehealth across states. For example, according to Gutierrez (2015), some states define only telehealth or only telemedicine, whereas others define both terms in law or policy regulations. Forty-seven states have written policies regarding Medicaid reimbursement for telehealth, whereas 29 states have laws governing private-payer telehealth reimbursement. The most commonly reimbursed form of telehealth is clinic-to-clinic live video. In addition, other restrictions, such as the originating or distant site, informed consent, and licensure laws, vary by state. The patient's home is often a nonreimbursable site; most states require informed consent; and payers reimburse service provision out of state only if the provider meets specific conditions.

## APPLICATIONS OF TELEHEALTH

We focus in the current chapter on the application of synchronous and asynchronous telehealth during consultation, diagnosis, training, and intervention services. In the first subsection below, we briefly describe pediatric subspecialty services, to provide applied behavior analysts with a greater context for understanding telehealth services. In the next section, we describe applications of telehealth involving applied behavior analysis (ABA), with specific examples from services we deliver in Iowa.

### Selected Applications across Pediatric Subspecialties

Many subspecialties in pediatrics—including radiology, dermatology, cardiology, neonatalogy, pathology, emergency services, child abuse, chronic disease, mental health, and dentistry—have embraced telehealth, with services spanning consultation, diagnosis, training, and intervention (Burke et al., 2015; Spooner, Gotlieb, the Steering Committee on Clinical Information Technology, & the Committee on Medical Liability, 2004). In addition, health care providers have delivered telehealth services in schools and homes to expand the breadth and quality of pediatric services while decreasing other factors, such as school absenteeism and medical risk for homebound patients (Spooner et al., 2004).

### Consultation

During *telehealth consultation*, a provider (often a specialist) gives care or advice to a client or patient (e.g., a child, parent, or teacher) who is in a different geographic location from the provider (Telehealth Resource Centers, 2016). Health care professionals have used telehealth to provide consultation to caregivers, teachers, and other professionals. As an example, the University of California Davis Medical Center developed a telehealth consultation program to manage pediatric obesity. A pediatrician and a registered dietician provided consultation to children and their caregivers who traveled to their nearby community clinics. Researchers at University of California Davis Medical Center compared the effectiveness of the synchronous telehealth consultation program to typical face-to-face consultation, and the results demonstrated that telehealth consultation showed (1) greater improvement in nutrition, (2) increases in activity level, and (3) decreases in screen time (Santiago Lipana, Bindal, Nettiksimmons, & Shaikh, 2013).

Medical professionals also have provided consultation via telehealth to parents directly in their children's schools. Langkamp, McManus, and Blakemore (2015) developed a program called Tele-Health Kids for children with developmental disabilities and their parents to receive asynchronous consultation for minor illnesses from primary care physicians directly in the children's schools. Parents rated their satisfaction with the school-based telehealth consultation as high. The benefits from the telehealth consultation included decreases in travel time, decreases in parent and child stress, increases in successful examinations, and fewer occurrences of problem behavior during the examination. Research has shown that similar school-based consultation is effective with teen parents (Nelson, Citarelli, Cook, & Shaw, 2003) and for children with complex medical needs (Looman et al., 2015) and behavioral needs (Bassingthwaite et al., 2018).

Professionals have used telehealth for peer-to-peer consultation. Callahan, Malone, Estroff, and Person (2005) evaluated the impact of a store-and-forward teleconsultation system on children's access to specialty care, quality of care received, and cost savings. The Electronic Children's Hospital of the Pacific is a teleconsultation system for military treatment facilities in the Pacific, in which a primary care physician requests consultation with pediatric subspecialists by entering information about the patient and uploading any still or motion images to a secure, encrypted website. Subspecialists receive notification of the consultation submission; review the patient's information; and provide recommendations on diagnosis, intervention, or both on the website. Results of this study demonstrated that primary care physicians received consultations from 33 different pediatric subspecialists, and that the median consult response time was 12 hours. In addition, the quality of care improved (as shown by changes in diagnosis, the diagnostic plan, or the intervention plan) for 15%, 21%, and 24% of cases, respectively. Finally, costs decreased because patients avoided travel to the medical center (typically a 5-hour plane flight and 1-week hospital stay) for 12% of cases. Similar peer-to-peer consultations conducted in real time have demonstrated changes in diagnosis, diagnostic plans, or intervention plans for children with obesity (Shaikh, Cole, Marcin, & Nesbitt, 2008), and have produced decreased patient transfers and costs for children presenting to rural emergency departments with acute illness or injury that required immediate physician involvement (Yang et al., 2015).

## Diagnosis

During *telehealth diagnosis*, a specialist makes or assists another provider to make a diagnosis for a patient (American Telemedicine Association, 2016), using synchronous and asynchronous formats. An off-site pediatric cardiologist, for example, might watch and listen to a live heart study in real time while guiding the on-site provider to obtain additional views of the heart during synchronous diagnostic consultation. By contrast, an off-site cardiologist using asynchronous diagnostic consultation might receive still, motion, or both kinds of images to review and interpret later (Sable, 2003). Research has shown that these telehealth diagnostic methods in pediatric cardiology are effective for many pediatric populations, including fetuses and neonates (Gomes et al., 2010), and for diagnoses ranging from no heart disease to pathological heart disease (Gomes et al., 2010; Mahnke et al., 2008). Specifically, results of these studies indicated that health care providers made or confirmed accurate diagnoses via telehealth, which in turn guided treatment plan initiations or changes and contributed to decisions regarding the necessity of emergency patient transfers. Research has produced similar results in pediatric dermatology, in which health care professionals provided accurate diagnoses for many dermatological issues via telehealth (Heffner, Lyon, Brousseau, Holland, & Yen, 2009).

## Training

*Telehealth training* refers to using technology to conduct specialized training on specific topics and to engage in online discussions with groups to provide peer-to-peer support and education (American Telemedicine Association, 2016). The primary example of training in medicine has been the Extension for Community Healthcare Outcomes project or Project ECHO, which was "designed to improve patient care by developing and supporting the competence of primary care providers in underserved areas to manage complex disorders" (Arora et al., 2007, p. 154). Researchers first developed Project ECHO at the University of New Mexico to address high rates of the Hepatitis C virus, which is amenable to treatment but time-consuming to treat and often beyond the scope of practice for many primary care physicians. The Project ECHO training model focuses on case-based, disease-specific learning during weekly 2-hour virtual visits in which primary care physicians present relevant cases from their practices, and specialists instruct and guide these physicians through appropriate care management (Arora et al., 2011). The benefits of this training model are twofold. First, primary care physicians develop content knowledge and skills for managing specific illnesses, as well as a network of colleagues to consult with on arising issues (Arora et al., 2011). Second, patients receive safer and more comprehensive care for illnesses that typically require specialty services often not available readily in the patients' communities (Arora et al., 2007). After the initial success of Project ECHO, others have applied the program to many specialty health care needs, including pediatric obesity (Arora et al., 2007), early detection of autism spectrum disorder (ASD) (Arora et al., 2011), treatment for ASD symptoms (Mazurek, Brown, Curran, & Sohl, 2017), and children and youth with epilepsy (American Academy of Pediatrics, 2016).

## Intervention

*Telehealth intervention* refers to an off-site professional providing intervention services, often indirectly via remote patient monitoring (American Telemedicine Association, 2016). For example, Ghio et al. (2002) used telehealth with two children who were receiving automated peritoneal dialysis treatment. The system transmitted and stored the peritoneal dialysis data from the children's peritoneal dialysis cycler to a computer in the dialysis lab. Thus the physician could remotely monitor skipped or shortened treatment, changes to the therapy parameters, skipped phases or cycles, or reduced fill volumes, which indicated whether the patients and families were complying with the dialysis treatment. In addition, real-time telehealth visits occurred at least every 3 days to follow up on collected data, compliance with treatment, additional clinical problems, and technical problems. Results of the remote-monitoring data demonstrated that the children in this study always complied with the dialysis treatment. Overall, these results demonstrated the effectiveness of telehealth for home dialysis patients. Izquierdo et al. (2009) produced similar results for children with Type 1 diabetes, in which the nurses at the children's school connected with the diabetes center via telehealth to obtain consultation and education. Researchers observed decreases in hemoglobin A1c and emergency visits to the nurses.

## Selected Applications across ABA Services

Clinical behavior-analytic researchers have integrated telehealth into ongoing delivery of services, such as those in pediatric subspecialties. Wacker et al. (2016) conceptualized the research and application of telehealth in ABA in a generational framework. The first generation included research and applications on consultation, diagnosis, training, and intervention (see bottom panel of Figure 31.1), and the second generation of research and applications extended these four broad areas to further identify best practices for ABA telehealth.

### Consultation

We began providing outpatient services to children and adults with developmental disabilities who displayed severe problem behavior at the Center for Disabilities and Development in Iowa during the mid-1980s (see Wacker et al., 2016, and Wacker, Schieltz, & Romani, 2015, for descriptions). When we initiated the outpatient clinic, we scheduled roughly two children or adults every other week, and this was sufficient to meet the need for this service. Over time, however, the demand for the service continued to grow, just as the demand for ABA services has grown throughout the United States. The ability of universities and training programs to produce trained applied behavior analysts has not matched the demand for these services. For example, Iowa had 77 certified applied behavior analysts in 2016 (Behavior Analysis Certification Board, 2016). Currently, our center continues to be the only provider of function-based assessment and treatment services in Iowa. The current wait time for services is 8 months from the time we schedule the clinic visit to the time when we conduct the evaluation. Most families receiving the services live within 100 miles of the tertiary-level hospital where the clinic is located, leaving most of Iowa without access to these services.

We launched our telehealth services in the mid- to late 1990s to increase access to ABA services for Iowans (Lee et al., 2014). Our outpatient clinic, the Biobehavioral Service, initiated telehealth services as part of a much larger telehealth grant to The University of Iowa Hospitals and Clinics (Kienzle, 2000). We conducted only consultation services for the first several years, meaning that we consulted with local pediatricians, nurse practitioners, and school teams regarding the problem behavior they were encountering in their clinics and classrooms. These were "talking heads" conversations, and we never saw the clients or practitioners in action. The local service providers appreciated the functional approach and expertise we brought to managing behavior.

The telehealth center at the Center for Disabilities and Development currently has four computer workstations devoted to telehealth services. Partitions seclude these spaces (see Lee et al., 2014, for a description), and our telehealth providers use headphones to maintain patient privacy. Our biobehavioral telehealth service assesses and treats problem behavior displayed by persons with developmental disabilities. Consultation continues to be the most common type of telehealth service this clinic provides. We have scheduled appointments routinely to consult via telehealth with specific school teams, ASD centers, and group homes. Most consultations involve the discussion of clients that we have never seen in the clinic, and we advise professionals how to proceed with on-site assessment and treatment. Increasingly, we are using telehealth to follow up with patients in their homes after initial evaluations in the clinic. We advise caregivers on proceeding with treatment, on incorporating treatment into their daily routines, and on promoting the generalization and maintenance of treatment effects. We have not obtained reimbursement from insurance companies for these services. We recently received information suggesting that we may be able to charge for these services soon, including clinic-to-home consultations. We also have begun to expand telehealth-delivered consultation and training to school teams that work with students with problem behavior (Bassingthwaite et al., 2018).

## Diagnosis

Behavior analysts provide behavioral diagnoses for problem behavior, using behavioral assessments such as functional analysis, preference assessment, and descriptive assessment. Our biobehavioral service relies primarily on functional analysis (Northup et al., 1991), which is why this was the first procedure we conducted via telehealth using the Iowa Communications Network. The Iowa Communications Network provides fiber-optic connections among hospitals, high schools, and many other service agencies statewide. The Iowa Communications Network clinic rooms consisted of tables, microphones, and desks, and were perfect for talk consultation or didactic instruction. To conduct functional analyses in real time, however, we had to move the tables and chairs, and we had to adjust our communication methods across sites because the existing microphones often were not useful. After several attempts, we successfully completed two functional analyses, one in a school and the other in a foster care state office (Barretto et al., 2006).

After our initial success in conducting functional analysis procedures entirely by telehealth, our biobehavioral service clinic continued to conduct these procedures, but on a limited basis due to funding challenges. Insurance companies have been reluctant or unwilling to reimburse psychologists for providing telehealth services, especially when we provide those services in non-health-care settings such as schools or homes. Although this is beginning to change, the immediate future for telehealth in Iowa appeared to be clinic to clinic, which was what we accomplished beginning in 2009 with a grant funded by the National Institute of Mental Health (Lindgren & Wacker, 2009).

Using an Internet-based teleconferencing network, we conducted functional analyses with 20 young children diagnosed with ASD in regional outpatient clinics that were located an average of 200 miles from our hospital (Wacker et al., 2013b). We implemented functional analyses based on the procedures Iwata, Dorsey, Slifer, Bauman, and Richman (1982/1994) described, as we have done in our biobehavioral service and in our in-home studies (e.g., Wacker et al., 2011). We conducted a series of controlled analogue conditions that tested the role of caregiver attention, access to preferred items or activities, and escape from demands on the continued occurrence of problem behavior. We alternated these test conditions with a control condition (play). The clinical goals were (1) to identify the social reinforcers maintaining problem behavior, and (2) to help caregivers see how predictably problem behavior "turned on and off" as they conducted the conditions.

Because caregivers conducted every session, they could see how responsive their children were to their behavior and how important their behavior was relative to their children's behavior. When we started our telehealth projects with caregivers, we had not anticipated how important this latter aspect of the functional analysis would be to so many caregivers. Conducting the controlled functional analysis described by Wacker et al. (2013b) permitted caregivers and consultants to learn how to communicate with each other. Each play and test condition in a functional analysis was highly structured and systematic, and we repeated each condition at least three times. Conducting multiple conditions multiple times permitted the consultants to learn (1) how to provide direction to the caregivers, (2) which fidelity errors consultants were likely to encounter (Suess et al., 2014), and (3) what challenges caregivers experienced at home. Caregivers learned about how the telehealth system worked and how to present questions to the consultants before treatment started. Our experience suggested that the importance of conducting an analogue-based functional analysis increased with the use of telehealth. The identification of the function of problem behavior was only one of several important goals. Outside of Iowa, Machalicek, O'Reilly, Chan, Lang, et al. (2009) also demonstrated this importance by showing the effectiveness of behavior intervention plans based on the results of functional analyses conducted via telehealth for reducing problem behavior displayed by children in a school.

## Training

Staff and caregiver training via telehealth has been the primary focus of several groups of applied behavior analysts, who have reported success training even complex skills (e.g., Fisher et al., 2014; Frieder, Peterson, Woodward, Crane, & Garner, 2009; Gibson, Pennington, Stenhoff, & Hopper, 2010; Hay-Hansson & Eldevik, 2013; Heitzman-Powell, Buzhardt, Rusinko, & Miller, 2014; Machalicek, O'Reilly, Chan, Rispoli, et al., 2009; Machalicek et al., 2010). The telehealth modalities used during training have ranged from online instruction (e.g., online training modules) to real-time didactic training and real-time coaching. Researchers have developed and tested web-based tutorials to train users on intervention techniques. For example, Kobak et al. (2011) developed a web-based educational program for caregivers of young children with ASD to increase their children's social communication skills and to manage problem behaviors. Behavior management strategies targeted in the web-based modules included reinforcement, modeling, and prompting. The modules contained videos demonstrating child behavior and caregiver models implementing the behavior management strategies. Caregivers completed the web-based modules at their own pace. Pre- and posttest measures demonstrated an increase in the caregivers' knowledge of behavior-analytic principles, as well as high caregiver satisfaction with technology-based training.

An alternative to online instruction is providing real-time didactic training via telehealth. The trainer connects remotely with the user (usually a caregiver, therapist, or teacher) to provide real-time instruction. Xie et al. (2013) conducted a randomized clinical trial of didactic training via telehealth with caregivers of young children with attention-deficit/hyperactivity disorder (ADHD). The investigators assigned caregivers to either the telehealth or face-to-face training groups. Training targeted basic behavior management strategies (e.g., establishing a token economy, using time out effectively, delivering demands appropriately). The trainers provided instruction only on the targeted skills, and they did not incorporate real-time coaching with the children. The results demonstrated that the caregivers' disciplinary practices improved, and that ADHD and problem behavior symptoms decreased on standardized rating scales. Treatment effects did not differ between training groups. Reese, Slone, Soares, and Sprang (2015) produced similar results when they trained caregivers of children with ADHD in their homes via telehealth to establish positive parenting practices.

Although online instruction and real-time didactic training allow users to acquire new skills, they have some limitations, such as the amount and quality of feedback received during training if researchers do not incorporate real-time coaching with confederates or children in the program. Researchers have used real-time coaching via telehealth to train caregivers, teachers, and therapists on specific skills, and the trainees have practiced the skills with confederates or children while receiving immediate feedback from the trainers. For example, Hay-Hansson and Eldevik (2013) used telehealth to train staff to implement discrete-trial training with young children with ASD. They conducted a randomized clinical trial, with participants assigned to a telehealth or an *in vivo* group. Participants practiced implementing the discrete-trial training procedures with the children and received real-time coaching (e.g., instructions, modeling) and feedback on their performance. Results showed improvements in discrete-trial training implementation skills across both groups, with no significant difference between groups on fidelity of implementation, suggesting that telehealth was an effective modality for providing staff training. Studies using telehealth to train novice graduate students to conduct preference assessments (Machalicek, O'Reilly, Chan, Rispoli, et al., 2009), and novice teachers to conduct functional analysis (Frieder et al., 2009; Machalicek et al., 2010) and functional communication training (Gibson et al., 2010), with children with ASD in school settings have produced similar findings.

Researchers have used telehealth to train caregivers to implement intervention programs. McDuffie et al. (2013) used real-time coaching via telehealth to train caregivers of children with ASD to implement a play-based intervention to facilitate language development. The researchers first provided the caregivers with *in vivo* didactic training on component skills of the intervention, followed by *in vivo* coaching in which the caregivers practiced the skills with their children while a therapist coached them. The researchers then coached the caregivers via telehealth while the caregivers practiced the procedures in their homes. Results showed that caregivers' use of the targeted skills increased after the *in vivo* coaching, and that skills were maintained when researchers provided coaching via telehealth.

More recently, telehealth studies have combined modalities (e.g., online instruction with remote coaching) into one training program. Fisher et al. (2014) developed a virtual program to train participants on ABA principles and procedures in discrete-trial and play-based formats. Participants first completed online modules with videos that described and demonstrated ABA principles and procedures. Each participant then practiced the procedures with a confederate while a therapist provided coaching and feedback via telehealth. Participants significantly improved their knowledge and implementation of ABA principles and procedures after the completion of the virtual training program, again suggesting that telehealth is an effective way to provide training. A study conducted by Heitzman-Powell et al. (2014) also demonstrated the effectiveness of a telehealth training program that incorporated online instruction and real-time coaching to train caregivers of children with ASD to implement ABA-based procedures.

We have combined modalities for our training project for school professionals, in which we provide real-time didactic instruction via telehealth on behavioral principles and assessment procedures as a supplement to the in-person training each professional receives from our team (Bassingthwaite & Wacker, 2015). Over the years of this project, this didactic instruction has evolved from the experts' providing the instruction to the school professionals to the school professionals' providing the instruction to each other, which may be like the premise of Project ECHO mentioned earlier. In addition to didactic instruction, we provide real-time training. Project staff members observe the performance of school teams while they evaluate a child. As with the didactic training, school staff members that our research team initially trained are now training other school staffers while our project staff members monitor them in real time via telehealth. In one case, a school team conducted a functional analysis at a school site while project staffers observed and coached the school team, as needed, from a remote location (Bassingthwaite et al., 2018).

### Intervention

The treatment procedure that we conduct most often via telehealth is functional communication training (FCT), for several reasons (Wacker et al., 2013a). First, when we initiated our in-home (Wacker et al., 1998), outpatient (Northup et al., 1991), and inpatient (Wacker et al., 1990) treatment programs, we most often used FCT for treatment. As research by our team and others has shown (Greer, Fisher, Saini, Owen, & Jones, 2016; Tiger, Hanley, & Bruzek, 2008), FCT is often effective in reducing problem behavior, and caregivers have rated it as highly acceptable. The goal of replacing problem behavior with an appropriate communicative response has made good sense to caregivers, and we based the treatment directly on the results of the functional analysis. Given both the reductions in problem behavior and the high acceptability ratings, we have continued to use FCT as our treatment of choice.

We conducted our first systematic effort to implement FCT via telehealth in regional outpatient clinics with 17 families of young children with ASD who displayed problem behavior (Wacker et al., 2013a). Seventeen children received FCT, and the mean decrease in levels of problem behavior

was 94%. Caregivers rated telehealth delivery of FCT very highly on the Treatment Acceptability Rating Form—Revised. Ratings were comparable to those obtained when trained applied behavior analysts traveled to the caregivers' homes and worked directly with them (Reimers, Wacker, Cooper, & DeRaad, 1992).

In a more recently completed project (Lindgren & Wacker, 2011, 2015), we implemented these procedures via telehealth, but in caregivers' homes. Our previous clinic-to-clinic results had established that we could conduct the procedures effectively via telehealth, which was important for establishing insurance reimbursement and expanding access to care. However, determining whether we could obtain the same results in caregivers' homes with no *in vivo* assistance, and when the caregivers had never met the applied behavior analysts working with them, was important. As summarized in Lindgren et al. (2016), we worked with 30 families and achieved a 97% mean reduction in levels of problem behavior. As in prior studies, caregivers rated the acceptability of the procedures very highly. Statistical analyses showed that the in-home *in vivo*, clinic telehealth, and home telehealth groups showed (1) no significant differences in reductions of problem behavior, (2) equivalent improvement in adaptive behavior such as task completion, and (3) equivalent caregiver acceptability ratings. Thus these results indicated that functional analysis and FCT conducted via telehealth in caregivers' homes were as effective as those conducted *in vivo* and in regional outpatient clinics, respectively, in at least some cases. In addition, the costs associated with the in-home telehealth services were lower than those of other treatment delivery methods.

Monitoring procedural fidelity is a critical aspect of behavioral treatments delivered via telehealth. Applied behavior analysts have begun systematically evaluating the impact of different levels of fidelity on the effects of behavioral treatments, and the results to date suggest that treatment fidelity can play a large role in the initial effects of treatment and in the maintenance of treatment effects over time (Bergmann, Kodak, & LeBlanc, 2017; Carroll, Kodak, & Fisher, 2013; St. Peter Pipkin, Vollmer, & Sloman, 2010; Volkert, Lerman, Call, & Trosclair-Lasserre, 2009). Telehealth severely restricts the way behavior analysts can implement and model the recommended treatments; therefore, close monitoring of treatment implementation fidelity by caregivers and other service providers is critical.

Suess et al. (2014) evaluated caregiver fidelity during FCT in the home with applied behavior analysts conducting remote coaching. Suess et al. showed that caregivers could conduct the procedure in their homes with good integrity, and that they could achieve clinically significant reductions in their children's problem behavior. Although Suess et al. produced good fidelity in the home via telehealth, the results of other studies suggest that errors in implementation integrity can negatively affect treatment (Schieltz et al., 2018; St. Peter Pipkin et al., 2010). Researchers are conducting studies to identify the best procedures for in-home caregiver training via telehealth (e.g., Fisher et al., 2014), and the results of those studies will be important to the success of future applications and extensions of telehealth services.

## Current Applications

Lindgren et al. (2016) showed that we can conduct behavioral assessment and treatment procedures effectively via telehealth. Suess, Wacker, Schwartz, Lustig, and Detrick (2016) suggest that the next generation of questions will focus on timing and dose of services. Relative to *in vivo* clinical procedures, when should we use telehealth, for how long, and on what schedule in relation to clinic, home, and school-based procedures?

We have incorporated telehealth evaluations into our biobehavioral service to provide brief behavioral assessment and treatment services to caregivers of children with ASD, who previously often waited up to 6 months for an in-person evaluation in our clinic (see Suess et al., 2016). Five caregiver–child dyads received brief behavioral diagnosis, intervention, and consultation via telehealth. Each child participated in four telehealth visits, one 60-minute visit for a functional analysis, and three 15-minute FCT visits. The total time for the telehealth assessment, 105 minutes, compared favorably to the length of our 90- to 120-minute clinic evaluations. However, rather than implementing functional analysis and FCT in one visit as we do during in-clinic evaluations, we implemented the procedures during four telehealth visits. Implementing frequent but brief visits allowed us to integrate telehealth services more efficiently into our existing clinic caseload. This integration was important, because we still had not received reimbursement for our telehealth services.

One question that researchers should address in future studies is how best to incorporate telehealth into existing services. For example, we wonder whether more frequent but brief sessions will be more effective and efficient than longer sessions distributed over a longer period.

For the telehealth visits, the caregivers and children traveled to a regional ASD center near their homes. The caregivers implemented the functional analysis and the FCT procedures, with an applied behavior analyst providing coaching via Skype™. The applied behavior analysts were in the telehealth center located at the University of Iowa Children's Hospital, which was approximately 170 miles from the regional ASD center (Wacker et al., 2013b). The director of the regional ASD center also participated in the telehealth visits by helping the caregivers as needed (e.g., making sure that appropriate toys and materials were available).

During the visit for the functional analysis, our team completed a behavioral diagnosis. That is, we conducted tests for positive-reinforcement functions (tangibles and attention) and negative-reinforcement functions (escape) in a multielement design for each child. We targeted negative-reinforcement functions during treatment, based on the functional analysis results. We implemented and evaluated treatment in a nonconcurrent multiple-baseline design across participants. Treatment was FCT in a two-step chain of task completion and manding described by Wacker et al. (2013a). We encouraged caregivers to practice the FCT procedure with their children outside of scheduled telehealth visits (Suess et al., 2014), and our applied behavior analysts provided additional brief consultation via telehealth.

The results from the brief behavioral diagnoses via telehealth showed social functions of problem behavior for four out of five children. Problem behavior decreased relative to baseline by a mean of 65% across children by the end of the third FCT visit. A statistical analysis showed a statistically significant reduction in levels of problem behavior from the functional analysis to the end of FCT (Hedge's $g = 1.3$, $z = 3.15$, $p < .001$). Mean increases in independent manding and task completion were 88% and 34%, respectively.

These results extended previous telehealth studies (Wacker et al., 2013a, 2013b) by showing that behavior analysts could incorporate brief behavioral assessment and treatment procedures via telehealth into an existing outpatient service. Brief behavioral assessment and treatment via telehealth may provide a means to initiate services while families remain on the wait list for clinic services. If the treatment initiated via telehealth is sufficient to reduce problem behavior, then we can cancel the clinic evaluation and decrease the size of our clinic wait list. However, if problem behavior continues, we can conduct a more extensive behavioral assessment and treatment in the clinic, and we can tailor the clinic services directly to the telehealth results.

One concern with behavioral telehealth relates to their security and ability to protect patient confidentiality. We have used Skype as the video-conferencing software in some of our previous telehealth studies, but we informed the caregivers in those studies of the security limits of telehealth and had them provide written consent before starting telehealth visits. More recently, we have collaborated with the e-health group at the University of Iowa Hospitals and Clinics to pilot-test video-conferencing software that is compliant with the Health Insurance Portability and Accountability Act (HIPAA) and directly connected to the patients' electronic medical records. This software allows patients to log into their medical records from their homes and initiate telehealth visits with providers at the University of Iowa Hospitals and Clinics. We used this new software initially to provide behavioral consultation for feeding-related concerns, but we hope to expand it soon to the myriad of telehealth-based services we have summarized in this chapter. Other behavior analysts who wish to deliver ABA services via telehealth should be aware of the health information privacy issues that are specific to this service delivery mode.

The results of Lindgren et al. (2016) suggest that behavior analysts can conduct research and clinical services successfully via telehealth. Research conducted via telehealth can potentially increase the access that families have to relevant research protocols and can increase the diversity of participants enrolling in projects at The University of Iowa. We recently completed a randomized clinical trial of FCT via a project funded by the Health Resources and Services Administration (HRSA) Maternal and Child Health Bureau (Lindgren & Wacker, 2011). In this project, participants received FCT either immediately after we completed the functional analysis or 3 months later. We successfully completed this study entirely via telehealth and in a much shorter period than if we had conducted the project in the home or the clinic (Lindgren et al., 2020).

We have received funding from the National Institute of Mental Health to conduct a randomized clinical trial of functional analysis (Lindgren & Wacker, 2015). We will randomly assign families of young children with ASD who display problem behavior to a group receiving either *standard* or *pragmatic* functional analysis. The standard group will receive the functional analysis Iwata et al.

(1982/1994) described. The pragmatic group will receive a 1-hour descriptive assessment that does not manipulate conditions in a single-case design. Our goal is to determine whether the potential clinical benefits of the standard functional analysis are significantly better than a more pragmatic version that we will evaluate in a systematic and quantitative fashion.

We believe that behavior analysts can conduct clinical and translational research via telehealth (e.g., Suess, Schieltz, Wacker, Detrick, & Podlesnik, 2020). We hope that these and other studies support the merits of using telehealth as a practical means to study problem behavior and deliver effective interventions to families affected by such behavior.

## LINGERING QUESTIONS AND CONCERNS

Behavior analysts have studied telehealth only as a means for directly delivering behavioral assessment and treatment via single-case designs since 2006, and Internet access has been available widely for only the last several years. Numerous questions and concerns regarding the future delivery of these services remain.

Questions that researchers need to address immediately relate to the timing and dose of services. Although researchers like Suess et al. (2016) showed what we can accomplish via telehealth, we also need to identify the limitations that warrant *in vivo* services (see Schieltz et al., 2018). Wacker et al. (2016) offered a flowchart of questions to ask to determine when behavior analysts should select either telehealth or *in vivo* service delivery. For example, the first three questions were these: (1) Can we assess and treat the target behavior remotely? (2) Does the family have the necessary equipment? and (3) Will insurance reimburse the service? Researchers need to determine, study, evaluate, and resolve these and many other questions as they consider wider clinical applications of telehealth. Similarly, we need to evaluate whether telehealth components, such as the visual presence of a consultant or the caregiver's wearing earbuds, functions as an inadvertent independent variable and alters behavior. If so, then further analysis of its impact on various dependent variables seems warranted.

Professional organizations have outlined ethical guidelines for providing services via telehealth (American Psychological Association, 2013; Behavior Analysis Certification Board, 2014), but this remains an area for professional discussion (Pollard, Karimi, & Ficcaglia, 2017; Romani & Schieltz, 2017). For example, under what conditions can we use family-friendly systems such as Skype or FaceTime™ with informed consent to assess and treat problem behavior? Are different levels of security needed for talking consultation versus direct implementation of procedures when children appear on screen, for example? If we record such sessions for later viewing using store-and-forward methods, how should we store and protect those video files? How can we best use telehealth in settings such as schools, day care centers, and group homes?

Behavior analysts may need a different skill set for telehealth services than for in-person services. Many applied behavior analysts model the skills they are trying to teach a caregiver. We frequently use gestures, such as pointing, and may have caregivers watch us implement a procedure several times before asking the caregivers to try it. We frequently work directly with the children during meltdowns or extinction bursts. Telehealth service delivery requires a different set of strategies, relying more on vocal instructions or video models. We need to provide clear and specific vocal instructions during telehealth services, and we often must prompt desired caregiver behavior to prevent fidelity errors. Caregivers are likely to implement procedures differently than we do, and as consultants, we must quickly discriminate whether variations in procedures are acceptable or constitute fidelity errors. Thus we need to consider the skills applied behavior analysts need to have and the best ways to teach those skills.

In providing training to caregivers, we need to consider how best to use procedures such as video modeling and interactive webpages. Suess et al. (2014) asked caregivers to practice the procedures between appointments, and an applied behavior analyst reviewed recordings of those sessions before the next appointment with a caregiver. As we have done with the dosage and timing questions raised earlier for delivering services via telehealth, we need to address questions for what occurs during times when an applied behavior analyst is not present. How much practice should caregivers conduct, and is this a function of their skills? For example, should caregivers practice a procedure several times per day at the beginning of treatment, or should they wait until treatment effects have occurred in session before they practice procedures in the home? Should we schedule additional but briefer sessions early in treatment? Suess

et al. (2016) scheduled three 15-minute treatment sessions rather than one 45-minute session. But are more frequent but briefer sessions easier or more effective for caregivers?

Another issue that we have considered concerns a child's behavior and a family's situation. Children who scream loudly and live in an apartment may not be good candidates for telehealth-based functional analyses, for example. Children with problem behavior that presents a danger to themselves, to others, to property, or a combination may also be difficult to assess and treat via telehealth. Caregivers who cannot follow a consultant's vocal instructions or who do not have support at home may not be candidates for telehealth, either. Most of our telehealth-based treatments have been for problem behavior maintained by social reinforcement. Reducing problem behavior maintained by automatic reinforcement has been more challenging with telehealth (Schieltz et al., 2018).

A final consideration is that of reinforcers for the applied behavior analysts who are conducting telehealth. Over the past 10 years that we have been conducting telehealth, not a single staff member or student has indicated that he or she would prefer to conduct sessions exclusively via telehealth. Most of us find working directly with clients and caregivers reinforcing. As supervisors, we find watching how skilled our trainees become reinforcing. We cannot completely remove these sources of positive reinforcement without considering what will replace those sources. As we consider telehealth options in the future, we will need to conduct research to address timing and dosage issues for the providers as well as the patients.

In general, the right mix of telehealth with clinic, in-home, center-based, and school-based programs warrants further consideration. The results to date certainly support telehealth, but we need further research to determine how best to implement services via telehealth.

## FUTURE DIRECTIONS

The options available for future telehealth applications and extensions appear to be limited only by the resourcefulness of applied behavior analysts who are implementing those services. Most medical subspecialties have embraced telehealth, and insurance providers have increasingly accepted this approach. We are embarking on three sets of future directions for our services in Iowa.

A doctoral dissertation (Lee, 2016) showed that a consultant in the United States could deliver functional analysis and FCT to families in Korea. Five young children with ASD who displayed problem behavior participated in the study. The children's caregivers conducted assessment and treatment procedures in their homes. The functional analysis identified social functions for the children's problem behavior, and FCT reduced problem behavior by 100% of baseline. We obtained these results by using smartphones for the telehealth consultations.

Similarly, Tsami, Lerman, and Toper-Korkmaz (2019) conducted functional analyses and FCT via telehealth with 12 children with ASD who resided across eight countries. Behavior analysts in the United States served as the families' coaches, and when needed, used interpreters who had been raised in the countries of the families. Across all participants, results were positive. Specifically, problem behavior was reduced by at least 80% from baseline levels and appropriate communication increased to at least 90% across opportunities. Additionally, parent procedural fidelity was accurate (average of at least 90%), parent ratings of treatment acceptability were high (average of 6.6 on a 7 point Likert scale), and the telehealth connections between the United States and the families' homes in other countries remained high (at least 92% of the scheduled appointment times occurred without connection issues).

There are many implications of these studies, and we mention two here. First, telehealth permits applied behavior analysts to work efficiently and immediately internationally. If future studies replicate Lee (2016) and Tsami et al. (2019), we will be able to show the international appeal of ABA and to meet the worldwide need for the service. Second, we have most often used laptop computers for in-home telehealth services to date, but Lee and Tsami et al. obtained equally positive results with smartphones and other electronic devices (e.g., tablets). As part of our routine outpatient clinical services, we now use smartphones to conduct sessions via our electronic medical records. Within 10 years, we have moved from a telehealth system involving fiber-optic cables that connected only a few locations to smartphones that can connect almost everywhere. We need to consider carefully how to maximize our use of telehealth to reach as many families as possible with state-of-the-art equipment and procedures.

A related future direction involves determining how to combine telehealth services into packages that maximally benefit families. Service teams across many disciplines have been studying how to consult, diagnose, train, and treat via telehealth. Many caregivers will need access to each of these services, which means that we need to consider how to blend services into an efficient and effective package. We need studies, for example, that identify (1) the conditions under which caregiver-training needs require in-home service delivery of behavioral treatment, (2) the need for ongoing consultation after treatment, and (3) the need for functional analysis before treatment. We need research to identify how to incorporate telehealth services into existing service delivery programs.

A final direction for the future is to determine how to use telehealth to expand our research programs. Telehealth offers opportunities for more diverse groups of families to participate in research, including clinical trials. We have recently initiated a randomized clinical trial of preceding FCT with either a standard functional analysis or a brief functional assessment. Three research centers at Iowa, Atlanta, and Houston are working jointly on the project; we will conduct assessment and treatment procedures via telehealth in the homes of the participating families. We can conduct this large-N trial using single-case designs, because telehealth permits us to work with far more families than would be possible if we needed to travel to the families' homes. Families do not need to live near any of the centers conducting the study, potentially increasing the overall diversity of participating families.

As we discussed in Schieltz and Wacker (2020), the current COVID-19 crisis has dramatically increased the relevance of telehealth-delivered services. The good news is researchers in behavior analysis have laid the foundation of how to effectively deliver these services across consultation, diagnosis, training, and intervention. The not so good news is there is still much to learn relative to how best to utilize this service delivery method. Although not systematically planned for, this health crisis has pushed more behavior analysts into using telehealth, and we hope that this encourages these researchers and practitioners to contribute to our understanding of the use of telehealth in behavior analysis.

## REFERENCES

American Academy of Pediatrics. (2016). Epilepsy in pediatrics: Project ECHO. Retrieved from www.

aap.org/en-us/advocacy-and-policy/aap-health-initia-tives/Coordinating-Center-on-Epilepsy/Pages/Project-ECHO.aspx.

American Psychological Association. (2013). *Guidelines for the practice of telepsychology*. Washington, DC: Author.

American Telemedicine Association. (2016). What is telemedicine? Retrieved from *www.americantelemed. org/about-telemedicine/what-is-telemedicine#.Vsky1ce-0GsI.*

Arora, S., Geppert, C. M., Kalishman, S., Dion, D., Pullara, F., Bjeletich, B., et al. (2007). Academic health center management of chronic diseases through knowledge networks: Project ECHO. *Academic Medicine, 82*(2), 154–160.

Arora, S., Kalishman, S., Dion, D., Som, D., Thornton, K., Bankhurst, A., et al. (2011). Partnering urban academic medical centers and rural primary care clinicians to provide complex chronic disease care. *Health Affairs, 30*(6), 1176–1184.

Barretto, A., Wacker, D. P., Harding, J., Lee, J., & Berg, W. K. (2006). Using telemedicine to conduct behavioral assessments. *Journal of Applied Behavior Analysis, 39*, 333–340.

Bassingthwaite, B. J., Graber, J. E., Weaver, A. D., Wacker, D. P., White-Staecker, D., Bergthold, S., et al. (2018). Using teleconsultation to develop independent skills of school-based teams in functional behavior assessment. *Journal of Educational and Psychological Consultation, 28*, 297–318.

Bassingthwaite, B., & Wacker, D. (2015). *Statewide behavioral consultation services*. Des Moines: Iowa Department of Education, Bureau of Special Education.

Behavior Analysis Certification Board. (2014). *Professional and ethical compliance code for behavior analysts*. Littleton, CO: Author.

Behavior Analysis Certification Board. (2016). Find/ contact certificants. Retrieved from *http://info.bacb. com/o.php?page=100155&by=state.*

Bergmann, S. C., Kodak, T. M., & LeBlanc, B. A. (2017). Effects of programmed errors of omission and commission during auditory–visual conditional discrimination training with typically developing children. *Psychological Record, 67*, 109–119.

Burke, B. L., Jr., Hall, R. W., & the Section on Telehealth Care. (2015). Telemedicine: Pediatric applications. *Pediatrics, 136*, e293–e308.

Callahan, C. W., Malone, F., Estroff, D., & Person, D. A. (2005). Effectiveness of an Internet-based store-and-forward telemedicine system for pediatric subspecialty consultation. *Archives of Pediatrics and Adolescent Medicine, 159*, 389–393.

Carroll, R. A., Kodak, T., & Fisher, W. W. (2013). An evaluation of programmed treatment-integrity errors during discrete-trial instruction. *Journal of Applied Behavior Analysis, 46*, 379–394.

Center for Connected Health Policy. (2016). What is telehealth? Retrieved from *http://cchpca.org/what-is-telehealth.*

Committee on Pediatric Workforce. (2015). The use of telemedicine to address access and physician workforce shortages. *Pediatrics, 136*(1), 202–209.

Fisher, W. W., Luczynski, K. C., Hood, S. A., Lesser, A. D., Machado, M. A., & Piazza, C. C. (2014). Preliminary findings of a randomized clinical trial of a virtual training program for applied behavior analysis technicians. *Research in Autism Spectrum Disorders, 8*, 1044–1054.

Frieder, J. E., Peterson, S. M., Woodward, J., Craine, J., & Garner, M. (2009). Teleconsultation in school settings: Linking classroom teachers and behavior analysts through web-based technology. *Behavior Analysis in Practice, 2*(2), 32–39.

Ghio, L., Boccola, S., Andronio, L., Adami, D., Paglialonga, F., Ardissino, G., et al. (2002). A case study: Telemedicine technology and peritoneal dialysis in children. *Telemedicine Journal and e-Health, 8*(4), 355–359.

Gibson, J. L., Pennington, R. C., Stenhoff, D. M., & Hopper, J. S. (2010). Using desktop videoconferencing to deliver interventions to a preschool student with autism. *Topics in Early Childhood Special Education, 29*, 214–225.

Gomes, R., Rossi, R., Lima, S., Carmo, P., Ferreira, R., Menezes, I., et al. (2010). Pediatric cardiology and telemedicine: Seven years' experience of cooperation with remote hospitals. *Revista Portuguesa de Cardiologia, 29*, 181–191.

Greer, B. D., Fisher, W. W., Saini, V., Owen, T. M., & Jones, J. K. (2016). Improving functional communication training during reinforcement schedule thinning: An analysis of 25 applications. *Journal of Applied Behavior Analysis, 49*, 105–121.

Gutierrez, M. (2015). *State telehealth laws and Medicaid program policies: A comprehensive scan of the 50 states and District of Columbia*. Retrieved from *http:// cchpca.org/sites/default/files/resources/STATE%20 TELEHEALTH%20POLICIES%20AND%20RE-IMBURSEMENT%20REPORT%20FINAL%20 %28c%29%20JULY%202015.pdf.*

Hay-Hansson, A. W., & Eldevik, S. (2013). Training discrete trials teaching skills using videoconference. *Research in Autism Spectrum Disorders, 7*, 1300–1309.

Heffner, V. A., Lyon, V. B., Brousseau, D. C., Holland, K. E., & Yen, K. (2009). Store-and-forward teledermatology versus in-person visits: A comparison in pediatric teledermatology clinic. *Journal of the American Academy of Dermatology, 60*, 956–961.

Heitzman-Powell, L. S., Buzhardt, J., Rusinko, L. C., & Miller, T. M. (2014). Formative evaluation of an ABA outreach training program for parents of children with autism in remote areas. *Focus on Autism and Other Developmental Disabilities, 29*(1), 23–28.

Iwata, B. A., Dorsey, M. F., Slifer, K. J., Bauman, K. E., & Richman, G. S. (1994). Toward a functional analysis of self-injury. *Journal of Applied Behavior Analysis, 27*, 197–209. (Reprinted from *Analysis and Intervention in Developmental Disabilities, 2*, 3–20, 1982)

Izquierdo, R., Morin, P. C., Bratt, K., Moreau, Z., Meyer, S., Ploutz-Snyder, R., et al. (2009). School-centered telemedicine for children with Type 1 diabetes mellitus. *Journal of Pediatrics, 155*(3), 374–379.

Kienzle, M. (2000, March). Rural–academic integration: Iowa's national laboratory for the study of rural telemedicine. Retrieved from *http://collab.nlm.nih.gov/tutorialspublicationsandmaterials/telesymposiumcd/UIowaFinalReport.pdf*.

Kobak, K. A., Stone, W. L., Wallace, E., Warren, Z., Swanson, A., & Robson, K. (2011). A web-based tutorial for parents of young children with autism: Results from a pilot study. *Telemedicine and e-Health, 17*(10), 804–808.

Langkamp, D., McManus, M. D., & Blakemore, S. D. (2015). Telemedicine for children with developmental disabilities: A more effective clinical process than office-based care. *Telemedicine and e-Health, 21*(2), 110–114.

Lee, G. (2016). *The application of telehealth procedures to provide behavior assessment and treatment to families with young children with autism spectrum disorder in Korea*. Unpublished doctoral dissertation, The University of Iowa, Iowa City, IA.

Lee, J. F., Schieltz, K. M., Suess, A. N., Wacker, D. P., Romani, P. W., Lindgren, S. D., et al. (2015). Guidelines for developing telehealth services and troubleshooting problems with telehealth technology when coaching parents to conduct functional analyses and functional communication training in their homes. *Behavior Analysis in Practice, 8*, 190–200.

Lindgren, S. D., & Wacker, D. P. (2009). *Behavioral treatment for autism in community settings using a telehealth network*. Washington, DC: U.S. Department of Health and Human Services, National Institute of Mental Health.

Lindgren, S. D., & Wacker, D. P. (2011). *Behavioral treatment through in-home telehealth for young children with autism*. Washington, DC: U.S. Department of Health and Human Services, Health Resources and Services Administration, Maternal and Child Health Bureau.

Lindgren, S. D., & Wacker, D. P. (2015). *Comparing behavioral assessments using telehealth for children with autism*. Washington, DC: U.S. Department of Health and Human Services, National Institute of Mental Health.

Lindgren, S., Wacker, D., Schieltz, K., Suess, A., Pelzel, K., Kopelman, T., et al. (2020). A randomized controlled trial of functional communication training via telehealth for young children with autism spectrum disorder. *Journal of Autism and Developmental Disorders*. [Epub ahead of print]

Lindgren, S., Wacker, D., Suess, A., Schieltz, K., Pelzel, K., Kopelman, T., et al. (2016). Telehealth expands access and reduces costs for treating challenging behavior in young children with autism spectrum disorders using applied behavior analysis. *Pediatrics, 137*(Suppl. 2), S168–S175.

Looman, W. S., Antolick, M., Cady, R. G., Lunos, S. A., Garwick, A. E., & Finkelstein, S. M. (2015). Effects of telehealth care coordination intervention on perceptions of health care by caregivers of children with medical complexity: A randomized controlled trial. *Journal of Pediatric Health Care, 29*(4), 352–363.

Machalicek, W., O'Reilly, M., Chan, J. M., Lang, R., Rispoli, M., Davis, T., et al. (2009). Using videoconferencing to conduct functional analysis of challenging behavior and develop classroom behavioral support plans for students with autism. *Education and Training in Developmental Disabilities, 44*, 207–217.

Machalicek, W., O'Reilly, M., Chan, J. M., Rispoli, M., Lang, R., Davis, T., et al. (2009b). Using videoconferencing to support teachers to conduct preference assessments with students with autism and developmental disabilities. *Research in Autism Spectrum Disorders, 3*, 32–41.

Machalicek, W., O'Reilly, M. F., Rispoli, M., Davis, T., Lang, R., Hetlinger Franco, J., et al. (2010). Training teachers to assess the challenging behaviors of students with autism using video tele-conferencing. *Education and Training in Autism and Developmental Disabilities, 45*, 203–215.

Mahnke, C. B., Mulreany, M. P., Inafuku, J., Abbas, M., Feingold, B., & Paolillo, J. A. (2008). Utility of store-and-forward pediatric telecardiology evaluation in distinguishing normal from pathologic pediatric heart sounds. *Clinical Pediatrics, 47*(9), 919–925.

Mazurek, M. O., Brown, R., Curran, A., & Sohl, K. (2017). ECHO autism: A new model for training primary care providers in best-practice for children with autism. *Clinical Pediatrics, 56*, 247–256.

McDuffie, A., Machalicek, W., Oakes, A., Haebig, E., Weismer, S. E., & Abbeduto, L. (2013). Distance video-teleconferencing in early intervention: Pilot study of a naturalistic parent-implemented language intervention. *Topics in Early Childhood Special Education, 33*(3), 172–185.

Nelson, E., Citarelli, M., Cook, D., & Shaw, P. (2003). Reshaping health care delivery for adolescent parents: Healthy steps and telemedicine. *Telemedicine Journal and e-Health, 9*(4), 387–392.

Northup, J., Wacker, D., Sasso, G., Steege, M., Cigrand, K., Cook, J., et al. (1991). A brief functional analysis of aggressive and alternative behavior in an outclinic setting. *Journal of Applied Behavior Analysis, 24*, 509–522.

Pollard, J. S., Karimi, K. A., & Ficcaglia, M. B. (2017). Ethical considerations in the design and implementation of a telehealth service delivery model. *Behavior Analysis: Research and Practice, 17*, 298–311.

Reese, R. J., Slone, N. C., Soares, N., & Sprang, R. (2015). Using telepsychology to provide a group parenting program: A preliminary evaluation on effectiveness. *Psychological Service, 12*(3), 274–282.

Reimers, T., Wacker, D., Cooper, L., & DeRaad, A. (1992). Clinical evaluation of the variables associated with treatment acceptability and their relation to compliance. *Behavioral Disorders, 18*, 67–76.

Romani, P. W., & Schieltz, K. M. (2017). Ethical considerations when delivering behavior analytic services for problem behavior via telehealth. *Behavior Analysis: Research and Practice, 17,* 312–324.

Sable, C. (2003). Telemedicine applications in pediatric cardiology. *Minerva Pediatrica, 55*(1), 1–13.

Santiago Lipana, L., Bindal, D., Nettiksimmons, J., & Shaikh, U. (2013). Telemedicine and face-to-face care for pediatric obesity. *Telemedicine and e-Health, 19*(10), 806–808.

Schieltz, K. M., Romani, P. W., Wacker, D. P., Suess, A. N., Huang, P., Berg, W. K., et al. (2018). Single-case analysis to determine reasons for failure of behavioral treatment via telehealth. *Remedial and Special Education, 39,* 95–105.

Schieltz, K. M., & Wacker, D. P. (2020). Functional assessment and function-based treatment delivered via telehealth: A brief summary. *Journal of Applied Behavior Analysis, 53,* 1242–1258.

Shaikh, U., Cole, S. L., Marcin, J. P., & Nesbitt, T. S. (2008). Clinical management and patient outcomes among children and adolescents receiving telemedicine consultations for obesity. *Telemedicine and e-Health, 14*(5), 434–440.

Spooner, S. A., Gotleib, E. M., the Steering Committee on Clinical Information Technology, & the Committee on Medical Liability. (2004). Telemedicine: Pediatric applications. *Pediatrics, 113*(6), e639–e643.

St. Peter Pipkin, C., Vollmer, T., & Sloman, K. (2010). Effects of treatment integrity failures during differential reinforcement of alternative behavior: A translational model. *Journal of Applied Behavior Analysis, 43,* 47–70.

Suess, A. N., Romani, P. W., Wacker, D. P., Dyson, S. M., Kuhle, J. L., Lee, J. F., et al. (2014). Evaluating the treatment fidelity of parents who conduct in-home functional communication training with coaching via telehealth. *Journal of Behavioral Education, 23,* 34–59.

Suess, A. N., Schieltz, K. M., Wacker, D. P., Detrick, J., & Podlesnik, C. A. (2020). An evaluation of resurgence following functional communication training conducted in alternative antecedent contexts via telehealth. *Journal of the Experimental Analysis of Behavior, 113,* 278–301.

Suess, A. N., Wacker, D., Schwartz, J. E., Lustig, N., & Detrick, J. (2016). Preliminary evidence in the use of telehealth in an outpatient behavior clinic. *Journal of Applied Behavior Analysis, 49*(3), 686–692.

Telehealth Resource Centers. (2016). Types of telemedicine specialty consultation services. Retrieved from *www.telehealthresourcecenter.org/toolbox-module/types-telemedicine-specialty-consultation-services.*

Tiger, J. H., Hanley, G. P., & Bruzek, J. (2008). Functional communication training: A review and practical guide. *Behavior Analysis in Practice, 1,* 16–23.

Tsami, L., Lerman, D., & Toper-Korkmaz, O. (2019). Effectiveness and acceptability of parent training via telehealth among families around the world. *Journal of Applied Behavior Analysis, 52,* 1113–1129.

Volkert, V. M., Lerman, D. C., Call, N. A., & Trosclair-Lasserre, N. (2009). Evaluation of resurgence during treatment with functional communication training. *Journal of Applied Behavior Analysis, 42,* 145–160.

Wacker, D. P., Berg, W. K., Harding, J. W., Derby, K. M., Asmus, J. M., & Healy, A. (1998). Evaluation and long-term treatment of aberrant behavior displayed by young children with disabilities. *Journal of Developmental and Behavioral Pediatrics, 19,* 260–266.

Wacker, D. P., Harding, J. W., Berg, W. K., Lee, J. F., Schieltz, K. M., Padilla, Y. C., et al. (2011). An evaluation of persistence of treatment effects during long-term treatment of destructive behavior. *Journal of the Experimental Analysis of Behavior, 96,* 261–282.

Wacker, D. P., Lee, J. F., Padilla Dalmau, Y. C., Kopelman, T. G., Lindgren, S. D., Kuhle, J., et al. (2013a). Conducting functional communication training via telehealth to reduce the problem behavior of young children with autism. *Journal of Developmental and Physical Disabilities, 25,* 35–48.

Wacker, D. P., Lee, J. F., Padilla Dalmau, Y. C., Kopelman, T. G., Lindgren, S. D., Kuhle, J., et al. (2013b). Conducting functional analyses of problem behavior via telehealth. *Journal of Applied Behavior Analysis, 46,* 31–46.

Wacker, D. P., Schieltz, K. M., & Romani, P. (2015). Brief experimental analyses of problem behavior in a pediatric outpatient clinic. In H. S. Roane, J. E. Ringdahl, & T. S. Falcomata (Eds.), *Clinical and organizational applications of applied behavior analysis* (pp. 151–177). Amsterdam: Elsevier.

Wacker, D. P., Schieltz, K. M., Suess, A. N., Romani, P. W., Padilla Dalmau, Y. C., Kopelman, T. G., et al. (2016). Telehealth. In N. N. Singh (Ed.), *Clinical handbook of evidence-based practices for individuals with intellectual disabilities* (pp. 585–614). New York: Springer.

Wacker, D. P., Steege, M. W., Northup, J., Sasso, G., Berg, W., Reimers, T., et al. (1990). A component analysis of functional communication training across three topographies of severe behavior problems. *Journal of Applied Behavior Analysis, 23,* 417–429.

Xie, Y., Dixon, F., Yee, O. M., Zhang, J., Chen, A., DeAngelo, S., et al. (2013). A study on the effectiveness of videoconferencing on teaching parent training skills to parents of children with ADHD. *Telemedicine and e-Health, 19*(3), 192–199.

Yang, N. H., Dharmar, M., Yoo, B. K., Leigh, J. P., Kuppermann, N., Romano, P. S., et al. (2015). Economic evaluation of pediatric telemedicine consultation to rural emergency departments. *Medical Decision Making, 35*(6), 773–783.

# CHAPTER 32

# Organizational Behavior Management

## David A. Wilder and Nicole E. Gravina

Behavior analysts have used behavioral principles successfully in a range of settings and with a variety of populations. We refer to the application of these principles to individuals and groups in business, industry, government, and human-service settings as *organizational behavior management* (OBM). In this chapter, we first provide a description of OBM and its relation to applied behavior analysis and industrial–organizational psychology. Next, we briefly review the history of OBM. Finally, we examine the various subdisciplines of OBM. In doing so, we focus on common assessment and intervention strategies in each.

## OBM AND RELATED DISCIPLINES

OBM is a branch of applied behavior analysis, which is a branch of the discipline of behavior analysis or the science of behavior. Behavior analysis also includes the experimental analysis of behavior (the basic science branch of the discipline) and behaviorism (the conceptual or theoretical branch of the discipline). Applied behavior analysis consists of the application of operant and, to a lesser extent, respondent principles to behaviors of social significance. Unlike mainstream psychology, behavior analysis has a unified theoretical approach, behaviorism, and uses an inductive model of investigation. The more traditional hypothetical/deductive model of research, in which an investigator tests a hypothesis to determine the likelihood of its validity, is generally not the focus in behavior analysis. Instead, behavior-analytic researchers focus on manipulation of individual environmental variables of interest. Subsequent studies are based on the results of previous research with no formal tested hypothesis (Wilder, Austin, & Casella, 2009).

OBM is also related to the field of industrial–organizational psychology, in that the focus of both disciplines is the application of psychological or behavioral knowledge to work settings (see Bucklin, Alvero, Dickinson, Austin, & Jackson, 2000, for a comparison). The Hawthorne studies, conducted in the 1920s at an electric power plant in Illinois, influenced the two fields. One of the main findings of the Hawthorne studies was that a variety of environmental changes in work settings, including simply observing employees, can affect worker performance and productivity.

Beyond these similarities, however, the two fields differ in several ways. First, industrial–organizational psychology has an eclectic conceptual background. It derives the concepts on which it is based from several theoretical orientations. By contrast, OBM has a strictly behavior-analytic orientation. A second difference between the two disciplines is the techniques in which the practitioners of the two fields engage. Industrial–organizational psychologists spend much of their professional time on selection and placement of employees in organizations. By contrast, OBM practitioners spend most of their time assessing the variables contributing to employee performance deficits and developing programs to improve performance for individual employees and systems. A third difference between the two disciplines is the topics that each discipline studies. Industrial–organizational psychologists typically study personnel selection and placement, organizational culture, and leadership/decision making, and often use correlational or between-participants designs in their research. OBM researchers typically study performance management (Griffin, Gravina, Matey, Pritchard, & Wine, 2019), safety (Gravina, King, & Austin, 2019), and organizational systems (Kelley & Gravina, 2018), and often use within-participants designs in their research (Bucklin et al., 2000; Vergason & Gravina, 2020). The disciplines also differ in size. The Society for Industrial and Organizational Psychology represents industrial–organizational psychology and has more than 9,600 members (*www.siop.org/benefits*). The Organizational Behavior Management Network represents OBM, is a special-interest group of the Association for Behavior Analysis International, and has fewer than 500 members (H. McGee, personal communication, May 11, 2016).

## A BRIEF HISTORY OF OBM

The precursors to OBM as a discipline date as far back as the 1950s (see Dickinson, 2001). B. F. Skinner's 1953 text *Science and Human Behavior* included a chapter on "Economic Control" and introduced ideas about wage schedules and differentially reinforcing high-quality work performance. Many magazines and journals in the1960s, including the *Harvard Business Review* and the *Journal of Advertising Research*, published articles on managing performance. In addition, a formal organization devoted to performance improvement, the International Society for Performance Improvement, was established in 1962. Many founding International Society for Performance Improvement members were behavior analysts (Dickinson, 2001).

Perhaps the most widely publicized application of OBM took place at Emery Air Freight in the late 1960s. Edward Feeney, a sales manager at Emery, used a behavioral-systems package that he learned about in an OBM workshop to increase Emery

sales by over $2 million in a single year (O'Brien, Dickinson, & Rosow, 1982, p. 459). *Fortune* magazine featured a story about this success, which did much to expand familiarity with OBM in the business world. The discipline expanded rapidly in the late 1960s and 1970s, with professionals founding consulting firms such as Praxis and Behavioral Systems, Inc., and researchers founding the flagship journal in the field, the *Journal of Organizational Behavior Management*. The first editor of the *Journal of Organizational Behavior Management*, Aubrey Daniels, was also the founder of one of the first OBM consulting firms, Behavioral Systems, Inc. Interestingly, Fran Tarkenton, a famed quarterback for the Minnesota Vikings and New York Giants, cofounded this company. Daniels later left Behavioral Systems and founded Aubrey Daniels and Associates, which eventually became Aubrey Daniels International. Aubrey Daniels International remains one of the top OBM consulting firms (Dickinson, 2001).

The mission of the *Journal of Organizational Behavior Management* was and still is to publish articles on "scientific principles to improve organizational performance through behavior change" (*http://obmnetwork.com/publications/journal-of-organizational-behavior-management-jobm*). The journal publishes both conceptual and applied articles, highlights reports from the field, and invites both academics and practitioners to contribute. *Journal of Organizational Behavior Management* is the official journal of the Organizational Behavior Management Network.

A few specific topic areas have developed throughout OBM's history, to the point that we now consider them subdisciplines. These include performance management (Daniels & Bailey, 2014), behavioral safety (McSween, 2003), and behavioral-systems analysis (Rummler & Brache, 2012).

## PERFORMANCE MANAGEMENT

Although some use the terms *performance management* and OBM synonymously, we consider performance management a subdiscipline of OBM. The focus in performance management is on assessing and changing the performance of individuals or groups of employees to increase productivity and efficiency. Performance management is often conducted in a step-by-step fashion. The major steps include pinpointing or operationally defining a target performance; developing a system to measure the target performance; assessing the environmental variables that contribute to the occurrence of the target performance; intervening on the target performance; assessing the social validity, costs, and benefits of the intervention; and evaluating the maintenance of performance change. This step-by-step process has produced substantial performance improvements in organizations large and small, in the public and private sector, and in many industries (Daniels & Bailey, 2014).

## Assessment

Assessment in performance management consists of evaluating the reinforcers supporting both the performance targeted for change and the alternative or desired performance. Consultants commonly use the *PIC/NIC analysis* (Daniels & Bailey, 2014). In a PIC/NIC analysis, the consultant analyzes whether the target performance and an alternative performance produce positive, immediate, and certain consequences versus negative, future, and uncertain consequences. The *PIC* in the PIC/NIC analysis represents *positive, immediate,* and *certain;* the *NIC* represents *negative, immediate,* and *certain.* When conducting a PIC/NIC analysis, the manager or consultant categorizes the possible performance consequences as either positive, immediate, and certain, or negative, future, and uncertain. Those consequences that are positive, immediate, and certain are highly likely to influence performance. The consultant's job is to adjust the positive, immediate, and certain consequences so that they occur after the desired performance.

A study by Doll, Livesey, McHaffie, and Ludwig (2007) nicely illustrates this tool. The researchers analyzed cleaning performance by employees at a ski shop. Their PIC/NIC analysis found that the consequences for cleaning were often negative, in that cleaning the store took time away from interacting with customers and required physical labor. The researchers implemented an intervention that reversed the PIC/NIC analysis results. After the intervention, cleaning produced positive consequences, such as comments from a supervisor and a graph depicting cleaning performance.

Another common form of assessment in performance management is an informant-based tool called the Performance Diagnostic Checklist (Austin, 2000). Austin developed the Performance Diagnostic Checklist by asking expert OBM consultants what they do when initially assessing a performance problem. He arranged their responses into four categories: antecedents and information; equipment and processes; knowledge and skills; and consequences. Austin created a list of three to six questions for each category and a dichotomous response system. Austin intended that consultants, managers, or supervisors would use the tool to identify targeted interventions to improve employee performance. The first empirical demonstration of the Performance Diagnostic Checklist took place in a store in a shopping mall. The store was experiencing chronic cash shortages for each cash register at the end of shifts. The researchers used the Performance Diagnostic Checklist to examine potential variables that explained the cash shortages. Eight customer-service representatives at the store served as participants. The Performance Diagnostic Checklist identified the equipment and processes and the consequence categories as problematic. Using these results, the researchers changed employee assignments during shifts and delivered verbal and posted feedback. The intervention reduced the cash shortage at the store dramatically (Rohn, Austin, & Lutrey, 2003).

Researchers have used the Performance Diagnostic Checklist since then to identify the variables responsible for poor employee performance in many settings, including a coffee shop (Pampino, Heering, Wilder, Barton, & Burson, 2004), a department store (Eikenhout & Austin, 2005), a retail framing and art store (Pampino, MacDonald, Mullin, & Wilder, 2004), restaurants (Amigo, Smith, & Ludwig, 2008; Austin, Weatherly, & Gravina, 2005; Rodriguez et al., 2006), and a health clinic (Gravina, VanWagner, & Austin, 2008). The Performance Diagnostic Checklist has become a common assessment tool in performance management and has recently been adapted for specialized settings, topics, and populations (e.g., Smith & Wilder, 2018).

Researchers have recently adapted the Performance Diagnostic Checklist for human-service settings (Carr, Wilder, Majdalany, Mathisen, & Strain, 2013). Although performance management in particular and OBM in general can be applied in any setting, Carr et al. (2013) argued that human-service settings are sufficiently different from for-profit settings to warrant a specialized version of the Performance Diagnostic Checklist. The Performance Diagnostic Checklist—Human Services includes questions designed specifically for employee performance problems likely to be encountered in schools, clinics, group homes, and hospitals. Unlike the original Performance

Diagnostic Checklist, it also includes a direct-observation component and a list of suggested interventions matched to the results. Carr et al. used the Performance Diagnostic Checklist—Human Services to evaluate poor preparation of therapy rooms by therapists at a university-affiliated clinic for early, intensive behavior intervention. The results suggested that a lack of proper training and insufficient feedback were responsible for the performance deficits. During the intervention, the researchers trained the therapists to prepare therapy rooms adequately. They also provided graphed feedback on the therapists' performance. The intervention was effective; mean correct preparation of therapy rooms greatly improved during the intervention. Interestingly, the researchers also implemented an intervention that was not based on Performance Diagnostic Checklist—Human Services results, and it was ineffective, suggesting that the Performance Diagnostic Checklist—Human Services correctly identified an appropriate intervention. Ditzian, Wilder, King, and Tanz (2015) replicated this study with a different dependent variable and obtained similar results.

## Intervention

We can divide performance management interventions into two broad categories: *antecedent-based* and *consequence-based* procedures. Antecedent-based interventions include task clarification, training, manipulation of the effort required to perform a task, and goal setting. Consequence-based interventions include feedback and incentives or contingent access to money or work perks.

Researchers commonly use antecedent-based interventions to address performance problems in performance management. Task clarification consists of reviewing employee responsibilities related to the deficient target performance. Sometimes the tasks an employee is responsible for are posted in a salient location. Rice, Austin, and Gravina (2009) used task clarification to improve the customer-service behaviors of employees at a grocery store. The researchers taught the manager to clarify how employees were supposed to greet customers and what to say to them at the end of an interaction. Researchers taught the manager to deliver social praise contingent on correct employee performance. The intervention was effective; correct employee performance improved from a mean of fewer than 15% of opportunities to more than 60% of opportunities. In addition, the researchers collected follow-up data 48 weeks after the initial

task clarification meeting and found that the employees who received the intervention performed well, but those who did not performed poorly. Researchers have used task clarification in many other studies, with similar results (e.g., Austin et al., 2005; Choi, Johnson, Moon, & Oah, 2018; Durgin, Mahoney, Cox, Weetjens, & Poling, 2014; Palmer & Johnson, 2013).

Another common antecedent-based intervention in performance management is training. Sasson and Austin (2005) evaluated the effects of training to increase correct ergonomic performance among office workers. The training consisted of a one-on-one meeting in which the instructor first described correct wrist, neck, and shoulder positions when typing on a keyboard. Next, the instructor modeled the correct positions. Finally, each participant demonstrated the correct performance, and the instructor provided feedback. Training in performance management often follows this three-step model of description, modeling, and feedback. In addition, training in performance management is often criterion based, which means that the learner or employee must meet a mastery criterion before completing training (Howard & DiGennaro Reed, 2015). Notably, although researchers commonly use training, its effectiveness without other performance management interventions is often modest. For example, Sasson and Austin (2005) added feedback and employee involvement in conducting observations of peer performance to increase performance to high levels. Other performance management studies (Nordstrom, Lorenzi, & Hall, 1991) and reports from the field (Haberlin, Beauchamp, Agnew, & O'Brien, 2012) have also used training.

Reducing the effort required to perform a task, often called *reduced response effort*, is another antecedent-based performance management intervention. Abellon and Wilder (2014) reduced the distance that employees had to travel to use protective eyewear in a manufacturing facility, thereby reducing the effort of accessing the eyewear. They found that employees used protective eyewear much more often when it was close to their workstations. Brothers, Klantz, and McClannahan (1994) manipulated the proximity of recycling containers to office workers, thereby reducing the effort required to recycle documents. They found that recycling increased substantially when recycling containers were close to employees. Other studies have also demonstrated using reduced response effort to improve employee performance (Casella et al., 2010; Ludwig, Gray, & Rowell, 1998).

Goal setting is another strategy researchers have used to improve employee performance. Goals for improving performance should be challenging but achievable and should be set in collaboration with the employees. Several studies have evaluated goal setting. For example, Downing and Geller (2012) used goal setting with feedback to increase the frequency with which cashiers in a large grocery store checked customer identification to prevent identity theft. Identification checks increased from under 1% to nearly 10% due to the intervention. The researchers used participative goal setting, which means that they asked each cashier for assistance in setting individual goals. Other performance management studies also have used goal setting effectively (Amigo et al., 2008; Loewy & Bailey, 2007).

By far the most common consequence-based intervention in performance management is feedback (Alvero, Bucklin, & Austin, 2001). Although feedback can be an antecedent, such as when it is presented immediately before a performance opportunity, we review it here as a consequence-based procedure. Researchers have evaluated many characteristics of feedback, such as the person who delivers feedback (peer, supervisor, consultant), the frequency of feedback delivery (immediate, daily, weekly, monthly), and the format in which feedback is delivered (oral, written, graphic). In general, research has found that feedback is most effective when someone with authority over an employee, such as a supervisor, delivers feedback; when the feedback provider uses it frequently, ideally immediately, daily, or weekly; and when the feedback is in an easy-to-understand graphic format (Alvero et al., 2001). Ludwig, Biggs, Wagner, and Geller (2002) used publicly posted feedback to increase the correct driving performance of 82 pizza delivery drivers. Specifically, the researchers targeted using turn signals, using safety belts, and coming to a complete stop at intersections. Researchers posted employees' driving scores on a public graph that included each driver's name. Correct driving increased by 17–22% above baseline levels. Other performance management studies have used feedback to improve performance (Palmer & Johnson, 2013; So, Lee, & Oah, 2013).

Researchers have used feedback to improve performance in many settings with a variety of employees. For example, researchers have used feedback to improve the performance of supervisors and animal trainers in a nongovernmental organization in east Africa (Durgin et al., 2014), to increase credit card use in a retail setting (Loughrey,

Marshall, Bellizzi, & Wilder, 2013), and to improve employee performance in an aluminum smelt manufacturing facility (Jessup & Stahelski, 1999). Pampino, Wilder, and Binder (2005) evaluated feedback as a component of an intervention to increase accurate record keeping and submission of time sheets by construction foremen building a neighborhood. The feedback was part of a training procedure that required foremen to practice the correct performance repeatedly; they received immediate feedback on several aspects of their performance. These and other applications of feedback illustrate the robust nature of this intervention.

One common and popular form of feedback is the *sandwich method*, in which a supervisor provides positive comments about an employee's performance, followed by a comment describing what the employee is doing incorrectly, followed by another positive comment. Research does not support the effectiveness of sandwich feedback. Henley and DiGennaro Reed (2015) compared the feedback sandwich (positive–corrective–positive) to other sequences of feedback (positive–positive–corrective and corrective–positive–positive), and found that the corrective–positive–positive sequence was most effective, although the differences among the sequences were small. Interestingly, these authors also looked at the timing of feedback delivery. They delivered feedback either immediately after performance or just before the next opportunity participants had to perform the task. They found no differences in performance based on the timing of the feedback.

Another consequence-based performance management intervention consists of incentives or access to money or other work perks contingent on improved performance. Several studies have found that incentive or pay-for-performance systems result in more productive performance than salary-based or hourly pay systems (Long, Wilder, Betz, & Dutta, 2012; Oah & Lee, 2011; Slowiak, Dickinson, & Huitema, 2011). Thurkow, Bailey, and Stamper (2000) compared the effects of three types of incentive pay systems on the performance of telephone company employees. The researchers found that both individual and group incentives produced better performance than that during baseline. Individual incentives produced the highest rate of employee performance.

Although we have been describing each performance management intervention individually, most performance management interventions include more than one component. So-called *pack-*

*age interventions* increase the likelihood of the interventions' effectiveness. Unfortunately, the specific component or components most responsible for the effectiveness of the package intervention are often difficult to identify. For that reason, we encourage performance management researchers and practitioners to introduce intervention components systematically, one at a time.

## BEHAVIORAL SAFETY

*Behavioral safety* is the use of behavior-analytic principles and techniques to improve safe performance (Krause, 1997). The *Journal of Organizational Behavior Management* published the first OBM study addressing safety in 1978 (Komaki, Barwick, & Scott, 1978). Shortly afterward, Fox, Hopkins, and Anger (1987) began working on one of the longest-running evaluations of a behavioral approach to improving safety in a coal mine and in a uranium ore mine. Many other behavior analysts have contributed to the development and evolution of behavioral safety since then, including Sulzer-Azaroff (1980), McSween (1995), Geller (1996), and Daniels and Agnew (2010). Today, behavioral safety is one of the most popular approaches to increasing safe performance in many industries (e.g., Hagge, McGee, Matthews, & Aberle, 2017).

The U.S. Bureau of Labor Statistics (BLS) reported that nearly 4 million workplace injuries and illnesses and over 4,600 workplace fatalities in the United States occurred in 2014 (BLS, 2014a). Safety-related incidents and injuries have been on the decline for many years, due to a greater understanding of ways to prevent them and an increased focus on reducing them. Although workplace injuries are declining, fatalities have flat-lined (BLS, 2014b), which has produced a new focus on process safety (Occupational Health and Safety Administration, 2000). Process safety includes identifying strategies to influence safe behaviors and noticing and reporting safety concerns—things that behavioral safety is well suited to address (Bogard, Ludwig, Staats, & Kretschmer, 2015).

The popularity of behavioral safety is likely due to its effectiveness for increasing safe behaviors and reducing injuries (Krause, Seymour, & Sloat, 1999). Many studies have demonstrated a reduction in injuries, and even more have demonstrated an increase in safe behaviors after the use of behavioral-safety techniques (Grindle, Dickinson, & Boettcher, 2000; Sulzer-Azaroff & Austin,

2000). One meta-analysis of behavioral-safety applications reported a reduction in injuries in 32 of 33 studies reviewed (Sulzer-Azaroff & Austin, 2000). The settings included construction sites, utility companies, manufacturing plants, mines, and shipyards; most were in the United States, but some were in other countries. A more recent behavioral-safety meta-analysis with more stringent inclusion criteria found a reduction in injuries in 12 of 13 studies evaluated (Tuncel, Lotlikar, Salem, & Daraiseh, 2006). The techniques researchers use in behavioral-safety applications can vary, depending on the unique needs of a site and assessment findings. Therefore, Tuncel et al. (2006) have recommended that researchers clearly report assessment methods and results in behavioral safety, so that they can more closely link assessment to intervention selection.

### Assessment

One of the first activities that usually occurs in a behavioral-safety implementation is a safety assessment. A safety assessment has several objectives, including (1) identifying behaviors and conditions to target that are likely to have an impact on safety and injury reduction, (2) identifying variables that influence the targets, (3) understanding the context in which those behaviors and conditions occur, (4) identifying existing safety programs, and (5) building employee and management support (Agnew & Snyder, 2008; McSween, 2003).

A consultant reviews workplace practices and policies and current safety initiatives and programs in a behavioral-safety assessment (McSween, 2003). Initiatives and programs often emphasize areas the organization views as deficient and may provide clues for behavioral targets. In addition, the consultant gathers information about the site, including number of employees, supervisors, managers, nature of the work, union affiliation, worker age, rate of turnover, and shift scheduling.

The consultant reviews data on injuries; incidents; close calls; and environmental issues, when applicable (e.g., spills at a chemical manufacturing site) for the previous 2–5 years (McSween, 2003). The goal is to uncover trends in how, when, where, and why injuries and incidents occur. This may require grouping the data by area, job, body part injured, task, shift, and other variables, to determine behaviors that may be valuable safety targets and situations in which injuries are more likely to occur. In addition to the site-specific data, safety information on the specific industry or job may provide more ideas for safety targets. For example, certified nursing assistants often have back injuries while transferring patients; therefore, patient lifting may be an important target for reducing these employees' back injuries (BLS, 2011).

The assessment should also include interviews, a survey, and direct observation to gather more information on the workplace's context, potential targets, and safety culture. The consultant should conduct interviews with front-line workers, supervisors, managers, and leaders, to learn about safety challenges at the site from multiple perspectives (McSween, 2003). Using an anonymous survey with behaviorally oriented questions is a low-effort way to identify safety concerns that may warrant further investigation. For example, most workers disagreeing with the statement "All injuries on this site are reported" may indicate that someone has punished injury reporting in the past, and that gathering accurate data in this area may require concerted effort. Or employees reporting that their supervisor talks to them about safety less than once per month may indicate that engaging supervisors in the behavioral-safety process will be important. Surveys are often followed by direct observation to verify accuracy.

The consultant may include several OBM tools in an assessment to facilitate a better understanding of why at-risk behaviors are occurring. For example, the Performance Diagnostic Checklist—Safety provides a list of questions aimed at identifying potential factors impeding safe performance and directions for intervention selection (Martinez-Onstott, Wilder, & Sigurdsson, 2016). Like similar assessments in OBM, the questionnaire covers four areas: antecedents and information; knowledge and skills; equipment and processes; and consequences. Research has shown that interventions selected from the results of a performance diagnostic checklist are effective (Johnson, Casella, McGee, & Lee, 2014).

An antecedent–behavior–consequence (A-B-C) analysis can also provide valuable insight for understanding antecedents and consequences that may influence safe and at-risk behaviors (Health and Safety Executive, 2012). A typical A-B-C analysis examines both the desired and undesired behaviors and lists antecedents and consequences for each. The consultant scores each behavior as positive or negative, immediate or future, and certain or uncertain (Daniels & Bailey, 2014). Positive, immediate, and certain consequences encourage behaviors, and negative, immediate, uncertain

consequences discourage behaviors. Often, safety-related behaviors do not have positive, immediate, certain consequences, or may even have negative, immediate, uncertain consequences. The reverse is often true for at-risk behavior. For example, wearing a hard hat may feel hot and uncomfortable, which are negative, immediate, and certain consequences. Working without it may produce social support for being "tough" and completing work faster, which are positive, immediate consequences. Changing this behavior involves attempting to adjust the consequences it produces. This level of analysis for safety targets allows for a more customized behavioral-safety process.

The safety assessment should produce a report that lists behaviors and conditions that a behavior-based safety intervention can target and recommendations for intervention components. In addition, the assessment may indicate the starting point for intervention, who to involve in the process, the cultural challenges, and when to start. We describe the steps in behavioral-safety interventions next.

### Intervention

Although there is some variation, practitioners and consultants use the following steps in the behavioral-safety process: (1) Form a safety committee; (2) identify behaviors and conditions to target; (3) develop a measurement system; (4) create a feedback, reinforcement, and problem-solving plan; and (5) continually improve the process (Austin, 2006; Agnew & Snyder, 2008; McSween, 2003). The safety committee usually consists of representatives from the workforce, supervisors, safety department (if one exists), and leadership (McSween, 2003). The safety committee manages the behavioral-safety process, which is often described as employee-led (Krause, 1995). Research in OBM suggests that participation by employees may increase the impact of the intervention (Sigurdsson & Austin, 2006), and behavioral-safety practitioners suggest that employee participation increases acceptance and maintenance of behavioral-safety programs (Geller, 2002). Research has also demonstrated that participation in setting safety goals may have a positive impact on performance (Fellner & Sulzer-Azaroff, 1985). The safety committee is one way that the behavioral-safety process increases employee engagement.

The consultant uses the safe behaviors and conditions the safety assessment has identified to create an observations checklist. Such checklists often include a space for describing barriers to performance (Austin, 2006). The observations can improve worker safety, produce better hazard recognition, produce improved feedback on safe performance, provide information for more focused safety intervention targets, and create social consequences for performing safely (McSween, 2003). Additionally, the observation process may leverage the observer effect, which occurs when a person conducting an observation improves his or her own safe behaviors (Alvero & Austin, 2004). Peer observations are the most common, but research has shown that self-observations increase safe behaviors and are a good alternative for employees who work alone (e.g., Hickman & Geller, 2005; Olson & Austin, 2001). Employees only (e.g., Cooper, Phillips, Sutherland, & Makin, 1994), supervisors only (e.g., Chhokar & Wallin, 1984), both, everyone in the organization, or outside observers only (e.g., Ludwig & Geller, 1997) can conduct the observations. The observation checklist serves as the basis for the measurement system.

The observation and feedback process can also focus on supervisory and leader behavior. For example, Cooper (2006) evaluated the impact of management support in a behavioral-safety process in a paper mill. Cooper asked employees to complete a checklist that indicated whether leaders with whom they interacted that week provided visible ongoing support. An exploratory analysis showed statistically significant correlations between visible ongoing support from leaders and safety performance of employees, ranging from .47 to .72 in the three areas included in the study, although the effects seemed to diminish over time. Zohar and Luria (2003) examined an intervention to increase line supervisors' safety-related interactions and found that safe behaviors and safety climate scores increased as safety interactions increased. Although research on the importance of manager engagement in safety observations and interactions is still limited, this is clearly an avenue worthy of further investigation and is potentially an important part of the observation system.

After a consultant establishes an observation system, he or she uses the data to provide feedback to employees and to reinforce progress. Feedback delivery often includes graphic, publicly posted feedback on safe behaviors. For example, Komaki et al. (1978) used publicly posted graphic feedback updated after each observation period to improve the safe practices of employees in a bakery. This intervention, plus goal setting and supervisor praise, produced a dramatic improvement in safe performance. The researchers also trained an employee to continue the intervention.

An intervention package can also include incentives for improving safety. McSween (2003) suggests offering a menu of awards and incentives in a tiered fashion based on effort. Hickman and Geller (2005) provided a small incentive ($1 per self-observation form) to short-haul truck drivers for completing self-observations before or after each shift. Participation in the prebehavior group was 42%, and participation in the postbehavior group was 75%. Both groups demonstrated an improvement in overspeed and extreme braking. At the other end of the spectrum, Fox et al. (1987) created an elaborate token-economy reward system for behaving safely *and* avoiding injuries at two mines. Workers could exchange the tokens in the local community to purchase products and services. The intervention produced a substantial reduction in injuries. Although it cost between $9,000 and $22,000 per year per site, the return on investment was substantial, ranging from 13:1 to 28:1 depending on the year. The intervention had been in place for 10 years when the study was published, demonstrating long-term maintenance of a behavioral-safety program.

There are several other considerations in designing a behavioral-safety intervention. For example, conducting observations can be mandatory or voluntary and can be scheduled daily, weekly, monthly, or even less frequently. Observation checklists can be lengthy or brief. Observers can announce their presence and give feedback, or can observe discreetly and not provide feedback in the moment. Unfortunately, the research available to inform these decisions is limited. One study suggested that mandatory behavioral-safety processes produced higher participation and satisfaction with behavioral-safety interventions than voluntary ones (DePasquale & Geller, 2000). Behavioral-safety interventions could benefit from more research on these and related topics.

Although behavioral safety has had a significant impact on improving safe practices and reducing injuries in the workplace, opportunities to strengthen and refine the practice exist. For example, the field needs more research to determine the best strategies for implementing a peer observation system. Whether overt or discrete observations, long or short checklists, or supervisor-to-employee or peer-to-peer observations yield the most accurate data and greatest behavior change is unclear. In addition, we need to focus on leadership behavior and design, to evaluate interventions that have a positive impact on leader behavior, and to evaluate the impact of changes in leader behavior on worker behavior and safe performance. Also, although research has demonstrated the efficacy of behavioral safety, some behavioral-safety processes are short-lived or meet resistance and never fully take hold in practice. Further investigation into the factors that produce active, well-received, and sustained behavioral-safety processes will allow OBM to have an even more substantial impact on workplace safety in the years to come. Finally, we need additional research on safety belt use and safe driving in general (see Wilder & Sigurdsson, 2015, for a review).

## BEHAVIORAL-SYSTEMS ANALYSIS

Another subdiscipline of OBM is *behavioral-systems analysis*, which involves understanding an organization by outlining the system's parts and processes and determining how they interact. Behavioral-systems analysis developed through the work of many pioneers in the fields of OBM and human performance improvement (e.g., Brethower, 1982; Gilbert, 1996; Glenn, 1988; R. W. Malott, 1974; M. E. Malott, 2003). OBM tends to focus on specific behaviors. By contrast, behavioral-systems analysis emphasizes the broader context in which the behaviors occur and is more likely to focus on results such as sales, expenses, and customer service (Abernathy, 2014; Hyten, 2009). Some researchers have suggested that OBM should adopt a more systemic approach to increase the durability of its interventions and its attractiveness and relevance to business; behavioral-systems analysis incorporates this approach (Abernathy, 2014; Hyten, 2009).

Rummler and Brache (2012) argue that the greatest opportunities for improving overall performance and results arise in the handoffs between employees or departments, which are often not the focus of OBM consultations or research. Unless the entire system is considered, an intervention that strengthens performance in one area could be detrimental to another (Abernathy, 2014; Rummler & Brache, 2012). To illustrate, if manufacturing triples production and sales are unable to keep up, the organization will have spent more money than necessary on products that it is now forced to store. Additionally, behavior targets identified without a

systems lens may not improve intended results. For example, Johnson and Frederiksen (1984) conducted a study in a mental health institution in which they compared the provision of feedback on process (behavioral) versus outcome (results) measures. The process intervention increased process behaviors but did not affect outcome; the outcome intervention did not improve outcome or process behaviors. This suggests that the researchers did not identify the correct behaviors that would have improved outcomes. Redmon (1991) suggests that OBM interventions should clearly link to key organizational goals. Behavioral-systems analysis helps OBM to place its effective interventions in the context of the whole business and align behavior targets with important goals and results.

### Assessment

Many tools exist in behavioral-systems analysis to assess organizational systems and processes, although research has empirically evaluated few of them (Johnson et al., 2014). Rummler and Brache (2012) examined organizations at three levels: the organization, the process, and the job and performer. The *organizational* level describes the organization in the greater context in which it exists, highlighting inputs, primary processes, outputs, and outside influences and sources of feedback (such as competitors, regulations, and stakeholders). The *process* level describes how the work gets done from first input to final output in a step-by-step fashion; it includes information about tools, quality checks, and decision points. The *job and performer* level focuses on factors affecting job completion that could cause and reduce human error and increase worker efficiency.

Assessments at each of these levels are designed to describe the current or *is* state of a system or process, and to identify opportunities for improving efficiency, reducing costs, reducing cycle time, and increasing quality (Sasson, Alvero, & Austin, 2006). An assessment often involves using a tool to create a visual depiction of the level, such as the Total Performance System Relationship Map described by Brethower (1982) or the Process Map described by Rummler and Brache (2012), and a list of performance deficiencies or opportunities for improving the system. In addition, the consultant gathers data on current performance levels and performance potentials (Gilbert, 1996). The upper panel of Figure 32.1 depicts an example of an *is* process map for an employee's trip approval process.

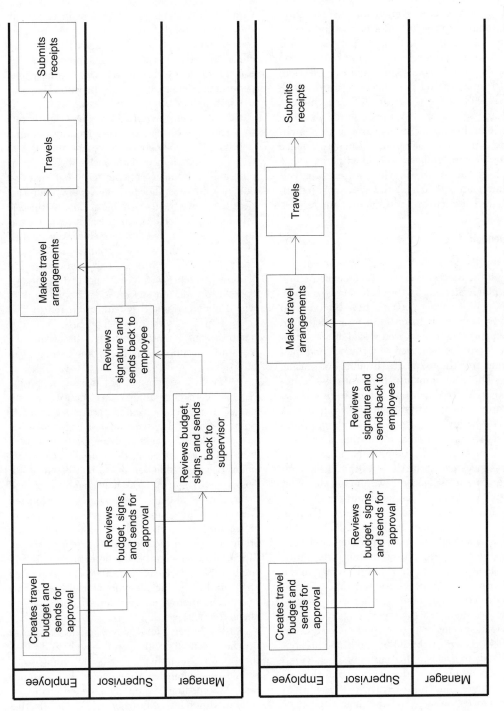

**FIGURE 32.1.** The upper panel depicts an *is* process map for an employee's trip approval process. The lower panel depicts a *should* process map for the same process. The consultant determined that manager approval was unnecessary.

Assessments in behavioral-systems analysis also involve collecting information in six areas, to identify root causes of process problems and opportunities for improvement: (1) information and expectations; (2) equipment, tools, and resources; (3) consequences and incentives; (4) knowledge and skills; (5) capacity, ability, and employee selection; and (6) motives and preferences (Austin, 2000; Binder, 1998; Sasson & Austin, 2003). In this way, these assessments are like the Performance Diagnostic Checklist (Austin, 2000), which researchers and consultants commonly use in performance management to evaluate individual performance as discussed above. In behavioral-systems analysis, this information then leads to a systemic intervention aimed at improving performance and results.

## Intervention

In behavioral-systems analysis, assessment involves using tools to create a visual depiction and greater understanding of the current or *is* state of a system or process in an organization. Intervention involves using tools to create a visual depiction and supports for an improved *should* or ideal state that will produce improved performance and then implementing those changes (Rummler & Brache, 2012). The consultant usually identifies the improved state by examining industry knowledge, the current state, and associated performance issues, and by interviewing people working in and around the system or process (Austin, 2000; Rummler & Brache, 2012). Using behavioral-systems analysis gives people in the organization a common and useful language to communicate about performance issues, which facilitates the development and implementation of solutions (Binder, 1998). The lower panel of Figure 32.1 depicts an example of a *should* process map for an employee's trip approval process. The consultant determined that manager approval, shown in the *is* map in the upper panel, was unnecessary and time-consuming, so the consultant omitted it in the *should* map.

The research on interventions devised via behavioral-systems analysis is sparse (Johnson et al., 2014). Sasson et al. (2006) conducted an analogue study to evaluate the impact of a behavioral intervention, a process intervention, and the two interventions combined. Participants completed a word-processing task, and the main dependent variables were completion speed and errors. The process differences were manual (physically picking up and dropping off the task) and electronic (receiving and sending the task by e-mail). The

behavioral intervention was a graduated monetary bonus for performance on each of the dependent variables. Data analysis showed main effects for the process and the behavioral interventions, but the combined intervention produced the greatest effect. The researchers concluded that process-level *and* performer-level interventions may maximize performance improvements in the workplace.

Cunningham, Geller, and Clarke (2008) compared a computerized provider order-entry system to a paper process for ordering medications in a hospital. The study goal was to determine the effects on compliance with medication-ordering protocols and time to patients' receiving their first dose of antibiotics. The hospital's goal was for a patient to receive the first antibiotic dose within 240 minutes of the medication order's arrival. Results showed that compliance with medication-ordering protocols was 60% with the computerized system, compared to 47% with the paper process. Additionally, patients received their first antibiotic dose within 240 minutes on 78% of opportunities with the computerized system, compared to 55% of opportunities with the paper process. This study demonstrated that process changes alone can have a significant impact on important outcomes in business.

Although research and practice support using behavioral-systems analysis to improve performance in organizations, an opportunity to incorporate behavioral-systems analysis into OBM research exists, even at the job and performer level. In a systematic review of the *Journal of Organizational Behavior Management* from 1992 to 2001, Sasson and Austin (2003) evaluated published interventions to determine how many considered the six areas listed above when selecting intervention components. The authors found that only one study considered the six areas (LaFleur & Hyten, 1995). Most only considered up to three (see Figure 9 of Sasson & Austin, 2003). They suggested that OBM could include more behavioral-systems analyses to improve intervention selection, even at the performer level.

Although behavioral-systems analysis focuses on the effects of context on behavior, and OBM focuses on the individual, the two frameworks should be synergistic. An employee will have difficulty succeeding in a poorly designed process or system (Rummler & Brache, 2012), but effective processes and systems require employees to behave productively. Therefore, a synergistic approach is likely to produce the best outcomes for business and increased recognition for the field.

## CONCLUSION

OBM is the application of behavioral principles to improve the performance of employees in organizations and is a branch of applied behavior analysis. In contrast to industrial–organizational psychology, OBM has a theoretically unified orientation and focuses on the direct manipulation of variables that have an important impact on employee well-being and the organization's bottom line. Three OBM subdisciplines exist: performance management, behavioral safety, and behavioral-systems analysis. Each of these includes assessment techniques and intervention procedures for a variety of organizational problems.

## REFERENCES

Abellon, O. E., & Wilder, D. A. (2014). The effect of equipment proximity on safe performance in a manufacturing setting. *Journal of Applied Behavior Analysis, 47,* 628–632.

Abernathy, B. (2014). Beyond the Skinner box: The design and management of organization-wide performance systems. *Journal of Organizational Behavior Management, 34*(4), 235–254.

Agnew, J., & Snyder, G. (2008). *Removing obstacles to safety: A behavior-based approach.* Atlanta, GA: Performance Management.

Alvero, A. M., & Austin, J. (2004). The effects of observing on the behavior of the observer. *Journal of Applied Behavior Analysis, 37,* 457–468.

Alvero, A. M., Bucklin, B. R., & Austin, J. (2001). An objective review of the effectiveness and essential characteristics of performance feedback in organizational settings. *Journal of Organizational Behavior Management, 21*(1), 3–29.

Amigo, S., Smith, A., & Ludwig, T. (2008). Using task clarification, goal setting, and feedback to decrease table busing times in a franchise pizza restaurant. *Journal of Organizational Behavior Management, 28*(3), 176–187.

Austin, J. (2000). Performance analysis and performance diagnostics. In J. Austin & J. E. Carr (Eds.), *Handbook of applied behavior analysis* (pp. 321–349). Reno, NV: Context Press.

Austin, J. (2006, January–February). An introduction to behavior-based safety. *Stone, Sand, and Gravel Review,* 38–39.

Austin, J., Weatherly, N. L., & Gravina, N. E. (2005). Using task clarification, graphic feedback, and verbal feedback to increase closing-task completion in a privately owned restaurant. *Journal of Applied Behavior Analysis, 38,* 117–120.

Binder, C. (1998). The Six Boxes™: A descendent of Gilbert's behavior engineering model. Retrieved from *www.binder-riha.com/sixboxes.pdf.*

Bogard, K., Ludwig, T. D., Staats, C., & Kretschmer, D. (2015). An industry's call to understand the contingencies involved in process safety: Normalization of deviance. *Journal of Organizational Behavior Management, 35*(1–2), 70–80.

Brethower, D. M. (1982). The Total Performance System. In R. M. O'Brien, A. M. Dickinson, & M. P. Rosow (Eds.), *Industrial behavior modification: A management handbook* (pp. 350–369). New York: Pergamon Press.

Brothers, K. J., Krantz, P. J., & McClannahan, L. E. (1994). Office paper recycling: A function of container proximity. *Journal of Applied Behavior Analysis, 27,* 153–160.

Bucklin, B. R., Alvero, A. M., Dickinson, A. M., Austin, J., & Jackson, A. K. (2000). Industrial organizational psychology and organizational behavior management. *Journal of Organizational Behavior Management, 20*(2), 27–75.

Bureau of Labor Statistics (BLS). (2011, October 20). Workplace injuries and illnesses—2010 (News release USDL-11-1502). Retrieved from *www.bls.gov/news.release/pdf/osh.pdf.*

Bureau of Labor Statistics (BLS). (2014a). Employer-related workplace injuries and illnesses—2014. Retrieved from *www.bls.gov/news.release/pdf/osh.pdf.*

Bureau of Labor Statistics (BLS). (2014b). National census of fatal occupational injuries. Retrieved from *www.bls.gov/news.release/pdf/cfoi.pdf.*

Carr, J. E., Wilder, D. A., Majdalany, L., Mathisen, D., & Strain, L. A. (2013). An assessment-based solution to a human-service employee performance problem: An initial evaluation of the Performance Diagnostic Checklist—Human Services. *Behavior Analysis in Practice, 6,* 16–32.

Casella, S. E., Wilder, D. A., Neidert, P., Rey, C., Compton, M., & Chong, I. (2010). The effects of response effort on safe performance by therapists at an autism treatment facility. *Journal of Applied Behavior Analysis, 43,* 729–734.

Chhokar, J. S., & Wallin, J. A. (1984). A field study of the effect of feedback frequency on performance. *Journal of Applied Psychology, 69*(3), 524–530.

Choi, E., Johnson, D. A., Moon, K., & Oah, S. (2018). Effects of positive and negative feedback sequence on work performance and emotional responses. *Journal of Organizational Behavior Management, 38*(2–3), 97–115.

Cooper, M. D. (2006). Exploratory analyses of the effects of managerial support and feedback consequences on behavioral safety maintenance. *Journal of Organizational Behavior Management, 26*(3), 1–41.

Cooper, M. D., Phillips, R. A., Sutherland, V. J., & Makin, P. J. (1994). Reducing accidents using goal setting and feedback: A field study. *Journal of Occupational and Organizational Psychology, 67,* 219–240.

Cunningham, T. R., Geller, E. S., & Clarke, S. W. (2008). Impact of electronic prescribing in a hospital setting: A process-focused evaluation. *International Journal of Medical Informatics, 77,* 546–554.

Daniels, A. C., & Agnew, J. (2010). *Safe by accident?* Atlanta, GA: Performance Management.

Daniels, A. C., & Bailey, J. (2014). *Performance management: Changing behavior that drives organizational effectiveness* (5th ed.). Tucker, GA: Performance Management.

DePasquale, J. P., & Geller, E. S. (1999). Critical success factors for behavior-based safety: A study of twenty industry-wide applications. *Journal of Safety Research, 30*(4), 237–249.

Dickinson, A. M. (2001). The historical roots of organizational behavior management in the private sector. *Journal of Organizational Behavior Management, 20*(3), 9–58.

Ditzian, K., Wilder, D. A., King, A., & Tanz, J. (2015). An evaluation of the Performance Diagnostic Checklist—Human Services to assess an employee performance problem in a center-based autism treatment facility. *Journal of Applied Behavior Analysis, 48,* 199–203.

Doll, J., Livesey, J., McHaffie, E., & Ludwig, T. D. (2007). Keeping an uphill edge: Managing cleaning behaviors at a ski shop. *Journal of Organizational Behavior Management, 27*(3), 41–60.

Downing, C. O., & Geller, E. S. (2012). A goal-setting and feedback intervention to increase ID-checking behavior: An assessment of social validity and behavioral impact. *Journal of Organizational Behavior Management, 32*(4), 297–306.

Durgin, A., Mahoney, A., Cox, C., Weetjens, B. J., & Poling, A. (2014). Using task clarification and feedback training to improve staff performance in an east African nongovernmental organization. *Journal of Organizational Behavior Management, 34*(2), 122–143.

Eikenhout, N., & Austin, J. (2005). Using goals, feedback, reinforcement, and a performance matrix to improve customer service in a large department store. *Journal of Organizational Behavior Management, 24*(3), 27–62.

Fellner, D. J., & Sulzer-Azaroff, B. (1985). Occupational safety: Assessment the impact of adding assigned or participative goal setting. *Journal of Organizational Behavior Management, 7,* 3–23.

Fox, D. K., Hopkins, B. L., & Anger, W. K. (1987). The long-term effects of a token economy on safety performance in open-pit mining. *Journal of Applied Behavior Analysis, 20,* 215–224.

Geller, E. S. (1996). *Working safe: How to help people actively care for health and safety.* Boca Raton, FL: CRC Press.

Geller, E. S. (2002). *The participation factor: How to increase involvement in occupational safety.* Chicago: ASSE.

Gilbert, T. F. (1996). *Human competence: Engineering worthy performance.* Amherst, MA: HRD Press.

Glenn, S. S. (1988). Contingencies and metacontingencies: Toward a synthesis of behavior analysis and cultural materialism. *Behavior Analyst, 11*(2), 161–179.

Gravina, N., King, A., & Austin, J. (2019). Training leaders to apply behavioral concepts to improve safety. *Safety Science, 112,* 66–70.

Gravina, N., VanWagner, M., & Austin, J. (2008). Increasing physical therapy equipment preparation using task clarification, feedback, and environmental manipulations. *Journal of Organizational Behavior Management, 28*(2), 110–122.

Griffin, M., Gravina, N. E., Matey, J., Pritchard, J., & Wine, B. (2019). Using scorecards and a lottery to improve the performance of behavior technicians in two autism treatment clinics. *Journal of Organizational Behavior Management, 39*(3–4), 280–292.

Grindle, A. C., Dickinson, A. M., & Boettcher, W. (2000). Behavioral safety research in manufacturing settings: A review of the literature. *Journal of Organizational Behavior Management, 20*(1), 29–68.

Haberlin, A. T., Beauchamp, K., Agnew, J., & O'Brien, F. (2012). A comparison of pyramidal staff training and direct staff training in community-based day programs. *Journal of Organizational Behavior Management, 32*(1), 65–74.

Hagge, M., McGee, H., Matthews, G., & Aberle, S. (2017). Behavior-based safety in a coal mine: The relationship between observations, participation, and injuries over a 14-year period. *Journal of Organizational Behavior Management, 37,* 107–118.

Health and Safety Executive. (2012). Leadership and worker involvement toolkit: The ABC analysis. Retrieved from *www.hse.gov.uk/construction/lwit/assets/downloads/abc-analysis.pdf.*

Henley, A. J., & DiGennaro Reed, F. (2015). Should you order the feedback sandwich?: Efficacy of feedback sequence and timing. *Journal of Organizational Behavior Management, 35*(3), 321–355.

Hickman, J. S., & Geller, E. S. (2003). Self-management to increase safe driving among short-haul truck drivers. *Journal of Organizational Behavior Management, 23*(4), 1–20.

Howard, V. J., & DiGennaro Reed, F. (2015). An evaluation of training procedures for animal shelter volunteers. *Journal of Organizational Behavior Management, 35*(3), 296–320.

Hyten, C. (2009). Strengthening the focus on business results: The need for systems approaches in OBM. *Journal of Organizational Behavior Management, 29*(2), 87–107.

Jessup, P. A., & Stahelski, A. J. (1999). The effects of a combined goal setting, feedback, and incentive intervention on job performance in a manufacturing environment. *Journal of Organizational Behavior Management, 19*(3), 5–26.

Johnson, D. A., Casella, S. E., McGee, H., & Lee, S. C. (2014). The use and validation of preintervention diagnostic tools in organizational behavior management. *Journal of Organizational Behavior Management, 34*(2), 104–121.

Johnson, R. P., & Frederiksen, L. W. (1984). Process vs. outcome feedback and goal setting in a human service organization. *Journal of Organizational Behavior Management, 5*(3–4), 37–56.

Kelley, D. P., & Gravina, N. (2018). Every minute counts: Using process improvement and performance feedback to improve patient flow in an emergency department. *Journal of Organizational Behavior Management, 38*, 234–243.

Komaki, J., Barwick, K. D., & Scott, L. R. (1978). A behavioral approach to occupational safety: Pinpointing and reinforcing safe performance in a food manufacturing plant. *Journal of Applied Psychology, 63*, 424–445.

Krause, T. R. (1995). *Employee-driven systems for safe behavior: Integrating behavioral and statistical methodologies.* New York: Van Nostrand Reinhold.

Krause, T. R. (1997). *The behavior-based safety process: Managing involvement for an injury-free culture.* New York: Van Nostrand Reinhold.

Krause, T. R., Seymour, K. J., & Sloat, K. C. M. (1999). Long-term evaluation of a behavior-based method for improving safety performance: A meta-analysis of 73 interrupted time-series replications. *Safety Science, 32*, 1–18.

LaFleur, T., & Hyten, C. (1995). Improving the quality of hotel banquet staff performance. *Journal of Organizational Behavior Management, 15*(1–2), 69–93.

Loewy, S., & Bailey, J. (2007). The effects of graphic feedback, goal setting, and manager praise on customer service behaviors. *Journal of Organizational Behavior Management, 27*(3), 15–26.

Long, R. D., Wilder, D. A., Betz, A., & Dutta, A. (2012). Effects of and preference for pay for performance: An analogue analysis. *Journal of Applied Behavior Analysis, 45*, 821–826.

Loughrey, T., Marshall, G., Bellizzi, A., & Wilder, D. A. (2013). The use of video modeling, prompting, and feedback to increase credit card promotion in a retail setting. *Journal of Organizational Behavior Management, 33*(3), 200–208.

Ludwig, T. D., Biggs, J., Wagner, S., & Geller, E. S. (2002). Using public feedback and competitive rewards to increase the safe driving of pizza deliverers. *Journal of Organizational Behavior Management, 21*(4), 75–104.

Ludwig, T. D., & Geller, E. S. (1997). Assigned versus participatory goal setting and response generalization: Managing injury control among professional pizza deliverers. *Journal of Applied Psychology, 82*(2), 253–261.

Ludwig, T. D., Gray, T. W., & Rowell, A. (1998). Increasing recycling in academic buildings: A systematic replication. *Journal of Applied Behavior Analysis, 31*, 683–686.

Malott, M. E. (2003). *Paradox of organizational change.* Reno, NV: Context Press.

Malott, R. W. (1974). A behavioral systems approach to the design of human services. In D. Harshbarger & R. F. Maley (Eds.), *Behavior analysis and systems analysis: An integrative approach to mental health programs* (pp. 318–343). Kalamazoo, MI: Behaviordelia.

Martinez-Onstott, B., Wilder, D., & Sigurdsson, S. (2016). Identifying the variables contributing to at-risk performance: Initial evaluation of the Performance Diagnostic Checklist—Safety (PDC-Safety). *Journal of Organizational Behavior Management, 36*(1), 80–93.

McSween, T. E. (1995). *The values-based safety process: Improving your safety culture with a behavioral approach.* New York: Van Nostrand Reinhold.

McSween, T. E. (2003). *The values-based safety process: Improving your safety culture with behavior-based safety* (2nd ed.). Hoboken, NJ: Wiley.

Nordstrom, R., Lorenzi, P., & Hall, R. V. (1991). A behavioral training program for managers in city government. *Journal of Organizational Behavior Management, 11*(2), 189–212.

Oah, S., & Lee, J. (2011). Effects of hourly, low-incentive, and high-incentive pay on simulated work productivity: Initial findings with a new laboratory method. *Journal of Organizational Behavior Management, 31*(1), 21–42.

O'Brien, R. M., Dickinson, A. M., & Rosow, R. P. (Eds.). (1982). *Industrial behavior modification.* New York: Pergamon Press.

Occupational Health and Safety Administration. (2000, reprinted). Process safety management. Retrieved from *www.osha.gov/Publications/osha3132.html.*

Olson, R., & Austin, J. (2001). Behavior-based safety and working alone: The effects of a self-monitoring package on the safe performance of bus operators. *Journal of Organizational Behavior Management, 21*(3), 5–43.

Palmer, M. G., & Johnson, M. (2013). The effects of task clarification and group graphic feedback on early punch-in times. *Journal of Organizational Behavior Management, 33*(4), 265–275.

Pampino, R. N., Heering, P. W., Wilder, D. A., Barton, C. G., & Burson, L. M. (2004). The use of the Performance Diagnostic Checklist to guide intervention selection in an independently owned coffee shop. *Journal of Organizational Behavior Management, 23*(2), 5–19.

Pampino, R. N., MacDonald, J. E., Mullin, J. E., & Wilder, D. A. (2004). Weekly feedback versus daily feedback: An application in retail. *Journal of Organizational Behavior Management, 23*(2), 21–43.

Pampino, R. N., Wilder, D. A., & Binder, C. (2005). The use of functional assessment and frequency building procedures to increase product knowledge and data entry skills among foreman in a construction organization. *Journal of Organizational Behavior Management, 25*(2), 1–36.

Redmon, B. (1991). Pinpointing the technological fault in applied behavior analysis. *Journal of Applied Behavior Analysis, 24*(3), 441–444.

Rice, A., Austin, J., & Gravina, N. (2009). Increasing

customer service behaviors using manager-delivered task clarification and social praise. *Journal of Applied Behavior Analysis, 42,* 665–669.

Rodriguez, M., Wilder, D. A., Therrien, K., Wine, B., Miranti, R., Daratany, K., et al. (2006). Use of the Performance Diagnostic Checklist to select an intervention designed to increase the offering of promotional stamps at two sites of a restaurant franchise. *Journal of Organizational Behavior Management, 25*(3), 17–35.

Rohn, D., Austin, J., & Lutrey, S. M. (2003). Using feedback and performance accountability to decrease cash register shortages. *Journal of Organizational Behavior Management, 22*(1), 33–46.

Rummler, G. A., & Brache, A. P. (2012). *Improving performance: How to manage the white space in the organizational chart* (3rd ed.). San Francisco: Jossey-Bass.

Sasson, J. R., Alvero, A. M., & Austin, J. (2006). Effects of process and human performance improvement strategies. *Journal of Organizational Behavior Management, 26*(3), 43–78.

Sasson, J. R., & Austin, J. (2003). Performer-level systems analysis. *Journal of Organizational Behavior Management, 22*(4), 27–58.

Sasson, J. R., & Austin, J. (2005). The effects of training, feedback, and participant involvement in behavioral safety observations on office ergonomic behavior. *Journal of Organizational Behavior Management, 24*(4), 1–30.

Sigurdsson, S. O., & Austin, J. (2006). Institutionalization and response maintenance in organizational behavior management. *Journal of Organizational Behavior Management, 26*(4), 41–77.

Slowiak, J. M., Dickinson, A. M., & Huitema, B. E. (2011). Self-solicited feedback: Effects of hourly pay and individual monetary incentive pay. *Journal of Organizational Behavior Management, 31*(1), 3–20.

Smith, M., & Wilder, D. A. (2018). The use of the Performance Diagnostic Checklist—Human Services to assess and improve the job performance of individuals with intellectual disabilities. *Behavior Analysis in Practice, 11*(2), 148–153.

So, Y., Lee, K., & Oah, S. (2013). Relative effects of daily feedback and weekly feedback on customer service behavior at a gas station. *Journal of Organizational Behavior Management, 33*(2), 137–151.

Sulzer-Azaroff, B. (1980). Behavioral ecology and accident prevention. *Journal of Organizational Behavior Management, 2*(1), 11–44.

Sulzer-Azaroff, B., & Austin, J. (2000). Does BBS work?: Behavior-based safety and injury reduction: A survey of the evidence. *Professional Safety, 45*(7), 19–24.

Thurkow, N. M., Bailey, J. S., & Stamper, M. R. (2000). The effects of group and individual monetary incentives on productivity of telephone interviewers. *Journal of Organizational Behavior Management, 20*(2), 3–25.

Tuncel, S., Lotlikar, H., Salem, S., & Daraiseh, N. (2006). Effectiveness of behaviour based safety interventions to reduce accidents and injuries in workplaces: Critical appraisal and meta-analysis. *Theoretical Issues in Ergonomics Science, 7*(3), 191–209.

Vergason, C. M., & Gravina, N. E. (2020). Using a guest- and confederate-delivered token economy to increase employee–guest interactions at a zoo. *Journal of Applied Behavior Analysis, 53*(1), 422–430.

Wilder, D. A., Austin, J., & Casella, S. (2009). Applying behavior analysis in organizations: Organizational behavior management. *Psychological Services, 6*(3), 202–211.

Wilder, D., & Sigurdsson, S. (2015). Applications of behavior analysis to improve safety in organizations and community settings. In H. S. Roane, J. E. Ringdahl, & T. S. Falcomata (Eds.), *Clinical and organizational applications of behavior analysis* (pp. 583–604). San Diego, CA: Academic Press/Elsevier.

Zohar, D., & Luria, G. (2003). The use of supervisory practices as leverage to improve safety behavior: A cross level intervention model. *Journal of Safety Research, 34*(5), 567–577.

# PART VIII

# PROFESSIONAL ISSUES IN APPLIED BEHAVIOR ANALYSIS

Behavior analysis began as a subfield of psychology, but over time it has developed its own philosophy, scientific methods, applications, journals, organizations, credentialing board, and even a set of Current Procedural Terminology (CPT) codes approved and published by the American Medical Association so that applied behavior analysts can bill for the services they provide. Because behavior analysis has evolved into a discipline separate from psychology, it has become increasingly important for applied behavior analysts to develop ethical and professional standards that address the unique features of their subfield; those standards are topics addressed in this section of the handbook.

In Chapter 33, O'Donohue and Ferguson examine the relation between the fields of behavior analysis and ethics at the levels of meta-ethics, normative ethics, and descriptive ethics. Their thoughtful discussion of current ethical guidelines relative to Skinner's contingency analysis of moral and ethical behavior should be of interest to applied behavior analysts. Carr, Nosik, Ratcliff, and Johnston discuss the history and development of professional certification in applied behavior analysis in Chapter 34. They describe the amazing growth in the number of behavior analysts certified by the Behavior Analyst Certification Board® to over 35,000 certificants, and they explain how the standards for certification have changed in accordance with the progress of the profession of applied behavior analysis.

# CHAPTER 33

# Behavior Analysis and Ethics

## William O'Donohue and Kyle E. Ferguson

Behavior analysis has a complex relationship with the field of ethics. In this chapter, we describe the general structure of this relationship, and some of its major complexities and unsettled issues. We typically construe ethical discourse as occurring at three distinct levels:

1. *Meta-ethics* addresses questions including these: What kind of thing is ethical discourse? Is it the same or different from empirical discourse? If it is the same, what kinds of discourse does ethical discourse belong to? If different, what kind of thing is ethical discourse, and how do we evaluate the *truth value* of ethical claims?
2. *Normative ethics* addresses questions of which ethical claims, among many possible candidates for ethical principles, are correct. Is doing X, for example, morally right, wrong, or indifferent, where X can range from being culturally insensitive (Benuto, Casas, & O'Donohue, 2018), to prescribing facilitated communication for a child with autism spectrum disorder, to eating an orange? Normative ethics tries to address the questions of which moral prohibitions, permissions, or mandates are correct and how we justify them.
3. *Descriptive ethics* addresses empirical questions

of what ethical claims or beliefs some individuals hold. This is an interesting empirical question, and we might conduct research to see what ethical claims behavior analysts hold. Because we could find no research on this issue, we do not examine this dimension of ethics in this chapter.

## BEHAVIOR ANALYSIS AND CONTROVERSIES AT THE META-ETHICAL LEVEL

Behavior analysis has paid most attention to two key meta-ethical problems. First, behavior analysts have followed Skinner and have responded to the meta-ethical question "Is ethical discourse even possible in a deterministic worldview?" in the affirmative, although it becomes a somewhat different kind of discourse than that in common folk discourse. Folk perspectives assume points in which an individual is free to choose morally bad or morally good alternatives. Skinnerians do not. Second, behavior analysts have answered the question "What kind of thing is ethical discourse?" with the response that it is naturalistic discourse, such as talk of observable properties of the world (e.g., color, smell). We first turn our attention to the issue of morality from a deterministic standpoint.

## Meta-Ethical Question 1: Determinism and Kant's Dictum "Ought Implies Can"

The moral philosopher Immanuel Kant (1997) asserted, "Ought implies can"; that is, asserting that someone ought to have done something makes no sense unless this person could have performed the action. For example, asserting that Jane ought to have jumped 6 meters in the air makes no sense when Jane cannot physically do so. Therefore, moral discourse presupposes choice: A person can do something because he or she is free to choose to do this. Thus morality presupposes free will.

Skinner, particularly in *Beyond Freedom and Dignity* (1971/2002), discussed the conflict between a scientific worldview and a view based on choice and free will. Science assumes some form of determinism because it assumes order, and it assumes that there are causal relations to discover (Fischborn, 2018). Science assumes that the world is orderly, and we can characterize this order as lawful relationships. A scientific law, however, describes an impossibility. According to the law of gravity, for example, for two objects to behave other than according to the law is simply impossible. Objects are neither free to choose other ways to behave, nor free to choose different relationships with other objects. The law describes the only way that the objects can behave. Skinner points out that if people are free to choose their behavior, then a science of behavior is not possible. Thus Skinner aptly titled his book *Beyond Freedom and Dignity* to argue that the scientific enterprise, when applied to human behavior, must move beyond the notion of free choice. Therefore, if they take Kant seriously, behavior analysts must assume that ethical discourse does not make sense.

How can behavior analysts come to terms with this issue? Behavior analysts, of course, can take the stance that adopting an ethical code for behavior analysts is just more determined behavior. However, behavior analysts must see that to remain consistent, they must accept that a deterministic view of ethical codes and discourse diverges greatly from normal ethical discourse. Behavior analysts do not choose to behave in one way or another; thus we should not praise or punish them for their behavior, because they could have done nothing else. That is, to remain consistent, they must be seen as compelled to emit the behavior in question. Normal ethical discourse takes choice seriously and is a kind of argument for individuals to make good choices when they are at a moral crossroad. Behavior analysts do not countenance

the existence of moral choices. Thus meta-ethical morality is fundamentally different for the determinist than for any libertarian.

Ringen (1996) addresses this question as follows:

> The scientific account of human action requires that every event is determined causally, so there are no acts that are free of determining causal influences. The conclusion is that the causal determinism involved in the scientific account of human action is incompatible with the account of autonomy and self-determinism that legal, political, and ethical arguments require. . . . (p. 356)

This view means that we cannot accept scientific determinism and the traditional concept that human beings act in a self-determining way. The reason is that if determinism is true, no human act is free of controlling influences. Accordingly, if we presume determinism in the science of behavior, does an ethics code for behavior analysts even make sense? If "ought implies can," then how can we hold an individual morally culpable when he or she could not have behaved otherwise (O'Donohue & Ferguson, 2003, p. 7)? As we shall see later, if we want behavior analysts to behave ethically, we need to understand the controlling influences or contingencies (i.e., antecedents and consequences) of which ethical and unethical behavior is a function.

## Meta-Ethical Issue 2: Skinner's Naturalistic Approach to Ethics and Moral Reasoning

Philosophers have made many claims about what kind of entity ethical discourse is. A brief list follows:

1. Ethical discourse derives from some divine source, usually resulting in some divine commandments, and is a kind of religious discourse. This view has held wide sway in the history of humankind and still has a significant number of proponents. We can argue that much of the founding discourse of Western civilization is based on this view; witness the theological–ethical connection in the U.S. Declaration of Independence and the Constitution. However, behavior analysis clearly does not ascribe to this view, and we may regard its emphasis upon naturalistic, evolutionary accounts as critical of the view that ethical discourse is based fundamentally on theological precepts.

2. Ethical discourse is meaningless. It is "language gone on holiday," to use Wittgenstein's (1953) phrase. The logical positivists held this view. They offered an *emotivist* meta-ethical theory and claimed that "X is bad" has no direct observational basis; it violates their verifiability principle and is meaningless. Their positive claim, though, was that humans tend to make these utterances because humans are not only logical, rational animals but also emotional ones, and their emotional capacity causes them to make these utterances. "Murder is bad" is equivalent to "Uck!" or "I hate murder," and nothing more. Logical positivism has not influenced behavior analysis to the extent that many distant observers think (see Smith, 1986). At the same time, it does not hold an emotivist view of ethics, either.

3. Ethical discourse refers to an entirely empirical, natural phenomenon maintained by its consequences, like other empirical, descriptive discourse or even causal discourse. "X is bad" is equivalent to "I have observed that X has some empirical property." Skinner (1971/2002) held this view; thus this view has been most influential in behavior analysis. We regard Skinner as an authority on this and many other topics in the science of behavior. In brief, Skinner held that "X is good" means that "X is reinforcing," where reinforcing is an empirical matter (i.e., a reinforcer increases the response rate of the behavior it is contingent on). Skinner argued that ethics is a completely natural discourse. This view, of course, is not above criticism.

4. Ethical discourse is *sui generis*. Ethical utterances and claims are not like descriptive, empirical discourse. In fact, they are not like any other kind of discourse: Ethical discourse is wholly unique. This is the view of many ethical theorists, such as Immanuel Kant (1997) and G. E. Moore (1903/1988). There is an ethical realm, and ethical claims have a wholly different status from that of empirical claims in the observable world. The exact status of ethical discourse depends on the specific ethical theorist. Behavior analysis has generally disagreed with this position in favor of naturalizing the normative.

Although Skinner originally maintained that ethics and moral reasoning are beyond the purview of behavior analysis (e.g., Skinner, 1953, p. 328), in his later writings he adopted a position akin to naturalism (e.g., Skinner, 1953). According to Skinner (1971/2002),

> Good things are positive reinforcers. . . . When we say that a value judgment is a matter not of fact but how someone feels about a fact, we are simply distinguishing between a thing and its reinforcing effect. Physics and biology study things themselves, usually without reference to their value, but the reinforcing effects of things are the province of behavioral science, which is a science of values to the extent that it focuses on operant reinforcement. (pp. 103–104)

*Naturalism* is the theory that we can derive moral values from facts about the world (MacIntyre, 1998). From this perspective, *is* can imply *ought*. Presumably, one ought to behave in ways that produce reinforcement from a Skinnerian point of view. Or, conversely, one ought not to behave in ways that produce punishment. One should escape or avoid aversive stimulation, as in the case of negative reinforcement. Skinner (1971/2002) added:

> Things are good (positively reinforcing) or bad (negatively reinforcing) presumably because of the contingencies of survival under which the species evolved. . . . It is part of the genetic endowment called "human nature" to be reinforced in particular ways by particular things. (p. 104).

Thus natural processes select human beings to know right from wrong, good from bad, which is part of our genetic endowment. What follows, therefore, is that "all reinforcers eventually derive their power from evolutionary selection" (Skinner, 1971/2002, pp. 104–105). Simply, individuals whose behavior is maintained by certain types of reinforcers live to reproduce; those insensitive to comparable reinforcers do not. Thus morality evolved insofar as our species evolved.

One inherent problem with Skinner's naturalistic position is that the concept of reinforcement is not clear. Early accounts were entirely functional. If animals were appropriately deprived (e.g., 80% of *ad libitum* weight), certain events were highly likely to function as reinforcers for many behaviors (e.g., delivery of food pellets). Thus we also must understand reinforcing effects by contextualizing the behavior in a matrix of variables that affect reinforcement. Ethical statements become somewhat complex in this view. For example, when X is deprived of Y to extent Z and emits behavior B, R is reinforcing—morally correct—to X. When the subject reaches satiation point $S$, $R$ becomes punishing—morally wrong (see Allison & Timberlake's [1975] response deprivation model of reinforcement). How many parameters need to be a part of such sentences because the field's understanding of the mechanisms of reinforcement is incomplete or is unclear? Thus a problem with this view is that the construct of reinforcement is by no means clear, and the controversies surrounding this construct are germane to ethical pronouncements from a naturalistic standpoint.

In addition, problematic counterexamples exist. Take pedophilia as a case in point. *Pedophilia* is sexual attraction to prepubescent children. Few would argue that pedophiles' behavior is not morally wrong, blameworthy, and so forth. However, stimuli associated with prepubescent children, such as child pornography or contact with children, are highly reinforcing for certain behaviors of such individuals. According to Skinner's position, therefore, the pedophiles' sexual behavior is morally good, at least for the pedophiles. They might like pedophilic stimuli (i.e., those stimuli serve as reinforcers), but can we say nothing else here? Does Skinner's naturalistic account force us into a relativism in which we can say that child pornography is good for $X$ because it functions as a reinforcer for $X$? Certainly, the problem is clear. $X$ can be a reinforcer, but still can be morally wrong in a broader sense.

The problem with Skinner's approach is due to what Moore (1903/1988) called the *naturalistic fallacy*. Moore stated:

"Good," then, if we mean by it that quality which we assert to belong to a thing, when we say that the thing is good, is incapable of any definition, in the most important sense of that word. The most important sense of definition is that in which a definition states what are the parts which invariably compose a certain whole; and in this sense good has no definition because it is simple and has no parts. It is one of those innumerable objects of thought which are themselves incapable of definition because they are the ultimate terms of reference to which whatever is capable of definition must be defined. . . . There is, therefore, no intrinsic difficulty in the contention that good denotes a simple and indefinable quality. . . .

Consider yellow, for example. We may try to define it by describing its physical equivalent. We may state what kind of light vibrations must stimulate the normal eye so we may perceive it. But a moment's reflection is sufficient to show that those light vibrations are not what we mean by yellow. They are not what we perceive. Indeed, we should never have been able to discover their existence unless we had been struck first by the difference of quality between the different colors. The most we can say of those vibrations is that they are what corresponds in space to the yellow that we perceive. (Section 10, Paragraphs 1 and 2, emphasis in original)

To the extent that yellow does not possess the property of yellowness, reinforcers do not possess the property of goodness. We must make such value judgments regardless of their reinforcing properties; otherwise, we run into the same problem as in our pedophilia example. Labeling behavior good or bad, right or wrong, seems to concern aspects of consequent stimuli unrelated to their reinforcing characteristics.

## NORMATIVE ETHICS: CONTROVERSIES CONCERNING AN ETHICAL CODE

The Florida Association for Behavior Analysis (1987) was the first chapter of what was then the Association for Behavior Analysis to develop an ethical code. The Texas Association for Behavior Analysis (1995) soon followed in the early 1990s, followed by the California Association for Behavior Analysis (1996). The Association for Behavior Analysis International (as it now is) adopted the American Psychological Association's (2002) Ethics Code, thus obviating those developed under individual chapters. Likewise, the Behavior Analyst Certification Board (BACB) by and large adopted the American Psychological Association's 2002 Ethics Code in 2004, with some modification. Accordingly, criticisms of the American Psychological Association's Ethics Code are relevant with respect to the Association for Behavior Analysis International's code, because they are virtually the same.

Ethical codes are not above criticism (O'Donohue, 2016; O'Donohue & Ferguson, 2003). Ethical codes are the product of human behavior and are fallible, like all human activity. The American Psychological Association's (2002) Ethics Code is no exception.

The Ethics Code is a fallible document. How fallible and in what ways constitute the crux of the matter. Of concern is that we pronounce individual behavior as unethical or ethical on the basis of a flawed code. The code's fallibility is easy to discern. First, why would it have undergone nine revisions since its inception if it were infallible? Of course, the American Psychological Association can argue that the code has morphed in accordance with changing ethics, and that successive iterations have accommodated these changes accurately. However, the American Psychological Association has not made this argument, and professional morality generally remains largely static over time. That is, the standards of beneficence and nonmaleficence, fidelity, responsibility, integrity, justice, and respect for individual rights and dignity do not change appreciably (O'Donohue & Ferguson, 2003).

Second, the American Psychological Association used fallible procedures to develop the code. Committee members voted for or against the codes, and no committee members were behavior analysts. Knowledge by way of authority is fallible due to the committee members' imperfect judgment, heuristic biases (e.g., representative biases), and the like. We did not conduct experimental analyses; hence no safeguards were there to mitigate against these biases, which probably were operating at some level during committee meetings.

Third, other professional organizations in the behavioral sciences have their own ethics codes, some of which differ on fundamental points in relation to the American Psychological Association (2002) Ethics Code. For example, what was then the Association for Advancement of Behavior Therapy (1977; now Association for Behavioral and Cognitive Therapies) long ago adopted a higher standard of evidence clinicians must use before they select interventions. Ethical codes of individual chapters, such as the California Association for Behavior Analysis (1996) and the Florida Association for Behavior Analysis (1987), also have inconsistencies relative to the Ethics Code. The question then becomes "Which one is right?" Although no hard and fast rules exist in determining this experimentally, we can evaluate these standards by following their lines of reasoning and turning to the empirical literature for support or counterevidence.

Let us take the BACB's (2004) Guidelines for Responsible Conduct for Behavior Analysts as a case in point. Consider Code 1.4.2 (Exploitative Relationships): "Behavior analysts *do not engage* in *sexual relationships* with *clients*, students, or supervisees in training over whom the behavior analyst has *evaluative* or *direct authority*, because such relationships *easily impair judgment* or become *exploitative*" (emphasis added). A likely interpretation of this guideline is that behavior analysts should not engage in sexual relationships with clients (ever), because authority never ends, although the code

does not explicitly state this. Namely, behavior analysts have special knowledge and skill sets that clients typically do not, and that place them at an unfair advantage. Thus the relationship is unilateral; there is a power differential. This specialized knowledge puts therapists in the role of authority. Behavior analysts, therefore, should not engage in sexual relationships with clients under any circumstances or at any time, because "such relationships easily impair judgment and become exploitive (due to this power differential)."Now consider the BACB's (2017) most recent version of its ethical guidelines, Code 1.0.7.b: "Behavior analysts refrain from any sexual relationships with clients, students, or supervisees, for at least two years after the date the professional relationship has formally ended." (p. 6). This, of course, is vastly different from the BACB's prior guidelines regarding such dual relationships. Ignoring the power differential mentioned earlier, Code 1.0.7.b states that such sexual relationships are not a problem if either party holds out for a minimum of 2 years. "Why 2 years?" is a reasonable question to ask. The BACB has not provided any empirical evidence why 2 years is better than 1 year, 6 months, or 10 years, for example. Nor has it provided any evidence to support that even having sexual relationships with former clients, irrespective of the time interval, is beneficial to either party or does no harm at the very least (i.e., *primum non nocere*).

Reason would suggest that the BACB's (2017) more recent standard is patently wrong. Once behavior analysts begin having sex with former clients, they might start viewing current clients differently. For example, they might view current clients as potential conquests. This, of course, can obfuscate professional boundaries and compromise the therapeutic alliance.

A fourth problem concerns the relation between the American Psychological Association (2002) Ethics Code and justification for these standards. Simply making the claim that one action is ethical and another is unethical, without alluding to some ethical theory or general ethical standard, is insufficient for several reasons (O'Donohue & Ferguson, 2003). First, how can we know if we are interpreting a given standard correctly? For example, deontological theory judges the rightness or wrongness of an action based solely on the nature of the act itself or its structural characteristics, irrespective of its consequences. We deem some actions unethical, even though they bear functional similarities to actions that are not. For example, we might view stealing from a client's purse as unethical, but not view charging excessive professional fees as unethical. Utilitarian ethics, by contrast, judge the rightness or wrongness of an act based solely on its consequences. If no one got hurt, we would not view the act as unethical, even if malicious intent was involved. Accordingly, deontic and utilitarian ethical theories provide different interpretations of the same code. Given that the BACB has not stated its position on this matter explicitly, either interpretation is defensible. Furthermore, the decision to take disciplinary steps would differ considerably, depending on the theoretical orientation of individual committee members, should the BACB investigate an alleged ethical violation. There has been much controversy in the American Psychological Association over the ethical propriety of psychologists involved in interrogation, but whether these arguments are based on deontic ethics, utilitarian ethics, virtue ethics, or some other normative theory is unclear (see O'Donohue et al., 2014).

A second problem is determining whether a behavior analyst has violated a standard (O'Donohue & Ferguson, 2003). For example, does the motive to do harm, as opposed to actual harm, constitute an ethical violation? The American Psychological Association (2002) and the BACB (2017) are both silent on this matter. Technically speaking, these contrasting views concern motivist ethical theory and utilitarian ethics, respectively. The intent of wrongdoing warrants disciplinary action from a motivist perspective, but not from a utilitarian perspective. The utilitarian perspective requires evidence that a client was harmed. Accordingly, because both the American Psychological Association and the BACB do not explain the morality upon which they based the Ethics Code, how can they ensure due process of ethical inquiries (O'Donohue & Ferguson, 2003, p. 7)? The answer is that they cannot, based on the arguments discussed above.

## SKINNER'S CONTINGENCY ANALYSIS OF MORAL AND ETHICAL BEHAVIOR

Although Skinner's science of behavior is inadequate in helping us determine what is moral or ethical behavior (i.e., normative ethics), his analysis of the contingencies by which people behave ethically is useful in helping us understand why people behave as they do (i.e., meta-ethics). By identifying the contingencies of which ethical behavior is a function, we can create conditions that foster ethical behavior and avoid conditions that promote unethical behavior.

According to Skinner (1972), "We cannot choose a way of life in which there is no control. . . . We can only change the controlling conditions" (pp. 97, 99, 194–195). What he meant by this is that our behavior is always under the control of genetic and environmental determinants (i.e., antecedent and consequential stimuli). Skinner's views on promoting ethical behavior, therefore, entail changing these controlling conditions. The most important aspect of these controlling conditions is the presence of countercontrol (Skinner, 1972).

*Countercontrol* is the "emotional reaction of anger . . . including operant behavior," on the part of the controllee (i.e., the person whose behavior is under the control of another), that "injures or is otherwise aversive to the controller" (Skinner, 1953, p. 321). In other words, countercontrol is the controllee's attempt at changing the aversive contingencies of which his or her behavior is a function. Several examples of countercontrol are as follows: An abused woman murders her abuser; an incarcerated criminal escapes from prison; citizens protest against their government; and the volunteers who served as inmates in the infamous Stanford prison rebelled against the volunteers who were randomly assigned to be guards.

The following passage summarizes how countercontrol relates to ethics:

> The consequences responsible for benevolent, devoted, compassionate, or public-spirited behavior are forms of countercontrol, and when they are lacking, these much-admired features of behavior are lacking. . . . The point is illustrated by five fields in which control is not offset by countercontrol and which have become classical examples of mistreatment. They are the care of the very young, of the aged, of prisoners, of individuals diagnosed with psychosis, and of individuals with intellectual disabilities. Critics often say that those who have these susceptible people in their charge lack compassion or a sense of ethics, but the conspicuous fact is that vulnerable individuals are not subject to strong countercontrol. The young and the aged are too weak to protest, prisoners are controlled by police power, and individuals diagnosed with psychosis or intellectual disabilities cannot organize or act successfully. Little or nothing is done about mistreatment unless external agencies introduce countercontrol from outside. (Skinner, 1971/2002, pp. 196–197)

Here Skinner was very clear about what professionals need to do to ensure ethical behavior. In circumstances where individuals are so disadvantaged that they have no effective mechanisms of countercontrol, external agencies need to step in to offset this imbalance. In recent times, no other area in health care illustrates the role of countercontrol and ethics better than the care of elderly persons with neurocognitive disorders (dementia) and other intellectual impairments.

## Countercontrol and Elder Abuse

Persons with cognitive and behavioral disorders who receive elder care are at particularly high risk of abuse, due to the burden their caregivers experience (Lachs, Williams, O'Brien, Hurst, & Horowitz, 1997; Pillemer, Burnes, Riffin, & Lachs, 2016). *Elder abuse* is physical, psychological, sexual, and/or financial exploitation; neglect; or a combination of these that may result from the actions of others, such as caregivers (Dyer, Pavlik, Murphy, & Hyman, 2000). The prevalence of elder abuse ranges from 1 to 12%, although these figures likely underestimate the problem, due to methodological weaknesses and to both recipients' and caregivers' reluctance to report abuse (Burnes et al., 2015; Tueth, 2000). After all, elder abuse is a felony and can result in criminal charges. Moreover, care recipients may be reluctant to report abuse for fear of being moved out of their homes to alternative living arrangements (e.g., assisted living or skilled nursing facilities).

Characteristics that place care recipients with dementia at risk for abuse include challenging behaviors, such as physical aggression, and their need for increasingly intense hands-on care with activities of daily living, such as bathing, toileting, and dressing, as they deteriorate (Dong, 2015; Lachs et al., 1997; Wangmo, Nordström, & Kressig, 2017). Physical abuse is most likely to occur in the context of hands-on caregiving. When a caregiver has direct contact with aggressive behavior, noncompliant behavior, or both from an elderly person with dementia, the caregiver is likely to be emotionally distressed, possibly angry, and in physical pain if injured by the elderly person (Paveza et al., 1992; Teri et al., 1992). Most importantly, care recipients with dementia are unable to exert effective countercontrol, given their overall impairment and often frail condition.

Although elder abuse has received widespread attention in the media lately (Roberto, 2016), the treatment of those who receive elder care has improved considerably over the last several decades as states have stepped in to ensure that better countercontrol mechanisms are in place. Reporting and documentation have become increasingly stringent. Moreover, skilled nursing facilities are subject to random checks by government agencies.

## CLOSING REMARKS

Behavior analysis has a complex relation with ethical discourse. This chapter has described the complexities of this relation and some unresolved issues. One of the major unsettled issues is this: Is it even possible to reconcile a scientific view of behavior with an indeterministic view or the notion of free will, which presupposes the most recent versions of the codes of ethics for the American Psychological Association (2002) and the BACB (2017)? Does it even make sense to have an ethics code for behavior analysts who espouse a scientific view of behavior? If indeed "ought implies can," then how can we hold a professional morally and ethically responsible when he or she could not have behaved otherwise (O'Donohue & Ferguson, 2003, p. 7)? The professional's unethical behavior was beyond his or her personal control. That is to say, the unethical behavior was due to genetic variables and deficiencies in the prevailing contingencies of which such behavior and other, incompatible ethical behavior are a function.

In *Beyond Freedom and Dignity*, Skinner (1971/2002) discussed this conflict between a scientific worldview and a view based on choice and free will. Science presupposes determinism because it assumes order in the universe. Based on the presupposition that the world is orderly, science then can elucidate those lawful relations (e.g., contingencies of survival and reinforcement) that enable our species to better predict and control or influence natural phenomena. Insofar as matter does not get to choose what natural forces operate on it, organisms do not get to choose what behavior gets emitted. Accordingly, the answer to the earlier question is no. The codes of ethics for the American Psychological Association (2002) and the BACB (2017) are incompatible with the science of behavior. Therefore, we should abandon them entirely.

Skinner's contingency analysis of moral and ethical behavior should supplant those codes of ethics. Although Skinner's science of behavior is inadequate in helping us determine *what* is moral or ethical behavior, his analysis of the contingencies by which people behave ethically could be instrumental in promoting ethical behavior among professionals. Although individuals might disagree about particulars, we can all agree about what is and is not ethical in most instances. For example, striking patients under any circumstances is unethical. Likewise, an ethical practice might be to maximize a patient's independence, while decreasing his or her dependence on other people. By identifying the contingencies of which ethical behavior is a function, psychology and behavior analysis can create the conditions that foster ethical behavior and obviate those conditions that evoke unethical behavior.

In closing, the wholesale adoption of the American Psychological Association's (2002) Ethics Code should come as a surprise to the behavior-analytic community, given that it is antithetical to the tenets of the science of behavior. Surprisingly, the community has remained largely silent about this change.

We might assume two things from the behavior-analytic community's lack of response. First, behavior analysts are silent on this issue because the American Psychological Association's (2002) Ethics Code is acceptable to them; hence they have no criticisms. This, of course, does not seem to be the case. Most behavior analysts would have been outraged by the Association of Behavior Analysis International's adoption of the American Psychological Association's Ethics Code, had they considered this action carefully. Second, they have not read the Ethics Code; they consider ethics only superficially at best. Although this remains an empirical question, we might safely assume that this is indeed the case. This attitude notwithstanding, members of the behavior-analytic community should note that accepting the American Psychological Association's Ethics Code has serious implications or consequences. The Ethics Code has no safeguards to ensure due process if a behavior analyst should ever be the subject of an ethical inquiry (O'Donohue & Ferguson, 2003, p. 7). Simply, there are no contingencies or countercontrol mechanisms to ensure a fair trial.

## REFERENCES

Allison, J., & Timberlake, W. (1975). Response deprivation and instrumental performance in the controlled-amount paradigm. *Learning and Motivation*, 6, 112–142.

American Psychological Association. (2002). Ethical principles of psychologists and code of conduct. Retrieved from *www.apa.org/ethics/code*.

Association for Advancement of Behavior Therapy. (1977). Ethical issues for human services. *Behavior Therapy*, 8, v–vi.

Behavior Analyst Certification Board (BACB). (2004). Behavior Analyst Certification Board guidelines for responsible conduct for behavior analysts. Retrieved from *www.bacb.com*.

Behavior Analyst Certification Board (BACB). (2017). Professional and ethical compliance code for behavior analysts. Retrieved from *www.bacb.com*.

Benuto, L. T., Casas, J., & O'Donohue, W. T. (2018). Training culturally competent psychologists: A systematic review of the training outcome literature. *Training and Education in Professional Psychology*, 12, 125–134.

Burnes, D., Pillemer, K., Caccamise, P. L., Mason, A., Henderson, C. R., Berman, J., et al. (2015). Prevalence of and risk factors for elder abuse and neglect in the community: A population-based study. *Journal of the American Geriatrics Society*, 63, 1906–1912.

California Association for Behavior Analysis. (1996). *Cal-ABA's code of ethics*. Morro Bay, CA: Author.

Dong, X. Q. (2015). Elder abuse: Systematic review and implications for practice. *Journal of the American Geriatrics Society*, 63, 1214–1238.

Dyer, C. B., Pavlik, V. N., Murphy, K. P., & Hyman, D. J. (2000). The high prevalence of depression and dementia in elder abuse or neglect. *Journal of the American Geriatrics Society*, 48, 205–208.

Fischborn, M. (2018). Questions for a science of moral responsibility. *Review of Philosophy and Psychology*, 9, 381–394.

Florida Association for Behavior Analysis. (1987). *Code of ethics of the Florida Association for Behavior Analysis*. Tallahassee, FL: Author.

Kant, I. (1997). *Lectures on ethics* (P. Heath & J. B. Schneewind, Trans.). Cambridge, UK: Cambridge University Press.

Lachs, M. S., Williams, C., O'Brien, S., Hurst, L., & Horowitz, R. (1997). Risk factors for reported elder abuse and neglect: A nine-year observational cohort study. *Gerontologist*, 37, 469–474.

MacIntyre, A. (1998). *A short history of ethics* (2nd ed.). Notre Dame, IN: University of Notre Dame Press.

Moore, G. E. (1988). *Principia ethica*. New York: Prometheus Books. (Original work published 1903)

O'Donohue, W. T. (2016). Oppression, privilege, bias, prejudice, and stereotyping: Problems in the APA code of ethics. *Ethics and Behavior*, 26(7), 527–544.

O'Donohue, W. T., & Ferguson, K. E. (2003). *Handbook of professional ethics for psychologists*. New York: SAGE.

O'Donohue, W., Snipes, C., Dalto, G., Soto, C., Maragakis, A., & Im, S. (2014). The ethics of enhanced interrogations and torture: A reappraisal of the argument. *Ethics and Behavior*, 24(2), 109–125.

Paveza, G. J., Cohen, D., Eisdorfer, C., Freels, S., Semla, T., Ashford, J. W., et al. (1992). Severe family violence and Alzheimer's disease: Prevalence and risk factors. *Gerontologist, 32,* 493–497.

Pillemer, K., Burnes, D., Riffin, C., & Lachs, M. S. (2016). Elder abuse: Global situation, risk factors, and prevention strategies. *Gerontologist, 56*(Suppl. 2), S194–S205.

Ringen, J. (1996). The behavior therapists' dilemma: Reflections on autonomy, informed consent and scientific psychology. In W. O'Donohue & R. F. Kitchener (Eds.), *The philosophy of psychology* (pp. 352–360). Thousand Oaks, CA: SAGE.

Roberto, K. A. (2016). The complexities of elder abuse. *American Psychologist, 71,* 302–311.

Skinner, B. F. (1953). *Science and human behavior.* New York: Macmillan.

Skinner, B. F. (1972). *Cumulative record* (3rd ed.). New York: Appleton-Century-Crofts.

Skinner, B. F. (2002). *Beyond freedom and dignity.* New York: Hackett. (Original work published 1971)

Smith, L. (1986). *Behaviorism and logical positivism.* Stanford, CA: Stanford University Press.

Teri, L., Rabins, P., Whitehouse, P. V., Berg, L., Reisberg, B., Sunderland, T., et al. (1992). Management of behavior disturbance in Alzheimer disease: Current knowledge and future directions. *Alzheimer Disease and Associated Disorders, 6,* 77–88.

Texas Association for Behavior Analysis. (1995). *Texas Association for Behavior Analysis code of ethics.* Denton, TX: Author.

Tueth, M. J. (2000). Exposing financial exploitation of impaired elderly persons. *American Journal of Geriatric Psychiatry, 8,* 104–111.

Wangmo, T., Nordström, K., & Kressig, R. W. (2017). Preventing elder abuse and neglect in geriatric institutions: Solutions from nursing care providers. *Geriatric Nursing, 38,* 385–392.

Wittgenstein, L. (1953). *Philosophical investigations.* New York: Macmillan.

# CHAPTER 34

# Professional Certification for Practicing Behavior Analysts

James E. Carr, Melissa R. Nosik, Christine L. Ratcliff, and James M. Johnston

Holding a professional credential is the traditionally recognized way for an individual to demonstrate to the public that he or she has met specific and recognized standards of competence in a profession. Consumers generally use a profession's credential as a necessary qualification when selecting a professional. For example, most of us would not obtain the services of a surgeon, attorney, or dentist unless that person was properly credentialed. Likewise, if we moved to a new city and needed the services of an attorney, we might begin our search by obtaining a list of attorneys who have the proper professional credential. If we needed a specialized service, such as a real estate lawyer, we might seek an attorney who also held a specialty credential in that area. Of course, we might do many other things to be sure of hiring a competent attorney (e.g., obtain references, talk with community members, review pubic records about the attorney's practice), but verifying that the attorney was properly credentialed would be a reasonable and customary first step in the selection process. Employers and government agencies use a similar approach because it is an efficient and effective means of hiring professionals or designating the required qualifications for a position. Although merely having a credential may not be sufficient for an individual to obtain a given professional position, it is most often a prerequisite. Thus, a professional credential has become the primary means of identifying qualified professionals.

Behavior analysts had no specific and widely recognized professional credential until the late 1990s. Consumers seeking a qualified behavior analyst before that did not have a credential on which they could rely to aid their search: rather, they were forced to use less reliable means of assessing practitioner qualifications, such as word of mouth, a review of the practitioner's curriculum vitae, and practitioner advertisements. Employers and government agencies found themselves in a similar predicament and were forced either to develop their own criteria for a *qualified* behavior analyst or to specify that individuals possess credentials from other professions (e.g., a psychology license, teacher certification). Neither of these options was particularly beneficial for consumers, due to their lack of specificity in relation to behavior analysis.

## TYPES OF PROFESSIONAL CREDENTIALS

Professional credentials sometimes take the form of a license issued by the state, provincial, or national government. These licenses are usually established through a law that limits either the use of a professional title or engagement in specified professional practice to those holding the appropriate license (Green & Johnston, 2009; Redbird, 2017). Under a title law, for example, individuals may identify themselves as licensed behavior analysts only if they are licensed by the government. Similarly, under a practice law, individuals may practice behavior analysis only if they are licensed as a behavior analyst. If the law combines title and practice features, individuals may not use the title or engage in the practice of behavior analysis unless they are appropriately licensed or explicitly exempted from the law. Usually the licensure law also establishes a professional board to oversee the licensing process and review disciplinary matters involving licensed professionals.

A second form of credential is professional certification. Although licensure and professional certification take fundamentally the same approach to the credentialing process, professional certification differs from licensure in these ways: A private organization rather than a government usually issues it; most often it is not limited to a single governmental jurisdiction; and it can be voluntary for practice. The profession rather than the government usually drives certification; thus, it is not as subject to the idiosyncrasies of a politically influenced governmental process, because a private organization develops and issues professional certification. In addition, because professional certification can cross state borders, it is more *portable* for certificants than local government licensure is (Hall & Lunt, 2005). Although licensure and professional certification differ in many respects, one parallel requirement is that both must adhere to the same legal, psychometric, and professional standards in the development of their credentials and assessment instruments, and in the operation of their credentialing programs. One of the ways that professional certification programs demonstrate their adherence to established credentialing standards is to obtain accreditation from a national standard-setting organization such as the American National Standards Institute (ANSI, n.d.) or the National Commission for Certifying Agencies (NCCA; Institute for Credentialing Excellence, n.d.).

## CREDENTIALING PROGRAM COMPONENTS AND REQUIREMENTS

A professional credentialing program, whether for licensure or professional certification, consists of four main components: eligibility standards, a written examination, continuing education for credentialed individuals, and disciplinary oversight. Applicants must first meet specific eligibility standards to qualify for examination. These standards usually require the applicant to have a minimum educational degree, specific university coursework, and some form of supervised experience. The cornerstone of any professional credentialing program, however, is the professionally developed written examination. To be viable, the written examination must meet both psychometric and legal standards; that is, the examination must separate "those who know" from "those who do not know" and must also be defensible in a court of law. To these ends, examinations must be constructed following established psychometric and legal standards, which are often promulgated by standards-setting bodies (American Educational Research Association, American Psychological Association, & National Council on Measurement in Education, 2014; ANSI, n.d.; Institute for Credentialing Excellence, n.d.; U.S. Equal Employment Opportunity Commission, 1978). Next, individuals who become credentialed must usually obtain continuing education (CE) to maintain their credential's currency. The purpose of a CE requirement is to help ensure that a credentialed professional continues to grow professionally and keeps abreast of new developments and techniques in the field. Finally, most credentialing organizations include a fourth step of disciplinary or ethical compliance based on a published code of ethics.

## THE HISTORY OF BEHAVIOR ANALYST CREDENTIALING

There have been several attempts to establish professional credentials for practicing behavior analysts (Johnston, Carr, & Mellichamp, 2017). For example, Minnesota initiated a certification program in the 1970s for practitioners working in the state developmental disabilities system, but it eventually fell victim to changes in philosophy and priorities in the state (Thomas, 1979). The Association for Behavior Analysis[1] sponsored a certification program in the mid-1980s, but later dissolved it for legal and practical reasons (Shook et al., 1988). In addition, Florida implemented a certification program based on a professionally de-

---

[1] The Association for Behavior Analysis was later renamed the Association for Behavior Analysis International (ABAI).

veloped examination in the mid-1980s (Johnston & Shook, 1993; Starin, Hemingway, & Hartsfield, 1993) because of misuse of behavioral procedures (Bailey & Burch, 2016; Johnston & Shook, 1987). Oklahoma, Texas, California, Pennsylvania, and New York followed suit in the 1990s with programs based on Florida's successful model and using Florida's examination. One state's providing an examination to another state was highly unusual, but in the case of applied behavior analysis (ABA), this is exactly what happened. Florida paved the way for other states to follow, and they did. As additional states and governments became interested in Florida's program, the need for a broader credentialing program for the profession became clear.

## THE BEHAVIOR ANALYST CERTIFICATION BOARD

The Behavior Analyst Certification Board® (BACB®) was founded as a 501(c)(3) nonprofit corporation in 1998 to meet the credentialing needs of the profession. In 1999, the BACB entered into an agreement with Florida to use the well-developed Florida examination and held its first examination administration in May 2000. In response to the successful implementation of the BACB certification program, Florida transferred the examination to the BACB, and all state-operated certification programs, including Florida's, ceased operation and transferred their certification responsibilities to the BACB (Johnston & Shook, 2001). Almost immediately, the interest in certification outside the United States became apparent, and the BACB subsequently increased its international activities to be responsive to this growing interest (Hughes & Shook, 2007; Martin & Carr, 2020; Virués-Ortega et al., 2009).

### BACB Certifications

The BACB offers two professional certification programs for behavior analysts:[2] Board Certified Behavior Analyst® (BCBA®) and Board Certified Assistant Behavior Analyst® (BCaBA®) (see Figure 34.1). Individuals who hold BCBA certification are graduate-level, independent practitioners

---

[2] The BACB also offers a certification program for paraprofessional behavior technicians who are supervised by behavior analysts, the Registered Behavior Technician® (RBT®) credential. The current chapter, however, focuses exclusively on professional credentials for *behavior analysts*.

of behavior analysis. Individuals who hold BCaBA certification may practice behavior analysis under the supervision of a BCBA. In addition, behavior analysts who hold BCBA certification and meet certain doctoral-degree requirements may qualify for a doctoral designation: Board Certified Behavior Analyst–Doctoral™ (BCBA-D™). Since 2007, both the BCBA and BCaBA certification programs have been accredited by NCCA continuously, which indicates that the BACB adheres to established testing and legal standards for boards that grant professional credentials.

Both BCBA and BCaBA certification have specific requirements for degree, coursework, and supervised experience (see Figure 34.2) that ap-

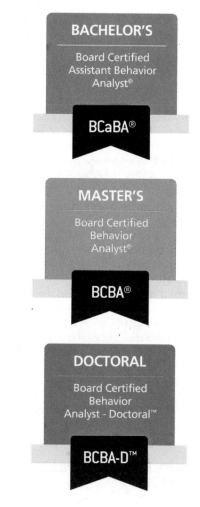

**FIGURE 34.1.** Behavior analyst certifications available from the BACB.

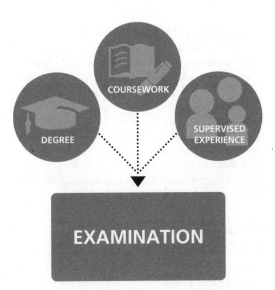

**FIGURE 34.2.** A visual depiction of the examination eligibility process for BCBA and BCaBA certification.

plicants must meet to qualify for the appropriate written examination. Applicants for the BCBA examination need at least a master's degree in an acceptable academic domain, graduate coursework in specific behavior-analytic content, and supervised professional behavior-analytic experience[3] to qualify. Applicants for the BCaBA examination need at least a bachelor's degree, undergraduate or graduate coursework in specific behavior-analytic content, and supervised professional behavior-analytic experience to qualify.

## BACB Examinations

The BACB's examinations are developed and reviewed routinely through processes that adhere to best-practice guidelines for credentialing, nationally accepted examination development standards, and NCCA requirements (Johnston, Mellichamp, Shook, & Carr, 2014). The BACB uses multiple workgroups of carefully selected subject-matter experts to write and revise examination items and make recommendations for ongoing changes to the BCBA and BCaBA task lists: this input serves as the basis of examination content. Task list revisions are content-validated through a large-scale

survey of certificants, known as the *job task analysis*. Thus the *profession* under the guidance of the BACB *staff* develops the task list and examinations (see also Johnston et al., 2014; Shook, 2005; Shook, Johnston, & Mellichamp, 2004).

The BACB has increased the availability of examinations to meet the demand for its certification programs. Over 300 sites worldwide administer examinations through Pearson VUE's network of secure, computer-based centers. The BCBA and BCaBA examinations are currently offered on a continual basis throughout the year (i.e., "on demand").

## Certification Maintenance

BCBA or BCaBA certification is granted only after an individual has met the eligibility requirements mentioned above and passed the appropriate examination. After obtaining a BACB credential, a certificant must meet maintenance requirements to help maintain an acceptable level of professional currency and competence in behavior analysis.

Professionals with BCBA and BCaBA certifications must obtain CE, which can be earned in several ways. These include passing university courses in behavior analysis, teaching such courses, attending state and national conferences, taking online tutorials, presenting approved sessions at conferences, and engaging in certain scholarly activities (such as editorial reviews and publication of journal articles). Certificants must dedicate a portion of the required CE to ethics content and to supervision content for those providing supervision to ensure continued development in particularly important areas.

## Ethics and Discipline

In addition to the maintenance requirements described above, the BACB employs a disciplinary system for ethical and professional behavior for certification applicants and certificants. The BACB's disciplinary system is based on the BACB's ethics code, the Professional and Ethical Compliance Code for Behavior Analysts (hereafter referred to as the Code; BACB, 2014a). The Code covers the wide range of ethical and professional situations faced by practicing behavior analysts. It also serves as a reference for consumers and employers when they are trying to determine what manner of behavior is appropriate and should be expected from a behavior analyst faced with ethi-

---

[3]There are currently two other eligibility options for BCBA certification for faculty members and senior, doctoral-level practitioners.

cal and professional issues. The BACB enforces the Code through a process designed to provide consumer protection, appropriate due process for the certificant involved, mentorship where appropriate, and consequences to the certificant for violations. Disciplinary sanctions, including the suspension or revocation of an individual's certification, are posted on the BACB's website (*www. bacb.com*).

## Growth of BACB Certification

The profession of behavior analysis has grown substantially in recent years (Carr & Nosik, 2017). As one example, the total number of individuals who hold BCBA or BCaBA certification worldwide has increased more than sevenfold since 2008 when there were 6,636 certificants (i.e., 4,747 BCBAs and 1,889 BCaBAs; Shook & Favell, 2008). As of August 2020, the total number of certificants is 48,219 (i.e., 43,476 BCBAs and 4,743 BCaBAs). As demand for the BACB's certification programs has increased, there has also been substantial growth in the number of educational programs providing behavior-analytic training. For example, there are currently over 300 institutions worldwide offering coursework identified as meeting the requirements for BCBA or BCaBA eligibility (i.e., verified course sequences). As the number of institutions with verified course sequences has grown, so has the need for feedback regarding students' performance on BACB examinations. The BACB provided data in the early years for each verified course sequence on the percentage of its graduates who passed a BACB examination on the first attempt. Since 2014, the BACB has publicly posted pass rates online. These changes are efforts to assist prospective students in making informed decisions about their training before enrollment, and to provide feedback for faculty about one outcome of their training. Beginning in 2019, ABAI assumed responsibility for administering the verified course sequence system.

The increase in the number of BACB certificants has created a corresponding increase in demand for CE opportunities in behavior analysis. The BACB operates a process for identifying providers of BACB-approved CE content at the organizational and individual levels (Authorized Continuing Education providers). Although CE opportunities were previously difficult to find outside of a few annual conventions, they are now plentiful. There are currently over 1,000 Autho-

rized Continuing Education providers worldwide. A marked increase in the availability of CE content on ethics and professional behavior has occurred after the 2008 implementation of the BACB's requirement that every certificant obtain a proportion of CE in that area. A similar phenomenon occurred in response to the BACB's training and CE requirements for certificants who wish to provide supervision (BACB, 2012). These data suggest that the BACB's CE requirements have influenced the landscape of available training for behavior analysts.

## Standards Changes

Regulatory standards change in any profession according to the progress of the profession, such as available training programs, consumer needs, and published research findings. The BACB addresses this need for behavior analysts by reviewing and revising its standards periodically using processes mandated by the NCCA. These processes involve workgroups of subject-matter experts who make recommendations regarding standards and their revision to the BACB's Board of Directors. For illustrative purposes, the following paragraphs describe changes to three standards areas.

Eligibility standards for the BCBA and BCaBA certification include specific requirements for qualifying degree, coursework, and supervised experience. Unlike the coursework and experience requirements, which have always been behavior-analytic, the original degree requirement was not limited to any specific field of study. The BACB restricted the BCBA-level requirement in 2011 to degrees from certain academic domains. It further restricted the BCBA degree requirement in 2016 to degrees in behavior analysis, education, psychology, or degree programs in which an applicant completed a verified course sequence. The primary pathway toward BCBA certification will require a graduate degree from a program accredited by ABAI beginning in 2022, although a secondary pathway will allow degrees from other academic domains.

The BACB convened a workgroup in 2017 to review the supervised experience standards that apply to individuals pursuing BCBA or BCaBA certification (BACB, 2017). The recommendations of that workgroup produced changes to several features of the experience standards, which will take effect in 2022. First, new BCBAs will need to wait 1 year before supervising individuals pursuing BCBA or BCaBA certification. The BACB revised acceptable activities to limit direct implementation of behavioral programs to no more than 40% and 60% of the total supervised experience for BCBAs and BCaBAs, respectively. It increased the amount of supervised experience from 1,500 to 2,000 and from 1,000 to 1,300 hours for BCBA and BCaBA trainees, respectively. Finally, it clarified the standards regarding the nature and structure of supervision, appropriate activities, and supervision documentation.

The BACB convened a workgroup in 2014 to review several standards, including the standards for the ongoing supervision of BCaBAs. Originally developed in 2007 and implemented in 2009, the policy at that time required every BCaBA to obtain 1 hour of supervision per month from a BCBA. The new policy, which went into effect in 2017, requires BCaBAs to be supervised for 2% of the time they spend providing ABA services. The policy also addresses many issues that the previous version did not, such as supervisory caseload, supervisor qualifications, the supervisor's responsibility for the BCaBA's clinical work, contracts, and group supervision (BACB, 2014b).

## Autism Spectrum Disorder Practice Guidelines

In response to the growing demand for ABA services for autism spectrum disorder, the BACB published practice guidelines in 2012 for healthcare funders and managers, consumers, and service providers. It later revised the practice guidelines in 2014 (BACB, 2014c). The purpose of the guidelines is to support ABA treatment for individuals diagnosed with autism spectrum disorder that is consistent with the best available scientific evidence and expert clinical opinion. Some of the unique features of ABA treatment that the guidelines address include: training and credentialing of behavior analysts; assessment, formulation of treatment goals, and measurement of client progress; service authorization and dosage; tiered service delivery models; behavior technicians; and case supervision. In addition, the document provides general guidance and basic descriptions of typical ABA service delivery that can be tailored to fit individual, local, and regional requirements and needs. As of 2020, these practice guidelines have been transferred to the Council of Autism Service Providers (CASP, 2020), who will be responsible for managing and updating the document in the future.

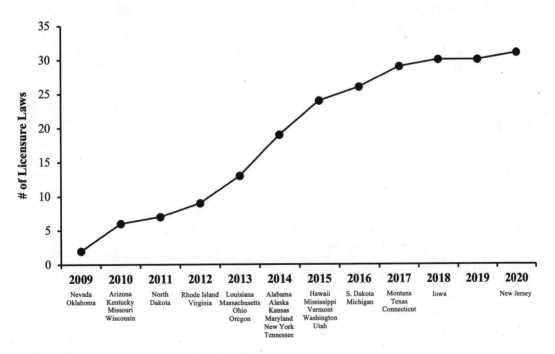

**FIGURE 34.3.** Cumulative number of U.S. licensure laws enacted through 2020 (*N* = 31). The states are indicated below the *x*-axis.

## U.S. STATE LICENSURE OF BEHAVIOR ANALYSTS

Since 2009, 31 U.S. states have enacted laws to regulate the practice of ABA through licensure (Association of Professional Behavior Analysts, n.d.; see Figure 34.3 on p. 575). Thirty-one states currently provide a pathway to licensure for behavior analysts with a graduate degree (Alabama, Alaska, Arizona, Connecticut, Hawaii, Iowa, Kansas, Kentucky, Louisiana, Maryland, Massachusetts, Michigan, Mississippi, Missouri, Montana, Nevada, New Jersey, New York, North Dakota, Ohio, Oklahoma, Oregon, Rhode Island, South Dakota, Tennessee, Texas, Utah, Vermont, Virginia, Washington, Wisconsin), and 24 of those states provide a pathway to licensure for assistant behavior analysts with an undergraduate degree (Alabama, Alaska, Iowa, Kansas, Kentucky, Louisiana, Massachusetts, Michigan, Mississippi, Missouri, Montana, Nevada, New Jersey, New York, North Dakota, Oklahoma, Oregon, Rhode Island, Tennessee, Texas, Utah, Vermont, Virginia, Washington)[4]. The BACB's credentials or standards constitute a pathway to licensure in these states, which assists behavior analysts who hold BACB credentials to move to different states and still qualify for licensure. We have yet to determine the impact of licensure on the practice of behavior analysis, because these legislative activities have occurred in the last decade, and several other states are still pursuing licensure. However, the existence and growth of licensure constitutes another indicator of the profession's increasing maturity.

## CONCLUSION

As a profession, ABA has undergone substantial growth in recent years. The growth is evident in the increasing number of credentialed behavior analysts, behavior-analytic training programs, and laws for the practice of behavior analysis; the increasing demand for behavior analysts (BACB, 2019); and the development of behavior-analytic infrastructure around the world. The BACB's professional certification programs, which provide a foundation for U.S. state licensure, represent current standards *for* behavior analysts developed *by* behavior analysts around the world. The BACB's systems for developing new standards and revising existing ones and the other resources the BACB has been able to provide will continue to serve as an important resource to the profession as it continues to mature.

## ACKNOWLEDGMENT

Gerald L. Shook contributed to the version of this chapter in the first edition of the *Handbook of Applied Behavior Analysis*.

## REFERENCES

American Educational Research Association, American Psychological Association, & National Council on Measurement in Education. (2014). *Standards for educational and psychological testing* (2014 ed.). Washington, DC: American Educational Research Association.

American National Standards Institute. (n.d.). Accreditation program for personnel certification bodies under ANSI/ISO/IEC 17024. Retrieved from *https://anab.ansi.org/credentialing/personnel-certification*.

Association of Professional Behavior Analysts. (n.d.). Licensure and other regulation of ABA practitioners. Retrieved from *www.apbahome.net/general/recommended_links.asp*.

Bailey, J. S., & Burch, M. R. (2016). *Ethics for behavior analysts* (3rd ed.). New York: Routledge.

Behavior Analyst Certification Board (BACB). (2012, September). Special edition on supervision. *BACB Newsletter*. Retrieved from *https://www.bacb.com/wp-content/Sep2012_Newsletter*.

Behavior Analyst Certification Board (BACB). (2014a). Professional and ethical compliance code for behavior analysts. Retrieved from *www.bacb.com/ethics/ethics-code*.

Behavior Analyst Certification Board (BACB). (2014b, December). Special edition on BCaBA supervision standards. Retrieved from *https://www.bacb.com/wp-content/Dec2014_Newsletter*.

Behavior Analyst Certification Board (BACB). (2014c). *Applied behavior analysis treatment of autism spectrum disorder: Practice guidelines for healthcare funders and managers* (2nd ed.). Littleton, CO: Author.

Behavior Analyst Certification Board (BACB). (2017, October). Revised BCBA and BCaBA experience and supervision requirements. *BACB Newsletter*. Retrieved from *https://www.bacb.com/wp-content/Oct2017_Newsletter*.

Behavior Analyst Certification Board (BACB). (2019). *U.S. employment demand for behavior analysts: 2010–2018*. Littleton, CO: Author.

Carr, J. E., & Nosik, M. R. (2017). Professional credentialing of practicing behavior analysts. *Policy Insights from the Behavioral and Brain Sciences, 4*, 3–8.

---

[4]Some states use the titles *certified* or *registered* instead of *licensed* for their behavior analyst or assistant behavior analyst credentials.

Council of Autism Service Providers. (2020). *Applied behavior analysis treatment of autism spectrum disorder: Practice guidelines for healthcare funders and managers* (2nd ed.). Retrieved from *casproviders.org/asd-guidelines.*

Green, G., & Johnston, J. M. (2009). A primer on professional credentialing: Introduction to invited commentaries on licensing behavior analysts. *Behavior Analysis in Practice, 2*(1), 51–52.

Hall, J. E., & Lunt, I. (2005). Global mobility for psychologists: The role of psychology organizations in the United States, Canada, Europe, and other regions. *American Psychologist, 60,* 712–726.

Hughes, J. C., & Shook, G. L. (2007). Training and certification in behaviour analysis in Europe: Past, present, and future challenges. *European Journal of Behavior Analysis, 8,* 239–249.

Institute for Credentialing Excellence. (n.d.). National Commission for Certifying Agencies (NCCA) standards. Retrieved from *https://www.credentialingexcellence.org/page/ncca.*

Johnston, J. M., Carr, J. E., & Mellichamp, F. H. (2017). A history of the professional credentialing of applied behavior analysts. *Behavior Analyst, 40,* 523–538.

Johnston, J. M., Mellichamp, F. H., Shook, G. L., & Carr, J. E. (2014). Determining BACB examination content and standards. *Behavior Analysis in Practice, 7,* 3–9.

Johnston, J. M., & Shook, G. L. (1987). Developing behavior analysis at the state level. *Behavior Analyst, 10,* 199–233.

Johnston, J. M., & Shook, G. L. (1993). A model for the statewide delivery of programming services. *Mental Retardation, 31,* 127–139.

Johnston, J. M., & Shook, G. L. (2001). A national certification program for behavior analysts. *Behavioral Interventions, 16,* 77–85.

Martin, N. T., & Carr, J. E. (2020). Training and certification of behaviour analysts in Europe. *European Journal of Behaviour Analysis, 21,* 9–19.

Redbird, B. (2017). The new closed shop?: The economic and structural effects of occupational licensure. *American Sociological Review, 82,* 600–624.

Shook, G. L. (2005). An examination of the integrity and future of Behavior Analyst Certification Board credentials. *Behavior Modification, 29,* 562–574.

Shook, G. L., & Favell, J. E. (2008). The Behavior Analyst Certification Board and the profession of behavior analysis. *Behavior Analysis in Practice, 1*(1), 44–48.

Shook, G. L., Johnston, J. M., Cone, J., Thomas, D., Greer, D., Beard, J., et al. (1988). *Credentialing, quality assurance and right to practice.* Kalamazoo, MI: Association for Behavior Analysis.

Shook, G. L., Johnston, J. M., & Mellichamp, F. (2004). Determining essential content for applied behavior analyst practitioners. *Behavior Analyst, 27,* 67–94.

Starin, S., Hemingway, M., & Hartsfield, F. (1993). Credentialing behavior analysts and the Florida behavior analysis certification program. *Behavior Analyst, 16,* 153–166.

Thomas, D. R. (1979). Certification of behavior analysts in Minnesota. *Behavior Analyst, 2*(1), 1–13.

U.S. Equal Employment Opportunity Commission. (1978). *United States Equal Employment Opportunity Commission guidelines on employment testing procedures.* Washington, DC: Author.

Virués-Ortega, J., Shook, G. L., Arntzen, E., Martin, N., Rodríguez-García, V., & Rebollar-Bernardo, M. A. (2009). Campo profesional y procedimientos de certificación en análisisaplicado del comportamiento en España y Europa [Professional field and certification in applied behavior analysis: Spain and Europe]. *Papeles del Psicologo, 30,* 1–10.

# Author Index

# Subject Index

Note. *f* or *t* following a page number indicates a figure or a table.